Geriatric Surgery

Geriatric Surgery

Comprehensive Care of the Elderly Patient

edited by

Mark R. Katlic, M.D.
Chief of Thoracic Surgery
Co-Director, Surgical Intensive Care Unit
Wilkes-Barre General Hospital
Wilkes-Barre, Pennsylvania

with 71 contributors

Urban & Schwarzenberg • Baltimore-Munich

Urban & Schwarzenberg, Inc.
7 E. Redwood Street
Baltimore, Maryland 21202
USA

Urban & Schwarzenberg GmbH
Landwehrstrasse 61
D-8000 München 2
West Germany

Printed in the United States

Notices

The Editors (or Authors) and the Publisher of this work have made every effort to ensure that the drug dosage schedules herein are accurate and in accord with the standards accepted at the time of publication. The reader is strongly advised, however, to check the product information sheet included in the package of each drug he or she plans to administer to be certain that changes have not been made in the recommended dose or in the contraindications for administration.

The Publishers have made an extensive effort to trace original copyright holders for permission to use borrowed material. If any have been overlooked, it will be corrected at the first reprint.

5 4 3 2 1
94 93 92 91 90

SANS TACHE

Library of Congress Cataloging-in-Publication Data

Geriatric surgery : comprehensive care of the elderly patient/edited by Mark R. Katlic ; with 71 contributors.
p. cm.
Includes bibliographical references.
ISBN 0-8067-1061-6
1. Aged—Surgery 2. Therapeutics, Surgical. I. Katlic, Mark R., 1951–
[DNLM : 1. Aging. 2. Postoperative Care—in old age. 3. Preoperative Care—in old age. 4. Surgery, Operative—in old age. WO 950 G369]
RD145.G48 1990
617.9'7—dc20
DNLM/DLC
for Library of Congress 90-12080
CIP

Sponsoring Editor: Charles W. Mitchell
Managing Editor: Kathleen C. Millet
Manuscript Editor: Teresa Tamargo
Design and Production: Stony Run Publishing Services, Inc., Baltimore, Maryland
Compositor: Brushwood Graphics, Inc., Baltimore, Maryland
Printer: John D. Lucas Printing Co., Baltimore, Maryland

ISBN 0-8067-1061-6 Baltimore
ISBN 3-541-71061-6 Munich

Contents

Contributors

William H. Adler, M.D.
Chief, Clinical Immunology Section
National Institutes of Health,
National Institute on Aging
Gerontology Research Center
Baltimore, Maryland 21224

Martin L. Albert, M.D.
Professor of Neurology
Boston University School of Medicine
Director, Behavioral Neurosciences
Veterans Administration Medical Center
Boston, Massachusetts 02130

Robert G. Atnip, M.D.
Assistant Professor of Surgery
Section of Vascular Surgery
The Pennsylvania State University
College of Medicine
Hershey, Pennsylvania 17033

Anita Beckerman, A.R.N.P., Ed.D.
Associate Professor, School of Nursing
Florida International University
Bay Vista Campus at North Miami
North Miami, Florida 33181

George L. Blackburn, M.D., Ph.D.
Associate Professor of Surgery
Harvard Medical School
Chief, Nutrition Metabolism Laboratory
New England Deaconess Hospital
Boston, Massachusetts 02215

Lawrence F. Borges, M.D.
Assistant Professor of Surgery (Neurosurgery)
Harvard Medical School
Assistant Visiting Neurosurgeon
Massachusetts General Hospital
Boston, Massachusetts 02114

Zeno N. Chicarilli, M.D., D.M.D.
Clinical Associate Professor of Surgery
Section of Plastic and Reconstructive Surgery
Yale University School of Medicine
New Haven, Connecticut 06510

Nonyelu Chukwuogo, M.D.
Research Fellow
State University of New York Health Science
Center at Brooklyn
Brooklyn, New York 11203

Donna Cohen, Ph.D.
Professor of Gerontology, School of Public Health
Associate Director, Gerontology Center
University of Illinois at Chicago
Chicago, Illinois 60612

Francis L. Delmonico, M.D.
Assistant Professor of Surgery
Harvard Medical School
Transplantation Unit, Department of Surgery
Massachusetts General Hospital
Boston, Massachusetts 02114

James E. Devitt, M.D.
Professor of Surgery
Director, Continuing Medical Education
University of Ottawa
Ottawa, Ontario, Canada K1Y-4E9

R. Bruce Donoff, M.D., D.M.D.
Professor of Surgery
Harvard School of Dental Medicine
Chief of Oral and Maxillofacial Surgery
Massachusetts General Hospital
Boston, Massachusetts 02114

Norig Ellison, M.D.
Professor of Anesthesia
Director, Cardiac Anesthesia Bloc
University of Pennsylvania School of Medicine
Philadelphia, Pennsylvania 19104

John T. Farrar, M.D.
Professor of Medicine
Medical College of Virginia
Chief of Staff, Hunter Holmes McGuire
Veterans Administration Center
Richmond, Virginia 23249

Nalton F. Ferraro, M.D., D.M.D.
Instructor in Surgery
Harvard School of Dental Medicine
Section of Oral and Maxillofacial Surgery
Division of Plastic and Reconstructive Surgery
Brigham and Women's Hospital
Children's Hospital
Boston, Massachusetts 02115

Marsha Fretwell, M.D.
Head, Program in Geriatric Medicine
Brown University, Program in Medicine
Roger Williams General Hospital
Providence, Rhode Island 02908

Randall D. Gaz, M.D.
Assistant Professor of Surgery
Harvard Medical School
Assistant Surgeon
Endocrine Surgical Unit, Department of Surgery
Massachusetts General Hospital
Boston, Massachusetts 02114

Philip B. Gorelick, M.D.
Assistant Professor of Neurology
University of Chicago Pritzker School of Medicine
Director, Stroke Service
Michael Reese Hospital and Medical Center
Chicago, Illinois 60616

Leonard Hayflick, Ph.D.
Professor of Anatomy
School of Medicine
University of California, San Francisco
San Francisco, California 94121

Mark S. Hochberg, M.D.
Associate Professor of Surgery
University of Medicine and Dentistry of New Jersey
Director of Cardiac Surgery
Newark Beth Israel Medical Center
Newark, New Jersey 07112

Frederick F. Holmes, M.D.
Hashinger Professor of Medicine and Gerontology
University of Kansas Medical Center
Kansas City, Kansas 66103

Chang-Zern Hong, M.D.
Assistant Professor of Physical Medicine
and Rehabilitation
University of California Irvine Medical Center
Orange, California 92668

James R. Horning, M.D.
Chief of Geriatrics
Assistant Professor of Medicine
University of South Dakota School of Medicine
Sioux Falls, South Dakota 57105

Laura F. Hutchins, M.D.
Assistant Professor of Medicine
University of Arkansas School for Medical Sciences
Little Rock, Arkansas 72205

Kenneth M. Janis, M.D.
Department of Anesthesiology
University of New Mexico School of Medicine
Albuquerque, New Mexico 87100

Albert R. Jonsen, Ph.D.
Professor of Ethics in Medicine
Department of Medical History & Ethics
University of Washington
Seattle, Washington 98195

Richard A. Josephson, M.D.
Department of Cardiology
Akron City Hospital
Akron, Ohio 44314

Fran E. Kaiser, M.D.
Associate Professor of Medicine
Associate Director, Division of Geriatric Medicine
St. Louis University School of Medicine
St. Louis, Missouri 63104

Marshall B. Kapp, J.D., M.P.H.
Professor and Course Director
Department of Community Health
Director, Office of Geriatric Medicine
and Gerontology
Wright State University School of Medicine
Dayton, Ohio 45401

Mark R. Katlic, M.D.
Chief of Thoracic Surgery
Co-Director, Surgical Intensive Care Unit
Wilkes-Barre General Hospital
Wilkes-Barre, Pennsylvania 18764

Ian Kellman, M.D.
Department of Radiology
Tyler Memorial Hospital
Tunkhannock, Pennsylvania 18657

Kevin Kiwak, M.D.
Chief Resident in Neurosurgery
Massachusetts General Hospital
Boston, Massachusetts 02114

Janice F. Knoefel, M.D.
Director of Geriatric Neurology
Assistant Professor of Neurology,
Boston University School of Medicine
Chief, Geriatric Evaluation Unit
Veterans Administration Medical Center
Boston, Massachusetts 02130

Charles F. Koopmann, Jr., M.D.
Associate Professor
Otolaryngology, Head and Neck Surgery
University of Michigan School of Medicine
Ann Arbor, Michigan 48109

Harry B. Kram, M.D.
Department of Surgery
Martin Luther King, Jr./Charles B. Drew Medical Center
UCLA School of Medicine
Los Angeles, California 90059

Edward G. Lakatta, M.D.
Chief, Laboratory of Cardiovascular Science
National Institutes of Health, National Institute on Aging
Gerontology Research Center
Baltimore, Maryland 21224

Peter P. Lamy, Ph.D.
Professor and Director
Center for the Study of Pharmacy and Therapeutics for the Elderly, School of Pharmacy
Research Professor, Epidemiology and Preventive Medicine, School of Medicine
University of Maryland
Baltimore, Maryland 21201

David A. Lipschitz, M.D.
Professor of Medicine
University of Arkansas for Medical Sciences
Director, Geriatric Research, Education, and Clinical Center
John L. McClellan Veterans' Hospital
Little Rock, Arkansas 72205

Daniel K. Lowe, M.D.
Associate Professor of Surgery
Yale University School of Medicine
New Haven, Connecticut 06510

Ali Mansouri, M.D.
Associate Professor of Medicine and Biochemistry
University of Arkansas School for Medical Sciences
Little Rock, Arkansas 72205

Charles H. McLeskey, M.D.
Associate Professor of Anesthesiology
Director of Academic Affairs
University of Colorado Health Sciences Center
Denver, Colorado 80262

William F. McManus, M.D.
Colonel, Medical Corps
Chief, Clinical Division
United States Army Institute of Surgical Research
Brooke Army Medical Center, Fort Sam Houston
San Antonio, Texas 78234

Anne E. Missavage, M.D.
Assistant Professor of Surgery
Director, Burn Unit
University of California at Davis
Sacramento, California 95817

John E. Morley, M.B., B.Ch.
Dammert Professor of Gerontology
Director, Division of Geriatric Medicine
St. Louis University School of Medicine
St. Louis, Missouri 63104

James E. Nagel, M.D.
Senior Surgeon, Clinical Immunology Section
National Institutes of Health, National Institute on Aging
Gerontology Research Center
Baltimore, Maryland 21224

Satish Patel, M.D.
Department of Radiology
Wilkes-Barre General Hospital
Wilkes-Barre, Pennsylvania 18764

Gregory J. Paveza, M.D.
Assistant Professor, School of Public Health
University of Illinois Medical Center
Chicago, Illinois 60612

Russell K. Portenoy, M.D.
Assistant Professor of Neurology
Cornell University Medical College
Director of Analgesic Studies, Pain Service
Assistant Attending Neurologist
Memorial Sloan Kettering Cancer Center
New York, New York 10021

Douglas C. Powers, M.D.
Medical Fellow, Geriatrics and Immunology
National Institutes of Health, National Institute on Aging
Gerontology Research Center
Baltimore, Maryland 21224

Basil A. Pruitt, Jr., M.D.
Colonel, Medical Corps
Commander and Director
United States Army Institute of Surgical Research
Brooke Army Medical Center, Fort Sam Houston
San Antonio, Texas 78234

Ronnie Ann Rosenthal, M.D.
Associate Professor of Clinical Surgery
Department of Surgery
University of Chicago
Chicago, Illinois 60637

Alan Rubin, M.D.
Clinical Associate Professor of Obstetrics and Gynecology
University of Pennsylvania School of Medicine
Chief, Department of Gynecology
Graduate Hospital
Philadelphia, Pennsylvania 19103

Stephen C. Rubin, M.D.
Associate Attending Surgeon
Gynecology Service
Memorial Sloan Kettering Cancer Center
New York, New York 10021

Paul S. Russell, M.D.
John Homans Professor of Surgery
Harvard Medical School
Visiting Surgeon and Chief, Transplantation Unit
Massachusetts General Hospital
Boston, Massachusetts 02114

Anthony G. Salem, M.D.
Chief of General Internal Medicine Section
Associate Professor of Medicine
University of South Dakota School of Medicine
Sioux Falls, South Dakota 57105

Thomas M. Scalea, M.D.
Associate Professor of Surgery
State University of New York Health Science Center at Brooklyn
Brooklyn, New York 11203

Robert B. Scott, M.D.
Professor of Medicine
Division of Geriatrics
Medical College of Virginia
Virginia Commonwealth University
Richmond, Virginia 23298

Robert D. Shamburek, M.D.
Research Fellow
Division of Gastroenterology
Medical College of Virginia
Virginia Commonwealth University
Richmond, Virginia 23298

William C. Shoemaker, M.D.
Professor of Surgery
Vice-Chairman for Academic Affairs
Martin Luther King, Jr./Charles R. Drew Medical Center
Los Angeles, California 90059

Denise Smith-Fraser, Ed.D.
President, Elderhelp, Inc.
Mount Vernon, New York 10552
Former Director, Graduate Gerontology and Psychology Programs
College of New Rochelle
New Rochelle, New York 10805

Jeffrey M. Spivak, M.D.
Senior Resident in Orthopaedic Surgery
Hospital for Joint Diseases Orthopaedic Institute
New York, New York 10003

Kenneth J. Storch, M.D., Ph.D.
Metabolic Support Specialist
Department of Medicine
Overlook Hospital
Summit, New Jersey 07901
Boston, Massachusetts

Jerome S. Tobis, M.D.
Professor of Physical Medicine and Rehabilitation
Founding Director, Program in Geriatric Medicine and Gerontology
University of California Irvine Medical Center
Orange, California 92668

Melvyn S. Tockman, M.D., Ph.D.
Associate Professor of Environmental Health Services
Johns Hopkins University School of Medicine
Department of Pulmonary Medicine and Epidemiology
Johns Hopkins Hospital
Baltimore, Maryland 21205

Donald D. Trunkey, M.D.
Professor and Chairman
Department of Surgery
Oregon Health Sciences University
Portland, Oregon 97201

Gary Victor, M.D.
Department of Medicine
Queensway Carleton Hospital
Ottawa, Ontario, Canada

Frank J. Weinstock, M.D.
Associate Professor of Ophthalmology
Northeastern Ohio Universities College of Medicine
Clinical Assistant Professor of Ophthalmology
Ohio State University College of Medicine
Department of Surgery, Aultman Hospital Timken Mercy Medical Center
Canton, Ohio 44708

Thomas H. Wiser, Pharm.D.
Professor and Chairman
Department of Pharmacy Practice
Campbell University School of Pharmacy
Buies Creek, North Carolina 27506

Harold C. Yang, M.D., Ph.D.
Assistant Professor of Surgery
Transplantation Surgery
The Pennsylvania State University College of Medicine
Hershey, Pennsylvania 17033

Kim Shiu-Chin Yang, M.D.
Pain Fellow, Unified Pain Service
Department of Neurology
Albert Einstein College of Medicine
Bronx, New York 10461

Edward T. Zawada, Jr., M.D.
Freeman Professor and Chairman
Department of Internal Medicine
University of South Dakota School of Medicine
Sioux Falls, South Dakota 57117

Joseph D. Zuckerman, M.D.
Director, Geriatric Trauma Program
Chief, Shoulder Clinic
Hospital for Joint Diseases Orthopaedic Institute
New York, New York 10003

Foreword

Scientists continue to pursue the elusive causes of aging. Why cells in culture media should wither and die after a few generations or why the human body deteriorates are unsolved problems. Meanwhile the number of oldsters continues to increase and thereby initiates further social, economic, and philosophical dilemmas. Practical methods must be devised to aid in their solution.

Medical disciplines offer enormous help. Assuming that ultimately deterioration and death are certain, it is an important goal to maintain every individual functioning in a reasonably physiologic fashion as long as possible. Abilities to use eyes, ears, and digestive tract, and to move hands and legs without pain unfortunately often have a propensity to deteriorate one by one rather than simultaneously. It is the task of the physician and the surgeon to shore up each of these functions in such a way that when they fail, they do so at about the same time.

In past centuries relief from the ills of the aged came chiefly from clerics and philosophers, who brought solace to those who left this mortal world by bits and pieces. From time to time physicians discovered a few drugs that were of great value to oldsters: laxatives, opiates, and foxglove are examples.

Until recently, surgeons had comparatively little to offer. But consider what the last few decades have witnessed! Eyesight is restored by lens implants, hearing by stapedectomy, and the horrible persistent pain of degenerated hip joints ameliorated by hip replacement. The number of amputations has been lessened spectacularly by arterial grafts. Carotid endarterectomies have reduced the expected number of strokes. Operations that for many years were restricted to the young, such as those on the heart and even organ transplantation, now occasionally are indicated for the old. Calendar age no longer is the prime determinant of therapy; aging is not merely a function of time.

In this volume the contributors have collated the advantages that can accrue to old individuals from the application of surgical techniques from all specialties. The amazing progress that is portrayed should be compared to information in the very rare books that appeared on the same subject a few years ago. No longer are surgical procedures in the aged restricted chiefly to such emergencies as broken bones, amputations, and strangulated hernias. Even prophylactic operations have their place.

Nevertheless, such exuberance must be tempered. Operations are more hazardous in the elderly. Furthermore, many problems are insoluble today. When senile dementia occurs, attempted prolongation of life by heroic measures is of questionable value. Thus philosophical and social problems will persist, and choices must be made in individual cases.

The chapters deal with these global problems. They document the increased risks that must be assessed carefully by the patient, by the doctor, and by the family as they attempt to keep the patient's most essential body systems in reasonable working order until sudden dissolution occurs.

Merely because they know little about the advantages of surgery, many physicians and others tend to view all operations with alarm. This book should provide all interested persons with enough information to replace emotional reactions with knowledge, and to make informed decisions based upon modern concepts.

Claude E. Welch, M.D.

Preface

With a few obvious exceptions, all surgeons are geriatric surgeons. Surgical problems abound in the elderly, and in 1990 the bulk of an average surgeon's time is devoted to the care of these older patients in the operating room, on the wards, and in the office. Our care of the elderly will become an even more prominent part of our practices in the future, a prophecy that has reverberated recently through both the medical literature and lay press. The number of people over age 85 years, for example, will double by the end of the century and those 65 years or older soon will exceed 20% of the population in the United States, as they have currently in Pennsylvania; the proportion in Wilkes-Barre is already closer to 25%. It is therefore not this book's intention to promulgate the notion of yet another surgical subspecialty, but rather to improve the care of the elderly surgical patient by all who care for him or her.

As this project evolved it became apparent that its audience should not be limited to surgeons. Geriatric physicians will benefit from the breadth of surgical knowledge that is condensed into one chapter in most geriatric medicine texts. Internists and family physicians will be able to discuss the risks and benefits of operation with their elderly patients and to improve their perioperative care. Anesthesiologists and intensivists will augment their comprehension of physiology in the elderly surgical patient. Surgeons and anesthesiologists will likely benefit more from the first sections of the book (physiologic changes in the elderly) and others from the last sections (specific operations and perioperative care).

The underlying premise of this text is that increased scientific knowledge leads to better surgical care. Superior surgery has always been rooted in superior science and the best surgeons are not only dexterous technicians but also questioning physiologists. Many surgeons, however, take for granted that they can care for the elderly since they have always done so; also, much of the research on altered physiology and results of surgery in the elderly has not reached the wider clinical audience. As Jonsen notes in his chapter, "In modern surgery, age enters into the assessment as a scientific datum, not as a prejudice." Not only can we all afford to improve our care of the elderly, but we must.

Patients in the extremes of age or debility have always challenged us, and we have learned the most from them. The man or woman who is a consistently good geriatric surgeon is likely to be a consistently good surgeon. So, let us all become good geriatric surgeons.

Mark R. Katlic, M.D., F.A.C.S.

Acknowledgments

I wish to extend sincere gratitude to the following individuals: to Charles Mitchell, Editor-in-Chief, and Kathleen Millet, Managing Editor, of Urban & Schwarzenberg for their patience and uncompromising standards; to my secretary Frances Stosek, whose compulsion and attention to detail exceed my own; and to my wife Diane and son Adam for sharing me with both the dawn operating room and the midnight desk.

To two of my mentors, J. Alex Haller, Jr., M.D., and Hermes C. Grillo, M.D.,
who taught and showed that all patients, regardless of age, deserve our best

Geriatric Surgery

SECTION I

Special Aspects of Geriatric Surgical Care

1

Biologic and Theoretical Perspectives of Human Aging

Leonard Hayflick

The common belief that the triumphs of modern biomedical research and its application to medical practice have lengthened the human life span is not supported by either vital statistics or biologic evidence. There is no proof that the maximum human life span has changed from what it was several hundred thousand years ago. No authentic record exists of a human ever living longer than about 115 years.

Medical achievements in this century simply have allowed more people to reach what appears to be the fixed upper limit of the human life span. That is, *life expectation* has increased but *life span* has not. Successful prevention and treatment of illnesses that formerly led to many deaths in the early years are yielding life tables that are simply becoming more rectangular (Fig. 1-1). In many privileged countries, one can now expect to grow old, which is a relatively new phenomenon.

The Rectangular Curve

More than 60 years ago, the pioneer gerontologist, Raymond Pearl, recognized that with the elimination of deaths in the early years, survival curves constructed over intervals were becoming more rectangular (1). This phenomenon subsequently was discussed extensively by Comfort, Strehler, Kohn, and Hayflick (2–7). More recent views on the accuracy of rectangular survival curves and their interpretation for future geriatric planning (8–11) have met with considerable controversy (12–15).

Fries has argued that the growing rectangularization of human survival curves for developed countries is compressing the period of time during which most mortality and morbidity occurs in later life (16). As the increase in life expectation and delayed clinical manifestations of chronic diseases approach the limit of our fixed life span, then compression occurs. This could mean that: (*a*) the number of very old people will increase; (*b*) the average period of diminished vigor will decrease; (*c*) chronic diseases will occur in a smaller proportion of the total life span; and (*d*) this will result in a reduction in the need for medical care in the elderly (8).

If the human life span is fixed and the diseases causing death occur at increasingly older ages, then morbidity and mortality will occupy an increasingly smaller proportion of the human life span. If true, this scenario has important implications for planning present and future allocations of health care resources. The probability that it is true, however, is questionable.

Is the Human Life Span Fixed?

The first premise on which this scenario rests is that the human life span is fixed. Although what little data exists have been interpreted (16) in support of a fixed human life span, there are important qualifications.

Most gerontologists will not accept a maximum human life span that exceeds about 115 years of age. The reason for skepticism is simple. First, unlike tree rings and fish scales, there are no reliable markers for accurately determining the chronological or biologic age of

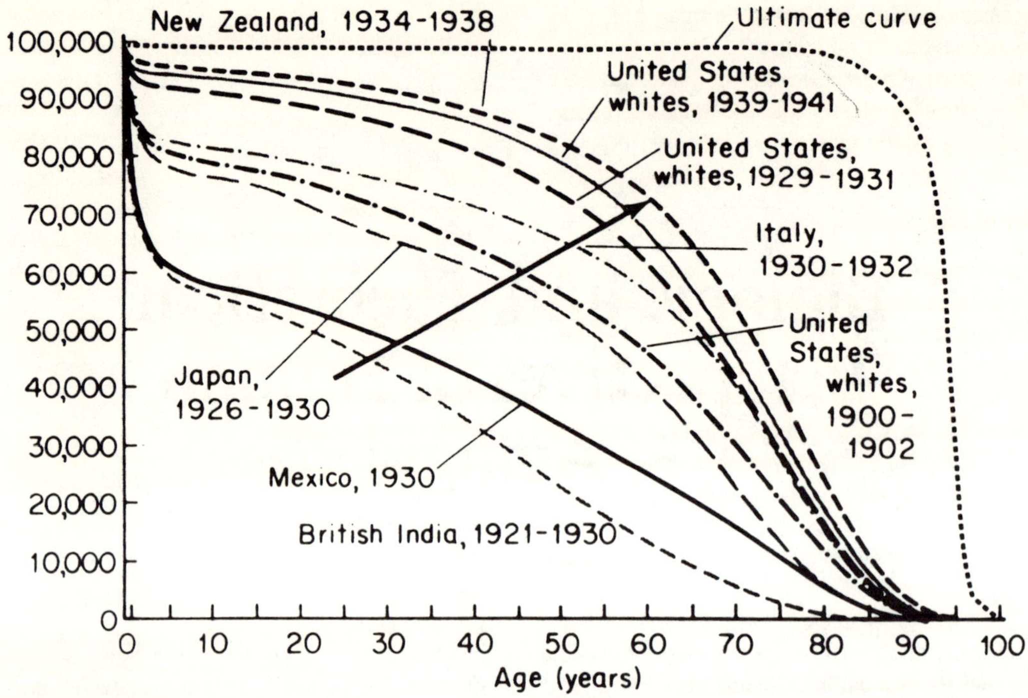

Figure 1-1. Human survival curves for various countries and times show that as medical care and hygiene improve, fewer deaths occur in the earlier years. This has the effect of rectangularizing the survival curves, as depicted by the direction of the arrow. Elimination of all causes of death, now attributable to diseases and accidents, would result in the hypothetical ultimate curve. Here individuals would die only from the physiologic decrements that lead to normal age changes or what were once called "natural causes." Virtually all successful medical research and patient care tends to increase life expectation in the direction of the ultimate curve. Little, if any, serious effort is now made to increase the human life span or to move the point of convergence of all of the lines further to the right. (Adapted from Comfort A: *Aging: The Biology of Senescence*, Holt, Rinehart and Winston, Inc., New York, 1964.)

humans. Therefore, it is necessary to assess written, or worse, oral records. If the scientific method is applied, few, if any, birth records for Americans older than, say 110, can be authenticated. Records that are accepted prove that cherished beliefs or faith are more persuasive forces than is scientific evidence (17, 18).

Because there are so few authentic centenarians, a correct determination of the maximum human life span is impossible. The reliability of noncontemporaneous records is even more questionable. Thus, the uncertainty of birth dates for old people and the small number of them conspire against accuracy.

This uncertainty of very old ages and the small cohort number not only compromises a determination of the maximum human life span itself, but it also prevents knowing whether it is, in fact, changing. For example, if the human life span increased by as much as 5 or even 10 years during this century, it could not be detected because reliable baseline data for the last century is virtually unobtainable. Consequently, as good an argument could be made for a fixed human life span as could be made for one that has increased or even decreased.

Evolution of Life Span

In spite of these uncertainties, on an evolutionary scale, there is good evidence that the human life span increased rapidly until about 100,000 years ago, when it slowed considerably. The evidence for this is the remarkable concordance found to occur when the ratio of the weight of the adult mammalian brain to the weight of the adult body is expressed as a function of life span (19–22). By this criterion, it is possible to say confidently that early hominids had a life span far shorter than modern humans because their brains were considerably smaller than ours in relation to body weight.

The brain weight/body weight ratio of humans slowed considerably about 100,000 years ago when the human life span presumably became what it is today. On an evolutionary scale, however, the human life span still may be increasing because the sensitivity of brain weight/body weight measurements are insufficient to detect small differences that may have occurred over the last 100, 1,000, or even 10,000 years. Nevertheless, on an evolutionary scale, the human life span *has* increased. This fact is important because it implies that the human life span, even if it has been fixed for millennia, has the potential to increase in the future. Of great interest in this respect are animal studies, showing clearly that life span can be extended by reducing caloric intake (23–25).

Demography of Life Span

Tantalizing evidence that the human life span may be increasing comes from the recent work of several demographers. Myers and Manton (13) have argued that the population dynamics of the very old have *not* been subject to the effects of the rectangularization of the survival curve. Survival curves for the United States, made at intervals during the period from 1900 to the present, show a large gain in life expectation. The greatest increases have occurred in the younger age groups, up to about 1960. Since 1960, there has been a substantial increase in life expectation in the older age groups.

How to Increase Human Life Expectation

If cardiovascular disease, which is now the leading cause of death in the United States and other developed countries, is successfully eliminated, approximately 14 years of additional life can be expected at birth (Table 1-1). If the second greatest cause of death—cancer—is eliminated, about 3 years of additional life expectation will result. From 1900 to 1978, the increase in life expectancy at birth achieved in the United States was 24.1 years. This increase resulted from the decrease in the large number of deaths that occurred before the age of 65; however, the gain in life expectancy at 65, 75, and 80 years of age from 1900 to 1978 was, respectively, only 4.4, 3.3, and 2.8 years (26).

What effect would there be on human longevity and the human life span if all causes of death reported on death certificates (not "natural causes") were totally eliminated (Table 1-1)? The effect on human longevity would be to realize the ultimate rectangular curve (Fig. 1-1) in which citizens would live out their lives free of the fear of premature death, but with the certain knowledge that their normal physiologic decrements would result in death on or about their 100th birthday.

These concepts force the conclusion that the disease-oriented approach to medical research might increase life expectation, but it will have little impact on increasing the human life span. If such an increase is desirable (and there is considerable doubt that it is), one must first separate the disease-related causes of death from the age-dependent normal physiologic decrements that give rise to the manifestations of old age. The diseases of old age are simply superimposed on these normal physiologic decrements but must be regarded separately to consider ways of increasing the human life span. Although age-associated physiologic decrements surely increase vulnerability to disease, the fundamental causes of death are not pathologies, but the physiologic decrements that make their occurrence more likely.

Table 1-1. Gain in expectation of life at birth and at age 65 due to elimination of various causes of death (1978)

Cause of death	Gain in years of life expectation if cause is eliminated: At birth	At age 65
Major cardiovascular diseases	13.9	14.3
Disease of the heart	7.0	6.6
Cerebrovascular diseases	1.1	1.2
Arteriosclerosis	0.2	0.2
Malignant neoplasms[a]	3.1	1.9
Influenza and pneumonia	0.4	0.3
Diabetes mellitus	0.2	0.2
Motor vehicle accidents	0.6	—
All accidents excluding motor vehicle accidents	0.6	0.2
Bronchitis, emphysema, and asthma	0.1	0.1
Cirrhosis of the liver	0.3	0.1
Nephritis and nephrosis	0.1	—
Infective and parasitic diseases	0.2	0.1

[a]Includes neoplasms of lymphatic and hematopoietic tissues.

Source: Das Gupta, P: "Cause-of-Death Analysis of the 1978 Mortality Data by Age, Sex and Race," U.S. Bureau of the Census, 1981 (unpublished manuscript), and U.S. Public Health Service, National Center for Health Statistics. Also in U.S. Bureau of the Census, Current Population Reports, Series P-23, No. 138, Demographic and Socioeconomic Aspects of Aging in the United States, USGPO, Washington, D.C. 1984.

Biomedical research has focused almost exclusively on the pathologies that cause death. Scant attention has been paid to the underlying causes of biologic aging—that is, the functional decrements that increase vulnerability to pathology. Unless more attention is given to these fundamental biologic causes of aging, the most likely fate of all those who are fortunate to become old will be death on or about their 100th birthday.

Prospects for Increasing Human Longevity

There are two ways in which biomedical research can be expected to extend human longevity in the next 25 years. The first is by reducing or eliminating the major causes of death. For most developed countries, this would mean eliminating cardiovascular disease and cancer. In the developing countries, (and in some areas of developed countries), life expectancy can be extended by simply motivating the political and economic infrastructure to provide citizens with the necessary food, hygienic conditions, and medical care that are commonplace in most developed countries. Minimal results will be obtained by reducing the effect of minor diseases in developed countries. For example, in the United States, if influenza, pneumonia, and other infectious-disease causes of death were completely eliminated, the gain in life expectation at birth would be less than 6 months (Table 1-1).

Thus, it could be argued that if an increase in life expectation becomes the main goal of biomedical research in the developed countries, all such research should be directed toward the elimination of the two major causes of death. This position, although less than humane and not likely to attract many adherents, is nonetheless the most logical conclusion to be drawn from life-table studies and the projections dealt with in Table 1-1.

The second way in which biomedical research can affect human longevity is to address itself specifically to the underlying normal physiologic decrements that increase vulnerability to pathology and death. This approach, then, does not directly concern itself with increasing human life expectation but is aimed at extending what appears to be a fixed life span.

Comparative Efforts

Current efforts directed toward these two approaches can be measured by the funds spent in the United States on cardiovascular disease and cancer research. They are about 20 times greater than the funds spent in biogerontology. It is also probable that the number of researchers, and consequently the amount of effort, in both of these areas also differs by 20-fold. The amount to be spent on AIDS research is also several fold more than what is to be spent in biogerontology. Yet the former has a long way to go before it results in as many deaths as those caused annually by highway accidents. Consequently, the likelihood that any significant increase in human longevity will occur in the next 25 years depends on (*a*) significantly better cure rates for cardiovascular disease or cancer or both, and (*b*) significant advances in our understanding and ability to manipulate the biological clocks that set a maximum life span for each species.

If potential success in either of these endeavors can be measured by the current attitudes and priorities of the biomedical research establishment in the United States and elsewhere, then clearly the search for cures for cardiovascular disease and cancer are much more likely to affect human longevity than is biogerontological research. A further conclusion is that by resolving these two diseases, a maximum of 14 years of additional life expectation can be attained, but with successful efforts to increase the life span itself, no fixed end point can be ruled out. Furthermore, the resolution of the two leading killers will in no way reverse or halt the decline in normal physiological decrements that are characteristic of old age, whereas efforts to increase the life span could lead to such a reversal. Clearly, research in cardiovascular diseases and cancer should not be stopped. Nevertheless, if our goal is to maximize opportunities to increase human longevity effectively, then our current priorities are seriously out of balance. If this imbalance continues unchanged, there is little likelihood that the research accomplishments of a handful of underfunded biogerontologists will ever increase the human life span.

Biology of Aging

The phenomenon of biologic aging is generally believed to be a universal property of all living things. It is a manifestation of the sum of a multitude of biologic decrements that occur after sexual maturation. Yet this concept cannot be accepted without qualification.

There are animals in which aging is rare or has never been demonstrated. Some fish and amphibians that have an indeterminate size may also have an indeterminate life span (2). Thus the universality of aging, even in vertebrates, remains unproven. These animals are not immortal. Although normal age changes may not occur, they will die eventually of disease, predation, or accidents at an annual rate similar to the half-life curve of radioactive decay. This is not true aging.

In fact, the occurrence of aging arguably is restricted to humans and the domestic and zoo animals that we choose to protect. The extreme manifestations of old age that are found to occur in humans simply do not occur in feral animals. If aging occurs at all in wild animals, its expression is brief because the physiologic decrements of aging quickly make these animals vulnerable to disease and predation. Few feral animals live long enough after sexual maturation to experience old age. As soon as they incur even slight decrements in, for example, running speed or jumping ability, they are culled by predators. Similarly, as soon as their immune system becomes less capable, they may die of disease. Or, what is more likely, they will be culled by predators when disease has reduced their ability to elude capture. As a result, the likelihood is remote that evolution could have selected for the aging process. There are simply too few feral animals on which selective pressure could have been applied. Thus, aging cannot be viewed as an adaptation.

In developed countries, humans have been so successful in resolving causes of death attributable to acute diseases in youth that their aging is expressed to an extreme unattainable by wild animals. Civilization has produced life expectations that were unknown in prehistoric times, revealing a plethora of physiologic decrements that perhaps, teleologically, never were intended to be revealed. Aging may be an artifact of civilization or domestication because the "unnatural" circumstance of greater life expectation has permitted the expression of aging, which otherwise would not have occurred (Fig. 1-2).

Aging and Disease

Aging must be distinguished from disease. Biologic changes attributable to aging are frequently referred to as "normal age changes," as if there was a category of "abnormal age changes." Age changes are not diseases, they are natural losses of function. Loss and graying of the hair, reduced exercise capacity and stamina, wrinkled skin, menopause, presbyopia, presbycusis, loss of short-term memory, and hundreds of other similar decrements of old age are not diseases. They do not increase our vulnerability to die. Other "normal" decrements in vital organs do produce increased vulnerability to pathologic change. For example, normal age-related decrements in immune system functions increase vulnerability to diseases that in youth would be easily resolved. Or perhaps, antigens recognized as self in youth might be recognized by an aging immune system as non-self, thus producing many of the chronic autoimmune diseases of old age.

Etiology of Aging

What is the cause of the aging phenomenon? This question, which is fundamental in the science of gerontology, might well be analogous to asking: "What is the cause of development?" Similarly, the frequently asked question: "How can aging be stopped or slowed?" is equivalent to asking: "How can development be stopped or slowed?"

There is no good reason why aging has to happen. August Weismann believed that aging occurs to benefit the species by removing less fit animals from an environment, where limited space and other resources should be conserved for the young (27). This is an illogical argument, because if chronologically older animals continued to remain fit, their deaths would not benefit younger members. Thus, there would be no basis for an aging process to evolve in the first place. Weismann's notion also can be discredited because with few, or no, old feral animals surviving, there is little possibility that evolution could have selected for the aging process.

Furthermore, there is no selective advantage for a species to have its members live much beyond the age of sexual maturity and child rearing. For example, from the standpoint of simple survival of the species, there is no advantage for humans to live much beyond 30 years. This would permit sufficient time for production of new progeny and rearing of that progeny to sexual maturation. Since life expectation at birth in prehistoric times was about 18 years, it is apparent that the human species has

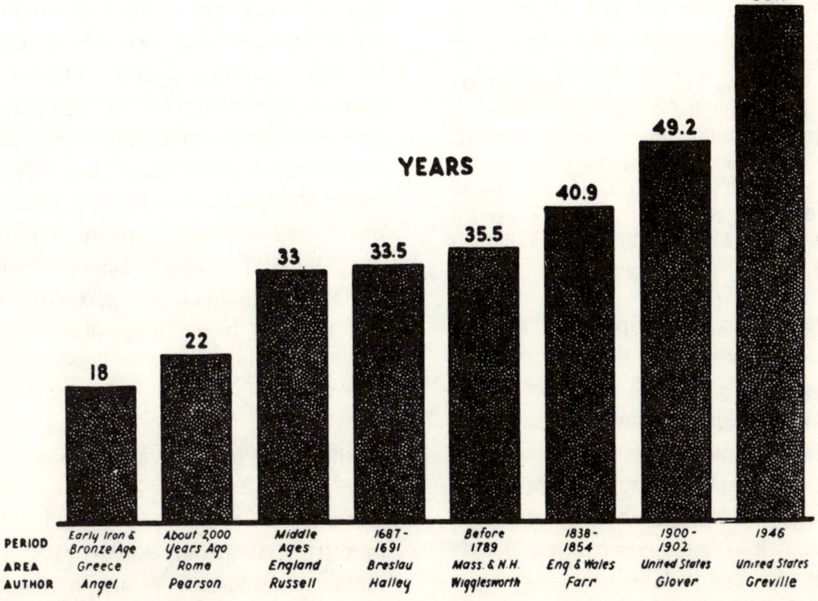

Figure 1-2. Average length of life from ancient to modern times. (From Dublin, LI, Lotka, AJ, and Spiegelman, M. 1949. *Length of Life*. New York: Ronald Press.)

survived far longer with an 18-year-life expectation than it has with the current 75-year expectation. Thus, the human species has survived for a much longer period of time with few, or no, old members than it has with many old members.

Weismann, however, was prescient on one major point. He surmised correctly that the ability of normal somatic cells to replicate and function was limited, despite the fact that the opposite was believed for decades. This dogma was finally upset by Hayflick and Moorhead in 1961 (33). Thus, the limited ability for normal human and animal cells to replicate and function may represent a fundamental reason why the lives of individual animals are finite. In fact, many of the multitude of functional decrements, reported to occur in cultured normal human cells as they reach the end of their life span, are identical to the changes that occur in humans as they age.

Emergence of Biogerontology

Despite the virtual universality of biologic aging, its study has been, perhaps, the most neglected area of biologic inquiry. The reasons for this are complex but are undoubtedly manifestations of the convergence of at least three separate phenomena.

First, the field has suffered more from a lunatic fringe than has, perhaps, any other area of biological research. Claims for increasing human longevity are probably as old as civilization itself. They have ranged from more recent dietary fads, inoculations with monkey testicular extracts, and "cell therapy" to the biblical admonition to King David who "was old and stricken in years . . . " In an effort to increase his longevity,

> His servants said unto him: 'Let there be sought for my lord the king a young virgin; and let her stand before the king, and be a companion unto him . . . that the lord the king may get heat' . . . So they sought for a fair damsel throughout all the borders of Israel . . . and brought her to the king. And the damsel was very fair; and she became a companion unto the king, and ministered to him; but the king knew her not. (28)

Yet like modern yogurt eaters and recipients of monkey testicle and lamb tissue extracts," . . . the days of David drew nigh that he should die . . . " (28).

Modern scientists are loathe to enter fields reputed to be dominated by charlatans and practitioners of the black arts. Young scientists would be foolhardy to attempt to begin a career against such odds and established investigators would prefer not to risk a reputation made in a "legitimate" field to enter one held in disdain.

A second reason for neglect of biogerontology has been the lack of a sufficient factual basis or testable theoretical foundation that could lead to the design of good experiments. This is, of course, the classic "Catch 22" because without good science, the insufficient factual base and unimpressive theoretical underpinning will not improve. And because of this few scientists will willingly enter.

A third reason why biogerontology has been passed over by the mainstream of biologic scientists is that minute amounts of research funds have been available. The few people who have worked in the field obtained financial support in the name of those basic disciplines that underpin biogerontology. These are biochemistry, physiology, cell biology, and, in fact, virtually any traditional field of basic biologic science. This also holds, of course, for other multidisciplinary fields, such as embryology and developmental biology. Yet to identify oneself as an embryologist or a developmental biologist has been far more acceptable than to identify oneself as a gerontologist. Thus, what progress has been made in biogerontology has occurred by identifying the research with a basic field of biology but interpreting the results in a gerontologic context. In this way, a few biogerontologists learned how to obtain research support and maintain their scientific reputations while conducting research on aging. Even to this day, many biogerontologists would prefer to be identified first as an immunologist, molecular biologist, biochemist, or cell biologist and secondly as a gerontologist.

In the past decade, all of these circumstances have radically changed. Perhaps the most important reason for this was the establishment of the National Institute on Aging at the National Institutes of Health. The handful of gerontologists who dedicated themselves to the establishment of this institute resolved, virtually with one stroke, all of the aforementioned reasons for lack of progress in the field. Gerontology suddenly became respectable and reasonably well funded. Instant gerontologists appeared and even some established researchers in the field began to publicly identify themselves as gerontologists. Thus, the field probably has advanced more in the past decade than it had in the entire previous 100 years.

One of the major benefactors of this dramatic change has been the field of "cytogerontology" (29), which holds that the cell is the main arena in which fundamental knowledge of the aging process is most likely to be found.

Foundations of Cytogerontology

The origin of age changes in multicellular organisms can be attributed to only three possibilities, which are not mutually exclusive. Aging in metazoans can only result from: (*a*) perturbations within individual cells; (*b*) changes in the extracellular matrix; or (*c*) influences of more highly organized cell hierarchies on other tissues or organs.

An essential element in considering the role of the cell as the origin of age changes is whether or not cells are capable of normal function, including division, for an indefinite period of time. That is, are normal somatic cells intrinsically immortal? If they are immortal, then age changes must result from initiating factors that are extrinsic to the cell.

Centennial of the Controversy

The controversy that arose in efforts to answer this fundamental question actually began about 100 years ago. But even this fact has been brought to light only recently (30). In 1881, the great German biologist August Weismann proposed that the somatic cells of higher animals would be found to have a limited doubling potential. Although he provided no experimental evidence for his conjecture, Weismann stated " . . . death takes place because a worn-out tissue cannot forever renew itself, and because a capacity for increase by means of cell division is not everlasting but finite (27)."

There are at least two ways in which the immortality of normal cells can be determined. First, vertebrate cells can be serially cultured in laboratory glassware, and second, similar cells, containing specific markers allowing them to be distinguished from host cells, can be serially transplanted in isogenic laboratory animals. The transplanted tissue is regrafted to a younger host when the previous host becomes old. The goal of such studies has been to answer this fundamental question: Can normal vertebrate cells that function and replicate under ideal conditions escape from the inevitability of aging and death that is obligatory for the animal from which they were derived?

Immortal Heart Cells?

With respect to studies undertaken in cell culture, one investigation stood out as the classic response to this question before 1960. In the early part of this century, Alexis Carrel, a noted cell culturist, surgeon, and Nobel Laureate, described experiments purporting to show that fibroblasts derived from chick heart tissue could be cultured serially indefinitely. The culture was voluntarily terminated after 34 years (31). This finding created worldwide interest not only among the scientific community but among the lay press as well.

Its importance to gerontologists was clear. If true, it strongly implied that cells released from in vivo control could divide and function normally for a period of time in excess of the life span of the species. Thus, either the types of cells cultured play no role in the aging phenomenon, or aging results from changes in the intracellular matrix or at higher levels of cell organization. That is, aging could result from physiologic interactions between cells only when they are organized as tissues or organs. In any case, Carrel's results and their interpretation were of vital concern to biogerontologists because they strongly suggested that aging is not the result of events occurring within individual cells.

In the years that followed Carrel's observations, support for his experimental results seemed to be forthcoming from many laboratories in which it was observed that several cell populations seemed to have the striking ability to replicate apparently indefinitely. Immortal cell populations derived from various human and animal tissues were reported to occur spontaneously in dozens of laboratories in the 20-year period from the early 1940s to the early 1960s. These cell populations, numbering in the hundreds, are best known by the prototype cell lines, HeLa (derived from a human cervical carcinoma in 1952) and L cells (derived from mouse mesenchyme in 1943). They continue to flourish even to this day in cell culture laboratories throughout the world.

Immortal cell populations still arise spontaneously from normal cell cultures by a mysterious process; however, now they can be created, albeit at low efficiency, by exposure to radiation, chemical carcinogens, or certain oncogenic viruses. More recently, this process of "immortalization," as it has come to be called, can be accomplished routinely by fusing mortal antibody-producing lymphocytes to immortal myeloma cells. The resulting hybrid, known as a hybridoma, will continue to express specific monoclonal antibodies indefinitely (32). Use of this technique is one important cause of the current revolution in biotechnology.

Nevertheless, what seemed to be incontrovertible evidence for the existence of immortal cells soon fell to new insights and a preponderance of opposing information.

Aging Under Glass

Of central importance to the question of cell immortality as it relates to biogerontology is whether the cell populations studied in vitro are composed of normal or abnormal cells. Clearly, the aging of animals occurs in normal cell populations. If we are to equate the behavior of normal cells in vivo with that of similar cells in vitro, then the latter must be shown to be normal as well. In 1961, Moorhead and I postulated that all immortal cell populations are abnormal in one or more important property (33). As such, they are not proper subjects for the study of aging and indeed are not proper subjects for the study of many other biologic phenomena, for which they are frequently incorrectly used. All immortal cell lines vary in chromosome number, morphology, or banding pattern from the original animal or human cells from which they were derived. Most, but not all, produce tumors when inoculated into experimental animals. They have other properties that distinguish them from normal cells. Yet, they are frequently used by researchers as normal cells.

Aging Is Inevitable

Moorhead and I described the finite replicative capacity of normal human fibroblasts and interpreted the phenomenon as aging at the cellular level (33). We demonstrated that when normal human embryonic cells were grown under the most favorable conditions, aging and death were inevitable consequences after about 50 population doublings. We called this the Phase III phenomenon. We also showed that the death of our cultured normal human cells was not due to some trivial cause involving medium components or culture conditions but was an inherent property of the cells themselves (33, 34). This observation now has been confirmed in hundreds of laboratories where variations in medium components and cultural conditions have been as numerous as the laboratories themselves.

Since our observations and interpretations were made in 1961, no normal human or animal cell population has been shown to be immortal. Immortality is defined as continuous serial cultivation in vitro or in vivo, in which at least 100 population doublings occur over a minimum of at least 2 years. Cultured or transplanted normal cells are defined as those having properties identical to the cells that compose the tissue of origin.

Conceptual Origins

Although there were many previous reports that described the failure of most cultured cells to proliferate indefinitely, none characterized the cells as normal, ruled out artifacts as the cause, or suggested that the phenomenon might be associated with aging (35–37). In fact, the observation that cultured cells frequently failed to replicate indefinitely was probably made hundreds of times from the genesis of cell culture techniques in the early 1900s to our report 60 years later.

Those prior failures went unreported because existing dogma insisted that the failure of cells to proliferate indefinitely in vitro must be attributable to errors in the "art" required to keep cells dividing forever. That dogma was so well entrenched that our original manuscript (33) was rejected by *The Journal of Experimental Medicine* with the statement that "The largest fact to have come out from tissue culture in the last fifty years is that cells inherently capable of multiplying will do so indefinitely if supplied with the right milieu in vitro." That belief was tantamount to the belief that, given the right milieu in vivo, human beings also will live forever.

The finding that cultured normal cells have a finite capacity to replicate has had important implications in gerontologic theory. But before considering these implications it is necessary to discuss how Carrel was misled into believing that he had successfully cultured chick fibroblasts for 34 years.

Alexis Carrel and the Myth of His Immortal Chick Cells

By the late 1960s, it became apparent to me and others that Carrel's claim to have cultured chick fibroblast cells for 34 years was spurious (38, 39). It had to be assumed that Carrel's chick cultures consisted of normal cells, because until quite recently no one had ever found an immortal chick fibroblast population (40). One of these immortal cell lines was produced by exposure of the chick cells to the carcinogen *N*-methyl-*N*′-nitro-*N*-nitrosoguanidine and the other arose spontaneously. In both cases, the immortal cells were shown to be abnormal and to produce retroviruses.

It has been 50 years since the voluntary termination of Carrel's alleged immortal chick fibroblasts, and this is the first authentic report of a spontaneous transformation of normal chick fibroblast. The rarity of this event can be appreciated when one considers that chick tissue has been one of the most frequently cultured tissues in the past 50 years. Thus, the likelihood that Carrel had found such a population is remote, especially since, until now, all attempts to repeat his findings have been negative (41–44). Furthermore, even if his observation were legitimate, the immortal cells must have been abnormal. Thus, they cannot be used as evidence that normal cells had escaped the inevitability of aging in vitro.

I have proposed one explanation for Carrel's findings in which the method of preparation of chick embryo extract, used as a source of nutrients for his culture, allowed for the introduction of new, viable fibroblasts into the so-called "immortal" culture at each feeding (39). Although we believed that Carrel was unaware of this artifact, Witkowski, in a lengthy study of Carrel's immortal cells, suggests otherwise (45–47).

Inverse Relationship Between Donor Age and Cell Population Doublings

In the decade that followed our first report (33), further evidence appeared from studies in cytogerontology that provided important new insights into cellular aging. In 1965, we reported that cultured fibroblasts derived from older humans replicated fewer times than those derived from embryos (34). Because the technique for determining population doublings was crude at that time, a direct relationship between donor age and population doubling potential was difficult for us to establish. Subsequent studies by others not only confirmed the principle that we had observed but extended it significantly.

Martin and his colleagues derived cultures from human donors ranging from fetuses to those 90 years of age (48). Although the data reveal considerable scatter, they observed a regression coefficient, from the 1st to the 9th decade, of −0.2 population doublings per year of life with a standard deviation of 0.05 and a correlation coefficient of −0.50. The scatter found is not unlike that reported to occur with virtually any age-related change that is measured cross-sectionally and not longitudinally. Nevertheless, at least nine more studies have confirmed the finding that the number of population doublings of cultured human cells is inversely proportional to donor age. This inverse relationship has now been shown to occur in normal human cells derived from such diverse tissue as lung (34), skin (48–51), liver (52), arterial smooth muscle (53), lens (54), and T-lymphocytes (55, 56).

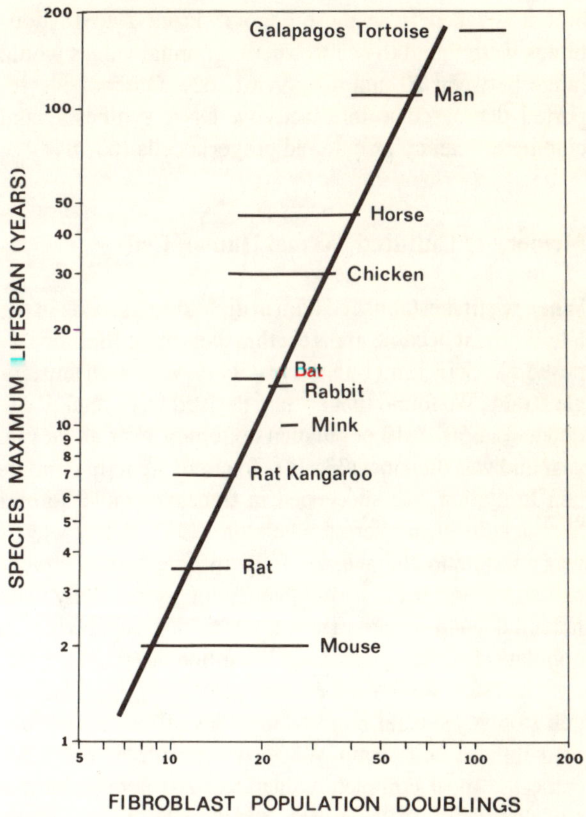

Figure 1-3. Fibroblasts from the embryos of 10 different species multiply in culture to a maximum number of population doublings that is roughly proportional to the life span for that species. Galapagos tortoise cells were derived from a juvenile animal.

Direct Relationship Between Maximum Species Life Span and Population Doublings of Their Cultured Cells

Several years ago we suggested that the population doubling potential of cultured fibroblasts from several animal species revealed a surprisingly good direct correlation with maximum species life span (5). In the years that followed, several other reports have added substantially to this idea, especially the work of Röhme (57). One report in which several marsupial species were studied does not support this finding; however, the authors did not determine population doublings by conventional means, nor is the maximum life spans of the species they studied known (58). Figure 1-3 shows the direct proportionality between different species maximum life spans and the population doubling potential of their cultured fibroblasts. Embryonic fibroblasts were used in nine of the ten species studied. Juvenile tissue was used in the study on the Galapagos tortoise.

If this relationship can be extended and confirmed, it will suggest the presence of a chronometer or pacemaker within all normal cells, which is characteristic for each species and which dictates maximum cell doubling or functional capacity with an apparent evolutionary basis. The postulated chronometer may or may not be the same one that we suggest might control the inverse relationship between donor age and population doubling potential.

Progeria and Werner's Syndrome

Progeria (Hutchinson-Gilford syndrome) is a human condition leading to a severe deceleration of growth in patients as young as 9 years of age (59). A very rare disease, it is thought by many to represent a model for precocious aging, in which individuals at the end of the 1st decade of life manifest the physical signs of aging typical of their normal counterparts at the 7th decade of life. Werner's syndrome is similar to progeria in many ways, although its salient manifestations occur in later years. The full clinical picture shows early graying and loss of hair, short stature, juvenile cataracts, a tendency to develop diabetes, atherosclerosis, calcification of the blood vessels, osteoporosis, and a high incidence of malignancy (60).

If Werner's syndrome and progeria are examples of accelerated aging, when does aging occur in cultured fibroblasts taken from these donors? From 2 to 18 doublings were found to occur, whereas normal values would range between 20 and 40 (49, 61, 62). Others have reported decreased mitotic activity, DNA synthesis, and cloning efficiency of cultured progeria cells (63, 64).

Memory of Cultured Normal Human Cells

When we first established human diploid cell strains in the late 1950s, it became apparent that their finite lifetime imposed a serious limit on the capacity to work with any single strain. We found that a strain derived from fetal tissue underwent 50 ± 10 population doublings over about one year and was then lost (33, 34). To circumvent this important limitation, we succeeded in freezing viable normal human cells at sub-zero temperatures (33). In this way, it was possible to characterize fully a single human diploid cell strain and have it available for long-term study. The potential yield of cells from a population capable of 50 population doublings is about 20 million metric tons (34).

In 1962, we developed, and placed into liquid nitrogen storage, several hundred ampules of our normal human diploid cell strain WI-38 which subsequently became the most completely characterized normal human cell population in the world. Today, it is the prototypic normal human fibroblast and is used worldwide in biologic research, virus isolation and identification, and the production of several human virus vaccines.

For 28 years, WI-38 has been in cryogenic storage, the longest period of time a viable normal human cell population has been stored. The ability to preserve normal cell strains has permitted experimentation directed toward answering a fundamental question in cytogerontology: If cells are frozen at various population doubling levels up to Phase III, how many population doublings will the cells undergo when they are thawed or reconstituted? Do they have a "clock" that is arrested in the cold at the population doubling level at which they were frozen? If so, then the total sum of doublings, both before and after freezing, would be about 50 in the case of a fetal strain. Or does freezing reset the "clock" to zero or to some random number?

In the 28 years since 1962 we have shown that WI-38 and other human cell strains have a remarkable memory. Even after 28 years WI-38 cells remember the population doubling level at which they were frozen and, upon reconstitution, undergo the number of population doublings that remain from the time they were frozen to 50. More than 130 ampules have been reconstituted by us in the past 28 years; the memory of these cells is as accurate today as it was in 1962.

Functional Failure as Cultured Normal Human Cells Reach Phase III

The probability that animals age because one or more cell type loses its ability to proliferate is unlikely. It is more likely that decrements in physiologic function that appear before cells lose their capacity to replicate are the true causes of age changes. In 1971, we reported the first functional decrement in a normal human cell population before its loss of proliferative capacity (65). We found that WI-38 cells lost much of their ability to synthesize collagen and to induce collagenolytic activity after almost 40 population doublings.

In the next decade, almost 200 functional changes have been found to occur in cultured normal human cells prior to their loss of replicative capacity. A full tabulation is presented in a review (66). The changes reported to occur cover virtually all aspects of cell biochemistry, morphology, and behavior. They include changes in lipids, carbohydrates, amino acids, proteins, RNA, DNA, enzymes, cell cycle dynamics, cell size and morphology, synthesis, incorporation, and stimulation.

It is more likely that these changes, which herald the approaching loss of division capacity, play the central role in expressing aging and result in the death of the individual animal well before its cells fail to divide.

Of great importance is the realization that many of these same changes that have been reported to occur in cultured normal human cells as they age in vitro are identical to changes that are known to occur in cells in vivo as humans age (66). This finding adds considerable weight to our contention that intrinsic limited life span of cultured normal cells is indeed an expression of aging at the cellular level.

Clearly, there are several classes of cells that are incapable of division in mature animals and it is just as likely, if not even more likely, that these cells play a greater role in the expression of age changes than those cells that are capable of dividing. Examples of nondividing cells would be neurons and muscle cells. It is important to emphasize that the cessation of mitotic activity is only one functional decrement whose genetic basis may be similar to those functional decrements known to occur in aging, nondividing cells. We have proposed, therefore, that the same kind of gene action that results in physiologic decrements in aging, nondividing cells also occurs in aging cells that can still divide. It is not our belief that age changes result necessarily from loss of the function to divide, but simply in the loss of any function characteristic of an aging cell. The basis for loss of any of these functions is thought to be similar.

If these conclusions are accurate, an understanding

of the mechanism by which normal cells lose their capacity to replicate could provide insights into the causes of decrements in other functional properties, such as those that occur in aging neurons or muscle cells.

Finite Lifetime of Normal Cells In Vivo

As indicated earlier, a determination of cell immortality can be made in two ways. The first method is to grow normal cells in culture. That has been discussed and the conclusion is that under these conditions normal cells do have a finite capacity to replicate and function. The second way in which this question can be answered is to determine whether normal cells can proliferate indefinitely in vivo.

If all cell types were continually renewed without loss of function or capacity for self-renewal, organs composed of such cells would be expected to function normally indefinitely; their host would live forever. Regrettably, renewal cell populations do not occur in most tissues, and when they do, cell proliferation is not indefinite.

Is it possible, then, to circumvent the death of normal animal cells that results in the death of the "host" by transferring marked cells to younger animals seriatim? Such experiments would provide an in vivo counterpart to the in vitro experiments described above. If the analogy is accurate we would predict that normal cells transplanted serially to proper inbred hosts would, like their in vitro counterparts, age. Such experiments would largely rule out objections to in vitro studies that are based on the artificiality of the in vitro environment. The question could be answered by serial orthotopic transplantation of normal somatic tissue to new, young, inbred hosts each time the recipient approaches old age.

Data reported from many different laboratories in which rodent mammary tissue (67), skin (68), and hematopoietic cells (69–74) were employed demonstrate that normal cells serially transplanted to inbred hosts do not survive indefinitely. Studies done with hematopoietic cells to investigate this point actually number in the dozens (75, 76).

The trauma of transplantation does not appear to influence the results; in heterochronic transplants survival time is related to the age of the grafted tissue (68). Cancer cells, on the other hand, frequently can be transplanted indefinitely. Thus the immortality of cancer cells in vitro is also demonstrable in vivo.

Many grafts transplanted in vivo have been found to survive much longer than the life span of the host or donor species before aging and dying. This fact has been erroneously interpreted by some to mean that normal cells can replicate continuously for periods of time in excess of the species' known life span. However, grafted tissue behaves quite differently from cultured cells. The latter are usually kept in a state of continuous proliferation. The cells in grafted tissue are not dividing continuously, nor are the number of cells in the dividing pool as great as that in cell cultures. If fibroblasts in grafted tissue replicated to the extent that comparable cells do in vitro, the graft would quickly weigh more than its host. Thus, it is important to appreciate that long survival time is not equivalent to proliferation time or rounds of division. Cells in grafts have a very low reproductive turnover rate. This is analogous to holding normal cell cultures at room temperature, which extends calendar time for cell survival but does not result in increased population doublings.

Theories of Biologic Aging

What then are the most likely causes of biologic aging? The relative newness of the field of gerontology as a seriously studied science and the consequent lack of an extensive and reliable data base has encouraged speculation on the theoretical underpinnings of the field. An additional reason for the plethora of biogerontologic theories is that manifestations of biologic changes over time affect virtually all components of living systems from the molecular level up to that of the whole organism. These hierarchical changes have made it possible to construct theories of aging based on events that occur over time at the level of the molecule, cell organelle, cell, tissue, organ, or whole animal.

Depending more upon the bias of the theorist than actual fact, a selected age-associated change within this hierarchy will often be defended with great vigor and emotion. Nevertheless, most current theories of biologic aging suffer from the criticism that they are or may be mere expressions of the effect of some more fundamental change. There is common failure to realize that changes more fundamental to the one observed may induce the effect that was chosen for study.

Since all fundamental life processes depend on genetic events, theories of aging that depend on these events have attracted the most attention.

Essential Concepts

Evidence for the proposition that *longevity* is somehow determined by genetic events is overwhelming, but evidence that *age* changes, which occur after maturity, are the result of gene expression is quite another matter. In order to dissect this concept and, indeed, all other theories of aging, it is essential to distinguish between what Sacher calls "the biology of the finitude of life, in its three aspects of longevity, aging, and death" (77).

Expressions of Longevity

I will add a fourth concept to Sacher's triad by introducing the notion that two forms or expressions of longevity exist and these must be distinguished for all species. I believe this to be a fundamental concept in deliberations on theories of the finitude of life.

The expression of longevity that is most familiar refers to the maximum period of time that members of a species live under optimum circumstances. For man this would be about 115 years. I propose that this maximum longevity or life span is the sum of two components.

The first component is the elapsed time from conception to the point of sexual development, which coincides with the beginning of postmaturational aging events. The biologic events that occur during this span of time result in what is commonly referred to as development. I will call this span of time *developmental longevity*. For humans this period is about 30 years.

The second component of maximum longevity or life span is the time that elapses from completed development of an organism to the achievement of the maximum life span characteristic for that species. I will call this period of time *postdevelopmental longevity*. Many of the biologic changes that occur during this period of time are what we call aging. For humans, this period of time, measured from age 30, is not known to exceed 85 years.

The sum of the span of time for developmental longevity and for postdevelopmental longevity to occur I will call *total longevity*.

With these distinctions in mind, developmental longevity must be genetically programmed but postdevelopmental longevity, during which time age changes occur, cannot. I will not discuss the fourth part of the finitude of life—the biology of death—because it is beyond the scope of this chapter.

Necessary Criteria for Theories of Aging or Longevity

Generalizations about theories of longevity or aging important to state at the outset are the criteria that must be satisfied if any theory of aging or longevity is to be tenable (78). The criteria most frequently applied are the four first expressed by Strehler (79). A theory of aging must explain changes that are:

1. Deleterious (i.e., reduce function)
2. Progressive (i.e., take place gradually)
3. Intrinsic (i.e., not due to modifiable environmental agents)
4. Universal (i.e., all members of a species, given the opportunity, should reveal the deficits).

In respect to universality, however, it is important to be mindful of the fact that, as indicated earlier, there are animals in which aging is rare or has never been demonstrated. Some fish and amphibians that have an indeterminate size may also have an indeterminate life span (2). Thompson (80) observes, "It is the rule in fishes and other cold-blooded vertebrates that growth is asymptotic and size indeterminate, while in warm-blooded animals, growth comes, sooner or later, to an end."

With respect to the criteria of deleteriousness, progression, and intrinsicality, aging must be distinguished from disease. The decrements (and some increments) characteristic of aging are not diseases, but rather are natural losses of function.

Other "normal" decrements of aging in vital organs do increase the likelihood of death by increasing vulnerability to diseases or pathologic change. For example, normal age-related decrements in immune system functions increase vulnerability to diseases that in youth would be easily thwarted.

With few exceptions, no one over the age of 65 ever dies directly from what is written on their death certificate. They die from the *normal* decrements of old age that have *increased their vulnerability* to what was written on the certificate.

History of Aging as a Genetically Programmed Phenomenon

Advocates of what has been called "Programmed Aging," unlike proponents of such probability-based theories as error accumulation, gene mutation, or free-radical reactions, postulate a purposeful sequence of events written into the genome.

The conceptual simplicity of this idea is part of its allure, but it cannot be defended in light of the driving force of natural selection and evolution. Although events occurring from conception to sexual maturity may be programmed, all of the postdevelopmental decrements that are characteristic of aging cannot be purposely determined by the genome.

Origins of Concept of Programmed Aging

In 1891 August Weismann apparently was the first to present an argument for natural selection that favored a program for age changes (27):

> . . . and thus we have the origin of old age, decay and death; for it is evident that when one or more individuals

> have provided a sufficient number of successors they themselves, as consumers of nourishment in a constantly increasing degree, are an injury to those successors. Natural selection therefore weeds them out, and in many cases favours such races as die almost immediately after they have left successors.

In 1908 Minot (81) suggested that aging is a continuation of development, " . . . the condition of old age, is merely the culmination of changes which have been going on from the first stage of the germ up to the adult, the old man or woman. All through life these changes continue. The result is senility." Minot did not attribute this continuum that he suggested to be governed by the genetic apparatus, but it is implied.

In 1925 Bidder (82) postulated that aging in mammals was an unimportant byproduct of an important positive adaptation, the limitation of size. In his view, aging was a side effect of a genetic program that dictated optimum size. Bidder was first to recognize, in 1932, that there is no selective advantage for a species to have its members live much beyond the age of sexual maturity and child rearing.

> If primitive man begat a son, the species had no more need of him by 37, when his son could hunt for food for the grandchildren. Therefore the dwindling of cartilage, muscle, and nerve cell, which we call senescence, did not affect the survival of the species, the checking of growth had secured that by ensuring a perfect physique between 20 and 40. Effects of continued negative growth were of indifference to the race; probably no man ever reached 60 years old until language attained such importance in the equipment of the species that long experience became valuable in man who could neither fight nor hunt (82).

As the molecular biology of development became better understood in subsequent years, a class of theories based on a putative genetic program for aging arose. The first idea, offered by Jacob and Monod in 1963 (83), suggested that essential genes required for continued existence are switched off as a result of a repression of their transcription.

A second hypothesis, the codon restriction theory suggested by Strehler, maintained that " . . . the site of control of gene expression is not primarily at the points of transcription initiation, but rather that programmed changes in the translational capacities of cells limits the kinds of products synthesized at each stage of the life cycle (79)."

A third hypothesis holds that errors in transcription and/or translation can lead to a self-amplification of errors in either or both processes resulting in an accumulation of faulty products (84, 85, 86).

In contention here is the extent to which gene expression governs age changes in an animal in ways comparable to the genetic determination of its development.

Why Aging Is Not Genetically Programmed

Before considering in detail the role of the genome in aging, it is important to appreciate that aging in its extreme manifestations occurs only in humans or the domestic and zoo animals that we choose to protect.

Feral animals old enough to have decrements in physiologic function comparable to that of a middle-aged human simply do not survive. As soon as they incur even slight decrements in, for example, running speed, jumping ability, or visual acuity, they are culled by predators. Similarly, as soon as vital organs or the immune system become less efficient, feral animals will soon die of disease or other pathology. Or more likely, they will be culled by predators when disease reduces their ability to elude capture. If aging occurs at all in wild animals its expression is quantitatively small and temporally brief.

Is Aging a Result of Natural Selection?

Because few feral animals become old, natural selection could not have favored the development of a genetically programmed aging process. Thus, aging cannot be viewed as a phenomenon that has been selected for by evolution. This is true even for humans. In the 2 or 3 million years of human existence, there have been too few old humans in any generation to have provided a selective advantage favoring the development of a genetic program that would determine age changes.

Furthermore, there is no selective advantage for animals to live much beyond the age of sexual maturity and rearing of progeny. In humans, there is no advantage for species survival for members to live much beyond age 30, which is generally believed to be the time when age changes become detectable and the Gompertz equation begins its exponential rise (87). Thirty years, as Bidder (88) observed, is sufficient time for humans to produce new progeny and to rear that progeny to sexual maturation.

Since life expectation at birth in prehistoric times was about 18 years, it is apparent that the human species has survived for a much longer period of time with an 18-year life expectation than it has with the current 75-year life expectation and 115-year life span. Thus, humans have survived far longer with few, or no, old members than they have with many old members. Natural selection for a genetic program that would express age changes could not have occurred in human evolution because most humans were killed by predation and disease before age 30.

Today, the application of knowledge obtained by biomedical research has produced life expectations in developed countries that were unknown in prehistoric times and even at the turn of this century. The magnitude of age changes expressed by humans who today live long enough to experience them is unattainable by feral animals.

Teleology and Aging

Aging, therefore, may be thought of as an aberration of civilization. It has permitted the expression of physiologic decrements, called aging, that otherwise would not have been revealed. Aging, in effect, has been eliminated in feral animals. It could be eliminated in humans also if we all chose to die at the age of 30.

In summary, since evolution could not have selected directly for age changes, it is impossible to account for the evolution of a genetic program that could produce those changes. Hence, the theory that a purposeful genetic program expressing age changes exists, as a comparable program might code for developmental changes, is untenable.

Other Criticisms of the Theory of Programmed Aging

Sacher has criticized the program theory of aging for what he believes to be other errors in logic (89). He illustrates his argument by comparing the life histories of annual plants and mammals. Annual plants are semelparous: that is, they are characterized by a single reproductive effort, completed at the end of the life span and frequently not until somatic cell death. The final step of the reproductive process, seed dispersal, depends on the death of the plant, and this requires that senescence be closely integrated with prior stages. The stages are known to be under the specific control of hormones and end with formation of specific hydrolytic enzymes.

Sacher restricts programmed aging to such cases, where there is specific control of onset either by internal or external signals, presence of a specific enzyme mechanism, and finally, a functional role for senescence and/or death in a specific temporal relationship with other life processes. The rapid aging and death of the Pacific salmon after spawning is a good example of this event occurring in a vertebrate. The same "big bang" reproduction effort followed by death has been reported to occur in male marsupial mice (90). These animals express developmental longevity but little or no postdevelopmental longevity.

Mammals, on the other hand, are examples of iteroparous reproduction, in which reproductive success depends on producing a number of litters over an extended reproductive span. Sacher argues that this offers no functional role for senescence and death. On the contrary, he maintains that this would place a premium on the maintenance of physiological vigor and survival. Most mammals, therefore, express both developmental and postdevelopmental longevity.

Genetic Basis for Determination of Longevity

While it is unlikely that a genetic program has evolved to program *age* changes, the evidence that genetic factors determine total longevity is quite convincing. Some of that evidence follows:

1. The life spans of individuals in each species are remarkably constant and species specific. For example, the maximum life span of a fruit fly is about 1 month, a mouse about 3 years, and a human about 115 years.

One exception to the constancy of species life spans is the extraordinary difference in longevity of certain social insects. The queen honey bee (*Apis mellifera*) may live for as long as 6 years. Workers live from 3 to 6 months. The determination of life span cannot be a fundamental difference in the genetics of these organisms since their genomes are identical. The difference is simply the result of whether or not they were fed royal jelly during the larval stage. There is no other example in nature in which a dietary supplement results in, among other profound changes, a 12- to 24-fold increase in longevity.

2. In humans, for example, the mean difference in total longevity between fraternal twins is twice as great as that in identical twins (91). The ancestors of centenarians and nonagenarians have significantly greater total longevity when compared with ancestors of individuals not selected for great longevity (1).

3. In many animal species the female is more longevous than the male, but this is by no means true for all animal species (2).

4. In the past decade it has become apparent that some single gene changes result in reduced life spans in humans, as in the case of progeria and the Werner's syndrome. In these conditions several age-related phenomena appear to be accelerated. Polygenic changes are also thought to influence the rate and characteristics of age changes in normal individuals. However, there is considerable skepticism that these conditions actually represent accelerated aging (92).

5. Genotoxic effects, the effect of mutagens (e.g. radiation) on total longevity, are virtually proven to be the result of effects on the cell genome.

6. A direct correlation has been reported to occur between the efficiency of certain kinds of DNA repair processes and species longevity. More long-lived species are found to have more efficient DNA repair capabilities (93).

7. The Lansing effect suggests that in some animals, including humans, the progeny of older mothers have a shorter life expectation. This effect may extend through several generations (2, 3, 94).

8. In a study of inbred mouse strains it has been estimated that half of the variance associated with total longevity was due to genetic factors (95).

9. Recombinant inbred lines of two varieties of the nematode *Caenorhabditis elegans* reveal large variances in life span. Some are in excess of the life spans of the parent organisms. Molecular genetic analyses of the control of total longevity in these animals thus becomes possible (96).

10. Cultured normal human and animal cells and those transplanted seriatim in vivo have a limited capacity to divide and function (33, 34, 97, 98). Fibroblasts derived from different animal species have a potential for population doublings that suggests a direct relationship with species longevity (99).

Longevity Assurance or Longevity Determinant Genes

The selective advantage to an organism of maintaining its physiologic vigor for as long as possible to ensure maximum reproductive success may be the essential indirect force that influences longevity.

For example, to ensure maximum parental vigor for survival of slowly maturing human progeny, there would be a selective advantage for parents to maintain their physiologic vigor for longer periods of time. Thus, the necessity for assuring the maintenance of vital life processes for longer periods of time would have strong survival value. There is some evidence for this since it has been shown recently that the variations in age at first reproduction among female mammals is correlated strongly with life expectation at birth even after the effects of body size have been eliminated (100).

Evolution of Longevity

Thirty years ago, some imaginative ideas were put forth by two theorists who attempted to explain how longevity may have evolved through a process of natural selection of gene expression.

Medawar suggested that the expression of deleterious genes in a species might be thwarted by a selection process that would postpone their manifestations if it were impossible to eliminate them by natural selection (101). This strategy would result in the accumulation of deleterious genes in the postreproductive period when their expression would do less harm.

A variation on this theme was made by Williams who postulated pleiotropic genes having both favorable and unfavorable actions (102). If the favorable gene expression is able to increase fecundity, that gene might be selected even though it might express a deleterious action later in life. Deleterious age changes then would be the penalty paid by individuals for the expression of beneficial genes early in life. An accumulation of such late-acting genes in various organ systems would behave like late-programmed events and give rise to the entire constellation of age changes. The postponement of the expression of late-acting deleterious genes would also have the effect of increasing total longevity.

Sacher (77, 89, 103) and Cutler (104) have suggested the existence of what the former calls "longevity assurance genes" and what the latter calls "longevity determinant genes" to account for the genetic basis for longevity determination. It is *not* postulated as a mechanism for aging.

The central hypothesis is that the appearance and evolution of regulatory genes that maintain vital life processes longer provides a selective advantage to the species. Thus, evolution of the genome could account for species longevity independent of the necessity for a genetic program that codes for age changes.

Developmental longevity in mammals, therefore, may be the result of selection for an extended period of assured physiologic performance. A great whale that lives 30 times longer than a mouse has a million times more cells at risk for age changes. Nevertheless, a comparable whale cell is orders of magnitude more stable than a mouse cell.

"It would be expected," says Sacher, "that the selective process acts on mechanisms for *increasing* the stability of the organism at all levels, from the molecular to the systemic." Sacher emphasizes the more evolutionary logical role of genetic systems that maintain life rather than theories that these systems might program age changes. Since evolution cannot select directly for total longevity, the study of life maintenance systems or "longevity assurance genes" may be more productive than the current emphasis on a search for the causes of age-associated physiologic decrements (89, 103).

There is no direct evidence for the existence of longevity assurance genes, although some indirect clues exist. Cutler (104) estimates that, in general, the longevity of species has increased. As indicated earlier, that old feral animals are unknown is consistent with the conclusion that longevity, not aging, has evolved. Cutler regards the rate of evolution of longevity to be closely linked to the environmental hazards that an animal is exposed to in its ecological niche. He argues that a species' mean life span in the wild "defines the point where further longevity would have little benefit." A reduction in those hazards presumably would be the prerequisite force needed to stimulate longevity assurance genes, thus enhancing reproductive capacity.

One mechanism that might account for the expression of longevity assurance might be the suggestion of Medvedev (84, 105) that the repeated DNA nucleotide sequences in the genome of eukaryotic organisms may be (*a*) a reserve of information for evolutionary change, (*b*) a means of increasing functional expression, and (*c*) a reserve mechanism for protecting vital information from random errors that occur in functioning DNA sequences.

Medvedev (84, 105) proposed that the loss of unique, nonrepeated DNA sequences could produce age decrements and that selected reiterated sequences may be an evolved means for delaying the inevitability of failure by providing the redundancy necessary for maintenance of vital information. The degree of redundancy, established by natural selection, would determine total life span by backing up vital functioning DNA sequences from random errors. This notion has the merit of simplicity because it does not require the formation of new genes.

Rate of Evolution of Longevity Assurance Genes

The rate of evolution of longevity assurance genes was determined by Sacher (106), who used the brain weight/body weight ratio of mammalian species that correlates so well with their total longevity. It has predictive value when the adult body and brain weight of fossil species can be determined. In this way, the maximum life span of fossil hominids has been determined.

The results of these studies indicate clearly that longevity has increased throughout the entire period of evolution for all mammalian species. Most important was the finding that the rate of increase was especially rapid for human hominid ancestors.

Causes of Aging

If age changes are not purposefully determined by the genome, why and how do they occur?

The forces of natural selection have provided sexually mature animals with an extraordinary reserve capacity in virtually all organs. This phenomenon has been neglected with respect to its role in aging where, I believe, it may be the determinant process in our understanding of the genesis of biologic aging.

Reserve capacity undoubtedly has been achieved by natural selection to better guarantee that animals will survive long enough to reach sexual maturity. That guarantee is best achieved by a selective process favoring animals with greater reserve capacity in vital systems. Redundancy is the most effective means of ensuring that systems perform accurately for specific periods of time. The forces that select and maintain redundant capacity are presumed to be the same forces that underlie the evolution of longevity assurance mechanisms. Indeed, longevity assurance mechanisms may be identical to the mechanisms that are hypothesized to produce redundancy.

All of natural selection is directed toward favoring animals that survive long enough to reproduce. Survival to the point of reproduction is best assured by selecting for overcapacity or redundancy in vital systems. As indicated earlier there is no survival value for a species to have its members live much beyond the period of sexual maturation hence there is no selective pressure favoring survival much beyond the period of developmental longevity.

Once sexual maturity is reached, animals will continue to function by utilizing the reserve capacity that evolved to ensure that they would reach the earlier stage of reproductive ability. The magnitude of reserve capacity is an essential element in determining postdevelopmental longevity. It could have been determined earlier by the action of hypothetical longevity assurance genes or simply by the production of redundant messages.

Thus the evolution of longevity assurance mechanisms that guarantee vigor in animals until sexual maturation indirectly may determine their postdevelopmental longevity.

In this way, age changes begin and continue to occur as organ systems "coast" or "free-wheel" on the reserve capacity that was "overengineered" during earlier development. This period of "coasting," defined earlier as postdevelopmental longevity, is characterized by a shift in energy balance that increases entropy in the same biochemical processes that earlier gave rise to the development and maturation of the organism.

Dysdifferentiation

Cutler (104) calls postdevelopmental decrements "dysdifferentiation" to distinguish them from dedifferentiation to the embryonic state or differentiation to a more specialized state. Dysdifferentiation would encompass all possible changes that might occur in cells after maturation and implies only the slow loss of the differentiated state. It does not require the acquisition of damage to cells, which is a prerequisite for most other hypotheses of aging.

Cutler argues that the "longevity determinant genes act to stabilize the cells' proper state of differentiation against the destabilizing effects of the pleiotropic by-products of energy metabolism and development" (107). Thus, the cells in longer living species would be inherently more stable in maintaining the proper differentiated state in the presence of destabilizing insults. The degree of stability, governed by longevity assurance genes, is therefore the indirect determinant of species longevity.

A manifestation of this event at the cellular level has been the observation made in the cultured normal cells of species with different life spans. Cells derived from longer living species undergo more rounds of division, maintain function longer, and are therefore inherently more stable than are cells derived from shorter living species (99).

Cell Death

One potential problem with the dysdifferentiation concept and the effect of longevity determinant genes on the rate of cell destabilization is that the destabilization of differentiated cells is a process not restricted to aging. It occurs early in embryogenesis and continues on a massive scale throughout development.

The death of cells and the cataclysmic destruction of tissues and organs is a normal part of morphogenic or developmental sequences in animals. It is the common method for eliminating organs and tissues that are useful only in the larval or embryonic stages of many animals. Cell degeneration is an important part of development and is a widespread occurrence in vertebrate cells (108, 109).

The processes of dysdifferentiation leading to cell aging that occur after maturation in an organism are identical to the processes by which cells are lost during embryogenesis and development. It is almost universally believed that the loss of cell function that ultimately leads to cell death in embryogenesis and development is a programmed event, yet Cutler (104) and others view what appears to be an identical event as a chance process when it occurs after maturation.

Conclusion

"Why do we age?" may be the wrong question. The right question may be, "Why do we live as long as we do?"

References

1. Pearl, R, and Pearl, RD. 1934. *The ancestry of the long-lived.* Baltimore: The Johns Hopkins Press.
2. Comfort, A. 1979. *The Biology of Senescence,* ed. 3. London: Churchill Livingstone.
3. Strehler, BL. 1977. *Time, Cells, and Aging*. ed. 2. New York: Academic Press.
4. Kohn, RR. 1971. *Principles of mammalian aging*. Englewood Cliffs, NJ: Prentice-Hall, Inc.
5. Hayflick, L. 1973. The biology of human aging. *Am J Med Sci* 265:433–445.
6. Hayflick, L. 1974. The strategy of senescence. *Gerontologist* 14:37–45.
7. Hayflick, L. 1976. The cell biology of human aging. *N Engl J Med* 295:1302–1308.
8. Fries, JF. 1980. Aging, natural death, and the compression of morbidity. *N Engl J Med* 303:130–135.
9. Fries, JF, and Crapo, LM. 1981. *Vitality and Aging: Implications of the Rectangular Curve*. San Francisco: WH Freeman.
10. Fries, JF. 1983. The compression of morbidity. *Milbank Memorial Fund Quarterly/Health and Society* 61:397–418.
11. Fries, JF. 1984. The compression of morbidity: Miscellaneous comments about a theme. *Gerontologist* 24:354–359.
12. Manton, KG. 1982. Changing concepts of morbidity and mortality in the elderly population. *Milbank Memorial Fund Quarterly/Health and Society* 60:183–244.
13. Myers, GC, and Manton, KG. 1984. Compression of mortality: Myth or reality? *Gerontologist* 24:346–353.
14. Schneider, EL, and Brody, JA. 1983. Aging, natural death, and the compression of morbidity: Another view. *N Engl J Med* 309:854–856.
15. Crimmins, EM. 1984. Life expectancy and the older population. *Res Aging* 6(4):490–514.
16. Fries, JF. 1985. The biological constraints on human aging: Implications for health policy. In: *Health Care for the Elderly*, Eds., KG Andreoli, LA Musser, and SJ Reiser. New York: The Haworth Press.
17. Mazess, RB. 1978. Health and longevity in Vilcabamba, Ecuador. *JAMA* 1781.
18. Medvedev, ZhA. 1974. Caucasus and Altay longevity: A biologic or social problem? *Gerontologist* 14:381.
19. Sacher, GA. 1959. Relation of lifespan to brain weight and body weight. In *The Lifespan of Animals*, Eds., GEW Wolstenholme and M O'Conner, pp. 115–141. Boston: Little, Brown & Co.
20. Sacher, GA. 1975. Maturation and longevity in relation to cranial capacity in hominid evolution. In *Interdisciplinary Topics in Gerontology*, Ed., RH Tuttle, vol 9, pp. 69–83, Basel: Karger.
21. Friedenthal, H. 1910. Ueber die Giltigkeit des Massenwirkung fur den Energieumsatz der lebendigen Substanz. *Zentralbl Physiol* 24:321–327.
22. Hofman, MA. 1983. Energy metabolism, brain size and longevity in mammals. *Q Rev Biol* 58(4):495–512.
23. McKay, CM, Crowell, MF, and Maynard, LA. 1935. The effect of retarded growth upon the length of life span and upon the ultimate body size. *J Nutr* 10:63–79.
24. Masoro, EJ. 1985. Extending the mammalian life span. In *Aging 2000:Our Health Care Destiny*, Eds., C Gaitz and T Samorajski. New York: Springer Publishing Co.
25. Weindruch, R, and Walford, RL. 1982. Life span and spontaneous cancer incidence in mice dietarily restricted beginning at one year of age. *Science* 215:1415–1418.
26. Siegel, JS, and Davidson, M. *Current Population Re-*

ports, Special studies, series P-23, no. 138, Issued August 1984. Demographic and Socioeconomic Aspects of Aging in the United States. U.S. Dept. of Commerce, Bureau of the Census.

27. Weismann, A. 1891. *Essays upon heredity and kindred biological problems*. Ed. 2. Oxford, Clarendon Press.
28. Ezra and Nehemiah: First Kings. 1944. Ch. 1, v. 1–4 and Ch. 2, v. 1, 5704. In *The Holy Bible*, Philadelphia: The Jewish Publication Society of America.
29. Hayflick, L. 1974. Cytogerontology. In *Theoretical Aspects of Aging*, Ed., M Rockstein. New York: Academic Press.
30. Kirkwood, TBL, and Cremer, T. 1982. Cytogerontology since 1881: A reappraisal of August Weismann and a review of modern progress. *Hum Genet* 60:101–121.
31. Parker, RC. 1961. *Methods of tissue culture*. New York: Harper & Row.
32. Kohler G, and Milstein, C. 1975. Continuous cultures of fused cells secreting antibody of predefined specificity. *Nature* 256:495–497.
33. Hayflick, L, and Moorhead, PS. 1961. The serial cultivation of human diploid cell strains. *Exp Cell Res*, 25:585–621.
34. Hayflick, L. 1965. The limited in vitro lifetime of human diploid cell strains. *Exp Cell Res* 37:614–636.
35. Puck, TT, Cieciura, SJ, and Fisher, HW. 1957. Clonal growth in vitro of human cells with fibroblastic morphology. *J Exp Med* 106:145–158.
36. Puck, TT, Cieciura, SJ, and Robinson, A. 1958. Genetics of somatic mammalian cells. III. Long-term cultivation of euploid cells from human and animal subjects. *J Exp Med* 108:945–956.
37. Swim, HE, and Parker, RF. 1957. Culture characteristics of human fibroblasts propagated serially. *Am J Hyg* 66:235–243.
38. Hayflick, L. 1970. Aging under glass. *Exp Gerontol* 5:291–303.
39. Hayflick, L. 1972. Cell senescence and cell differentiation in vitro. In *Aging and Development*. Academy of Science and Literature, Mainz, Germany. Stuttgart: FK Schattauer Verlag.
40. Ogura, H, Fujiwara, T, and Namba, M. 1984. Establishment of two chick embryo fibroblastic cell lines. *Gann* 75:410–414.
41. Harris, M. 1957. Quantitative growth studies with chick myoblasts in glass substrate cultures. *Growth* 21:149–166.
42. Hay, RJ, and Strehler, BL. 1967. The limited growth span of cell strains isolated from the chick embryo. *Exp Gerontol* 2:123–135.
43. Lima, L, and Macieira-Coelho, A. 1972. Parameters of aging in chicken embryo fibroblasts cultivated in vitro. *Exp Cell Res* 70:279–284.
44. Ponten, J. 1970. The growth capacity of normal and Rous-virus-transformed chicken fibroblasts in vitro. *Int J Cancer* 6:323–332.
45. Witkowski, JA. 1979. Alexis Carrel and the mysticism of tissue culture. *Med Hist* 23:279–296.
46. Witkowski, JA. 1980. Dr. Carrel's immortal cells. *Med Hist* 24:129–142.
47. Witkowski, JA. 1985. The myth of cell immortality. *Trends in Biochemical Sciences* 10:258–260.
48. Martin, GM, Sprague, CA, and Epstein, CJ. 1970. Replicative life span of cultivated human cells. Effect of donor's age, tissue, and genotype. *Lab Invest* 23:86–92.
49. Goldstein, S, et al. 1978. Chronologic and physiological age effect replicative life span of fibroblasts from diabetics, prediabetics, and normal donors. *Science* 199: 781–782.
50. Schneider, EL, and Mitsui, Y. 1976. The relationship between in vitro cellular aging and in vivo human aging. *Proc Nat Acad Sci USA* 73:3584–3588.
51. Vracko, R, and McFarland, BM. 1980. Life span of diabetic and nondiabetic fibroblasts in vitro. *Exp Cell Res* 129:345–350.
52. LeGuilly, Y, et al. 1973. Long-term culture of human adult liver cells: Morphological changes related to in vitro senescence and effect of donor's age on growth potential. *Gerontologia* 19:303–313.
53. Bierman, EL. 1977. The effect of donor age on the in vitro lifespan of cultured human arterial smooth-muscle cells. *In Vitro* 14:951–955.
54. Tassin, J, Malaise, E, and Courtois, Y. 1979. Human lens cells have an in vitro proliferative capacity inversely proportional to the donor age. *Exp Cell Res* 123:388–392.
55. Walford, RL. 1982. Studies in immunogerontology. *J Am Geriat Soc* 30:617–625.
56. Walford, RL, Jawaid, SQ, and Naeim, F. 1981. Evidence for in vitro senescence of T-lymphocytes cultured from normal human peripheral blood. *Age* 4:67–70.
57. Röhme, D. 1981. Evidence for a relationship between longevity of mammalian species and life spans of normal fibroblasts in vitro and erythrocytes in vivo. *Proc Natl Acad Sci USA* 78:5009–5013.
58. Stanley, JF, Pye, D, and MacGregor, A. 1975. Comparison of doubling numbers attained by cultured animal cells with the life span of species. *Nature* 255:158–159.
59. Reichel, W, Garcia-Bunuel, R, and Dilallo, J. 1971. Progeria and Werner's syndrome as models for the study of normal human aging. *J Am Geriatr Soc* 19:369–375.
60. Epstein, CJ, et al. 1966. Werner's syndrome: A review of its symptomatology, natural history, pathologic features, genetics and relationship to the natural aging process. *Medicine* 45:177–221.
61. Goldstein, S. 1969. Life span of cultured cells in progeria. *Lancet* 1:424.
62. Goldstein, S. 1971. The biology of aging. *N Engl J Med* 285:1120–1129.
63. Danes, BS. 1971. Progeria: A cell culture study on aging. *J Clin Invest* 50:2000–2003.
64. Nienhaus, AJ, DeJong, B, and Tenkate, LP. 1971. Fibroblast culture in Werner's syndrome. *Humangenetik* 13:244–246.
65. Houck, JC, Sharma, VK, and Hayflick, L. 1971. Functional failures of cultured human diploid fibroblasts after continued population doublings. *Proc Soc Exp Biol Med* 137:331–333.
66. Hayflick, L. 1980. Cell aging. In *Annual Review of Gerontology and Geriatrics*. Ed., C Eisdorfer. New York: Springer Publishing Co.
67. Daniel, CW, deOme, KB, Young, JT, et al. 1968. The in vivo life span of normal and preneoplastic mouse mammary glands: A serial transplantation study. *Proc Natl Acad Sci USA* 61:53–608.

68. Krohn, PL. 1962. Review lectures on senescence. II: Heterochronic transplantation in the study of aging. *Proc R Soc Lond (Biol)* 157:128–147.
69. Cudkowicz, G, et al. 1964. Lymphocyte content and proliferative capacity of serially transplanted mouse bone marrow. *Nature* 201:165–167.
70. Ford, CE, Micklem, HS, and Gray, SM. 1959. Evidence of selective proliferation of reticular cell-clones in heavily irradiated mice. *Br J Radiol* 32:280.
71. Harrison, DE. 1973. Normal production of erythrocytes by mouse marrow continuous for 73 months. *Proc Natl Acad Sci USA* 70:3184–3188.
72. Harrison, DE. 1975. Normal function of transplanted marrow cell lines from aged mice. *J Gerontol* 30:279–285.
73. Hellman, S, et al. 1978. Proliferative capacity of murine hematopoietic stem cells. *Proc Natl Acad Sci USA* 75:490–494.
74. Siminovitch, L, Till, JE, and McCulloch, EA. 1964. Decline in colony-forming ability of marrow cells subjected to serial transplantation into irradiated mice. *J Cell Comparat Physiol* 64:23–31.
75. Hayflick, L. 1984. Immortality. *Science* 225:268.
76. Effros, R, and Walford, L. 1984. T Cell Cultures and the Hayflick Limit. *Hum Immunol* 9:49–65.
77. Sacher, GA. 1980. Theory in gerontology, Part 1. In *Annual Review of Gerontology and Geriatrics*, Ed., C Eisdorfer, pp. 3–25. New York: Springer Publishing Co. Inc.
78. Hayflick, L. 1985. Theories of biological aging. *Exp Gerontol* 20:145–159.
79. Strehler, BL. 1982. Aging: Concepts and Theories. In *Lectures on Gerontology*, Ed., A Viidik, pp. 1–57. New York: Academic Press.
80. Thompson, DW. 1942. *On Growth and Form*, New Edition, p. 199. Cambridge, England: Cambridge University Press.
81. Minot, CS. 1908. *The problem of age, growth, and death*. New York: GP Putnam's Sons, The Knickerbocker Press.
82. Bidder, GP. 1925. The mortality of plaicc. *Nature* 115:495.
83. Jacob, F and Monod, J. 1963. In: *Cytodifferentiation and Macromolecular Synthesis*, Ed., M Locke, pp. 30–64. New York and London: Academic Press.
84. Medvedev, ZhA. 1961. *Aktual Vopr Sovr Biol* 51:299.
85. Medvedev, ZhA. 1972. Repetition of molecular-genetic information as a possible factor in evolutionary changes of lifespan. *Exp Gerontol* 7:227–238.
86. Orgel, LE. 1963. The maintenance of the accuracy of protein synthesis and its relevance to aging. *Proc Natl Acad Sci USA* 49:517–521.
87. Gompertz, B. 1825. On the nature of the function expressive of the law of human mortality and on a new mode of determining life contingencies. *Philos Trans R Soc Lond Ser A* 115:513–585.
88. Bidder, GP. 1932. Senescence. *Br Med J* 115:5831.
89. Sacher, GA. 1968. Molecular versus systemic theories on the genesis of aging. *Exp Gerontol* 3:265–271.
90. Diamond, JM. 1982. Big-bang reproduction and aging in male marsupial mice. *Nature* 298:115.
91. Kallman, EJ, and Jarvik, LF. 1959. Individual differences in constitution and genetic background. In *Handbook of Aging and the Individual*, Ed., JE Birren, pp. 216–263. Chicago: University of Chicago Press.
92. Epstein, CJ. 1985. Werner's syndrome and aging: A reappraisal. In: *Werner's Syndrome and Human Aging* Advances in Experimental Medicine and Biology, Eds., D Salk, Y Fujiwara, and GM Martin, vol. 190, pp. 219–228. New York and London: Plenum Press.
93. Hart, RW, and Setlow, RB. 1974. Correlation between DNA excision repair and life-span in a number of mammalian species. *Proc Natl Acad Sci USA* 71:2169–2173.
94. Lansing, AI. 1947. A transmissible, cumulative, and reversible factor in aging. *J Gerontol* 2:228–239.
95. Goodrick, CL. 1975. Life-span and inheritance of longevity in inbred mice. *J Gerontol* 30:257–264.
96. Johnson, TE, and Wood, WB. 1982. Genetic analysis of life span of the nematode, *Caenorhabditis elegans*. *Proc Natl Acad Sci USA* 79:6603.
97. Hayflick, L. 1984. The coming of age of WI-38. In *Advances in Cell Culture*, Ed., K Maramorosch, vol. 3, pp. 303–316. New York: Academic Press, Inc.
98. Hayflick, L. 1980. The cell biology of human aging. *Sci Am* 242:58–66.
99. Hayflick, L. 1985. The cell biology of aging. In *Clinics in Geriatric Medicine*, The Aging Process, 1(1):15–27.
100. Harvey, PH, and Zammuto, RM. 1985. *Nature* 315:319–320.
101. Medawar, PB. 1957. *The Uniqueness of the Individual*. London: Methuen.
102. Williams, GC. 1957. Pleiotropy, natural selection, and the evolution of senescence. *Evolution* 11:398–411.
103. Sacher, GA. 1982. Evolutionary theory in gerontology. *Perspect Biol Med* 25:339.
104. Cutler, RG. 1982. Longevity is determined by specific genes: Testing the hypothesis. In *Testing the Theories of Aging*, Eds., RC Adelman and GS Roth, pp. 25–114. Boca Raton, FL: CRC Press Inc.
105. Medvedev, ZhA. 1972. Possible role of repeated nucleotide sequences in DNA in evolution of life spans of differentiated cells. *Nature* 237:453–472.
106. Sacher, GA. 1960. The dimensionality of the life span. In *The Biology of Aging*, Ed., BL Strehler, pp. 251. Washington, DC: AIBS.
107. Cutler, RG. 1984. Free radicals and aging. In *Molecular Basis of Aging*, Eds., AK Roy and B Chatterjee, pp. 263–352. Orlando, FL: Academic Press, Inc.
108. Saunders, JW, Jr. 1966. Death in embryonic systems. *Science* 154:604–612.
109. Whitten, JM. 1969. Cell death during early morphogenesis; Parallels between insect limb and vertebrate limb development. *Science* 163:1456–1457.

2

Ethical Approach to Surgery for the Geriatric Patient

Albert R. Jonsen

The ethics of surgical practice is not essentially different from the ethics of medicine in general. The surgeon must "be of benefit and do no harm." The surgeon must approach the patient respectfully, seeking informed consent for the recommended procedure, and must perform competently, assessing the relative risks and benefits of that procedure and carrying it out with skill. As are all physicians, the surgeon is bound to confidentiality and responsible for the well-being of his or her patient, even before the welfare of society. These are fundamental tenets of the ethics of medicine (1). Still, there are certain characteristics of surgical practice that call for special interpretation, and surgical problems that require special applications of these general tenets. Surgical care of the elderly patient presents some of these problems.

Ethical principles are, in themselves, quite definite and clear, but ethical problems, in which the principles must be applied to particular cases, are often ill defined. They are marked by a vagueness that can be frustrating to persons trained to be precise and definite. Thus, some surgeons will take refuge in the generality of principles rather than flounder in the uncertainties of ethical perplexity. They will refuse to acknowledge an ethical problem and plunge ahead, certain that their skill will see them through. Surgery is not a meditative specialty; it is more geared to action than to reflection. In addition, the typical surgeon likes to operate and may find the task of reviewing the ethical pros and cons onerous and obfuscating. Nevertheless, the responsible surgeon will sometimes feel the need to pause and think through the complexities of an ethical problem.

When such an occasion arises, it is useful to have in mind a pattern or a logic that can guide one's thinking in an orderly way through the myriad and often arguable considerations. Giving order to the problem may not solve it, but can clarify it, so that the key issues become more obvious and the options more manifest. An orderly pattern of thinking can be imposed on an ethical problem by considering in turn four features that are inevitably present: (*a*) the medical indications for treatment, (*b*) the patient's preferences about treatment, (*c*) the patient's quality of life, and (*d*) certain external socioeconomic factors. This pattern constitutes a sort of ethical "review of systems." It can help to locate precisely where the problem is and often illuminate the proper approach. This chapter will present the ethics of surgical intervention in the elderly patient according to that pattern (2).

Medical Indications

Medical indications refer to the physical and physiologic facts about a patient that suggest the utility of a diagnostic or therapeutic intervention. In every case, the competent surgeon obtains these facts and analyzes the risks and benefits associated with any procedure. For example, radiologic evidence of a fracture indicates that the bone should be set or pinned. An acute right upper quadrant pain, a palpable gallbladder, a spiking fever, and Murphy's sign suggest acute cholecystitis and radiographic confirmation of this indicates cholecystectomy. This is the standard stuff of medical and surgical decision making. In addition, this strictly medical information is also essential to the understanding of any *ethical* problem that might occur in clinical decision making. The nature of the patient's physical problem, various options for intervention, and the prognosis, with or without intervention, must be made as clear as possible. It is strange that, in a setting so attuned to discussing medical interventions, they are so often neglected when the discussion turns ethical.

The discussion becomes ethical whenever there is a question of whether a procedure that is technically possible should be done on a person of a certain age. For example, a 72-year-old man suffers from angina that is unresponsive to medical management. He has a history of previous myocardial infarction, hypertension, and diabetes mellitus. Studies reveal triple vessel disease. Coronary artery bypass surgery is an available therapy. Is this patient's age relevant to the decision to recommend such surgery? The answer depends on the present knowledge of the efficacy and the risks associated with this procedure in patients over the age of 65. This information may or may not be available in scientific form (3). If it is, the patient's age may be relevant to the decision: high rates of intra- or perioperative mortality, low survival rates, etc. obviously determine the recommendation.

Such information is often unavailable, due to the paucity of controlled studies; when it is, it is often controversial. Nevertheless, the ethical import of such information is noteworthy. It is, in effect, the practical application of the ancient ethical adage, "be of benefit and do no harm." The mere fact that a procedure is technically possible does not ethically indicate that it ought to be recommended. An informed assessment of the expected burdens and benefits must be added to the technical possibility, and age is an essential ingredient in such an assessment. In modern surgery, age enters into the assessment as a scientific datum, not as a prejudice.

A prejudice is a judgment without regard to, or prior to hearing, the facts of the case. In the past, age often disqualified patients from surgery. "Persons of this age do not do well." That kind of judgment was made without regard to or before hearing the facts. Clearly, without surgery, death precluded further evaluation of these patients. But many unproven assumptions tainted such judgments. It was necessary to undertake suitable trials to discern precisely how well persons of a certain age did. Prejudice, in the sense used here, need not be a vicious bias; it simply depends on plausible assumptions that can be dispelled or refined by making the effort to do careful studies. For example, plausible assumptions about the limited physical capacity of the elderly govern thinking about anesthetic management of the aged patient. Those assumptions, based on physiologic fact, need to be tested clinically and refined for application to clinical care. Thus, it can now be said that, while the elderly patient presents special challenges, "age alone is almost never the sole contraindication to anesthesia and surgery (4)."

Age, of course, has a somewhat ambiguous reference. It can refer to the chronological span of a human life measured in years or to the biologic condition of a human being who has lived a certain period. It is commonly said that, in making clinical decisions, age is relevant only in the second sense: the patient may be a "very young 75-year-old." Good clinicians pride themselves on being able to discern the general health of their patients. Thus, caution is recommended that biologic, not chronologic age, is relevant. Still, it must be noted that the careful studies designed to inform about the efficacy and risks of surgery and anesthesia depend, in large part, on cohorts broken down into chronological age. Of course, factors such as concurrent morbidity and health history are included, but the results are reported in terms of "patients over 65, over 70, and over 80." Thus, while it is true that each patient must be assessed individually, even the best data will report in categories and in statistical terms. My "healthy 75-year-old" may fall into the high-risk category of "over 70." Thus, a delicate balance of enthusiasm about my patient and skepticism about all patients "over 70" is required.

The key ethical question in the evaluation of medical indications is "Is it likely that this recommendation will lead to a realization of the goals of good medicine, namely, restoration of health, relief of pain, and enhancement of impaired function?" Preservation of life, often cited among these goals, is ambiguous at best. Implantation of an artificial heart into a 70-year-old dying of cardiomyopathy may preserve his life, but that life may be hardly worth living if marred by mental deficits due to cardiovascular accidents and if dependent on a machine. This issue will be discussed in the section on "Quality of Life." Here, note that preservation of life is not considered, by most contemporary ethicists, to be a goal of medicine in the absence of attainment, to some degree, of the other goals (5).

Preferences of the Patient

It is the duty of the surgeon to recommend to the patient the approach judged most beneficial for the patient's health. In recent years, the doctrine of informed consent has emerged in the law and in ethics (6). That doctrine is based upon the fundamental ethical and legal obligation to respect the autonomy of the patient. Informed consent requires the surgeon to inform the patient about the nature of the morbid condition, the various possibilities for treatment, and the risks and benefits of the various alternatives. While some surgeons find these obligations onerous, most now accept them as an integral part of their duty to the patient. Indeed, there are particular problems: how does one deal with risks of great magnitude but very low probability? Should one refrain from telling a fearful patient certain frightening risks? How can the surgeon be sure that the patient comprehends the information? These are problems familiar to all practitioners.

Surgeons do, however, have a problem that is characteristic of their practice: they rarely have a very thorough acquaintance with their patient. Unlike the internist or family practitioner, who may deal with a patient over time, the surgeon is called in on relatively short notice. The opportunity to come to know the patient well before the surgery is limited; the opportunity to follow the patient very long after the surgery is curtailed. Thus, the most basic problem about informed consent, namely, effecting a meeting of minds, is an acute one for the surgeon (as well as for the anesthesiologist and the radiologist). There is a temptation to let informed consent be a mechanical recitation of fact.

In such circumstances, it is not uncommon to omit a very important element of informed consent, namely, the presentation of alternatives. Studies have shown that this element is frequently omitted by practitioners (7). Surgeons may be the worst offenders, not because they are callous, but because they are often convinced of the validity of their work. This may be so because they have a vivid impression of immediate operative and postoperative success and a dimmer perception of how their patient lives beyond the perioperative time. It may also be because the surgeon may not be well acquainted with the benefits of medical management or the advisability of no intervention at all. It is ethically important that the surgeon carefully review the alternatives to surgical procedures.

This has been recommended in the previous section; it is an essential element of sound decision making. However, in considering patient preferences there is another reason for careful review of alternatives. An operative procedure that might be quite commonly accepted by the majority of patients may be quite unacceptable to the elderly patient. Some elderly persons have settled ideas about the way they wish to spend their final years and the way they prefer to die. Given the choice of continued angina or the risk of intra- or postoperative morbid events, requiring intubation and a long, distressing period of intensive care, some elderly persons may reject cardiac surgery. The elderly diabetic in need of amputation of a gangrenous limb may prefer death from sepsis to mutilation. Generalizations are not possible, but careful and sympathetic inquiry about the elderly patient's preferences may elicit such sentiments. Obviously, those based on objective error should be corrected and occasionally ignored (as is quite appropriately done when a recent surgical patient, suffering great pain but with an excellent prognosis for recovery, asks to be allowed to die). Nevertheless, the preferences of the elderly are often very well considered and deeply held. They must be respected.

Often, however, it is difficult or impossible to ascertain the preferences of the elderly patient. Dementia may deprive them of the ability to formulate or express preferences. Confusion or foreshortened memory may make difficult the assessment of information (8). In the past, much reliance was placed on the decisions of next-of-kin, even though law has generally accorded them little authority to make health care decisions for their disabled relative (5). In addition, the family's decisions may not be judicious due to their deep concern for their elderly relative or to the absence of such concern. In recent years, various devices, such as the living will, its legal counterpart, the Natural Death Act, and the Durable Power of Attorney have been developed in an effort to extend a person's preferences past their loss of competence. These devices, which many elderly persons make use of, should be viewed with respect, although they may not always be followed literally (9). It is essential that the surgeon discuss the meaning of any such document with the patient who presents one or inquire of the patient's internist or family practitioner, should the patient no longer be competent.

The key ethical issue in dealing with a patient's preferences is the autonomy of the patient. It is clear in ethics and in law that persons have the right to make their own decisions about medical treatment: they have the right of informed consent and the right to refuse. The elderly patient, however, suffers peculiar threats to personal autonomy. They may be losing physical mobility and agility of mind; they may be more dependent socially and economically. They are often treated as children, even while still competent. It is incumbent upon their physicians and surgeons to assist them in the realization of their preferences and to enhance, when possible, their autonomy.

Quality of Life

Quality of life is a phrase fraught with peril. In its best sense, it refers to the goal of all medical and surgical care: to improve the patient's quality of life by curing illness and relieving pain and disability. In its more dubious sense, it refers to the evaluation of an individual's capacities and life-style, which basically relies on the subjective judgments of onlookers. The surgeon in the prime of life looks at the weak and confused elder as one with poor quality of life; the elder may find life, even in that debilitated state, acceptable in terms of certain small pleasures unimaginable to the surgeon. Ideally, each person is the judge of the quality of his or her own life. However, many elderly persons have lost the ability to so judge or to express their judgment. It is in these cases that others, often their physicians and surgeons, must assess the quality of life on their behalf (10).

In the first section of this chapter, it was noted that preservation of life alone, in the absence of other qualities, was not an independent goal of medical treatment. The question is, "What other qualities?" For the competent patient, those qualities are those that they choose for themselves. An elderly patient, faced with the loss of speech following a laryngectomy, might prefer to accept death from his disease. This choice is his own by right. More frequently, however, the patient may undergo a radical transformation of life quite unexpectedly: an elderly patient in sound health undergoes elective hernia surgery, suffers a cardiopulmonary arrest, and is left in a chronic vegetative condition; an asymptomatic patient with a carotid bruit elects an endarterectomy and suffers a cerebral vascular accident. These patients now live a life dramatically different from their previous one. Does this change in quality of life justify a decision to forego some form of life support?

This question can arise for patients of any age. For the elderly patient, the added question arises: "Does the fact of their being aged make any difference in the decision?" Does the estimate that they will not have much longer to live, under any circumstances, modify the judgment? Does the diminished quality of aged life itself add any weight to the diminished quality due to their deficit? Difficult as these questions are, some reasonable responses can be offered. First, the obligation of physicians and surgeons is to contribute to restoration of health and relief of pain and discomfort. If any procedure can effect these goals, it is the ethical responsibility of health care providers to propose it. Thus, relief of bowel obstruction or hip replacement may be appropriate in the elderly, demented patient, since the immediate effect will be relief of pain. Surgical excision of a slow-growing tumor may not be appropriate, if the patient is likely to die before the tumor becomes fatal or if the manner of death expected from such a tumor would be without excessive distress.

A second consideration about quality of life bears on the probability that some patients suffer a life of "negative quality" or have nothing that can even be called quality. The first are those patients who apparently experience none of the pleasures and joys of being alive and only the pain and distress of living. The very demented, hallucinating person, bedridden, restrained, force-fed, not amenable to comforting touch or soothing word, may have only "negative" quality. The patient in a persistent vegetative condition, who presumably has no organized experience either of pleasure or pain, may be said to have no quality at all, since quality seems to presuppose some ability to experience.

In such a case, the obligation of others to do those things that sustain life is drastically reduced. The questions about foregoing life support are treated in general medical ethics (1, 2, 5). The peculiarly surgical questions, regarding whether to attempt operative procedures in such patients, seem relatively clear: if no improvement in the quality of life is possible, no procedure is indicated. Many ethicists today, although not all, maintain that even the provision of nutrients for such patients is not obligatory. Thus, even inserting a gastrostomy tube would not be indicated (11, 12).

The primary ethical issue raised by quality of life has to do with the nature of the benefits that can be conferred upon the patient by any medical or surgical intervention. It is important to recognize that the benefit is not to be measured in terms of physical and physiologic improvement but in terms of how the patient will live and experience the results of that improvement. So, for example, the repair of an aortic aneurysm in a patient over 80 may promise 8.2 years of life, but, should the patient be otherwise debilitated or demented, those 8.2 years may be of such poor quality as to suspect that the patient, if able, would reject them (13). Similarly, the prospect of serious deterioration after a major surgical procedure for a patient incapable of consent can also suggest the ethical propriety of refraining from the surgery. It is the duty of the responsible surgeon to consider the future quality of life of the patient without bias and prejudice.

External Socioeconomic Factors

The fourth set of considerations relevant to ethical decisions is a complex of factors external to the patient's own welfare, such as the costs of care, the allocation of resources, and the impact of the growing geriatric population on the society. At present, these matters are the subject of widespread debate. Some influential commentators have broached the controversial opinion that our society cannot afford to expend its resources on the elderly at the expense of other groups with equally serious need and greater potential for contribution (14). This is a genuine question of social priorities. However, it cannot readily become a question of clinical care. The surgeon facing the patient has neither the knowledge, nor the authority, to integrate social policy into the decisions required for that patient's care.

The integration of the issues mentioned in the first three sections is possible and can, to some extent, affect the broad issues of social policy. A careful and discriminating assessment of medical indications, a respect for patient's preferences, and an appreciation of the importance of quality of life does lead to a limitation of expensive care. These factors counter the uncritical assumption that whatever can be done must be done. Their serious consideration will often lead to the conclusion that some things that can be done ought not be done. However, they do so with an eye to the benefits accruing to the patient, rather than an eye on the utilization of social resources.

Occasionally, the broad social question may become a clinical question, as when a triage must be made under circumstances of constrained resources. The principles of triage were developed by surgeons faced with a flood of wounded from the battlefield. In this and other disastrous situations, focusing on the social benefit rather than the particular patient becomes legitimate, since the disaster itself is destroying the fabric of society. It is difficult to affirm that the increased number of elderly persons will destroy the fabric of our society, although it may force it to change its priorities. When the operating suites are at peak capacity and the critical care unit is so crowded as to compromise care, selection of younger patients over older ones may be a legitimate principle of triage. The older patients are more sick and require more care; the probability of survival is lower and of recurrent morbidity high. Unlikely as this scenario is, it represents one of the few occasions in which external socioeconomic factors may legitimately affect a clinical decision.

Conclusion

The ethical principles pertaining to surgery for the geriatric patient are, then, an amalgam of the standard principles of medical ethics, the particular capabilities of the surgeon and the physical, psychologic, and social status of the elderly person. The ancient maxim, "be of benefit and do no harm" deserves special attention. The capabilities of the surgeon are great, but the benefits that can come to the elderly patient from use of those capabilities are sometimes small. This disparity may arise from the patient's general disability, diminished awareness, and short life expectancy. The ethical surgeon will carefully match the great capabilities of surgical art to the limited capacities of the elderly patient, discerning where genuine cure of disease, relief of pain, and enhancement of function are more likely to result than increased debilitation, reduced function, and diminished quality of life.

References

1. Beauchamp, TL, and Childress, JF. 1985. *Principles of Biomedical Ethics*, ed. 2. New York: Oxford University Press.
2. Jonsen, AR, Siegler, M, and Winslade, WJ. 1986. *Clinical Ethics*, ed. 2. New York: MacMillan.
3. Gersh, BJ, et al. 1983. Coronary arteriography and coronary artery bypass surgery: Mortality in patients ages 65 or older. *Circulation* 67:483–491.
4. Freund, PR, and Ward, RJ. 1985. Anesthesia for geriatric patients. In *Principles of Geriatric Medicine*, Eds., R Andres, EL Bierman, and WR Hazzard. New York: McGraw-Hill.
5. President's Commission for the study of ethical problems in medicine. 1983. Deciding to forego life-sustaining treatment. Washington, DC: Government Printing Office.
6. Beauchamp, TL, and Faden, RR. 1986. A History and Theory of Informed Consent. New York: Oxford University Press.
7. President's Commission for the study of ethical problems in medicine. 1982. Making health care decisions. Washington, DC: Government Printing Office.
8. Taub, HA. 1980. Informed consent, memory and age. *Gerontologist* 206:686–690.
9. Eisendrath, S, and Jonsen, AR. 1983. The living will. *JAMA* 249:2054–2058.
10. Pearlman, R, and Jonsen, AR. 1985. Use of quality of life considerations in medical decision making. *J Am Geriatr Soc* 33:344–352.
11. Lynn, J. 1984. Deciding about life-sustaining treatment. In *Geriatric Medicine*, Eds., CK Cassell and JR Walsh, Vol II. New York: Springer.
12. Lynn, J (Ed). 1986. *By No Extraordinary Means*. Bloomington: University of Indiana.
13. Treiman, RL, et al. 1982. Aneurysmectomy in the octagenarian. *Am J Surg* 144:194–197.
14. Callahan, D. 1986. Adequate health care and an aging society: Are they morally compatible? *Daedalus* 115:247–267.

3

Legal Aspects of Geriatric Surgical Care

Marshall B. Kapp

Legal considerations pervade the modern practice of medicine. Certain legal doctrines and requirements take on particular importance where surgical intervention for a patient is contemplated or performed. Although most of these legal factors apply generically regardless of the chronologic age of the patient, in the case of geriatric surgical patients special considerations may affect the manner in which the surgeon's legal responsibilities are fulfilled. Just as the patient's age may be relevant to the surgeon in making and carrying out clinical decisions, so too may the patient's age influence the legal context of surgery.

This chapter outlines a few of the significant legal doctrines relevant to surgery today, both generally and with specific reference to the geriatric patient. Particular issues included are professional malpractice, informed consent, substitute decision making, confidentiality, record keeping, and the potential legal implications of health care cost control efforts.

Professional Malpractice

In a typical malpractice lawsuit based on allegations of substandard patient care, the plaintiff must prove each of four essential elements in order for professional liability to be found. Failure to establish any one of these defeats the plaintiff's entire claim. The four elements are: (*a*) **duty**, (*b*) **breach** or violation of that duty; (*c*) **damage** or injury; and (*d*) **causation**. A helpful mnemonic device for remembering these elements is the Law of D Cubed—A **D**ereliction of **D**uty must **D**irectly **D**amage. Let us now examine each of these four elements.

Duty/Standard of Care

To succeed in a malpractice lawsuit, a plaintiff must first demonstrate that the defendant physician owed the plaintiff some enforceable legal duty. The type and extent of duty to which a physician is held responsible depends upon the applicable **standard of care**. In the health delivery setting, this standard is generally stated as the duty to use "due or reasonable care under the circumstances," or the duty to have and to use the degree of knowledge and skill that is usually possessed and used by competent, prudent similar physicians in like or similar circumstances.

The degree of knowledge and skill that is "usually possessed and used" refers to a broad range of acceptable ways to provide care for the same person. The range of acceptable conduct may be defined by a defendant's entire profession or by a majority of that profession. Moreover, as long as even a "respectable minority" of a defendant's professional peers support the mode of conduct chosen, in terms of arguing that it was reasonable and did not unnecessarily expose the patient to foreseeable risk, the defendant's position is legally defensible. Support for a defendant's chosen course of conduct may be drawn from such sources as usual clinical practice, professional literature, conference presentations, voluntary standards (set by the medical profession itself) (1), government regula-

The author acknowledges with appreciation the careful review of an earlier draft of this chapter and the thoughtful comments of Daniel W. Elliott, M.D., former Chair (retired), Department of Surgery, Wright State University School of Medicine.

tions, and curriculum content being taught in educational settings.

The concepts of respectable minority and due or reasonable care defy mathematical precision; this fuzziness is intentional, to allow as much latitude for professional discretion as possible, within broad parameters necessary for the protection of the consumer (2). It can be stated with certainty, though, that a physician is not held legally liable for every mistake or error in judgment, or for every unfortunate patient outcome, but only for patient injuries that are directly caused by the provision of care that falls below the due or reasonable range.

The "similar physicians" whose degree of knowledge and skill set the standard of care against which the defendant's conduct will be measured in any particular case are that defendant's peers—that is, practitioners of the same profession and specialty as the person whose actions are being reviewed. Thus, a general surgeon is measured against other general surgeons, an orthopedic surgeon would be evaluated according to standards set by other orthopedic surgeons, a nurse in the operating room by nursing standards, and so forth. The only exception to this rule occurs when a health care provider steps outside of his or her own usual professional boundaries. Thus, for example, a general surgeon who performs thoracic surgery on a patient will be judged, for purposes of evaluating the legal acceptability of the care, according to the standards of thoracic surgeons who ordinarily provide that kind of care. This is because the general surgeon in this situation has at least tacitly represented to the patient that he or she possesses sufficient expertise and skill to provide such care. Since the patient, unknowledgeable and dependent as he or she is, reasonably relied on the surgeon's representation, it would be unfair to hold that surgeon to a lesser standard of care than that which the patient was led to expect.

As noted earlier, legal fact-finders look in various places for sources of the standard of care to be enforced in any case. (In the typical civil trial, there is a jury that serves as the fact-finder, while the judge rules only on questions of law. In some cases, the parties waive or give up their right to be heard by a jury, and the judge then both rules on legal issues and acts as the fact-finder.) Among these sources of the standard of care, customary practice among a majority or at least a respectable minority of similar health care providers is ordinarily the most weighty, although not necessarily the conclusive determinant. Relevant statutes and regulations, such as those pertaining to licensure and discipline, may also be carefully considered, as are voluntarily adopted standards (1, 3, 4) and professional codes of ethics. Voluntary standards may be the product of professional organizations and specialty societies or may be established by the Joint Commission on Accreditation of Healthcare Organizations (5) and other similar accrediting or certifying bodies. In many situations, violation of a legal rule or internal guidelines may, by itself, establish negligence per se, thereby shifting to the defendant the burden of justifying the deviation (6).

The source of the physician's duty of due care has two roots. First, a level of acceptable care is an implied, if not expressed, condition of the physician/patient contract that is reaffirmed each time that care is provided. Second is the tort rationale. A tort is a civil wrong based on violation (intentional or by neglect) of some duty that arises from a source other than a promise. A duty of due care is the logical outgrowth of the fiduciary or trust nature of the relationship that is formed between the relatively powerful (because of expertise and skill) physician and the relatively powerless (because of lack of needed expertise and skill, as well as physical and psychologic dependency) patient. This relationship and the faith that the patient puts in it imposes upon the physician the legal and ethical obligation to act always in a manner that promotes the patient's best interests, even if that is accomplished at the expense of the physician's own self-interest.

Along these lines, the particular condition, needs, and capacities of a patient are central in determining the standard of care that is owed. How much care is "due" will depend in large part on what the provider knew or should have known about the patient involved. Thus, the patient's age may be relevant in several ways.

Although the elderly are a highly heterogeneous group in all respects except chronological age, they do on the whole—both collectively and individually—have important physical (as well as mental, psychologic, social, economic, legal, and spiritual) characteristics and needs that tend to distinguish them from the younger population. The aged are special in many senses, including health care delivery. The physician must be thoroughly sensitive to and knowledgeable regarding any particular age-based characteristics or needs that may affect diagnostic or therapeutic decision making or activity for an older patient (7). One who undertakes to deliver services to an older patient also undertakes, explicitly or implicitly, to develop and maintain a significant data base in the physical (as well as mental, psychologic, social, economic, legal, and spiritual) realities of aging in contemporary America and to develop and maintain appropriate concomitant clinical abilities. To do less—that is, to fail to take age-related factors into account in caring for an older person—is to flirt dangerously with a deviation from the legally acceptable standard of care.

For instance, surgeons frequently write prescriptions for older patients in conjunction with surgical care. The area of drug therapeutics exemplifies the importance of developing and maintaining particular sensitivity to and knowledge and skills for addressing the special characteristics and needs of the elderly. People change physically as they age (although these changes occur at very differing rates among individuals), and these changes immensely affect the way that certain pharmaceuticals act on the body and mind of an older person. Geriatric pharmacology is a comparatively recent, specialized, and rapidly developing field of professional study. The legal significance of this phenomenon is exacerbated by the fact that statistically the elderly are disproportionately high consumers of both prescription and over-the-counter medications. The centrality of licit drug usage in both the chronic and the acute health care of many older persons underscores the physician's responsibility to gain particular familiarity with reasonably foreseeable effects of specified pharmaceutical interventions on geriatric patients. This knowledge must be assiduously assimilated into practice and made a part of each decision concerning the appropriate drug(s), dosage(s), and route(s) of administration to be prescribed or recommended in the course of the older person's therapy.

Another important example of the need for this age-specific knowledge is in the realm of risk appraisal for surgery (8). Morbidity and mortality from surgery increase in the elderly, although many older patients tolerate surgery well and benefit greatly from it (9). Therefore, age alone cannot be the basis for surgical decisions. The ability to use age and its risks as one of many factors in arriving at reasonable (although not necessarily perfect) surgical decisions and corresponding actions is part of the physician's duty of due care.

Breach/Violation of Duty

The second necessary element of proof in any negligence-based malpractice lawsuit is that there has been a breach or violation of the applicable standard of care. This concept, that a defendant may be held legally liable only where shown to be at fault, is fundamental to the traditional American tort system. Although there have been and continue to be proposals made to move health care malpractice toward some form of a no-fault system, the success of such "reform" efforts in the foreseeable future is highly problematic for several reasons.

First, fault as a cornerstone of professional malpractice is entrenched in our legal tradition. Second, our current malpractice system exists to serve at least two quite distinct purposes: (*a*) the just financial compensation of innocent, injured patients, and (*b*) the maintenance of a high level quality of care by deterring undesirable provider practices (10). While a no-fault system might serve the first of these functions very well, it could seriously undermine the latter one by removing the legal, and hence financial, incentive for health care providers to exercise due care in their treatment of patients. Legal carte blanche, unfortunately, is inconsistent with effective quality assurance. Third, there is considerable doubt about whether movement to a no-fault system is likely to achieve its prime goal of cutting health care costs, since it would open the door to the filing and collection of many small, questionably meritorious patient claims that are now filtered out by the current tort system.

Negligence may occur in one of three general circumstances. **Nonfeasance** is fault through inaction or omission—failing to do something that should have been done. **Misfeasance** consists of performing an act that should have been done, but performing it in a substandard manner. Finally, **malfeasance** is the performing of an act that should not have been done in the first place.

A breach or violation of duty may occur at any time during the course of the physician/patient relationship. Negligence (defined as an accidental or unintentional breach of duty) may happen at any time between the two points of formation and termination of a legal relationship between a physician and a patient.

In the surgical context, this means that the surgeon is legally bound to properly assess the patient before surgery, both in terms of need for the surgery vis-à-vis other alternatives and in terms of the likely risks for that patient, and to perform the actual surgery competently. It also means that the surgeon's duty of due care extends to engaging in reasonable preoperative maneuvers to reduce risks and to handling postoperative care involving somatic problems, pain control, and postoperative confusion (8). The surgeon's responsibilities do not end when the patient leaves the hospital. Allegations are made that many surgeons fail to follow-up older patients after surgery, instead "dumping" them back on their primary care physicians (11). If true, this conduct exposes the surgeon to substantial risk for foreseeable and avoidable patient problems that develop following an otherwise uneventful operation.

A hospital or physician may be held **personally liable** for its own substandard acts or omissions. Additionally, in certain circumstances, the providers may also be held legally responsible, **vicariously**, or **corporately**, for the faulty conduct of others (12).

Damage or Injury

For the third requisite element of proof in a malpractice action, the plaintiff must show that damage or injury has taken place. The legal system recognizes and compensates for injuries of three types: (*a*) physical, (*b*) emotional, and (*c*) invasion of **autonomy**.

Physical injury represents by far the largest number of filed claims, with severity of the injury frequently being the most important single factor in the decision to sue. Particularly in claims involving the elderly, the patient's death is frequently the injury claimed. It behooves physicians, legally as well as ethically, to do a better job of communicating with the family after a patient's death. Such communication is especially important where the patient's death happened unexpectedly (e.g., in the operating room where a good result had been predicted) (13).

Claims for emotional injuries are usually raised in conjunction with physical injury complaints, although there is a trend among courts in many jurisdictions toward permitting emotional injury claims to stand on their own merits (14). Increasingly, courts also are showing receptivity toward claims raised by parties *other than the patient* (e.g., close family members), alleging that the other party has suffered serious emotional and/or physical damage stemming from the intentional or unintentional mistreatment of a patient with whom they have a special relationship (15). Lastly, invasion of autonomy or the right to self-determination, which is seldom cited by itself but is often coupled with claims for physical or emotional injuries, generally involves a claim that the health care provider has somehow invaded and intervened in the patient's life (e.g., by performing surgery) in the absence of the patient's valid consent.

Once a meritorious malpractice claim has been established to the jury's satisfaction, the defendant(s) is ordinarily ordered to pay a specific amount of money to the injured plaintiff. (In actual practice, this money is usually supplied by the defendant's liability insurer.) This is referred to as a damage **award**. Damage awards fall into three categories: (*a*) nominal, (*b*) compensatory, and (*c*) punitive.

Nominal damages are rarely involved in malpractice cases, since they are negligible in amount and intended only to publicly signify that the patient's rights have been technically invaded. This is why relatively few violation of autonomy cases are brought on that theory alone. Our current legal system discourages (successfully but not completely) the bringing of lawsuits based solely on matters of principle, encouraging people to sue instead in cases where they seek and expect to obtain significant dollars.

The vast percentage of successful malpractice lawsuits involve the awarding of **compensatory damages**. This money is intended to compensate the victim for his or her harms, to make the victim "whole" again (to the extent that money can accomplish this). Compensatory damages are of two types. **Pecuniary**, economic, or **special** compensatory damages entail mathematically measurable out-of-pocket expenditures or lost opportunity costs, such as extra medical bills, special equipment needs, and lost wages. **Non-pecuniary**, non-economic, or **general** compensatory damages encompass more subjective losses, such as pain and suffering. When one hears today about very large malpractice awards, in most cases a large percentage of the award is attributable to this pain and suffering component, and many proposals to reform the malpractice system involve calls for a limitation or abolition of general damages.

Punitive or **exemplary damages** are rarely awarded in malpractice cases, since they are intended to punish defendants for egregious, intentional wrongs (such as patient abuse) and to set an example to deter others from engaging in similar misconduct. Since negligence, by definition, consists of unintentional wrongdoing, punitive or exemplary damages generally would not make sense. It should be remembered, however, that such damages are available for intentional wrongs and are unlimited in amount, not necessarily bearing any relationship to the extent of the plaintiff's actual injuries. It is also noteworthy that, as a strategic maneuver, many plaintiffs will include a claim for punitive damages solely to introduce before the jury what otherwise would be inadmissible evidence concerning the financial status of the defendant.

Although it is unusual, a plaintiff may also ask the court for injunctive relief as well as money damages. An injunction is a court order compelling (under threat of a contempt of court sanction) the defendant to do a particular act (e.g., let the patient stay in the hospital) or to refrain from doing some act (e.g., refrain from preventing a patient from leaving).

Causation

The fourth, and generally most difficult, element for the plaintiff to prove in a typical malpractice lawsuit is that the injury suffered was caused by the defendant's breach of duty. This is a particularly large evidentiary obstacle for many older persons to overcome, since it can often be counterargued that any adverse reactions they sustain are the result not of physician negligence, but rather of the elder's underlying illnesses and disabilities.

Unlike the scientific perspective, which tends to characterize cause and effect relationships in terms of absolute certainty, the legal system accepts as sufficient proof of this element that, to a degree of "reasonable medical certainty," it is more likely (more probable than not) that A caused B. This difference in the concept of causation is the law's practical accommodation to its need to work with the facts available, and the realization that it cannot afford the scientist's luxury of waiting until all other potential causes have been positively eliminated.

Nevertheless, a malpractice plaintiff must establish

that the physician's negligence was a **cause in fact** or **substantial factor** in bringing about the injury. Put differently, it must be shown that "but for" (the Latin term for this legal principle is ***sine qua non***) the physician's negligence, the injury would not have happened.

But that is not enough. The plaintiff is required to show that the physician's negligence not only was a substantial factor, but that it was the most direct or **proximate cause** of the injury sustained. That is, there can be no intervening, superceding, unforeseeable causes that occur to break the causal link between physician negligence and patient injury. Take, for example, the case of a surgeon who performs an operation improperly. As a result of the surgeon's mistake, it is necessary for the patient to undergo additional surgery the next day. On the way from the patient's hospital room to the operating room, the patient falls out of a wheelchair in which he was not properly tied by the orderly, hits the floor, and suffers additional injuries. The surgeon's error the previous day in the patient's operation would be a substantial factor causing those new injuries; "but for" the physician's negligence, the patient would not have been in the process of being transported to the operating room and the injuries would not have occurred. However, the physician would not be liable for those additional injuries here because the orderly's failure to transport the patient properly was an intervening, superceding, unforeseeable event that broke the proximate causal link.

Defenses

This section outlines in brief some of the more common defenses that may be available to physicians who are accused of malpractice. This information is not provided for the purpose of making the reader a more skillful malpractice defendant; once a lawsuit has been filed, preparing a defense is the job of the physician's attorney, and should be left to him or her. Rather, a word about defenses is mentioned so that physicians may better anticipate and prepare for—the better to avoid or mitigate at the outset—situations that may lead to potential legal trouble.

There are two basic categories of legal defenses to civil (or criminal, for that matter) charges of wrongdoing: (*a*) denials and (*b*) affirmative defenses. A **denial** is a direct refutation of the charge itself, an "I did not do what I am accused of doing" kind of defense. By comparison, an **affirmative defense** admits the truth of the substance of the allegation but claims that there was a good reason that should justify the defendant's actions in this case. It takes the form of "Yes, I did what I am accused of doing, but here are the reasons why I should not be held legally accountable this time." In most jurisdictions it is permissible for a defendant to raise both denials and affirmative defenses in the same lawsuit, although generally this tactic is not strategically desirable.

Several types of denial defenses are frequently raised in malpractice cases. First, the defendant may challenge the way that the plaintiff has defined the duty owed, as not applicable to the specific facts of that case. Second, the defendant may argue that there was no violation of duty, or fault, either because the defendant's conduct did meet the plaintiff's definition of duty, or because the defendant pursued an alternate course of conduct that still fell within the range of acceptable conduct as defined by the defendant's professional peers. Third, a defendant may dispute the element of proximate causation, arguing that the plaintiff relied on an inapposite theory of causation under the facts, that the patient's injury was inevitable with or without the defendant's negligence (probably the most commonly interposed defense where the plaintiff is elderly), or that some other intervening, superceding, unforeseeable force occurred to break the causal link between defendant and plaintiff. Fourth, the defendant may question the plaintiff's request for damages, either in terms of their computation or their existence at all.

Among affirmative defenses, one of the most immediately relevant to the surgical sphere would be **contributory** or **comparative negligence**. Under the traditional contributory negligence theory, if the plaintiff's own negligence has contributed to (helped to proximately cause) the plaintiff's injuries, then the plaintiff's entire claim is defeated. Take, for instance, the case of a mentally competent patient who tries to get out of bed, against the physician's expressed orders, and falls and becomes injured in the process. Under the contributory negligence rationale, the negligence of the nurse and hospital in failing to put up guard rails for that patient would be excused because of the patient's own deviation from the standard of conduct that society expects from a reasonable, prudent patient. Where the patient is not mentally competent, this affirmative defense would be much less available, since the court may impose a relaxed standard of care on the older patient (6, 16).

Because of a belief that strict application of the contributory negligence doctrine unfairly penalizes plaintiffs while giving guilty defendants an undeserved windfall, in the last decade many jurisdictions have moved toward a comparative negligence test instead (17). Under this doctrine, the degree to which the defendant's fault caused plaintiff's injury is measured against the extent to which the plaintiff's own negligence may have contributed to the injury. The defendant is then ordered to pay only for that percentage of the damages that he or she was directly responsible for causing, but (unlike the situation in contributory negligence states) the plaintiff at least is not completely precluded from any recovery.

Another frequently raised affirmative defense is **assumption of risk**. Here, the defendant submits that the plaintiff voluntarily, knowingly, and competently accepted the risk that eventually materialized to cause the injury. For instance, a mentally competent patient who, after being fully informed of the possible consequences, voluntarily refuses to undergo recommended surgery and suffers the adverse effects about which he was warned, has legally assumed the risk. The physician would not be held liable in that scenario for failure to perform the surgery. The key to a successful assumption of risk defense, it must be stressed, lies in the presence of three elements: (*a*) the plaintiff was mentally competent to assume the risk; (*b*) the plaintiff's decision to accept the risk was voluntarily made; and (*c*) the plaintiff was adequately informed about the potential risks to be encountered as a result of the decision (often a major evidentiary stumbling block). The assumption of risk doctrine is explored further in the "Informed Consent" section of this chapter.

An affirmative defense that has not been well received by the courts so far is the attempt by some physicians to include an **exculpatory clause** in the provider/patient contract. Such a provision seeks, before the relationship has even begun, to excuse the physician from legal liability for patient injuries that might be incurred in the course of care. Courts faced with this issue have tended for the most part to invalidate the exculpatory clause on the grounds that it violates public policy. This is because, unlike in the usual business setting, in health care the parties to a relationship generally bring to the table a great difference in bargaining power. Since the prospective patient (and this would be especially true for most older surgical candidates) ordinarily lacks equal footing with the physician in negotiating the terms and conditions of their relationship, most courts deem it unfair to enforce against the patient an exculpatory clause that likely was not—at least in psychologic terms—voluntarily and knowingly agreed upon (18).

Finally, affirmative defenses to malpractice claims are often founded on procedural rules. Most states now require a malpractice plaintiff to go through some form of preliminary notice, arbitration, or pretrial screening process. A plaintiff's failure to do so is grounds for dismissal of the claim. Likewise, the plaintiff's failure to file the claim within the applicable statute of limitations time frame is grounds for dismissal. However, most courts tend to construe this requirement liberally, allowing the available time to begin running from the point at which the patient discovers or should (using reasonable diligence) have discovered the existence of the injury, rather than from the moment that the negligence actually occurred. Where a plaintiff, *after* becoming aware of an injury, agrees to release the physician from liability (generally with some type of negotiated compensation in return), courts usually recognize such a **release of liability** as a defense to subsequent claims arising from the same injury. **Prior related litigation** (technically called ***res judicata*** or **collateral estoppel**) is also a defense; once an issue has been tried and decided by a court, a plaintiff is not entitled to a new "bite" at the identical "apple." Lastly, some governmental (federal, state, or county) health care facilities may be protected against any lawsuits by the doctrine of **sovereign immunity**, although most jurisdictions have enacted statutes in recent years limiting or abolishing completely that defense.

Informed Consent

Legal Basis and Ethical Values

Older persons face important decisions every day of their lives (19). These decisions may concern matters of mundane living, such as what clothes to wear, what food to eat, what television show to watch, and in what activities to partake. These decisions may also involve difficult and fundamental medical issues, such as which physician to select (20), whether to take one's medicine, and whether to submit to a recommended surgical procedure.

As a general legal and ethical principle, such decisions should regularly be made by the person most directly affected by the consequences of that decision. Such a rule best respects and promotes the dignity and autonomy of the individual (21). This doctrine of informed consent is fully applicable to older persons who are candidates for surgery. Requirements concerning informed consent for older persons stem from common law court decisions, state statutes and regulations, and various voluntary guidelines.

Knowledge of bare legal requirements in this sphere is not, however, enough. If the informed consent principle is truly to do its job in fostering more complete, humane, trusting, and compassionate interaction between care provider and care receiver (22–25), those responsible for fulfilling it must also understand the ethical values that underpin the legal rules. Briefly stated, these are the values of autonomy (every person should be as free as possible to make personal choices concerning his or her own life, with a minimum of outside interference) and beneficence (allowing a person to make choices for himself or herself is most likely to result in "better" choices, as far as that individual is concerned, and therefore best promotes that person's own well-being) (26, 27).

What is needed in health care delivery generally, and

in the geriatric sphere particularly, is a practical way to balance the altruistic goals of autonomy and beneficence with the pragmatic need of physicians and other providers to be legally protected within the confines of their resources. It is toward this balance that the chapter now turns.

Elements of Valid Consent

Voluntariness

The first requirement for a valid legal consent is that the patient's participation in the decision-making process and ultimate decision must be voluntary. The usual definition of voluntariness in the context of consent is that the person giving or withholding consent must be "so situated as to be able to exercise free power of choice without the intervention of any element of force, fraud, deceit, duress, overreaching or other ulterior form of constraint or coercion" (28). It means simply that the person must be free to reject participation in the proposed intervention. Voluntariness in decision making is best understood as a matter of degree (29).

Informed

The second essential requirement for valid consent is that the patient's agreement be informed. "Patients are persons generally unlearned in the medical sciences and therefore, except in rare cases, courts may safely assume the knowledge of patient and physician are not in parity" (30). Therefore, the legal doctrine of informed consent requires that the physician, before undertaking an intervention, disclose certain information to the individual who is the subject of the proposed intervention.

The legal disclosure requirement is justified not just on ethical grounds of autonomy and beneficence, but for therapeutic reasons as well (31). In most instances, thorough provision of information to the patient is good clinical practice as well as good legal and ethical conduct. A patient on powerful medication, for instance, who is warned of possible symptoms he or she may experience will be able to better cooperate with the physician and nurses in treating these side effects, and the therapeutic process is facilitated.

A number of studies show that informed surgery patients tend to experience less anxiety, are more compliant with instructions, cope better with complications, and express greater satisfaction with the results of surgery than do less well-informed patients (32–41). This link between sufficient information and real and perceived quality is very positive from a legal risk management perspective (42). Additionally, risk management objectives are promoted by adequate information disclosure to the patient even where the medical intervention turns out to be less than successful (43).

General admonitions that consent must be informed offer little concrete guidance. The following sections comment on the amount, scope, content, and impact of required disclosures.

Standards for disclosure. There are several competing standards detailing the amount and type of information that the physician should convey to a patient (27, 44–46). The test selected has practical, as well as philosophical, ramifications.

The most complete and hence most cautious and safe standard for informed consent is full disclosure; all known or knowable significant information concerning the proposed intervention would be required to be communicated to the patient. Thus, if the physician were considering performing a specific procedure on a patient primarily for its placebo effect, a full disclosure standard would require that the physician disclose the placebo intent to the patient (47). Although no jurisdiction has yet adopted this standard, full disclosure coupled with sufficient documentation is the best defense a physician could have against a claim of lack of informed consent. No higher standard can be expected than full disclosure.

The disclosure standard currently enforced in the majority of American jurisdictions is referred to as the "professional," "reasonable physician" (45, 46), or "community" (48) standard. Under this test, the adequacy of disclosure is judged against the amount and type of information that a reasonable, prudent physician would have disclosed under similar circumstances. Where persuasive proof is adduced that the customary practice within the medical professional community, at least for a respectable minority if not the majority of the profession, would be to withhold the questioned facts from the patient, a defense is established in a professional standard jurisdiction.

As physicians become more familiar with the informed consent doctrine and more concerned about maximum protection against malpractice claims based on negligence for lack of informed consent, the customary practice has evolved, and continues to evolve, to one of ever-widening disclosure. As the acceptable standard of care evolves toward disclosure, it will become increasingly difficult to locate even a respectable minority of physicians that practices widespread nondisclosure.

A growing, although lately slowing (49), minority of jurisdictions have accepted a more expansive standard of information disclosure: the "reasonable patient" or "material risk" standard (45, 46, 50). This standard dictates that the physician communicate the information that a "reasonable patient" in the same situation would need to make a voluntary and intelligent decision. Under this test, the patient must be told about all material risks—that is, those factors that might make a difference to a reasonable, average patient under similar circumstances. This certainly includes answering fully and truthfully any questions asked by the patient (51). The determinative element is the resident's informational needs.

Since the focus is on a "reasonable" patient, this is sometimes referred to as an "objective" (52) or "prudent person" (48) standard. A "subjective" or "individual patient" standard, asking what the particular (rather than a hypothetical "reasonable") patient would have wanted to know under the circumstances, has been advocated by some (53, 54) and accepted by a few state courts (49). Otherwise, though, the subjective, idiosyncratic standard has been rejected as unfair to the physician.

Arguments that have been put forward on behalf of the consumer-oriented or material risk standard of informed consent, as opposed to the professional or community standard, include: (*a*) patient autonomy, (*b*) enhanced communications, (*c*) better health consumer awareness, (*d*) less litigation, and (*e*) improvement in the quality of care (55, 56). Underlying these arguments is empirical evidence suggesting that most patients and their families wish to receive more information than many physicians would willingly choose to disclose (57, 58).

The patient's desire for information is not diminished even in situations where the patient trusts the physician fully and wishes him or her to make the ultimate choices (59). As noted earlier, studies demonstrate a positive correlation between degree of patient involvement in care (through, among other things, more information) and improved functional outcomes (60).

The age of a patient may be relevant in affecting what information is material to that patient's medical decision making (61). For instance, a likely side effect that will not manifest itself for another 20 years probably will not be very important to an older person. However, the probability that a particular intervention will be accompanied by a great amount of physical pain or discomfort may make quite a difference to an old, frail individual. Also, the likelihood that surgery may be riskier with advanced age should be considered in the informed consent calculus (8). Among numerous other factors, physicians and other health care professionals should always consider the physical and mental effects of aging when deciding whether information regarding an intervention might be material to the specific individual. The physician should begin as early as possible in the preoperative period to "feel out" the particular patient's informational preferences (62).

Where the physician has purposely withheld information about the nature of an intervention, the plaintiff's burden of proof under the reasonable patient standard would be much more easily satisfied than under the professional standard. Under the latter, an expert witness would be necessary to establish the appropriate conduct; under the former, no expert witness is needed, since figuring out what information a reasonable patient (or the particular patient, in a subjective standard jurisdiction) would want to know is a matter well within the capabilities of lay jurors (45). The jury's tendency to identify with the patient in a material risk jurisdiction is likely to lead to a finding that failure to disclose the nature of an intervention was a culpable professional omission.

Even where the defendant physician develops strong evidence that the information withheld did not create, in his or her professional opinion, an undue risk of physical or mental harm, this could be dismissed as irrelevant on the issue of the materiality of the information to the patient. The legal test is whether the disclosure might make a difference to the patient, not to the treating physician.

The obvious corollary to the materiality standard is the proposition that information that is immaterial need not be provided (63). That is, the physician is not obligated to disclose facts and opinions that would not make a difference in the decision.

Elements of disclosure. With these standards of disclosure in mind, I now move to an enumeration of the specific informational items that fall within any of these standards. The particular elements of disclosure have usually been listed as follows (31, 45, 46, 50):

1. Diagnosis—The patient should know what the "problem" is that the physician intends to pursue, to identify, and to treat.

2. Nature and purpose of the proposed intervention—In medical terms, this equates to the indications for its use. The physician should discuss the diagnostic or therapeutic rationale with the patient, in language that is clear, nontechnical, and understandable to the patient. This information should pertain not only to the surgery itself, but also to its follow-up requirements (64).

3. Risks, consequences, or perils of the intervention—Whether one is in a professional or a patient standard jurisdiction may influence the decision whether or not to disclose specific risks. In general, patients are most interested in risks associated with death, disability, or discomfort. For the elderly, risks of discomfort may be especially weighty. As either the potential severity or the likelihood of a risk's occurrence (the incidence rate) increases, the balance tips more toward disclosure. As a matter of legally defensive practice, it is always wise to err on the side of more disclosure (65).

4. Probability of success—In medical terms, what would the prognosis be if the particular recommended intervention is undertaken (competently, of course)? In other words, what are the expected benefits of the intervention?

5. Alternatives—What options are reasonable and available?

6. Result anticipated if nothing is done—In any situation, one of the alternatives to any plan of intervention is to let nature take its course. But this, too, may entail specific risks and consequences of which the patient must be told. Just as consent must be informed, so also must refusal of proferred intervention be informed if it is to represent a legally valid patient choice (66–69).

7. Limitations on professional or facility—It has been suggested that any relevant legal, clinical, ethical, or other limitations on the ability of a physician or facility to serve a particular patient should be clearly delineated (70).

8. *Advice*—While most persons strongly desire sufficient information and the right to make ultimate decisions, most also want (and expect) advice and recommendations from the physicians in whose hands they entrust their well-being. This is likely to be especially true for the older patient, who tends to be more dependent and more respectful of authority (71). The giving of an opinion is not necessarily coercion or the exercise of undue influence (72). Rather, if done in an objective yet compassionate way, mindful of the human characteristics and values of the particular patient, it is the proper fulfillment of one's professional duties (73). The physician is not a mere technician, but a counselor and manager (63). The health care professional's doubts regarding the proposed intervention should also be shared frankly with the patient and family (74), for both therapeutic and legal reasons (43).

Even if the patient's attorney can establish the absence of informed consent, no civil recovery can be had unless the patient's attorney can also prove that the physician's failure to inform was a proximate or direct cause of some injury suffered (45, 46, 50). "Such a causal connection arises only if it is established that, had the revelation been made, consent to the treatment would not have been given" (30). Put differently, if the patient would have proceeded with the intervention anyway, he or she cannot subsequently complain about a risk that he or she would have found unpersuasive (49, 140, 141).

In judging causation, whether a jurisdiction follows a (*a*) "subjective", individual patient or (*b*) "objective", prudent patient standard is very significant. As alluded to earlier, a handful of states have adopted a subjective test, asking whether this particular patient would have judged a specific risk material and would have rejected the intervention if disclosure had been made. Most courts and legislatures that have considered the question, however, have rejected or abandoned the subjective test in favor of an objective one—whether a reasonable, average person in the patient's position would have undergone the proposed intervention if he or she had been more fully informed. Under such a test, the patient's testimony, if offered, is relevant to the proximate cause issue, but such testimony is neither necessary nor controlling (50).

Effectiveness of disclosure. The informed consent doctrine has been criticized by certain commentators and empirical researchers on the grounds that it is virtually impossible for the vast majority of nonprofessionally educated patients to adequately understand, assimilate, and utilize the often extensive and detailed information that must be disclosed (75, 76). This argument is made with special vehemence in the case of elderly patients, some of whom suffer from some form of mental dysfunction, particularly depression and dementia. Thus far, the courts and legislatures have generally managed to avoid confronting this problem head-on, by focusing their inquiries almost exclusively on the quantitative and qualitative nature of the information disclosed by the health care professional, while essentially ignoring what is done with that information by the patient (51, 77). In other words, in practice "informed" consent has not usually been equated with "understanding" consent, although the terms are often used (inaccurately) interchangeably.

Thoughtful commentators from both the legal (76, 77) and medical (23, 78) communities contend that both informed and understanding consent, while perhaps seldom achieved today, is a realistic possibility for most patients and should be the standard that is legally enforced. This author supports this view and the notion that comprehension is less a function of patient characteristics or the complexity of the medical problem than it is dependent on the commitment and effort of the communicator and the method of communication used to inform the patient (29, 63, 78–80). There needs to be a shift away from the mere disclosure model of informed consent to a more interactive, participatory model (26, 62). A dialogue that is open, nontechnical, compassionate, receptive to questions, and involves significant family members can, in many cases, bring about meaningful patient comprehension and can serve a valuable therapeutic purpose at the same time (12).

Presenting surgical information with audiovisual aids, such as videotapes and specially prepared pamphlets and written materials, can be useful, as long as these devices are used to reinforce, not substitute for, a face-to-face discussion with the surgeon (62). Especially when the elderly are involved, simple cost-free techniques, like speaking more slowly and loudly and repeating information on different occasions, can have a significant impact on the ability of the patient to take an active part in medical decision making (81).

Another misplaced but frequently cited criticism of the informed consent doctrine is that the disclosure of information tends to frighten and dissuade many patients from agreeing to undergo clinically indicated interventions. In fact, empirical research shows that ample disclosure not only does not increase the patient refusal rate, but that most refusals are based on inadequate disclosure; the refusal rate actually decreases as the amount and kind of information disclosed increases (82, 83).

The connection between the foregoing discussion and the prevention of malpractice lawsuits is clear. Talking *with* (but not at) patients and their families—informatively and compassionately—contributes mightily to patient satisfaction and well-being. Technical legal doctrine aside, fostering the patient and family's attitude that the physician cares deeply enough to relinquish some of his or her own traditional power and involve them meaningfully in the decision-making process is the best form of risk management achievable (84). It is preferable for all concerned that information be timely and appropriately discussed, rather than that its nondisclosure subsequently have to be defended.

Competent

The third essential element of legally effective consent is that the patient must be mentally competent to give valid consent regarding personal care. Where the patient lacks sufficient mental capacity, a substitute or proxy decision maker must be involved.

Incapacity and questionable capacity of patients is a fundamental and widespread issue for every surgeon who serves geriatric patients. Because this dilemma is so important and complex, a section that appears later in this chapter is devoted to its discussion.

Exceptions to the Consent Requirement

Several well-recognized exceptions exist to the general informed consent requirements (85). In appropriate circumstances, almost all of these are applicable to geriatric surgery patients. They include: (*a*) emergencies, (*b*) waiver, (*c*) therapeutic privilege, and (*d*) commonly known risks.

Emergency Exception

The emergency exception applies in the following situations: (*a*) when immediate medical treatment is required to preserve life or to prevent a serious permanent impairment to health, but (*b*) consent cannot be obtained from the patient (or from someone legally empowered to authorize treatment on the patient's behalf), and (*c*) when there is no serious indication that the treatment would be refused were the patient then able to make his or her own wishes known. It is sometimes said that consent in such situations is "implied by law," by analogy to situations in which a patient by his or her conduct implies consent without putting it into words. This terminology is misleading in the emergency context. More accurately, in an emergency the law sets aside the requirement of consent, based on the presumption that a reasonable person would want emergency aid to be rendered and that a particular patient has such wishes unless he or she has definitively indicated otherwise previously (45, 46, 50, 86, 87).

To justify reliance on the emergency exception, the physician has the burden of proving the presence of two factors in the case at issue (86–88). First, it must be shown that it was not reasonably possible prior to the intervention to obtain the express consent of the patient or the consent of a person authorized to decide for the patient. Second, it must be established that there was an immediate threat of death or of serious, permanent injury.

Since the establishment of these factors is the physician's responsibility, every reasonable effort should be made to document the facts in such a situation. Adequate notations should be included in the medical record, explaining the immediate threat to life or health and what efforts were made, if any, to obtain express consent. Consultation with other health care professionals, if they are available and time permits, is most helpful in justifying the treating physician's action (88).

Defense of Waiver

Just as personal autonomy is the primary ethical underpinning of the patient's right to make decisions, it is also the foundation for the physician's defense of waiver. Ever since the earliest judicial recognition of the doctrine of informed consent, it has also been acknowledged that, if the patient has a right to know a proposed medical intervention's nature, risks, alternatives, and probability of success, then the patient must also possess the prerogative to waive or relinquish that right (50). It is not legally required that physicians oversupply patients with unwanted information or "truth-dump." Allowing the patient the opportunity to waive the right to be informed is "paternalism with permission" (63, 89), and is a necessary part of the full recognition of the patient's claim to self-determination.

Patient waiver of informed consent undoubtedly reflects the tacit understanding in a considerable percentage of professional/patient encounters. This is especially true for older patients, who are often in even greater awe of the status of physicians than are most others (90). Many patients are content to have the specifics of their medical treatment remain a mystery, as long as it "works," and the expectations about what qualifies as an intervention "working" may be severely diminished for the elderly. Health, as a "good," is judged by many people as more important than the seemingly esoteric concept of rights (91).

However, to prevent the waiver defense from becoming the exception that rapidly obliterates the rule, it has been strongly urged in some quarters that the patient's right to decide not to be informed must be exercised unambiguously if it is to be given effect. Consequently, the waiver should ideally be expressed rather than implied and should be recognized only in circumstances where the physician has made clear that there are risks and alternatives associated with the advised intervention and that he or she is willing to discuss them fully with the patient and family if so requested (29, 51, 53, 54).

Therapeutic Privilege

The most controversial exception to compliance with informed consent requirements is the doctrine of "therapeutic exception," generally known as the defense of "therapeutic privilege" (45, 46). Therapeutic privilege is recognized expressly in many states by statute or common law decision.

The defense of therapeutic privilege to a claim of nondisclosure of material information about a patient's diagnosis, prognosis, or treatment is applicable when, in the physician's good faith judgment, disclosure would be likely to complicate or hinder necessary treatment, cause severe psychological harm, and be so upsetting as to render a rational decision by the patient impossible. In such circumstances, it is permissible to proceed with the intervention in the absence of disclosure and informed consent (92).

Therapeutic privilege has been construed extremely narrowly by the courts (50, 93), which have implied that it only applies when the patient is severely and emotionally unstable, and where some "dread disease" would imminently imperil the patient's life. Moreover, the privilege, in any event, cannot last longer than the condition that justifies it. Once the patient has improved, disclosure must take place. In light of the weighty limitations that have been placed on the therapeutic privilege defense by the courts, the widespread use of this defense must be viewed with substantial skepticism.

The preferred rule is a presumption (rebuttable in rare and limited circumstances) that the physician must inform the patient of all material information (94), but that the manner in which the information is conveyed (encompassing such factors as time, place, language used, and other people present) be permitted to vary depending on the patient's particular characteristics (51, 93). While some physicians insist that they might be held liable for telling the patient too much, no court has ever found a physician liable for giving a patient an excessive amount of accurate and relevant information (31, 51).

Intervention without adequate disclosure cannot be justified merely because the physician thinks that the intervention would be in the patient's best interest. "A doctor might well believe that an operation or form of treatment is desirable or necessary, but the law does not permit him to substitute his own judgment for that of the patient by any form of artifice or deception" (95). To argue that a physician is justified in withholding information because a patient would, on the basis of those facts, decline therapy that the physician deems desirable would be a complete perversion of the principle of therapeutic privilege. Besides, empirical research demonstrates that the patient consent rate actually tends to increase in direct proportion to the amount of relevant information disclosed to the patient (29, 83), and that even for severely mentally compromised patients the giving of complete information does not impair the course of treatment (96).

Before opting to treat a patient under therapeutic (or "medically contraindicated") privilege, the physician would be wise to consult other physicians to secure independent support for the determination that there is a clinical basis to act under the privilege. The physician must document exactly what information is being withheld from the patient's knowledge and why, and this notation should be done completely and contemporaneously (97). Once the decision to withhold information is made and documented, the physician is best advised to disclose the facts to the appropriate next of kin, when available, and to document that disclosure (45, 70).

The general restrictions discussed regarding use of the therapeutic exception apply to all types of competent patients and all types of interventions, including surgery. They apply with particular force to older patients, for whose personal values and preferences the physician should have the highest respect (98, 99). The elderly should not be treated differently from other persons regarding therapeutic privilege; in no case will advanced age by itself automatically justify this exception to the usual informed consent requirement.

Commonly Known Risks

The final notable exception to informed consent requirements comes into play when the foreseeable risks are of a commonly known variety. In general, a physician is not required to disclose a risk of which a particular patient is already aware on the basis of past experience. This exception to informed consent requirements also is recognized where a risk is so widely known that the average patient would be aware of it (70). For example, it might be argued that almost everyone knows that there is a slight chance of infection whenever a blood sample is drawn, and therefore, there is no need to so specifically inform the patient. What is "commonly known" is determined in most jurisdictions by an objective standard, namely, whether a "reasonable patient" would have knowledge of the risk in question. Where a patient claims that he or she was not personally aware of a particular risk, juries often tend to react sympathetically, and so, physicians should withhold information on this basis only with great care. This admonition should be underscored in the case of major bodily invasions, such as surgery.

Responsibility to Assure Consent

Each health care professional who seeks to do some medical intervention to a patient has a personal legal responsibility to obtain effective consent from the patient for that intervention, although the patient education process should be a team effort (27). Thus, if surgery is contemplated, it is the involved surgeon who has the legal obligation to assure that the patient has been adequately informed and has authorized the surgery; this obligation may be fulfilled through a combination of the surgeon's personal efforts and those of other team members.

Timing of Consent

What is the appropriate time for obtaining informed consent? For how long is a patient's consent legally valid? Does it "expire" at some point? Conversely, is there a minimum required time-lag between the giving of the consent and the performance of the intervention for which the consent was given? Must consent be repeated or reaffirmed at specific time intervals?

While these are interesting philosophical questions, neither statutes nor judicial decisions have provided much in the way of concrete legal guidance regarding the timing of consent. As a general proposition, a physician would do best to focus less on days and hours than on the function and purpose of consent. Particularly, the timing of consent will be held proper where it is shown to be far enough in advance of the intervention to allow for meaningful comprehension and reflection (i.e., not while the patient is being wheeled into the operating room), yet close enough to accurately reflect the patient's decision concerning that particular intervention. General consents to standard, nonintrusive, nonrisky kinds of care are valid for longer than consents to particular, intrusive, risky sorts of interventions, such as surgery. Any time that new circumstances arise that alter anticipated benefits, risks, or alternatives, a new consent is necessary.

Significance of Refusal

Most patients generally accept the advice of their physicians and consent to undergo recommended medical interventions. Such cases present few legal (or ethical) dilemmas, as the physician almost invariably acts as though the consenting patient (by virtue of agreeing with the physician) must be competent and has understood the physician's explanation of the intervention.

Some patients, though, at certain times reject specific suggested medical interventions, particularly surgery. This may occur for various reasons, including misunderstanding; religious objections; fear of embarrassment, invasion, or physical pain; machoism; cost concerns; or any number of other rational or irrational motivations (100). In the face of patient refusal, there are several possible physician responses: (*a*) to accept this, (*b*) to convince the patient to change his or her decision, or (*c*) to informally override or attempt to formally override the patient's decision.

One possible physician response to patient refusal of a suggested intervention is simply to accept the patient's choice and not proceed any further with the intervention. A competent and informed adult, certainly including an older patient, has the fundamental right voluntarily to refuse any suggested medical intervention (even if lifesaving), subject only to competing compelling state interests that are rarely germane to elderly patients in need of surgery. A physician who relies on the voluntary refusal of a competent, informed patient is generally on firm legal ground.

However, complete acceptance of a patient's refusal to have recommended medical intervention should not ordinarily be automatic or unquestioning. Acceptance of patient refusal should never be used merely to avoid caring for an older patient, whom the physician and the hospital would rather not care for anyway. In such cases, refusal may be taken at face value and used as a pretext to abandon a patient when abandonment may be neither justified morally nor consistent with the patient's legal rights. In the current era of Diagnosis Related Groups (DRGs) (101) and other cost control strategies, both health care facilities and individual physicians may have a financial incentive to terminate or not initiate expensive treatment, such as surgery and its follow-up care. It is vital that such incentives not be the main basis for uncritical acceptance of a patient's treatment refusal (102).

Although the patient has a right to refuse medical interventions, it remains the legal responsibility of the physician to ensure that the patient understands the consequences of that refusal. Many treatment refusals may be interpreted as really requests for more personal attention by the physician, and, as noted earlier, patient consent actually increases with greater physician attention and disclosure (82). Physicians have an ethical and legal obligation to strenuously seek to persuade recalcitrant patients and their families to consent to clinically indicated interventions (103). Every effort should be made to explain to the patient and family, in a gentle and warm way, why the particular intervention is desirable. (If the physician has difficulty in articulating this point, then perhaps the intervention is not so desirable after all!)

If the attempt at persuasion fails, the patient and family should be reminded that by refusing, they now accept the responsibility—clinical, ethical, and legal—for the consequences (100). Failure to try one's best to convince the patient and family is an indictment of the physician's persuasive ability and might be construed by others as an attitude of indifference to the patient that could place the physician in subsequent legal jeopardy (104).

Despite one's best persuasive efforts, some patients and their families will persist in their refusal. In such circumstances, several options are possible.

First, once he or she has verified that the patient is competent to make treatment decisions and that adequate explanations have been given that the patient understood, the physician may and ordinarily should respect the patient's refusal and refrain from performing the proposed intervention. This general rule regarding competent patients applies to emergency as well as nonemergency health care (86, 87, 105), and extends to refusals made by properly appointed substitute decision makers in the case of incompetent patients. The Uniform Health Care Consent Act drafted by the National Conference of Commissioners on Uniform State Laws (106–108) would codify the prevailing common law principle that a physician declining to intervene, in reliance on the refusal of consent by an individual whom the physician in good faith believes is legally authorized to make health care decisions, is not subject to criminal prosecution, civil liability, or professional disciplinary action on the basis of that reliance. When the physician relies on treatment refusal, such refusal should be thoroughly documented.

An option available to a private physician who finds a patient's refusal of treatment personally objectionable in a particular case is to terminate his or her relationship with that patient. To avoid legal liability for abandoning a patient in distress, the physician should formally notify the patient and family of the relationship termination and the reasons for it, and should make all reasonable efforts to refer the patient to another competent physician who agrees to care for the patient and whom the patient and family agree to accept as a caregiver (31, 103).

Faced with treatment refusal, some hospitals formally override or attempt to formally override the patient choices. Although in most cases legally perilous, nonconsensual or involuntary treatment, especially for mentally impaired or confused but not legally declared incompetent persons, is fairly widespread (82). Involuntary treatment most often involves imposition of physical restraints and psychotropic medications (as well as intravenous fluids and nutrients).

Formal legal mechanisms exist for overriding the choices of a patient. For most patients, the only legal basis for transferring decision-making authority to someone other than the patient himself or herself would be the patient's mental incompetence. It should be emphasized here that every health care facility should have in place a written policy detailing its avenues of response to patient refusal of treatment recommendations, with special reference to what circumstances will trigger resort to formal legal attempts to transfer decision-making authority from the patient (109).

Documentation of Consent

The prevalent confusion concerning the legal significance of written consent forms is unfortunate, as it leads in far too many cases to a tendency for the written form to be equated with and substituted for the consent itself (29, 110). The error of this thinking and this practice cannot be stressed strongly enough; valid legal consent is not achieved by a piece of paper, but rather requires compliance with the communicative process detailed in the preceding pages of this chapter (96, 109, 111, 112).

A written consent is not even legally required in most states except when the proposed intervention is part of a biomedical or behavioral research protocol (70). Even when a written form has been signed by the patient, its legitimacy can be attacked in numerous ways (113, 114).

Nevertheless, almost all health care facilities and many physicians regularly utilize written consent forms in everyday practice, especially for interventions that are considered nonroutine, intrusive, or risky (such as surgery) (115). This is largely a result of the confusion between form and substance described above. The liberal use of written consent forms, however, can serve various legitimate purposes for both the hospital and its physicians and their patients (109).

First, the regular use of consent forms is required by the standards of the Joint Commission on Accreditation of Healthcare Organizations (JCAHO). Strictly speaking, these standards do not represent legal authority; however, voluntary JCAHO accreditation is valuable to a hospital from a quality assurance and professional prestige perspective, as well as for third-party reimbursement purposes.

Second, the written form can and should serve as a valuable source of information and education for the patient and family. It should be written in clear, understandable, nontechnical language and given to the patient and family in advance of the proposed intervention, allowing for its study in a nonstressful, relaxed way. It should be orally supplemented by thorough, responsive explanations by all concerned health care professionals (116). Thus, the written form can become an integral part of the physician/patient relationship and can perform a tremendous cognitive as well as therapeutic function for the patient and family (110, 111, 117). Additionally, as alluded to earlier, an increasing number of audiovisual educational aids are now being marketed to supplement this function of consent forms (118), and many of these are appropriate for surgical candidates.

Third, the written consent form does provide some measure of legal protection for the hospital and physician (118). Although it does not by itself constitute the totality of the required consent, the written form does have status, based either on state statute (50, 119) or court decision, as an important piece of evidence that the required process of communication did take place (50, 52). The existence of a written form signed by the patient (or proxy) creates a legal presumption that valid consent was obtained; the burden then shifts to the patient to rebut or overcome that presumption by persuasively showing that one or more of the essential elements (voluntariness, competence, adequate information) were missing.

Specific techniques of documentation are really secondary. The important thing is to make sure that the information set forth in the documentation has in fact been communicated to the patient, in a way that is understandable to the patient. If the objective is to fill paper with signatures, the whole point of patient consent is lost, and the forms become legally and ethically meaningless. If the objective is to recognize and respect the principle that a patient, even one who is elderly, should be presumed the rightful determiner of his or her own destiny, then the consent form becomes a meaningful documentation of the patient's legitimate authorization.

Substitute Decision Making

As explained in the previous section, there is a strong legal, as well as ethical, presumption toward respect for the individual patient's autonomous right to make decisions concerning his or her own life, including choices about undergoing surgery. Ordinarily, observing and fostering the exercise of patient informed consent is the physician's and hospital's best protection against allegations of improper interference with a patient's physical or mental integrity.

For some older patients, however, the combination of illness and the hospital environment may substantially impair the ability to make and communicate autonomous choices on important matters. While it is always important to try to informally involve family members, friends, and other relevant persons to assist patients with their decisions, sometimes the patient's own judgment or capacity to communicate becomes so compromised that the actual power to make major life decisions must be shifted from the patient to a substitute decision maker (often referred to as a surrogate or proxy). The legal basis for permitting a patient's rights to devolve to and be exercised by another person is the doctrine of *parens patriae*, which is the inherent authority of a society to act to protect the interests of someone who cannot or will not protect himself or herself. It is predicated on the ethical principle of beneficence, which is our desire to help those who are in need or to do good for others.

The physician responsible for a patient's well-being needs to know who has the legal authority to speak on behalf of that patient. As a follow-up to the previous section's discussion of informed consent, this section discusses the rationale, the means, and the consequences of substitute decision making for patients of destroyed or questionable decision-making capacity when surgical intervention is contemplated.

Determinations of Competency

Concept of Competency

Competence is the most crucial issue in the decision making realm, since a lack of competence or even the questioning of an individual's competence may deprive the individual of the liberty to make personal decisions (102). As a practical matter, an individual's competence is often questioned for the first time when that person refuses a physician's recommendation, although in theory the same considerations should also be raised where the resident accepts the physician's medical proposal (120, 121). If a person understands and appreciates the information needed to give an informed consent, then that individual is competent to give both an informed consent and to refuse consent.

It is vital to remember that legal competency refers to a relative, rather than an absolute, degree of ability scale (121). To say that a person is legally incompetent implies that the individual is below some minimum level of capacity and range of opportunity, and not simply that the person has less capacity and opportunity than certain other people.

While courts generally (in the minds of critics of the guardianship system *too* routinely) grant petitions for appointment of substitute decision makers for older persons, in seriously contested cases, there is a strong judicial preference for and deference toward letting older persons make and live (or die) with their own decisions (122). However, the great majority of situations in which the decision-making capacity of a patient is called into question is handled on a *de facto* rather than *de jure* basis. That is, most such cases are quite properly—and without adverse legal consequence—managed by the physician, usually in conjunction with the family, without formal court involvement in deciding and acting upon the patient's decision-making impairment. When judicial involvement is sought by the parties, it is often because ethical issues concerning autonomy versus benevolence have been disguised as clinical/legal questions, to shift the focus of responsibility from the family and the caregivers to the legal system (123).

In most circumstances, competency should be addressed as an ethical matter by those who are closest to the patient. Resort to the courts is neither necessary nor desirable, since it is expensive, time-consuming, and emotionally draining. Initiation of judicial involvement in competency determinations should be the exception instead of the rule. It will depend on a variety of factors in any case, but elements that might point toward the advisability of advance, formal legal clarification include (109): (*a*) the incapacity is great and likely to be prolonged, and there is no obvious surrogate; (*b*) the capacity of the patient is questionable, and the decision to be made is significant; (*c*) the views of the surrogate are strongly at variance with medical judgment or the patient's known views; or (*d*) the choice of the individual to serve as surrogate is controversial and all efforts to resolve the matter at the hospital level have failed; and (*e*) family members radically disagree about the course of action for a patient who lacks adequate decision-making capacity.

Standards of Competency

In some situations, such as the patient in a long-term coma or a persistent vegetative state (PVS), the determination of incompetence is fairly straightforward. In most circumstances, though, clinical presentations of potential incompetence are more cloudy: transient incapacity, due to acute illness or side effects of medication; mental retardation; mental illness or emotional problems; or physical handicap (124). Determining legal status requires more information than the clinical diagnosis.

There exists no single, uniform standard of competence, although the potential value of such a model has been noted (125). Instead, competence to engage in decision making has been only rarely and vaguely defined in statutes and court decisions. In daily practice, it is frequently the attending physician acting alone who decides when a person is incapable of making decisions and a substitute should be involved, without any explicit standards for that determination being employed. Although the proposed (but not yet in any state adopted) Uniform Law Commissioners' "Model Health Care Consent Act" (106) endorses this ad hoc, "seat-of-the-pants" approach, the absence of clearly stated substantive standards for determining competency is a disservice to the patient and places the physician and hospital in an awkward legal predicament. The patient would be better protected and physicians and hospitals placed on firmer legal ground if competency determinations were based on enunciated and documented substantive standards.

While there is no global definition of competence, various approaches to determining its presence or absence have been suggested (27, 61, 102, 120, 126). The three main approaches that have been proposed are: outcome, status, and function. Under the outcome approach, decisions that are inconsistent with the values of the caregivers are conclusive of the person's incompetence; a "wrong" decision is, by definition, incompetently made. Under the status approach, an individual's competence is judged by his or her physical or mental status (e.g., age, place of residence) or diagnosis (e.g., dementia or depression), without further inquiry about how that status or diagnosis actually affects the person. This is sometimes called the membership approach, since the resident's membership in a particular class of persons is deemed controlling. The functional approach focuses on the individual's personal ability to function in decision-making situations.

Although in everyday practice most older patients are probably subjected to the outcome or status tests, virtually all legislators, judges, and commentators who have thought about the issue favor a functional orientation, emphasizing individual abilities or dysfunctions. The most thoughtful analyses urge that emphasis not be placed on the "objective" nature of the patient's clinical categorization (e.g., elderly) or of the specific choice made by the patient, but rather on the capacity of the individual patient and the subjective thought process followed in arriving at the "good" or "bad" decision (103, 127). The outcome and status approaches tend to take insufficient account of the particular values, goals, and perspectives of the patient actually affected by a decision. Thus, for instance, an elderly patient who chooses short-term comfort over longer-term survival may not be acting irrationally, even though the same decision made by a younger, otherwise vibrant person would seem irrational in the physician's value scheme.

There may certainly be a connection between a patient's clinical diagnosis and that patient's competence to make specific decisions. Factors, such as dementia or depression, may negatively affect the patient's functional capacity. However, the physician cannot go automatically from one finding to the other, assuming that the status equals the functional impairment. Where a clinical condition accounts for functional impairment rising to the level of incompetence, it is still the functional impairment—not the diagnosis—which necessitates a substitute decision maker.

Under a functional inquiry, the fundamental questions suggested are these: (*a*) Can the person make and communicate (by spoken words or otherwise) (128) choices concerning his or her life? (*b*) Can the person offer any reasons for the choices made? (*c*) Are the reasons underlying the choice "rational?" For instance, the person who declines amputation of a gangrenous leg because she does not wish to continue living with only one leg is acting more rationally than someone making the same decision out of fear that with an amputation she will not be able to run away from invading Martians fast enough; (*d*) Is the person able to understand the implications (i.e., the likely risks and benefits) of the alternatives presented and the choices that are made and the fact that those implications apply to that person? (*e*) Does the person actually understand the implications of those choices for him or her? (54, 127, 129). More elaborate versions of this psycholegal construct are available elsewhere, which examine the capacity to: (*a*) understand the relevant information which needs to be considered in reaching a decision; (*b*) deliberate about the information which needs to be considered in reaching a decision; and (*c*) decide to accept, reject, or modify a proposed plan of action (121).

Under this functional approach, the patient need not understand the scientific theory underlying the physician's recommendations in order to be deemed competent, as long as the patient comprehends the general nature and likely consequences of the choices presented. Also under this approach, competency must be determined on a decision-specific basis; that is, a resident may be capable of rationally making certain sorts of decisions, but not others (120). The minimally necessary degree of intellectual and emotional capacity may be visualized as falling somewhere on a sliding scale that depends on the nature of the decision being faced (130–132). Thus, competency should not be treated as an all-or-nothing affair. Partial competence is not the same thing as incompetence. The patient may be competent "enough" to make the decision in question.

Additionally, competency may wax or wane for a particular patient according to environmental factors, such as time of day, day of the week, physical location, acute, transient medical problems, other persons involved in supporting or pressuring the patient's decision, or medication reactions. Physicians are under an obligation to manipulate, whenever possible, environmental barriers to capacity in an attempt to maximize the decision-making capacity of a patient. Thus, if a decision can be delayed until a patient is in a more lucid state (i.e., after medications have been altered), this is preferable to proceeding unnecessarily on the basis of substituted decision-making. Also, many acute physical or mental problems of elderly patients, which impinge on decision-making capacity, can be sucessfully medically treated, and that course should be vigorously pursued before considering the patient incompetent (122).

Many elderly patients are capable of "assisted" consent with a little extra time and effort on the part of health care providers (61). For example, an elderly patient, who may not be able to process complex information as swiftly and efficiently as a younger person, may nevertheless be able to understand the complexities of a proposed treatment if given enough time to fully process the information. Physicians should be aware that elderly patients may need more time to process complex information regarding treatment and accordingly should not equate the speed with which an elderly patient processes information with level of competency.

Even where a patient is determined to be incapable of giving legally sufficient consent to or refusal of care in a particular situation and a surrogate decision maker must be involved, the patient should still be consulted and encouraged to participate in the decision-making process (though not to ultimately and exclusively make the decision) to the greatest extent possible.

Even patients with severe cognitive or emotional difficulties are capable of understanding more information and holding preferences to a larger extent than is generally supposed (96). Besides respecting individual autonomy, involving (although not in a binding way) even the legally incompetent patient tends to enhance that person's morale and feelings of control, which may in turn yield positive mental and physical health consequences (133).

Alternative Forms of Substitute Decision Making

Once it has been determined that a patient lacks sufficient capacity to independently make legally binding medical choices, an acceptable means of substitute decision making must be achieved, both to protect the well-being of the patient and the legal security of involved health care professionals and institutions. Alternative ways of delegating what would ordinarily be the patient's authority to make decisions to someone else to exercise that power on behalf of the patient, may be categorized as follows: (*a*) delegation of authority beforehand by the patient himself or herself, through methods of advance planning, such as a living will or durable power of attorney; (*b*) delegation of authority to a substitute by operation of statute, regulation, or broad judicial precedent; (*c*) informal delegation of authority to a substitute (usually a family member) by custom; and (*d*) delegation of authority to a substitute by a court order in the specific case (e.g., guardianship appointment) (134, 135).

Consequences of Substitute Decision Making

Any substitute decision-making scheme will necessarily involve a certain deprivation of a patient's decision-making autonomy. In this area, as in others discussed in this chapter, the physician's and hospital's legal interests will be best served by sincere concern for the patient's well-being and basic human dignity. Here, as elsewhere, good risk management depends on: (*a*) a clear, written institutional policy, (*b*) good faith and honest implementation of that policy, involving effective communication with and input from all affected parties, and (*c*) thorough documentation of processes and outcomes.

Other Issues

An almost endless variety of generic medicolegal issues have potential applicability to geriatric surgery. Three of the most important of these issues are confidentiality, medical record keeping, and the possible impact of health care cost containment efforts on legal liability.

The usual rules of confidentiality concerning information derived through the physician/patient relationship apply with full force to the surgeon who is caring for an elderly patient (27). If anything, the privacy of personal, intimate information may take on added significance for the older patient. Where the patient is mentally competent, the surgeon should be sure to obtain his or her permission to discuss matters with others, including relatives, before actually sharing any patient information. It should not be presumed automatically that every older patient wishes his or her personal medical information to be shared with spouse, children, siblings, etc. When the patient is temporarily or permanently incompetent, the surgeon should share relevant information with the person or persons who are formally or informally being relied on to make health care decisions for the patient. After a patient's death, information should be freely shared with the family (13), unless the patient had left prior express instructions not to reveal information to the family.

Medical record keeping is an essential aspect of quality patient care. In addition to its clinical importance, the medical record also has potentially substantial legal purposes. It is the process and the product of tangible documentation for later scrutiny of the nature and quality of medical services delivered. The medical record may become a central piece of evidence in resolving various legal issues in a panoply of legal contexts involving older surgical patients.

The final issue that will be mentioned briefly here concerns the possible legal liability implications of various health care cost control strategies that are currently in place or are likely to be the subject of experimentation in the near future. Cost-containment efforts definitely exert an impact on contemporary surgical practice (136). There has been much speculation that many of the cost-control strategies now in vogue will result in diminished access to and quality of medical (including surgical) services for many older individuals, as manifested by things such as premature hospital discharge, less than optimum care while in the hospital (i.e., withholding diagnostic and therapeutic interventions from a clinically appropriate candidate in order to save money), performing procedures on an outpatient basis that could be provided with less risk and hardship to the patient on an inpatient basis, and the like. Further, there has been much speculation that the resulting diminution in access to and quality of services to the elderly will result in greater exposure to the risk of legal liability for physicians and hospitals (101, 137–139).

Although political charges abound, there is no definitive evidence available yet regarding the accuracy of these predictions, either generally or as applied to geriatric surgery particularly. At the least, surgeons (both collectively as a profession and as individual practitioners) should be motivated to re-examine and eliminate practices and interventions of questionable or absent clinical benefit, to limit proven interventions to appropriate candidates (with age as only one criterion of appropriateness), and generally to practice cost-conscious, efficient medicine for all patients, including the elderly. At the same time, attention to the particular patient's wishes and best interests must be given foremost attention in the surgeon's decision making.

Conclusion

Surgical intervention for an older patient often entails increased clinical risks for the patient, and therefore heightened legal risks for the surgeon, other involved health care professionals, and the health care facility where the surgery is contemplated and/or performed. Physical and mental risks to the older patient, and legal risks to the health care providers, may result from either too little or too much surgical intervention or surgery that is performed improperly. As the legal issues discussed in this chapter illustrate, law can act as a valuable societal instrument in pushing toward a proper balance in geriatric surgery, where the patient's age is an essential—but only one of many essential—considerations in the planning, performance, and post operative provision of services by those in whose hands older patients and their families place their welfare and their lives.

References

1. Hornbein, TF. 1986. The setting of standards of care. *JAMA* 256:1040–1041.
2. Necheles, T. 1982. Standards of medical care: How does an innovative medical procedure become accepted? *Law Med Health Care* 10:15–18.
3. Brown, R. 1975. An appraisal of the nursing home enforcement process. *Arizona Law Review* 17:304–356.
4. Dornette, W. 1977. The legal impact of voluntary standards in civil actions against the health care provider. *New York Law School Review* 22:925–942.
5. Joint Commission on Accreditation of Healthcare Organizations. 1989. *Accreditation Manual for Hospitals*. Chicago: JCAHO.
6. LeGrand, C. 1984. Mental hospital regulation and the safe environment: Liability for sexual assault. *Law Med Health Care* 12:236–242.
7. Kapp, MB. 1985. Legal and ethical standards in geriatric medicine. *J Am Geriatr Soc* 33:179–183.
8. Koin, D. 1984. Surgical concerns. In *Geriatric Medicine: Fundamentals of Geriatric Care*, Eds., CK Cassel and JR Walsh, vol. II. New York: Springer-Verlag.
9. Samet, J, et al. 1986. Choice of cancer therapy varies with age of patient. *JAMA* 255:3385–3390.
10. Schwartz, W, and Komesar, N. 1978. Doctors, damages, and deterrence: An economic view of medical malpractice. *N Engl J Med* 298:1282–1289.
11. Ginzberg, E. 1985. *American Medicine: The Power Shift*. Totowa, NJ: Rowman & Allanheld.
12. Kapp, MB. 1985. *Legal Guide for Medical Office Managers*. Chicago: Pluribus Press.
13. Tolle, SW, et al. 1986. Communication between physicians and surviving spouses following patient deaths. *J Gen Intern Med* 1:309–314.
14. Stevens, G. 1982. Negligent infliction of emotional distress by physicians and hospitals. *Med Trial Technique Q* 1982:233–241.
15. Werthmann, B. 1984. *Medical Malpractice Law: How Medicine is Changing the Law*. Lexington, MA: Lexington Books.
16. Barrett, C. 1984. Negligence and the elderly: A proposal for a relaxed standard of care. *John Marshall Law Review* 17:873–893.
17. Miller, L. 1982. Comparative negligence. *JAMA* 248:1443–1444.
18. Berg, R, and Harpur, T. 1981. Should health care practitioners be allowed to exculpate themselves from liability? You be the judge. *J Med Assoc Ga* 70:273–276.
19. Doudera, AE. 1985. Decisionmaking and patients' rights. *Am Health Care Assoc J* 11:5–8.
20. Lehrer, S. 1985. Rights of autonomy and freedom of choice. *Am Health Care Assoc J* 11:26–28.
21. Jameton, A. 1984. Ethical dimensions of the physician-patient relationship. In *Geriatric Medicine: Fundamentals of Geriatric Care*, Eds., CK Cassel and JR Walsh, volume II. New York: Springer-Verlag.
22. Furrow, B. 1984. Informed consent: A thorn in medicine's side? An arrow in laws' quiver? *Law Med Health Care* 12:268–273, 278.
23. Katz, J. 1984. *The Silent World of Doctor and Patient* New York: Free Press.
24. Kapp, MB. 1985. Medical discourse: Recent contributions on the patient's role. *J Leg Med* 6:283–292.
25. Wertheimer, MD, et al. 1985. Ethics and communication in the surgeon-patient relationship. *J Med Educ* 60: 804–806.
26. Hollander, R. 1984. Changes in the concept of informed consent in medical encounters. *J Med Educ* 59:783–788.
27. Kapp, MB, and Bigot, A. 1985. *Geriatrics and the Law: Patient Rights and Professional Responsibilities*. New York: Springer.
28. Turnbull, HR. 1977. *Consent Handbook*. Washington, DC: American Association on Mental Deficiency.
29. President's Commission for the Study of Ethical Problems in Medicine and Biomedical and Behavioral Research. 1982. *Making Health Care Decisions: The Ethical and Legal Implications of Informed Consent in the Patient-Practitioner Relationship*. Washington, DC: GPO.
30. *Cobbs v. Grant*, 1972. 8 Cal. 3d 299, 502 P. 2d 1, 104 Cal. Rptr. 505.
31. Halleck, S. 1980. *Law in the Practice of Psychiatry: A Handbook for Clinicians*. New York: Plenum.
32. Andrew, JM. 1970. Recovery from surgery with and without preparatory instruction for three coping styles. *J Pers Soc Psychol* 15:223–226.
33. Becker, M, et al. 1979. Patient perceptions and compliance: Recent studies of the health belief model. In *Compliance in Health Care*, Eds., D Haynes, D Taylor, and D Sackett, pp. 78–109. Baltimore: Johns Hopkins University Press.
34. Davis, M. 1968. Variations in patients' compliance with doctors' advice: An empirical analysis of patterns of communication. *Am J Public Health* 58:274–288.
35. Hulka, BS, et al. 1976. Communication, compliance, and concordance between physicians and patients with prescribed treatment medications. *Am J Public Health* 66:847–853.
36. Stone, GC. 1979. Patient compliance and the role of the expert. *J Soc Issues* 35:34–59.
37. Egbert, LD, et al. 1964. Reduction of post-operative pain by encouragement and instructions to patients. *N Engl J Med* 270:825–827.
38. Bertakis, KD. 1977. The communication of information from physician to patient: A method for increasing patient retention and satisfaction. *J Fam Pract* 5:217–222.

39. Denney, MK, Williamson, D, and Penn, R. 1976. Informed consent: Emotional responses of patients. *Postgrad Med* 60:205–209.
40. Leydhecker, W, Gramer, E, and Krieglstein, GK. 1980. Patient information before cataract surgery. *Ophthalmologica* 1810:241–246.
41. Rittersma, J, Casparie, AF, and Reerink, E. 1980. Patient information and patient preparation in orthognathic surgery: A medical audit study. *J Maxillofac Surg* 8: 206–209.
42. Bremer, LH, and Gerken, E. 1986. Informed consent: Myths and risk management alternatives. In *Risk Management and Quality Assurance: Issues and Interactions*, Ed., G Chapman-Cliburn, pp. 142–147. Chicago: Joint Commission on Accreditation of Hospitals.
43. Gutheil, T, Bursztajn, H and Brodsky, A. 1984. Malpractice prevention through the sharing of uncertainty. *N Engl J Med* 311:49–51.
44. Halligan, P. 1980. The standard of disclosure by physicians to patients: Competing models of informed consent. *Louisiana Law Review* 41:9–67.
45. Rosoff, AJ. 1981. *Informed Consent: A Guide for Health Care Providers*. Rockville, MD: Aspen Systems.
46. Rozovsky, FA. 1984. *Consent to Treatment: A Practical Guide*. Boston: Little, Brown.
47. Kapp, MB. 1983. Placebo therapy and the law: Prescribe with care. *Am J Law Med* 8:371–405.
48. Christoffel, T. 1982. *Health and the Law: A Handbook for Health Professionals*. New York: Free Press.
49. LeBlang, T. 1983. Informed consent—duty and causation: A survey of current developments. *Forum* 18: 280–289.
50. Miller, L. 1980. Informed consent I, Informed consent II, Informed consent III, Informed consent IV. *JAMA* 244:2100–2103, 2347–2350, 2556–2558, and 2661–2662, respectively.
51. Somerville, M. 1981. Structuring the issues in informed consent. *McGill Law J* 26:740–808.
52. Pozgar, G. 1983. *Legal Aspects of Health Care Administration*, ed. 2. Rockville, MD: Aspen Systems.
53. Annas, GJ, Glantz, L, and Katz, B. 1977. *Informed Consent to Human Experimentation: The Subject's Dilemma*. Cambridge, MA: Ballinger.
54. Meisel, A. 1981. *Informed consent: Who decides for whom*? In Ed., M Hiller. *Medical Ethics and the Law: Implications for Public Policy*. Cambridge, MA: Ballinger.
55. Trichter, JG. 1980. Informed consent: The patient as individual. *Forum* 15:455–465.
56. Trichter, JG, and Lewis, P. 1981. Informed consent: The three tests and a modest proposal for the reality of the patient as an individual. *South Texas Law J* 21:155–170.
57. Faden, R, et al. 1981. Disclosure of information to patients in medical care. *Med Care* 19:718–733.
58. Faden, R, et al. 1981. Disclosure standards and informed consent. *J Health Politics Policy Law*. 6:253–284.
59. Strull, W, Lo, B, and Charles, G. 1984. Do patients want to participate in medical decision making? *JAMA* 252:2990–2994.
60. Greenfield, S, Kaplan, S, and Ware, J. 1985. Expanding patient involvement in care: Effects on patient outcomes. *Ann Intern Med* 302:900–902.
61. Schwartz, R, et al. 1984. *Medical treatment and physicians' legal duties*. In *Geriatric Medicine: Fundamentals of Geriatric Care*, Eds., CK Cassel and JR Walsh, vol. II. New York: Springer-Verlag.
62. Redden, EM, Baker, DC, and Meisel, A. 1985. The patient, the plastic surgeon, and informed consent: New insights into old problems. *Plast Reconstr Surg* 75: 270–276.
63. Perry, C, and Applegate, W. 1985. Medical paternalism and patient self-determination. *J Am Geriatr Soc* 33:353–359.
64. Romang, L. 1986. Patient education before discharge from the hospital. *South Med J* 79:998–1001.
65. Alton, W. 1977. *Malpractice: A Trial Lawyer's Advice for Physicians (How to Avoid, How to Win)*. Boston: Little, Brown.
66. Friedman, D. 1981. Informed dissent: A new corollary to the informed consent doctrine? *Chicago-Kent Law Review* 57:1119–1144.
67. Hasty, FE, III, 1985. When the patient takes over, the doctor can get sued. *Med Econ* 62:111–125.
68. Kold, E, and Ramseyer, N. 1981. Informed refusal in simple diagnostic testing. *Univ Calif Davis Law Review* 14:1105–1120.
69. Ryan, JM. 1981. Expansion of physician's duty to warn—an "informed refusal" malpractice action. *Univ Bridgeport Law Review*. 2:155–173.
70. Annas, GJ, Glantz, L, and Katz, B. 1981. *The Rights of Doctors, Nurses and Allied Health Professionals*. New York: Avon Books.
71. Klein, L, et al. 1982. Aging and its relationship to health knowledge and medication compliance. *Gerontologist* 22:384–387.
72. Devlin, M. 1983. Informed consent. *JAMA* 249:815.
73. O'Donnell, W. 1982. Let's stop ducking decisions on patient care. *Med Econ* 59:32–42.
74. Bursztajn, H, et al. 1981. *Medical Choices, Medical Chances: How Patients, Families, and Physicians Can Cope With Uncertainty*. New York: Delacorte Press.
75. Cassileth, P, et al. 1980. Informed consent—why are its goals imperfectly realized? *N Engl J Med* 302:896–900.
76. Meisel, A, and Roth, L. 1981. What we do and do not know about informed consent. *JAMA* 246:2473–2477.
77. Meisel, A. 1977. The expansion of liability for medical accidents: From negligence to strict liability by way of informed consent. *Nebraska Law Review* 56:51–152.
78. Rennie, D. 1980. Informed consent by 'well-nigh abject' adults. *N Engl J Med* 302:917–918.
79. Gregory, D. 1981. Informed consent: An overview. *Leg Aspects Med Pract* 9:4–6.
80. Siegler, M. 1982. The physician-patient accommodation: A central event in clinical medicine. *Arch Intern Med* 142:1899–1902.
81. Weiner, M, and Lovitt, R. 1984. An examination of patients' understanding of information from health care providers. *Hosp Community Psychiatry* 35:619–620.
82. Appelbaum, P, and Roth, L. 1983. Patients who refuse treatment in medical hospitals. *JAMA* 250:1296–1301.
83. Johnson, B. 1980. *An overview of informed consent: majority and minority rules*. In *Legal Medicine—With Special Reference to Diagnostic Imaging*. Ed., JA Everitt, Jr. Baltimore: Urban & Schwarzenberg.
84. Wadlington, W. 1984. Breaking the silence of doctor and patient. *Yale Law J* 93:1640–1651.

85. Meisel, A. 1979. The 'exceptions' to the informed consent doctrine: Striking a balance between competing values in medical decisionmaking. *Wisconsin Law Review* 1979:413–488.
86. George, J. 1980. *Law and Emergency Care*. St. Louis: C. V. Mosby.
87. Mancini, M, and Gale, A. 1981. *Emergency Care and the Law*. Rockville, MD: Aspen Systems.
88. Southwick, A. 1978. *The Law of Hospital and Health Care Administration*. Ann Arbor, MI: Health Administration Press.
89. Cross, AW, and Churchill, LR. 1982. Ethical and cultural dimensions of informed consent. *Ann Intern Med* 96: 110–113.
90. Norman, A. 1980. *Rights and Risks: A Discussion Document on Civil Liberties*. London: National Corporation for the Care of Old People.
91. Thomasma, D. 1983. Beyond medical paternalism and patient autonomy: A model of physician conscience for the physician-patient relationship. *Ann Intern Med* 98:243–248.
92. Vogel, J, and Delgado, R. 1980. To tell the truth: Physicians' duty to disclose medical mistakes. *Univ California-Los Angeles Law Review* 28:52–94.
93. Annas, GJ. 1975. *The Rights of Hospital Patients*. New York: Avon Books.
94. Somerville, M. 1984. Therapeutic privilege: Variation on the theme of informed consent. *Law Med Health Care* 12:4–12.
95. Simmons, B. 1978. Problems in deceptive medical procedures: An ethical and legal analysis of the administration of placebos. *J Med Ethics* 4:172–181.
96. Munetz, M, and Roth, L. 1985. Informing patients about tardive dyskinesia. *Arch Gen Psychiatry* 42:866–871.
97. Buford, A. 1984. *Residents' Rights: A manual for Long Term Care Facility Administrators and Supervisors* Washington, DC: American Health Care Association.
98. Gaylin, W. 1982. The competence of children—no longer all or none. *Hastings Center Report* 12:33–38.
99. May, W. 1982. Who cares for the elderly? *Hastings Center Report* 12:31–37.
100. Chapman, S. 1981. Refusal of consent: What the doctor must do. *Physician's Management* 21:84–87, 90, 92.
101. Kapp, MB. 1984. Legal and ethical aspects of health care reimbursement by diagnosis related groups. *Law Med Health Care* 12:245–253.
102. Annas, GJ, and Densberger, J. 1984. Competence to refuse medical treatment: Autonomy vs. paternalism. *Toledo Law Review* 15:561–596.
103. Jonsen, A, Siegler, M, and Winslade, W. 1986. *Clinical Ethics*, ed. 2. New York: MacMillan.
104. Pollack, R. 1980. *Clinical Aspects of Malpractice*. Oradell, NJ: Medical Economics Co.
105. Besdine, RW. 1983. Decisions to withhold treatment in nursing home residents. *J Am Geriatr Soc* 31:602–606.
106. LeBlang, T. 1983. Uniform law commissioners' model health-care consent act: An overview. *J Leg Med* 4: 479–500.
107. Pickle, J. 1983. Uniform law commissioners' model health-care consent act: Considerations in favor of adoption. *J Leg Med* 4:501–512.
108. Capron, AM. 1983. Uniform law commissioners' model health-care consent act: Considerations against adoption. *J Leg Med* 4:513–524.
109. American Hospital Association, Special Committee on Biomedical Ethics. 1985. *Values in Conflict: Resolving Ethical Issues in Hospital Care*. Chicago: American Hospital Association.
110. Victor, M. 1980. Informed consent. *Med Trial Technique Q* 27:138–175.
111. Burdett, R, Jr. 1981. Consent is authorization—not a form. *Top Health Rec Manage* 1:61–66.
112. Vaccarino, J. 1978. Consent, informed consent and the consent form. *N Engl J Med* 298:455.
113. Belli. 1983. Don't let informed consent backfire. *Med Econ* 60:78.
114. Heller, J. 1982. The question of informed consent: A progress report. *MD Magazine* 26:165–181.
115. Redden, EM, and Baker, DC. 1984. Coping with the complexities of informed consent in dermatologic surgery. *J Dermatol Surg Oncol* 10:111–116.
116. Cushing, M. 1984. Informed consent—an MD responsibility? *Am J Nurs* 84:437–440.
117. Grundner, T. 1980. On the readability of surgical consent forms. *N Engl J Med* 302:900–902.
118. Malone, M. 1983. Informed consent and hospital consent forms: Paper chasing in a video world. *J Urban Law* 61: 105–125.
119. Ludlam, J. 1978. *Informed Consent*. Chicago: American Hospital Association.
120. Culver, C. 1985. The clinical determination of competence. In *Legal and Ethical Aspects of Health Care for the Elderly*, Eds., MB Kapp, H Pies, and AE Doudera, pp. 277–285. Ann Arbor, MI: Health Administration Press.
121. Tepper, A, and Elwork, A. 1984. Competence to consent to treatment as a psycholegal construct. *Law Human Behavior* 8:205–223.
122. Douglas, D, et al. 1985. Rx for the elderly: Legal rights (and wrongs) within the health care system. *Harvard Civil Rights-Civil Liberties Law Review* 20:425–483.
123. Caplan, A. 1985. Let wisdom find a way. *Generations* 10: 10–14.
124. Munetz, M, Lidz, C, and Meisel, A. 1985. Informed consent and incompetent medical patients. *J Fam Pract* 20:273–279.
125. Select Committee on Aging, U.S. House of Representatives. 1985. *Dying With Dignity: Difficult Times, Difficult Choices*. Committee Print, Committee Pub. No. 99–518, 99th Congress, 1st Session.
126. Robertson, J. 1983. *The Rights of the Critically Ill*. Cambridge, MA: Ballinger.
127. Meisel, A, Roth, L, and Lidz, C. 1977. Toward a model of the legal doctrine of informed consent. *Am J Psychiatry* 134:285, 289.
128. Steffen, G, and Franklin, C. 1985. Who speaks for the patient with locked-in syndrome? *Hastings Center Report* 15:13–15.
129. Gutheil, T, and Appelbaum, P. 1982. *Clinical Handbook of Psychiatry and the Law*. New York: McGraw-Hill.
130. Drane, J. 1984. Competency to give an informed consent: A model for making clinical assessments. *JAMA* 252:925–927.
131. Drane, J. 1985. The many faces of competency. *Hastings Center Report* 15:17–21.

132. Harris, S. 1985. Protecting the rights of questionably competent long-term care facility residents. In: *Legal and Ethical Aspects of Health Care for the Elderly*. Eds., MB Kapp, H Pies, and AE Doudera. Ann Arbor, MI: Health Administration Press.

133. White, C, and Janson, P. 1985. *Helplessness in institutional settings: Adaptation or iatrogenic disease* In M. Baltes and P Baltas Eds., *Aging and the Psychology of Control*. Hillsdale, NJ: Lawrence Erlbaum.

134. Fowler, M. 1984. Appointing an agent to make medical treatment choices. *Columbia Law Review* 84:985–1031.

135. Kapp, MB. 1987. *Preventing Malpractice in Long-Term Care: Strategies for Risk Management*. New York: Springer.

136. Smits, HL, and Watson, RE. 1984. DRGs and the future of surgical practice. *N Engl J Med* 311:1612–1615.

137. Kapp, MB. 1986–1987. Health care delivery and the elderly: Teaching old patients new tricks. *Cumberland Law Review* 17:437–467.

138. Marsh, FH. 1985. Health care cost containment and the duty to treat. *J Leg Med* 6:157–190.

139. Mehlman, MF. 1985. Rationing expensive lifesaving medical treatments. *Wisconsin Law Review* 1985:239–303.

140. Bernstein, A. 1981. *A Trustee's Guide to Hospital Law*. Chicago: Teach'em, Inc.

141. Koopersmith, E. 1984. Informed consent: The problem of causation. *Med Law* 3:231–236.

4

Sociologic Aspects of Geriatric Surgical Care

Denise Smith-Fraser and Anita Beckerman

Nearly 30 million people in the United States are over the age of 65 years, one in every eight Americans. Comprising 12.3% of the population, they accounted for 31% of all hospital stays and 42% of all days of care in hospitals in 1987 (1). Various age-related changes in the 3rd quarter of life and beyond make surgical hospital stays for the elderly different enough from other groups to warrant discussion of their treatment.

The case of Raymond Jones, a composite patient with a successful rehabilitation, follows. What encompassed that success and the part physicians played in pre- and post-care is the focus of this chapter.

Case Study

Chief Complaint

This is the first hospital admission for Raymond Jones, a 66-year-old male with a history of peripheral vascular disease who presents with an oozing inflamed lesion on the lateral aspect of his left calf.

History of Present Illness

Mr. Jones has a 15-year history of heart disease and arteriosclerosis. He was a 2-pack per day smoker for 10 years and only recently stopped when an influenza infection left him with some shortness of breath. He first developed small leg ulcers about 5 years ago when he found himself becoming somewhat unsteady on his feet, frequently banging his legs when ambulating. Five years prior to this, he experienced intermittent calf pain when on his feet for an extended period of time, especially when walking. Diagnosed with intermittent claudication secondary to peripheral vascular disease, he has been treated with vasodilators since then. He did not at that time stop smoking, even though he was warned of the increased risks of complications if he continued. He has been self-managing the care of his leg with warm soaks and dry dressings. The lesion has now affected his ability to ambulate and care for himself.

Past Medical History

Hypertension for 20 years
Decreased visual acuity:
Etiology: Vision changes secondary to aging
Hypertensive changes

Present Medications

Minoxidil 10mg OD
Hydrochlorothiazide 50 mg ÷ OD
Methyldopa 250 mg ÷ BID

Allergies

None known

Personal/Family/Social History

Mr. Jones and his wife of 40 years live in Cleveland in a two-level private home with bedrooms and bathroom on the second level. They have two children who live nearby and four grandchildren. There is frequent contact with their children, who are very concerned about their father's health status. He and his wife enjoy taking short trips, especially to visit relatives in various parts of the country. Mr. Jones still drives short distances, but mostly during the daytime hours. His vision has somewhat decreased and he finds it very tiring to drive for any extended period of time. He does wear glasses for distance, but finds that his poor response to changes in light perception, especially at night, is too stressful. He is a retired construction worker, currently receiving social security and pension benefits. His income is limited, but sufficient for his present needs, barring any crisis. He keeps himself busy doing small repair jobs around his house, and, as a hobby, has recently begun doing small wood carvings.

Physical Examination

Mr. Jones is a well-nourished white male, somewhat overweight for his height and build. He appears his stated age, 66 years, and is in moderate distress.

Vital Signs: B/P = 145/90; P = 90; R = 20; T = 100.6° F (0)
Weight: 200 lbs.
Height: 5′ 7″
Extremities: Right leg pale in color, with decreased hair and shiny skin.
Palpable dorsalis pedis pulse.
Left leg has a 4 cm × 4 cm ulceration on lateral aspect of calf.
Ulcer is oozing yellow purulent drainage and eschar is present at the edges.
An extended area of bluish discoloration, measuring about 3 cm, surrounds the entire ulcer. There are no palpable pulses below the diminished femoral pulse.
Eyes: Extraocular movements are intact. Sclerae are clear and conjunctivae are pink. Pupils are equal, round, and react to light and accommodation. Funduscopic examination revealed arteriolar constriction with AV nicking bilaterally. Visual acuity is slightly diminished.

Mental Status

Mr. Jones is alert, oriented to person, time, and place, and appears to be of normal intelligence. He is somewhat anxious and complains of pain whenever his left leg is moved or touched.

Laboratory Data

Positive for active infection; WBC 15,000 with shift to left.

Impressions

Acutely infected ulcer on left leg, secondary to peripheral vascular disease
Bilateral retinal changes secondary to hypertension
Moderate obesity

Treatment Plan

Surgical consult, with possible consideration of amputation of left leg below the knee.

Hospital Course

A below the knee (BKA) amputation was performed on the left leg. A multidisciplinary care plan was formulated, involving staff members from medicine, nursing, psychiatry, nutrition, physical therapy, occupational therapy, social services, and therapeutic recreation.

Goal of Treatment

Maximal independence in activities of daily living (ADLs)

Outcome

Prothesis fitted
Ambulatory status achieved
Patient discharged to home after hospital stay of 45 days

General Considerations for Successful Recovery

Preadmission counseling, if appropriate
Rehabilitation beginning immediately after surgery
Physical therapy
Occupational therapy
Recreational therapy
Psychiatry involvement
Social services and discharge planning involvement
Evaluation of home environment
Possible discharge from hospital to rehabilitation center to home
Visiting nurse supervision
Teaching re: Right leg generally and good foot care
Graduated walking program to develop collateral circulation for right leg
Home-delivered meals program
Senior housing consideration
Safety considerations—Patient is at increased risk secondary to visual changes
Outpatient support group for amputees

Senior center involvement

Meeting with professional social gerontologist to discuss possibilities for future, i.e., volunteer or employment opportunities, support groups, senior center involvement, etc.

Goals of Rehabilitation

In conceptualizing and formulating rehabilitation goals, of utmost importance is the prevention of further disability or related deterioration. Any approach therefore should include setting realistic goals for patients and, equally important, for their families. This program should involve both groups in giving direct physical care and providing the necessities for patient comfort.

It is also important to acknowledge the fact that the elderly of today often have multiple health problems in addition to normal age-related changes. Providers of health care must ensure that patients receive rehabilitation after surgery to aid medical or surgical treatment.

Assessment

Normal aging changes can impact upon pathologic processes, making it essential that these changes are considered in any assessment and plan of care of the elderly patient. Omitting these considerations can result in goals and plans that are unrealistic, unreachable, demoralizing, and debilitating.

Decisions regarding the treatment environment are critical determinants of the kind and amount of care an older person will receive. Rarely can they be made on the basis of medical knowledge alone. Nahemow and Pousada state that for geriatric patients, decisions regarding hospitalization and discharge are complicated, especially where functional disabilities, rather than the presenting medical problem, may become the critical issue (2).

Evaluative measures that address the individuality of the elderly patient should be used to achieve successful rehabilitation after surgery. To ensure success, evaluative measures that identify self-care ability prior to hospitalization must be employed in forming the basis for a plan of care, one that would develop and adjust for strengths of the patient while in the hospital and upon discharge.

Lorensen states that the self-care activities and conditions that make it possible for the elderly person to remain at home after hospitalization can be found in the patient's self-care activities before admission. Focusing on this aspect of health care, that is, the assessment of self-care abilities or activities of daily living (ADLs) as currently labeled, would also identify what resources would be needed upon discharge (3).

Kane and Kane point out that measures of functional and social status, which examine the ability to function independently despite disease, physical and mental disability, and social deprivation, are the most useful overall indicators to assist those who care for the elderly (4). All care delivered to elderly persons with multiple disabilities should be planned in the context of each individual's functional abilities and not be based simply upon standardized norms of the general aged population. Such assessments provide baselines for understanding a patient's postoperative behavior.

The assessment of ADLs, which includes levels of ability in bathing, dressing, going to the toilet, transferring, continence, and feeding, should be made in a structured interview, with a specific format. The Katz Index of ADL is just one instrument that provides such an index of independence (5). Widely used and tested, it not only gives invaluable information to the health provider for formulating a baseline of patient functioning, but also provides data on changes over time.

In that physical and mental functioning are interdependent, the degree of the latter has implications for self-care abilities. For this reason, in addition to the need for a baseline assessment, there is also a need for measuring change in mental function. This is especially so when planning care for the elderly surgical patient. Psychosocial effects of hospitalization and surgery, while secondary to the physiologic condition, can be serious. Assessment of psychologic status is necessary and essential for consideration of appropriate interventions (6). The short portable mental status questionnaire (SPMSQ) developed at Duke University in 1978 as a screening tool for mental status is one such instrument. It is simple to administer and reliable, and includes available norms (4).

In addition to assessment of ADLs and mental status before and after surgery, it is recommended that one acquire information on the social functioning of the patient. Kane and Kane divide social functioning into three component concepts: (*a*) social interactions and resources; (*b*) personal coping and subjective well-being; and (*c*) environmental fit (4). Tools for this purpose are generally untested for validity and reliability, requiring the health professional to utilize careful judgment in the selection of an instrument and in analysis of the data.

Comprehensive Planning

Any planning for rehabilitation of the elderly surgical patient must take an approach that is comprehensive and all-inclusive. This can be achieved by using a multidisciplinary team arrangement, including all disciplines that are deemed necessary for the successful realization of formulated patient rehabilitation goals. Such a team would encompass staff members from the medical, nursing, psychosocial and social services, occupational therapy, physical therapy, nutrition, recreational, and other departments, depending upon the functional assessment outcomes of the patient on admission and during the postoperative and discharge planning periods.

In talking about the need for social services, Nahemow and Pousada emphasize that the patient can have many problems, only some of which are medical (2). Because there are more medical problems of longer duration in this age group, they are often considered separately from the social ones, a tendency which is often detrimental, leading to lack of appropriate care, as with rehabilitation of elderly surgical patients. They also state that physicians who do not understand the role of the social worker or other health team members in both the hospital and the community will be unable to utilize available services to the fullest extent.

Assuming a comprehensive approach is taken, the next consideration is that of time, specifically, the onset of the active rehabilitation process. The importance of quickly establishing a program of rehabilitation for the older patient has a basis in both physical as well as psychologic well-being. First, the elderly are at greater risk than any other age group of developing additional disabilities if rehabilitation treatment is delayed. Secondly, patients who undergo rehabilitation treatment as soon as possible are most likely to remain at home and not be institutionalized and/or be rehospitalized (6). These measures also lessen the increased risk of postoperative immobility and, as a positive byproduct, increase self-esteem and independence.

The comprehensive care plan that is developed should address all three phases: preoperative, postoperative, and discharge. Dealing with preoperative measures, Demmerle discusses the importance of taking into account sensory changes in the elderly, suggesting a tour of the hospital facility, as is done with prenatal patients, to increase familiarity with the environment (7). Skeet also advocates this approach, stating that the elderly individual, because of possible disorientation when moved away from familiar surroundings and personal support systems, is in a most vulnerable position (8). This preadmission hospital orientation is also helpful in reducing anxiety-related stress. During this visit, a "dry run" of what actually will take place can be offered to the patient and key family members or friends. Having the latter two groups involved is important for the psychologic well-being of the patient, especially following surgery and upon discharge.

The positive impact of instructive information on upcoming surgery for the older adult and family members cannot be overemphasized. Kathol (1984) has done research on the outcomes of using videotapes preoperatively for teaching purposes (9). She found that the tapes decreased family anxiety regarding surgery, and consequently, patient anxiety was reduced. This coincides with what has been known for years: that teaching that incorporates visual aids is more effective than discussion alone. Considering, however, the multiple sensory changes of normal aging, perhaps coupled with disease changes, it is imperative that assessment of functional abilities of sensory organs be completed before any teaching is initiated.

As with other age groups in this society, independence is valued by the elderly as a sign of control. At the same time, the present approach to hospitalized clients tends to require some surrender of autonomy. For the elderly, this surrender of autonomy and identity, coupled with possible disorientation upon hospitalization, can result in a serious risk to positive rehabilitation (8). Being cursed with as poor an image of old age as other age groups and behaving the way they think old people are supposed to act, all too often the elderly do themselves and society great harm by adopting behaviors of dependency and helplessness. It is therefore important to directly involve the patient in the care plan, thus increasing their feeling of control. Individualizing the assessment and plan is also key to planning each patient's abilities regarding independence (i.e., the plan should take into account the individual's strengths and weaknesses, demands and resources). Independence also can be encouraged and the recovery process greatly aided through simple verbal assurances by each member of the health care team and family members. Jackson (10) and Brawley (11) both advocate involvement of the patient in what they call a "wellness" atmosphere. This type of atmosphere can be created by having the patient involved in small tasks as soon as possible. This can include talking to others early in recovery, wearing one's own clothes, eating with others as a group, and participating in group activities, such as reality orientation or recreational therapy. This kind of approach improves the quality of life and care, by focusing on the elderly patient's abilities rather than disabilities. It increases reactivation, reintegration, and socialization back into an independent lifestyle.

Discharge Planning

Elderly individuals discharged from hospital to home must make major adjustments. While the boost in morale provided by going home can be great, they remain vulnerable until rehabilitation back to their own normal lifestyles is complete (8). The goals of discharge planning are to smooth the transition back to home living and to prevent readmission to the hospital, while providing continuity of care (12). To accomplish this, it is necessary to accurately document the current level of functional abilities, as discussed earlier, as well as to assess the home environment for consideration of at-home needs.

Rosenblatt suggests a rehabilitation home visit for the purpose of assessing the patient in his own environment (13). He found that this type of visit smoothed the transition back to home living for hospitalized patients and often improved a patient's motivation by reducing anxiety in both patient and family. It can provide reassurance to the patient who fears not being able to function at home and at the same time reveal problems not previously anticipated by the patient, caregivers, or hospital staff.

When home-based rehabilitation is possible, all resources identified as being needed are brought to the home, in the true sense of comprehensive rehabilitation: occupational therapy, physical therapy, etc. Koren states that planned rehabilitation in the home can enhance recovery by eliminating the "artificial," well-structured hospital environment (14). All aspects of the home environment are taken into account and any adjustments are made as needed.

While support systems are an integral part of positive rehabilitation, this is especially so when designing a plan of care for the elderly surgical patient. The "old-old," those persons 75 years and older, are a rapidly increasing segment of the population. Often there is an absence of available, competent support persons to care for them, be they paid or natural supports. For the "old-old" and those health care professionals responsible for them, this represents a genuine dilemma. But the differences between this group of elderly and their younger aged counterparts are significant in this and many other ways. Physicians and other health care professionals must take a fresh look at the aging process, paying keen attention to biologic changes, the presence of pathologic conditions, and the sociologic implications of a growing aged population with diverse needs. Multidisciplinary health teams interested in this population should explore new avenues for providing needed help, in this case, for the recovering elderly surgical patient. This will mean that community services must be fully incorporated into the planning of care. It will also mean that in cases in which neither paid nor natural supports are available, consideration for short-term nursing home rehabilitation will become a normal part of the rehabilitation steps taken.

As with most groups, the quality of life of the elderly is greatly improved when and where they can assume the utmost level of independence and functioning. Ensuring this can take a good deal of time, caring, and involvement, both directly and indirectly, in the assessment and care of the elderly patient. In situations, however, where steps are not taken to enhance maximum independence and functioning, a kind of learned helplessness can result, leaving the patient more dependent than ever before. This is particularly true after the patient has experienced the trauma of surgery.

The Recovery Process

Once physical recovery is successfully progressing, ways to enhance this process and a patient's life in general become of greatest importance. At this point, the assumption cannot be made that recovery is an end unto itself. It is extremely important to suggest or support meaningful goals beyond physical recovery. Keeping in mind what is realistic, there are possibilities in several areas, including employment, volunteerism, and continuing education.

With the work ethic as strong as it is among today's elderly population, after allowing appropriate recovery time, a return to work can assist an individual in making a good recovery. If not full-time, then perhaps part-time work would be appropriate. In cases where work was a source of stress to the patient, however, it might be recommended that either a different kind of job be sought or that volunteerism be considered. There are also those elderly who need work to supplement their incomes. Communities across the country have private senior employment agencies as well as public ones, the latter frequently being run by local and/or county offices on aging.

Whether it is tutoring children, running the gift shop in a hospital, or teaching reading in a prison literacy program, volunteers are always a welcome sight in major institutions across the United States. Agencies exist for the sole purpose of matching people with places. Again, it is the local or county offices on aging, many of which also serve as the federally designated area agencies on aging (AAAs), that can give information on how to locate a volunteer bureau or agency. Appendices A and B at the end of this chapter provide information on how to get the name and address of local and state offices on aging.

Deep personal satisfaction can be achieved by older adults who choose to take advantage of one of the many continuing education programs available to people of all ages across the country today. Courses on practically every conceivable topic can be found in adult evening programs in high schools and in 2- and 4-year colleges. Many of these courses offer a reduced rate or free tuition to persons over 60 years who are not seeking any course credit. They can vary greatly from the highly technical to the very practical, but all are extremely enjoyable. A few colleges across the country, particularly at the 2-year college level, have clubs, courses, and programs geared specifically to older adults.

Conclusion

Ingenuity and persistence are required to look beyond the immediate frustrations of one's own life and mortality and at the possibilities remaining for each elderly patient. Focus must be placed on the frequently small rewards of caring for elderly patients, while helping them to recover as much of their independent status as possible. In return, what is gained is a fuller understanding of those things found to be unique about the aged, individuals who are much like our future selves. As their special needs are acknowledged, the door begins to close on a period when the specific needs of this population went unmet.

For some physicians, it will become increasingly necessary to pass along the kind of information provided in this chapter. It represents a body of information about which all health care professionals must be aware. Recent national census reports indicate that the fastest growing age group in the United States today is made up of individuals over 85 years of age. Having achieved this, the issue of quality of life for the aged has become equally challenging for gerontologists and society at large. For the caregiver who is most often looked to for answers, this information will be helpful both today and in the years to come, but only if it is used and only if interaction among all professionals with knowledge of the aged—the social and psychologic as well as medical aspects—takes place.

What the elderly need to hear, particularly from the highly trained health care professionals whom they trust, is that life does more than just go on. It can and should be enjoyed in as active a way as possible, and one or even two chronic illnesses does not make an invalid.

Appendix A: Resources

The following information gives definitions for some of the most commonly available community services in the United States serving the elderly. It is followed by a listing of agencies throughout the United States where any interested individual can get further information.

Commonly Available Community Services for the Elderly

Congregate or Assisted Housing

This type of housing includes services, such as meals and housekeeping, and can also include health and personal services, transportation, special architecture, communication devices and more. Frequently, such sites are a senior citizen apartment building or retirement hotel, each of which would have appropriate space on the main floor for communal dining as well as recreational and other activities. While some congregate housing is for "private-pay" persons only, there is also federally subsidized housing available.

Geriatric Day Care Centers

For many frail older persons living at home with their adult children, the senior day care center offers a safe place during daytime hours where socialization and planned activities can take place. Besides the director and a recreational therapist, there is usually a nurse on site who can give any needed medications and do things such as giving periodic blood pressure checks. Adult children can bring a relative to a site in the morning before going to work and pick up that person as they return from work in the evening. Under the provisions of the Older Americans Act, funds are available nationwide for the establishment of these senior day care centers. Some day care center programs specialize (e.g., Alzheimer's day care).

Home-Delivered Meals Programs

For the older person who is either temporarily or permanently confined to home and cannot prepare a meal, this program, also called Meals on Wheels in some places, can provide one hot home-delivered meal, usually five days per week, with the Friday delivery often including additional food for the weekend. In addition to the national, federally funded programs that are either free of charge or have a minimal fee, many states, counties, and privately funded local programs provide the same or similar services.

Nutrition Sites/Senior Centers

Also called congregate meals programs, the goal of nutrition sites, whether federally or privately funded, is to provide nutritionally sound meals and to reduce isolation. Eligible participants are persons 60 years of age and older and their spouses of any age. Frequently, nutrition sites provide a tie-in with other social service programs at the site. Senior centers are usually funded at a higher level than nutrition sites and offer greater recreational and educational programs.

Senior Employment Services

For the individual who cannot afford to retire or who equates work with self-esteem, senior employment agencies can assist in finding part-time or full-time jobs, often short-term or seasonal work. Such agencies usually maintain a file of the qualifications of older adults interested in work, as well as a file of job openings. Recruiters within the agency work to let each group know about the other and to update and maintain the files. There are for-profit and non-profit agencies in large cities throughout the country as well as government-sponsored programs. Many of the government-sponsored programs are designed specifically to assist low-income elderly. The local area agency on aging can usually direct a person to the various types.

Several national employment programs are available specifically for seniors. The U.S. Department of Labor has three programs that offer part-time employment to older adults who serve as aides in various community agencies, such as child care centers, vocational training centers, homemaker services, and building security. The Senior Community Aides Program is sponsored by the National Retired Teachers Association and the American Association of Retired Persons. The Senior Aides Program is administered by the National Council of Senior Citizens, and the Senior Community Service Aides is sponsored by the National Council on the Aging. Other federally sponsored employment programs include Green Thumb, administered in more than 20 states by the National Farmers' Union, and the Seniors in Community Service Program, administered by the National Urban League.

Volunteer Bureaus

In addition to the many community volunteer jobs older adults perform, either independently or through local volunteer programs, there are quite a few that are federally funded and provide administrative and transportation supports. They include the Retired Senior Volunteer Program (RSVP), the Service Corps of Retired Executives (SCORE), the Senior Companion Program, and the Foster Grandparents Program. Additionally, persons of all ages are eligible to volunteer with the Literacy Volunteers of America, Volunteers in Service to America (VISTA), sometimes called the domestic Peace Corps, the Peace Corps itself, and many others. The federal agency that coordinates each of these programs and others is called ACTION.

Appendix B: National Organizations

ACTION
806 Connecticut Avenue, NW
Washington, DC 20525

Administration on Aging
Office of Public Information
330 Independence Avenue, SW
Washington, DC 20201

Write them to get a copy of the directory of addresses and phone numbers of every state office on aging in the country as well as each area agency on aging within each state. As the document is close to 200 pages, you may prefer to ask only for selected states.

Al-Anon (for families and friends of alcoholics)
PO Box 182, Madison Square Station
New York, NY 10010

Alzheimer's Disease and Related Disorders Association
360 North Michigan Avenue
Chicago, IL 60601

American Association for Geriatric Psychiatry
230 North Michigan Avenue
Suite 2400
Chicago, IL 60601

American Association of Homes for the Aging
1050 17th Street, NW
Washington, DC 20036

American Association of Retired Persons
National Retired Teachers Association
1909 K Street, NW
Washington, DC 20049

American Cancer Society
777 Third Avenue
New York, NY 10017

American Diabetes Association
1660 Duke Street
Alexandria, VA 22314

American Foundation for the Blind
15 West 16th Street
New York, NY 10011

American Geriatrics Society
10 Columbus Circle
New York, NY 10019

American Health Care Association
(American Nursing Home Association)
1025 Connecticut Avenue, NW
Washington, DC 20036

American Heart Association
7320 Greenville Avenue
Dallas, TX 75321

American Lung Association
1740 Broadway
New York, NY 10019

American Parkinson's Disease Association
Room 602
47 East 50th Street
New York, NY 10022

Arthritis Foundation
1314 Spring Street, NW
Atlanta, GA 30309

Association of Rehabilitation Facilities
5530 Wisconsin Avenue, NW
Washington, DC 20015

Center for the Study of Mental Health of the Aging
National Institute of Mental Health
Parklawn Building
5600 Fishers Lane
Rockville, MD 20857

Deafness Research Foundation
Suite 705
366 Madison Avenue
New York, NY 10017

Gray Panthers
3700 Chestnut Avenue
Philadelphia, PA 19104

House Select Committee on Aging
House Office Building
Annex 1, Room 712
Washington, DC 20515

International Federation on Aging
1909 K Street, NW
Washington, DC 20006

National Amputation Foundation
12–45 150th Street
Whitestone, NY 11357

National Association for the Deaf
814 Thayer Avenue
Silver Spring, MD 20910

National Center and Caucus on the Black Aged
1424 K Street, NW
Washington, DC 20036

National Clearinghouse on Aging
Administration on Aging
330 Independence Avenue, SW
Washington, DC 20201

National Council on Aging
600 Maryland, SW
West Wing 100
Washington, DC 20024

National Council of Senior Citizens
925 15th Street, NW
Washington, DC 20005

National Federation of the Blind
1346 Connecticut Avenue, NW
Washington, DC 20036

National Hearing Aid Society
20361 Middlebelt Road
Livonia, MI 48152

National Indian Council on Aging
P.O. Box 2088
Albuquerque, NM 87103

National Institute on Aging
Department of Health and Human Services
Public Health Service
National Institutes of Health
Building 31
Bethesda, MD 20205

National Pacific/Asian Resource Center on Aging
811 First Avenue
Coleman Building, Suite 210
Seattle, WA 98104

National Policy Center on Women and Aging
University of Maryland
Cole Field House, Room 1150
College Park, MD 20742

National Self-Help Clearinghouse
Graduate School and University Center/CUNY
33 West 42nd Street, Room 1227
New York, NY 10036

National Self-Help Resource Center
2000 S Street, NW
Washington, DC 20009

Senate Special Committee on Aging
Dirksen Senate Office Building
Room G233
Washington, DC 20510

United Ostomy Association
111 Wilshire Boulevard
Los Angeles, CA 90017

References

1. American Association for Retired Persons/Administration on Aging. 1988. *A Profile of Older Americans: 1988*. Washington, D.C.
2. Nahemow, L, and Pousada, L. 1983. Social aspects of aging. In *Geriatrics Diagnostics*, 39. New York: Springer.
3. Lorensen, M. 1985. Effects on elderly females' self-care in case of acute hospitalization as compared with men. *Health Care for Women International* 6:247–265.
4. Kane, RL, and Kane, R. 1981. *Assessing the Elderly*. Lexington, MA: Lexington Books.
5. Katz, S, Ford, AB, and Moskowitz, RW. 1963. Studies of illness in the aged. The index of ADL: A standardized measure of biological and psychosocial function. *JAMA* 185:94–98.

6. Williams, FT, and Jones, PW. 1985. Rehabilitation in our aging society. *Aging* 350:2–3.
7. Demmerle, B. 1982. Nursing care. *Geriatric Nurs* Sept/Oct: 316–321.
8. Skeet, M. 1983. When elderly people go into hospital: Planning care. *Nurs Focus* May:15–16.
9. Kathol, DK. 1984. Anxiety in surgical patients' families. *Am Operating Room Nurs J* 40(1):131–137.
10. Jackson, MF, 1984. Geriatric rehabilitation on an acute-care medical unit. *J Adv Nurs* 9:441–448.
11. Brawley, J. 1983. The aged require attention. *Curatonis* 6(1):31–32.
12. Feeney, E, Williams, MP, and Doyle, GC. 1986. Meeting the needs of the hospitalized elderly. *Nurs Management*, 17(9):35–42.
13. Rosenblatt, DE, Campion EW, and Mason, M. 1962. Rehabilitation home visits. *J Am Geriatr Soc* 34:441–447.
14. Koren, MJ, and Bills, D. 1985. Home may be the best place for rehabilitation. *Aging* 350:14–17.

SECTION II

Physiologic Changes in the Elderly

5

Cardiovascular Changes in the Elderly

Richard A. Josephson and Edward G. Lakatta

A complete description of the changes that occur in the cardiovascular system with aging requires consideration of three different processes: the presence of disease, both clinically apparent and occult, the effect of changes in life-style that often occur with advancing age, and alterations in cardiovascular function that may rightly be attributed to aging per se. It is only after the first two processes are excluded that one may properly ascribe changes in the cardiovascular system that are seen in the elderly to aging itself. This chapter delineates what is presently understood about those changes in the cardiovascular system that occur with aging and illustrates how our concept of "normal" cardiovascular function must change when evaluating individuals of different ages. The major emphasis is on left ventricular function, but the related and important processes of coronary heart disease, dysrhythmias, valvular heart disease, and systemic blood pressure are discussed as well. Baseline characterics are described as well as alterations induced by "stress" and pharmacologic interventions, for the latter circumstances are often of prime concern to surgeons. Thereafter, a rational approach to the preoperative evaluation of the elderly surgical patient is outlined.

Coronary Artery Disease and the Elderly

It is apparent to physicians and laymen alike that many pathologic processes increase in incidence and/or prevalence with age. Coronary artery disease is one such process. While a surgeon would clearly wish to know if an elderly patient had clinically significant coronary artery disease, this is not always as straightforward as one might think.

Autopsy data indicate that coronary artery disease increases exponentially with advancing age. The International Atherosclerosis Project collected numerous specimens from 1960 to 1965. That study indicates that while the earliest definitive atherosclerotic intimal lesion, the fibrous plaque, occurs in 30% of those aged 15 to 24, its prevalence increases to greater than 85% by age 35 to 44. More important is the prevalence of more advanced atherosclerotic lesions. The prevalence of coronary artery stenosis resulting in greater than 50% luminal diameter narrowing likewise increases with age, resulting in a prevalence of 50% by ages 55 to 64 (1). Elveback et al. (2) reported the autopsy findings from Olmstead County, Minnesota from the period 1950 to 1979 (Fig. 5-1). Their data confirm that of the International Atherosclerosis Project, namely, that there is a significant and increasing prevalence of coronary artery stenosis with advancing age. Their study also indicates that the age-specific prevalence of coronary artery stenosis has risen from the late 19th century to the mid-20th century (2).

Clinical evaluation tends to underestimate the above figures. One reason is due to the inherent selection bias of autopsy studies. Another major reason is the frequent insensitivity of clinical data. The Baltimore Longitudinal Study on Aging (BLSA) has examined community-dwelling individuals for over 25 years, and much information on the epidemiology and pathophysiology of the cardiovascular system has resulted from this. Figure 5-2 shows that when one employs conventional "resting" criteria (history of angina pectoris or documented myocardial infarction, or abnormal resting 12-lead electrocardiogram), the prevalence of suspected coronary artery disease is estimated to increase from 10% at ages 51 to 60

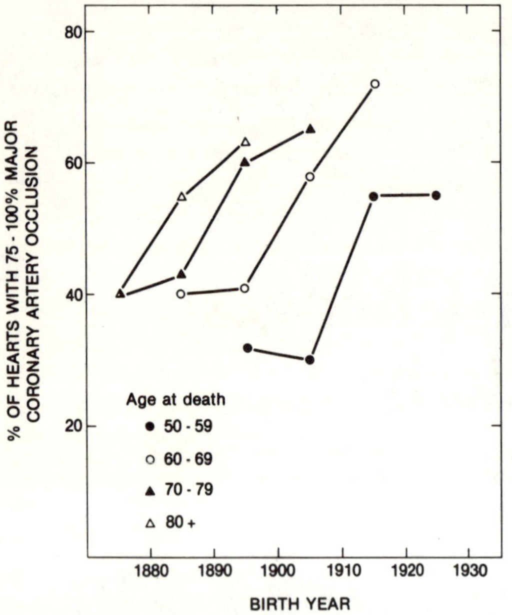

Figure 5-1. Prevalence of significant atherosclerotic coronary artery stenosis as a function of age and birth year. (From Elveback et al. [2].)

to 20% at ages 71 to 90 (3). These figures are in general agreement with those of the Framingham Heart Disease Epidemiology Study (The Framingham Study), which indicate an average annual incidence of coronary morbidity (i.e., clinically overt coronary artery disease) at ages 65 to 74 of 17 per 1,000 (4, 5). However, when the BLSA participants were also screened with symptom-limited exercise tests, the suspected prevalence of coronary artery disease is seen to be much higher, especially when thallium-201 scintigraphy is used in addition to electrocardiography. Thallium-201 is a radionuclide that is given intravenously during the test and aids in the detection of underperfused myocardium. The additional data gained during such stress tests increase the estimate of the prevalence of coronary artery disease to 25% at ages 51 to 60 and 55% at ages 71 to 90 (3). These figures, obtained antemortem, are in close agreement with the described autopsy data. Of particular note is that the positive predictive value of stress testing increases with increasing age (i.e., the prevalence of occult coronary artery disease increases with advancing age): at ages 51 to 60, stress testing roughly doubles the measured prevalence of coronary artery disease from 15% to 25%, while at ages 71 to 80 the figures more than triple, from 18% to 58%. Clearly, one could argue that rather than using advanced age as a relative contraindication to stress testing, the stress test, because of its demonstrated sensitivity, may be particularly valuable in detecting occult coronary artery disease in the aged. Confirmation of this hypothesis awaits additional study of the positive and negative predictive value of exercise stress testing in the elderly.

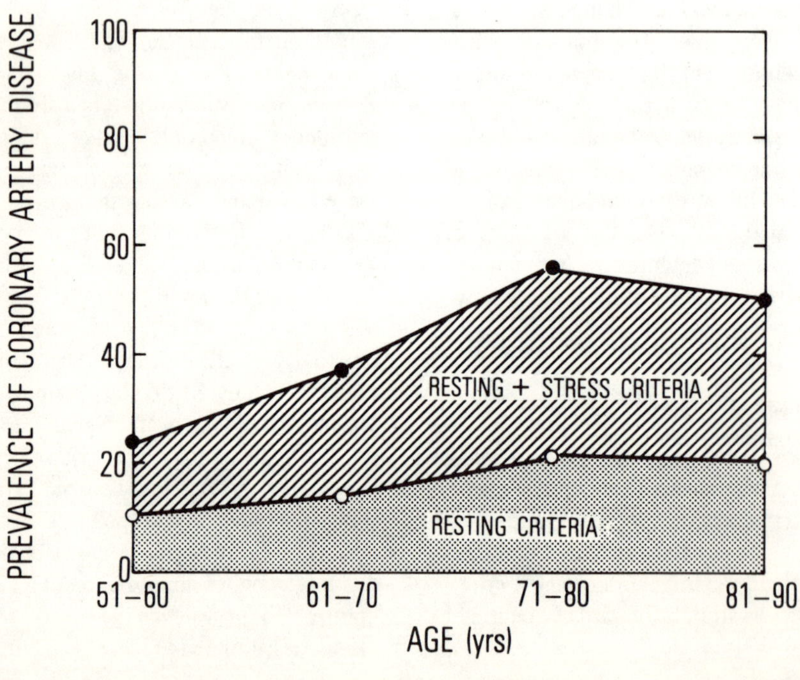

Figure 5-2. Prevalence of ischemic coronary artery disease in BLSA participants as assessed by resting (history and resting electrocardiogram) and stress (symptom limited exercise test) criteria as a function of age.

Life-Style

The study of the aging cardiovascular system entails unraveling the interactions of aging per se, the presence of overt and occult disease, and variations in life-style, as described above. While we can now separate those individuals with suspected clinically significant coronary artery disease from those without, as discussed previously, it is much more difficult to separate the effects of life-style. Numerous studies have documented that physical activity declines with age. Therefore, when one investigates an elderly patient population, even one that may be considered healthy by the criteria previously enumerated, and discerns differences in cardiovascular function with increasing age, one usually is really investigating the combined effects of aging and declining physical activity. The definitive human studies examining age-related changes while controlling for the level of physical activity have not been done. This chapter delineates those changes in the cardiovascular system that are known to occur with a more sedentary life-style (within a given age). These changes are compared with the studies of normal human aging, so that the effects of aging per se may be better appreciated. There is a dearth of information on how other age-associated life-style variables, (i.e., nutrition, tobacco consumption, alcohol consumption, and personality) affect the elderly cardiovascular system on either an acute or chronic basis, and we will elaborate on only two of these points.

A sedentary versus a more active (or physically trained) life-style has been shown to result in characteristic changes in the cardiovascular system. The resting heart rate increases while stroke volume decreases, resulting in little or no change in cardiac output. Left ventricular end diastolic volume decreases, and there is conflicting data on the alterations in end systolic volume and contractility. The ability to respond to exercise stress is reduced, whether measured as the amount of work performed (watts or metabolic equivalent of resting energy expenditure [METS]) or as the maximum aerobic capacity (VO_2 max). A sedentary life-style also produces significant changes in the skeletal musculature. Total muscle mass declines, and the ultrastructure of individual muscles is altered, with a prominent decrease in mitochondrial number. This diminished muscle and mitochondrial mass is largely responsible for the decline in VO_2 max noted above (6).

Because of the inherent difficulties with human investigation, some researchers have studied in vitro measures of cardiac muscle function. Peak tension, time to peak tension, and rate of tension development are unchanged with exercise training, at least in the adult rat model. Two recent papers describe a differential effect of exercise on adult versus senescent rats: exercise prolonged the contraction duration of papillary muscles from adult rats but shortened the contraction duration of papillary muscles from senescent rats (7, 8). Thus, one must consider the effects of life-style on the cardiovascular system, but it also appears that a similar life-style variable, such as exercise, may have different effects on the elderly than on younger individuals. Clearly, more work is needed in this important area.

Dietary intake of salt is epidemiologically associated with an increase in arterial blood pressure and arterial wall stiffness. Avolio et al. (9) studied two Chinese populations (an urban population with a high dietary intake of salt and a rural population with a lower dietary intake of salt). They found that those individuals with a high salt intake had higher systemic blood pressures and arterial pulse wave velocities (a measure of arterial stiffness) than age-matched individuals from the population with low salt intake (Fig. 5-3). These findings are important in two regards. One, the data suggest that dietary composition or physical activity level may affect cardiovascular function in the elderly. Two, it raises the question of whether the finding of increased arterial stiffness and systemic blood pressure with advancing age (discussed at length below) is purely an age-associated alteration, or whether it represents the consequences of excess sodium intake or diminished physical activity level, independent of age per se.

Cardiovascular Changes Associated with Normal Human Aging

Cardiac Rate, Rhythm, and Conduction

Cardiac dysrhythmias are common in the elderly. Investigation of 98 participants in the BLSA, aged 60 to 85, who were screened for the absence of cardiac disease by both resting and exercise criteria, revealed that the majority of them had single supraventricular or ventricular beats, a third had multiform ventricular ectopy, 11% had ventricular couplets, and 4% had nonsustained ventricular tachycardia (10). Table 5-1 provides a more detailed listing of these data. These findings have been confirmed by others. Thus, elderly individuals who have been extensively screened for the absence of cardiovascular disease may still have considerable tachyarrhythmias. It is tempting to consider these individuals "healthy" and not requiring therapy; confirmation of this hypothesis will require additional study and follow-up data.

Conduction abnormalities are more prevalent in the elderly, and several studies have found that while left bundle branch block is usually associated with intrinsic cardiac disease (*e.g.*, ischemic, hypertensive) right bundle

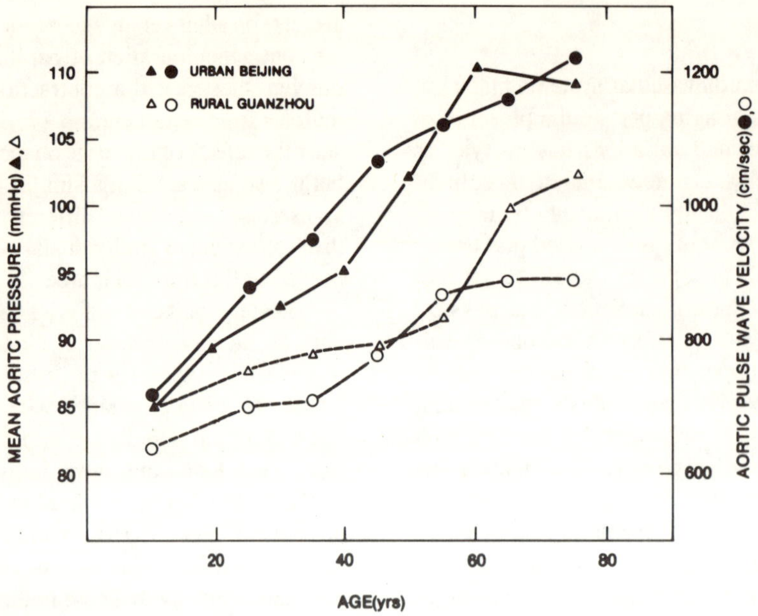

Figure 5-3. Arterial stiffness as assessed by pulse wave velocity and blood pressure as a function of age and sodium intake. (From Avolio et al. [9].)

Table 5-1. Supraventricular and ventricular arrhythmias observed in 98 healthy elderly subjects

	No. subjects	Percentage of total
Supraventricular		
Any	86	88
Isolated ectopic beats	86	88
⩾ 30 beats in any hour	22	22
⩾ 100 beats in 24 hours	25	26
Benign slow atrial tachycardia	27	28
Paroxysmal atrial tachycardia	13	13
Atrial flutter	1	1
Accelerated junctional rhythm	1	1
Ventricular		
Any	78	80
Isolated ectopic beats	76	78
⩾ 5 in any hour	37	38
⩾ 30 in any hour	12	12
⩾ 60 in any hour	7	7
⩾ 100 in any hour	17	17
Multiform	34	35
Ventricular couplets	11	11
Ventricular tachycardia	4	4
R on T phenomena	1	1
Accelerated idioventricular rhythm	1	1

branch block is not infrequently seen in apparently healthy older men (11). Left anterior fascicular block is more common in the elderly than in middle-aged adults, and it is not generally associated with progression to more severe abnormalities. Though the majority of studies have shown that the resting heart rate is not age related, it appears that the mean heart rate is lower in elderly men than in elderly women. The elderly may manifest less cardioacceleration during either routine daily activities or a formal exercise stress test. Frank episodes of sinus arrest or extreme bradycardia (< 40 beats per minute) appear to be rare in healthy elderly, and their presence ought to be taken as a sign of underlying disease (12). Asymptomatic prolongation of the PR interval or true first degree heart block is more common in the elderly than in younger individuals. It is secondary to the age-associated increase in atrio-His bundle conduction time, with the conduction time from the His bundle to the ventricle being relatively unaffected. Like other instances of supra-Hisian atrioventricular block, the prognosis is good, and prophylactic pacemaker insertion is not warranted.

Cardiovascular Function at Rest

There is a stiffening of the media of large vessels with advancing age (9, 13–15). This contributes to an increase in the aortic input impedance. When the heart ejects a given volume of blood into the aorta, there will be a greater systolic blood pressure in the elderly than in younger individuals. This decrease in vascular distensibility presumably is clinically related to the epidemiologic finding of an increase in systolic blood pressure with advancing age. Furthermore, by Laplace's law (wall stress $\propto$ pressure/[2 $\times$ wall thickness]), this increase in left ventricular systolic pressure would increase left ventricular wall stress. There appears to be a compensatory left ventricular hypertrophy with aging (Fig. 5-4), and this increase in left ventricular wall thickness normalizes wall stress (16). This "compensatory" hypertrophy in turn has certain functional consequences: peak left ventricular filling rate as measured by radionuclide ventriculography or left ventricular early diastolic filling as measured by M-mode echocardiography is decreased with advancing age (these data were obtained in participants in the BLSA, screened for the absence of cardiovascular disease with rest and stress criteria, as outlined above). In conjunction with this decline in early diastolic filling, there is an increase in the atrial contribution to ventricular filling (16, 17).

Exercise and Cardiac Reserve

There have been many studies to suggest that maximum aerobic capacity, as measured by VO_2 max, declines significantly with age (18). Recent studies indicate that some of this measured decline may be secondary to the inclusion of individuals with clinically occult cardiac disease. Furthermore, if one considers that the purpose of the cardiovascular system is to supply blood containing oxygen and nutrients to metabolically active tissue and remove wastes from same, it is reasonable to normalize measured VO_2 max for muscle mass. This normalization is employed because both body weight and percentage of body weight that is muscle change with advancing age. The result of this normalization is that the decline in VO_2 max with advancing age is less than previous studies have shown (19). These data suggest that much of the decline in VO_2 max with advancing age may be secondary to peripheral rather than primary cardiac alterations.

The pumping ability of the heart, as measured by cardiac output, is often said to decline with age (20). Studies using the well-screened BLSA participants have found that cardiac output at rest, with positional changes, and with exercise is fairly constant over the age range of 40 to 80 years (21). These studies, which employed radionuclide angiography, indicate that the mechanism of cardiovascular adaptation to exercise is different in the elderly and the nonelderly. Whereas middle-aged individuals augment their cardiac output with a large increase in heart rate and a modest increase in stroke volume, the elderly tend to increase their heart rate less but increase their stroke volume more. Furthermore, the mechanism underlying this increase in stroke volume is different in the elderly and nonelderly. Younger individuals increase stroke volume principally by a decrease in end-systolic volume, with a modest increase in end-diastolic volume. In contrast, the elderly increase stroke volume by a modest decrease in end-systolic volume and a significant increase in end-diastolic volume (Fig. 5-5). That is, the elderly tend to employ the Frank-Starling mechanism to compensate for a diminished heart rate response to exercise.

Given that the sympathetic nervous system, via beta-adrenergic receptors, mediates arterial dilation, increased

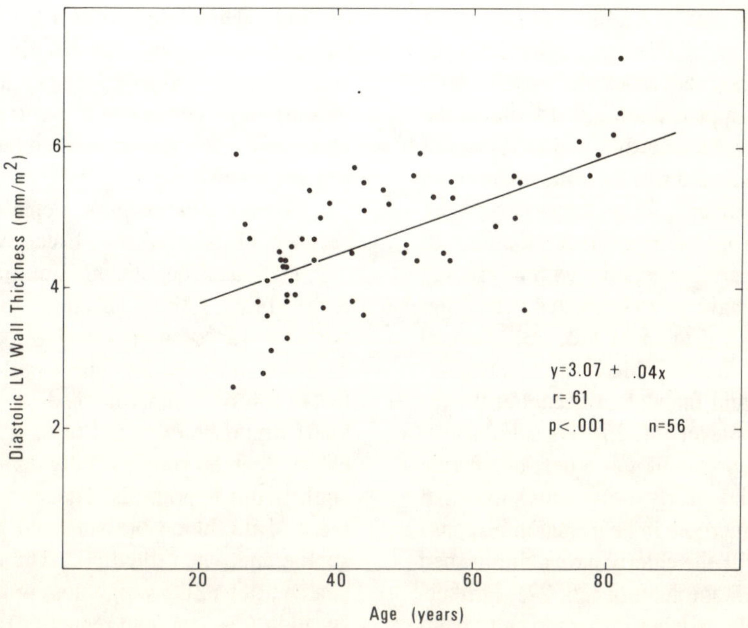

Figure 5-4. Left ventricular wall thickness measured by M-Mode echocardiography as a function of age.

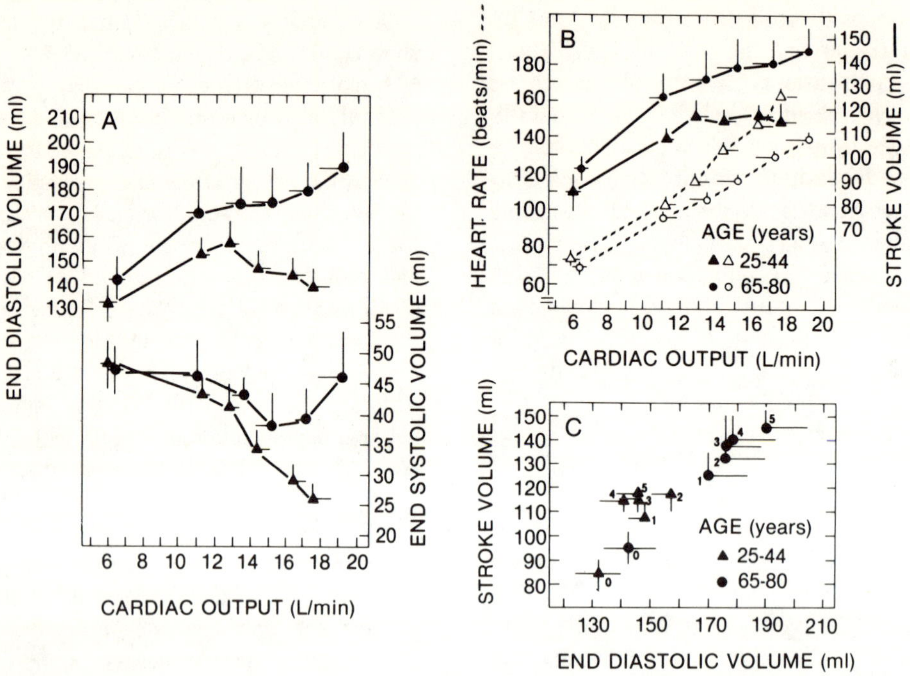

Figure 5-5. Cardiac response to exercise stress in young and elderly BLSA participants. Note the diminished heart rate response in conjunction with an augmented stroke volume in the elderly (*panel B*). This augmentation of stroke volume is achieved principally by an increase in end-diastolic volume with less change in end-systolic volume, the Frank-Starling mechanism (*panel A*). The potency of the Frank-Starling mechanism appears unchanged with age however (*panel C*).

heart rate, and increased contractility (i.e., diminution in end-systolic volume without a change in preload, or end-diastolic volume) one might characterize senescence as a relative "hyposympathetic" state. Indeed, pharmacologic studies have suggested just that. The administration of the beta-blocker, propanolol, to middle-aged individuals results in the behavior of their cardiovascular system, both at rest and with exercise, approximating that found in the elderly (maintenance of exercise cardiac output via less of an exercise-induced tachycardia and a greater reliance on the Frank-Starling mechanism). This "hyposympathetic state" does not appear to be due to a decreased ability of the nervous system to secrete catechols with advancing age. In fact, the elderly have an exaggerated catecholamine response to exercise (Fig. 5-6) (22, 23). Several lines of evidence suggest that the elderly are less responsive to catecholamines, and this defect occurs at the receptor and/or postreceptor level (24, 25). The administration of equal dosages of isoproterenol, a beta-adrenergic agonist, to middle aged and elderly individuals shows that the latter have less of an increase in heart rate in response to this drug (14). Similarly, the elderly have a diminished vasodilatory response to isoproteronol (26, 27). Furthermore, data suggest that the number of high-affinity beta-adrenergic receptors decreases with advancing age in human noncardiac tissue; the corresponding experiments on heart muscle have yet to be done. In vitro animal studies suggest that there is also a defect in postreceptor events involved in catecholamine action in senescent myocardium. Therefore, while basal cardiac output is unchanged with aging, the elderly are less responsive to catecholamine-induced augmentation of function, and thus are more dependent on ventricular dilation (preload) to increase cardiac output when required (the Frank-Starling mechanism).

Intravascular volume depletion, which may occur because of poor intake, excessive diuresis, fever, decreased plasma oncotic pressure, increased microvascular permeability ("third spacing"), or pharmacologic vasodilation (a common effect of volatile anesthetics), is common in the perioperative period. The deleterious effect of intravascular volume depletion (a reduction in preload) would be expected to have a greater affect on the elderly than on younger individuals. A recent study helps confirm this hypothesis. The study involved the measurement of the blood pressure and pulse of subjects while supine and when tilted 60°. The measurements were repeated after a 2-kg weight loss induced by diuretic administration (*i.e.*, preload reduction). Prior to diuresis, both the young and elderly subjects maintained their systolic

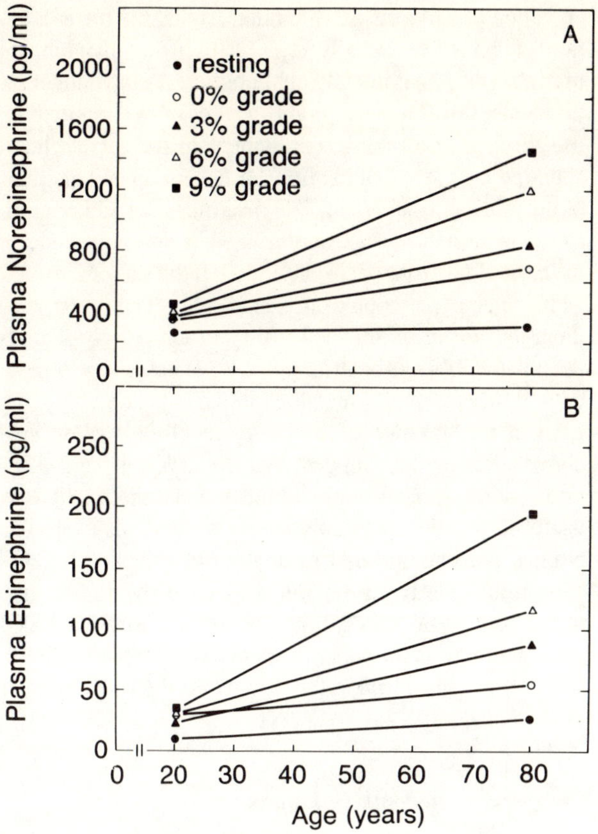

Figure 5-6. Plasma catecholamine level in BLSA participants as a function of age and work load. Note that resting catecholamine level is not age related, while exercise-induced augmentation of plasma catecholamines is increased with advancing age.

blood pressure in response to tilt. After diuresis, the young subjects were still able to maintain their systolic blood pressure when stressed by tilt, while tilt stress resulted in a significant decline in systolic blood pressure in the elderly. In half the elderly subjects, this decline was symptomatic. After diuresis, the elderly subjects did not manifest as great a tachycardia as the younger subjects in response to tilt. This defect in cardioacceleration was believed to underlie the orthostasis in the elderly (28) (Fig. 5-7).

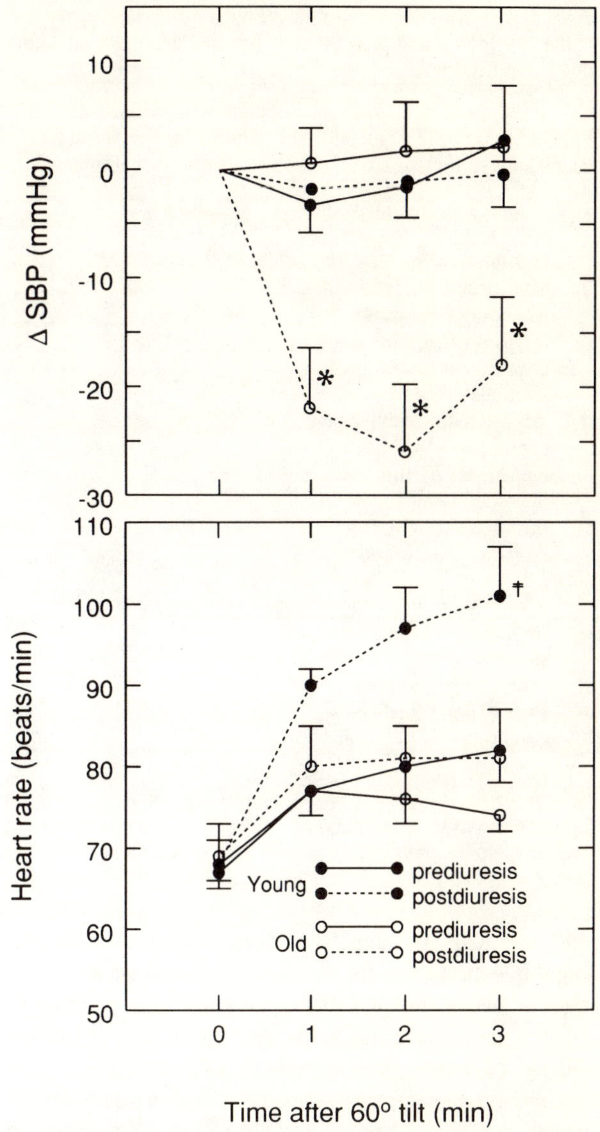

Figure 5-7. Alterations in systolic blood pressure (*top panel*) and heart rate (*bottom panel*) induced by 60° tilt. Note that both the young and old do not become orthostatic in the basal (prediuresis) state. The elderly, in contrast to the young, manifest a significant decline in systolic blood pressure when subjected to tilt in the volume depleted state (*, $p < .05$). This is related to the ability of the young to raise the heart rate when so stressed (†, $p < .05$), while the elderly cannot mount this tachycardia. (From Shannon et al. [28].).

Clinical Guidelines

Evaluation

Coronary Artery Disease and Left Ventricular Function

A landmark study, "Multifactorial Index of Cardiac Risk in Noncardiac Surgical Procedures" identified several clinical characteristics that were of prognostic importance for the risk of cardiovascular complications in noncardiac thoracic or abdominal surgery (Table 5-2) (29, 30). Other investigators have attempted to assess the perioperative cardiac risk of the elderly in particular (31). The findings of these important studies may be summarized as follows. Clinically evident left or right ventricular failure (as evidenced by an S_3 gallop or a jugular venous pressure greater than 9 cm water), hemodynamically significant

Table 5-2. Multivariate analysis: Preoperative factors related to the development of postoperative life-threatening or fatal cardiac complications

Factors (in order of decreasing significance)	Stepwise significance level when added to previous factors in column
1. S_3 gallop or jugular-vein distention on preoperative examination	$p<.001$
2. Myocardial infarction in preceding 6 months	$p<.001$
3. Rhythm other than sinus or premature atrial contractions	$p<.001$
4. >5 premature ventricular contractions/min documented at any time before operation	$p<.001$
5. Intraperitoneal, intrathoracic or aortic operation	$p<.001$
6. Age > 70 yr	$p=.001$
7. Important valvular aortic stenosis	$p=.007$
8. Emergency operation	$p=.007$
9. Poor general medical condition[a]	$p=.027$

[a]Partial pressure of oxygen <60 mm Hg, partial pressure of carbon dioxide >50 mm, potassium <3.0 or bicarbonate <20 mEq liter, blood urea nitrogen >50 or creatinine > 30 mg/dl, elevated transaminase, signs of chronic liver disease, or patient bedridden from noncardiac causes.

aortic stenosis, or a myocardial infarction within the preceeding 6 months were all associated with an increased risk of perioperative cardiac complications in middle-aged adults. These risk factors were less sensitive in the elderly. However, the inability to perform 2 minutes of supine bicycle exercise (a maximum work load of only 50 watts) or to obtain a maximal heart rate of greater than 99 beats per minute (levels achieved by all of 51 elderly individuals in the BLSA who were free of cardiovascular disease) was highly predictive (sensitivity of 85%, specificity of 64%) of an adverse clinical outcome in the elderly. Thus, it has been recommended that preoperative screening of elderly individuals begin with assessment of the aforementioned risk factors, followed by exercise stress testing of those who would otherwise be considered to be at low perioperative cardiac risk. Preliminary data indicate that this sequential technique has the potential to identify the vast majority of elderly individuals likely to experience a significant perioperative cardiac complication.

Valvular Heart Disease

Murmurs are common in the elderly, occurring in upwards of 50% of individuals. While the origin is usually "benign" and secondary to fibrous thickening and/or calcification of valve cusps or annular tissue, the differentiation of hemodynamically significant from insignificant murmurs may be clinically challenging. As in younger individuals, the diagnosis of aortic stenosis is supported by the absence of an aortic component to the second heart sound, the presence of cardiomegaly, and certain qualities of the murmur (harshness, late peaking) (32). Other clinical characteristics, such as the timing and amplitude of the carotid upstroke, an S_4 gallop, and the presence of left ventricular hypertrophy on a resting 12-lead electrocardiogram, are of diminished utility in the elderly. This is due to alterations in arterial pulse wave velocity and myocardial hypertrophy, which are known to occur with aging even in the absence of aortic valve disease (described above). Recent data suggest that the noninvasive evaluation of aortic stenosis with doppler echocardiography is as useful in the elderly as in younger individuals (33). The clinical presentation and evaluation of mitral valve disease in the elderly has been less extensively studied than that of the aortic valve. In the absence of more detailed information, it is probably prudent to evaluate the elderly individual with mitral valve disease in the same manner as the nonelderly.

Preoperative Recommendations

Therefore, presently the following approach is suggested for the preoperative cardiovascular evaluation of the elderly for noncardiac surgery. For essentially all surgical procedures, it would be prudent to perform a thorough history and physical examination to discern evidence suggestive of significant valvular, coronary artery, or myopathic disease. If the planned surgery is one that is generally considered to have low cardiac risk, such as transurethral prostatectomy or distal amputation, the history and physical examination is probably sufficient preoperative evaluation. For higher risk operations, such as thoracic or abdominal procedures, a more thorough preoperative evaluation may be required. In the elderly, the absence of positive findings in the history or physical examination is often insufficiently sensitive to exclude the possibility of a perioperative cardiac complication. Strong consideration should be given to exercise testing of those elderly individuals initially considered to be at low risk, to detect those who are truly high risk as determined by the inability to achieve a maximum work load greater than 50 watts (5 METS) or a maximum pulse rate greater than 99 per minute. In those elderly who are unable to exercise (either because of chronic debility or the acute illness necessitating surgery) noninvasive determination of potentially ischemic myocardium by techniques such as dipyridamole thallium scintigraphy may be employed. While the efficacy of such an approach has not been confirmed by additional studies, it appears a reasonable one. We would certainly recommend exercise testing of any elderly patient in whom there was a question as to the limitation of exercise ability because of coronary artery disease. The benefits of such testing would be manifest not only in terms of perioperative risk reduction but perhaps also in improvement in quality or quantity of life. It must be recalled that a large percentage of elderly individuals will indeed have a positive exercise test. The important point of the study described above, as well as literally dozens of related studies, is the occurrence of "positive" findings at a low work load. Furthermore, in those individuals in whom the need for noncardiac surgery arises within 6 months of a myocardial infarction, an exercise stress test is quite helpful in differentiating those with evidence of continued ischemia (and presumably at relatively high surgical risk) from those without (and presumably at low surgical risk).

Treatment Recommendations

The management of individuals who according to the above paradigm are considered at increased risk of cardiovascular complications requires clinical judgment; one must balance the risks associated with delaying or foregoing needed noncardiac surgery with the documented risks of subjecting such individuals to the stress of surgery. Therapy for those felt to be at high cardiac risk may include not only medical treatment or coronary artery bypass grafting (CABG), but percutaneous transluminal coronary angioplasty (PTCA) as well. PTCA has been shown to be both successful and relatively low risk in the elderly, and because the recuperation period is brief, may not significantly delay the desired noncardiac surgery. Data indicate that some high-risk individuals who undergo CABG may then undergo needed noncardiac surgery at significantly reduced risk (34–36). While it appears logical that effective preoperative therapy of high-risk individuals with drugs and/or PTCA would likewise result in risk reduction, there has not been any prospective clinical trial to confirm this hypothesis.

The risks of cardiac catheterization, coronary artery bypass surgery, and valve replacement, while higher in the elderly than in younger individuals, are sufficiently low that age itself should seldom be considered a contraindication to otherwise indicated invasive diagnostic or therapeutic maneuvers (37–41). The newly described technique of percutaneous balloon valvuloplasty holds much promise for the therapy of aortic and mitral stenosis in elderly individuals. The balloon dilation is performed under local anesthesia in a well-equipped cardiac catheterization laboratory. The entire procedure takes only a couple of hours, and recuperation requires only 1 or 2 days. Immediate and short-term results appear encouraging in appropriately selected patients, although the eventual role of this promising technology will require study over the next few years.

Perioperative invasive hemodynamic monitoring of high-risk patients undergoing major surgery is accepted clinical practice for adults in general, and presumably, would be of benefit to the elderly in particular. Prospective randomized data addressing this issue are unavailable, however. It would appear prudent to maintain an adequate left ventricular filling pressure (preload) as assessed by physical examination or invasive techniques if necessary, because of the greater dependence of cardiac output on preload in the elderly. Similarly, postoperative atrial fibrillation with the resultant loss of the atrial contribution to ventricular filling may be more deleterious in the elderly and should be treated aggressively.

There is a considerable body of data to suggest that the incidence of perioperative myocardial infarction is increased in the elderly, probably even in those considered at low risk according to the previously described paradigm. The time frame of this risk includes not only the operation itself, but the first 3 to 5 postoperative days (42). Therefore, we would recommend a preoperative electrocardiogram in all geriatric surgical patients, not only to serve as a screening test for cardiac disease, but also to serve as a baseline for the future. For patients whose surgical procedure and postoperative course have been uneventful, daily electrocardiograms for the first 3 postoperative days would appear to be prudent and have a favorable risk/benefit ratio. If significant perioperative hemodynamic instability occurs, then the measurement of serum "cardiac" enzymes (total creatinine phosphokinase and its MB fraction) is indicated. These recommendations are based in large measure on the knowledge that approximately one-third of postoperative myocardial infarctions are unassociated with anginal chest pain, and therefore laboratory diagnosis is crucial.

In general, a fairly aggressive approach to the preoperative evaluation and therapy of cardiac disease is recommended in the elderly. A thorough knowledge of normal cardiovascular physiology and its alteration with advancing age is necessary for interpreting the results of various diagnostic studies as well as for judging the patient's ability to adapt to the stress imposed by the contemplated surgery. The data presented above support the view that the elderly in general, and especially those with cardiovascular disease, may have a diminished ability to compensate for the stresses imposed by surgery and that both diagnostic testing (e.g., echocardiography, doppler echocardiography, cardiac catheterization, and exercise stress testing) and medical or surgical therapy (including percutaneous transluminal coronary angioplasty, coronary artery bypass grafting, and valve replacement) usually have favorable risk/benefit ratios in the elderly. Therefore, rigorous preoperative evaluation and therapy may allow the elderly to undergo needed surgery with minimal risk of perioperative morbidity and mortality, the goal of cardiologists and surgeons alike.

References

1. Tejada, C, et al. 1968. Distribution of coronary and aortic atherosclerosis by geographic location, race, and sex. *Lab Invest* 18:49–66.
2. Elveback, LR, Connolly, DC, and Melton, LJ, III. 1986. Coronary heart disease in residents of Rochester, Minnesota. VII. Incidence, 1950 through 1982. *Mayo Clin Proc* 61:896–900.
3. Gerstenblith, G, et al. 1980. Stress testing redefines the prevalence of coronary artery disease in epidemiologic studies. *Circulation* 62(Part III):111–308.
4. Dawber, TR. 1980. The Framingham Study: The epidemiology of atherosclerotic disease. Cambridge: Harvard University Press.
5. Abrams, WB, and Frohlich, ED. 1986. Arteriosclerotic heart disease in the elderly. *Geriat Cardiol* 4:253–283.
6. Schaible, TF, and Scheuer, J. 1985. Cardiac adaptations to chronic exercise. *Prog Cardiovasc Dis* 27:297–324.
7. Li, YX, et al. 1986. Age-related differences on cardiac muscle function in rats. *Am J Physiol* 251:(20)H12–H18.
8. Lakatta, EG, and Spurgeon, HA. 1987. Effect of exercise on cardiac muscle performance in aged rats. *Fed Proc* 46:1844–1849.
9. Avolio, AP, et al. 1985. Effects of aging on arterial distensibility in populations with high and low prevalence of hypertension: comparison between urban and rural communities in China. *Circulation* 71:202–210.
10. Fleg, JL, and Kennedy, HL. 1982. Cardiac arrhythmias in a healthy elderly population. Detection by 24-hour ambulatory electrocardiology. *Chest* 81:302–307.
11. Fleg, JL, Das, DN, and Lakatta, EG. 1983. Right bundle branch block: Long-term prognosis in apparently healthy men. *J Am Coll Cardiol* 1:887–892.
12. Tresch, DD, and Fleg, JL. 1986. Unexplained sinus bradycardia: Clinical significance and long-term prognosis in apparently healthy persons older than 40 years. *Am J Cardiol* 58:1009–1013.
13. Chadwick, RS, Goldstein, DS, and Keiser, HR. 1986. Pulse-wave model of brachial arterial pressure modulation in aging and hypertension. *Am J Physiol* 251:H1–H11.
14. Yin, FCP, et al. 1976. Age associated decrease in chronotropic response to isoproterenol. *Circulation* 54(40, Suppl2):II–167.
15. Murgo, JP, et al. 1980. Aortic input impedance in normal man: Relationship to pressure wave forms. *Circulation* 62:105–116.
16. Gerstenblith, G, et al. 1977. Echocardiographic assessment of a normal adult aging population. *Circulation* 56:273–278.
17. Arora, RR, et al. 1987. Atrial kinetics and left ventricular diastolic filling in the healthy elderly. *J Am Coll Cardiol* 9:1255–1260.
18. Bruce, RA. 1985. Functional aerobic capacity, exercise, and aging. In *Principles of Geriatric Medicine*. Ed., R Andres, EL Bierman, and WR Hazzard, pp. 87–103. New York: McGraw-Hill.
19. Fleg, JL, and Lakatta, EG. 1987. Role of muscle loss in the age-related reduction in maximal oxygen consumption. *Fed Proc* 46:319.
20. Port, S, et al. 1980. Effect of age on the response of the left ventricular ejection fraction to exercise. *N Engl J Med* 303:1133–1137.
21. Rodeheffer, RJ, Gerstenblith, G, and Becker, LC. 1984. Exercise cardiac output is maintained with advancing age in healthy human subjects: Cardiac dilation in increased stroke volume compensates for a diminished heart rate. *Circulation* 69:203–213.
22. Fleg, JL, Tzankoff, SP, and Lakatta, EG. 1985. Age-related augmentation of plasma catecholamines during dynamic exercise in healthy males. *J Appl Physiol* 59: 1033–1039.
23. Lehman, M, and Keul, J. 1986. Age-associated changes of exercise-induced plasma catecholamine responses. *Eur J Appl Physiol* 55:302–306.
24. Guarnieri, T, et al. 1980. Contractile and biochemical correlates of β-adrenergic stimulation of the aged heart. *Am J Physiol* 239:H501–H508.
25. Kyriakides, ZS, et al. 1986. Systolic functional response of normal older and younger adult left ventricles to dobutamine. *Am J Cardiol* 587:816–819.
26. Van Brummelen, P, et al. 1981. Age-related decrease in cardiac and peripheral vascular responsiveness to isoprenaline. Studies in normal subjects. *Clin Sci* 60: 571–577.
27. Pan, HY-M, et al. 1986. Decline in beta adrenergic receptor-mediated vascular relaxation with aging in man. *J Pharmacol Exp Ther* 228:802–807.
28. Shannon, RP, Wei, JY, and Rosa, RM. 1986. The effect of age and sodium depletion on cardiovascular response to orthostasis. *Hypertension* 8:438–443.
29. Goldman, L, et al. 1977. Multifactorial index of cardiac risk in noncardiac surgical procedures. *N Engl J Med* 297:845–850.
30. Goldman, L, et al. 1978. Cardiac risk factors and complication in non-cardiac surgery. *Medicine* 57:357–370.
31. Gerson, MC, et al. 1985. Cardiac prognosis in noncardiac geriatric surgery. *Ann Intern Med* 103:832–837.
32. Aronow, WS, Schwartz, KS, and Koengsberg, M. 1986. Correlation of aortic cuspal and aortic root disease with aortic systolic ejection murmurs and with mitral anular calcium in persons older than 62 years in a long-term health care facility. *Am J Cardiol* 58:651–652.
33. Hatle, L. 1981. Noninvasive assessment and differentiation of left ventricular outflow obstruction and Doppler ultrasound. *Circulation* 64:381–387.
34. Scher, KS, and Tice, DA. 1976. Operative risk in patients with previous coronary bypass. *Arch Surg* 111:807–809.
35. Crawford, ES, et al. 1978. Operative risk in patients with previous coronary artery bypass. *Ann Thorac Surg* 26:215–221.
36. McCollum, CH, Garcia-Rinaldi, R, and Graham, JM. 1977. Myocardial revascularization prior to subsequent major surgery in patients with coronary artery disease. Surgery 81:302–304.
37. Copeland, JG, et al. 1978. Isolated aortic valve replace-

ment in patients older than 65 years. *JAMA* 237: 1578–1582.

38. Dorros, G, et al. 1987. Coronary artery bypass surgery in patients over age 70 years: Report from the Milwaukee Cardiovascular Data Registry. *Clin Cardiol* 10:377–382.
39. Naunheim, KS, et al. 1987. Coronary artery bypass surgery in patients aged 80 years or older. *Am J Cardiol* 59:804–807.
40. Rahimtoola, SH, Grunkemeier, GL, and Starr, A. 1986. Ten-year survival after coronary artery bypass surgery for angina in patients aged 65 years and older. *Circulation* 74:509–517.
41. Stephenson, LW, MacVaugh, H III, and Edmunds, LH Jr. 1978. Surgery using cardiopulmonary bypass in the elderly. *Circulation* 58:250–254.
42. von Knorring, J. 1981. Postoperative myocardial infarction: A prospective study in a risk group of surgical patients. *Surgery* 90:55–60.

6

Aging of the Respiratory System

Melvyn S. Tockman

Pathophysiology of Aging Lung

Common pulmonary problems are found with increased frequency in the elderly. The altered pulmonary physiology associated with aging impairs the ability of the lung to clear infectious and environmental insults once handled easily by the more youthful lung. In addition to diminished lung function, the geriatric patient loses important nonpulmonary defense mechanisms. Neurological disorders and sedation lead to an increased tendency for aspiration through altered swallowing and impaired cough. Diminished activity of effector T cells, perhaps due to enhancement of suppressor cells or reduced capacity for functional differentiation, reduces the likelihood of containing a pulmonary insult.

The changes in pulmonary function with age are of fundamental importance, since impaired function (airways obstruction) is associated with increased rates of death from all causes (primarily cardiovascular disease and chronic obstructive pulmonary disease, COPD) (1, 2). Further, ventilatory obstruction is associated with risk of subsequent lung cancer mortality (3). *Thus, impaired pulmonary function on spirometric testing can identify increased risk for three of the five leading causes of death in men and for three of the seven leading causes of death in women* (4). These observations, made after adjustment for other risk factors including cigarette smoking, provide compelling reasons to assess pulmonary function even in "normal" elderly individuals.

Following the end of adolescent growth and development, the age-related increase in lung volumes slows (after age 17 in females, after age 19 in males); forced expiratory airflows reach a maximum between 20 and 24 years of age in both sexes (5). Further aging leads to a progressive decline in lung function, although until 40 years of age, the age-related decrease in forced vital capacity (FVC) and maximal expiratory flow rate are thought to be due to changes in body weight and strength rather than to attrition of tissues (6).

This subsequent loss of lung function accelerates slightly as age increases (7) but is remarkably consistent across populations (8), averaging for nonsmoking males 14 to 30 cc/year of FVC and 23 to 32 cc/year of 1-second forced expiratory volume (FEV_1). Nonsmoking females show slightly lesser rates of decline (FVC, 15 to 24 cc/year; FEV_1, 19 to 26 cc/year) (see Tables 6-1 and 6-2). The relatively constant rate of decline of lung function associated with aging suggests that (in the absence of additional respiratory insult) the most important factor determining whether individuals fall below the threshold of pulmonary impairment with advancing age is the level of forced expiration they reach at the completion of their growth (9).

Effect of Aging on Interaction Between Lung and Chest Wall

The volume of the resting lung (functional residual capacity, FRC) is determined by the equilibrium between the inward elastic tissue forces of the lung and the outward forces of the ribs and muscles of respiration. The loss of inward elastic recoil seen with increased age (especially

Reprinted with permission from *Principles of Geriatric Medicine and Gerontology,* ed 2. Ed., Hazzard et al. © 1990. New York: McGraw-Hill.

Table 6-1. Predicted changes in normal pulmonary function for males (as determined by the age coefficient term from male reference value prediction equations)

Pulmonary function	Equation	95% Confidence interval	Loss of function per year of age	Reference
TLC	0.0795*H + 0.0032*Age − 7.333	1.61	(increase) 3 ml	Morris et al. (26)
FRC	0.0472*H + 0.0090*Age − 5.290	1.46	(increase) 9 ml	Morris et al. (26)
RV	0.0216*H + 0.0207*Age − 2.840	0.76	(increase) 20 ml	Morris et al. (26)
FVC	0.0600*H − 0.0214*Age − 4.650	1.115	21 ml	Crapo et al. (8)
FEV_1	0.0414*H − 0.0244*Age − 2.190	0.842	24 ml	Crapo et al. (8)
FEV_1/FVC	−0.1300*H − 0.152*Age + 110.49	8.28	0.15%	Crapo et al. (8)
Pa_{O_2}	− 0.323*Age − 100.10		0.32 torr	Sorbini et al. (18)
N_2P_{111}	+ 0.010*Age + 0.710	0.84	(increase) 0.01% N_2/liter	Buist and Ross (15)
DLco − SB	0.4160*H − 0.219*Age − 26.34	8.20	0.2 ml CO/min/mmHg	Crapo and Morris (16)
Hgb corr. (Cotes)	0.4100*H − 0.210*Age − 26.31	8.20	0.2 ml CO/min/mmHg	Crapo and Morris (16)
$Vo_{2\ max}$	− 0.032*Age + 4.2 (SD ± 0.4)		32 ml O_2/min	Jones et al. (23)
Expressed per kg	− 0.550*Age − 60 (SD ± 7.5)		0.55 ml/kg/min	Jones et al. (23)

*Note lower boundary of normal determined by calculating predicted value from equation, then subtracting the 95% confidence interval.

after age 55) is usually evenly matched by a reduction of respiratory muscle strength and increased rib stiffness (6, 10). This balance is shown by the lack of change in total lung capacity (TLC) and the minimal increase of the FRC with increasing age (see Table 6-1 and Fig. 6-1).

During forced expiration, increasing contraction of chest wall voluntary muscles increases intrathoracic pressure and expiratory airflow until dynamic compression of the airways limits further expiratory flow (after approximately 25% of the vital capacity has been exhaled). Collapse of the airways (at the equal pressure point) is prevented only by intraalveolar (upstream) pressure, generated by elastic recoil within the lung (11). The inward elastic recoil of the lung results from the combina-

Table 6-2. Predicted changes in normal pulmonary function for females (as determined by the age coefficient term from female reference value prediction equations)

Pulmonary function	Equation	95% Confidence interval	Loss of function per year of age	Reference
TLC	0.0590*H + 0.0000*Age − 4.537	1.08	(increase) 00 ml	Morris et al. (26)
FRC	0.0360*H + 0.0031*Age − 3.182	1.06	(increase) 3 ml	Morris et al. (26)
RV	0.0197*H + 0.0201*Age − 2.421	0.78	(increase) 3 ml	Morris et al. (26)
FVC	0.0491*H − 0.0216*Age − 3.590	0.676	22 ml	Crapo et al. (8)
FEV_1	0.0342*H − 0.0255*Age − 1.578	0.561	26 ml	Crapo et al. (8)
FEV_1/FVC.	−0.2020*H − 0.252*Age + 126.58	9.06	0.25%	Crapo et al. (8)
Pa_{O_2}	− 0.323*Age − 100.10		0.32 torr	Sorbini et al. (18)
N_2P_{111} (<60 yr old)	+ 0.009*Age + 1.036	1.12	(increase) 0.01% N_2/liter	Buist and Ross (15)
N_2P_{111} (≥60 yr old)	+ 0.058*Age + 1.777	2.55	(increase) 0.06% N_2/liter	Buist and Ross (15)
DLco − SB	0.256*H − 0.144*Age − 8.36	6.0	0.1 ml CO/min/mmHg	Crapo and Morris (16)
Hgb corr. (Cotes)	0.282*H − 0.157*Age − 10.89	6.1	0.1 ml CO/min/mmHg	Crapo and Morris (16)
$Vo_{2\ max}$	− 0.014*Age + 2.6 (SD ± 0.4)		14 ml O_2/min	Jones et al. (23)
Expressed per kg	− 0.370*Age − 48 (SD ± 7.0)		0.37 ml/kg/min	Jones et al. (23)

*Note lower boundary of normal determined by calculating predicted value from equation, then subtracting the 95% confidence interval.

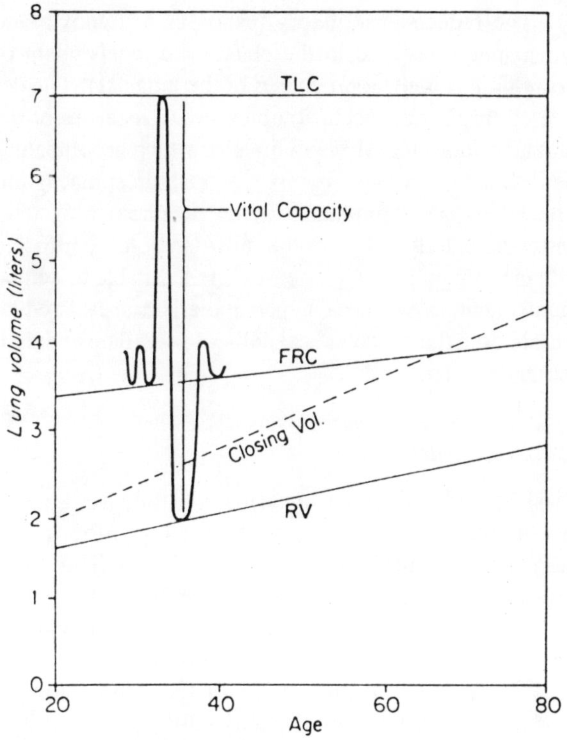

Figure 6-1. The effect of age on subdivisions of lung volume: TLC, total lung capacity; FRC, functional residual capacity; RV, residual volume. Values shown are for men of average height; the changes with age are similar for women.

tion of parenchymal elastic fibers and the surface forces generated at the air–fluid interface of the terminal respiratory units. The elastic fibers within alveolar walls are tethered to the respiratory and terminal bronchioles, helping to maintain the patency of these small conducting airways at low lung volumes. There is no evidence for an aging change in the length or diameter of these fibers (12), but rather for an age-associated disruption of elastic fiber attachments (13). The loss of these elastic attachments leads to increased compliance of affected alveoli, collapse of the small conducting airways, nonuniformity of alveolar ventilation, and air trapping. There is no evidence for an aging effect on either the inward directed air–fluid surface forces or on the effectiveness of surfactant which mitigates these forces (14).

The residual volume (RV) is the amount of air that remains in the lungs after a maximal exhalation. During younger years while peripheral airways are patent, the RV is determined by the minimum size reached by the bony thorax and the maximum ascent of the diaphragm. External compression of the young chest can, in fact, expel additional air from the lungs. The RV increases with age (Fig. 6-1), reflecting air trapped in peripheral airways following loss of the elastic fiber attachments described above. As the TLC remains constant with increasing age, the increase in RV comes at the expense of the vital capacity (VC), reducing the amount of air that can be blown from the lungs after a maximal inhalation (Fig. 6-1).

Distribution of Ventilation

The distending force of the thoracic wall is modified by gravity. The erect individual has a declining gradient of distending (pleural) pressure from the apex to the base of the lung. As a result of this distending pressure gradient, airways at the apex of the lung are more widely patent than those at the base. As the lung empties from maximum to minimum distension during a normal expiration, the narrower airways at the base of the lung close first, and closure progresses from base to apex. The single-breath nitrogen (SBN_2) washout technique has been used to determine the uniformity of alveolar ventilation and the lung volume at which small conducting airways collapse (the closing volume, CV; see Fig. 6-1) (15). Non-uniformity of ventilation is shown by an increased slope of the SBN_2 phase III (alveolar plateau), while the volume at which the terminal respiratory units begin to close is demonstrated by elevations of the SBN_2 phase IV (closing volume). With advancing age, the slope of the N_2P_{III} increases (see Tables 6-1 and 6-2) and the closing capacity (closing volume plus residual volume) may exceed the FRC, indicating that closure of terminal respiratory units occurs before the end of a normal tidal breath. Closing capacity begins to exceed the supine FRC at about 44 years of age and the sitting FRC at approximately 65 years of age.

Diffusing Capacity

Diffusion of gas from the alveoli into the blood depends upon two factors: the total area and thickness of the alveolar-capillary membrane, and the ability of the blood elements to absorb the gas. Progressive age-related decreases in total pulmonary diffusing capacity are usually due to both morphologic changes (loss of surface area of the alveolar-capillary membrane) and increasing inhomogeneities in ventilation and/or blood flow (6).

The single-breath carbon monoxide diffusing capacity (DLco) increases to a maximum in the early twenties and thereafter undergoes a gradual decline with age. This reduction has been estimated to be approximately 0.5% (0.2 ml CO/min/mmHg)/year (see Tables 6-1 and 6-2). The age-related decline in DLco is not linear, although linear prediction regressions are used (16). Women are found to have 10% lower diffusion capacity values than men for the same age and height (17).

Arterial O_2 Tension

Although at rest airways and alveoli at the base are more nearly closed than are apical structures, at maximum inspiration all alveolar units distend to approximately equal size. Thus, a greater proportion of the inhaled breath must go to the basal airways. In a fortunate arrangement, the greater proportion of blood circulates also to the bases of the lung providing, in the normal individual, a ventilation–perfusion ratio of near unity. This matching of ventilation and perfusion leads to optimal gas exchange.

Inflammatory destruction or aging of alveolar structures leads to deterioration of the match of ventilation with perfusion. While collapse of peripheral airways decreases ventilation to alveoli, perfusion remains unaffected. These changes are accentuated by factors that reduce the FRC (e.g., the supine posture, obesity, small airway closure from inflammation/edema). A ventilation–perfusion imbalance results in regional shunting of blood, impaired oxygen uptake, and arterial oxygen desaturation. Arterial O_2 tension follows a linear deterioration with age of approximately 0.3% Pa_{O_2} per year (see Tables 6-1 and 6-2) (18). Transfer of the more rapidly diffusable carbon dioxide is limited only by the rate of alveolar ventilation.

For the elderly individual, the consequences of a ventilation–perfusion mismatch are particularly harsh. The Pa_{O_2} (and thus O_2 delivery) may be further compromised by age-associated reductions in cardiac output (19). When ventilation and perfusion are evenly matched, changing cardiac output has no effect on Pa_{O_2}. However, as ventilation–perfusion inequalities worsen, the Pa_{O_2} at any given cardiac output decreases; the further loss of cardiac output magnifies the reduction of O_2 delivery. It is possible, therefore, that the association (described above) between airways obstruction and mortality may be mediated partly by mechanical limitations of ventilation and a lowered arterial O_2 tension.

Control of Breathing

Otherwise healthy older persons may be more vulnerable to transient reductions in levels of arterial oxygen tension (e.g., during pneumonia, exacerbation of COPD) due to age-related diminished responsiveness to hypoxia and hypercapnia (20). The ventilatory response to hypoxia is reduced by half in healthy older men (64 to 73 years of age) compared with young healthy men (22 to 30 years of age), while the ventilatory response to CO_2 is reduced by approximately 40%. Although the reasons for this suppression of breathing are still under study, it appears that age attenuates chemoreceptor function, either at peripheral chemoreceptors or in the integrating central nervous system pathway.

The reduced ventilatory responses to hypoxia and hypercapnia observed in the elderly are independent of the aging mechanical properties of the lung (21). The decreased inspiratory occlusion pressure (a measure of the total neuromuscular drive to breath), which accompanies the decreased drives of hypoxia and hypercapnia, is unaffected by the compliance of the respiratory system. Thus, the elderly, who are the most likely to be afflicted with chronic pulmonary diseases, are least able to defend against acute hypoxia or hypercapnia because of reductions in both their mechanical ability to ventilate and their neural drive to breathe.

Exercise Capacity

Physical work capacity (fitness) is generally assessed by measurement of the ability to deliver O_2 to the tissues (maximal O_2 consumption, or $Vo_{2\ max}$) (22). Three systems must interact to transport O_2 from the outside air to the working muscles: pulmonary ventilation, blood circulation, and muscle tissue. At any age the $Vo_{2\ max}$ is related to the physical dimensions of these three components: pulmonary (vital capacity, diffusing capacity), cardiovascular (heart volume, blood volume, red blood cell mass), and skeletal muscle mass. The importance of body size to the measurement of $Vo_{2\ max}$ is reflected by the inclusion of weight in the measurement (expressed as maximal O_2 uptake per kilogram of body weight, or $Vo_{2\ max}$/kg). Cardiorespiratory performance is even more closely related to lean body mass than to weight (especially in obese subjects). Lean body mass may be obtained from body weight by correcting for body fat, as estimated from skinfold measurements or underwater weighing.

The increase in work capacity ($Vo_{2\ max}$) observed during childhood and adolescence is due to the growth of lungs, heart, and muscle. Following a plateau in the mid-twenties, the $Vo_{2\ max}$ gradually declines due to reductions in two of these three components (cardiac output and muscle mass) seen with advancing years (23). The gradual linear decline of O_2 delivery (32 ml/min/year in men and 14 ml/min/year in women) can be described by a prediction equation (see Tables 6-1 and 6-2) dependent only upon body size and age (which correlates with cardiac output and muscle mass).

Although ventilatory function also declines with age, reduced ventilation seldom limits exercise in healthy subjects. However, in patients with a ventilatory capacity reduced sufficiently to limit exercise performance, the FEV_1 is a reasonably accurate indicator of maximal ventilation in exercise. More typically, the reduced $Vo_{2\ max}$ seen in elderly individuals with mild to moderate airways obstruction is due to cardiovascular deconditioning associated with lowered levels of habitual physical activity.

The differences in exercise performance between similarly aged men and women largely disappear when factors such as size (lean body mass), hemoglobin level, and levels of training are taken into account. Regular training can substantially slow the decline in maximal oxygen delivery due to age-related cardiovascular deconditioning (6). Commenting on the results of a period of exercise training of sedentary subjects, a recent study concluded "the increase in V_E/V_{O_2} (ventilatory response for a given oxygen uptake) during submaximal exercise observed with aging can be reversed by endurance training, and that after training, previously sedentary older individuals breathe at the same percentage of MVV during maximal exercise as highly trained (master) athletes of similar age" (24).

Defense Mechanisms

Clearance

An intact cough reflex is a necessary defense under conditions of dysphagia and impaired esophageal motility, which are more frequently encountered in old age. While cough is not essential for normal clearance of the respiratory tract, it is a powerful adjunct when normal mucociliary clearance is overloaded by foreign materials or secretions. Loss of an effective cough reflex (and subsequent aspiration) also contributes to an increased susceptibility to pneumonia in the elderly. While there seems to be an inverse relationship between age and the rate of mucociliary transport, the importance of mucous transport as a pulmonary defense mechanism has not yet been demonstrated experimentally (25). Nevertheless, clinical observations of patients with primary ciliary immotility of Kartagener's syndrome (situs inversus, chronic sinusitis, and bronchiectasis) demonstrate recurrent respiratory tract infections, chronic bronchitis, and bronchiectasis (25).

Humoral Immunity

Humoral immune competence is only roughly predicted by immunoglobulin levels in the bloodstream. Despite the lack of age-related change in IgA and IgG concentrations, the antibody response to extrinsic antigens, such as pneumococcal and influenza vaccines, is reduced considerably in old age. It is possible that this diminished antibody response reflects age-related reductions in T-cell helper activity, increases in T-cell supressor activity, or the reduced ability of B cells to produce normal high-affinity antibodies in response to antigen (all of which have been observed). The increased circulating immunoglobulin seen in older individuals may reflect increased production of antibody to various intrinsic antigens (i.e., autoantibodies), which replaces production of specific antibodies (6).

Cellular Immunity

An age-related decline in functional ability has most clearly been seen in cell-mediated immunity. There is a reduced blastogenic response (to plant mitogens phytohemagglutinin and pokeweed mitogen) of lymphocytes from elderly adults (75 to 90 years old) compared with younger adults (25 to 50 years old). As measured by delayed hypersensitivity (the number of positive skin test reactions to five common antigens), reduced cellular immunity among individuals over 60 years of age has been correlated with increased mortality over the subsequent 2 years. Finally, the decline of cell-mediated immunity with increasing age correlates with an increasing frequency of reactivation tuberculosis.

Use of Tests of Pulmonary Function

Initial Assessment of Normality

A test such as spirometry should be obtained at baseline for every patient and at 5-year intervals thereafter (in the absence of occupational or environmental exposure) or more frequently if the patient is potentially exposed to inhaled toxins. A young normal lung should be able to expel 80% of its vital capacity in the first second (a FEV_1/FVC ratio of 80%). Normalizing to the VC is an excellent way to standardize ventilatory function in healthy individuals. However, with the onset of pulmonary impairment, not only the 1-second forced expiratory volume, but also the forced vital capacity, are both likely to deteriorate. In the absence of a constant VC, investigators have standardized their patients' results to spirometry from cross-sectional surveys of "normal" ("healthy," nonsmoking) individuals. These "normal" results are expressed as linear regression functions of age and height, separately for males and for females (see Tables 6-1 and 6-2).

There are a variety of prediction equations in the literature, and, until recently, their selection has been somewhat arbitrary. The research populations studied to develop these prediction equations are often quite different from the populations encountered in a chest clinic. The 1988 Snowbird conference now recommends that directors of pulmonary function laboratories select the equation that best predicts as normal a sample of the clinically normal individuals tested in their laboratories. Since few of these prediction equations have included sufficient numbers of normal elderly individuals, it is advisable to inquire regarding the origin of the prediction equation used by the lab.

The prediction equation estimates the average function for individuals of similar sex, age, height, and race.

The variation in normal pulmonary function is relatively constant across the range of adult ages and heights so that the normal 95% of the population will fall within a fixed interval of the predicted range. The lower limit of normal can be calculated by subtracting a constant quantity from the predicted value for each test. Prediction equations and the appropriate subtraction constants for white males and females are given in Tables 6-1 and 6-2.

This method for determining the lower limit of normal replaces the commonly used 80% of predicted. If 80% of predicted were taken as the lower limit of normal, then as the predicted value got smaller with increasing age, the range of normal would become spuriously narrower. Several examples should clarify the point. From the FEV_1 prediction equation (Table 6-1), a 25-year-old man of 170 cm would be expected to have an FEV_1 of 4.2 liters. A male of similar age and height would still be considered to have a normal FEV_1 if he exhaled 4.2 − 0.842 liters (95% confidence interval constant determined from table) or 3.4 liters. For a young man, this lower limit is 80% of the predicted value. Similarly, a 60-year-old man of 165 cm would be expected to have an FEV_1 of 3.2 liters. The lower limit of normal for this predicted value is 2.3 liters (3.2 − 0.842 liters) or 74% of predicted value. These considerations are particularly important for the elderly, where progressively smaller normal values would increase the likelihood of misclassification.

Blacks have a similar pulmonary geometry to whites, and their lungs have similar mechanical emptying characteristics. For any given standing height, however, blacks have a smaller trunk (smaller trunk/height ratio). A reduction of 12% from the white predicted value accommodates the racial difference in pulmonary function somewhat better than a regression based upon "sitting height."

Assessment of Risk for Morbidity and Mortality

The risks for heart disease, chronic obstructive lung disease, and lung cancer are not limited to the small proportion of the population with "abnormal" pulmonary function. Rather, there is a continuous increase in risk associated with progressively lower (although still normal) levels of ventilatory function. It is therefore of great importance to assess not only the initial pulmonary function, but the trend of pulmonary function with advancing age. Considerable pulmonary function may be lost before an individual crosses into the clinically abnormal range.

At the end of pulmonary growth and development the ranking (percentile) of an individual's pulmonary function within the population might be ascertained in the same way that pediatric growth curves plot the percentile of height and weight for age (27). Thereafter, at subsequent evaluations, it can be determined whether an individual's lung function is maintaining its expected ("normal") rate of decline or describes a more rapid rate of decline by crossing percentiles. Examples of these pulmonary function percentile curves (for FEV_1 and FVC for males and females) are provided in Figures 6-2 and 6-3. Elderly individuals with a more rapid rate of decline in pulmonary function may be correctly perceived to be at risk for mortality from several causes well in advance of developing "abnormal" pulmonary function.

Assessment of Type and Extent of Pulmonary Disorder

Finally, the common respiratory diseases—restrictive pattern, asthma, chronic bronchitis, and emphysema—can be distinguished by simple pulmonary function tests. Once a pulmonary function is recognized as abnormal (Tables 6-1 and 6-2), the abnormality may be quantified by the guidelines in Table 6-3.

The inability to inhale a normal volume of air is recognized as a "restrictive pattern" on the spirogram by the presence of a normal FEV_1/FVC and a reduced FVC. Restriction may be due to a scarring of the lung, to weakness or loss of neural stimuli to chest wall muscles, or to changes in the shape of the bony thorax. Substantial obstruction with air trapping may produce a "mixed" pattern, but the underlying obstruction is often obvious if the forced expiration is carried out for at least 10 seconds. If the appearance of restriction persists, lung volume measurement is appropriate.

The obstructive diseases—asthma, chronic bronchitis, and emphysema—all demonstrate a reduction of the FEV_1/FVC on spirometry. Reversible obstruction is the hallmark of asthma (conventionally defined as an increase in FEV_1 equal to or greater than 15% of baseline). Bronchodilator reversibility may be absent when the pulmonary function is normal or severely abnormal. Incomplete reversibility suggests a component of "asthmatic bronchitis." The chronic (nonreversible) obstructive pulmonary diseases (chronic bronchitis and emphysema) both manifest a low FEV_1, but the destruction of the alveolar-capillary membrane associated with emphysema produces a lowered D_{LCO} in that condition.

Approach to Geriatric Patient with Disorders of Respiratory System

Lung disease in the elderly has certain unique features. First, some importance must be attached to the setting in which the elderly patient is seen. Pneumonia is 50 times more frequent among residents of chronic care facilities than expected in the population at large. In contrast, el-

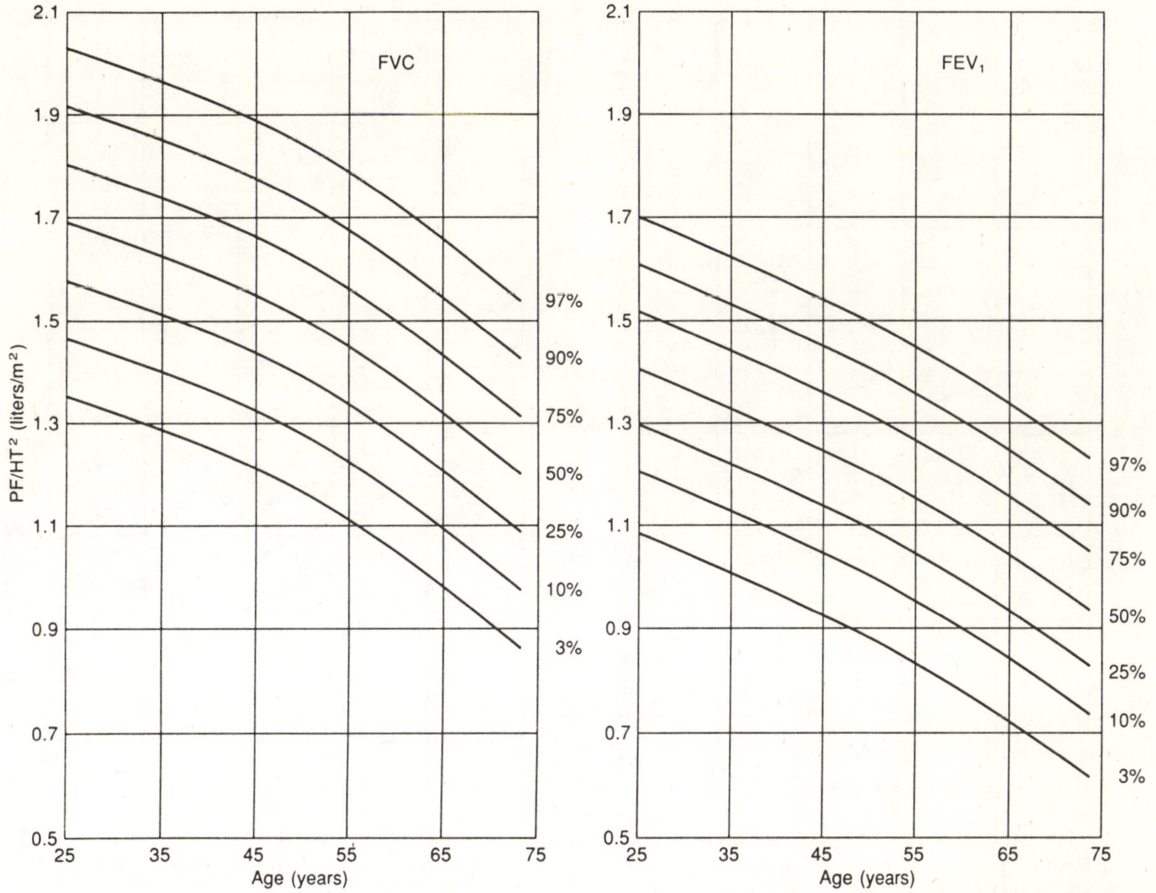

Figure 6-2. Percentile charts for height standardized pulmonary function of men. The "percentiles" of pulmonary function (liters) divided by height (meters) squared (PF/HT^2) presented here and in Figure 6-3 are based upon measurements of white nonsmokers who reported no respiratory symptoms, and who were drawn from a random sample of adults in six U.S. cities. (Redrawn from Dockery DW et al. 1985. Distribution of forced expiratory volume in one second and forced vital capacity in healthy, white, adult never-smokers in six U.S. cities. *Am Rev Respir Dis* 131:511.)

derly individuals residing in the community seem not to have an increased prevalence of pneumonia but do more poorly than younger individuals when pulmonary infections develop. Even with appropriate antibiotic therapy, elderly patients with pneumonia sustain a 15% to 20% mortality. Advanced age also modifies the organisms likely to be responsible for a pneumonic infiltrate.

Obviously, such factors as depressed level of consciousness and reduced level of self-care, which have been shown to contribute to the risk of pneumonia, also enhance the likelihood that such individuals will be institutionalized. Thus, the increased risk of pneumonia observed in institutionalized patients is certainly due in some part to the underlying reasons for which the individual remains in the institution. Yet, the institutional setting itself adds to the risk of pulmonary infection in the elderly patient. In the closed populations of chronic care facilities, the attack rates among nonvaccinated or immune-depressed elderly for both influenza and tuberculosis are striking.

It must be appreciated that the clinical presentation of elderly individuals may be different from that of younger adults. The blunted inflammatory response in the presence of infection is often a source of missed diagnoses in the aged patient. The presentations of pneumococcal pneumonia as a bronchopneumonia (instead of lobar consolidation) or tuberculosis as a miliary disease (instead of an apical infiltrate) are both more common in the elderly patient.

In contrast, the obstructive airways diseases have been so closely associated with advanced age that their presence often evokes little interest in the physician. Nevertheless, since 1968 there has been a progressive increase in the age-adjusted death rate for chronic obstructive pulmonary disease (COPD). In the United States, more than 4 million persons are estimated to have COPD,

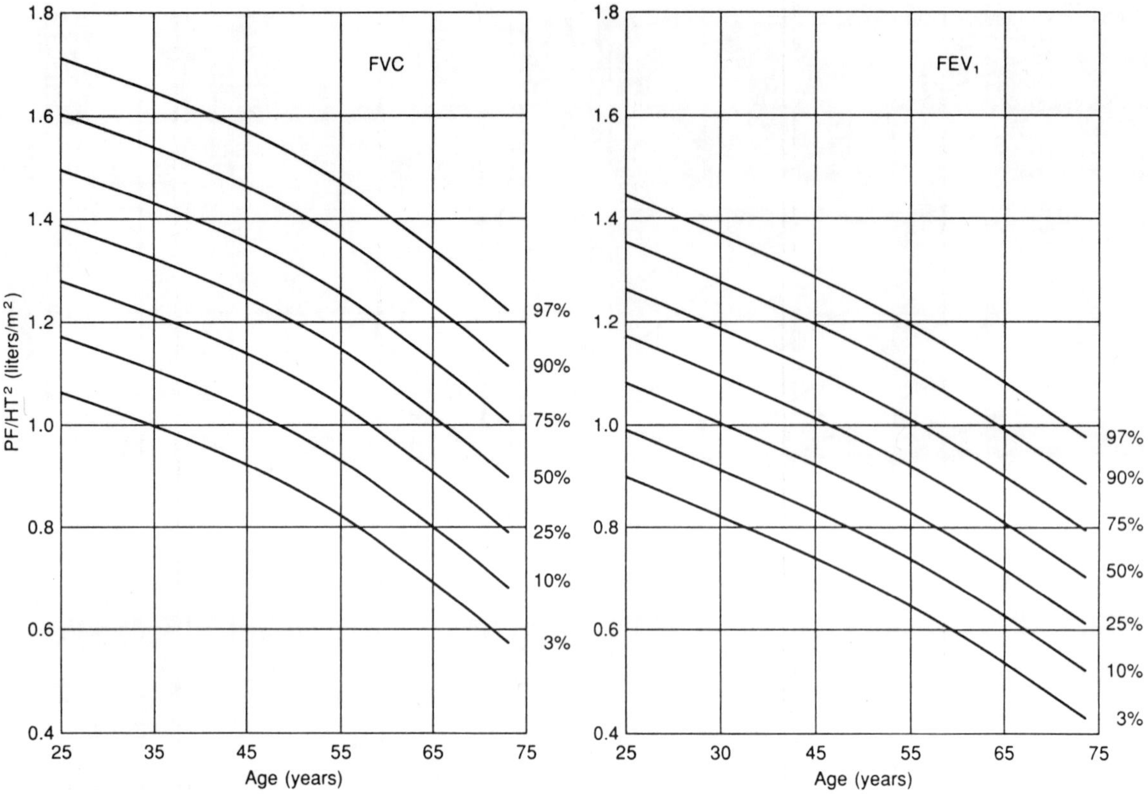

Figure 6-3. Percentile charts for height standardized pulmonary function of women. (Redrawn from Dockery DW et al. 1985. Distribution of forced expiratory volume in one second and forced vital capacity in healthy, white, adult never-smokers in six U.S. cities. *Am Rev Respir Dis* 131:511.)

and in 1979 $5 billion was spent for direct and indirect costs arising from COPD. The ease with which this condition can be detected by spirometry and the observation of slowing of ventilatory deterioration following smoking cessation strongly support the clinical recommendation that older smokers be routinely evaluated with this test.

Other conditions that might be responsible for dyspnea in the elderly patient, such as congestive heart failure, interstitial lung disease, or pulmonary emboli, should be routinely included in the differential diagnosis. However, diminished reserve in the elderly patient limits the vigor with which diagnosis and therapy can be pursued. The use of exercise to evaluate dyspnea must be limited to those elderly in otherwise good clinical condition. Agents affecting both the sympathetic and parasympathetic nervous systems used in the diagnosis and treatment of lung disorders may affect the aging heart. Antibiotics required for pulmonary infection may lead to further compromise through nephrotoxicity of elderly kidneys with diminished reserve. Steroid and anticoagulation therapy may lead to a myriad of complications. Perhaps more than at any other time of adulthood, the geriatric pulmonary patient must be evaluated and treated in the context of *primum non nocere*.

One of the great challenges facing the physician responsible for the care of the elderly is ensuring that com-

Table 6-3. Quantitation of impaired pulmonary function

	FVC	FEV_1/FVC	TLC or RV	DLco
Normal	Within 1 CI	Within 1 CI	Within 1 CI	Within 1 CI
Slight (minimal)	1–1.75	1–2	±1–1.5	1–1.75
Moderate	>1.75–2.5	2–4	±>1.5–2.0	>1.75–2.5
Severe	>2.5	>4	±>2.0	>2.5

Expressed as numbers of confidence intervals (CI) to be subtracted from predicted value.

Source: Miller (28).

Table 6-4. Services needed for comprehensive respiratory outpatient care

1. Comprehensive evaluation
   a. Complete medical evaluation
   b. Evaluation of patient and family financial and emotional support
2. Interval medical attention
3. Pulmonary function studies
4. Chest radiography
5. General laboratory services
   a. Bacteriology
   b. Hematology
   c. Chemistry
   d. Cytology
6. Electrocardiography
7. Immunization services
8. Drugs, medical supplies, and equipment
9. Routine transportation and communication
10. Emergency services (mobile unit with expertise) to bring patient from remote area to intensive care facility
11. Bronchial hygiene
12. Breathing instruction
13. Physical conditioning
14. Nutrition
    a. Counseling
    b. Provision of adequate nourishment
15. Homemaker and housekeeping services
16. Personal hygiene services (bathing, shampooing, etc.)
17. Psychosocial counseling
18. Financial support and planning
19. Vocational counseling
    a. For patient, family, or both
    b. Job training and placement
20. Environmental control
    a. Occupational exposures
    b. Household exposures
21. Education
    a. Patient
    b. Family
    c. Professional
22. Patient interaction groups

prehensive medical care does not begin and end at the hospital door. This is especially true for chronic respiratory disease. The fluctuating respiratory impairment associated with seasonal change, episodic upper respiratory tract infections, and other intercurrent illness will require a variety of medical and nonmedical responses to maintain the health of the elderly respiratory patient. The physican must both recognize the need for respiratory outpatient support services and appreciate that other professionals, including a respiratory nurse, a respiratory therapist, and a social worker, will often be required to provide them. There should be someone in the physician's office whom the patient can call regarding access to support services. A list of outpatient services, which have been required by outpatients with chronic obstructive lung diseases, is shown in Table 6-4. It is important that the physician's representative not only be knowledgeable about obtaining such services, but also be able to recognize when such services are needed and make recommendations to both physician and patient. Unfortunately, delivery of adequate outpatient care to the aged respiratory patient has not kept pace with the improvements in diagnosis and therapy. The recognition of geriatric pulmonary disease and its appropriate treatment in the context of the diminished physiological, emotional, and social reserves of the elderly make the practice of geriatric pulmonary medicine particularly challenging.

References

1. Beaty TH, Newill CA, Cohen BH, Tockman MS, Bryant SH, and Spurgeon HA. 1985. Effects of pulmonary function on mortality. *J Chronic Dis* 38:703.
2. Tockman MS, and Comstock GW. 1989. Respiratory risk factors and mortality: Longitudinal studies in Washington County, Maryland. *Am Rev Respir Dis* (Suppl) 139.
3. Tockman MS, Anthonisen NR, Wright EC, and Donithan MG. 1987. Airways obstruction and the risk for lung cancer. *Ann Intern Med* 106:512.
4. Silverberg E, and Lubera J. Cancer statistics, 1986. 1986. *CA* 36:9.
5. Schwartz JD, Katz SA, Fegley RW, and Tockman MS. 1988. Analysis of spirometric data from a national sample of healthy 6- to 24-year-olds (HNANES II). *Am Rev Respir Dis* 138:1405.
6. Murray JF. 1986. Aging. In *The Normal Lung*, ed. 2. Philadelphia: Saunders, pp. 339–360.
7. Fletcher CM, Peto R, Tinker C, and Speizer FE. 1976. *The Natural History of Chronic Bronchitis and Emphysema: An Eight-Year Study of Early Chronic Obstructive Lung Disease in Working Men in London*. New York: Oxford University Press.
8. Crapo RO, Morris AH, and Gardner RM. 1981. Reference spirometric values using techniques and equipment that meet ATS recommendations. *Am Rev Respir Dis* 123:659.
9. Dockery DW, Speizer FE, Ferris BG Jr, Ware JH, Louis TA, and Spiro A. 1988. Cumulative and reversible effects of lifetime smoking on simple tests of lung function in adults. *Am Rev Respir Dis* 137:286.
10. Turner JM, Mead J, and Wohl ME. 1968. Elasticity of human lungs in relation to age. *J Appl Physiol* 25:664.
11. Mead J, Turner JM, Macklem PT, and Little JB. 1967. Significance of the relationship between lung recoil and maximum expiratory flow. *J Appl Physiol* 22:95.
12. Niewoehner DE, and Kleinerman J. 1977. Morphometric study of elastic fibers in normal and emphysematous human lungs. *Am Rev Respir Dis* 115:15.
13. Petty TL, Silvers GW, and Stanford RE. 1987. Mild emphysema is associated with reduced elastic recoil and increased lung size but not with air-flow limitation. *Am Rev Respir Dis* 136:867.
14. Rooney SA. 1985. State of art. The surfactant system and lung phospholipid biochemistry. *Am Rev Respir Dis* 131:439.
15. Buist AS, and Ross BB. 1973. Quantitative analysis of the alveolar plateau in the diagnosis of early airway obstruction. *Am Rev Respir Dis* 108:1078.

16. Crapo RO, and Morris AH. 1981. Standardized single breath normal values for carbon monoxide diffusing capacity. *Am Rev Respir Dis* 123:185.
17. Forster RE, Dubois AB, Briscoe WA, and Fisher AB. 1986. *The Lung,* ed 3. Chicago: Year Book Medical Publishers, p. 213.
18. Sorbini CA, Brassi V, Solinas E, and Muiesan G. 1968. Arterial oxygen tension in relation to age in healthy subjects. *Respiration* 25:3.
19. West JB, and Wagner PD. 1977. Pulmonary gas exchange. In *Bioengineering Aspects of the Lung,* Eds., JB West and PD Wagner. New York: Marcel Dekker, pp. 361–457.
20. Kronenberg RS, and Drage CW. 1973. Attenuation of the ventilatory and heart rate responses to hypoxia and hypercapnia with aging in normal men. *J Clin Invest* 52:1812.
21. Peterson DD, Pack AI, Silage DA, and Fishman AP. 1981. Effects of aging on ventilatory and occlusion pressure responses to hypoxia and hypercapnea. *Am Rev Respir Dis* 124:387.
22. Davies CTM. 1972. The oxygen-transporting system in relation to age. *Clin Sci* 42:1.
23. Jones NL, Moran Campbell EJ, Edwards RHT, and Robertson DG. 1975. *Clinical Exercise Testing.* Philadelphia: Saunders.
24. Yerg JE, Seals DR, Hagberg JM, and Holloszy JO. 1985. Effect of endurance exercise training on ventilatory function in older individuals. *J Appl Physiol* 58:791.
25. Wanner A. 1980. Pulmonary defense mechanisms: Mucociliary clearance. In *Current Pulmonology,* vol. 2. Ed., DH Simmons. Boston: Houghton Mifflin, pp. 325–356.
26. Morris AM et al. 1984. *Clinical Pulmonary Function Testing: A Manual of Uniform Laboratory Procedures,* ed. 2. Salt Lake City: Intermountain Thoracic Society.
27. Dockery DW, Ware JH, Ferris BG Jr, Glicksberg DS, Fay ME, Spiro A, and Speizer FE. 1985. Distribution of forced expiratory volume in one second and forced vital capacity in healthy, white, adult never-smokers in six U.S. Cities. *Am Rev Respir Dis* 131:511.
28. Miller A (ed). 1986. *Pulmonary Function Tests in Clinical and Occupational Lung Disease.* New York: Grune & Stratton.

7

Renal, Fluid, Electrolyte, and Acid-Base Problems During Surgery in the Elderly

Edward T. Zawada, Jr., James R. Horning, and Anthony G. Salem

The changing world population, which is comprised of an ever increasing number of not only elderly individuals but the "extreme" old—over the age of 80 years, has been alluded to previously in this textbook. There is now greater awareness of the problems of the elderly, including both the primary and subspecialty medical problems. The field of geriatrics is being accompanied in its growth by the birth and development of expertise in geriatric internal medicine, geriatric surgery, and now in areas such as geriatric cardiology and geriatric nephrology. On the one hand, the successes of surgery and invasive procedures in the elderly are prolonging life; on the other hand, as expected, the complications are high in many elderly patients. Hospitalization and perioperative management of geriatric patients are a great challenge to the physician because the kidney's ability to correct fluid, electrolyte, and acid-base disturbances and hemodynamic insults lessens with age.

This chapter describes the disordered renal anatomy and physiology of senescence that alerts the primary care physician (i.e., internist and surgeon) to the pitfalls of fluid, electrolyte, and acid-base management in the elderly patient undergoing surgery. It reviews renal diseases that may be encountered in the elderly undergoing surgery. It describes factors contributing to acute renal failure in the elderly and management of acute renal failure in the elderly patient recovering from surgery. This chapter also focuses on urologic problems and especially renal surgery in the aged.

Histopathology of the Aging Kidney

Autopsy material, biopsy material from kidney donation, and nephrectomy for tumor and trauma have led to a careful series of measurements called morphometrics of the aged glomerulus and tubules (1). The glomerular changes have been called sclerosis. On light microscopy (Fig. 7-1), there is an acellular obliteration of glomerular capillary architecture with resultant loss of functional tissue available to perform ultrafiltration of plasma. The difference between the "swiss cheese" open capillary loops (Fig. 7-2) in normal kidneys and the sclerosis of aged kidneys is readily apparent.

The cause of the sclerosis of the aged glomerulus is problematic although several theories have been postulated. It is difficult to dissect change due to age alone from that due to common diseases of late middle life, such as hypertension, diabetes, and atherosclerosis. It appears that even in the absence of these diseases such changes occur. The consequence of reduced filtration area is a reduced glomerular filtration rate. The glomerular changes and functional loss of glomerular filtration rate are responsible for many complications of perioperative management of the elderly patient.

The most widely accepted theory to explain the development of this glomerular problem has been summarized as the "hyperfiltration" theory. It was originally described in an animal model of reduced renal mass prepared to study the syndrome of chronic renal insuffi-

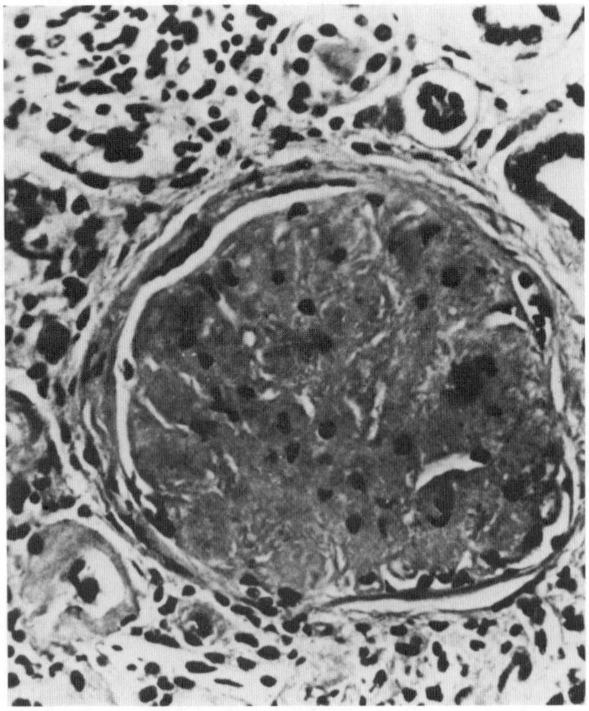

Figure 7-1. Light microscopy showing glomerular sclerosis, the glomerular "lesion" of senescence.

ciency. The remnant tissue did not remain normal but deteriorated with the development of glomerulosclerosis. Further studies revealed that the glomerulosclerosis resulted from intraglomerular hypertension, which was an attempt to increase the glomerular filtration rate per nephron as an adaptation to compensate for reduced total glomerular filtration rate (2). In addition, these studies showed that the intraglomerular hypertension was worse with a normal protein diet, which obligated the kidney to attempt to excrete nitrogenous wastes with reduced excretory units. The efferent arteriole appeared to increase its resistance to accomplish the pathologic adaptation. These glomerular pressures and pathologic anatomy did not occur on reduced protein intake. In individuals with renal diseases that reduce renal mass, continuation of normal protein intake can result in this deterioration of glomerular filtration rate. Elderly individuals who have hypertension or diabetes may have more deterioration of renal function than elderly people who do not have these underlying medical problems; however, even in the absence of diseases affecting the kidney, such intraglomerular hypertension occurs daily after every episode of protein intake. After decades of episodic glomerular hyperfiltration, such glomerulosclerosis develops and eventually causes deterioration of renal function by this same pathophysiology. It appears that renal glomerular senescence begins in the 4th decade and progresses linearly with age, reducing glomerular filtration rate by 1 cc/min for every year over 40 years of age (3). This predictable reduction of glomerular filtration rate (GFR) is one of the main factors responsible for morbidity in the elderly surgical patient. The decreased filtration reserve makes acute renal failure more likely with any nephrotoxic or ischemic renal insult, and fluid and electrolyte and acid-base problems a challenge to avoid. Reduced filtration of sodium, water, acid, and base loads is the first factor to consider in the perioperative setting by injudicious use of intravenous fluid therapy.

Reduction of glomerular filtration due to aging is inapparent in the day-to-day observation of aged patients. The serum creatinine, which is our usual marker of glomerular filtration rate, is often normal despite marked reductions of filtration in the elderly. The explanation is that in addition to reduced excretion of creatinine, there is a simultaneous reduction of creatinine production in the elderly. Despite reduced GFR, serum creatinine remains in the normal range because of parallel reduction of muscle mass in the elderly, which leads to reduced creatinine production. It is the normal serum creatinine level which makes glomerular senescence occult to the clinician in the superficial surveillance of renal function solely by the chemistry panel. The serum creatinine will often be in the normal range on the panel result even when glomerular filtration is markedly decreased.

In addition to glomerular senescence, there is also tubular senescence with advancing age (4). Tubular length decreases, interstitial fibrosis between tubules occurs, and tubular basement membrane constitution and anatomy change. Atherosclerosis of nutrient peritubular capillaries contributes in part to the latter. The consequence of tubular senescence is reduced tubular function, (i.e., reduced tubular flexibility to reabsorb or secrete an electrolyte load). For example, there is reduced tubular reabsorption of glucose in the elderly tubules. Again, the clinician is usually unaware of this tubular insufficiency because such tubular function is not routinely evaluated preoperatively to assess potential surgical risks. Such tubular dysfunction is hidden because reduced tubular reabsorption of glucose is not manifested by glycosuria: the parallel reduction of GFR leads to a reduced filtered glucose load with less glucose presenting itself to the senescent tubule. The clinician is likely to overestimate renal function by the failure to appreciate such tubular insufficiency preoperatively.

Renal Physiology in the Elderly

The glomerular changes ascribed to aging lead to a linear reduction of GFR beginning at age 40. The slope of the

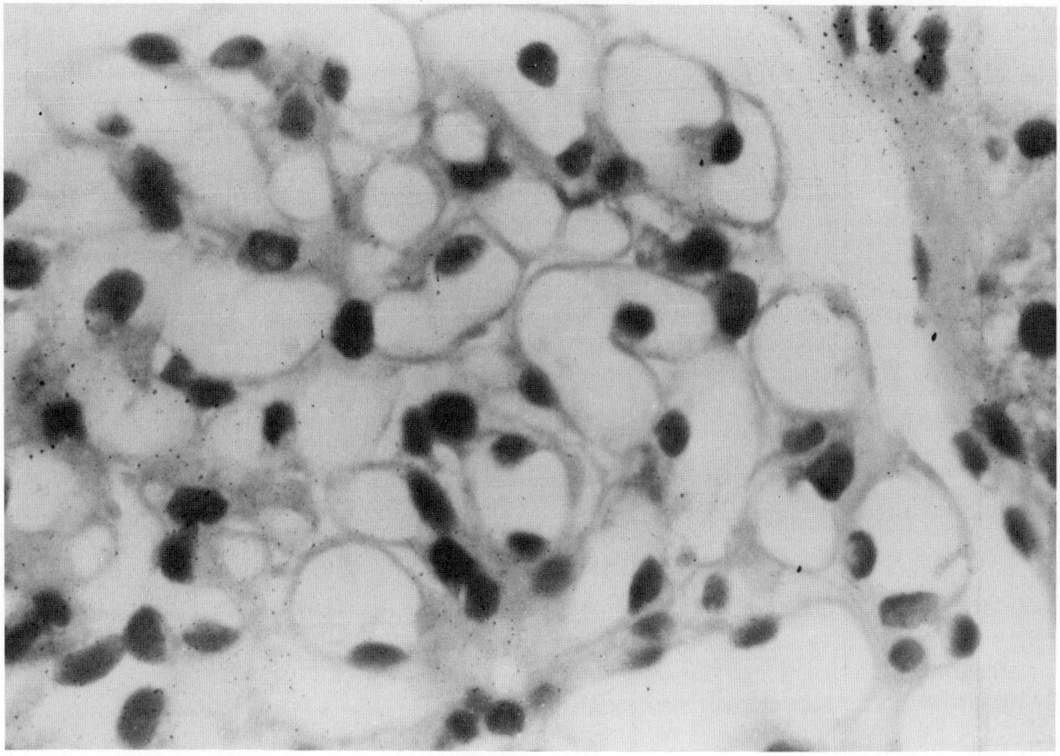

Figure 7-2. Normal glomerulus by light microscopy.

decline is 1 cc/min/year. Any substance whose excretion is dependent in part upon filtration is affected by aging. The excretion rate of these substances is reduced in the elderly. Tubular dysfunction cannot be quantitated as accurately. Tubular senescence results in disordered reabsorption and secretion of solutes (5). There is reduced ability to reabsorb and thus conserve sodium. There is impaired secretory capacity for potassium and hydrogen ion.

Clinical Assessment of Renal Function in the Elderly

There are two simple strategies to predict the reduction of renal function in the elderly surgical candidate. The first is to reduce the glomerular filtration rate by 1 cc/min for every year of age over 40 and to compare the resultant filtration rate to a normal of 100 cc/min as a percentage of normal. For example, in the 90-year-old patient, the probable percentage of GFR is (90 − 40)/100 = 50% of normal.

The second strategy is to use a urine-free formula to calculate GFR. These formulas utilize the fact that urine creatinine excretion remains constant under conditions of reduced renal function at the expense of a rise in serum creatinine. The urine creatinine excretion can be estimated from the age and weight of the patient quite accurately, which will predict the muscle mass of the patient from which the urine creatinine will be produced and excreted as a constant amount under steady-state conditions. The 24-hour urinary creatinine excretion is approximated by the formula $U_{creat}V = [(140 - \text{Age}) \times \text{Weight (KG)}]/72$. The creatinine clearance can then be estimated by using the above urinary creatinine excretion divided by the serum creatinine of the patient which should be measured preoperatively in the elderly patient. The final formula (6), which does not require the actual collection of the 24-hour urine, is: Creat. Clearance = [(140-Age) × Weight (kg)]/(72 × Serum Creat.) For women the above calculation should be multiplied by 0.85 because they have less muscle mass and, therefore, less creatinine generation and urinary excretion at any age and weight.

Two examples can be used to illustrate these formulas. If a 68-year-old woman weighs 40 kg and has a serum creatinine of 2 mg/dl, it may seem that the patient has mild renal insufficiency since the serum creatinine level is elevated. Using the formula:

$$\text{Creat. Clearance} = [(140 - 68) \times 40]/(72 \times 2) \times 0.85.$$
$$\text{Creat. Clearance} = (72 \times 40)/(72 \times 2) \times 0.85$$
$$\text{Creat. Clearance} = (40/2) \times 0.85 = 20 \times 0.85$$
$$\text{Creat. Clearance} = 17 \text{ cc/min}$$

Thus in an older woman with little muscle mass (40 kg), a serum creatinine as high as 2 mg/dl reflects a reduction of filtration to 17% of normal.

The second case involves a "healthy," athletic 68-year-old male who weighs 110 kg and has a serum creatinine of 2 mg/dl. It would appear that such a patient has mild renal insufficiency as the serum creatinine is abnormally elevated. Using the formula:

$$\text{Creat. Clearance} = [(140 - 68) \times 110]/(72 \times 2)$$
$$\text{Creat. Clearance} = (72 \times 110)/(72 \times 2)$$
$$\text{Creat. Clearance} = 110/2 = 55 \text{ cc/min}$$

In this case, there is only mild renal insufficiency. In the first case, the filtration reduction was somewhat occult because the serum creatinine was not markedly elevated due to concomitant muscle loss in an elderly, slightly built woman.

Drug-Dose Modification in the Elderly

Drugs that are eliminated from the body by renal excretion require dose modifications in the aged. Usually, these dose modifications require calculation of less frequent doses by a mathematical calculation involving the serum creatinine. Since the serum creatinine does not accurately reflect reduced renal function in the elderly, the dose of toxic drugs, such as the aminoglycosides, requires adjustments based on creatinine clearance and calculated by the 24-hour urine collection or by the estimate of creatinine clearance using the urine-free formula described above. The dose interval (DI) can be calculated from the following:

$$\text{DI} = (100/\text{estimated creatinine clearance}) \times \text{Usual interval}$$

If the 68-year-old woman described above required a course of gentamycin, a loading dose would be given at the usual 2 mg/kg. Then 1 mg/kg would be given every (100/17) × 8 hours. Thus, the interval would be every 47 hours. This would lessen the likelihood that the trough level would be elevated, which has been associated with aminoglycoside toxicity in several studies (7).

Survey of Renal Diseases of the Elderly

A prospective study was conducted in the United Kingdom on the causes of chronic progressive renal disease leading to admission to a renal unit for initiation of end-stage renal disease (ESRD) management (8). It revealed that the leading causes in patients over 60 years of age were pyelonephritis (20%), nephrosclerosis (16%), post-renal causes (15%), glomerulonephritis (11%), urolithiasis (6%), polycystic disease (2%), and diabetes (2%). Post-renal causes ranked high on the list.

In the surgical setting, it would behoove the clinician to search for obstructive symptoms and signs in the elderly patient with chronic azotemia. Rectal exam of the prostate, post-void residual volume of urine in the bladder, and renal ultrasound are all quite helpful and minimally invasive. Bladder catheterization may necessitate earlier consideration of antibiotics for endocarditis prophylaxis in patients with heart valves or prosthetic joints. The choice of antibiotics to cover genitourinary organisms should cover *enterococcus* as well as gram-negative organisms. Diabetics may have genitourinary colonization with gram-positive organisms. Broad-spectrum prophylaxis is thus likely to be necessary. Such surveillance for occult obstructive uropathy should be considered preoperatively in elderly patients. The etiology of the chronic azotemia might become apparent from these tests, and postoperative oliguria might be avoided by routine bladder catheterization prior to surgery in the patient with borderline compensation for benign prostatic hypertrophy (i.e., residual volume 25–150 cc). It can also be seen that parenteral management of hypertension might be necessary in the elderly patient who undergoes surgery, as nephrosclerosis due to hypertension was a common cause of chronic renal disease in this age group.

Common glomerular diseases in the elderly include an idiopathic, rapidly progressive glomerulonephritis (9), whose light microscopy reveals crescents in Bowman's space (Fig. 7-3) and an indolent glomerular disease, the so-called idiopathic membranous nephropathy. The former is nephritic in its clinical presentation, which means that the patient has fever, myalgias, fatigue, and other severe systemic symptoms. The glomerular inflammation results in a marked reduction of glomerular filtration rate. The latter glomerular disease presents as the nephrotic syndrome. There is little active inflammation and thus no systemic symptoms. The glomerular pathology (Fig. 7-4) reveals capillary loops that are wide open, and so the glomerular filtration rate is not reduced. The pathologic changes in the glomerular capillary wall are caused by immune complex deposition, which alters wall permeability and causes a urinary protein leak into the final urine of greater than 3 grams per 24 hours. The resultant hypoalbuminemia accounts for the clinical finding and the complaint of edema.

In the authors' experience, another common category of chronic renal diseases in the elderly is vascular disease, such as renovascular hypertension due to atherosclerotic renal artery stenosis, renal thromboemboli from clots released from the heart during episodes of cardiac arrhythmias, and atheroemboli that develop spontaneously from severe generalized vascular atherosclerosis or are caused by manipulation of the aorta during diagnostic radiologic procedures or aortic surgery.

At the University of South Dakota Hospitals and

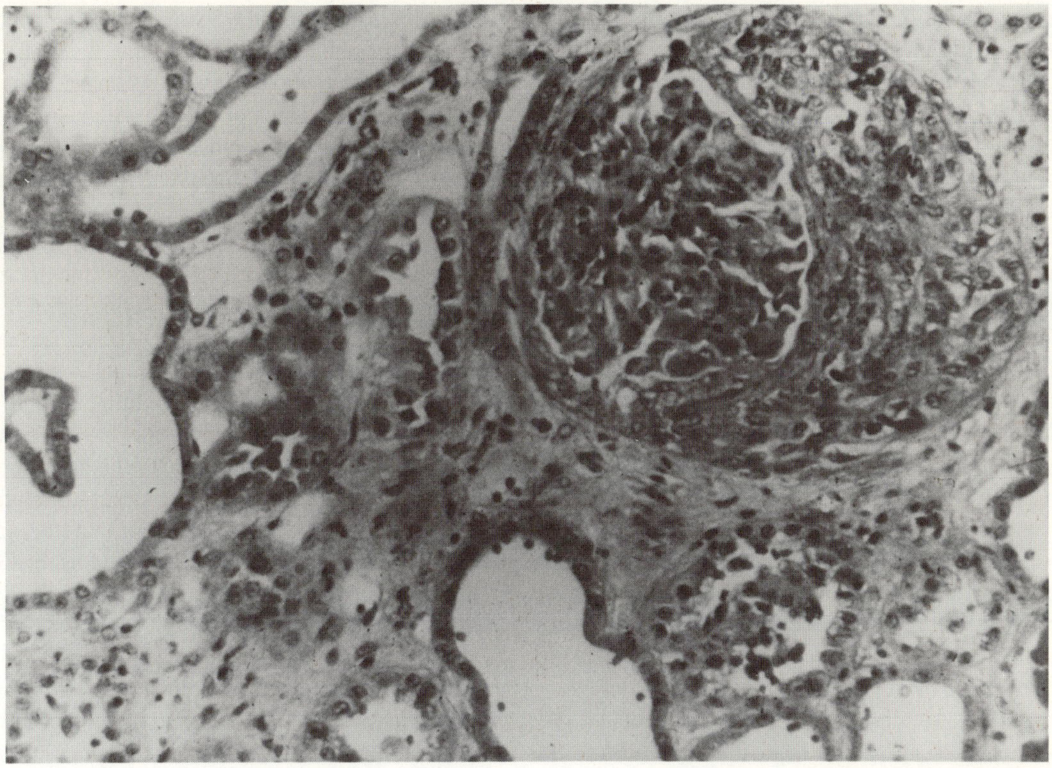

Figure 7-3. Crescentic glomerulonephritis, the most common cause of nephritic syndrome in the elderly. The crescent in Bowman's space is rapidly reducing the glomerular filtration rate.

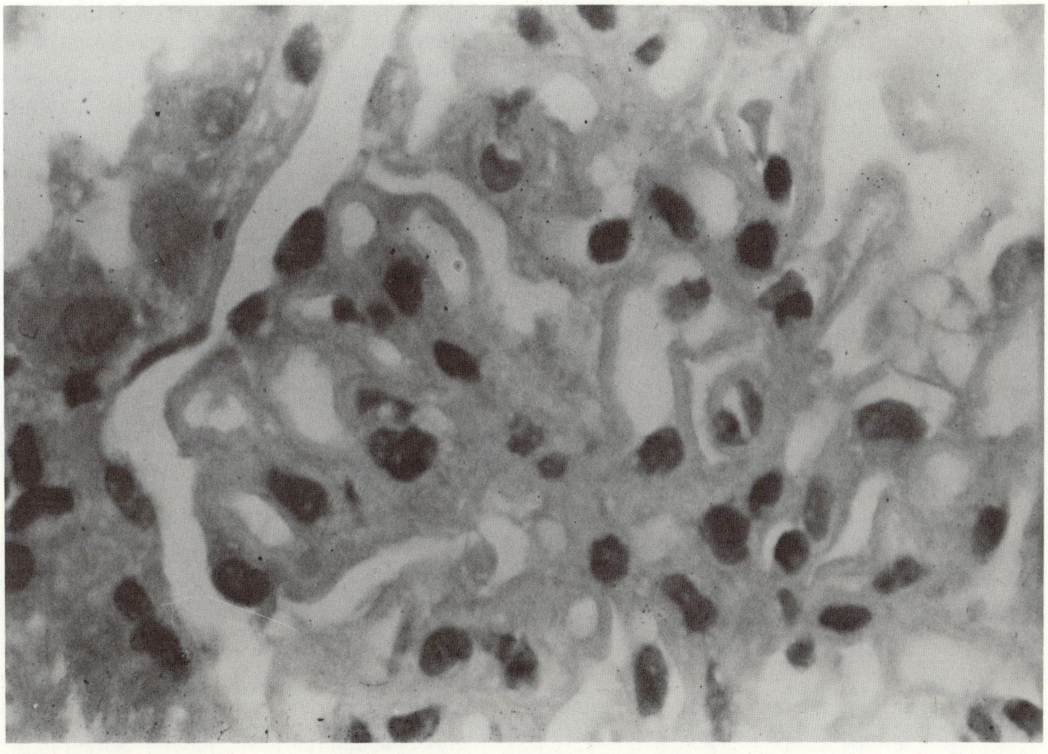

Figure 7-4. Membranous nephropathy, the most common cause of nephrotic syndrome in the elderly. The immune complexes are deposited in the basement membrane causing thickness and altered permeability to albumin.

Clinics in a series of 43 patients over the age of 60 with chronic renal failure, 50% had type II diabetes—by far the leading cause of chronic renal failure in this population of patients—but 25% had renovascular hypertension as the cause of their chronic renal failure. Thus, vascular disease made up the second largest group of patients with chronic renal failure in this series. The remaining causes of renal failure in this series included essential hypertension, tubulointerstitial disease, and glomerulonephritis.

Other common diseases in the elderly that can lead to chronic renal failure are amyloidosis and multiple myeloma (10). Multiple myeloma is the plasma cell malignancy that causes lytic lesions of bones and produces high levels of monoclonal immunoglobulins or their subunits. There is an increased incidence of multiple myeloma with advancing years. Multiple myeloma can affect the kidneys by five distinct mechanisms of injury: (*a*) "myeloma kidney" refers to direct parenchymal injury due to the immunoglobulins that are tubular cell toxins; (*b*) plasma cells can directly infiltrate the kidney, disturbing organ function much like any infiltrating tumor; (*c*) hypercalcemia resulting from bone dissolution due to the lytic lesions can lead to calcium deposits in the kidneys or stones; (*d*) uric acid crystals can deposit in the kidney during chemotherapy, which destroys the plasma cells, leading to release of nuclear material, such as purines and pyrimidines, which are then metabolized to uric acid; and (*e*) the immunoglobulins or their fragments can be woven into amyloid fibrils which deposit in the glomeruli and tubules, causing heavy proteinuria, glomerular obliteration, tubular dysfunction, and tubulointerstitial failure. Amyloidosis can result from multiple myeloma as just described, or it may develop in several other ways. The most treatable form of amyloidosis is that secondary to chronic inflammation in which a serum reactive protein or complement component is woven into the fibril. In these conditions, such as a chronic osteomyelitis, more aggressive therapy of the underlying condition stabilizes the renal deterioration by controlling the degree of amyloid fibril formation. One form of amyloidosis is not secondary to any other disturbance but is idiopathic and is called primary amyloidosis. This may involve the heart and/or the kidneys, can be an important cause of morbidity and mortality, and usually has a very poor prognosis (11).

Fluid and Electrolyte Disorders of the Elderly Undergoing Surgery

If an elderly individual is put on a low-salt diet with fluid restriction, the aging kidney will be less able to conserve sodium (12) and water (13) than the younger kidney. Geriatric patients who receive inadequate oral or intravenous fluid administration and who are undergoing diagnostic or surgical procedures, which require that the patient be given nothing by mouth (npo), will have greater sodium and water output than input. They will be in negative fluid balance and become volume contracted. The latter produces hypotension, predisposing to acute renal failure, prerenal azotemia, and a greater risk of insufficient coronary or cerebral blood flow. Conversely, the elderly patient, by virtue of reduced GFR, has difficulty excreting a salt and water load. Vigorous saline administration is likely to lead to intravascular and extracellular volume expansion, which results in edema and congestive heart failure with less total fluid administration than the younger surgical patient. Hypotonic intravenous solutions result in dilution of plasma tonicity if administered at high flow rates or in excessive amounts per 24 hours. Classic studies have revealed that such impaired free water clearance (CH_2O) disappeared when factored by the GFR, demonstrating that the impaired CH_2O is due to the reduced GFR of aging.

Elderly patients have reduced tubular function, including a reduction in secretory capacity. Excess potassium is excreted into the urine by tubular secretion under the influence of the hormone aldosterone (Fig. 7-5). Aldosterone is released from the adrenal gland when an increase in plasma renin levels causes an increase in circulating angiotensin II. Renin production by the juxtaglomerular apparatus is reduced in the elderly (14) as a consequence of renal tubular and vascular senescence. All of these circumstances put the elderly patient at risk for hyperkalemia after too rapid administration of potassium-containing intravenous solutions. Some diseases such as diabetes, which commonly affects the elderly, may have tubular injury as their predominant renal involvement. These patients will also be at risk for hyperkalemia because of potassium release from tissues injured during surgery as well as the use of maintenance intravenous solutions containing potassium.

Hypokalemia may develop at any age when a patient is npo after surgery and not receiving potassium by the intravenous route. The renal ability to conserve potassium under low intake is poor in any age group, but especially in the elderly. This can be explained by the obligate distal tubular sodium reabsorption under the influence of aldosterone. Sodium reabsorption obligates potassium excretion. Even without potassium intake, urinary potassium excretion will remain greater than 20 mEq/L of urine for many days, leading to negative potassium balance. Diarrhea, gastrointestinal bleeding, diuretic administration, nasogastric suction, and vomiting are all commonly encountered in the elderly patient perioperatively and result in additional gastrointestinal and urinary potassium losses.

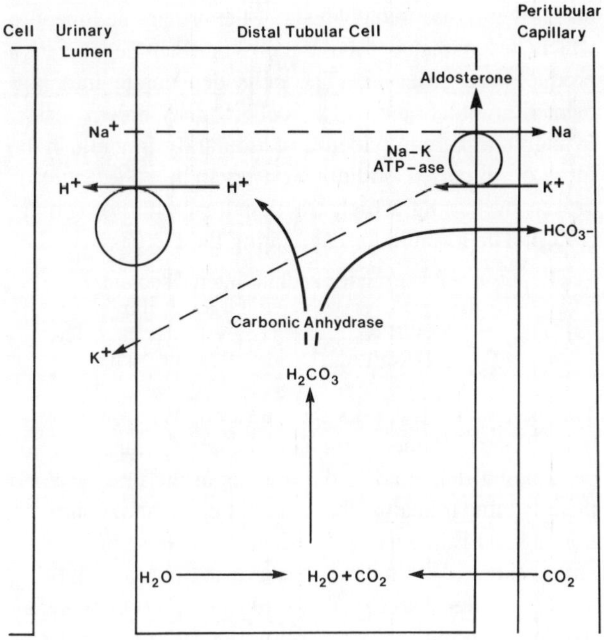

Figure 7-5. Schematic representation of distal tubular cell functions. Under the influence of aldosterone, which drives the sodium-potassium-ATPase pump on the basal membrane, a favorable environment is created for sodium entry into the cell at the luminal surface, allowing passive potassium transfer into the urine at the luminal surface, causing potassium to be pumped into the urine at the luminal surface with bicarbonate being regenerated and returned to the peritubular capillary.

Metabolic Acid-Base Disturbances in the Elderly Surgical Patient

Alkalosis

A reduction of the ability to excrete an alkaline load begins to occur at the age of 40 and progressively worsens thereafter (15). This may in part be due to reduced GFR. The importance of this finding is that in the perioperative period any alkalosis created by loss of acid (i.e., nasogastric suction or vomiting) can persist for longer periods of time. Alkalosis may be less well tolerated in the elderly patient because potassium will be drawn intracellularly. At the level of the distal tubule, the absence of hydrogen ion (titrated by the extra bicarbonate to CO_2 and blown off in the lungs) will obligate more potassium "exchange" for sodium under the influence of aldosterone as shown in Figure 7-5. The resultant hypokalemic alkalosis is a risk for cardiac arrhythmias in the elderly surgical patient, especially if the patient has ischemic heart disease or is on digitalis.

Lactated Ringer's solution is commonly used in surgical settings. The lactate is metabolized to bicarbonate. The lactate concentration in this solution is 28 mEq/L, which, if given too rapidly or in too great an amount, raises the serum bicarbonate level due to the impaired renal excretion of alkali in the elderly.

Acidosis

The elderly are more prone to metabolic acidosis. From the metabolism of the Western potash diet, 1 mEq of hydrogen ion per kilogram of body weight is created daily. The immediate buffering is accomplished by the bicarbonate ion, which accepts the proton, forming CO_2 that is then blown off in the lungs. As shown in Figure 7-5, to regenerate the lost bicarbonate, the distal tubule takes CO_2, and under the influence of aldosterone and carbonic anhydrase, delivers regenerated bicarbonate to the circulation and makes hydrogen ion available to be pumped into the urine where it will lower urinary pH. To enhance the hydrogen ion excretion, ammonia, filtered phosphate, and filtered sulfate accept hydrogen ions in the urine to reduce the concentration gradient of free hydrogen ion and thus lower the energy necessary for active transport of hydrogen ion against a concentration and charge gradient. Ammonia is produced in the renal tubular cell from glutamine, while phosphate and sulfate are generated from the metabolism of the potash diet. This releases sulfate and phosphate as sulfuric and phosphoric acid, which promptly release their hydrogen ion, leaving the phosphate and sulfate to be filtered into the urine. In the elderly, these tubular processes are less efficient. Also, the lower aldosterone levels lead to a decreased ability to excrete an acid load and to regenerate bicarbonate. The ability of the kidney to compensate for metabolic acidosis will thus be diminished.

Probably the two most common causes of metabolic acidosis in the elderly patient undergoing surgery are diarrhea and lactic acidosis. In diarrhea, bicarbonate-containing lower gastrointestinal fluids are lost, and the kidney is unable to keep pace by regenerating lost bicarbonate. Lactic acidosis occurs when the geriatric surgical patient has had a perioperative catastrophe, leading to tissue ischemia and/or hypoxia. Anaerobic metabolism releases lactic acid, whose hydrogen ion titrates down the existing bicarbonate level. The impaired GFR leads to less direct filtration of lactic acids, and the reduced tubular function and lower aldosterone levels lead to less regeneration of bicarbonate, already titrated by the lactic acid (3).

Suggestions for Fluid and Electrolyte Management in the Elderly Surgical Patient

From the discussion above, it is clear that intravenous therapy in the aged surgical patient is a double-edged sword. Generally, it is necessary to initiate intravenous therapy at the time of surgery or before surgery in many patients, because the acute illness necessitating the surgery frequently leads to poor fluid and food intake by the patient. In view of the impaired salt- and water-conserving ability of the aging kidney, such patients are likely to already be hypovolemic. Owing to the impaired ability to excrete a load of fluids and electrolytes, it is best to begin replacement slowly over a prolonged period. If the patient is already volume-contracted before surgery, 5% dextrose with 0.45% saline should be begun at 75 to 100 cc/hr. If the patient is to have a diagnostic study, such as an angiogram, but is currently euvolemic, then administration of 5% dextrose at 50 cc/hr is recommended.

If the patient is considerably hypovolemic postoperatively or is hypotensive, normal saline is the intravenous solution of first choice. Once urine output is assured at > 30 cc/hr, the addition of 10 to 20 mEq/L of KC1 is recommended. It is critical in this situation *not* to utilize a hypotonic solution such as 0.45% saline or, even worse, 0.2% (quarter normal) saline. Hypovolemia and/or hypotension will lead to decreased renal perfusion; this will aggravate the impaired free water clearance of the geriatric patient, which can result in hyponatremia and cerebral edema. The latter produces confusion, focal neurologic findings, seizures, aspiration, and respiratory arrest when it develops rapidly in the hospital setting (16). Lactated Ringer's solution is inappropriate, as it can cause alkalosis: the impaired renal perfusion aggravates the geriatric patient's already impaired ability to excrete an alkaline load (i.e., the lactate).

Acute Renal Failure and Its Prevention in the Elderly Surgical Patient

Acute renal failure is a disastrous complication of surgery in the elderly patient. In one series, major surgery was the second most common cause of acute renal failure in the elderly (17). In this group of 122 patients, the mortality rate was 57.3%. The causes of death were pneumonia, myocardial infarction and cardiac arrest, pulmonary embolism, and septicemia in decreasing order of frequency. Taken together, bronchopneumonia and septicemia led the authors to conclude that infectious complications were the single greatest mortality risk in the elderly patient with acute renal failure.

There are several types of acute renal failure in the elderly, but the most common (as in other age groups) is acute tubular necrosis (ATN). The tubular necrosis results from ischemia or nephrotoxicity, the latter most commonly due to aminoglycoside antibiotics, chemotherapy drugs, or intravenous contrast agents. The diagnosis is made by microscopic analysis of the urinary sediment in which desquamated tubular cells or their degenerative products are observed. The cells degenerate into pigmented granular casts, often called "dirty brown" casts. In addition, there is evidence of tubular dysfunction in the form of impaired sodium conservation. The latter is proven by finding a high fractional excretion of sodium (FE_{Na}). The formula for calculating the FE_{Na} is:

$$FE_{Na} \text{ (as a \%)} = \text{excreted sodium/filtered sodium} \times 100$$
$$FE_{Na} = \text{UNaV/(PNa} \times \text{GFR)} \times 100$$
$$FE_{Na} = \text{UNaV/[PNa} \times \text{(UCrest. V/PCrest.)]} \times 100$$
$$FE_{Na} = \text{(UNa/PNa)(UCrest./PCrest.)} \times 100$$

This calculated test asks the question: What are the tubules doing to influence the final urinary sodium excretion per amount delivered to the tubules in the first place? If there is tubular health, there should be sodium conservation, a low FE_{Na}, a value less than 1%. During tubular necrosis, there is a failure to conserve sodium, a high FE_{Na}, a value greater than 1%. In a typical case of volume contraction with reduced urine output but no tubular necrosis, the urine sodium is typically < 20 mEq/L, and the urine creatinine is greater than 40 mg/dl. Take, for example, a urine sodium of 15 mEq/L, a serum sodium of 140 mEq/L, a slightly elevated serum creatinine of 1.5 mg/dl, and a urine creatinine of 140 mg/dl (a not uncommon value in concentrated urine). Plugging these values into the formula for FE_{Na}, the following is derived:

$$FE_{Na} = (15/140)/(140/1.5) \times 100 = 0.107/93.3 \times 100 = 0.11\%$$

This value is less than 1%, reflecting healthy tubules that are effectively conserving sodium.

In the case of tubular necrosis, common values are likely to be:

UNa = 140 mEq/L, PNa = 140 mEq/L, Ucreat. = 15 mg/dl, and serum creat. = 1.5 mg/dl.

Using the formula:

$$FE_{Na} = (140/140)/(15/1.5) \times 100$$
$$FE_{Na} = 1/10 \times 100$$
$$FE_{Na} = 10\%$$

This high fractional excretion of sodium would indicate tubular dysfunction as evidenced by "salt wasting" instead of conservation.

A modification of the fractional excretion expression that is even simpler to apply is called the renal failure index (RFI). In this formula, the plasma sodium is felt to be a constant near 100, which cancels the multiplication by 100 to achieve a percent. Thus, the formula can be simplified:

$$FE_{Na} = \text{(UNa/PNa)/(Ucreat./Pcreat.)} \times 100$$
$$\text{RFI} = \text{UNa/(Ucreat./Pcreat.)}$$

Again, the value 1 is the cutoff between prerenal and tubular necrosis causes of oliguria.

Using the numbers from the examples above in the RFI formula:

Example 1: RFI = 15/(140/1.5) = 0.16

Since this is less than 1, it suggests renal conservation of sodium and normal tubular function.

Example 2: RFI = 140/(15/1.5) = 14

This value is much greater than 1, suggesting tubular necrosis and failure to conserve sodium.

This discussion of acute renal failure in the elderly has concentrated on the diagnosis of acute tubular necrosis. If the analysis described above as well as bedside evaluation, weight, orthostatic changes in vital signs, low central venous pressure, low pulmonary artery pressures, or low pulmonary capillary wedge pressures point to volume contraction as the cause of decreasing urine output and rising creatinine and blood urea nitrogen, the therapy is to restore plasma volume with normal saline and/or colloid, such as packed red blood cells (RBCs) or albumin.

In summary, from these theories it can be seen that prevention of the filtration failure in advance of a renal insult that might cause tubular cell necrosis is accomplished by avoiding nonsteroidal anti-inflammatory drugs and by hydrating to prevent volume contraction and to suppress the renin-angiotensin axis. At the time of the insult and if the volume status of the patient permits it, mannitol and furosemide should be given. If the volume status does not permit these drugs to be given, then low-dose dopamine (≤3 mg/kg/min) and an intravenous furosemide drip at 5–30 mg/hr should be started. When these measures are utilized, the filtration failure will be lessened in the setting of tubular necrosis. The patient will often not be oliguric and may have a rise of creatinine which reaches a level that does not require dialysis. Nonoliguric acute tubular necrosis has an improved prognosis with less morbidity and mortality.

Other types of acute renal failure that must be ruled out in the elderly include glomerular, vascular, and allergic interstitial causes. The glomerular cause of acute renal failure that occurs in the elderly is crescentic glomerulonephritis. These patients may have systemic symptoms, such as fever and hypertension. The diagnosis requires the finding of red blood cell casts in microscopic analysis of the urine sediment. Thus, it is strongly recommended that any patient with acute renal failure have the sediment reviewed by the clinician for the presence of these casts. Failure to do so may result in the failure to recognize this form of acute renal failure, which can be stabilized with high-dose corticosteroids. Failure to treat these patients with corticosteroids can result in permanent renal failure. It is recommended that such steroid treatment be carried out in consultation with an internist or nephrologist whenever possible.

Vascular causes of acute renal failure are suspected when acute renal failure develops in certain high-risk situations. For example, thromboemboli may develop in the elderly surgical patient who has a cardiac arrhythmia. Clots may form in the heart and be expelled into the systemic circulation. Hematuria, flank pain, and hypertension heighten the suspicion. Renal flow scan shows reduced flow and the areas of infarct on the static images. Renal lactic dehydrogenase (LDH) isoenzymes may be elevated. Atheroemboli may also occur in the setting of aortic manipulation, i.e., during surgery or angiography. An atherosclerotic plaque is dislodged and travels downstream into the renal arteries to occlude afferent arterioles.

Finally, allergic renal interstitial nephritis occurs in response to therapy with certain classes of drugs. There is filtration failure by mechanisms similar to that of tubular necrosis. The difference is that fever, rash, eosinophilia, and occasionally eosinophiluria are evidence of the allergic nature of this renal injury. In addition to stopping the offending drug, steroid therapy is often necessary to minimize the course of acute renal failure in these patients. The drug classes that are associated with allergic interstitial nephritis are: penicillins, anticonvulsants, antituberculous drugs, sulfa antibiotics, and sulfa-like diuretics (thiazide, furosemide, metolazone).

Once reduced glomerular filtration has occurred in acute tubular necrosis, it cannot be reversed until the tubular cells regenerate. This usually takes about 2 weeks. Hyperalimentation and aggressive dialysis, when necessary, have proven to shorten the duration of the acute renal failure when compared to intravenous fluid therapy (18).

Management of Hypertension in the Elderly Surgical Patient

Loss of control of hypertension in the elderly surgical patient can cause a great deal of morbidity. Poor control of blood pressure may result in exacerbation of angina due to increased afterload; it may precipitate congestive heart failure in the patient with borderline compensated contractility; finally, it may worsen postoperative bleeding. An exacerbation of hypertension may rarely cause a cerebrovascular accident in the perioperative setting, since the aged individual is at higher risk for this vascular complication of hypertension as well.

If any of the above complications occur or if the hypertension is quite severe (greater than 115 mm Hg diastolic), the usual forms of emergency management of hypertension should be employed as in any age group:

sublingual nifedipine or intravenous nitroprusside by pump infusion. Sublingual nifedipine has become the initial treatment of choice for hypertensive emergencies. A 10-mg capsule is opened, and the contents are placed under the tongue. Blood pressure is lowered within 10 to 15 minutes and rarely goes to frankly hypotensive levels; the treatment is effective in most cases. If ineffective, then nitroprusside should be initiated. For long-term therapy in the setting of an acute exacerbation of severe hypertension, nitroprusside therapy should be used since it has rapid onset and offset of action, so that titration of blood pressure is instantaneous. Two ampules are dissolved in 250 cc of normal saline or 5% dextrose, and the drip infusion is used to titrate the blood pressure to diastolic blood pressure levels of 95–100 mm Hg at the lowest. An arterial line should be in place to monitor the blood pressure reduction if at all possible. If not possible, a number of excellent accurate electronic blood pressure recording devices that use an arm cuff are routinely available in most hospitals. They allow frequent measurements and are an acceptable alternative to intra-arterial blood pressure monitoring.

It is important not to lower the diastolic pressure to normal (i.e., 80 mm Hg) since frank cerebral insufficiency may result from decreased perfusion pressure through vessels with extensive atherosclerotic narrowing. Both nifedipine and nitroprusside have favorable hemodynamic patterns for supply and demand of oxygenated blood to heart muscle and do not exacerbate angina or heart failure as blood pressure is lowered. Anesthesiologists often use a nitroglycerine drip infusion to lower blood pressure in the acute setting. In these authors' experience, the effectiveness of nitroglycerine is short-lived. Therefore, it is important to convert the patient to other therapy within a few hours. On the other hand, nitroprusside can be given for 2 to 3 days, while other antihypertensive therapy is instituted. Since nitroprusside has a cyanide moiety, thiocyanate may accumulate rapidly in the elderly because of their reduced GFR. Thiocyanate blood levels should be drawn regularly.

Other parenteral antihypertensive therapies that can be used for "maintenance therapy" in the perioperative setting include: intravenous methyldopa, intravenous hydralazine, transdermal clonidine, and the newest addition, intravenous labetalol. Drugs to be avoided in the elderly surgical patient with hypertension are intravenous beta blockers, intravenous diazoxide, intramuscular hydralazine, and intravenous ganglionic blockers. The lack of dependable control and the side effect profile make these drugs less desirable.

Intravenous hydralazine can be used in doses of 5–75 mg three times daily. Reflex tachycardia is a potential problem that can exacerbate angina. However, in the elderly patient cardiac conduction system senescence often makes this problem less common than in middle-aged patients with coronary artery disease. Intravenous methyldopa is accompanied by somnolence, but is otherwise effective and safe. Transdermal clonidine is administered as a patch in small, medium, and large sizes and is applied to the skin once weekly. This is an easy way to prevent exacerbation of hypertension in the mild hypertensive who goes to surgery (19). The patch should be applied 1–2 days preoperatively. When effective in controlling blood pressure, it is left on throughout the surgery and during the postoperative period.

Surgery in the Elderly Patient with Advanced Renal Failure

Acute renal failure in the elderly patient during the perioperative period is associated with a high mortality as described previously. By contrast, surgery in the patient with chronic renal failure (i.e., even a dialysis patient) is becoming more and more common. Further, it is clear that with some precautions these patients tolerate surgery with a low mortality rate. The good outcome of dialysis patients undergoing coronary artery bypass surgery has been previously reported (20). It was possible in that study to combine dialysis with cardiopulmonary bypass to delay postoperative dialysis for several days. There was no mortality in this small series. Thus, in the elderly patient with advanced renal failure, surgery can be performed provided precautions are taken to minimize uremia preoperatively and to perform dialysis easily postoperatively. In patients with chronic azotemia, placement of a Gore-Tex™ hemodialysis arteriovenous fistula 2 weeks before surgery allows it to be usable perioperatively at the first sign of fluid overload, electrolyte imbalance, or acid-base deterioration. This would obviate the need for central dialysis catheters or prolonged hemodynamic monitoring with catheters that predispose to the danger of serious nosocomial infections.

Renovascular Surgery in the Elderly

As described previously, renovascular disease and renovascular hypertension are common causes of blood pressure disturbances and renal insufficiency in the elderly. In the authors' experience, renal scan and digital subtraction angiography have been the best screening tests for renal artery stenosis. Surgical candidates are those patients with renovascular hypertension who have uncontrolled blood pressure while on potent antihypertensive therapy and/or who have azotemia attributable to the renovascular lesions. At the University of South Dakota, bypass graft, often in conjunction with aortoiliac surgery, has been the surgery of choice for this disease. The measurement of preoperative renal vein renin levels is no longer necessary, since these patients are frequently operated on to preserve renal function rather than to control hypertension. There have been reports of substantial long-term reductions of serum creatinine with revascularization, especially when there has been bilateral renal artery stenosis. Angioplasty affords an alternative for blood pressure reduction and preservation or even improvement of renal blood flow in the elderly patient with renal artery stenosis. The greatest success has been achieved with non-ostial lesions somewhat downstream from the take off of the renal arteries from the aorta.

Surgical Considerations in Obstructive Renal Disease in the Elderly

As described previously, obstruction of the urinary tract is a common cause of renal failure in the elderly. This is most often due to prostate disease in men and gynecologic pathology in women. Prostate diseases include benign prostatic hypertrophy and prostate cancer. The former is a fibromyoadenoma and consists of hypertrophy of glandular and supportive tissues. In the classic study by Franks, 100% of men reaching the age of 90 had autopsy evidence of prostate cancer (21). Additional causes of obstructive uropathy in the elderly include stone disease and bladder cancer. The most common causes of stone disease in the elderly are hypercalcemia due to malignancy, hyperuricemia due to chemotherapy for cancer, and hyperparathyroidism. Additionally, stones arise in patients who had idiopathic hypercalciuria at an early age and have survived to the latter decades. Magnesium ammonium phosphate stones arise from urinary tract infection with urea-splitting organisms. The infections are related to inadequate bladder emptying due to prostate disease, spinal cord injury, and detrusor insufficiency from diabetes. Surgical management of elderly patients' obstructive uropathy includes transurethral prostatectomy (TURP), open prostatectomy, radical prostatectomy, total cystectomy with creation of an ileal conduit, stone extraction through cystoscopy, and open surgical removal of urinary calculi. The mortality rate in patients over the age of 65 undergoing these types of urologic procedures ranges from 0.5% for TURP to 17% for the more invasive surgery, such as radical prostatectomy and cystectomy (22). Palliative measures, such as nephrostomy drainage followed by medical therapy, are available as alternatives. Extracorporeal lithotripsy is a less invasive alternative to open stone extraction in the elderly patients with obstructive nephropathy due to stones.

Renal Transplantation in the Elderly

For many years transplantation centers have had an upper age limit of 55 years for renal transplantation. More recently, the patient's physiologic age rather than chronologic age is used to help make the decision for transplantation. Several series have reported renal transplant results in older patients (23, 24). These studies documented good survival rates similar to those of younger age groups, attesting to the lack of technical problems with such surgery in aged individuals. However, the overall success rate at 1 year is most often reduced due to death of the patient. Causes of death include myocardial infarction, stroke, and infection. The first two are uncommon causes of death in younger nondiabetic transplant patients.

Summary

The elderly surgical patient represents a great management challenge due to reduced renal reserve. This is the result of glomerulosclerosis and senescence of tubules. Fluids and electrolytes must be administered carefully. Delay in their institution or too rapid administration of fluids will lead to morbidity. Acute renal failure is best prevented with preoperative hydration. Perioperative hypertension must also be managed definitively but carefully, avoiding "total normalization" of blood pressure. More surgery is being performed in the elderly, such as renal revascularization and renal transplantation. Surgical risks are higher in elderly patients than in younger patients, but the risk/benefit ratios are acceptable to most patients.

References

1. Tauchi, H, Tsuboi, K, and Okutoni, J. 1971. Age changes in the human kidney of the different races. *Gerontology* 17:87–97.
2. Brenner, BM, Meyer, GW, and Hostetter, TH. 1982. Dietary protein intake and the progressive nature of kidney disease: The role of hemodynamically mediated glomerular injury in the pathogenesis of progressive glomerular sclerosis in aging, renal ablation, and intrinsic renal disease. *N Engl J Med* 307:652–659.
3. Adler, S, et al. 1968. Effect of acute acid loading on urinary acid excretion by the aging human kidney. *J Lab Clin Med* 72:278–279.
4. Darmady, EM, Offer, J, and Wookhouse, MA. 1973. The parameters of the aging kidney. *J Pathol* 109:195–209.
5. Epstein, M. 1985. Renal physiologic changes with age. In *Geriatric Nephrology and Urology*, Ed., ET Zawada, Jr. and DA Sica, pp. 1–14. Littleton, MA: PSG Publishing Company, Inc.
6. Cockroft, DW, and Gault, MN. 1976. Prediction of

creatinine clearance from serum creatinine. *Nephron* 16:31–41.
7. Duchin, KL. 1985. Pharmacodynamics and pharmacokinetics of drugs in the elderly. In *Geriatric Nephrology and Urology*, Ed., ET Zawada, Jr. and DA Sica, pp. 215–229. Littleton, MA: PSG Publishing Company, Inc.
8. McGeown, MG. 1972. Chronic renal failure in Northern Ireland, 1968–70 (A prospective survey). *Lancet* 1:307–310.
9. Moorthy, AV, and Zimmerman, SW. 1980. Renal disease in the elderly: clinicopathologic analysis of renal disease in 115 elderly patients. *Clin Nephrol* 14:223–229.
10. Frocht, A, and Fillit, H. 1984. Renal disease in the geriatric patient. *J Am Geriatr Soc* 32:28–43.
11. Zawada, ET Jr, et al. 1987. An elderly male with deterioration of renal function and heavy proteinuria. *Am J Nephrol* 7:482–489.
12. Epstein, M, and Hollenberg, NK. 1976. Age as a determinant of renal sodium conservation in normal man. *J Lab Clin Med* 87:411–417.
13. Dontas, AS, Marketos, SG, and Papanayiotou, P. 1972. Mechanisms of renal tubular defects in old age. *Postgrad Med J* 48:295–303.
14. Weidman, P, et al. 1975. Effect of aging on plasma renin and aldosterone in normal man. *Kidney Int* 8:325–333.
15. Sica, DA, and Centor, RM. 1985. Tests of glomerular and tubular function in the elderly. In *Geriatric Nephrology and Urology*, Ed., ET Zawada, Jr and DA Sica, pp. 33–47. Littleton, MA: PSG Publishing Company, Inc.
16. Arieff, AI, Llack, F, and Massry, SG. 1976. Neurologic manifestations and morbidity of hyponatremia: Correlation with brain water and electrolytes. *Medicine* 55: 121–141.
17. Kumar, R, Hill, CM, and McGeown, MG. 1973. Acute renal failure in the elderly. *Lancet* 1:90–91.
18. Abel, RM, et al. 1973. Improved survival from acute renal failure after treatment with intravenous essential L-amino acids and glucose. *N Engl J Med* 288:695–699.
19. Horning, JR, et al. 1988. Efficacy and safety of two years of antihypertensive therapy with transdermal clonidine. *Chest*. 93:941–945.
20. Zawada, ET Jr., Stinson, JB, and Done, G. 1982. New perspectives on coronary artery disease in hemodialysis patients. *South Med J* 75:694–697.
21. Franks, LM. 1954. Latent carcinoma of the prostrate. *J Pathol Bacteriol* 68:603–616.
22. Stults, B. 1985. Surgical considerations in the elderly. In *Geriatric Nephrology and Urology*, Ed., ET Zawada, Jr. and DA Sica, pp. 397–428. Littleton, MA: PSG Publishing Company, Inc.
23. Baquero, A, and Goldman, MH. 1985. Renal transplantation in the elderly. In *Geriatric Nephrology and Urology*, Ed., ET Zawada, Jr. and DA Sica, pp. 253–263. Littleton, MA: PSG Publishing Co., Inc.
24. Wedel, N, Brynger, H, and Blohme, I. 1980. Kidney transplantation in patients 60 years and older. *Scand J Urol Nephrol* 54:106–108.

8

Gastrointestinal and Liver Changes in the Elderly

Robert D. Shamburek, Robert B. Scott, and John T. Farrar

Until recently, knowledge of age-related changes in the gastrointestinal tract, biliary tract, liver, and pancreas of man was sparse. Even now, the data are fragmentary and conclusions tentative.

One problem with assessing the effects of age on man is the extreme individual variation in function seen in elderly patients. This individual variation is part of the human species but is more obvious in the aged. Compare, if you will, the relative homogeneity of a group of children at age 10 with a group at age 80.

Each person is unique, but in the absence of severe congenital disease, there is a semblance of homogeneity in youth. At age 10, everyone can run, play, read, reason and joke. As individuals reach the age of 80 the differences between them are immense. These differences are due to the genetic programming of each person and each organ, as well as all environmental, psychologic, nutritional, toxic (tobacco, alcohol, atmospheric pollutants), and physical effects (damage to joints, ears and eyes).

Fortunately, the margin of safety provided to man by nature is very great, and in many gastrointestinal and liver functions, there is 10 to 20 times the quantitative functional capacity required for normal life.

There are two practical consequences to this very great variation between different aged individuals and the large functional reserve capacity in normal individuals. On the one hand, the variation renders studies on the effect of aging difficult to perform, because chronologic age is not a valid normalizer. Then, because of the great margin of safety, for instance, in absorptive capacity from the small intestine, it is difficult to detect changes in absorption in vivo due to aging even if such changes occur.

Theories of Aging in Relation to the Gut

An extensive literature exists on aging of both cellular and interstitial human tissues. At the risk of oversimplifying this literature, we propose to think of aging of the human gut and liver as caused by one or more of the following:

1. *Genetic Programming*—The DNA molecules of the genes apparently determine the upper limit of life span of all species. In addition, certain cells can only divide a finite number of times before the cell line dies out. It seems that genetic programming is the final determinant of the length of life and possibly of many processes affected by aging.
2. *Alterations in Function Consequent to the Vicissitudes of Life and Time*—In this category are such influences as radiation effects, environmental effects due to toxins, physical wear and tear, chromosomal abnormalities, and long-term psychologic influences. Many of these influences may themselves be modulated by genetic programming.
3. *Alterations Consequent to Intercurrent Disease*—These effects are different from those in category 2 above only insofar as there are demonstrable pathologic changes in an organ characteristic of a known disease entity. Examples are autoimmune atrophic gastritis and pancreatic atrophy due to chronic alcohol intake.

Whenever a decrease in function is demonstrated, the problem is to determine what proportion of the loss of function is due to genetic programming, environmental effects, or actual disease.

Epithelial Cell Functions

The Tongue and Taste

The tongue plays an important role in the gastrointestinal tract by aiding mastication and deglutition. Microscopically, connective tissue atrophy and surface epithelial thinning occurs throughout the tongue and oral mucosa in the elderly (1), but it is difficult to separate age-related changes from those due to systemic disease.

Taste perception is another important function of the tongue. Taste receptors reside within taste buds, primarily on three types of papillae on the tongue. Fungiform papillae are located on the anterior two-thirds of the tongue, and the taste receptors are innervated by the chorda tympani branch of the facial nerve. Taste receptors on the circumvallate papillae and foliate papillae are innervated by the glossopharyngeal nerve. The circumvallate papillae lie on the dorsal and the foliate papillae lie on the lateral aspects of the posterior one-third of the tongue.

Earlier reports of diminished taste and taste buds with aging have been questioned (2). Some elderly individuals show slightly elevated taste detection thresholds, which represent the lower range of concentrations required to provide stimuli, but food provides stimuli far above these thresholds (2). Therefore, the slight alterations in taste threshold have no clinical impact on the perception of what we eat or drink.

Taste perception of sweet, sour, salty, and bitter correlate with the distribution and number of taste buds stimulated. Stereomicrographic examination of fungiform papillae reveal no age-related changes in the number of taste buds per papillae (3). Wide variability occurs in the density of taste buds from person to person at all ages (4–6) and this variability may partially account for some of the conflicting data on taste changes in the elderly. Most investigators now believe that aging does not cause a significant decrease in the number of taste buds (3, 4, 6–8).

Food recognition also depends upon the olfactory system. Age-related declines occur in the olfactory system (9–11) and have important implications on taste. Complaints of loss of taste in the elderly often relate to the diminished sense of smell rather than a decrease in taste. Perceived flavor and food identification are influenced by many factors other than taste and olfactory receptors and include CNS integration, medications, poor nutrition, poor oral hygiene, and decreased salivary flow (9). These factors have not always been controlled in studies on aging.

To summarize the effects of aging on the tongue and taste:

1. Connective tissue atrophy and surface epithelial thinning occurs throughout the tongue with age.
2. The number of taste buds varies from person to person but does not change with aging.
3. Taste detection thresholds are elevated in the elderly, but this does not alter taste since food provides stimuli far above the threshold.
4. Taste perception may be altered by olfactory changes; olfactory sensation is decreased in aging.

Salivary Glands

Saliva is produced by three major pairs of glands (parotid, submandibular, sublingual) and several smaller glands (buccal, palatal, labial). Alterations in saliva production have an impact on lubrication, digestion, mucosal integrity, and antimicrobial resistance. Age-related changes in salivary secretion and composition must, if possible, be differentiated from those due to disease and drugs.

Salivary glands show an overall trend of loss of parenchyma with aging with replacement by fat and connective tissue (12, 13). Total gland volume remains constant (12, 13). Acinar cells are the major parenchymal cells replaced. In submandibular glands, 25% to 40% of the acinar cells are gradually replaced with adipose, fibrous, and ductal tissue (12, 13). Age-related increases in the extralobular and nonstriated intralobular ducts (14) account for up to a 30% increase in duct volumes (12). The replacement of acinar cells by ducts, fat, and fibrous tissue is accelerated in the extreme elderly (12).

Labial salivary glands have similar age-related decreases in acinar volume with ductal dilatation and fibrosis (15, 16). Fatty changes are not as marked as in submandibular glands (16). Unfortunately, the above autopsy findings have not been correlated with physiologic changes.

Slight changes in stimulated and unstimulated salivary flow have been found with aging depending on the stimulus, collection method, patient population, disease state, and medication usage. Whether there is a significant clinical impact remains unsettled. Unstimulated whole saliva flow rate diminishes slightly (17–19) with age or remains unchanged (20) depending on the collection device. Stimulated whole saliva flow rate does not decrease with aging (17, 20–22) even in individuals with a low unstimulated flow rate (17) suggesting that normal stimulated physiologic activity is preserved in the elderly. However, up to 11% of elderly persons have very low stimulated salivary flow rates (<0.3 ml/min), and 35% have hyposalivation (<0.7 ml/min). These decreases correlate better with the increased use of medications rather than age (22). Elderly patients on multiple medications, especially those that decrease secretions, will have lower stimulated salivary secretory rates (22). Chronic hyposalivation may lead to increased dental caries, increased oral infections, reduced denture retention, alteration in taste, and decreased sublingual drug absorption.

Variable flow rates are found in the different salivary glands. Unstimulated (20, 23) and stimulated parotid flow rates (20, 23–25) do not change with aging. However, both resting and stimulated submandibular flow rates are markedly reduced, 78% and 61% respectively, in healthy elderly individuals (26). A similar reduction (50%) of labial salivary gland stimulated flow rate has been described (20). This age-related reduction in flow rate has not yet been correlated with subjective complaints, histologic changes, or changes in oral health.

Xerostomia is the subjective complaint of dryness of the mouth. Dry mouth is a frequent complaint in the elderly, occurring in up to 60% of women and 37% of men (22). Medication is a common cause of dry mouth (22). Approximately half of institutionalized (27) and non-institutionalized (28) elderly individuals take at least one drug that causes hyposalivation or xerostomia. These include antihistamines, antipsychotics, antidepressants, anticholinergics, sedatives, diuretics, and many others (29). Thus, xerostomia is more likely due to medications or a systemic disease (22, 30, 31) than to normal aging.

The typical salivary gland consists of acinar cells that secrete a solution that is modified by an active transport mechanism in the salivary ducts to produce saliva. Resting and stimulated salivary flow results in different concentrations of sodium, potassium, bicarbonate, and digestive enzymes.

Little is known about the changes in salivary composition with aging. Age does not alter the pH of stimulated saliva (21, 22). However, the majority of elderly individuals have a resting and stimulated salivary buffer effect below normal (19, 22). Selective changes occur in electrolyte composition in saliva with aging. The sodium content of stimulated parotid saliva declines with age, while potassium content remains unaltered (25). Anionic proline-rich protein secretion by the parotid gland is unaffected by age (32). Age-related changes in salivary amylase content have not been described. Salivary amylase normally contributes 14% of the total amylase content in the small bowel (33). Salivary amylase is normally destroyed in the strongly acidic milieu of the stomach. In achlorhydria, amylase is not destroyed in the stomach, and 27% of the amylase in the small bowel is of salivary origin (33).

Salivary immunoglobulin levels and protein content remain unchanged in the aged. The opsonic activity of the saliva, however, is reduced in the elderly, and this may have relevance in the immune response to oral microbial pathogens (34). Because data on compositional changes of saliva with aging are fragmentary, the reported changes do not appear to be significant to some investigators (35).

To summarize the effects of aging on the salivary glands in man:

1. A decrease in acinar cell volume occurs with age, and the gland volume is maintained by replacement with fat, ducts, and fibrous tissue.
2. Slight decreases in stimulated and unstimulated salivary flow occur with aging, but most of this decrease may be due to concomitant drug usage.
3. Dry mouth is a frequent complaint in the elderly; this complaint is best correlated with drug usage but may also be due to age-related decreases in salivary flow.
4. Both the sodium and the buffer content of saliva are reported to decrease with age; in addition, the opsonic activity of saliva decreases with age. Whether these changes have clinical significance is not yet known.

Pancreas

The gross anatomic and histologic changes that occur with aging must be taken into account when interpreting ultrasonography, computerized tomography (CT), and pancreatography. The head, body, and tail varies markedly between individuals but progressively shrinks with age (36, 37). Autopsy studies, using retrograde pancreatography, show that the main pancreatic duct diameter increases 8% per decade after age 40 (38). The maximal duct diameter increases up to 1 cm without any evidence of obstruction and maintains the normal uniform tapering appearance with smooth margins (38, 39). Intralobular and interlobular duct dilatation as well as small cyst formation increase with age. Endoscopic retrograde cholangiopancreatography (ERCP) reveals smaller age-related increases in the diameter of the main duct. The diameter of the main pancreatic duct in the adult is 3 to 4 mm by ERCP and increases slightly in the elderly (37). Some discrepancy occurs in any radiographic test due to distention from instillation of contrast medium and radiographic magnification. High-resolution real-time ultrasonography of the main pancreatic duct does not reveal any variation of duct size with age (40). The diameter of the normal pancreatic ducts are 2 mm or less by ultrasound (41). These negative ultrasonographic results must be interpreted cautiously because the resolution of the method is not sufficient to detect slight changes in diameter.

Significant fatty infiltration occurs in the acini of the pancreas in the elderly (37). Abdominal CT scans of individuals without pancreatic disease reveal a significant increase in the lobulation of the external contour of the pancreas with age, which is felt to correspond to progressive fat replacement of the pancreatic parenchyma (36, 42). Age-related increases in pancreatic fat are felt to be reflected in increased echogenicity seen on ultrasonography (43). The histologic development of diffuse fine and patchy intra-acinar fibrosis increases with age (44). Increased inhomogenous and patchy structures in the pancreas on CT scans in the elderly are thought to be due to localized fibrosis, sclerosis, and lipomatosis (36, 42).

The pancreas has a major role as an exocrine and endocrine gland. The endocrine portion is responsible for secretion of many hormones including insulin, glucagon, somatostatin, vasoactive intestinal polypeptide (VIP), and pancreatic polypeptide, while the exocrine portion is important in the secretion of bicarbonate, water, digestive enzymes, and other electrolytes.

The acinar and duct cells form the basis of the exocrine system. Acinar cells make up more than 80% of the pancreas and are responsible for the secretion of the digestive enzymes. These cells are well organized for the production of large amounts of enzymes. Duct cells contribute bicarbonate, water, and other electrolytes to pancreatic juice. The main pancreatic duct may also contribute to the fluid and electrolytes secreted (45).

Secretin is a potent stimulant of duct cells to secrete bicarbonate and fluid, but it also is a weak inducer of acinar cell enzyme secretion. In contrast, cholecystokinin (CCK) primarily stimulates enzyme secretion, but it is also a weak inducer of bicarbonate and water. Age-related changes in the mechanisms controlling the secretion of pancreatic juice have not been described.

In vivo studies on elderly subjects are conflicting as to whether pancreatic output is decreased (46–48) or unchanged (49, 50). The reserve capacity is enormous since clinical malabsorption is not present until 90% of the gland is functionally absent (51). Acinar cells produce more than a dozen enzymes and coenzymes. The isotonic alkaline solution neutralizes acidic gastric chyme and maintains an optimal pH range for activation of digestive enzymes. Maximal pancreatic enzyme output is maintained for the first 2 to 3 hours after a solid or liquid meal. Reducing postprandial acid output by 50% with cimetidine does not change trypsin and lipase outputs (52). Reduced acid load delivery to the duodenum as in achlorhydria probably does not affect pancreatic enzyme secretion.

In vivo studies have been performed to obtain pancreatic juices by quantitative aspiration of duodenal contents after a variety of stimuli including a standard meal (53), a bolus dose of secretin (46, 49), a bolus dose of secretin and CCK (47), continuous stimulation by secretin and cerulein (50), the pancreolauryl test (50), or endoscopic catheterization of the pancreatic duct with stimulation by secretion and CCK (48). Some of these studies showed no change in bicarbonate or pancreatic enzymes with age (49, 50, 53–55), while others suggest a reduction in bicarbonate, pancreatic juice output, trypsin, chymotrypsin, and lipase (48) or a selective reduction in some enzymes (46). Another study using two repetitive bolus injections of secretin and CCK reported a diminished secretion of pancreatic juice bicarbonate and amylase, suggesting impaired pancreatic reserve or reduced sensitivity to stimuli (47). The limited number of subjects and possibly incomplete collection of duodenal juice casts some doubt on many of the above studies. In spite of these limitations, there appears to be a slight decrease in pancreatic exocrine secretion due to age, but this may not be clinically significant.

Age-related changes in serum pancreatic enzymes must be considered when evaluating a patient for possible pancreatic disease. The serum pancreatic amylase isoenzyme fraction but not the total serum amylase diminishes with aging (56). In contrast, pancreatic serum immunoreactive trypsin is markedly increased in healthy elderly persons (57–60). The serum level of trypsin is dependent upon renal clearance, but similar elevations are found in elderly persons with normal renal function (59). Data on serum lipase in the elderly are conflicting, revealing no changes (57) or increases up to 32% above normal (60).

To summarize the effects of aging on the pancreas and its exocrine function:

1. The pancreas shrinks with age, and there is an increase in fat and fibrous tissue and an increased ductal diameter.
2. Some studies show a decrease in pancreatic secretory output of bicarbonate and enzymes with age, but others show no changes. Age-related changes do occur but are slight and do not result in impaired digestion.
3. The fraction of normal serum amylase contributed by pancreatic isoamylases decreases with age.

Stomach

The stomach mucosa is composed of a single layer of columnar epithelial cells with intervening gastric pits containing gastric glands. The gastric glands are responsible for the secretion of HCL, pepsinogen, gastrin, intrinsic factor, mucus, and many gastrointestinal hormones. Age-related changes in the histology of the gastric mucosa and its secretion are frequently difficult to differentiate from the cumulative damage from ethanol, aspirin, nonsteroidal anti-inflammatory drugs (NSAID), stress, and toxins. The damage to the mucosa over time, due to all of these influences, may result in atrophic gastritis, gastric atrophy, achlorhydria, and intrinsic factor deficiency.

The simplest method to measure basal and stimulated acid output is by aspirating gastric contents through a radiopaque gastric tube. Maximal acid output (MAO) or peak acid output (PAO) can be determined by administering histamine, a histamine analog, betazole (Histalog), or a gastrin analog, pentagastrin. The limitations of this method include the difficulty with positioning the tube, intermixing with saliva, and loss of fluid into the duodenum. Despite these limitations, acid secretion can be quantified with considerable accuracy.

The overall trend of basal acid output (BAO) in aging is one of decline (61–65), although one study has found no change (66). In the early studies in patients with decreased basal acid output, morphologic damage to the gastric mucosa was not evaluated. Recently, decreases in BAO with aging were found in patients with a histologically normal fundic mucosa (64).

Maximal acid secretory capacity diminishes with aging (61–63, 65, 67, 68) with few exceptions (66). The decrease in maximal acid output (MAO) parallels the increased prevalence of superficial gastritis and atrophic changes with aging (67). In one study of a randomly selected population, no decrease in MAO, expressed as fat-free body weight, was present when the individuals with morphologically normal fundic mucosa were examined separately (67). However, the overall population trend still showed a decreased acid output with increasing age. Gastric output depends significantly on the morphologic state of the mucosa.

The incidence of true achlorhydria rises with age, but it remains uncertain if this represents normal or pathologic changes. Several earlier studies have cited a high percentage of achlorhydria in the elderly (69), but limitations of the test method, sensitivity of the testing reagents, and failure to account for the condition of the gastric mucosa may have overestimated the numbers. Many of the individuals probably had decreased acid secretion rather than true achlorhydria. In any case, the higher pH associated with achlorhydria or hypochlorhydria may have profound effects on the absorption of iron, folic acid, calcium, vitamins A and E, and cobalamin and may result in bacterial growth in the small intestine.

Pepsinogen secretion decreases with aging (65), but the decrease is not as marked as that of acid secretion (70). Serum pepsinogen levels correlate best with the morphologic appearance of the gastric mucosa but decline only after severe damage (70–73). The increased severity of chronic fundic gastritis results in the progressive decrease in the serum pepsinogen I to pepsinogen II ratio determined by specific radioimmunoassays (72).

Intrinsic factor (IF) is essential for the binding and absorption of cobalamin (B_{12}). Synthesis and secretion of IF occurs in the parietal cells of the oxyntic glands. Total gastrectomy is accompanied by cobalamin (B_{12}) malabsorption due to IF deficiency, but the deficiency does not occur for 3 to 5 years due to adequate B_{12} stores. The loss of gastric glands related to aging is difficult to differentiate from loss due to other causes such as autoimmunity, drugs, and environmental damage. Mild declines in IF secretion with normal aging (68) are probably offset by the enormous daily excess of IF secreted (74), so that B_{12} deficiency does not occur. Intrinsic factor deficiency is increased in the elderly. However, this occurs only after severe and almost total loss of gastric glands, which probably represents pathologic changes rather than normal aging.

Age-related changes in the morphology of the gastric mucosa are very common. However, the classification and etiology of such changes have defied rational explanation. The symptoms ascribed to chronic gastritis bear little relationship to the radiologic changes said to be due to gastritis, and neither radiologic changes nor symptoms correlate with histologic changes in the mucosa. For the purposes of this section, only histologic changes are discussed. The etiology of chronic gastritis is unknown. It seems likely that many factors are involved, and these probably include autoimmune mechanisms, infectious agents, other environmental factors, and aging.

Classically, chronic gastritis has been divided into chronic superficial gastritis, chronic atrophic gastritis, and chronic gastric atrophy. Superficial gastritis is characterized by inflammatory cells such as lymphocytes and plasma cells with or without polymorphonuclear leukocytes limited to the lamina propria of the gastric pits without involvement of the gastric glands. Atrophic gastritis is characterized by similar inflammatory cell infiltration but with extensive involvement of the entire lamina propria and progressive loss of gastric glandular cells. Total obliteration of gastric glands is seen in gastric atrophy, and the gastric mucosa may be replaced by an intestinal type columnar epithelium.

Atrophic gastritis has been classified into type A and type B (75). Type A chronic atrophic gastritis occurs throughout the body and fundus, and it is frequently associated with hypochlorhydria, pernicious anemia, and parietal cell antibodies. Type B chronic atrophic gastritis is more common and can occur as a patchy process in the antrum with variable involvement of the fundus. Unfortunately, many individuals with atrophic gastritis cannot be classified as belonging to type A or B (76).

Helicobacter pylori has added a new element in attempts to classify gastritis. The prevalence of *H. pylori* increases with age and *H.pylori* has been found in greater than 75% of individuals over the age of 60 (77, 78). *Helicobacter pylori* has been associated with chronic antral gastritis (79), particularly type B chronic gastritis (78). Despite the association of *H. pylori* with aging and gastritis, the causality remains to be determined.

The overall prevalence of chronic gastritis varies in different studies from 48% to 96% in populations in such different geographic locations as Estonia, Finland, Hungary, Italy, Japan, and New South Wales (80–83). All these authors agree that an increase in prevalence of chronic gastritis occurs with aging. No population studies have been done in North America, but similar increases with aging appear likely.

The natural history of chronic gastritis appears to be a slow progression from chronic superficial gastritis to chronic atrophic gastritis (84). Although the main trend is one of progressive damage, the process is actually a dynamic one, with progression and regression of superficial gastritis and atrophic gastritis (84, 85). In a long-term study over 23 to 27 years, fundic superficial gastritis improved in 18% and progressed to atrophic fundic gastritis in 42% (84).

Atrophic gastritis tends to extend proximally with aging, occurring more on the lesser curvature than on the greater curvature (82). In many cases, the superficial and atrophic changes are often more pronounced in the antrum rather than the fundus (84).

To summarize the effects of aging on the stomach:

1. Basal acid output (BAO) decreases with age in most studies, and this decrease may be unrelated to mucosal changes.
2. Maximal acid output (MAO) also decreases with age, and this decrease is positively correlated with gastritis and atrophic changes in the gastric mucosa.
3. Pepsinogen production decreases slightly with age and correlates with abnormalities in the gastric mucosa.
4. Intrinsic factor (IF) secretion decreases slightly with normal aging; clinically important decreases in IF secretion occur only when the mucosa is severely damaged by disease.
5. Chronic gastritis increases with age; atrophic gastritis tends to extend proximally with aging. The relative contributions of uncomplicated aging and disease on gastritis is simply unknown.

Liver and Biliary Tract

The importance of considerations of liver function and liver disease in patients anticipating surgery is not difficult to understand. Not only must the liver produce adequate amounts of clotting factors to make surgery possible, but underlying liver disorders may impair the metabolism of anesthetic agents, analgesics, and sedatives. When compounded by additional age-related alterations of hepatic capacities and functions, the considerations of the liver during surgery become even more important. The fact that commonly used liver function tests may change little with age despite age-related alterations in some important liver functions, especially drug metabolism, makes understanding of the present status of knowledge of these changes important for the internist, the surgeon, and the anesthesiologist.

There are some distinct changes in hepatic anatomy and physiology with aging, but their clinical importance has not been clearly delineated in many cases. Autopsy studies show that the liver decreases in size during aging (86, 87). This decrease is proportionately greater than the decrease in total body weight that normally is seen with aging. There is some evidence that there may be a compensatory hypertrophy of individual hepatocytes (88, 89), and there is an increase in the number of binucleated hepatocytes with age (90). Whether these histologic changes reflect any metabolic compensation for loss of liver mass is not known.

Blood flow to the liver distinctly decreases with age (91–93) and falls on the order of 1% per year. This is of potentially great importance in the metabolism of certain drugs in the elderly. The metabolism of drugs such as propranolol and isoproterenol, which are normally cleared from plasma by the "first pass" through the liver, is exquisitely dependent on changes in hepatic blood flow. This could be especially important if blood flow changes intraoperatively due to hypotension and cardiac decompensation, or postoperatively in the recovery room.

Hepatic drug metabolism is characterized by two general mechanisms, microsomal oxidation and hydrolysis (phase I reactions) and conjugation with glucuronide or other moieties (phase II reactions). Some drugs first require microsomal oxidation before they can be conjugated and excreted, while others merely require conjugation directly.

It is difficult to generalize about drug metabolism in the elderly since actual drug elimination studies often have unpredictable results. Frequently, however, those drugs which only require conjugation (an example is Lorazepam) are eliminated at a normal rate in the elderly. Drugs that require microsomal oxidation (such as acetaminophen) frequently are more slowly metabolized in the elderly. Knowing that hepatic clearance of some drugs is decreased and that age effects are not always predictable, the best rule is to use smaller doses of any drug in older patients.

One specific drug worth mentioning, the anticoagulant warfarin, is metabolized by the liver. The liver is also the site of action of the drug. Although the metabolism of the drug is normal in the elderly (normal clearance) (94), the aging liver cell is unusually sensitive to a given dose of the drug (pharmacodynamic effect) (95). Thus the older patient requires significantly smaller doses to obtain the accepted level of anticoagulation.

Commonly used liver function tests are surprisingly well maintained with age. In patients with biopsy-proven normal liver histology, there were little or no changes in transaminase, bilirubin, or alkaline phosphatase with age (96). The albumin level in plasma does fall slightly with age (97) and could influence the metabolism of drugs that depend on albumin binding. Bromsulphalein (BSP) excretion appears to decrease with age (98), suggesting a decreased capacity for transport and storage of organic anions in the elderly. When alkaline phosphatase elevation is the sole abnormality, the most likely cause is Paget's disease of the bone. Thus, abnormal liver function tests in the elderly require a search for disease, not age alone, as the cause.

There is general agreement that there is decreased activity of the cellular immune system in the aged. This may account for the observation that the clinical manifestations of acute viral hepatitis tend to be milder in the aged (99). In the older patient with hepatitis, there is a smaller increase in transaminase and serum bilirubin and a greater rise in alkaline phosphatase (100).

Secretion of cholesterol by the liver is reported to increase with age. This increase is coupled with a decrease in bile acid synthesis (101). These changes would appear to explain the increase in cholesterol saturation of bile in the elderly. Such an increase in cholesterol and decrease in bile acids predispose to the formation of gallstones, and these biochemical changes parallel the incidence of gallstones in the elderly.

Table 8-1 summarizes the effect of aging on the liver.

Table 8-1. Aging changes in the liver

1. Liver size	Decreased
2. Hepatocytes	Increased in size with increased polyploidy, pigment inclusions (lipofuscin)
3. Hepatic blood flow	Decreased
4. Hepatobiliary transport	Decreased for BSP
5. Microsomal drug metabolism	Normal to decreased
6. Glucuronidation	Generally unchanged
7. Serum albumin	Slightly decreased
8. Routine liver chemistries	Normal
9. Hepatic secretion of cholesterol	Increased
10. Bile acid synthesis	Decreased

Small Intestine

The principal function of the small intestine is to absorb nutrients, water, electrolytes, and minerals. Other functions are to secrete enzymes and hormones.

The absorbing surface of the small intestine in man is very great, estimated at 200 m^2, if one includes the surface of the microvilli. In animals, the morphology of the villi are reported by some investigators to be altered in old age (102). In man, the scanty evidence available would suggest that aging has a slight but definite effect on small intestinal morphology. In one study of 39 patients, ages 67–90 years, the villi were shorter than in a control group and in other published series. In addition, there was a suggestion that the villi were broader in the aged (103). In a preliminary report, the villous surface in well-nourished elderly patients was reduced when compared to younger patients (104). It should be noted that no studies of the microvilli have been done in the aged. Such studies may yield important information since microvilli are important both as an absorbing surface and as the locus of a number of functionally important enzymes.

The absorption of carbohydrates is decreased in elderly human subjects. Absorption of a standard meal, containing 100 g of carbohydrate, was monitored by breath hydrogen excretion. Subjects between 65 and 89 years of age had a decreased carbohydrate absorption, and this decrease was more striking the older the subject (102). Xylose was also less efficiently absorbed in a group of geriatric patients than in a younger group (105).

Protein absorption has not been well studied in the aged, but the consensus is that such absorption is well maintained (102).

Studies of fat absorption have not been adequate to enable us to know whether fat is malabsorbed. Several studies suggest that chylomicron responses to a standard meal are lower in the elderly (106), but the data are simply inadequate to permit a final conclusion.

Absorption of both calcium and iron are reported to be decreased in the aged (102). The calcium malabsorption may well be related to the low acid production in the elderly stomach (107).

Absorption of fat-soluble vitamins is said to be increased in the aged, but more studies need to be done to elucidate the possible mechanisms for hyperabsorption. Absorption of water-soluble vitamins are not changed in the aged, but again studies are sparse.

To summarize the data on the small intestine:

1. Surface area and villus height of the small intestine are slightly decreased in the aged.
2. Carbohydrate absorption is decreased in the aged.

3. Calcium and iron absorption are decreased in the elderly.
4. Vitamin, fat, and protein absorption have not been studied thoroughly enough to reach firm conclusions.

Connective Tissue Functions

Visceral Smooth Muscle

The digestive system is equipped with an intricate neuromuscular system that propels food down the digestive tract and promotes both digestion and absorption by control mechanisms that are both neural and endocrine.

Traditionally, this neuromuscular function has been referred to as "motility," but it is often unclear whether motility (or movement) refers to contractions of the muscle or movement of intraluminal contents. For simplicity, the effect of aging on three in vivo functions that are caused by smooth muscle activity are discussed: tone, phasic contractions, and intraluminal transit.

Tone in smooth muscle is the maintenance of active tension over a sustained period. This function is calcium and energy dependent but is quite economical of energy. Another way of defining tone is that it is the resistance of the muscle to stretch.

Phasic contractions in the esophagus, stomach, and small and large bowel are the active contractions that promote mixing, absorption, and/or transit. A measurement of intraluminal pressure is a way of detecting these contractions. Recordings of electropotentials with electrodes also indicate contractions (action potentials) and control potentials (slow waves, MMC).

Intraluminal movement is one final result of all contractions and is a simple, and probably simplistic, way to assess smooth muscle function. Transit times have the advantage of being the sum of all aboral and oral movements.

Esophagus

Swallowing disorders are very common in the elderly and result in significant morbidity and mortality. Presbyesophagus is the term given to esophageal motor dysfunction attributed to aging (108). Many manometric and cineradiographic changes attributed to aging are probably due to disease. Much confusion still exists as to the effect of aging on esophageal function.

The process of swallowing begins once food has been placed in the mouth. Initially, food needs to be moistened and broken down to allow a smooth passage. The absence of dentition, improperly fitting dentures, or alteration in salivary flow may impair an otherwise normal passage. Even when comparing young and elderly individuals with the same number of teeth, there is an age-related increase in the chewing time and the number of chewing strokes prior to swallowing (109, 110). The presence of dentures causes a further decline in the masticatory function (110). Accidental choking due to the diminished masticatory function may result during periods of altered mental status. Postoperative infections and medications are frequent causes of altered mental status in the elderly. The selection of foods that are softer and easier to chew will help minimize complications.

Limited information is known about the anatomic changes of normal aging in the pharynx and esophagus. The pharyngeal constrictors are primarily composed of Type II muscle fibers, while the proximal esophagus is primarily Type I muscle fibers. Age-related changes in the percent of Type I fibers and changes in the mean muscle fiber diameter have not been found to occur (111). However, a significant decrease in the density of muscle fibers occurs in the pharynx and proximal esophagus (111) with aging. The actual thickness of the longitudinal and circular smooth muscles of the distal esophagus does not change with advancing age (112). The increase of sliding hiatal hernias in the elderly has been postulated to be caused by the upward migration of the lower esophagus and lower esophageal sphincter due to muscular and ligamentous laxity (113, 114).

Very little is known about alterations in the neurologic control of the esophagus in aging. A decrease in the number of ganglionic cells per cm^2 occurs in the distal esophagus in the elderly, and this has been suggested as a possible cause for motor dysfunction (112). Most studies of the anatomic changes rely on autopsy specimens, which have not been correlated with function in life.

In the resting state, the upper esophageal sphincter (UES) and lower esophageal sphincter (LES) maintain a basal muscle tone. The length and resting pressure of the LES remains constant with aging (108, 115–117). With deglutition, the UES and LES relax to accommodate the passage of food. The relaxation phase allows passage of a bolus of food. This is followed by a contraction phase to close the LES with a gradual return to the basal muscle tone. In aging, a decrease in the amplitude of the contraction phase is seen, but there is no change in the relaxation phase (115). The duration of each phase remains constant. Inadequate LES response occurs in up to 5.9% of healthy young individuals. However, individuals over age 60 have up to 17.8% inadequate LES responses to deglutition mainly due to the absence of the contraction phase or total absence of both phases (115).

Conflicting data exist on alterations of esophageal contractions in aging. Differences in the techniques used in measuring these contractions and the use of elderly populations that frequently have a high rate of disease in the esophagus have added to the confusion. The onset of peristalsis after swallowing remains unchanged in asymptomatic elderly individuals (118). The amplitude of the primary peristaltic wave in elderly patients varies considerably from study to study and includes no change at all (108, 117). However, a 33% decrease in the amplitude of the peristaltic wave in the lower esophagus occurred in one group of asymptomatic elderly individuals over 60 years (115), while marked differences throughout the esophagus were not seen in another group until after age 80 (118). The peristaltic velocity remains constant (108, 118) or slows slightly in the lower third of the esophagus (115) with aging. The duration of the primary peristaltic pressure wave remains constant (108, 117, 118).

Aging may affect the chance that swallowing is followed by a primary peristaltic wave. Early cineradiographic studies showed that swallowing is followed by peristalsis in 85% of cases in all ages (119). However, peristalsis following swallowing was noted to occur in only 50% of octogenarians and 20% of nonagenarians. Early manometric studies, which included many individuals with neuromuscular diseases, found peristalsis in only 51% of nonagenarians following swallowing (108). Other studies in asymptomatic elderly individuals without neurologic disease reported that peristalsis resulted from swallowing 75% to 98% of the time (115, 117, 118). Primary peristalsis was absent in 25.3% of swallows in healthy individuals over the age of 60, as compared to 8.2% of swallows in healthy individuals under age 40 (115).

Secondary peristalsis, as measured by balloon distention of the esophagus, has not been adequately studied in healthy elderly individuals.

Conflicting data exist on whether tertiary contractions are normal phenomena (120), the consequence of aging, or the result of disease. Early studies using cineradiology revealed frequent tertiary contractions occurring in 60% of nonagenarians (108). However, most of these patients had neurologic diseases that frequently were associated with altered motility. Another study suggests that tertiary waves occur in all age groups and markedly increase only after age 71 (119). One manometric study on healthy elderly men reported no increase in tertiary contractions (118).

Esophageal clearance and neutralization of refluxed acid normally occurs after the first or second peristaltic wave in the presence of normal saliva (121). Esophageal clearance by cineradiographic measurement remains constant until after the age of 81 years, when it substantially decreases (119). Decreased peristalsis or a decrease in saliva may decrease acid clearance. Very little information is available on gastroesophageal reflux in the elderly (122). A slight increase in erect gastroesophageal reflux occurs with age, but the clinical significance is unknown (123). The presence of a sliding hiatal hernia does not appear to play an important role in the development of gastroesophageal reflux, but the association remains controversial (124–127).

To summarize the effects of aging on esophageal motor function:

1. Resting LES pressure does not change with age.
2. The amplitude of the contraction phase of the LES to deglutition decreases with age.
3. Inadequate LES response to deglutition increases in the elderly.
4. The amplitude of the primary peristaltic wave decreases with age.
5. Aging decreases the chance that a swallow will be followed by a primary peristaltic wave.
6. Tertiary waves in the body of the esophagus are more common in the aged. Whether this effect is due to uncomplicated aging or disease is not known.

Stomach

Gastric emptying results from a complex coordinated process involving the proximal stomach, distal stomach, pylorus, and duodenum. This is finely controlled by neurotransmitters, hormones, and paracrine substances. Gastric emptying can be affected by drugs, systemic disease, gastric surgery, particle size, and meal composition. Liquids empty from the stomach at a more rapid rate than solids. However, solutions that are hyperosmolar, acidic, or high in fatty acid concentrations are delayed in the stomach. The proximal stomach has a major role in determining gastric emptying of liquids. The emptying of solids from the stomach occurs primarily as a function of the antrum and the pyloric segment.

Changes in gastric emptying remain controversial due to the variability of methods for evaluating emptying. Limitations result from technical problems, uncontrolled studies with too few individuals, and different testing materials. The most frequent methods of measuring gastric emptying are gastroduodenal intubation, radiologic techniques involving a barium meal, real-time ultrasound, and radionuclide test meals. Radioisotope tests are currently the most reliable method due to the noninvasiveness, reduced radiation hazard, practicality, and the wide range of physiologic meals.

Gastric emptying of liquids by real-time ultrasound show that the elderly have an impaired early adaptive phase in which there is a rapid loss of liquid from the stomach during the first 5 minutes (128). However, no alterations are seen after the first 5 minutes of gastric emptying by real-time ultrasound. Radionuclide studies of the liquid phase of gastric emptying in elderly patients with multiple chronic diseases were associated with a significant delay (129). The delay is probably due to the disease state rather than aging. Another radionuclide study looking at the solid phase of gastric emptying showed a significant delay in the elderly (130). Dual radionuclide studies of gastric emptying of liquids and solids have shown either a delay of liquids emptying only (131) or a delay in emptying of both liquids and solids (132). The finding of a delay in both the solid and liquid phases of gastric emptying is real, but the differences from normal are not great and are unlikely to be clinically significant (131, 132) in the absence of systemic disease.

Conflicting data exist as to whether gender or menopause affects gastric emptying (132–135). Premenopausal and postmenopausal women on hormone replacement were shown to have slower liquid and solid phase gastric emptying than did men or postmenopausal women by dual radionuclide techniques (133, 135). However, no differences based on gender were found in the number of antral contractions, mean amplitude of contractions, or motility index (133).

None of the above studies examined the histology of the gastric mucosa to determine if it influenced gastric emptying. Gastric emptying in achlorhydric persons with atrophic gastritis and persons with hyposecretion of acid has been shown to be altered (136). Achlorhydria is associated with a marked delay in the solid phase of gastric emptying, while the liquid phase of emptying remains normal (137) or increases (136). The delay in solid-phase gastric emptying is felt to be due to a problem with antral motility and to the alkaline pH, since gastric emptying improves in 40% of the persons with metoclopramide and in 20% with the instillation of HCL (137).

To summarize the effects of aging on gastric emptying:

1. There is a mild delay in the emptying of liquids and solids from the stomach in the aged.
2. These delays may be related to decreased acid secretion or to disease.

Small Intestine

Movement of contents through the small intestine and the mixing of contents are mediated by myogenic mechanisms (the migrating myogenic complex or MMC), peptide hormones, and the autonomic nervous system.

Aging has been reported (138) to increase the length of the MMC cycle in the proximal jejunum, but no effect has been noted on the duration of phase III of the MMC or the propagation of the MMC. During the fed state, the frequency of phasic contractions of the small intestine decreased significantly (139), but no changes in amplitude of the contractions were noted.

The transit time of barium in the small intestine is quite variable, but no significant differences due to age or gender were observed in one study (140).

No good studies have been done to assess the effect of aging on the tone of the small intestine. However, on the basis of observation of plain films of the abdomen in elderly patients, the suspicion exists that the amount of air in the small bowel is often excessive, even in the absence of overt disease. A decrease in tone and a decrease in "clearing" of the bowel would account for this excess air. Admittedly, this is speculation.

To summarize the effect of aging on small intestinal motility:

1. The length of the MMC cycle increases slightly with age.
2. The frequency of phasic contractions decreases with age.
3. No changes in transit time have been reported; decrease in tone of the small intestine seems likely but evidence is not available to prove this.

Large Intestine

Information is still sparse on the limits of normality of colonic movements. In addition, the control of colonic motor function is still incompletely understood. Electrical control waves are readily recorded from distal colonic muscle, but the role of these waves in coordinating proximal colonic contractions is uncertain. Electrical control, neuropeptides, and autonomic neural function are all important in the control of colonic motility.

Gastrointestinal neuropeptide concentrations in the muscularis externa of the colon are unchanged in the aged (141). However, electrophysiologic studies of the circular muscle of the normal sigmoid colon suggest that a decrease in binding sites for inhibitory neuropeptides, or alternatively, a decrease in release of inhibitory neuropeptides might occur with aging (142).

The variation in normal motor patterns as indicated by intraluminal pressure recordings in the colon is very great. As a result, it is difficult to detect definite abnormalities, even if present. In one study of intraluminal pressures in the rectosigmoid colon, age and gender did not affect the patterns (143).

Total or segmental colonic transit times as indicated by gelatin capsules (144) or radiopaque markers (145, 146) are not affected by aging.

Anorectal Segment

Anorectal function has received considerable attention due to the easy accessibility. Numerous methods have been developed to study anorectal function. Normal continence depends on the integration of smooth muscle, striated muscle, and sphincters coordinated by mechanisms ranging from local reflexes to higher cortical input. Incontinence is prevented by the interaction of two anorectal sphincters and the pelvic diaphragm muscles. Two anal sphincters under tonic contraction help in the coordinated and timely passage of stool. The internal anal sphincter is a thickened, circular layer of smooth muscle under involuntary control. Surrounding the internal anal sphincter and slightly caudad is the external anal sphincter, which is composed of striated muscle under voluntary control. The puborectalis muscle, which is part of the pelvic diaphragm muscle, is important in the maintenance of continence of solid stool. A sling is formed around the rectum by the puborectalis muscle fibers. Contraction of the puborectalis muscle pulls the rectum forward, producing a 90-degree angle, aiding in the occlusion of the rectal lumen.

Feces entering the rectum cause distention of the wall, which triggers defecation reflexes. Distention results in the reflex relaxation of the internal anal sphincter and the initiation of contractions propelling feces toward the anus. Defecation is prevented by the voluntary contraction of the external anal sphincter and subsequent adaptation of the internal sphincter to the pressure. Defecation occurs when both anal sphincters relax and the puborectalis muscle relaxes, allowing the anorectal angle to straighten. Intact rectal and anal sensation is essential in differentiating solid, liquid, and gas in the distal rectum as well as in allowing for the appropriate timing and setting of defecation. Alterations in any of the anorectal functions can result in fecal incontinence or constipation.

Wide variations occur in the normal anorectal function, but significant changes occur with aging. The rectal diameter increases with aging (147, 148). Conflicting results exist for age-related changes in rectal pressure, with some having increases (147) and others decreases (149).

Resting anal pressure (RAP) mainly reflects the tonic contraction of the internal anal sphincter with a small contribution from the external anal sphincter. Most studies show a progressive decline in RAP with aging (149–153) or a decline only after the eighth decade (154). Elderly women have a more significant decline in RAP than elderly men (150, 151, 153, 154). Gender differences have been attributed to a stronger muscular system in men (149), a greater degree of perineal descent in elderly women as compared to young women, which does not occur in men (151), or neuropathic damage to the pudendal nerve due to multiparity (149, 152, 155), but this has been challenged (150).

The maximal squeeze pressure (MSP) in the anal canal is derived from the summed pressure of the voluntary maximal contraction of the external anal sphincter and pelvic diaphragm muscles. Elderly individuals have a significantly diminished MSP (149–151, 153, 154). Gender differences are not as consistent as in RAP. Elderly women have a greater decline in MSP than elderly men in some studies (150, 151, 153), but no difference in others (149, 154).

Balloon distention of the rectum produces higher rectal pressures (151) and lower anal canal pressures (149) in the elderly. This suggests a loss of elasticity. In addition, elderly women but not men require smaller rectal balloon volumes than young women to induce anal sphincter relaxation (151). The maximal tolerable volume but not maximal tolerable pressure during distention with a rectal balloon is significantly lower in the elderly (151). However, the rectal volume or pressure required to initiate rectal contractions does not change with aging (151).

Rectal sensory threshold to rectal distention does not vary with aging (151, 152). Normal defecatory sensation occurs in the nonconstipated elderly. However, older people require a longer time to pass a simulated stool (consisting of hard plastic spheres or a water-filled balloon), suggesting they may strain for longer periods when attempting to pass a stool (151).

To summarize the effects of aging on colonic and anorectal function:

1. Total or segmental transit times through the colon are not changed in the aged.
2. No consistent change in phasic motor activity in the proximal colon occurs with aging.
3. Rectal diameter increases with age.
4. Balloon distention of the rectum produces higher rectal pressures and lower anal canal pressures in the aged. This suggests a loss of elasticity with aging.
5. Resting anal pressure decreases with both sexes in the elderly, but to a much greater degree in females.
6. Maximal squeeze pressure in the anus decreases with aging.
7. Rectal sensory threshold to distention does not change with age.

Relation of colonic motility to constipation and diverticulosis. Interest in colonic and anorectal motility is considerably enhanced by the possibility that smooth muscle function contributes to the pathogenesis of two important conditions in the elderly, constipation and diverticulosis.

Constipation is a symptom rather than a clearly defined disease process. The subjective complaints of constipation include hard stools, small caliber stools, infrequent defecation, and incomplete evacuation. The frequency of bowel movements would seem a readily available objective measure, but the variation is very great in all ages. In a random sampling of people 62 to 90 years, 90% of women and 95% of men had a bowel movement between twice daily and once every 2 days (156). In spite of these apparently normal objective figures, most studies suggest that some of the above subjective symptoms are increased in the aged, and that some physiologic alterations probably coexist. According to a recent study (157), subjective constipation occurs in 0.5% of males under age 45 and 4.2% of males over age 65. In women, constipation occurs in 1.5% of those under 45 and in 8.4% of women over age 65.

The most likely causes of constipation in the elderly in this country are: 1) a diet low in fiber, 2) sedentary habits, and 3) disturbances in motility of the colon, including malfunction of the anorectal segment.

The contribution of diet to constipation became well known after the classical studies of Burkitt. The contribution of sedentary habits is less well appreciated. During the sleeping hours, the human colon is, fortunately, almost entirely quiescent. In addition, when a patient is awake but supine, motor activity in the colon is very slight. In many studies which report a high incidence of constipation, the patients are confined to bed, and this lack of activity undoubtedly contributes to an inactive colon.

The role of smooth muscle function or dysfunction in causing the symptoms and objective findings in constipation is not known. For years constipation was thought to be simply due to a sluggish colon with decreased contractions and virtual atony. Then there were reports (158, 159) that suggested that increased segmental colonic contractions impeded the passage of feces. The problem is made more difficult by our relative ignorance of the physiology of colonic transport. Many people still speak of "mass movements" as the predominant mechanism of transport, and there seems little evidence to support such a mechanism in man in the absence of a barium enema.

In spite of our global ignorance of colonic motor function, there are some findings in patients with constipation that may lead to a better understanding. Excess endogenous opioid activity has been reported (160, 161), which may increase segmental colonic contractions and impede fecal transit. Both reduced cholinergic nerve activity (162) and abnormal colonic myenteric plexuses (163) have been reported in the colon in patients with constipation.

Fecal impaction occurs as a consequence of impaired rectal sensation rather than as an alteration in the anal sphincters. Resting anal pressure and the maximal squeeze pressure in persons with fecal impaction are not decreased further from age-matched controls (164). In addition, the internal anal sphincter relaxes normally to rectal balloon distention but requires lower volumes to induce relaxation. In contrast, higher rectal distending volumes are necessary to induce rectal contractions, and larger volumes are needed to perceive rectal pain, fullness, and the urge to defecate in patients with fecal impaction (164). Seventy-four percent of the above individuals with fecal impaction had absent or impaired perianal sensation, and 77% had absent or impaired anal canal sensation. The impairment in rectal perception of feces leads to further accumulation of feces in the rectum and ultimately fecal impaction.

The second important condition in which colonic motility has been said to have a role is colonic diverticulosis. Whether motility plays a role or not is still controversial (165, 166). Abnormalities of colonic musculature (167, 168), elastic tissue (169), and collagen (165) have also been implicated in the formation of colonic diverticulosis. Diverticular disease of the colon in Western populations increases with age (168, 170–172), rising from 5% of individuals in the fifth decade to 50% in the ninth decade (171), but the true incidence is unknown because most patients are asymptomatic. Classically, diverticulosis was felt to result from low stool weight, increased intraluminal pressure, and prolonged transit time. Yet this remains controversial since normal stool weight (165) and normal luminal pressure (173) are frequently found in individuals with diverticulosis. An abnormally rapid electrical rhythm in colonic smooth muscle is found in some patients with symptomatic diverticular disease (174). This abnormally rapid rhythm was reduced by treatment with bran. However, the colonic transit time is not felt to be increased in patients with colonic diverticulosis (165).

In the absence of compelling data linking colonic motility abnormalities with diverticulosis, it can be tentatively concluded that colonic diverticula form as a result of normal intraluminal pressure, causing herniation through gaps in the muscularis that are protected only by fibrous tissue. This fibrous tissue and its principal protein, collagen, are less elastic in the aged and allow the creation of these pseudodiverticula.

Connective Tissue

Although connective tissue is not, strictly speaking, a part of this section, we must mention that age-related changes in connective tissue probably play a larger role in causing gastrointestinal disease than age-related changes in the mucosa or muscles of the gut or secretory organs.

The changes in connective tissue that make it less flexible may be due to the chemical nature of the collagen and other structural proteins. Whatever the cause, these changes occur throughout the body, including the human gut.

It seems likely that not only diverticulosis and hiatus hernia but also angiodysplasia of the gut (175, 176) are probably related to a failure of supporting connective tissue in the colon.

References

1. Shklar, G. 1966. The effects of aging upon oral mucosa. *J Invest Dermatol* 47:115–120.
2. Bartoshuk, LM. 1988. Clinical psychophysics of taste. *Gerodontics* 4:249–255.
3. Kullaa-Mikkonen, A, Koponen, A, and Seilonen, A. 1987. Quantitative study of human fungiform papillae and taste buds: Variation with aging and in different morphological forms of the tongue. *Gerodontics* 3:131–135.
4. Arvidson, K. 1979. Location and variation in number of taste buds in human fungiform papillae. *Scand J Dent Res* 87:435–442.
5. Miller, IJ. 1986. Variation in human fungiform taste bud densities among regions and subjects. *Anat Rec* 216: 474–482.
6. Miller, IJ. 1988. Human taste bud density across adult age groups. *J Gerontol* 43:B26–B30.
7. Bradley, RM. 1988. Effects of aging on the anatomy and neurophysiology of taste. *Gerodontics* 4:244–248.
8. Whitehead, MC. 1988. Neuroanatomy of the gustatory system. *Gerodontics* 4:239–243.
9. Chauhan, J, et al. 1987. Age-related olfactory and taste changes and interrelationships between taste and nutrition. *J Am Diet Assoc* 87:1543–1550.
10. Stevens, JC. 1984. Chemical senses and aging: Taste versus smell. *Chem Senses* 9:167–179.
11. Schiffman, S, and Pasternak, M. 1979. Decreased discrimination of food odors in the elderly. *J Gerontol* 34:73–79.
12. Scott, J. 1977. Quantitative age changes in the histological structure of human submandibular salivary glands. *Arch Oral Biol* 22:221–227.
13. Waterhouse, JP, et al. 1973. Replacement of functional parenchymal cells by fat and connective tissue in human submandibular salivary glands: An age-related change. *J Oral Pathol* 2:16–27.
14. Scott, J. 1977. A morphometric study of age changes in the histology of the ducts of human submandibular salivary glands. *Arch Oral Biol* 22:243–249.
15. Drummond, JR, and Chisholm, DM. 1984. A qualitative and quantitative study of the ageing human labial salivary gland. *Arch Oral Biol* 29:151–155.
16. Syrjanen, S. 1984. Age-related changes in structure of labial minor salivary glands. *Age Ageing* 13:159–165.
17. Ben-Aryeh, H, et al. 1984. Whole-saliva secretion rates in old and young healthy subjects. *J Dent Res* 63: 1147–1148.
18. Bertram, U. 1967. Studies on salivary secretion. *Acta Odontol Scand* (Suppl.) 49:1–126.
19. Heintze, U, Birkhed, D, and Bjorn, H. 1983. Secretion rate and buffer effect of resting and stimulated whole saliva as a function of age and sex. *Swed Dent J* 7: 227–238.
20. Gandara, BK, et al. 1985. Age-related salivary flow rate changes in controls and patients with oral lichen planus. *J Dent Res* 64:1149–1151.
21. Parvinen, T, and Larmas, M. 1982. Age dependency of stimulated salivary flow rate, pH, and lactobacillus and yeast concentrations. *J Dent Res* 61:1052–1055.
22. Thorselius, E, Emilson, CG, and Osterberg, T. 1988. Salivary conditions and drug consumption in older age groups of elderly Swedish individuals. *Gerodontics* 4:66–70.
23. Heft, MW, and Baum, BJ. 1984. Unstimulated and stimulated parotid salivary flow rate in individuals of different ages. *J Dent Res* 63:1182–1185.
24. Baum, BJ. 1981. Evaluation of stimulated parotid saliva flow rate in different age groups. *J Dent Res* 60: 1292–1296.
25. Baum, BJ, Costa, PT, and Izutsu, KT. 1984. Sodium handling by aging human parotid glands is inconsistent with a two-stage secretion model. *Am J Physiol* 246:R35–R39.
26. Pedersen, W, et al. 1985. Age-dependent decreases in human submandibular gland flow rates as measured under resting and post-stimulation conditions. *J Dent Res* 64:822–825.
27. Handelman, SL, et al. 1986. Prevalence of drugs causing hyposalivations in an institutionalized geriatric population. *Oral Surg Oral Med Oral Pathol* 62:26–31.
28. Levy, SM, et al. 1988. Use of medications with dental significance by the non-institutionalized elderly population. *Gerodontics* 4:119–125.
29. Sreebny, LM, and Schwartz, SS. 1986. Reference guide to drugs and dry mouth. *Gerodontology* 5:75–99.
30. Sreebny, LM, and Valdini, A. 1987. Xerostomia. *Arch Intern Med* 147:1333–1337.
31. Fox, PC, et al. 1985. Xerostomia: Evaluation of a symptom with increasing significance. *J Am Dent Assoc* 110:519–525.
32. Baum, BJ, Kousvelari, EE, and Oppenheim, FG. 1982. Exocrine protein secretion from human parotid glands during aging: Stable release of the acidic proline-rich proteins. *J Gerontol* 37:392–395.
33. Fried, M, Abramson, S, and Meyer, JH. 1987. Passage of salivary amylase through the stomach in humans. *Dig Dis Sci* 32:1097–1103.
34. Ganguly, R, et al. 1986. Defective antimicrobial functions of oral secretions in the elderly. *J Infect Dis* 153: 163–164.
35. Baum, BJ. 1986. Salivary gland function during aging. *Gerodontics* 2:61–64.
36. Heuck, A, et al. 1987. Age-related morphology of the normal pancreas on computer tomography. *Gastrointest Radiol* 12:18–22.
37. MacCarty, RL. 1986. Imaging of the pancreas. In *The Exocrine Pancreas: Biology, Pathobiology and Disease*, Ed., VLW Go. New York: Raven Press.
38. Kreel, L, and Sandlin, B. 1973. Changes in pancreatic morphology associated with aging. *Gut* 14:962–970.
39. Millbourn, E. 1960. Calibre and appearance of the pancreatic ducts and relevant clinical problems: A roentgenographic and anatomic study. *Acta Chir Scand* 118: 286–303.
40. Bryan, PJ. 1982. Appearance of normal pancreatic duct: A study using real-time ultrasound. *J Clin Ultrasound* 10:63–66.
41. Parulekar, SG. 1980. Ultrasonic evaluation of the pancreatic duct. *J Clin Ultrasound* 8:457–463.

42. Kreel, L, Haertel, M, and Katz, D. 1977. Computed tomography of the normal pancreas. *J Comput Assist Tomogr* 1:290–299.
43. Worthen, NJ, and Beabeau, D. 1982. Normal pancreatic echogenicity: Relation to age and body fat. *Am J Radiol* 139:1095–1098.
44. Pitchumoni, CS, et al. 1984. Pancreatic fibrosis in chronic alcoholics and nonalcoholics without clinical pancreatitis. *Am J Gastroenterol* 79:382–388.
45. Scratcherd, T, and Case, RM. 1973. The secretion of electrolytes by the pancreas. *Am J Clin Nutr* 26:326–339.
46. Fikry, ME. 1968. Exocrine pancreatic functions in the aged. *J Am Geriatr Soc* 16:463–468.
47. Bartos, V, and Groh, J. 1969. The effect of repeated stimulation of the pancreas on the pancreatic secretion in young and aged men. *Geront Clin* 11:56–62.
48. Laugier, R, and Sarles, H. 1984. Pancreatic function and diseases. In *Gastrointestinal Tract Disorders in the Elderly,* Eds., J. Hellemans and G Vantrappen. Edinburgh-London-Melbourne-New York: Churchill Livingstone.
49. Rosenberg, IR, et al. 1966. The effect of age and sex upon human pancreatic secretion of fluid and bicarbonate. *Gastroenterology* 50:191–194.
50. Gullo, L, et al. 1983. Exocrine pancreatic function in the elderly. *Gerontology* 29:407–411.
51. DiMagno, EG, Go, VLW, and Summerskill, WHJ. 1973. Relations between pancreatic enzyme outputs and malabsorption in severe pancreatic insufficiency. *N Engl J Med* 288:813–815.
52. Longstreth, GF, Go, VLW, and Malagelada, JR. 1977. Postprandial gastric, pancreatic, and biliary response to histamine H_2-receptor antagonists in active duodenal ulcer. *Gastroenterology* 72:9–13.
53. Thaysen, EH, et al. 1964. Amylase concentration of duodenal aspirates after stimulation of the pancreas by a standard meal. *Gastroenterology* 46:23–31.
54. Gullo, L, et al. 1986. Aging and exocrine pancreatic function. *J Am Geriatr Soc* 34:790–792.
55. Carrere, J, et al. 1987. Human serum pancreatic lipase and trypsin 1 in aging: Enzymatic and immunoenzymatic assays. *J Gerontol* 42:315–317.
56. Bossuyt, PJ, et al. 1981. Relation of age to isoenzyme pattern and total activity of amylase in serum. *Clin Chem* 27:451–454.
57. Kohn, HD, et al. 1982. Immunoreactive trypsin, amylase and lipase in serum—Is there an age-dependence? *Clin Biochem* 15:49–51.
58. Peterson, JM, and Pederson, S. 1982. Cathodic trypsin-like immunoreactivity in serum: Influence of sex, age, renal function, food, and diurnal variation. *Clin Chim Acta* 124:31–37.
59. Ammann, RW, Pei, P, Satz, N, and Woodfli, W. 1982. Variations with age of immunoreactive serum trypsin: Higher reference ranges in "healthy" elderly people. *Klin Wochenschr* 60:243–264.
60. Mohiuddin, J, et al. 1984. Serum pancreatic enzymes in the elderly. *Ann Clin Biochem* 21:102–104.
61. Grossman, MI, Kirshner, JB, and Gillespie, IE. 1963. Basal and Histalog-stimulated gastric secretion in control subjects and in patients with peptic ulcer or gastric cancer. *Gastroenterology* 45:14–26.
62. Baron, JH. 1963. Studies of basal and peak acid output with an augmented histamine test. *Gut* 4:136–144.
63. Brandt, LJ. 1984. The stomach. In *Gastrointestinal Disorders of the Elderly.* New York: Raven Press.
64. Krentz, K, and Jablonowski, H. 1984. Functional and histological gastric changes with age. In *Gastrointestinal Tract Disorders in the Elderly,* Eds., J. Hellemans and G Vantrappen. Edinburgh-London-Melbourne-New York: Churchill Livingstone.
65. Steinheber, FU. 1985. Aging and the stomach. *Clin Gastroenterol* 14:657–686.
66. Wormsley, KG, and Grossman, MI. 1965. Maximal Histalog test in control subjects and patients with peptic ulcer. *Gut* 6:427–435.
67. Kekki, M, et al. 1982. Age- and sex-related behaviour of gastric acid secretion at the population level. *Scand J Gastroenterol* 17:737–743.
68. Doscherholmen, A, et al. 1977. Influence of age and stomach function on serum vitamin B_{12} concentration. *Scand J Gastroenterol* 12:313–319.
69. Bird, T, and Schade, ROK. 1977. Gastric histology and its relation to anemia in the elderly. *Gerontology* 23: 309–321.
70. Bock, OAA, et al. 1963. The serum pepsinogen level with special reference to the histology of the gastric mucosa. *Gut* 4:106–111.
71. Glass, BGJ, et al. 1960. Gastric atrophy, atrophic gastritis, and gastric secretory failure. *Gastroenterology* 39:429–453.
72. Samloff, IM, et al. 1982. Relationship among serum pepsinogen I, serum pepsinogen II, and gastric mucosal histology. *Gastroenterology* 83:204–209.
73. Varis, K, and Isokoski, M. 1981. Screening of Type A gastritis. *Ann Clin Res* 13:133–138.
74. Jeffries, GH, and Sleisenger, MH. 1965. The pharmacology of intrinsic factor secretion in man. *Gastroenterology* 48:444–448.
75. Strickland, RG, and Mackay, IR. 1973. A reappraisal of the nature and significance of chronic atrophic gastritis. *Dig Dis* 18:426–440.
76. Bins, M, et al. 1983. Is discrimination between Type A and Type B atrophic gastritis clinically useful in achlorhydria? *J Clin Gastroenterol* 5:17–19.
77. Morris, A, et al. 1986. Seroepidemiology of *Campylobacter pyloridis. NZ Med J* 99:657–659.
78. Graham, DY, and Klein, PD. 1987 *Campylobacter pyloridis* gastritis: The past, the present, and speculations about the future. *Am J Gastroenterol* 82:283–286.
79. Blaser, MJ. 1987. Gastric campylobacter-like organisms, gastritis, and peptic ulcer disease. *Gastroenterology* 93: 371–383.
80. Villako, K, et al. 1976. Prevalence of antral and fundic gastritis in a randomly selected group of an Estonian rural population. *Scand J Gastroenterol* 11:817–822.
81. Ihamaki, T, Varis, K, and Siurala, M. 1979. Morphological, functional and immunological state of the gastric mucosa in gastric carcinoma families. *Scand J Gastroenterol* 14:801–812.
82. Kimura, K. 1972. Chronological transition of the fundic-pyloric border determined by stepwise biopsy of the lesser and greater curvatures of the stomach. *Gastroenterology* 63:584–592.
83. Andrews, GR, et al. 1967. Atrophic gastritis in the aged. *Aust Ann Med* 13:230–235.
84. Ihamaki, T, Saukkonen, M, and Siurala, M. 1978. Long-

term observations of subjects with normal mucosa and with superficial gastritis: Results of 23–27 years' follow-up examinations. *Scand J Gastroenterol* 13:771–775.
85. Rosch, W, Demling, L, and Elster, K. 1975. Is chronic gastritis a reversible process? Follow-up study of gastritis by step-wise biopsy. *Acta Hepato Gastro* 22: 252–255.
86. Boyd, E. 1933. Normal variability in the weight of the adult human liver and spleen. *Arch Pathol* 16:350–372.
87. Calloway, NO, Foley, CF, and Lagerbloom, P. 1965. Uncertainties in geriatric data. II. Organ size. *J Am Geriatr Soc* 13:20–28.
88. Schmucker, DL, Mooney, JS, and Jones, AL. 1978. Stereological analysis of hepatic fine structure in the Fischer 344 rat. *J Cell Biol* 78:319–337.
89. Tauchi, H, and Sato, T. 1975. Effect of environmental conditions upon age changes in the human liver. *Mech Aging Dev* 4:71–80.
90. Engelmann, GL, et al. 1981. Age-related changes in isolated rat hepatocytes. Comparison of size, morphology, binucleation, and protein content. *Mech Aging Dev* 16: 385–395.
91. Bender, AD. 1965. The effect of increasing age on the distribution of peripheral blood flow in man. *J Am Geriatr Soc* 13:192–198.
92. Vestal, RE, et al. 1979. Effects of age and cigarette smoking on propranolol disposition. *Clin Pharmacol Ther* 26:8–15.
93. Wood, AJJ, et al. 1979. Effect of aging and cigarette smoking on antipyrine and indocyanine green elimination. *Clin Pharmacol Ther* 26:16–20.
94. Shepherd, AMM, et al. 1977. Age as a determinant of sensitivity to warfarin. *Br J Clin Pharmacol* 4:315–320.
95. Routledge, PA, et al. 1979. Factors affecting warfarin requirements. *Eur J Clin Pharamcol* 15:319–322.
96. Kampmann, JP, Sinding, J, and Moller-Jorgensen, I. 1975. Effect of age on liver function. *Geriatrics* 30:91–95.
97. Greenblatt, DJ. 1979. Reduced serum albumin concentration in the elderly: A report from the Boston collaborative drug surveillance program. *J Am Geriatr Soc* 27:20–22.
98. Thompson, EN, and Williams, R. 1975. Effect of age on liver function with particular reference to bromsulphalein excretion. *Gut* 6:266–269.
99. Chiramonte, M, Floreani, A, and Naccarato, R. 1982. Hepatitis B virus infection in homes for the aged. *J Med Virol* 9:247–255.
100. Zauli, D, et al. 1985. Different course of acute hepatitis B in elderly adults. *J Gerontol* 40:415–418.
101. Einarsson, K, et al. 1985. Influence of age on secretion of cholesterol and synthesis of bile acids by the liver. *N Engl J Med* 313:277–282.
102. Holt, PR. 1985. The small intestine. *Clin Gastroenterol* 14:689–723.
103. Webster, SGP, and Leeming, JT. 1975. The appearance of the small bowel mucosa in old age. *Age Ageing* 4: 168–174.
104. Warren, PM, Pepperman, MA, and Montgomery, RD. 1978. Age changes in small intestinal mucosa (letter). *Lancet* II:849–850.
105. Webster, SGP, and Leeming, JT. 1975. Assessment of small bowel function in the elderly using a modified xylose tolerance test. *Gut* 16:109–113.
106. Webster, SGP, Wilkinson, EM, and Gowland, E. 1977. A comparison of fat absorption in young and old subjects. *Age Ageing* 6:113–117.
107. Recker, RR. 1985. Calcium absorption and achlorhydria. *N Engl J Med* 313:70–73.
108. Soergel, KH, Zboralske, FF, and Amberg, JR. 1964. Presbyesophagus: Esophageal motility in nonagenarians. *J Clin Invest* 43:1472–1479.
109. Feldman, RS, et al. 1980. Aging and mastication: Changes in performance and in the swallowing threshold with natural dentition. *J Am Geriatr Soc* 18:97–103.
110. Idowu, AT, Graser, GN, and Handelman, SL. 1986. The effect of age and dentition status on masticatory function in older adults. *Spec Care Dent* 6:80–83.
111. Hopwood, GL. 1986. Muscle fibre typing in the human pharyngeal constrictors and oesophagus: The effect of aging. *Acta Anat* 127:77–80.
112. Eckardt, VF, and LeCompte, PM. 1978. Esophageal ganglia and smooth muscle in the elderly. *Dig Dis Sci* 23:443–448.
113. Eliska, O. 1973. Phreno-oesophageal membrane and its role in the development of hiatal hernia. *Acta Anat* 86:137–150.
114. Sheth, N, and Diner, WC. 1988. Swallowing problems in the elderly. *Dysphagia* 2:209–215.
115. Khan, TA, et al. 1977. Esophageal motility in the elderly. *Dig Dis Sci* 22:1049–1054.
116. Zaninotto, G, et al. 1988. The lower esophageal sphincter in health and disease. *Am J Surg* 155:104–110.
117. Csendes, A, et al. 1978. Relation of gastroesophageal sphincter pressure and esophageal contractile waves to age in man. *Scand J Gastroenterol* 13:443–447.
118. Hollis, JB, and Castell, DO. 1974. Esophageal function in elderly men: A new look at "presbyesophagus." *Ann Intern Med* 80:371–374.
119. Mandelstam, P, and Lieber, A. 1970. Cineradiographic evaluation of the esophagus in normal adults. *Gastroenterology* 58:32–39.
120. Richter, JE, et al. 1987. Esophageal manometry in 95 healthy adult volunteers: Variability of pressures with age and frequency of "abnormal" contractions. *Dig Dis Sci* 32:583–592.
121. Helm, JF, et al. 1984. Effect of esophageal emptying and saliva on clearance of acid from the esophagus. *N Engl J Med* 310:284–288.
122. Mold, JW, and Rankin, RA. 1987. Symptomatic gastroesophageal reflux in the elderly. *J Am Geriatr Soc* 35:649–659.
123. Cheadle, WG, et al. 1988. Computerized ambulatory esophageal pH monitoring in 50 asymptomatic volunteer subjects: Results and clinical implications. *Am J Surg* 155:503–508.
124. Dodds, WJ, et al. 1981. Pathogenesis of reflux esophagitis. *Gastroenterology* 81:376–394.
125. Dodds, WJ. 1988. The pathogenesis of gastroesophageal reflux disease. *Am J Radiol* 151:49–56.
126. Richter, JE, and Castell, DO. 1982. Gastroesophageal reflux. *Ann Intern Med* 97:93–103.
127. Cohen, S, and Harris, LD. 1971. Does hiatal hernia affect competence of the gastroesophageal sphincter? *N Engl J Med* 284:1053–1056.
128. Kupfer, RM, et al. 1985. Gastric emptying and small-

bowel transit rate in the elderly. *J Am Geriatr Soc* 33: 340–343.
129. Evans, MA, et al. 1981. Gastric emptying rate in the elderly: Implications for drug therapy. *J Am Geriatr Soc* 29:201–205.
130. Hogan, DB, Lamki, L, and Cape, RDT. 1984. Gastric emptying and aging. *J Clin Exp Gerontology* 6:145–152.
131. Moore, JG, et al. 1983. Effect of age on gastric emptying of liquid-solid meals in man. *Dig Dis Sci* 28:340–344.
132. Horowitz, M, et al. 1984. Changes in gastric emptying rates with age. *Clin Sci* 67:213–218.
133. Hutson, WR, Roehrkasse, RL, and Wald, R. 1989. Influence of gender and menopause on gastric emptying and motility. *Gastroenterology* 96:11–17.
134. Datz, FL, Christian, PE, and Moore, J. 1987. Gender-related differences in gastric emptying. *J Nucl Med* 28:1204–1207.
135. Datz, FL, Christian, PE, and Moore, JG. 1987. Differences in gastric emptying rates between menstruating and postmenopausal women. *J Nucl Med* 28:604A–604B.
136. Halvorsen, L, Dotevall, G, and Walan, A. 1973. Gastric emptying in patients with achlorhydria or hyposecretion of hydrochloric acid. *Scand J Gastroenterol* 8:395–399.
137. Frank, EB, Lange, R, and McCallum, RW. 1981. Abnormal gastric emptying in patients with atrophic gastritis with or without pernicious anemia. *Gastroenterology* 80:1151.
138. Kellow, JE, et al. 1985. Human interdigestive motility: Variations in patterns from esophagus to colon. *Gastroenterology* 91:386–395.
139. Anuras, S, and Sutherland, J. 1984. Small intestinal manometry in healthy elderly subjects. *J Am Geriatr Soc* 32:581–583.
140. Kim, SK. 1968. Small intestine transit time in the normal small bowel study. *Am J Radiol* 104:522–524.
141. Koch, TR, Carney, JA, and Go, VLW. 1984. Effect of disease duration upon gut peptide concentrations in inflammatory bowel disease. *Dig Dis Sci* 29:43S.
142. Koch, TR, Go, VLW, and Szurszewski, JH. 1986. Changes in some electrophysiological properties of circular muscle from normal sigmoid colon of the aging patient. *Gastroenterology* 90:1497.
143. Loening-Baucke, V, and Anuras, S. 1984. Sigmoidal and rectal motility in healthy elderly. *J Am Geriatr Soc* 32: 887–891.
144. Brauer, PM, Slavin, JL, and Marlett, JA. 1981. Apparent digestibility of neutral detergent fiber in elderly and young adults. *Am J Clin Nutr* 34:1061–1070.
145. Melkersson, M, et al. 1983. Intestinal transit time in constipated and non-constipated geriatric patients. *Scand J Gastroenterol* 18:593–597.
146. Metcalf, AM, et al. 1987. Simplified assessment of segmental colonic transit. *Gastroenterology* 92:40–47.
147. Newman, HF, and Freeman, J. 1974. Physiologic factors affecting defecatory sensation: Relation to aging. *J Am Geriatr Soc* 12:553–554.
148. Loening-Baucke, V, and Anuras, S. 1985. Effects of age and sex on anorectal manometry. *Am J Gastroenterol* 80:50–53.
149. Poos, RJ, et al. 1986. Influence of age and sex on anal sphincters: Manometric evaluation of anorectal continence. *Eur Surg Res* 18:343–348.
150. McHugh, SM, and Diamant, NE. 1987. Effect of age, gender, and parity on anal canal pressures: Contribution of impaired anal sphincter function to fecal incontinence. *Dig Dis Sci* 32:726–736.
151. Bannister, JJ, Abouzekry, L, and Read, NW. 1987. Effect of aging on anorectal function. *Gut* 28:353–357.
152. Varma, JS, et al. 1988. Constipation in the elderly: A physiologic study. *Dis Colon Rectum* 31:111–115.
153. Read, NW, et al. 1979. A clinical study of patients with fecal incontinence and diarrhea. *Gastroenterology* 76: 747–756.
154. Matheson, DM, and Keighley, MRB. 1981. Manometric evaluation of rectal prolapse and fecal incontinence. *Gut* 22:126–129.
155. Snooks, SJ, et al. 1984. Injury to innervation of pelvic floor sphincter musculature in childbirth. *Lancet* II: 546–550.
156. Milne, JS, and Williamson, J. 1972. Bowel habits in older people. *Geront Clin* 14:56–60.
157. Sonnenberg, A, and Koch, TR. 1988. Age-related increase in the occurrence of constipation in the United States. *Gastroenterology* 94:A436.
158. Connell, AM. 1962. The motility of the pelvic colon. II. Paradoxical motility in diarrhea and constipation. *Gut* 3:342–348.
159. Bloom, AA, LoPresti, P, and Farrar, JT. 1968. Motility of the intact human colon. *Gastroenterology* 54:232–240.
160. Kaufman, PN, et al. 1988. Role of opiate receptors in the regulation of colonic transit. *Gastroenterology* 94: 1351–1356.
161. Kreek, M, et al. 1983. Naloxone, a specific opioid antagonist, reverses chronic idiopathic constipation. *Lancet* I:261–262.
162. Burleigh, DE. 1988. Evidence for a functional cholinergic deficit in human colonic tissue resected for constipation. *J Pharm Pharmacol* 40:55–57.
163. Krishnamurthy, S, et al. 1985. Severe idiopathic constipation is associated with a distinctive abnormality of the colonic myenteric plexus. *Gastroenterology* 88:26–34.
164. Read, NW, et al. 1985. Anorectal function in elderly patients with fecal incontinence. *Gastroenterology* 89: 959–966.
165. Eastwood, MA, Watters, DAK, and Smith, AN. 1982. Diverticular disease—Is it a motility disorder? *Clin Gastroenterol* 11:545–561.
166. Smith, AN. 1986. Colonic muscle in diverticular disease. *Clin Gastroenterol* 15:917–935.
167. Huizinga, JD. 1986. Electrophysiology of human colon motility in health and disease. *Clin Gastroenterol* 15: 879–901.
168. Hughes, LE. 1969. Postmortem survey of diverticular disease of the colon. *Gut* 10:336–351.
169. Whiteway, J, and Morson, BC. 1985. Elastosis in diverticular disease of the sigmoid colon. *Gut* 26:258–266.
170. Thompson, WG, and Patel, DG. 1986. Clinical picture of diverticular disease of the colon. *Clin Gastroenterol* 15:903–916.
171. Parks, TG. 1975. Natural history of diverticular disease of the colon. *Clin Gastroenterol* 4:53–69.
172. Horner, JL. 1958. Natural history of diverticulosis of the colon. *Dig Dis Sci* 3:343–350.
173. Weinreich, J, and Anderson, D. 1976. Intraluminal pres-

sure in the sigmoid colon: Patients with sigmoid diverticula and related conditions. *Scand J Gastroenterol* 11:581–586.
174. Taylor, I, and Duthie, HL. 1976. Bran tablets and diverticular disease of the sigmoid colon. *Br Med J* 1:988–990.
175. Meyer, CT, et al. 1981. Arteriovenous malformations of the bowel: An analysis of 22 cases and a review of the literature. *Medicine* 60:36–48.
176. Weaver, GA, et al. 1979. Gastrointestinal angiodysplasia associated with aortic valve disease: Part of a spectrum of angiodysplasia of the gut. *Gastroenterology* 77:1–11.

9

Endocrine Changes in the Elderly

Fran E. Kaiser and John E. Morley

The steadily increasing proportion of older persons has led to a marked awareness of the importance of aging and its interaction with various disease processes. As a person ages, the definitions that separate "wellness" and "disease" become less distinct. Furthermore, it has become increasingly apparent that "health" and "disease" exist as extremes on a continuum rather than as static, distinct entities. This chapter provides basic information on how aging interacts with the endocrine system; such knowledge is essential to allow adequate interpretation of endocrine function in the elderly, to logically modify therapy of the common endocrine disorders as the patient ages, and to review current thinking on those endocrine conditions that are peculiar to or most common in the aged, e.g., osteoporosis.

With age, the loss of functional reserve in many organs tends to lead to deficiency diseases, such as hypothyroidism, diabetes mellitus, and hypogonadism. This, coupled with the decreasing immune competence related to aging and the autoimmune basis of many endocrine disorders, leads to an increasing prevalence of hypoendocrine disease with increasing age and a tendency for more than one endocrine disorder to occur in the same person (polyglandular failure syndromes) (1). In the elderly, atypical presentations (e.g., apathetic thyrotoxicosis) and nonspecific presentations (e.g., weight loss, fatigue, depression, dementia) lead to delays in seeing a physician and often result in misdiagnosis. It needs to be remembered that most normal laboratory values have been developed from tests on young, healthy people, and abnormal results may reflect the aging process. This is further complicated by the presence of intercurrent disease in the elderly, which can per se alter basal and stimulated hormonal values. The hormonal changes commonly seen in the elderly and the effect of illness on them are outlined in Table 9-1.

Ectopic hormone production from neoplasms can mimic classic endocrine diseases. Since malignancies become more prevalent as people age, the incidence of ectopic hormone production increases. Awareness of ectopic hormone syndromes is important, as it can lead to the early diagnosis of an occult cancer or to the solution of a clinical problem; additionally, it can avoid inadequate or incorrect treatment of an endocrinopathy. Ectopic hormone production can also be used to monitor the effectiveness of therapy or to demonstrate recurrence after therapy. Ectopic production of hormones, such as bombesin and calcitonin, may play a role in the pathogenesis of cancer anorexia (2). Thus, in any elderly person in whom a hyperendocrine disease is developing, particularly where the biochemical parameters are disproportionately raised as compared to the clinical presentation, the clinician should have a high index of suspicion that an ectopic hormone syndrome is the culprit.

Aging and Anterior Pituitary Function

A growing but still limited number of studies have examined effect of aging on the human pituitary gland. There appears to be no change in pituitary weight, based on autopsy studies (3), but age-related changes in pituitary composition do occur. Decreased vascularity, altered distribution of cell types, and increased connective content can be found with a marked decrease in eosinophil content and a small increase in basophil and chromophobe cells.

Table 9-1. Hormonal changes of aging

	Aging	Aging + illness
GH (basal)	N	N
GH response to GRF	↓	?
GH response to surgery		↓
ACTH (basal)	N	N
ACTH response to CRF	N?	N?
LH, FSH (basal)	↑	N/ ↓
LH, FSH response to LRH	↑ ↑	N/ ↓
PRL (basal)	N	N/ ↑
TSH basal	N	N/ ↓
TSH response to TRH	N	N/ ↓
T_4	N	N/ ↓
T_3 RIA	N	N/ ↓
Cortisol	N	N
Aldosterone	↓	↓
Renin	↓	↓
Insulin	↑	↑
Glucagon	↑	? ↑
PTH	↑	?
Calcitonin	↓	?
1, 25 $(OH)_2D$	↑	?
GIP	N	?
Pancreatic Polypeptide	↑	?

N = normal; ↑ = increased; ↓ = decreased.

There is an increase in the occurrence of adenomas with age, but this does not appear to be of functional significance. An increase in the pituitary content of gonadotropins occurs in postmenopausal females and an increased content of luteinizing hormone (LH) in aged males has been found (4, 5). There appears to be no change in the pituitary content of growth hormone (GH), thyrotropin (TSH), prolactin, or adrenocorticotropin (ACTH). Despite this apparent lack of change in pituitary hormonal content, however, alterations of the secretory pattern or response to dynamic testing exist for some of these hormones as a normal concomitant of aging.

Basal GH concentration does not appear to change with age in males (6), but a slight decrease in basal levels can be seen in females (5). The response of growth hormone to growth hormone releasing hormone (GHRH) is markedly diminished with age in some studies (6), but more recent data (7) suggest the response to GHRH is normal. The response to insulin-induced hypoglycemia, a potent stimulator of growth hormone, has been variously reported to decrease or change little with aging (8, 9). Most of growth hormone secretion occurs during the first few hours of sleep; this does decrease after age 40, as does somatomedin C (insulin growth factor I), which mediates some of the actions of growth hormone (10–13).

A recent study of somatomedin C binding and action in fibroblasts of aged subjects concluded that in vivo aging does not appear to be associated with somatomedin C receptor alteration or decreased cellular responsiveness to the mitogenic effects of somatomedin C (14). The true significance of alterations in growth hormone and somatomedin C is unclear; however, reduced GH secretion and low concentrations of somatomedin C may cause atrophy of lean body mass and be responsible for some of the catabolic effects on muscle and bone that are associated with aging.

Corticotropin-releasing factor (CRF) and other factors, such as vasopressin and norepinephrine, stimulate beta endorphin and corticotropin (ACTH) secretion from the pituitary. Basal plasma ACTH remains unchanged with age, and a normal circadian rhythm of ACTH is maintained in men and women (15). The response to CRF shows no change with age (7). Unlike plasma concentrations, cerebrospinal fluid levels of beta-endorphins diminish with age, suggesting that a different regulatory mechanism exists in CSF for this opiate peptide (16).

A large body of data exists regarding this effect of illness on pituitary-thyroid function, but fewer data regarding changes with normal aging are available. Basal levels of TSH do not generally appear to change with aging (17). The response of TSH to thyrotropin releasing hormone has been varyingly reported as normal or decreased, especially in elderly males (18–20). This latter study also reported a slight increase in basal TSH in the elderly subjects. Ohara et al. found an increased responsiveness to TRH in the elderly, compared to young subjects, when a small dose of TRH (100 μg) was administered (21). Clearly, there is no consensus regarding the response to TRH in the aged population. Blunting of the TSH response to TRH can be seen with depression, fasting, uremia, and nonthyroidal illness, as well as with hypothalamic pituitary disease (22–28). The advent of newer immunoradiometric assays of TSH, with their increased sensitivity and specificity, may obviate the need for TRH testing (29). At present, however, a positive TSH response to TRH excludes hyperthyroidism, but a blunted response does not make the diagnosis in the elderly.

With aging, levels of LH and follicle stimulating hormone (FSH) increase in both men and women (30, 31). Deslypere et al. found a diminution of LH pulse frequency but unchanged pulse amplitude in healthy elderly men, raising the possibility of impaired hypothalamic-pituitary function (32). Harman et al. also found a diminution and delay in the response of gonadotropins to gonadotropin hormone releasing hormone (GnRH) in elderly men (30). With critical illness, a fall in gonadotropins occurs both in males and females (28, 33), and in a subset of postmenopausal, critically ill subjects, there is a loss of responsivity to GnRH (28). Further discussion of the menopause and male sexual function appears later in this chapter.

Prolactin is the only hormone under inhibitory control. The major inhibitory factor is dopamine. If the hypothalamus or pituitary stalk is disrupted, prolactin secretion will increase. Prolactin levels have been reported to decrease in elderly women (34). The response of prolactin to stimulation with TRH has been reported to be decreased in elderly subjects (35, 36) or delayed (37). In a study of healthy ambulatory elderly, stimulated prolactin levels showed differences primarily by gender (17). The circadian rhythm of prolactin is maintained with age.

Clinical features of hypopituitarism, or decreased secretion of pituitary hormones, are essentially the same in the elderly as in the young, but hypopituitarism may be more subtle in the elderly because some of the clinical features, such as loss of menstrual periods in females, decreased libido in males and females, and loss of body hair, may occur as normal concomitants of aging. Also, apathy, fatigue, muscle weakness, and anemia may erroneously be considered to be due to "old age" (ageist viewpoint). A high degree of suspicion and use of dynamic testing, such as TRH, metyrapone, and L-Dopa stimulation tests, as well as computerized tomography scans when appropriate, should help delineate whether pituitary failure is present.

In summary, some changes in the hypothalamic pituitary axis occur with normal aging. With illness, a further "turn off" of certain hormones that are unessential in maintaining life under a stress situation (FSH, LH, growth hormone, TSH) may occur; but ACTH, vital to responding to stress, is preserved. However, the positive anabolic effects of these hormones are also lost. At present, there are no data to suggest that hormonal intervention has any impact on the morbidity and mortality associated with critical illness.

Posterior Pituitary

Helderman (38) found rare, degenerative changes in the vasopressin-synthesizing cells of the hypothalamus, without evidence of cellular destruction, but rather with an increase in cellular size (even more so postoperatively). Elderly subjects have increased basal levels of arginine vasopressin (AVP) (39) but volume-pressure stimulation of AVP (baroreceptor mediated) decreases with age (38).

The institutionalized elderly are especially at risk for hyponatremia. Serum sodium should be closely watched in patients who are unable to have direct access to water or to verbalize their needs. In diabetic elderly patients, the use of chlorpropamide, which potentiates antidiuretic hormone, has been associated with diminished mental function in up to 15% of elderly patients (40).

Thyroid

With aging, the thyroid gland becomes more fibrotic; there is infiltration with small round cells and increased basophilic staining in the colloid (41). A decrease in follicular diameter and follicular epithelial height occurs. The prevalence of thyroid nodules also increases with age and reaches approximately 5% by age 60 (42). Controversy remains as to whether the size of the thyroid increases with age. The incidence of asymptomatic carcinoma of the thyroid is 2% to 13% in routine autopsies, but the age-specific incidence of thyroid carcinoma does not change with age. Thyroid carcinoma tends to be far more aggressive in older patients, and giant and spindle cell (anaplastic) carcinomas primarily occur in elderly patients.

Thyroxine levels have variously been reported to rise (43), decrease (20), or remain unaltered with aging (44, 45), in healthy elderly. Both plasma clearance and the production rate of thyroxine decrease with age (46), but thyroid binding globulin remains unaltered.

Changes in triiodothyronine (T_3) concentration among healthy elderly also remains the subject of controversy. Olsen et al. (47) and Azizi et al. (48) reported no decrease in T_3; Harman et al. (20) did find a drop in T_3 with age, but TSH concentration was not increased in that group of subjects. However, T_3 concentration in hospitalized elderly individuals is generally reduced 40% to 50% (49). These changes can be seen with various illnesses and with nutritional changes, such as fasting. In some patients with critical illness, T_4 may also drop. These hormonal changes are generally unaccompanied by a rise in TSH, and patients are clinically euthyroid. (For reviews of non-thyroidal illness, the following may be helpful: 49–51). Nonthyroidal illness can make the interpretation of thyroid function testing difficult, but primary hypothyroidism can be readily distinguished from nonthyroidal illness by using a TSH concentration greater than 20 μU/ml to make the diagnosis of hypothyroidism (Table 9-2).

The overall incidence of thyroid dysfunction is variously reported to be from 2.3% to 7% in several large studies, as reported by Burrows and Shenkman (52). Hypothyroidism in the elderly has been reported in up to 4% of the elderly populations screened in some studies.

Table 9-2. Comparison of the effect of primary hypothyroidism, illness, and aging on thyroid function tests

	Primary Hypothyroidism	Euthyroid sick syndrome	Aging
T_4	↓	N/↓ (in severe cases)	N
T_3 RU	↓	N/↓/↑	N
Free T_4 index	↓	N/↓	N
T_3 RIA	↓	↓↓	N
TSH	↑	N/↓	N

Hypothyroidism has an insidious onset and progresses slowly over several years. Symptoms such as fatigue, lethargy, mental confusion, dry skin, and constipation may be mistaken for "normal aging." Some patients may be asymptomatic. Weight loss and depression may occur, and "masked hypothyroidism" (in that patients may not appear or complain of symptoms generally attributable to thyroid dysfunction) may occur. Hypothermia, unexplained pleural or pericardial effusion, or muscle dysfunction should prompt a rapid investigation of thyroid function. Antibodies to thyroidal antigens can be detected in low titer in approximately 10% of the population. The prevalence of detectable antibodies to thyroidal antigens increases with age, but clinically significant thyroid disease does not seem to occur in most subjects with low levels of antibodies. Some subjects, with diffuse glandular involvement and high titers of antibodies (Hashimoto's thyroiditis), may go on to become hypothyroid (53).

Therapy should always utilize synthetic L-thyroxine. Since T_4 production does fall with age, the needed replacement dose of thyroid hormone is generally lower than that used with younger subjects (54). Most elderly hypothyroid patients, including those who had longstanding hypothyroidism or those with heart disease, are best started with small doses of thyroxine (12.5 to 25 μg per day) and gradually titrated up to replacement (an increment of 25 μg every 3 weeks until reaching a dose of approximately 100 μg). Thereafter, if further increments in dosage are required to achieve normalization of TSH concentration, they should be made in 12.5 μg increments. Full replacement doses may be difficult to achieve in patients with angina (55), and in fact, may not be desirable.

The prevalence of hyperthyroidism has been reported to be between 0.5% and 3.0%. Approximately 15% of patients are over 65 years of age at the time they present (56). Furthermore, only about 25% of elderly thyrotoxic patients have the typically restless, nervous appearance of younger thyrotoxic patients, and apathetic thyrotoxicosis with depression, weight loss, muscle weakness and cardiovascular symptoms may dominate the picture (57). The appearance of atrial fibrillation, heart block, or congestive heart failure should prompt an investigation of thyroid function. Thyroid function tests may be only minimally elevated in the elderly, but usually there are elevations of both T_3 and T_4 concentrations, although isolated elevation of either one may be seen. For example, in patients who are ill or who are taking medications that impair T_4 or T_3 conversion, T_4 may be the only thyroid hormone to be elevated. However, as pointed out by Mooradian et al. (58), high doses of beta blockers may artificially increase T_4 concentrations. With the newer, more sensitive, and more specific TSH assays, there appears to be the ability to distinguish between normal and very low levels of TSH, such as would be seen with hyperthyroidism (29). The presence of autoantibodies in the serum (which are common in the elderly) may artificially elevate the TSH level, producing a false negative in patients with hyperthyroidism. The diagnosis of hyperthyroidism, therefore, can be made with either an elevation of free T_4 index and/or free T_3 index and very low (less than normal) levels of TSH, using a radioimmunometric assay. The treatment of hyperthyroidism does not differ from that used in younger patients. However, if cardiovascular symptomatology is present—such as heart failure, arrhythmias, or embolic episodes—patients should be treated with thionamides before, and in most instances for a few months following, radioactive iodine therapy. In general, because of the frequent difficulty in clinically assessing thyroidal status in the elderly, we recommend screening for thyroidal dysfunction in the following settings: 1) acute hospital admission; 2) patients with unexplained lethargy or weight loss; 3) patients with deterioration of mental function; 4) new onset of atrial fibrillation; 5) tachyarrhythmias; and 6) proximal myopathy. A reasonably cost-effective screening measure is to obtain a serum T_4 and ask the laboratory to hold the serum (59). If the T_4 is low (less than 6.0 μg/dl), a TSH should be obtained. If the T_4 is greater than 10 to 12 μg/dl, a TSH by radioimmunometric assay should be obtained. If the T_4 is low and the TSH is greater than 15 μU/ml, primary hypothyroidism can be diagnosed. If the T_4 is elevated and the TSH is suppressed to less than normal, the diagnosis of hyperthyroidism may be entertained.

Parathyroids: Disorders of Calcium Metabolism, Hypercalcemia

Calcium metabolism undergoes some age-related alterations (Fig. 9-1). It is important to note that even in a sunny climate sun exposure may be limited, and with aging

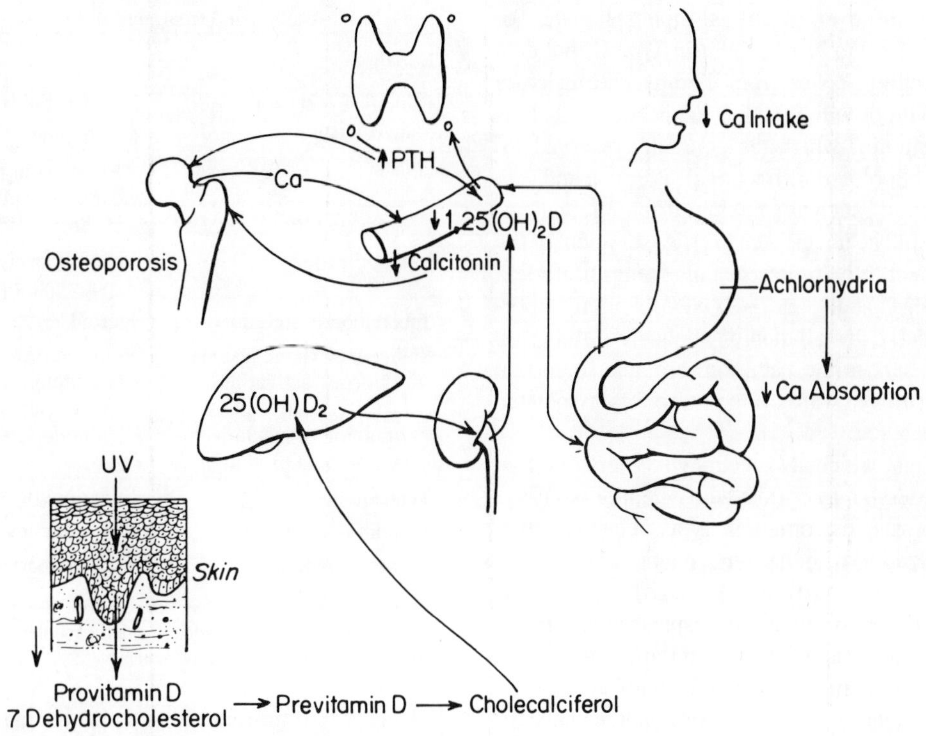

Figure 9-1. Age-related changes in calcium and vitamin D metabolism.

there appears to be a diminished ability of the elderly to synthesize vitamin D in the skin (60). As a result of lack of substrate, lower levels of 25(OH) vitamin D have been found in some elderly subjects (61, 62). The diminution in 25(OH) vitamin D correlates with alterations in renal function as well as diminution in bone mineral content (62). Although $1,25(OH)_2D$ has been reported as unchanged, the consensus is that with aging a decrease in $1,25(OH)_2D$ does occur, which can result in decreased calcium absorption from the intestine (63–65). Some subjects with low $1,25(OH)_2D$ have an increase in parathormone (PTH) concentration (65–67). These age-related PTH increases are also associated with changes in renal function and with diminished calcium absorption. Additionally, calcitonin in both basal and stimulated states decreases with age (68).

Osteoporosis remains a significant problem in the elderly. Among women over 70 years of age, 25% to 40% experience vertebral crush fractures and 10% suffer wrist fractures. The causes of osteopenia are multiple, involving nutritional, hormonal, and life style factors. There is a loss of both organic (mineralized) and inorganic multifactorial (nonmineralized) phases, resulting in bone that is normally mineralized but highly porous and very fragile. Osteoporosis has been divided into two forms by Melton and Riggs (69). Type I occurs in a small subset of postmenopausal women (50 to 65 years of age) and, rarely, in men of the same age. Type II occurs in large numbers of men and women over the age of 75 (Table 9-3). Vertebral and Colles' fractures seem to occur more frequently in Type I subjects and involve trabecular bone. Hip, pelvic, and humeral fractures are more common in Type II subjects. For Type I subjects, the relationship to menopausal onset implies estrogen deficiency as a major pathogenetic factor, and estrogen replacement (along with a progestational agent if the patent still has a uterus) is indicated. In the Type II patient, there appear to be two factors playing a role: impaired bone formation and secondary hyperparathyroidism with increased bone turnover (70). It is possible that therapies directed against

Table 9-3. Type of osteoporosis

Postmenopausal (Type I)	Age-related (Type II)
Age: 50–65	75+
Type of bone involved:	
Trabecular bone	Cortical bone
Common fractures:	
Vertebral	Hip
Colles' fracture	Pelvis, humerus
Etiology: Estrogen deficiency	? Secondary hyperparathyroidism
Treatment: Estrogen	Calcium

increased bone turnover, such as diphosphonates or calcitonin, may prove to be of benefit in Type II, but data are presently lacking. Aside from therapy with calcium and estrogen (with or without other medications, such as fluoride or calcitonin, which are generally reserved for those patients with recurrent fractures), exercise and cessation of risk factors, such as smoking, drinking, and caffeine usage, should be undertaken (71). Assessment of the home environment to help prevent falls from unsafe features—loose rugs, stairs, etc.—is also of vital importance in the elderly. Installation of adequate lighting on stairs and grab bars in the bathroom are also important preventive measures to ward off the morbidity associated with osteoporosis.

Osteomalacia, which also occurs with increased frequency in the elderly, may coexist with osteoporosis (72). Unlike osteoporosis, osteomalacia is associated with a loss of mineralization of bone, with maintenance of the organic matrix. X-rays may be identical to those seen with osteoporosis. Serum alkaline phosphatase may be elevated and phosphorus may be low, but these findings are inconsistent. Only a bone biopsy will distinguish osteoporosis from osteomalacia. In general, osteomalacia occurs due to alteration in vitamin D status (as occurs with drugs, such as anticonvulsants, or malabsorption) or depletion of phosphorus (73). The important factor to remember is that it is difficult to distinguish osteoporosis from osteomalacia clinically. In patients with osteomalacia as well as osteoporosis (particularly common in those with hip fractures), low-dose vitamin D therapy with careful monitoring of serum calcium levels is indicated.

Hypercalcemia in both young and elderly patients can be divided into two categories: hyperparathyroidism and everything else (Table 9-4). Hyperparathyroidism has a peak incidence between the 5th and 7th decades of life. Only 17% of patients with hyperparathyroidism are over the age of 60. It is important to remember that tuberculosis may be a cause of hypercalcemia (present in 28% of the series of Abbasi et al.) due to increased intestinal absorption and skeletal resorption (74). Other factors, such as immobilization with decreased bone formation and increased bone resorption (75) and malignancy-related hypercalcemia, should be thought of for elderly subjects (for reviews of the latter, see Refs. 76–78). Vitamin A and D supplements, which are commonly used in the elderly, may also lead to hypercalcemia.

Table 9-4. Causes and treatment of hypercalcemia

Etiology	Treatment
Primary hyperparathyroidism	Surgery, fluids, phosphorous, Calcitonin[a] ? Estrogen in postmenopausal women (Selby and Peacock, 1986)
Immobilization	Fluid replacement, phosphorous, diphosphonates[a]
Tuberculosis/sarcoidosis	Steroid
Malignancy (bone lesions, osteoclast activating factor, prostaglandins, ? binding of calcium by myeloma proteins)	Removal of tumor, saline, calcitonin, mithramycin, prostaglandin synthetase inhibitors, steroids
Thiazides	Stop diuretic therapy
Vitamin A or D	Stop vitamins
Addison's disease, hyperthyroidism	Treat endocrine disorders

[a]Furosemide is dangerous in elderly and never indicated unless concomitant renal failure is present.

Diabetes Mellitus

The prevalence of diagnosed diabetes in the United States is 6.9% in males and 8.9% in females over age 65. By the age of 80, 16% of the population has diabetes mellitus. Diabetes mellitus represents one of the major chronic disorders of the growing elderly population, and diabetic patients are particularly prone to disorders requiring surgery as well as hospitalization.

Mild glucose intolerance occurs with advancing age. After exclusion of patients with frank diabetes mellitus, one study found that 3% of patients aged 18 to 24 years had a plasma glucose greater than 160 mg/dl 1 hour after a glucose load, while elevated glucose levels occurred in 16% of those 45 to 54 years, in 36% of those 65 to 74 years, and in 42% of those 75 to 79 years (79). Thus, over the age of 50 there is a 1 to 2 mg/dl increase in fasting glucose and a 5 to 10 mg/dl increase in the 2-hour postprandial glucose with each decade. Diagnostic criteria for diabetes mellitus in the elderly require a random blood glucose above 200 mg/dl or two fasting blood glucose levels greater than 140 mg/dl.

Glycosylated hemoglobin levels are also elevated in normal elderly (80, 81), which suggests that protein glycosylation occurs in association with the hyperglycemia of aging. This protein glycosylation appears to play a role in the pathogenesis of cataracts and microvascular disease. The glucose intolerance of aging has also been associated with an increase in atherosclerotic cardiovascular disease (82).

The major cause of the glucose intolerance of aging is insulin resistance. This resistance is based on both changes in receptors and a postreceptor defect (83), leading to an increased insulin response seen following a glucose load or a mixed meal in the elderly. Additionally, there is a decrease in both insulin degradation and removal with advancing age (84). Finally, the elderly also show a defect in second beta-cell response (85) and an increase in circulating glucagon levels (86).

Patients with onset of diabetes mellitus prior to the age of 75 have an excessive mortality compared to the rest of the population (87); most of this excessive mortality is due to cardiovascular disease. Forty percent of all diabetics who are blind from retinopathy are over age 70, and cataract extraction is three to four times more common in diabetics over 70 than in nondiabetics. Further, hyperglycemia-induced changes in refraction can cause major problems in elderly patients with borderline vision. Diabetic patients have poorer neurological recovery following ischemic stroke, and this appears to be related to the level of glucose during the stroke (88).

Fifty percent of elderly men and eighty percent of elderly females with gangrene are diabetics. Soft tissue foot infections, with or without underlying osteomyelitis, are a major source of serious morbidity in elderly diabetics. The importance of careful foot care in such patients cannot be overemphasized. Physicians should examine the feet of diabetics at every office visit; patients with severe calluses or with other, even trivial, skin lesions should be referred to a podiatrist for treatment. Continuing education of the diabetic patient regarding foot care is of paramount importance.

Certain complications are more or less specific to the elderly diabetic (87). Cranial nerve palsies which resolve spontaneously within 3 months occur commonly in diabetes. Intracranial aneurysms must always be considered in the differential diagnosis of third nerve palsies. Glaucoma occurs with increased frequency in diabetics. Necrotizing infections of the external auditory canal caused by *Pseudomonas aeruginosa* occur exclusively in elderly diabetics; this condition is called malignant otitis externa. Approximately 50% of patients with renal papillary necrosis are over 60 years. Diabetic amyotrophy is a progressive and painful weakness of the pelvic girdle muscles, which is often asymmetrical and associated with minimal sensory changes; spontaneous resolution of this condition usually occurs within 12 months. Diabetic neuropathic cachexia is a severe form of this syndrome and is associated with anorexia and extreme weight loss. Both conditions and tuberculosis occur in the elderly diabetic. Choledochal pathology occurs three times more commonly in the elderly than in younger subjects. Diabetics appear to be at particular risk for developing cholecystitis associated with gallstones. Hypothermia can occur both as a complication of hypoglycemia and diabetic ketoacidosis in the elderly.

The elderly represent a group that is at particular risk for developing trace element deficiency (89), and diabetes can further aggravate this situation. For example, Type II diabetes mellitus is associated with hyperzincuria and impaired zinc absorption (90). In a recent study, zinc replacement in Type II diabetes with zinc depletion was found to improve T-cell function as measured by the T-lymphocyte response to phytohemagglutinin (91). Zinc has been shown to play a role in wound healing. In fact, zinc supplementation accelerated the rate of healing of leg ulcers in zinc-deficient elderly subjects (92). Hypomagnesemia occurs commonly in poorly controlled diabetics (93). Chromium deficiency has been suggested as a cause of poor glucose tolerance in some elderly. As many as 70% of the elderly take vitamin supplements; therefore, it is important to remember that vitamin C in large doses interferes with glucose measurements and can hamper the monitoring of diabetic control.

In the therapy of the elderly diabetics, a careful balance needs to be struck between the benefits of aggressive therapy and the complications associated with therapy. Lipson has enumerated the factors that interfere with optimum treatment of diabetes in the elderly: alterations in vision, taste, and smell; difficulties in food preparation and consumption secondary to tremor, arthritis, and poor dentition; hypodipsia; altered renal and hepatic function; cognitive and psychiatric impairment; decreased physical activity; interaction with multiple medications and other disease processes; and poverty (94). Thus, in the elderly, major changes of diet are often impossible to bring about and classical diabetic diets are often too expensive for pensioners. In many of the elderly, oral hypoglycemic agents appear to be the treatment of choice. However, a disproportionate percentage of patients who develop hypoglycemia while on oral agents are found among the elderly. Chlorpropamide, with its long half-life, produces twice as many episodes of hypoglycemia in the elderly when compared to other agents. It also produces an unacceptable incidence of hyponatremia in the elderly (95, 96).

Many elderly require insulin, and this therapy should not be withheld because of the misguided viewpoint that insulin injections represent an undue hardship. Certainly, reduction in the fatigue and frequent urination together with improvement in the reduced visual acuity associated with hyperglycemia represent important quality-of-life issues. Although the use of insulin in the elderly needs to be individualized, many patients who would benefit from this treatment are denied it by their physician. Older diabetics have been shown to make from a 10% to 20% error when drawing up their insulin (97).

Urine testing in the elderly is often misleading because of the high renal threshold in old age and, in males, the problem of inadequate bladder emptying associated with prostatic hypertrophy and bladder neuropathy. Home blood glucose monitoring is more accurate, but the benefits have to be weighed against the problems of adding this chore to the lives of the elderly.

Adrenal Disorders

With aging, the adrenal glands undergo degenerative changes, with capsular fibrosis and a tendency toward nodular hyperplasia, but their weight remains relatively unchanged (98, 99). Daily cortisol secretion and excretion decrease with age, but if cortisol excretion is expressed per gram creatinine, remain normal. The cortisol clearance rate is also diminished with age (100), reflecting alterations in plasma volume or alterations in hepatic steroid enzymes and generally resulting in normal cortisol levels. More recent data (101, 102) reveal a trend towards decreased plasma cortisol with age. It does, however, seem reasonable to consider lower dose steroid therapy when necessary to treat with steroids, in view of the diminished cortisol clearance.

The changes of adrenal androgen production are more marked than for glucocorticoids. There is a progressive decrease in plasma and urinary 17-ketosteroid levels. Dehydroepiandrosterone (DHEA) secretion declines linearly from 20 to 96 years of age (103), and these alterations cannot be corrected by reference to creatinine excretion. DHEA is undergoing increased scrutiny, as it may cause weight loss without altering food intake (104), and it appears to be inversely related to cardiovascular mortality (105). Also, DHEA and its metabolites exert a protective effect on the development of tumors, certain immune diseases, and diabetes in experimental animals (106, 107).

Plasma aldosterone, plasma aldosterone clearance, aldosterone secretory rate, and urinary excretion of aldosterone all decrease with age (5). An age-related decrease in renin also occurs (108), and the responses of both aldosterone and renin to salt restriction are diminished.

Fewer than 10% of the patients with Addison's disease are over age 60 (109). Hyponatremia, hypotension, and a propensity toward hypoglycemia should prompt consideration of adrenal insufficiency. In the elderly, tuberculosis and adrenal hemorrhage secondary to anticoagulant therapy should also be thought of as possible etiologies.

Cushing's disease in the elderly is also relatively uncommon, but hypertension, diabetes, and osteoporosis occurring in the same individual should also prompt an investigation of adrenal hyperfunction. However, elevated cortisol levels and nonsuppression of cortisol by dexamethasone occur in elderly patients with depression and Alzheimer's disease. These conditions need to be taken into account in the differential diagnosis. Iatrogenic Cushing's syndrome is probably the most common cause of adrenal dysfunction, and care should be exercised in the use of steroids in the elderly (45). Indeed, because of the diminished cortisol clearance with age, steroid doses for replacement and therapy should be lower in the elderly.

The occurrence of ectopic ACTH syndrome is also increased in the elderly, with the majority of patients being males over the age of 50. Here, the effects of carcinoma (such as cachexia) may overshadow the clinical features of Cushing's syndrome. One clue to ectopic ACTH may be found in electrolyte abnormalities: hypokalemic alkalosis. Once again, the subtlety of symptoms in the elderly makes it necessary to have a high index of suspicion in diagnosing these conditions in this population.

GI Hormones

Cholecystokinin (CCK), which stimulates pancreatic enzyme secretion and gallbladder contraction, has been shown to be increased in both fasting and fat-stimulated states (110). Gastrin, which stimulates gastric acid secretion and increases gastric antral motility and pepsin secretin, also increases with age (111, 112). Atrophic gastritis (due to decreased mucosal cell synthesis), which is common among the elderly, has been linked to gastric ulceration (113, 114). Changes in gastric motility can affect the rate and extent of drug absorption; whether this can be directly linked to changes in gastrin concentration remains to be documented. Gastrointestinal peptide (GIP) has an insulinotropic effect when given with glucose; that is, GIP potentiates insulin release and improves glucose tolerance. Surprisingly, however, GIP levels are elevated in both diabetes and obesity (115, 116). A defective feedback loop has been suggested as a possible cause of increased GIP levels. Circulating GIP concentrations appear to be unaltered with aging. Pancreatic polypeptide, which enhances intestinal motility and gallbladder tone, but whose true physiologic significance remains undefined, appears to increase with age (117, 118). The roles of these and other peptides, such as motilin and substance P, and the possible interrelationships of these hormones and age-related alterations in GI function remain fertile areas of investigation.

Menopause

The average age at the menopause is 51 years, with a range of 41 to 59. During the life span the human ovary transforms itself from a follicle-rich, stroma-poor organ at birth into a postmenopausal organ, consisting predominantly of corticomedullary stroma. The increasing stromal cells are an important source of postmenopausal hormones, accounting for up to 30% of androstenedione and 50% of testosterone (119). In the postmenopausal ovary, these steroidogenically active stromal cells result in a marked proliferation of ovarian surface epithelium. The common and lethal surface epithelial (germinal) cancer arises predominantly in the postmenopausal ovary and, as such, can be considered a sequela of ovarian aging (120). Hilar cells also increase markedly with advancing age (121).

Between the ages of 35 to 45, variations in menstrual cycles occur which may last 2 to 8 years before menopause. Premature menopause, before the age of 40, occurs in less than 1% of women and can be due to Turner's mosaicism, autoimmune disorders, resistant ovarian syndrome, 17-alpha-hydroxylase deficiency, chemotherapy, pelvic irradiation, or surgical removal (122). During the perimenopausal period, there is a fall in estrogen levels initially, a gradual rise in FSH, and then a rise in LH to postmenopausal levels. Estrone becomes the dominant estrogen being produced by conversion from ovarian and adrenal androgens in peripheral adipose tissue. Thus, obesity becomes a risk factor for endometrial cancer because it leads to excessive production of estrogens (123).

The hot flash is the most common postmenopausal complaint. In addition to increases in skin temperature, they are associated with tachycardia, tachypnea, and an increased basal metabolic rate. Flashes are associated with a pulsatile LH release (124). Estrogens are the most specific and effective therapy for the vasomotor symptoms.

The vaginal epithelium is rich in estrogen receptors. With menopause, vaginal epithelium thins, lubrication decreases, and the pH rises. Some vaginal shortening occurs, leading to increased susceptibility of the vagina to trauma. These physiologic changes can lead to pruritus, burning, dryness, dyspareunia, and some bleeding. The postmenopausal vagina is very responsive to low doses of estrogen. Topical estrogen is well absorbed from the vagina and cannot be used in patients who would not be candidates for systemic therapy.

The vulva shows age-related changes, consisting of subcutaneous fat regression, reduction in size of the labia majora, thinning of hair, and regression of epithelium that are poorly responsive to estrogens. Testosterone ointment, however, maintains epithelial thickness and gives good relief of dryness and itching (125). Vulvar dystrophy is common, but gross lesions require early biopsy as vulva cancers have a good prognosis when diagnosed and treated early.

The urethral mucosa, which contains estrogen receptors, atrophies postmenopausally, leading to prolapse and increased ascending urinary tract infections. Prolapse, which can be confused with carcinoma, usually responds well to treatment with local estrogen cream.

The aging female skin results from a decrease in collagen, a reduction in papillary capillaries, a decrease in the elastic network, reduction in tensile strength, and dry skin. In addition, depigmentation (vitiligo), hyperpigmentation ("aging spots"), and telangiectasia ("red spots") increase. Estrogens will delay some of these changes. The use of moisturizer and avoidance of excessive sunlight exposure will also decrease the aging changes in the skin.

Recently, much interest has been generated by transdermal estradiol patches. Absorption is excellent, with reduction in LH levels, though not to premenopausal levels (126). Transdermal estradiol decreases hot flashes, sleep disturbances, and irritability. Its advantage over oral preparations is that it appears not to alter estrogen-sensitive liver proteins. No matter what route of administration is used, estrogens should be given in a cyclic fashion; in a woman with a uterus, a progestational agent should be added. Monitoring should include biannual measurements of blood pressure and weight as well as breast, abdominal, and pelvic examinations. Mammograms should be obtained annually in women over 50 years.

Male Sexual Function

Sexual dysfunction occurs commonly in elderly males. One in three males over the age of 40 who comes to see a physician will have some difficulty in obtaining erections adequate for intercourse (127). While in younger patients psychological factors play a major role in the pathogenesis of impotence, in older patients organic factors are often the major factor (89). The major factors causing impotence in the elderly are listed in Table 9-5. In most cases, the cause of impotence in the elderly is multifactorial, and the exact role of hormonal factors is often controversial. Further, it is clear that many systemic diseases, which occur with increasing frequency with aging, will cause some degree of hormonal dysfunction (128).

From the physiologic perspective, a clearcut decline in sexual activity occurs with age. By the 8th decade, males have only 20% of the number of sexual events compared to those in the 3rd decade (129). Plasma testosterone levels decrease with advancing age, although they may be maintained in extremely healthy older males (130). In young males, testosterone levels peak at 6:00 to 8:00 A.M., while the morning peak is less predominant in the elderly, probably secondary to a decreased frequency in luteinizing hormone (LH) pulses (131). There is also

Table 9-5. Causes of impotence in the elderly

Vascular	Arterial insufficiency Venous incompetence (leakage)
Medications	Diuretics Other antihypertensives Drugs interfering with testosterone receptor (e.g., cimetidine, spironolactone) Psychiatric drugs Cytotoxic drugs
Hypogonadism	Primary Secondary
Other hormonal	Thyroid disease Increased prolactin
Diabetes mellitus	
Neurologic	Autonomic neuropathy Sensory neuropathy Spinal cord injury Pelvic surgery
Central nervous system disease	Cerebrovascular accident Multiple sclerosis Temporal lobe epilepsy
Nutritional	Zinc deficiency Protein caloric malnutrition
Depression	
Other psychogenic	Performance anxiety Widower's syndrome

a decreased testosterone response to human chorionic gonadotrophin in the elderly, suggesting some degree of primary testicular exhaustion. This is confirmed anatomically by the finding of decreased Leydig cell numbers with advancing age (132). This leads to an increase in LH and follicle stimulating hormone. The increased FSH level is associated with the degeneration of seminiferous tubular elements and a decrease in spermatids. Despite these changes, sperm counts do not markedly decrease with advancing age, attesting to the redundancy of the male reproductive system (133). With advancing age, there is a reduction in sperm motility and an increase in abnormal morphology.

Aging is accompanied by an increased plasma binding of circulating testosterone and a decrease in the bioavailable testosterone (134). A diminished accumulation of 5-alpha-reduced steroids occurs in reproductive tissues (135). Superimposed on these age-related physiologic changes is an increased incidence of both hypergonadotrophic and hypogonadotrophic hypogonadism (89).

With the increased prevalence of hypogonadism in the elderly, an increased awareness of the pharmacologic effects of testosterone becomes important. Testosterone can exert its effects on tissues either directly or following conversion to dihydrotestosterone by 5-alpha-reductase or secondary to aromatization to estrogens. Estradiol levels tend to increase with advancing age (136). Testosterone can cause an increase in prostatic tissue growth, making regular (biannual) rectal examinations essential in those receiving pharmacologic replacement. In the elderly, testosterone replacement, which leads to water retention, can precipitate heart failure or worsen hypertension. Testosterone therapy also increases the hematocrit and can lead to overt polycythemia. Finally, when testosterone is first administered, it is aromatized to estrogen, which can lead to the development of painful gynecomastia.

The majority of elderly males appear to have reduced male hormones when compared to their younger counterparts. The role of these changes in the declining sexual function associated with aging has not been clearly established. It needs to be remembered that with the availability of penile prostheses, vacuum devices, intracorporeal papaverine injections, and hormonal therapies, sexual dysfunction should not be considered an inevitable concomitant of aging, but rather a highly treatable condition that can have a major impact on the quality of life.

References

1. Trence, DL, Morley, JE, and Handwerger, BS. 1984. Polyglandular autoimmune syndromes. *Am J Med* 77:107–116.
2. Morley, JE, and Levine, AS. 1985. The pharmacology of eating behavior. *Annu Rev Pharmacol* 25:127–146.
3. Andres, R, and Tobin, JD. 1977. Endocrine systems. In *Handbook of the Biology of Aging*, Ed., CE Finch and L Hayflick, pp. 367–378. New York: Van Nostrand Reinhold Company.
4. Ryan, RJ. 1962. The luteinizing hormone content of human pituitaries I. Variations with sex and age. *J Clin Endocrinol Metab* 22:300–303.
5. Gregerman, RI, and Bierman, EL. 1981. Aging and hormones. In *Textbook of Endocrinology*, ed. 6, Ed., RM Williams, pp. 1192–1212. Philadelphia: WB Saunders Co.
6. Shibasaki, T, et al. 1984. Age-related changes in plasma growth hormone response to growth hormone releasing factor in man. *J Clin Endocrinol Metab* 58:212–214.
7. Pavlov, EP, et al. 1986. Responses of growth hormone (GH) and somatomedin C to GH releasing hormone in healthy aging men. *J Clin Endocrinol Metab* 62:595–600.
8. Laron, Z, Doron, M, and Amikam, B. 1967. Plasma growth hormone in old age. *Harefuah* 73:375–376.
9. Muggeo, M, et al. 1975. Human growth hormone cortisol response to insulin stimulation in aging. *J Gerontol* 30:546–551.
10. Bennett, A, et al. 1984. Insulin-like growth factors I and II on aging and bone density in women. *J Clin Endocrinol Metab* 59:700–705.
11. Rudman, D, et al. 1981. Impaired growth hormone secretion in the adult population. *J Clin Invest* 67:1361–1368.
12. Rudman, D, et al. 1986. Hyposomatomedinemia in the nursing home patient. *J Am Geriatr Soc* 34:427–430.

13. Ho, KY, et al. 1987. Effects of sex and age on the 24-hour profile of growth hormone secretion in man: Importance of endogenous estrogen. *J Clin Endocrinol Metab* 64:51–58.
14. Conover, CA, et al. 1985. Somatomedin C binding and actions in fibroblasts from aged and progeric subjects. *J Clin Endocrinol Metab* 60:685–691.
15. Blichert-Toft, M. 1971. Assessment of serum corticotropin concentrations and its nyctohemeral rhythm in the aging. *Gerontol Clin* 13:215–220.
16. Facchinetti, G, et al. 1983. Different patterns of central and peripheral beta EP, beta LPH and ACTH throughout life. *Peptides* 4:469–474.
17. Kaiser, FE. 1987. Variability of response to TRH in normal elderly. 1987. *Age Ageing* 16:345–354.
18. Snyder, PJ, and Utiger, RD. 1972. Response to thyrotropin-releasing hormone (TRH) in normal man. *J Clin Endocrinol Metab* 34:380–385.
19. Snyder, PJ, and Utiger, RD. 1972. Thyrotropin response to thyrotropin releasing hormone in normal females over forty. *J Clin Endocrinol Metab* 34:1096–1098.
20. Harman, SM, Wehman, RE, and Blackman, MR. 1984. Pituitary-thyroid hormone economy in healthy aging men: Basal indices of thyroid function and thyrotropin response to constant infusions of thyrotropin-releasing hormone. *J Clin Endocrinol Metab* 58:320–326.
21. Ohara, H, et al. 1974. Thyroid function of the aged as viewed from the pituitary thyroid system. *Endocrinol Japan* 21:377–386.
22. Prange, AJ, et al. 1972. Effects of thyrotropin releasing hormone in depression. *Br J Med* 2:999–1001.
23. Vinik, AL, et al. 1975. Fasting blunts the TSH response to synthetic thyrotropin releasing hormone levels in acute illness. *J Clin Endocrinol Metab* 40:509–511.
24. Ramirez, G, et al. 1976. Thyroid dysfunction in uremia: Evidence for thyroid and hypophyseal abnormalities. *Ann Intern Med* 84:672–676.
25. Weissel, M, et al. 1979. Basal and TRH stimulated thyroid and pituitary hormones in various degrees of renal insufficiency. *Acta Endocrinol* (Copenh) 90:23–32.
26. Kaptein, EM, et al. 1981. Thyroxine metabolism in the low thyroxine state of critical non-thyroidal illness. *J Clin Endocrinol Metab* 53:764–771.
27. Vierhapper, H, et al. 1982. Impaired secretion of TSH in critically ill patients with "low T_4 syndrome". *Acta Endocrinol* (Copenh) 101:542–549.
28. Quint, AR, and Kaiser, FE. 1985. Gonadotropin determinations and thyrotropin-releasing hormone and luteinizing hormone-releasing hormone testing in critically ill postmenopausal women with hypothyroxinemia. *J Clin Endocrinol Metab* 60:464–471.
29. Seth, J, et al. 1984. Sensitive immunoradiometric assay for serum thyroid stimulating hormone: A replacement for the thyrotropin-releasing hormone test? *Br Med J* 289:1334–1336.
30. Harman, SM, et al. 1982. Reproductive hormones in aging men. II. Basal pituitary gonadotropins and gonadotropin responses to luteinizing hormone-releasing hormone. *J Clin Endocrinol Metab* 54:547–551.
31. Siler, TM, and Yen, SS. 1973. Augmented gonadotropin response to synthetic LRF in hypogonadal state. *J Clin Endocrinol Metab* 37:491.
32. Deslypere, JP, et al. 1987. Influence of age on pulsatile luteinizing hormone release and responsiveness of the gonadotrophs to sex hormone feedback in men. *J Clin Endocrinol Metab* 64:68–73.
33. Woolf, PD, et al. 1985. Transient hypogonadotropic hypogonadism caused by critical illness. *J Clin Endocrinol Metab* 60:444–450.
34. Vekemans, M, and Robin, C. 1975. Influence of age on serum prolactin levels in men and women. *Br J Med* 4:738–739.
35. Arnetz, BB, Lahnborg, G, and Eneroth, P. 1986. Age-related differences in the pituitary prolactin response to thyrotropin releasing hormone. *Life Sci* 39:135–139.
36. Blackman, MR, et al. 1986. Basal serum prolactin levels and prolactin responses to constant infusions of thyrotropin releasing hormone in healthy aging men. *J Gerontol* 41:699–705.
37. Yamaji, T, et al. 1976. Effect of age and sex on circulating and pituitary prolactin levels in humans. *Acta Endocrinol* (Copenh) 83:711–719.
38. Helderman, JH. 1982. The impact of normal aging on the hypothalamic-neuro-hypophysical-renal axis. In *Endocrine Aspects of Aging*, Ed., SG Korenman, pp. 9–32. New York: Elsevier Biomedical.
39. Rondeau, E, et al. 1982. High plasma antidiuretic hormone in patients with cardiac failure: Influence of age. *Miner Electrolyte Metab* 8:267–274.
40. Sloan, RW, Kreider, RM, and Luderer, JR. 1983. The effect of chlorpropamide hyponatremia on mental status in a nursing home population. *J Fam Pract* 16: 937–942.
41. Irvine, RE. 1973. Thyroid disease in old age. In *Textbook of Geriatric Medicine* Ed., JC Brocklehurst, pp. 435–458. Edinburgh: Churchill Livingston.
42. Maxon, HR, et al. 1977. Ionizing irradiation and the induction of clinically significant disease in the human thyroid gland. *Am J Med* 63:967–978.
43. Britton, KE, et al. 1975. Is "T_4 toxicosis" a normal biochemical finding in elderly women? *Lancet* 2:141–142.
44. Melmed, S, and Hershman, JM. 1982. The thyroid and aging. In *Endocrine Aspects of Aging*, Ed., SG Korenman, pp. 33–54. New York: Elsevier Biomedical.
45. Kaiser, FE, and Doe, RP. 1984. Steroid use in the elderly. *Postgrad Med* 65–74.
46. Wenzel, KW, and Horn, WR. 1976. Triiodothyronine (T_3) and thyroxine (T_4) kinetics in aged men. In *Thyroid Research*, Ed., J Robins and RL Utiger, pp. 270–273. Amsterdam: Excerpta Medica.
47. Olsen, T, Laurberg, P, and Weeke, J. 1978. Low serum triiodothyronine in old age: An effect of disease not age. *J Clin Endocrinol Metab* 47:1111–1115.
48. Azizi, F, et al. 1975. Pituitary-thyroid responsiveness to intramuscular thyrotropin-releasing hormone based on analyses of serum thyroxine, triiodothyronine and thyrotropin concentrations. *N Engl J Med* 292:273–277.
49. Wartofsky, L, and Burman, KD. 1982. Alterations in thyroid functions in patients with systemic illness: The "euthyroid sick syndrome." *Endocrinol Rev* 3:164–217.
50. Tibaldi, JM, and Surks, MI. 1985. Effects of nonthyroidal illness on thyroid function. *Med Clin NA* 69:899–911.
51. Chopra, IJ, et al. 1983. Thyroid function in nonthyroidal illness. *Ann Intern Med* 98:946–957.
52. Burrows, V, and Shenkman, L. 1982. Thyroid function in the elderly. *Am J Med Sci* 283:8–17.
53. Tunbridge, WM, et al. 1977. The spectrum of thyroid

disease in a community. The Whickham survey. *Clin Endocrinol* 7:481–493.
54. Rosenbaum, RL, and Barzel, US. 1982. Levothyroxine replacement dose for primary hypothyroidism decreases with age. *Ann Intern Med* 96:53–55.
55. Levine, HD. 1980. Compromise therapy in the patient with angina pectoris and hypothyroidism: A clinical assessment. *Am J Med* 69:411–418.
56. Davis, PJ, and Davis, FB. 1974. Hyperthyroidism in patients over the age of 60 years. Clinical features in 85 patients. *Medicine* 53:161–181.
57. Tibaldi, JM, et al. 1986. Thyrotoxicosis in the very old. *Am J Med* 81:619–622.
58. Mooradian, AD, et al. 1983. Propranolol-induced hyperthyroxinemia. *Arch Int Med* 143:2193–2198.
59. Morley, JE, et al. 1983. The interpretation of thyroid function tests in hospitalized patients. *JAMA* 249:2377–2379.
60. McLaughlin, J, and Holick, MF. 1985. Aging decreases the capacity of human skin to produce vitamin D_3. *J Clin Invest* 76:1536–1538.
61. Alveoli, LV. 1982. Aging, bone and osteoporosis. In *Endocrine Aspects of Aging*, Ed., SG Korenman, pp. 199–230. New York: Elsevier Biomedical.
62. Orwoll, ES, and Meier, DE. 1986. Alterations in calcium, vitamin D and parathyroid hormone physiology in normal men with aging. *J Clin Endocrinol Metab* 63:1262–1268.
63. Riggs, BL, et al. 1978. A syndrome of osteoporosis, increased serum immunoreactive parathyroid hormone and inappropriately low 1,25 dihydroxyvitamin D. *Mayo Clin Proc* 53:701–706.
64. Gallagher, JC, and Wilkinson, R. 1973. Effect of ethinyl estradiol on calcium and phosphorus metabolism of postmenopausal women with primary hyperparathyroidism. *Clin Sci Mol Med* 45:785–802.
65. Dadona, P, et al. 1986. Low 1,25 dihydroxyvitamin D, secondary hyperparathyroidism, and normal osteocalsin in elderly subjects. *J Clin Endocrinol Metab* 63:459–462.
66. Clemens, TL, et al. 1986. Serum vitamin D_2 and vitamin D_3 metabolite concentrations and absorption of vitamin D_2 in elderly subjects. *J Clin Endocrinol Metab* 63:656–660.
67. Marcus, R, Madvig, P, and Young, G. 1984. Age-related changes in parathyroid hormone and parathyroid hormone action in normal humans. *J Clin Endocrinol Metab* 58:223–230.
68. Deftos, LJ, et al. 1980. Influence of age and sex on plasma calcitonin in human beings. *N Engl J Med* 30:1351–1353.
69. Melton, LJ, and Riggs, BL. 1983. Epidemiology of age-related fractures. In *The Osteoporotic Syndrome: Detection and Prevention*, Ed., LV Alvioli, pp. 45–72. New York: Grune and Stratton.
70. Delmas, PD, et al. 1983. Increase in serum bone Y-carboxyglutamic acid protein with aging in women: Implications for the mechanism of age-related bone loss. *J Clin Invest* 71:1316–1321.
71. Heaney, RP, et al. 1982. Calcium, nutrition and bone mass in the elderly. *Ann J Clin Nutr* 36:986–1013.
72. Aaron, JE, et al. 1974. Frequency of osteomalacia and osteoporosis in fractures of the proximal femur. *Lancet* 1:229–233.
73. Frame, B, and Parfitt, AM. 1978. Osteomalacia: Current concepts. *Ann Int Med* 89:966–982.
74. Abbasi, AA, et al. 1979. Hypercalcemia in active pulmonary tuberculosis. *Ann Intern Med* 90:324–328.
75. Minaire, P, Neunier, P, and Edouard, C. 1974. Quantitative histological data on disuse osteoporosis: Comparison with biological data. *Calcif Tissue Res* 17:57–73.
76. Mundy, GR, and Martin, TJ 1982. The hypercalcemia of malignancy: Pathogenesis and management. *Metabolism* 31(12):1247–1277.
77. Mundy, GR, Ibbotson, KJ, and D'Souza, SM. 1985. Tumor products and the hypercalcemia of malignancy. *J Clin Invest* 76:391–394.
78. Stewart, AF, et al. 1980. Biochemical evaluation of patients with cancer-associated hypercalcemia: Evidence for humoral and nonhumoral groups. *N Engl J Med* 303:1377–1383.
79. Bennett, PH. 1976. Report of work group on epidemiology (U S DHEW Publication No. NIH 76-1021), pp. 63–133, vol. 3, pt. 1. Washington, DC: National Commission on Diabetes.
80. Fink, RI, Kolterman, OG, and Olefsky, JM. 1984. The physiological significance of the glucose intolerance of aging. *J Gerontol* 39:273–278.
81. Arnetz, BB, Kallner, A, and Theorell, T. 1982. The influence of aging on hemoglobin Alc. *J Gerontol* 37:648–650.
82. Jarrett, RJ, McCartney, P, and Keen, H. 1982. The Bedford Survey: Ten year mortality rates in newly diagnosed diabetics, borderline diabetics and normoglycaemic controls and risk indices for coronary heart disease in borderline diabetics. *Diabetologia* 22:79–84.
83. Morley, JE, et al. 1987. Diabetes mellitus in the elderly. Is it different? *Am J Med* 83:533–544.
84. Minaker, KL, Rowe, JW, and Tonino, R. 1982. Influence of age on clearance of insulin in man. *Diabetes* 31:851–855.
85. Chen, M, et al. 1985. Pathogenesis of age-related glucose intolerance in man: Insulin resistance and decreased B-cell function. *J Clin Endocrinol Metab* 60:13–20.
86. Davidson, MB. 1982. The effect of aging on carbohydrate metabolism: A comprehensive review and a practical approach to the clinical problem. In *Endocrine Aspects of Aging*, Ed., SG Korenman, pp. 231–267. New York: Elsevier Biomedical.
87. Tattersall, RB. 1984. Diabetes in the elderly—a neglected area? *Diabetologia* 27:167–173.
88. Pulsinelli, WA, et al. 1983. Increased damage after ischemic stroke in patients with hyperglycemia with or without established diabetes mellitus. *Am J Med* 74:540–544.
89. Morley, JE. 1986. Impotence. *Am J Med* 80:897–905.
90. Kinlaw, WB, et al. 1983. Abnormal zinc metabolism in type II diabetes mellitus. *Am J Med* 75:273–277.
91. Niewoehner, CB, et al. 1986. The role of zinc supplementation in Type II diabetes mellitus. *Am J Med* 81:63–68.
92. Hallbrook, T, and Lanner, E. 1972. Serum-zinc and healing of venous leg ulcers. *Lancet* 2:780–782.
93. Mooradian, AD, and Morley, JE. 1987. Micronutrient status in diabetes mellitus. *Am J Clin Nutr* 45:877–895.
94. Lipson, LG. 1986. Diabetes in the elderly: Diagnosis, pathogenesis and therapy. *Am J Med* 80(Suppl 5A):20–21.
95. Kadowaki, T, et al. 1983. Chlropropamide-induced hyponatremia: Incidence and risk factors. *Diabetes Care* 6:468–471.

96. Feldman, JM. 1985. Review of glyburide after one year on the market. *Am J Med* 79:102–108.
97. Puxty, JAM, Hunter, DM, and Burr, WA. 1983. Accuracy of insulin injection in elderly patients. *Br Med J* 287:1762.
98. Calloway, NO, Foley, CF, and Lagerbloom, P. 1965. Uncertainties in geriatrics data II. Organ size. *J Am Geriatr Soc* 13:20–28.
99. Blichert-Toft, M. 1978. The adrenal glands in old age. In *Geriatric Endocrinology,* Ed., RB Greenblatt Aging Series, pp. 81–102, vol. 5. New York: Raven Press.
100. West, CD, Brown, H, and Simonset, AL. 1961. Adrenocortical function and cortisol metabolism in old age. *J Clin Endocrinol Metab* 21:1197–1207.
101. Drafta, D, et al. 1982. Age-related changes of plasma steroids in normal adult males. *J Steroid Biochem* 17:683–687.
102. Sherman, B, Wysham, C, and Pfohl, B. 1985. Age-related changes in the circadian rhythm of plasma cortisol in man. *J Clin Endocrinol Metab* 61:439–443.
103. Parker, LN, and Odell, WD. 1978. Decline of adrenal androgen production as measured by radioimmunoassay of urinary unconjugated dehydroepiandrosterone. *J Clin Endocrinol Metab* 47:600–602.
104. Yen, TT, et al. 1977. Prevention of obesity in Avyla mice by dehydroepiandrosterone. *Lipids* 12:409–413.
105. Barrett-Connor, E, Khaw, KT, and Yen, SSC. 1986. A prospective study of dehydroepiandrosterone sulfate, and cardiovascular disease. *N Engl J Med* 24:1519–1524.
106. Coleman, DL, Leiter, EH, and Applezweig, N. 1984. Therapeutic effects of dehydroepiandrosterone metabolites in diabetic mutant mice (C57BL/KsJ-db/db). *Endocrinology* 115:239–243.
107. Pashko, LL, and Schwartz, AG. 1983. Effect of food restriction, dehydroepiandrosterone or obesity on the binding of 3H-7, 12 dimethylbenz (a) anthracene to mouse skin DNA. *J Gerontol* 38:8–12.
108. Tuck, ML, Williams, GM, and Cain, JP. 1973. Relation of age, diastolic pressures and known duration of hypertension to presence of low renin essential hypertension. *Am J Cardiol* 32:632–637.
109. Irvine, WJ, and Barnes, EW. 1975. Addison's disease, ovarian failure and hypoparathyroidism. *Clin Endocrinol Metab* 4:379–434.
110. Khalil, T, et al. 1985. Effect of aging on gallbladder contraction and release of cholecystokinin-33 in humans. *Surgery* 98:423–429.
111. Reaven, E, et al. 1982. Functional homogeneity of cholecystokinin-33 in humans. *Surgery* 98:423–429.
112. Kitahara, A, and Adelman, RC. 1979. Altered regulation of insulin secretion in isolated islets of different sizes of aging rats. *Biochem Biophys Res Commun* 87:1209–1213.
113. Cox, AJ. 1983. Gastric mucosal changes in peptic ulcers. *Gastoenterology* 45:558–561.
114. Bird, T, Hall, MRP, and Schade, ROK. 1977. Gastric histology and its relation to anemia in the elderly. *Gerontology* 23:309–321.
115. Ross, SA, Brown, JC, and Dupre, J. 1977. Hypersecretion of gastric inhibitory polypeptide following oral glucose in diabetes mellitus. *Diabetes* 26:525–529.
116. Ebert, R, et al. 1976. Response of gastric inhibitory polypeptide (GIP) to test meal in chronic pancreatitis—relationship to endocrine and exocrine insufficiency. *Diabetologia* 12:609–612.
117. Floyd, JC, Jr, et al. 1978. A newly recognized pancreatic polypeptide plasma level in health and disease. *Recent Prog Horm Res* 33:519–570.
118. Berger, D, et al. 1978. Effects of age on fasting plasma levels of pancreatic hormones in man. *J Clin Endocrinol Metab* 47:519–570.
119. Chang, JR, and Judd, HL. 1981. The ovary after menopause. *Clin Obstet Gynecol* 24:181–191.
120. Nicosia, SV. 1987. The aging ovary. *Med Clin North Am* 71:1–8.
121. Bigelow, B. 1958. Comparison of ovarian and endometrial morphology spanning the menopause. *Obstet Gynecol* 11:487–513.
122. Zbella, EA, and Scommegma, A. 1986. Premature menopause. *Med Aspects Hum Sexuality* 20:118.
123. Cutler, WB, and Garcia, CR. 1982. *The Medical Management of Menopause and Perimenopause*. Philadelphia: J.B. Lippincott Co.
124. Casper, RF, Yen, SSC, and Wilkes, MM. 1979. Menopausal flushes: A Neuroendocrine link with pulsatile luteinizing hormone secretion. *Science* 205:823–825.
125. Friedrich, EG. 1985. Vulvar dystrophy. *Clin Obstet Gynecol* 28:178–187.
126. Huppert, LC. 1987. Hormonal replacement therapy: Benefits, risks, doses. *Med Clin North Am* 71:23–39.
127. Slag, MF, et al. 1983. Impotence in medical clinic outpatients. *JAMA* 249:1736–1740.
128. Morley, JE, and Melmed, S. 1979. Gonadal dysfunction in systemic disorders. *Metabolism* 28:1051–1073.
129. Martin, CE. 1977. Sexual activity in the aging male. In *Handbook of Sexology*, Ed., J Money and H Moustafi, pp. 813–924. Amsterdam: ASP Biol Med Press.
130. Swerdloff, RS, and Heber, D. 1982. Effects of aging on male reproductive function. In *Endocrine Aspects of Aging,* Ed., SG Korenman, pp. 119–135. New York: Elsevier Biomedical.
131. Bremner, WJ, Vitiello, MV, and Prinz, PN. 1983. Loss of circadian rhythmicity in blood testosterone levels with aging in normal men. *J Clin Endocrinal Metab* 56:1278–1281.
132. Tillenger, KC. 1957. Testicular morphology. *Acta Endocrinol* (Copenh) 24(Suppl):1–192.
133. Natoli, A, Riondeno, G, and Broniati, A. 1972. Studio della funizone gonadale ormoniei e spermatogeniticanel corso della sensecenza maschile. *G Gerontol* 20:1103–1119.
134. Nankin, HR, and Calkins, JH. 1986. Decreased bioavailable testosterone in aging normal and impotent men. *J Clin Endocrinol Metab* 63:1418–1420.
135. Mooradian, AD, Morley, JE, and Korenman, SG. 1987. The biological actions of androgens. *Endocr Rev* 8:1–28.
136. Pirke, KM, and Doerr, P. 1970. Age related changes in free plasma testosterone, dihydrotestosterone and estradiol. *Acta Endocrinol* 80:171–178.

10

Hematologic Changes in the Elderly

David A. Lipschitz

Effects of Aging on Normal Hematopoietic Function

The production of bone marrow cells is regulated by a complex set of interactions between hematopoietic cells, their stromal microenvironment, and a series of diffusible hormones that affect cell proliferation. Hematopoietic cells are initially derived from a small pool of pluripotential stem cells that have the ability, under the appropriate stimulation, to give rise to committed, more differentiated stem cells that follow a specific line of hematopoietic development. During the process of commitment an identical multipotential daughter cell is formed. This capacity for self-renewal allows a small pluripotential compartment to maintain its cell numbers, while simultaneously amplifying into large numbers of differentiated hematopoietic precursors. The pluripotent hematopoietic stem cell is termed colony forming unit-spleen (CFU-S), by virtue of its ability to produce colonies in spleens of lethally irradiated mice (1, 2). CFU-S is also capable of repopulating the marrow of irradiated recipients and preventing marrow failure. Being the earliest hematopoietic cell that can be satisfactorily assayed, it constitutes a powerful research tool for studying differentiation and growth control. The hierarchy of production of hematopoietic precursors from CFU-S is shown in Figure 10-1. There are two forms of erythroid stem cells. The more primitive precursor, which forms large colonies in cultures containing high concentrations of erythropoietin, is referred to as a burst forming unit-erythroid (BFU-E). This precursor is thought to give rise to a more mature stem cell that develops colonies in cultures at shorter intervals and requires lower erythropoietin concentration. It is the immediate precursor of the morphologically recognizable proerythroblast and is referred to as the colony forming unit-erythroid (CFU-E). A committed myeloid stem cell or colony forming unit culture (CFU-C) is the immediate precursor of the myeloblast. These committed stem cells are morphologically unrecognizable and can only be identified by appropriate in vitro culture techniques. Under the appropriate stimulation these stem cells divide and differentiate into morphologically recognizable precursors of the various hematopoietic lineages. These cells mature and their eventual terminally differentiated products leave the bone marrow and enter the peripheral blood where they participate in oxygen transport, hemostasis, and host defense against infection.

Because of the bone marrow's high proliferative rates, it seems likely that aging may adversely affect it. Although there is some evidence that the pluripotential hematopoietic stem cell has a finite replicative capacity, a series of animal studies have shown that this marrow compartment does not diminish with age (3). Recent animal studies have also examined the effect of age on the number of committed hematopoietic stem cells as well as the differentiated cell number (4, 5). In mice, no age-related reduction in the number of erythroid or myeloid stem cells occur. In addition, the number of differentiated erythroid and myeloid precursors in the bone marrow is unaffected by age in normal animals. Red cell survival and red cell blood mass is unchanged with aging. The apparent anemia, so frequently demonstrated in aged mice, appears to be due to an expansion of plasma volume.

These findings indicate that no change in basal hematopoiesis occurs with aging. The aging process is typically characterized by a reduction in reserve capacity. Thus, although basal function may be normal, the ability to respond to increased stimulation is frequently compromised. There is evidence that this principle applies to the

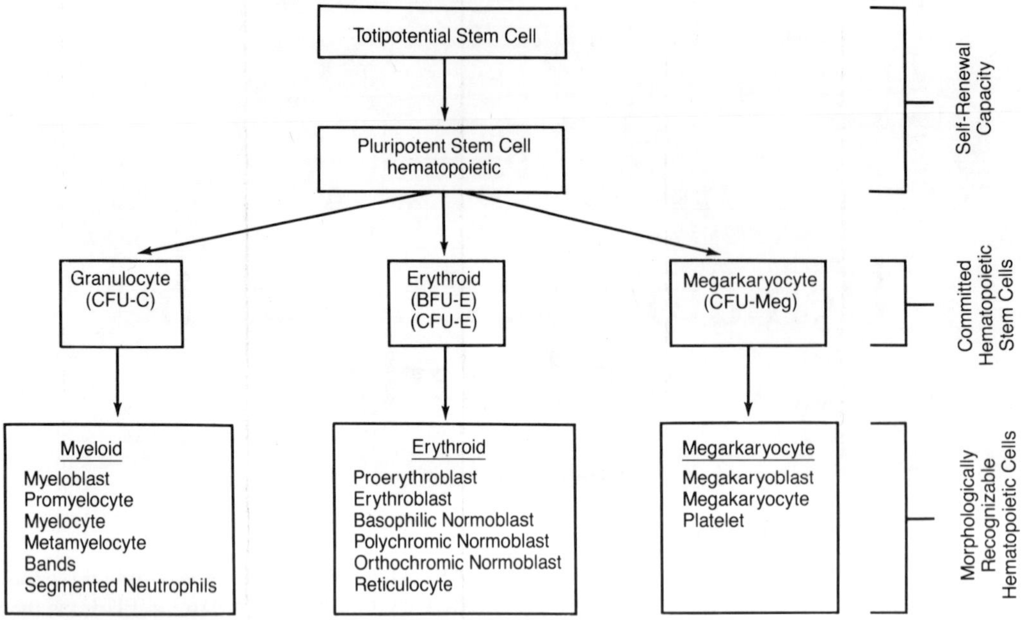

Figure 10-1. The hierarchy and production of hematopoietic precursors from primitive pluripotent stem cells.

aged hematopoietic system. For example, older mice recover their hemoglobin values more slowly after phlebotomy than do younger mice (4). Furthermore, when aged animals are placed in a high altitude chamber, the expected increase in hemoglobin levels is more variable. The levels tend to be lower in older than in younger animals (6). In vitro studies have also shown that hematopoietic stem cells and differentiated cells from old animals respond more slowly to stimulation than do cells from the young (7).

Does this diminished ability to respond to stimulation have any clinical relevance? If reserve capacity is compromised, it may be expected that an elderly subject's marrow would compensate less well for a given degree of acute or chronic disease than would a young subject's. This would make the elderly more prone to the development of disease-induced hematologic abnormalities. There is some evidence in an animal model that this may be true. When very old mice are housed in individual cages (1 animal per cage), no change in hematopoiesis is seen. Significant alterations in bone marrow function occur if they are housed in groups of 5 animals per cage, which is the common method employed for caging young animals (5). The aged animals become anemic and neutropenic, and the number of stem cells in the bone marrow decreases. Significant reductions also occur in the morphologically recognizable erythroid precursors. These findings are identical to hematopoietic changes previously described with overcrowding. The effects of overcrowding, however, are only seen when young mice are housed in groups of 10 or more per cage. This finding indicates that a minor stress, which does not affect hematopoiesis in young animals, causes a significant alteration in aged animals.

Another example of the relevance of age-related reduction in reserve capacity is illustrated by the effects of aging on neutrophil function. The killing of bacteria by the neutrophil occurs when phagocytized organisms are destroyed by exposure to highly toxic radicals and to secreted enzymes. During this reaction, a respiratory burst occurs in which oxidative metabolism and other neutrophil responses increase by 50–100 fold. This author and others have recently examined the effect of age on neutrophil function (8–10). As would be expected, basal function in the young and old is identical. In response to stimulation, however, the respiratory burst, enzyme secretion and other measurable metabolic responses is clearly reduced in the old. This diminution in function is not large enough to interfere with the ability of neutrophils of the elderly to phagocytose bacteria. However, the diminished neutrophil reserve capacity does have relevance. When mice are made protein deficient, a modest reduction has been shown to occur in neutrophil function, which is very similar to that seen with aging (11). In old mice, the effect of protein deficiency and aging are additive, so that in this circumstance neutrophil function decreases to a level where the ability of the cell to undertake its most critically important role of phagocytosis is severely compromised (Fig. 10-2). This finding is of particular importance, as it may help to explain the high prevalence of serious bacterial infection in hospitalized and older individuals who are

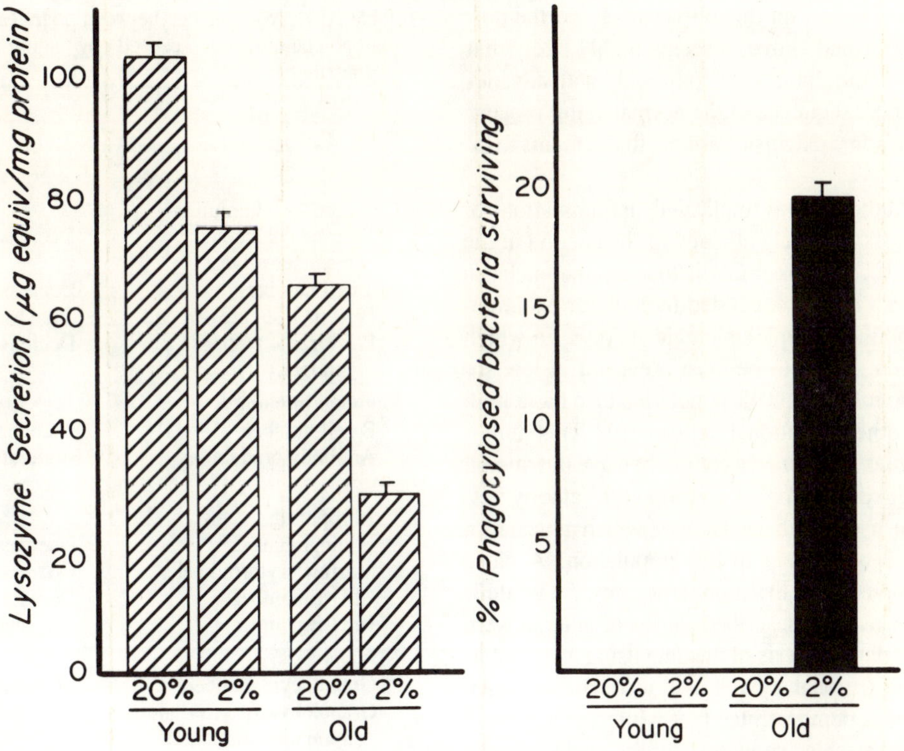

Figure 10-2. Secretion of the enzyme lysozyme (*left-hand panel*) following activation of neutrophils from young (6-month) or old (24-month) mice fed a 20% (normal) or 2% protein diet for 3 weeks prior to sacrifice. The *right-hand panel* shows the percentage of phagocytosed bacteria not killed by neutrophils from young and old mice fed a 2% or 20% protein diet. The results clearly demonstrate that neutrophils obtained from old mice fed a 2% protein diet are unable to kill all phagocytosed bacteria.

frequently malnourished. It also demonstrates the relevance of diminished reserve capacity, which results in increased susceptibility to disease.

Anemia in the Elderly

The most uniformly described hematopoietic change with aging in humans is a higher prevalence of anemia. This observation is primarily derived from epidemiologic studies in the United States, Canada, and Europe (12–16). The prevalence of anemia in women older than age 59 is approximately equal to that found in women of child-bearing age. In men, a definite increase in the prevalence of anemia is found in older age groups. Studies from Great Britain are important, as they have determined the incidence of anemia in large numbers of subjects older than 60 years. In both men and women, the prevalence of anemia increased significantly with each successive decade. A recent analysis of the second National Health and Nutrition Education Survey (NHANES 2) demonstrated a significant reduction in hemoglobin levels with advancing age in apparently healthy males and a minimal, although significant, decrease in elderly females (17). Based on a lower normal limit of 14 g/dl, a very large percentage of elderly males would be found to be anemic. This study proposed that the reduction for males was a consequence of aging and suggested that age-specific reference standards for hemoglobin concentration for the elderly be adopted.

A close evaluation of apparently healthy elderly subjects with mild anemia has revealed that the cause is not usually obvious (18). A careful assessment of hematopoiesis in these individuals revealed mild marrow failure as evidenced by reductions in bone marrow differentiated cell and stem cell number and modest decreases in peripheral leukocyte counts (19). A major unanswered question is whether or not this decline in hemoglobin with advancing age is a consequence of the normal aging process or reflects some yet to be defined abnormality. Of particular importance in this regard is the recent finding that anemia is extremely rare in an affluent, healthy elderly population examined in New Mexico (20). None of the elderly males and females in this group were anemic. Furthermore, longitudinal monitoring of these subjects over a 5-year period failed to demonstrate an increased prevalence of anemia. Based on this observation and the animals studies described above, it seems highly likely that the decrease in hemoglobin seen commonly with advancing age is not a consequence of the normal aging process and is related to some extrinsic variable that remains to be determined.

Recent studies have implicated inflammation or chronic disease as the likely etiology of the anemia in the elderly (21). A second possibility is that the anemia has a nutritional basis. This is suggested by a closer examination of data obtained in epidemiologic surveys, in which anemia has been shown to be most prevalent in low socioeconomic populations. This population also has a high prevalence of other nutritional deficiencies. This author and his colleagues performed a comprehensive nutritional and hematologic evaluation on a group of 73 elderly veterans living in a domiciliary facility, which revealed a high prevalence of anemia in this population. A close evaluation demonstrated that iron deficiency, folate deficiency, or other usually described causes of anemia were rare. A multivariate analysis of the data using age, hematopoietic and nutritional factors as covariants was then performed. It was demonstrated that while age appeared to be the major variable accounting for the decline in immunologic measurements observed in this elderly population, age did not appear to be an important factor in the prevalence of anemia. In contrast, serum albumin, transferrin, and pre-albumin, which assess nutritional status, appeared to be excellent predictors of anemia. This information provides indirect evidence that a nutritional variable may contribute to the anemia seen in these elderly populations.

Further evidence suggesting that a nutritional factor may contribute to the anemia comes from the observation that there is a marked similarity between the alterations in immunologic and hematopoietic function that occur with aging and those that occur with protein deprivation (Table 10-1). This raises the possibility that protein deprivation in some form may contribute to the hematopoietic changes normally ascribed to aging. There is evidence that correction of protein energy malnutrition in the hospitalized elderly can markedly improve hematopoietic function (22). In these subjects, interpretation of improvements in hematologic status is extremely difficult. Any hospitalized elderly person has coexisting diseases that affect hematopoietic function. Thus, the overall improvement seen with nutritional rehabilitation may reflect an overall improvement of the medical status of the patient. In a more recent study, the effect of increased feeding on hematopoietic status was examined in relatively healthy elderly subjects who lived at home and were ambulatory, but were underweight and had marginal evidence of protein energy deprivation. By providing polymeric dietary supplements to these subjects between meals, it was possible to correct nutritional deficiencies and obtain weight gain. Despite a positive impact on nutritional status, however, the anemia, which was invariably present in this population, did not improve (23).

Table 10-1. Similarities between changes in immune and hematopoietic function caused by aging or protein energy malnutrition

	Aging	Protein energy malnutrition
Cell-mediated immunity		
Delayed cutaneous hypersensitivity	Decreased	Decreased
T cell number	Decreased	Decreased
Percent T suppressor cell	Increased	Increased
Blastogenic response to mitogen	Decreased	Decreased
Humoral immunity		
B cell number	Unchanged	Unchanged
Antibody production	Moderately decreased	Moderately decreased
Erythropoiesis		
Hemoglobin	Decreased	Decreased
Marrow erythroid cells	Decreased	Decreased
CFU-E number	Decreased	Decreased
BFU-E number	Normal	Normal
Myelopoiesis		
Granulocyte number	Reduced	Reduced
Granulocytosis after endotoxin administration	Decreased	Decreased
CFU-C number	Decreased	Decreased

Some conclusions can be drawn from these observations. It is clear that significant nutritional deficiencies aggravate the hematologic abnormalities in the elderly. Even in apparently healthy older persons, it is possible that nutritional factors contribute to their hematopoietic changes, but alternative mechanisms, other than simple nutritional deficiency, must be considered. Marginal reductions of one or more nutrients acting alone or in combination over a prolonged period of time may modulate hematopoietic change usually ascribed to aging. Alternatively, nutrient delivery to the target organ may be altered with aging, or changes in nutrient target interaction may occur. These possibilities could account for the higher prevalence of anemia reported in epidemiologic studies; they remain no more than potential hypotheses that will require further research.

Evaluation of Anemia in the Elderly

For practical purposes, 12 g/dl is recommended as a lower limit of normal for hemoglobin for both elderly men and elderly women. Attempting to define the cause of anemia when the hemoglobin concentration is between

12 and 14 g/dl in elderly men rarely yields an etiology. Even with a borderline low hematocrit (at a level of 12 g/dl), a decision as to how aggressively to evaluate a patient must rest on clinical judgment. The complex nature of the problems that present in older individuals together with the high risk of multiple pathologies occurring simultaneously makes this even more critical. On the other hand, once a decision has been made to investigate a low hemoglobin in an older person, the principles involved in assessment and evaluation are very similar to that which would be used in subjects of any age group. The etiologies of the various anemias seen in the elderly are summarized in Table 10-2.

The initial approach to the patient with anemia must include a complete history and physical examination, as well as a complete blood count (CBC) to evaluate red blood cell size and red blood cell production rate. Microcytosis, defined as a mean corpuscular volume (MCV) of less than 84 fl (Coulter counter), indicates an impairment of hemoglobin synthesis. Macrocytosis, defined as an MCV of over 100 fl, may be caused by reticulocytes or more frequently by an abnormality in nuclear maturation. Red cell production is estimated from the reticulocyte production index. Hemolytic anemia usually has a reticulocyte index greater than 3, whereas a failure of production is indicated by a reticulocyte index of less than 2. Decreased production is caused by the hypoproliferative anemias or by ineffective erythropoiesis. The latter disorder is characterized by significant increases in erythroid cell proliferation. Due to maturation abnormalities, these cells are unable to exit the bone marrow and are destroyed by marrow reticuloendothelial cells in a process referred to as intramedullary hemolysis. The disorder may be associated with either macrocytosis or microcytosis. An elevated LDH and indirect hyperbilirubinemia result from the increased destruction of red cell precursors in the marrow and may be used to distinguish ineffective erythropoiesis from hypoproliferative anemia. After excluding hemolytic anemia by the absence of a high reticulocyte index, the next approach required to define the etiology of the anemia is outlined in Figure 10-3. Observation may be reasonable for those older individuals who have a mild decrease in hemoglobin (10.5–12 g/dl), a normal reticulocyte index, normochromic normocytic indices, no leukocyte or platelet abnormalities, and no occult blood in the stool. Further investigation is indicated if the anemia worsens or a change in the peripheral blood pattern occurs. For individuals with mild anemia and hypochromic microcytic indices, or more severe anemia with normochromic normocytic indices, a more extensive workup is required. Similarly, the presence of macrocytosis warrants additional investigation.

Hypoproliferative Anemias

The majority of anemias in the elderly will be of the hypoproliferative type, most commonly associated with inadequate iron supply for erythropoiesis. This is diagnosed by the presence of a decreased serum iron and a reduced transferrin saturation (serum iron divided by the total iron-binding capacity [TIBC] expressed as a percent). Absolute iron deficiency (blood loss) is the commonest cause of iron-deficient erythropoiesis in younger subjects. In the elderly, the etiology is more likely to be the "anemia of chronic disease" or anemia associated with inflammation. Iron-deficient erythropoiesis in these disorders results from a defective ability of the reticuloendothelial system to reutilize iron derived from senescent red cells. Thus, tissue iron stores are normal or increased, resulting in a serum ferritin concentration above 50 ng/ml and a reduction in the TIBC. This contrasts with a low serum ferritin and high TIBC, which reflect absent iron stores in blood loss anemia.

Blood loss, the anemia of inflammation and chronic disease, and that associated with protein energy malnutrition are the most prevalent anemias in elderly populations. In younger individuals, iron deficiency anemia is usually due to either blood loss or nutritional iron deficiency. In

Table 10-2. Physiologic classification of anemia

Hypoproliferative	Ineffective	Hemolytic
1. Iron-deficient erythropoiesis	1. Megaloblastic	1. Immunologic
a. Iron deficiency	a. Vitamin B_{12}	a. Idiopathic
b. Chronic Disease	b. Folate	b. Secondary to drug, tumor, or disease
c. Inflammation	c. Refractory	
2. Erythropoietin lack	2. Microcytic	2. Intrinsic
a. Renal	a. Thalassemia	a. Metabolic
b. Nutritional	b. Sideroblastic	b. Abnormal hemoglobin
c. Endocrine		
3. Stem cell dysfunction	3. Normocytic	3. Extrinsic
a. Aplastic anemia	a. Stromal disease	a. Mechanical
b. Red blood cell aplasia	b. Dimorphic	b. Lytic substance

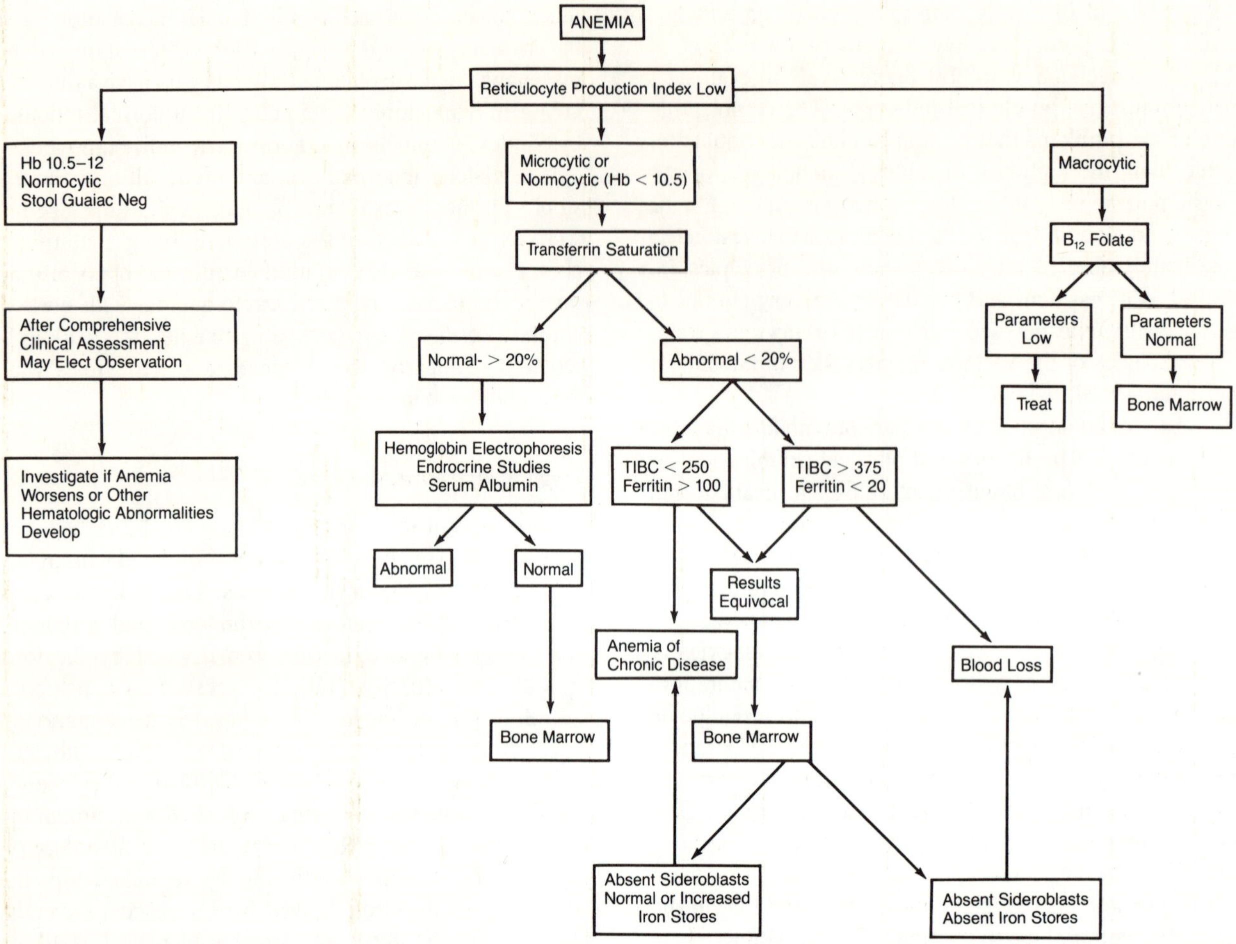

Figure 10-3. An approach to the evaluation of anemia in the elderly after hemolysis is excluded by the reticulocyte production index.

both men and women, a progressive increase in iron stores occurs with advancing age. In older men, tissue iron stores average 1200 mg and in women, iron stores increase from a mean of 300 mg to approximately 800 mg over the decade following menopause. Thus nutritional iron deficiency is rare in the elderly despite the preponderance of other nutritional problems. When unexplained iron deficiency does occur, it is almost exclusively due to blood loss from the intestinal tract, even if bleeding is undetected by repeated stool guaiac determinations. Other routes of bleeding may occur but are easily recognizable (epistaxis, abnormal bleeding from the uterus, hematuria). The causes of blood loss in the elderly include drugs (aspirin) and bleeding due to a neoplasm. Angiodysplasia of the large bowel and diverticular disease are frequent causes but should only be considered once a neoplasm has been excluded. Rarely, iron deficiency can result from malabsorption or urinary losses of iron which occur in the fact of intravascular hemolysis.

Inflammation is a second important cause of anemia in the elderly and is perhaps the more frequent. Inflammation may be the result of bacterial infection, immune reaction, tissue necrosis, or neoplasm. Usually, the decrease in hematocrit is moderate. Hematologic findings differ from iron deficiency in that the iron block is less severe, and microcytosis is usually minimal. In some instances, these hematologic findings may be present with little or no evidence of inflammation. Inadequate food intake and increased tissue breakdown may contribute to the severity of the anemia through decreased erythropoietin stimulation. Treatment is that of the underlying disease. Only rarely is anemia severe enough to require transfusion. Iron therapy is usually ineffective owing to the limited absorption of iron in the presence of inflammation and the trapping of parenteral iron in the macrophage.

Anemia of chronic disease is a label often used to explain an anemia associated with some other major disease process, such as cancer, collagen vascular disorders, rheumatoid arthritis, and inflammatory bowel disease. Occasionally, the anemia may be the initial manifestation of an occult disease. It is critical for the clinician to be aware of this possibility and to assure a rational and appropriate workup. Management of this type of anemia consists of ensuring adequate nutrition and treating the underlying disease process.

Nutritional deprivation in the aged generally results in a normocytic normochromic anemia with an essentially normal peripheral smear. In the hospitalized patient, evidence of iron-deficient erythropoiesis (low transferrin saturation) is common, and the serum ferritin is elevated. There is usually a history of weight loss, and laboratory studies indicate a reduced serum albumin and a decreased TIBC (< 240 g/dl). This disorder is particularly important, as there is evidence that correction of the nutritional deficiency and its underlying cause can result in significant improvement in the hemoglobin level and other hematopoietic parameters.

A multifactorial etiology of anemia is more likely in frail older subjects with multiple medical problems. A classic example is a patient with active rheumatoid disease who has lost blood from aspirin ingestion. Similarly, protein energy malnutrition or blood loss will markedly aggravate the anemia associated with neoplasia. The possibility of a multifactorial etiology, including blood loss, malnutrition, folate deficiency, or hemolytic disease, should be considered when the anemia of chronic disease or inflammation is associated with a hemoglobin below 10 g/dl. In this circumstance, laboratory investigations frequently give equivocal results, and hence, a bone marrow examination may be required.

Marrow failure due to interference with proliferation of hematopoietic cells occurs in the elderly. The disorder is generally associated with suppression of all marrow elements and is suggested by the presence of peripheral pancytopenia. Common causes include drugs, immune damage to the stem cell population, intrinsic marrow lesions, and marrow replacement by malignant cells or fibrous tissue. The latter is usually associated with a myelophthisic blood picture (nucleated red cells, giant platelets, and metamyelocytes on smear) as a reflection of the disruption of marrow stromal architecture. The presence of pancytopenia and the absence of iron-deficient erythropoiesis is an indication for bone marrow aspiration and biopsy. Occasionally, isolated suppression of erythropoiesis occurs; this is referred to as pure red cell aplasia. This disorder may be drug related or may be caused by benign or malignant abnormalities of lymphocytes, including thymoma. These subjects present with isolated anemia, an elevated serum iron, and absent erythroid precursors on bone marrow examination.

Ineffective Erythropoiesis

Macrocytic anemias in the elderly result from vitamin B_{12} and folate deficiency. The prevalence of pernicious anemia increases significantly with advancing age. The disorder results from malabsorption of vitamin B_{12} as a consequence of antibodies against gastric parietal cells and intrinsic factor. Atrophic gastritis and decreased secretion of extrinsic factor occur, which result in failure of vitamin B_{12} absorption. Pernicious anemia occurs most frequently in subjects over the age of 60 and is more common in women. The anemia may be very severe, the patient presenting with weakness and a lemon-yellow discoloration. Neurologic abnormalities, including peripheral neuropathy, ataxia, loss of position sense, and upper motor neuron signs, are frequent. Behavioral abnormalities and dementia are well described. Occasionally, there is evidence of a more generalized immunologic disorder, manifested by myxedema, hypoadrenalism, and vitiligo. The presence of pancytopenia, macrocytosis, hypersegmented polymorphonuclear leukocytes in the peripheral smear, a decreased reticulocyte index, and an increased LDH and indirect hypobilirubinemia suggest a diagnosis of megaloblastic anemia. The bone marrow classically shows giant metamyelocytes, hypersegmented polymorphonuclear leukocytes, and enlarged erythroid precursors with more hemoglobin than would be expected from the immaturity of their nuclei (nuclear cytoplasmic dissociation). The diagnosis is made by demonstrating serum vitamin B_{12} concentration of less than 100 pg/mL. Vitamin B_{12} deficiency may also be caused by diseases of the ileum. The Schilling test is able to distinguish a deficiency of intrinsic factor (malabsorption corrected by ingested vitamin B_{12} and intrinsic factor) from an abnormality in the ability of the ileum to absorb the vitamin B_{12} intrinsic factor complex (absorption still impaired with intrinsic factor plus vitamin B_{12}). Treatment consists of weekly or biweekly injection of 100 μg of vitamin B_{12} until stores are replenished. A maintenance dose at monthly intervals is then adequate.

Epidemiologic studies have generally shown an adequate folate nutriture in the elderly. Folate deficiency of sufficient severity to cause anemia in the elderly is most frequently found in association with protein energy malnutrition and excessive alcohol consumption. Alcohol and various other drugs are also known to interfere with folate absorption and internal metabolism. Vulnerability to deficiency is significantly greater when folate requirements are increased as a result of inflammation, neoplastic disease, or hemolytic anemia. The hematologic profile is identical to that described for vitamin B_{12} deficiency. The diagnosis is made by the demonstration of significant reductions in the serum (< 2 ng/ml) or red cell (< 100 ng/ml) folate concentration. Prior to commencement of therapy with folate, it is important to exclude vitamin B_{12} deficiency, as treatment with folate can aggravate the neurologic abnormalities in the latter disorder.

The major causes of ineffective erythropoiesis and microcytosis are thalassemia and the sideroblastic anemias. Although thalassemia is generally diagnosed at an earlier age, there are reports of its initial detection in older people. On the other hand, acquired sideroblastic anemia is primarily a disease of the elderly. It is a heterogeneous group of disorders, characterized by the presence of iron deposits in the mitochondria of normoblasts. The disorder is a consequence of impaired heat synthesis. It usually reflects an intrinsic marrow lesion (idiopathic) but may be secondary to inflammation, neoplasia, or drug ingestion. The common finding is the presence of a dimorphic red cell population. One population of red cells is markedly hypochromic, while the remainder are filled with hemoglobin. The diagnosis is made by the demonstration of ringed sideroblasts in the bone marrow as well as the presence of maturation abnormalities of myeloid and erythroid precursors. A fraction of elderly patients with sideroblastic anemia show some response to pharmacologic doses of pyridoxine (200 mg t.i.d.). This dose should be given to all patients until it becomes apparent that a rise in hemoglobin concentration will not occur. For those patients unresponsive to pyridoxine, the anemia must be treated symptomatically.

Di Guglielmo's syndrome is more common in older people who present with megaloblastic erythroid precursors. Frequently, abnormal sideroblasts will also be seen. The peripheral smear usually demonstrates pancytopenia with occasional nucleated red cells or immature myeloid and megakaryocytic precursors. The bone marrow is markedly hyperplastic. It is essential to exclude the presence of vitamin B_{12} and folate deficiencies, and a trial of pyridoxine may be indicated. Treatment is usually supportive. There is some evidence that these disorders are premalignant, evolving rarely into a subacute or acute myelogenous leukemia.

Hemolytic Anemias

The causes of hemolytic anemia in the elderly are somewhat different from those found in younger subjects. Although most patients with congenital disorders will have previously been identified, an occasional patient with congenital hemolytic anemia may present for the first time with symptoms related to cholelithiasis. Autoimmune hemolytic anemia is the most common cause in the elderly. The diagnosis is made by the presence of a positive Coombs test. In younger subjects, an etiology of the autoimmune hemolysis is rarely identified. In the elderly, on the other hand, the anemia is more likely to be associated with a lymphoproliferative disorder (non-Hodgkin's lymphoma or chronic lymphocytic leukemia), collagen vascular disease, or drug ingestion. Steroids and splenectomy are usually effective in patients with red cell antibodies of the IgG type. Patients with red cell antibodies of the IgM variety are more likely to be refractory to such treatment.

A disorder of some importance in the aged is microangiopathic hemolytic anemia. This is usually associated with severe infection or disseminated neoplasm and presents with not only hemolytic anemia but also a consumptive coagulopathy. The presence of red cell fragmentation, thrombocytopenia, a prolonged partial thromboplastin time, and hemosiderinuria should suggest this diagnosis.

Conclusion

There is evidence from both animal models and humans that basal hematopoiesis is either unchanged or only minimally altered with aging. Because of compromised reserve capacity, hematopoietic alterations are likely to occur with more subtle stresses in the elderly than in young persons. This reduced reserve capacity, so typical of the aging process, may contribute to the high prevalence of anemia in the elderly, to the increased susceptibility to infection, and to an elderly individual's decreased potential to recover from a relatively minor insult.

References

1. Till, JE, and McCulloch, EA. 1961. A direct measurement of the radiation sensitivity of normal mouse bone marrow cells. *Rad Res* 13:213–222.
2. Schofield, R. 1979. The pluripotent stem cell. *Clin Haematol* 8:221–237.
3. Chen, MG. 1971. Age related changes in hematopoietic stem cell population of a long lived hybrid mouse. *J Cell Physiol* 78:225–232.
4. Boggs, DR, and Patrene, KD. 1985. Hematopoiesis and aging III: Anemia and a blunted erythropoietic response to hemorrhage in aged mice. *Am J Hematol* 19:327–338.
5. Williams, LH, Udupa, KB, and Lipschitz, DA. 1986. An evaluation of the effect of age on hematopoiesis in the mouse. *Exp Hematol* 14:827–832.
6. Udupa, KB, and Lipschitz, DA. 1984. Erythropoiesis in the aged mouse I. Response to stimulation *in vivo*. *J Lab Clin Med* 103:574–580.
7. Udupa, KB, and Lipschitz, DA. 1984. Erythropoiesis in the aged mouse II. Response to stimulation *in vitro*. *J Lab Clin Med* 103:581–588.
8. Nagel, JE, et al. 1982. Oxidative metabolism and bacteri-

cidal capacity of polymorphonuclear leukocyte from young and aged adults. *J Gerontol* 37:529–534.
9. McLaughlin, B, O'Malley, K, and Cotten, TG. 1986. Age-related differences in granulocyte chemotaxis and degranulation. *Clin Sci* 70:59–62.
10. Lipschitz, DA, Udupa, KB, and Boxer, LA. 1988. The role of calcium in the age-related decrease in neutrophil function. *Blood* 71(3):659–665.
11. Lipschitz, DA, and Udupa, KB. 1986. Influence on aging and protein deficiency on neutrophil function. *J Gerontol* 41:690–694.
12. Parson, PL, Whithey, JL, and Kilpatrick, GS. 1965. The prevalence of anemia in the elderly. *Practitioner* 195:656–660.
13. Hill, RD. 1967. The prevalence of anemia in the over-65s in a rural practice. *Practitioner* 217:963–967.
14. Myers, MA, Saunders, CRG, and Chalmers, DG. 1968. The hemoglobin level of fit elderly people. *Lancet* 2:261–263.
15. McLennan, WJ, et al. 1973. Anemia in the elderly. *Q J Med* 52:1–13.
16. Nutrition Canada. 1973. National Survey. Ottawa, Canada: Information Canada.
17. Yip, R, Johnson, C, and Dallman, PR. 1984. Age-related changes in laboratory values used in the diagnosis of anemia and iron deficiency. *Am J Clin Nutr* 39:427–436.
18. Lipschitz, DA, Mitchell, CO, and Thompson, C. 1981. The anemia of senescence. *Am J Hematol* 11:47–54.
19. Lipschitz, DA, et al. 1984. Effect of age on hematopoiesis in man. *Blood* 63:502–509.
20. Garry, PJ, Goodwin, JS, and Hunt, WC. 1985. In *Nutrition, Immunity and Illness in the Elderly,* Ed., RJ Chandra, pp. 77–83. Oxford: Pergamon.
21. Dallman, PR, Yip, R, and Johnson, C. 1984. Prevalence and causes of anemia in the United States, 1976 to 1980. *Am J Clin Nutr* 39:437–445.
22. Lipschitz, DA, and Mitchell, CO. 1982. The correctability of the nutritional, immune and hematopoietic manifestations of protein calorie malnutrition in the elderly. *J Am Coll Nutr* 1:17–25.
23. Lipschitz, DA, et al. 1984. Nutritional evaluation and supplementation of elderly subjects participating in a "meals on wheels" program. *JPEN* 9:343–347.

11

Coagulation in the Elderly

Ali Mansouri and Laura F. Hutchins

Hemostasis is a complex process that requires the participation of various components of the blood vessel wall and the circulating blood. For the sake of easier description and understanding, hemostasis can be divided into three phases: (*a*) the vascular phase; (*b*) platelet participation; and (*c*) blood coagulation (fibrinogenesis and fibrinolysis). Each phase is equally important, and its malfunction may lead to bleeding tendency or thrombosis. The clinical presentation of various component abnormalities (quantitative or qualitative) varies not only because of the particular function of that component in the overall scheme of hemostasis, but also according to the type of trauma sustained. For example, both patients with hemophilia and low platelet counts bleed excessively during a surgical operation, but under the normal stress of life, the former might have massive bleeding, whereas the latter usually has easy bruising.

The hemostatic problems are either inherited or acquired. In general, the hereditary problems are due to the qualitative or quantitative abnormality of one protein, whereas the acquired problems are usually the result of multiple qualitative and quantitative abnormalities combined. In addition, the clinical picture of the latter is often complicated by the underlying disorder, which is the primary cause of the hemostatic abnormality. It is clear that, although the treatment of hereditary conditions includes replacement therapy and preventive measures, the treatment of acquired conditions necessitates measures taken to correct the underlying disorder.

Hemostatic disorders of the elderly can be managed in the same fashion as those of other age groups. There are no major biochemical differences in hemostatic process between the young and the old, although minor differences have been noted by some investigators. However, there are undeniable physiologic differences in the elderly. For example, older people are more prone to thromboembolism, regardless of the presence of any known disease. Diminished subcutaneous supportive tissue can lead to increased bleeding tendency. In addition, older people often suffer from a multitude of chronic diseases that can affect the hemostatic process. The association of cancer and its treatment with hemostatic abnormalities is well known. Diabetes, liver disease, renal insufficiency, and atherosclerotic vessels can all initiate or complicate a hemostatic problem. In addition, some hemostatic abnormalities, which do not cause any problems under normal conditions, will assume major importance when there is need for surgery. This article outlines a comprehensive diagnostic and therapeutic approach for the management of the hemostatic problems of the elderly. However, the treatment of thrombosis will not be covered since this theme is usually handled separately.

Overview of Hemostasis

The vascular endothelium is a nonthrombogenic surface, but the subendothelium reacts with strong affinity to the circulating platelets. Factor VIII von Willebrand (VIII vWf) serves as a connecting piece between a platelet surface receptor (glycoprotein Ib complex) and vascular subendothelium (1–3). The adherent platelets rapidly spread on the subendothelium. This function depends on the presence of fibronectin and platelet membrane glycopro-

The authors wish to express their gratitude to Mrs. Frances Lewandoski for her diligent and skillful secretarial assistance.

tein complex IIb/IIIa as well as calcium. Following adhesion, ADP is released, which recruits more platelets. Platelet adhesion and aggregation lead to the release of biologically active substances that promote vasoconstriction and blood coagulation.

Factor X plays a central role in blood coagulation. It is activated by the intrinsic or extrinsic system. The intrinsic system is activated when the blood comes into contact with subendothelium (4). This activates factor $XII \rightarrow XII_a$, which in turn activates prekallikrein to kallikrein. Kallikrein and high molecular weight (HMW) kininogen generate more factor XII_a, which in its turn activates factor $XI \rightarrow XI_a$. Factor XI_a activates factor $IX \rightarrow IX_a$. Factor IX_a activates factor $X \rightarrow X_a$ in the presence of factor VIII_a, Ca^{2+} and phospholipid (platelet surface). Alternatively, factor X activation takes place by the activation of factor VII in the presence of tissue factor and Ca^{2+} (the extrinsic system). The activation of factor $X \rightarrow Xa$ through intrinsic or extrinsic system, in the presence of factor Va, phospholipid, and Ca^{2+}, converts prothrombin to thrombin. Prothrombin in turn converts fibrinogen to fibrin. The stabilization of fibrin (cross linking) by factor XIII leads to insoluble fibrin with efficient tensile strength.

The blood coagulation is counterbalanced by several anticoagulatory reactions. In this respect, the endothelial surface plays a major role. The inhibition of platelet adhesion to endothelium is mediated by prostacyclin (PGI_2), which is a product of the arachidonic acid metabolism in these cells (5). The activation of protein C, a vitamin K-dependent, naturally occurring anticoagulant, is also dependent on the endothelial surface, since thrombomodulin, a cofactor of protein C that is activated by thrombin, is an endothelial cell surface protein (6, 7). The anticoagulatory properties of protein C are of significant clinical importance. Patients who lack this protein have strong predisposition to thrombosis (8). Antithrombin III is another naturally occurring anticoagulant that inhibits thrombin. The inactivation of thrombin by antithrombin III is significantly enhanced by heparin and heparin-like substances that are synthesized by the endothelial cells (9). The endothelium is also rich in plasminogen activator, which leads to the generation of plasmin and to fibrinolysis (10). All these reactions make the endothelial surface highly nonthrombogenic. However, recent studies have shown that perturbation of the endothelium can also induce tissue factor and promote coagulation (11). It is clear from these observations that the endothelium is highly active in promotion and retardation of clot formation. It is possible that alteration of the above reactions in the elderly can predispose this population to higher incidence of thrombosis. However, these putative changes cannot be measured in the clinical laboratory at the present time. Therefore, under the heading of "vascular abnormalities," only anatomical vascular abnormalities are included.

Vascular Abnormalities

Most vascular abnormalities are not specific for any age. However, some may develop or worsen in later life. One problem which is specific for the older age group is the atrophy of the supportive tissue around superficial vessels (12). This abnormality is of no great consequence but can occasionally lead to extensive subcutaneous bleeding after mild trauma. Another vascular abnormality that becomes more pronounced with age is hereditary hemorrhagic telangiectasia. This is an autosomal dominant disorder that is manifested by dilated capillaries and arteries, appearing as macular or nodular lesions on the skin and mucous membranes. These lesions blanch under pressure since they are blood vessels with very thin walls lacking smooth muscle. Chronic blood loss from the nose and gastrointestinal system characteristically leads to iron deficiency anemia (13). The diagnosis is not difficult since the triad of repeated hemorrhage, multiple telangiectases, and familial occurrence is so characteristic. Most patients have lesions on the face, around the mouth, and on the tongue. However, the telangiectases must be differentiated from similar lesions seen in the elderly, such as cherry angiomas, spider telangiectases of liver disease, and venous abnormalities. Gastrointestinal angiodysplasia is another vascular abnormality that is not uncommon in the elderly; this lesion may cause recurrent bleeding and anemia. These patients also often have other reasons for increased bleeding tendency, such as renal failure or acquired von Willebrand's disease (vWD). Awareness of this entity is important for treating the bleeding episodes early and effectively.

A large number of drugs can cause purpuric lesions unrelated to platelet or coagulation abnormalities. Although there is no bleeding problem per se, the clinical picture suggests bleeding disorder. The pathophysiology of this type of drug-induced purpura is ill understood and might differ from one drug to another or from one patient to another. However, in most cases it is of an allergic nature. The major offenders are antibiotics, analgesics, and sedatives. A similar picture can be caused by autoimmunity and dysproteinemia. Finally, a wide variety of infectious agents might cause purpura, probably directly by injuring the vascular endothelium or indirectly by depositing immune complexes on the endothelial surface, as in autoimmune processes.

Quantitative Platelet Disorders

Thrombocytopenia is the most common hemostatic abnormality in the elderly. It is most often mild to moderate but at times severe, causing bleeding. The normal venous blood platelet count is 140–440 $\times$ 10^9/L (14). Significant bleeding is rare if the platelet count is above 50 $\times$ 10^9/L, as long as the platelets remain functionally normal. Thrombocytopenia can be attributed to three processes or their combinations: (*a*) decreased platelet formation; (*b*) increased platelet distruction; and (*c*) abnormal platelet distribution (Table 11-1).

Decreased Platelet Production

Decreased platelet production could be caused by any process that temporarily or permanently damages the bone marrow megakaryocytic pool or interferes with its function.

Bone marrow hypoplasia can result from a number of physical or chemical agents. Ionizing radiation is a relatively common cause of bone marrow hypoplasia in elderly patients who are treated with radiotherapy. The effect of radiotherapy is dependent on the dose and extent of treatment. Patients who receive total nodal radiation or total or hemibody radiation develop moderate to severe thrombocytopenia, which can be of long duration. Chemical agents such as drugs, notably cancer chemotherapeutic agents, cause predictable thrombocytopenia. Radiation exposure and chemotherapeutic agents usually lead to pancytopenia and not to thrombocytopenia alone. However, anemia is not always apparent during the early course of treatment due to the long red cell life span. Certain drugs may selectively inhibit the production of platelets without significantly affecting the rest of the bone marrow cells. Kutti and Weinfeld (15) have reported that about one quarter of patients taking thiazide diuretics develop mild thrombocytopenia with reduced megakaryocytes. The decrease in the number of megakaryocytes in the bone marrow is probably due to direct suppression of these cells, but the exact cause of this remains unknown. Decreased thrombopoiesis has also been related to the use of diethylstilbestrol (DES). However, most patients who develop thrombocytopenia with the use of DES have normal numbers of megakaryocytes in the marrow (16, 17).

Table 11-1. Causes of thrombocytopenia

Decreased platelet production
- Decrease in all normal bone marrow cells
  - Bone marrow damage due to physical or chemical agents
  - Nutritional deficiency (ineffective thrombopoiesis)
- Selective decrease in megakaryocytes (drugs)

Increased platelet destruction
- Immune type
  - Idiopathic thrombocytopenic purpura (ITP)
  - Underlying lymphoproliferative or autoimmune process
  - Drug related
- Nonimmune type
  - Disseminated intravascular coagulation (DIC)
  - Infection
  - Microangiopathic (thrombotic thrombocytopenic purpura)
  - Drug related

Abnormal platelet distribution
- Splenomegaly
- Massive bank blood transfusion

Ineffective Thrombopoiesis

Ineffective thrombopoiesis can be described as inadequate platelet production in spite of a normal or an increased number of megakaryocytes in the bone marrow. This condition is usually due either to an intrinisic DNA abnormality, such as bone marrow dysplasia, or due to a deficiency of a nutrient, especially vitamin B_{12} or folic acid (18). Bone marrow dysplasia, also referred to as preleukemic syndrome, is a heterogeneous condition with unknown etiology, which has some morphologic features of megaloblastic hematopoiesis with ineffective cell production. Acquired DNA synthetic abnormalities usually involve all bone marrow cells, not just megakaryocytes. However, heavy consumption of alcohol suppresses or interferes predominately with thrombopoiesis (19).

Increased Platelet Destruction

Accelerated platelet destruction is divided into two subcategories, depending on whether an immune or a nonimmune process is at work.

Immune Thrombocytopenia

Immune thrombocytopenias of clinical importance are idiopathic thrombocytopenic purpura (ITP) and transfusion-related and drug-related thrombocytopenias.

Idiopathic thrombocytopenic purpura. Idiopathic thrombocytopenic purpura (ITP) is a common cause of thrombocytopenia in the adult, often starting insidiously. The diagnosis is made by excluding other causes of thrombocytopenia. In addition, the bone marrow should have a normal or increased number of megakaryocytes. The cause of thrombocytopenia is immune destruction of platelets by circulating antibodies. These antibodies can be demonstrated in about 65% of patients (20). However, with more sensitive tests, antibodies can be demonstrated in almost 100% of patients (21, 22). Although ITP is a disease of middle age, ITP-like conditions are not uncommonly observed in the elderly suffering from cancer, infection, or inflammatory processes. Patients often respond to the administration of prednisone. Since the treatment of ITP is not benign, one should diligently exclude other causes of thrombocytopenia before initiating treatment.

Post-transfusion thrombocytopenia. Post-transfusion thrombocytopenia is characterized by sudden onset of thrombocytopenia about 7 to 10 days after blood transfusion (23). Patients who receive repeated transfusions are at risk; however, about 3% of the population who are negative for PLA_1, are at higher risk (23). PLA_1 is a platelet specific antigen and is present in 97% of the population (24, 25). Other platelet-specific antigens are PLA_2 (24, 25), DUZO (26), Ko^aKo^b, PLE_1, and PLE_2 (25). These antigens are less involved as the cause of post-transfusion purpura. The possible mechanisms of post-transfusion thrombocytopenia have been described (27). Post-transfusion thrombocytopenia is usually a self-limited condition, but at times it can be severe enough to require treatment. Fatalities have been reported in a small percentage of cases (28).

Drug-related immune thrombocytopenia. Acute thrombocytopenia following the ingestion of quinine had been observed many years ago. In 1928, Rosenthal showed that thrombocytopenia could be reinduced after drug challenge (27). It was later shown that the platelets could in fact be lysed in the presence of quinine (29). This drug sensitivity was also transferable (30). Today, there are a large number of drugs that can lead to thrombocytopenia without bone marrow suppression. However, only occasionally is the platelet destruction mediated by an immune response. Some drugs induce thrombocytopenia by several different mechanisms. For example, heparin can induce thrombocytopenia shortly after its use (31). This type of thrombocytopenia is dependent on the preparation of heparin used. Heparin also causes delayed thrombocytopenia, which appears about 1 to 2 weeks after its administration. This type of thrombocytopenia is probably mediated by an immune mechanism.

Nonimmune Thrombocytopenia

There are many instances in which platelet destruction is accelerated but in which no platelet antibody can be found. It is believed that the platelet destruction takes place by a nonimmune reaction. The more common underlying disorders associated with these cases are administration of drugs, infection, and intravascular coagulation.

Drugs. There are many drugs that can occasionally cause thrombocytopenia by what is probably a nonimmune process. A good example is ristocetin, an antibiotic that is not used clinically now because it causes platelet aggregation. Aspirin and antibiotics, such as penicillin (32), streptomycin (33), and sulfonamides (34, 35) can cause a nonimmune type of thrombocytopenia (31–34). However, it is not always certain that there is no immune process at work, since the inability to demonstrate such a reaction does not necessarily exclude it.

Infections. Infection with certain viruses can cause thrombocytopenia. Influenza, rubella, cytomegalovirus disease, and infectious mononucleosis can all be associated with thrombocytopenia. Another viral illness that is associated with thrombocytopenia is the human immunodeficiency virus which is responsible for the acquired immune deficiency syndrome (AIDS).

Disseminated intravascular coagulation. Disseminated intravascular coagulation (DIC) is often associated with thrombocytopenia. This condition in its mild form in not uncommon and can be associated with various infections, trauma, carcinomatosis, etc. Thrombocytopenia can at times be severe, requiring immediate attention. This will be further discussed in association with coagulation abnormalities.

Abnormal Platelet Distribution

Under normal conditions, approximately one third of total platelets remain in the spleen (18, 36). In the case of splenomegaly, this fraction might increase (37, 38). However, the exact mechanism of thrombocytopenia associated with various types of splenomegaly is not well understood. Thrombocytopenia due to splenomegaly usually does not cause major clinical problems unless there are other processes complicating the situation. In Felty's syndrome, for example, there is immune destruction of platelets as well as splenomegaly. It should be noted that in many cases of splenomegaly, such as chronic lymphocytic or granulocytic leukemia or liver cirrhosis with portal hypertension, there are multiple etiologic factors that cause thrombocytopenia.

Qualitative Platelet Disorders

Except vWD, most hereditary causes of platelet functional abnormalities are quite rare.

von Willebrand's Disease

One of the hallmarks of vWD is impaired platelet adhesion to subendothelium (39). Although there is usually no intrinsic platelet abnormality, the abnormal vWf renders the platelet functionally deficient (40, 41). von Willebrand's disease is an autosomal dominant trait, males and females being equally affected. It is also compatible with long life and can be the cause of hemostatic abnormality in the elderly. Other hereditary platelet functional abnormalities are quite rare.

Drugs

Drugs may alter the platelet function and cause bleeding, especially if the platelet count is low. Most of the nonsteroidal anti-inflammatory agents affect platelet function. By inhibiting the cyclo-oxygenase enzyme, which is needed for the production of thromboxane A_2, aspirin or other similar agents impair platelet aggregation (42, 43). Other drugs that alter platelet function are antibiotics, such as penicillin, antidepressants such as imipramine, and antiarrhythmics such as propranolol. Complete lists of such drugs are available in textbooks of pharmacology.

Uremia

Uremia impairs platelet function (44, 45), which is manifested by decreased platelet subendothelium interaction and prolonged bleeding time. This is due to both plasmatic and platelet alterations. In addition, the low hematocrit in uremics is also a contributing factor to decreased platelet aggregation (45). Dialysis improves all these abnormalities (46). The qualitative platelet abnormalities in uremia have no relationship to the type of underlying renal disease.

Dysmyelopoiesis

Platelet structural and functional abnormalities are common in patients with myeloproliferative syndromes, such as polycythemia vera, chronic myelogenous leukemia, and preleukemia. The platelet abnormality is often manifested as decreased platelet aggregation with occasional significant bleeding tendency; however, thromboembolic phenomena have also been reported (47). Platelet dysfunction has also been described in patients with paraproteinemia (48), whether or not associated with dysmyelopoiesis. In such cases, the platelet abnormalities have been attributed to coating of platelets by paraprotein (49).

Liver Disease and Disseminated Intravascular Coagulation

The conversion of fibrinogen to fibrin is the mainstay of coagulation. However, fibrin formation stimulates fibrinolytic reactions, which degrade fibrin to smaller molecules (split products). Some of these molecules possess anticoagulant activity. The platelet function is also affected in DIC (50, 51). The exact biochemical events leading to platelet dysfunction are not well known but thc "by-products" of proteolysis of fibrinogen by plasmin have been postulated to interfere with the function of platelets (52). The causes of acquired platelet dysfunction are listed in Table 11-2.

Coagulation Abnormalities

Although occasionally the diagnosis of mild hereditary bleeding problems will be made in late adulthood, most of the hemorrhagic conditions in the elderly are acquired. These acquired conditions are due to decreased or abnormal synthesis, increased consumption or loss of coagulation factors, or the appearance of inhibitors of coagulation. It is understood that a combination of the above is also possible.

Defective or Decreased Synthesis

The liver synthesizes most coagulation factors, and vitamin K is responsible for the proper functional integrity of factors II, VII, IX, and X as well as protein C and protein S. For this reason, the use of vitamin K antagonists and liver disease are the most common causes of synthetic abnormalities. Since the naturally occurring vitamin K is fat soluble, the fat malabsorption (e.g., due to obstructive jaundice) also interferes with coagulation factor synthesis. Vitamin K is required for the carboxylation of specific glutamic acid residues of the above-mentioned factors. Its lack or antagonism by drugs leads to formation of poorly functional coagulation factors, which are inadequate for proper fibrin formation. Coagulation derangements due to liver failure are more complex than vitamin K deficiency since the liver plays such a major role in the blood coagulation process. The liver is not only the site of synthesis but also the site of clearance of coagulation proteins (53). In severe liver disease, all coagulation proteins except factors VIII and calcium are deficient. The severity of liver failure correlates with coagulation impairment. In severe liver disease, fibrinogen is low for two reasons. It is

Table 11-2. Causes of acquired platelet dysfunction

Disseminated intravascular coagulation (DIC)
Drugs
Liver disease
Uremia
Paraproteinemia
Myeloproliferative syndromes
Dyshemopoiesis

synthesized in deficient quantity and it is degraded by plasmin, since plasminogen activators are not effectively inactivated in the liver. Fibrinogen degradation products (FDP) inhibit blood coagulation, creating a situation somewhat similar to DIC.

Coagulation Protein Loss

Coagulation proteins can be lost by massive blood or plasma loss and replacement by bank blood which is deficient in labile coagulation factors. A more common situation is consumption of coagulation proteins by continuous DIC and fibrinolysis, which can be acute or chronic. It is increasingly apparent that a large number of clinical conditions can cause chronic DIC with consumption of coagulation factors and hemorrhagic tendency (Table 11-3). Disseminated intravascular coagulation is apparently initiated by release of tissue factor and proteolytic enzymes, which activate the coagulation process and lead to platelet aggregation and widespread fibrin deposition. This process results in thrombocytopenia and low level of coagulation proteins, expecially fibrinogen, factor V, and factor VIII, due to breakdown of these by plasmin. Contrary to normal coagulation, which is initiated by a short-lived stimulus and remains localized, in DIC the stimulus is prolonged and the coagulation process disseminated. It must be remembered that since the DIC process is secondary to an underlying disease process, any attempt to stop DIC should be aimed at the elimination of the primary disorder (54–61).

It is clear that DIC is always associated with fibrinolysis, but fibrinolysis can occur independently in "primary fibrinolysis" due to the release of plasminogen activators from normal tissue (e.g., prostate) or from tumors (e.g., leukemia). The outcome is decreased fibrinogen and a hemorrhagic tendency.

Acquired Coagulation Inhibitors

Acquired coagulation inhibitors are proteins (usually antibodies) that inhibit blood coagulation due to inhibition of one or more clotting factors. They are produced either appropriately due to antigenic stimulation in patients receiving blood, plasma, or plasma components therapy or inappropriately due to known or unknown immunologic disorders. The most common inhibitors are lupus anticoagulants and factor VIII inhibitors. However, inhibitors to most coagulation factors have been described.

Table 11-3. Causes of disseminated intravascular coagulation

Obstetric complications
Incompatible blood transfusion
Poisoning
Crush injuries
Burns
Hypoxemia
Carcinomatosis
Autoimmune disease

Lupus Anticoagulant

Anticoagulant activity in the plasma of patients with systemic lupus erythematosus (SLE) was described by Conley and Hartmann in 1952 (62). This was probably the condition which was referred to later as "Lupus Anticoagulant" (63). It should be emphasized that although 5% to 10% of patients suffering from SLE might have these anticoagulants, many other clinical conditions could also be associated with lupus anticoagulants (63). These conditions are various types of cancers, such as lymphoma and myeloma (64), drug-induced SLE (65), autoimmune diseases other than SLE, and the chronic ingestion of some drugs, notably chlorpromazine (66). A characteristic of lupus anticoagulants is lack of clinical bleeding. In fact, numerous patients with lupus anticoagulants have been described who did not have excessive bleeding in spite of major surgical operations (63).

When bleeding is clinically present, it is usually believed to be due to some other complicating factor, such as thrombocytopenia, which is not uncommon in SLE, or other immunologic problems or platelet dysfunction (e.g., due to uremia). It has been realized, however, that patients carrying the lupus anticoagulants with or without SLE have a significantly high incidence of thrombotic phenomena (venous or arterial) as well as recurrent abortions (67). The mechanisms of these phenomena are unclear, but it has been suggested from laboratory experimentation that these inhibitors can inhibit the release of prostacycline (PGI_2) from the endothelial cells (68). Since PGI_2 is an important factor rendering the endothelial surface nonthrombogenic, it is assumed that deficiency of PGI_2 plays an important role in the genesis of thrombotic phenomena seen in these patients. It has also been suggested that the inhibitors interfere with the release of arachidonic acid from the phospholipids in the cell membrane. Since arachidonic acid serves as substrate for PGI_2, deficiency of PGI_2 ensues (68). The mechanisms by which lupus anticoagulants appear in blood or their site of action are unknown. They are immunoglobulins of IgG or IgM class and in contrast to acquired factor VIII inhibitors, their action in vitro is usually instantaneous and is mainly inhibition of the interaction between two or more clotting factors that lead to deficient "prothrombinase complex" generation (69). In fact, it has been shown more recently that these inhibitors are directed against phospholipids (64).

Factor VIII Inhibitors

Factor VIII inhibitors appear in four different groups of patients: hemophiliacs, some postpartum patients, patients with known immunologic disorders, and some elderly patients without any known disease. The incidence of factor VIII inhibitors varies widely among reports but is probably about 5% to 10% among hemophiliacs (70). These inhibitors usually occur among hemophiliacs with severe disease and quite early in life. Although with modern therapy of hemophilia, some patients with severe disease reach old age, hemophilia is not a common problem among the elderly population. The inhibitors which occasionally occur postpartum are not a problem of the elderly either, since the inhibitors usually disappear after 12 to 18 months (71, 72). For this reason, this discussion focuses on the remaining two situations, which are more a problem of the elderly. Factor VIII inhibitors are either associated with an autoimmune disorder such as SLE, rheumatoid arthritis, etc., or they are not associated with any known disease conditions. Almost all factor VIII inhibitors are IgG antibodies; however, IgA and IgM antibodies have been described (73, 74).

The inhibitors are specific for factor VIII:C (procoagulant activity) and do not interact with vWf antigen or activity. It is then not surprising that the bleeding time is normal. Factor VIII inhibitors are neutralized by factor VIII, but the neutralization reaction is not instantaneous and it takes about 1 hour or more for completion.

It is possible to neutralize any amount of factor VIII inhibitor in vitro by the addition of appropriate quantities of factor VIII procoagulant. The kinetics of the reactions are those of antigen-antibody reaction. However, the inhibitors in nonhemophilic and nontransfused patients do not show anamnesis after transfusion of factor VIII, in contrast to inhibitors in hemophiliacs. This observation strengthens the view that their occurrence is not due to previous exposure to factor VIII antigen but rather to an immunologic disturbance.

Factor VIII inhibitors cause the activated partial thromboplastin time (aPTT) to be prolonged. The level of factor VIII inhibitors is measured in Bethesda units, each of which is equivalent to about 0.25 unit of factor VIII procoagulant (75).

Acquired inhibitors to other coagulation factors have been described. Inhibitors to factor IX have been described in patients with hemophilia B who have been transfused. It also occurs in nonhemophiliacs. These inhibitors are usually IgG immunoglobulins (76). Inhibitors to factor V have been reported occasionally in older patients. In some patients the inhibitor will disappear with or without therapy. Both prothrombin time (PT) and aPTT are abnormal with factor V inhibitors (77). Several cases of an acquired inhibitor to factors XI, XII and XIII and more recently a case of an acquired inhibitor of protein C have also been reported (78).

Acquired von Willebrand's Disease

Antibodies against vWf antigen have been reported in a small percentage of patients with severe vWD after numerous transfusions (79–81). These antibodies can occasionally pose a therapeutic problem. In addition, there is another class of patients who are usually older and have never had bleeding problems or transfusion. They develop a clinical syndrome similar to that of vWD with prolonged bleeding time and low vWf antigen. Some of these patients have an autoimmune disease or a lymphoproliferative disorder, but some others seem to have no known disease. Acquired vWD in conjunction with essential thrombocythemia and chronic myelocytic leukemia has been suggested to be related to proteolysis, which preferentially destroys the large vWf multimers (82).

Diagnosis

The diagnosis of bleeding disorders is unraveled by examining the history as well as the physical and laboratory aspects of the patient's condition. Features in the history and physical examination may help distinguish inherited versus acquired defects, platelet versus coagulation disorder, or systemic versus local abnormalities. Or, they may uncover an underlying causative condition or medication. The latter two are more likely with increasing age (83, 84). The history of previous trauma, surgery (including dental procedures, childbirth, menses, and family history can help uncover inherited defects not known to the patients. A silent, inherited abnormality is less likely to occur in the older patient than in children or young adults, but it is not impossible. Mild forms of hemophilia A and B can go undetected if the system has not been severely tested in the past (83, 84).

Bleeding caused by platelet or vessel wall abnormalities is usually manifested by prolonged superficial bleeding, due to relatively small amounts of blood from spontaneous bleeding vessels or vessels disrupted by another process, such as surgery, menses, penetrating gastrointestinal ulcers, and dental extractions. The physical examination frequently demonstrates petechiae in dependent areas and oozing blood from needle sticks and nasal and oral mucosae. The bleeding seen with coagulation disorders involves larger quantities of blood loss and is marked on physical examination by deep hematomas and hemarthroses. Patients who bleed either spontaneously or from multiple sites are more likely to have a systemic defect than those who bleed from a single site (83, 84).

A combined problem (open blood vessel and systemic clotting disorder) should not be dismissed in a patient whose bleeding appears to be diffuse, but in whom bleeding from a single site accounts for most of the blood loss. A patient with thrombocytopenia and massive upper intestinal bleeding is a case in point. In such a patient, it is very likely that an anatomic lesion exists in combination with the platelet abnormality, since large volumes of spontaneous blood loss due to a platelet disorder alone is unexpected.

The laboratory investigation of hemostatic problems would include a platelet count and if the count is normal, a bleeding time. Spontaneous hemorrhage does not usually occur with platelet counts above 10–20 × 10^9/L. Surgery and trauma can be tolerated with counts ≥ 50 × 10^9/L. A combined problem should be considered if bleeding occurs with counts ≥ 50 × 10^9/L. An abnormally low platelet count in a patient with no history or physical signs of bleeding should be confirmed by examination of the blood film to avoid error caused by the EDTA-induced pseudothrombocytopenia (85). The bleeding time measures overall platelet function and number. It requires normal platelet interaction with the vessel wall. It measures the time to achieve hemostasis following a standard incision in the skin, while venous pressure of 40 mm mercury is maintained (83, 84).

Defects in the coagulation system are usually detected by an abnormality in the aPTT. This test screens the intrinsic pathway and is prolonged with deficiencies or dysfunction of factors XII, XI, IX, VIII, X, V, II, fibrinogen, HMW kininogen, and prekallikrein. Coagulation inhibitors or heparin will also prolong this test. Abnormalities in factor VII are confirmed by obtaining a prolonged PT with a normal aPTT. Thrombin time (TT) is mainly affected by fibrinogen and heparin. Figure 11-1 illustrates the areas of the coagulation cascade that are evaluated by the aPPT, PT, and TT. The results of these initial tests provide some direction for more specific confirmatory tests.

The separate addition of a series of plasmas, each deficient in a known factor, to the patient's plasma and the measurement of the aPTT allows for the discovery of the missing factor since only the plasma lacking the same factor as the patient's plasma fails to correct the aPPT. Special tests that may measure the specific enzymatic conversion or the amount of the protein present are also available and add additional information. Care must be taken in interpreting tests that measure the amount of the protein without assessing its function, since some bleeding disorders are associated with normal quantities of dysfunctional protein. Communication with the laboratory should avoid this problem (84).

Between 30% and 40% of normal concentrations of most factors is adequate for hemostasis. Fibrinogen and factor XI are exceptions; only 100 mg/dl and 20% of normal, respectively, are needed for adequate hemostasis. Deficiencies or abnormalities of factor XII, prekallikrein, and HMW kininogen are associated with a marked prolongation of aPTT without any clinical bleeding (86).

The presence of coagulation inhibitors is suspected when the aPTT is prolonged and is not normalized by the addition of normal plasma. The screening test is carried out by mixing normal plasma with the patient's plasma in a 1:1 ratio and measuring the aPTT. It is recommended to incubate the mixture for 1 hour at 37°C since some inhibitors do not react immediately. The screening will not disclose factor XIII, alpha-2 plasmin inhibitor (alpha-2PI), or mild deficiencies of other factors. Factor XIII can be evaluated by the solubility of a fibrin clot in 6M urea. Plasminogin activator, plasmin, and alpha-2PI may be measured by specific immunologic or functional assays. Overall fibrinolytic activity can be assessed by measuring FDPs and a euglobulin clot lysis time. Mild factor deficiencies will require clinical suspicion and specific assays (83, 84). Figure 11-2 can serve as a practical guideline to approach patients with bleeding problems.

Treatment

The optimal treatment of bleeding requires the correct etiologic diagnosis, correction of underlying problems, and usually replacement of missing or dysfunctional components. Fresh frozen plasma (FFP), cryoprecipitate, platelet concentrate, and certain specific plasma components are the mainstay of transfusion therapy.

Fresh frozen plasma, which should be type specific, contains all coagulation factors. Factor VIII and V decrease in activity with prolonged storage. The usage of FFP is limited by the volume required for a therapeutic dose. The dose in adults is usually an initial dose of 100ml followed by 500 ml every 12 hours. If vascular overload is a problem, plasmapheresis may be a useful way of exchanging the patient's plasma for normal plasma. Some authors propose the use of single donor plasma or cryoprecipitate poor plasma in lieu of FFP to provide factors excluding V and VII (87).

Cryoprecipitate is rich in fibrinogen and factor VIII. It contains approximately 200 to 250 mg of fibrinogen per bag. Therefore, a hemostatic dose for hypofibrinogenemia would be one-half bag of cryoprecipitate per kg of body weight, followed by 1 bag/15 kg body weight daily. For hemophilia, between 15 and 50 units of factor VIIIC/kg are required, depending upon the severity of the hemorrhage. Cryoprecipitate contains between 70 and 100 units of factor VIIIC per bag. The dose would need to be re-

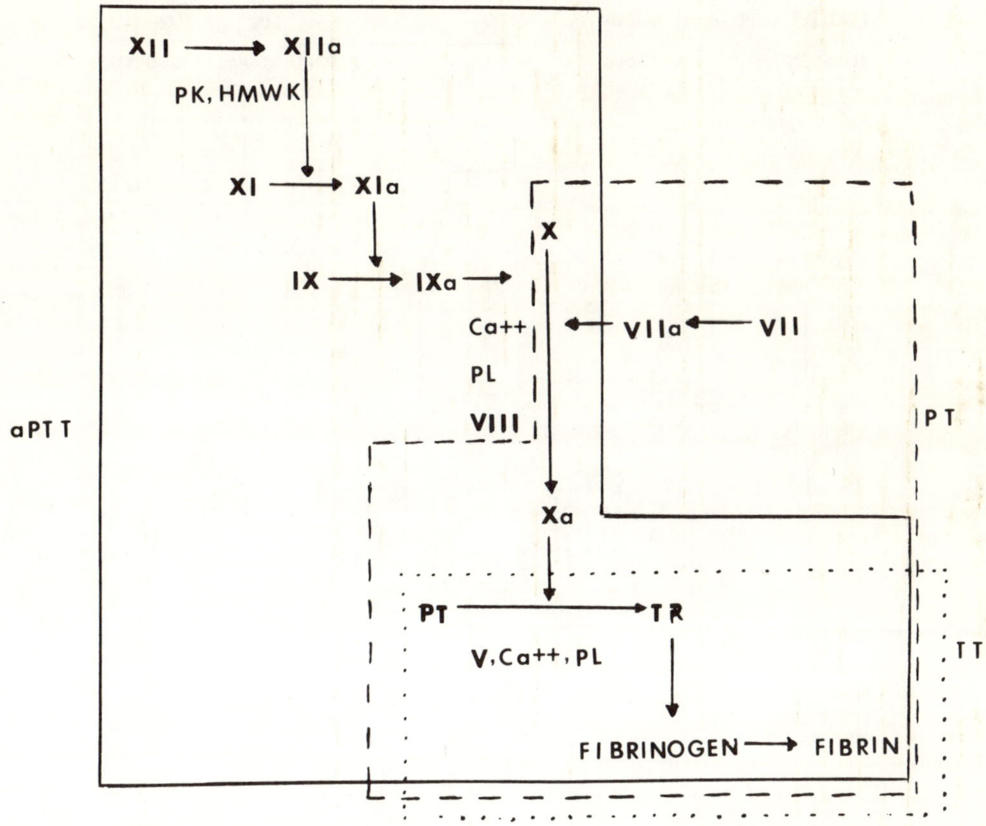

Figure 11-1. The assessment of the blood coagulation by the activated partial thromboplastin time (aPTT), ________; the prothrombin time (PT), ---------; and the thrombin time (TT), ... Prekallikrein, PK; high molecular weight kininogen, HMWK; calcium, Ca^{++}; phospholipid, PL.

peated every 12 hours for several days to several weeks for life-threatening bleeding (88).

Other special products include Konyne (Cutter) and Proplex (Hyland), both of which contain concentrates of the vitamin K dependent factors (II, VII, IX, X). These products have been used to treat hemophilia B, liver disease, and overdosage of oral anticoagulants. Their advantage is that they can be administered in small volumes, but they do carry a potential risk of thrombosis from activated factors. However, the presence of the activated factors presumably accounts for their effectiveness in the treatment of patients with hemophilia associated with factor VIII inhibitors (89–99).

So far, the use of plasma component therapy has been discussed but there are also some pharmacologic agents that are helpful in treating certain coagulopathies. These drugs are 1-deamino-8-d-arginine vasopressin (DDAVP), epsilon-aminocaproic acid (EACA), protamine sulfate, and some immunosuppressive agents. DDAVP increases the plasma levels of factor VIII, most likely by increasing its release from the vascular endothelium. It can be quite useful in patients with mild hemophilia A and vWD, in whom the factor VIII molecules are decreased but functionally normal. The dose is 0.4 to 0.5 μg/kg and can be repeated every 12 hours but becomes less effective with repeated administration. DDAVP has also been used in controlling bleeding in uremia and following coronary artery bypass surgery (100–105).

Epsilon-aminocaproic acid inhibits fibrinolysis and can be useful alone or more often in combination with replacement therapy for primary fibrinolysis, for iatrogenic fibrinolysis caused by streptokinase, urokinase, or tissue plasminogen activator, and for fibrinolysis after urologic, dental, or neurosurgical procedures. Hemophiliacs with inhibitors may also benefit from EACA used as an adjunct treatment. The dose is 8 to 36 g/day in divided doses depending upon the site of bleeding. The major complication is thrombosis. It should not be used in patients with DIC. Other side effects include nausea, vomiting, syncope, dizziness, and diarrhea (106–118).

Protamine sulfate can reverse the anticoagulant effect of heparin. One milligram will reverse the effect of 80 to 100 USP units of heparin. Therefore, the usual dose of protamine is 1 mg for each 100 units of the last dose of

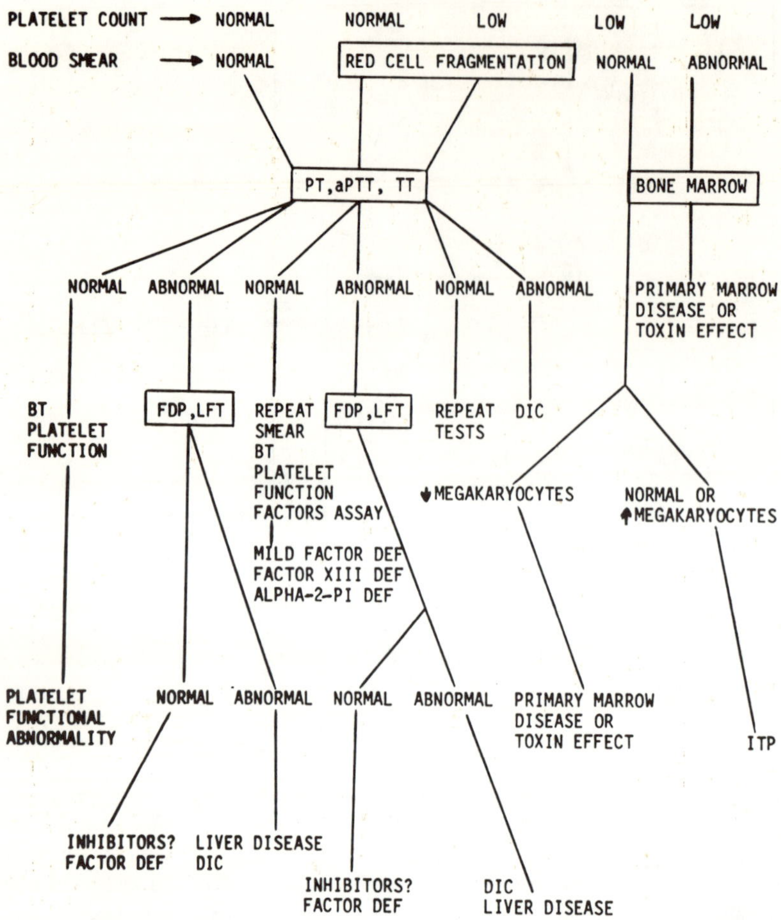

Figure 11-2. Guideline to solve a bleeding problem (examine CBC and blood smear). PT, prothrombin time; aPTT, activated partial thromboplastin time; TT, thrombin time; FDP, fibrin split products; LFT, liver function tests; DIC, disseminated intravascular coagulation; ITP, idiopathic thrombocytopenic purpura; BT, bleeding time; and alpha-2-PI, alpha-2 plasmin inhibitor.

heparin. For patients who are receiving continuous heparin infusion, 1 mg of protamine is given for each 100 units of heparin received in the preceding 4 hours. Watchfulness for rebound bleeding is necessary since protamine is cleared more rapidly than heparin (84, 116).

Immunosuppressive agents, such as azathioprine, 6-mercaptopurine, and cyclophosphamide, are useful in attempting to decrease the titers of coagulation inhibitors. Their usage must be individualized since the currently available data are difficult to interpret due to the diversity of concomitant clinical problems (119–121).

Patients with thrombocytopenia due to decreased production should be supported with prophylactic platelet transfusion to maintain their platelet count greater than 10×10^9/L. The appearance of isoimmune platelet antibodies in patients who have been previously transfused poses difficult problems.

The use of compatible single donors is at times quite helpful. Patients with platelet consumption should be treated for the underlying disorder and usually do not benefit from transfusion. Idiopathic thrombocytopenia may require therapy with corticosteroids, danazol, splenectomy, or vincristine (122–125). Patients with dysfunctional platelets due to lack of factor VIII, as seen in vWD, respond best to transfusion of cryoprecipitate or the administration of DDAVP. Uremic patients may also respond to these maneuvers as well as to dialysis. Estrogen has also been tried (126–131). Patients with intrinsically abnormal platelets, such as those with Glanzmann's thrombasthenia, can be managed with platelet transfusions in spite of a normal platelet count. The usual dose would be 4 to 6 units of random donor or 1 unit of single donor platelets. This dose could be repeated every 72 hours until the risk of bleeding has passed (132).

An approach to preoperative hemostatic evaluation of patients was published by Dr. Rapaport in 1983. Patients are divided into several groups based on the risk of surgery and the index of suspicion of a possible bleeding disorder. Patients undergoing minor surgery who have a negative history need no laboratory testing. Patients with a stressful surgery and a negative history should be screened with an aPTT and a platelet count. Patients undergoing major surgery and who have a questionable history should have a bleeding time, PT, and a clot solubility.

Patients with a positive history for bleeding or a predisposing condition, such as cirrhosis of the liver, should have a bleeding time, factors VIII and IX levels, and a thrombin time. If any of these screening tests are abnormal, further diagnostic studies would be required (133). Several other guidelines regarding preoperative hemostatic evaluation have been published (134–137).

References

1. Baumgartner, HR, Tschopp, TB, and Meyer, D. 1980. Shear rate dependent inhibition of platelet adhesion and aggregation on collagenous surfaces by antibodies to human factor VIII von Willebrand factor. *Br J Haematol* 44:127–139.
2. Meyer, D, and Baumgartner, HR. 1983. Role of von Willebrand factor in platelet adhesion to the subendothelium. *Br J Haematol* 54:1–9.
3. Berndt, MC, and Caen, JP. 1984. Platelet glycoproteins. *Prog Hemost Thromb* 7:111–150.
4. Kaplan, AP, and Silverberg, M. 1987. The coagulation-kinin pathway of human plasma. *Blood* 70:1–15.
5. Moncada, S. 1982. Biological importance of prostacyclin. *Br J Pharmacol* 76:3–31.
6. Esmon, CT. 1983. Protein C: biochemistry, physiology and clinical implications. *Blood* 62:1155–1158.
7. Esmon, CT. 1984. Protein C. *Prog Hemost Thromb* 7:25–54.
8. Griffin, JH, et al. 1981. Deficiency of protein C in congenital thrombotic disease. *J Clin Invest* 68:1370–1373.
9. Rosenberg, R, and Damus, P. 1973. The purification and mechanism of action of human antithrombin-heparin cofactor. *J Biol Chem* 248:6490–6503.
10. Levin, EG, and Loskutoff, DJ. 1982. Cultured bovine endothelial cells produce both urokinase and tissue-type plasminogen activators. *J Cell Biol* 94:631–636.
11. Nawroth, PP, and Stern, DM. 1985. An endothelial cell procoagulant pathway. *J Cell Biochem* 28:253–264.
12. Schuster, S, and Scarborough, H. 1961. Senile purpura simplex. *Lancet* 1:145–146.
13. Williams, GA, and Brick IB. 1955. Gastrointestinal bleeding in hereditary hemorrhagic telangiectasia. *Arch Intern Med* 95:41–51.
14. Wintrobe, MM, et al., Eds. 1981. In *Clinical Hematology* ed. 8, pp. 1078–1084. Philadelphia: Lee & Febiger.
15. Kutti, J, and Weinfeld, A. 1968. The frequency of thrombocytopenia in patients with heart disease treated with oral diuretics. *Acta Med Scand* 83:245–250.
16. Watson, CJ, Schultz, AL, and Wikoff, HM. 1947. Purpura following estrogen therapy with particular reference to hypersensitivity to diethylstilbestrol and with note on the possible relationship of purpura to endogenous estrogens. *J Lab Clin Med* 32:606–617.
17. Cooper, BA, and Bigelow, FS. 1960. Thrombocytopenia associated with the administration of diethylstilbestrol in man. *Ann Intern Med* 52:907–909.
18. Harker, LA, and Finch, CA. 1969. Thrombokinetics in man. *J Clin Invest* 48:963–974.
19. Lindenbaum, J, and Hargrove, RL. 1968. Thrombocytopenia in alcoholics. *Ann Intern Med* 68:526–532.
20. Karpatkin, S. 1980. Autoimmune thrombocytopenic purpura. *Blood* 56:329–343.
21. Dixon, R, Rosse, W, and Ebbert, L. 1975. Quantitative determination of antibody in idiopathic thrombocytopenic purpura. *N Engl J Med* 292:230–236.
22. Kelton, JG, et al. 1981. The development and application of a serum assay for platelet-bindable IgG (S-PBIgG). *J Lab Clin Med* 98:272–279.
23. Schulman, NR, et al. 1961. Immunoreaction involving platelets: *J Clin Invest* 40:1597–1620.
24. Loghem, JJ, et al. 1959. Serological and genetical studies on a platelet antigen (Zw). *Vox Sang* 4:161–169.
25. Schulman, NR. 1965. Platelet and leukocyte isoantigens common to man and other animals. In *Histocompatibility Testing,* Eds., H Balnor, et al., p. 113. Copenhagen: Munksgaard.
26. Moulinier, J. 1958. Iso-immunisation maternelle antiplaquettaires et purpura neo-natal: Le Systeme de groupe platquettaire "duzo" In *Proceedings of the Sixth Congress of the European Society of Haematology.* Basel: S Karger AG. 817.
27. Rosenthal, N. 1928. The blood picture in purpura. *J Lab Clin Med* 13:303–322.
28. Hoak, JC, et al. 1979. Post-transfusion purpura (PTP) A multifaceted enigma (abst). *Clin Res* 25:510A.
29. Grandjean, LC. 1948. Case of purpura haemorrhagica after administration of quinine with specific thrombocytolysis demonstrated *in vitro*. *Acta Med Scand* 131 (suppl 213):165–170.
30. Steinkamp, R, Moor, CV, and Doubek WG. 1955. Thrombocytopenic purpura caused by hypersensitivity to quinine. *J Lab Clin Med* 45:18–29.
31. Gollub, S, and Ulin, AW. 1962. Heparin-induced thrombocytopenia in man. *J Lab Clin Med* 59:430–435.
32. Hsi, YJ, Kuo, HY, and Ouyang. 1966. Thrombocytopenia following administration of penicillin. *Chin Med J* 85:249–251.
33. Oppenheim, M, and De Meyer, G. 1949. Granulo-und Thrombocytopenic in Folge Streptomycin Behandlung. *Schweiz Med Wochenschr* 79:1187–1190.
34. Hurd, RW, and Jacox, RF. 1943. Thrombocytopenic purpura developing as a complication of sulfathiazole and sulfadiazine therapy. *JAMA* 122:296–298.
35. Niewig, HO, et al. 1963. Haematological side effects of some antirheumatic drugs. *Ann Rheum Dis* 22:440–443.
36. Aster, RH, and Jandl, JH. 1964. Platelet sequestration in man: II. Immunological and clinical studies. *J Clin Invest* 43:856–869.
37. Amorosi, EL. 1965. Hypersplenism. *Semin Hematol* 2:249–285.
38. Rowley, PT, and Jacobs, M. 1972. Case Report: Hypersplenic thrombocytopenia in sickle cell-beta thalassemia. *Am J Med Sci* 264:489–493.
39. Tschopp, TB, Weiss, HJ, and Baumgartner, HR. 1974. Decreased adherence of platelets to subendothelium in von Willebrand's disease. *J Lab Clin Med* 83:296–300.

40. Wall, RT, et al. 1980. Binding and release of factor VIII/von Willebrand factor by human endothelial cells. *Br J Haematol* 46:287–298.
41. Tuddenham, EGD, Lazarchick, J, and Hoyer, LW. 1981. Synthesis and release of factor VIII by cultured human endothelial cells. *Br J Haematol* 47:617–626.
42. Roth, GJ, Stanford, N, and Majerus, PW. 1975. Acetylation of prostaglandin synthetase by aspirin. *Proc Natl Acad Sc USA* 72:3073–3076.
43. Majerus, PW, and Stanford, N. 1977. Comparative effects of aspirin and diflunisal on prostaglandin synthetase from human platelets and sheep seminal vesicles. *Br J Clin Pharmacol* 4 suppl 1:15S–18S.
44. Rabiner, SF, and Hrodek, O. 1968. Platelet factor III in normal subjects and patients with renal failure. *J Clin Invest* 47:901–912.
45. Castillo, R, et al. 1986. Defective platelet adhesion on vessel subendothelium in uremic patients. *Blood* 68: 337–342.
46. Stewardt, JH, and Castaldi, PA. 1967. Uremic bleeding: A reversible platelet defect corrected by dialysis. *Q J Med* 36:409–423.
47. Keenan, JP, et al. 1977. Defective platelet lipid peroxidation in myeloproliferative disorders. *Br J Haematol* 35:275–283.
48. Vigliano, EM, and Horowitz, HI. 1967. Bleeding syndrome in a patient with IgA myeloma: Interaction of protein and connective tissue. *Blood* 29:823–836.
49. Pachter, MR, et al. 1959. Bleeding, platelets and macroglobulinemia. *Am J Clin Pathol* 31:467–482.
50. Barnhart, MI, et al. 1967. Influence of fibrinogen split products on platelets. *Thromb Haemost* 17:78–98.
51. Fuster, V, et al. 1973. Assay of platelet factor-IV in plasma. *Mayo Clin Proc* 48:103–106.
52. Thomas, DP. 1972. Abnormalities of platelet aggregation in patients with alcoholic cirrhosis. *Ann NY Acad Sci* 201:243–250.
53. Roberts, HR, and Cederbaum, AI. 1972. The liver and blood coagulation, physiology and pathology. *Gastroenterology* 63:297–320.
54. Bachmann, F. 1969. Disseminated intravascular coagulation. DM 3–44.
55. Deykin, D. 1970. The clinical challenge of disseminated intravascular coagulation. *N Engl J Med* 283:636–644.
56. Pitney, WR. 1971. Disseminated intravascular coagulation. *Semin Hematol* 8:65–83.
57. Owen, CA, and Bowie, EJW. 1974. Chronic intravascular coagulation syndromes. A summary. *Mayo Clin Proc* 49:673–679.
58. Colman, RW, Minna, JD, and Robboy, SJ. 1974. Disseminated intravascular coagulation: A problem in critical care medicine. *Heart Lung* 3:789–796.
59. Colman, RW, Robboy, SJ, and Minna, JD. 1979. Disseminated intravascular coagulation: A reappraisal. *Ann Rev Med* 30:359–374.
60. Sharp, AA. 1977. Diagnosis and management of disseminated intravascular coagulation. *Br Med Bull* 33: 265–272.
61. Colman, RW, and Marder, VJ. 1987. Disseminated intravascular coagulation (DIC): Pathogenesis, pathophysiology and laboratory abnormalities. In *Hemostasis and Thrombosis: Basic Principles and Clinical Practice* Eds., RW Colman, et al., pp. 654–663. Philadelphia: J.B. Lippincott.
62. Conley, CL, and Hartmann, RC. 1952. A hemorrhagic disorder caused by circulating anticoagulant in patients with disseminated lupus erythematosus. *J Clin Invest* 31:621–622.
63. Feinstein, DI, and Rappaport, SI. 1972. Acquired inhibitors of blood coagulation *Prog Hemost Thromb* 1:75–95.
64. Thiagarajan, P, Shapiro, SS, and De Marco, L. 1980. Monoclonal immunoglobulin M lamda coagulation inhibitor with phospholipid specificity. *J Clin Invest* 66: 397–405.
65. Boxer, M, Ellman, L, and Carvalho, A. 1976. The lupus anticoagulant. *Arthritis Rheum* 19:1244–1248.
66. Canoso, RT, Hutton, RA, and Deykin, D. 1977. A chlorpromazine-induced inhibitor of blood coagulation. *Am J Hematol* 2:183–191.
67. Elias, M, and Eldor, A. 1984. Thromboembolism in patients with the "lupus"-type circulating anticoagulant. *Arch Intern Med* 144:510–515.
68. Carreras, LO, et al. 1981. Arterial thrombosis, intrauterine death and "lupus" anticoagulant: Detection of immunoglobulin interfering with prostacyclin formation. *Lancet* 31:244–246.
69. Schleider, MA, et al. 1976. A clinical study of the Lupus anticoagulant. *Blood* 48:499–509.
70. Biggs, R. 1978. Complications of treatment. In *Treatment of Hemophilia A and B and von Willebrand's Diseased* ed. 3, Eds., R Biggs and RG Macfarlane, pp. 181–203. London: Blackwell.
71. Voke, J, and Letsky, E. 1977. Pregnancy and antibody to factor VIII. *J Clin Pathol* 30:928–932.
72. Michiels, JJ, et al. 1978. Factor VIII inhibitor postpartum. *Scand J. Haematol* 20:97–107.
73. Glueck, HI, and Hong, R. 1965. A circulating anticoagulant in λ_1A multiple myeloma: Its modification by penicillin. *J Clin Invest* 44:1866–1881.
74. McKelvey, EM, and Kwaan, HC. 1968. Circulating anticoagulant in a macroglobulin with factor VIII inhibitory activity. *Ann Intern Med* 68:1170–1173.
75. Kasper, CK, et al. 1975. A more uniform measurement of factor VIII inhibitors. *Thromb Diath Haemorrh* 34: 869–872.
76. Shapiro, SS, and Hultin, M. 1975. Acquired inhibitors to the blood coagulation factors. *Semin Thromb Hemost* 1:336–385.
77. Chediak, J, et al. 1980. Successful management of bleeding in a patient with factor V inhibitor by platelet transfusion. *Blood* 56:835–841.
78. Mitchell, CA, et al. 1987. A fatal thromboembolic disorder associated with an acquired inhibitor of protein C. *N Engl J Med* 317:1638–1642.
79. Egberg, N, and Blomback, M. 1976. On the characterization of acquired inhibitors to ristocetin induced platelet aggregation found in patients with von Willebrand's disease. *Thromb Res* 9:527–531.
80. Maragall, S, et al. 1979. Inhibition of Willebrand's factor in von Willebrand's disease. *Thromb Res* 14:495–500.
81. Mannucci, PM, et al. 1981. Precipitating antibodies to factor VIII/von Willebrand factor in von Willebrand's disease: Effects on replacement therapy. *Blood* 57: 25–31.

82. Ruggeri, ZM, and Zimmerman, TS. 1987. von Willebrand factor and von Willebrand's disease. *Blood* 70: 895–904.
83. Bachmann, F. 1980. Diagnostic approach to mild bleeding disorders. *Semin Hematol* 17:292–305.
84. White, GC, et al. 1987. Approach to the bleeding patient. In *Hemostatis and Thrombosis, Basic Principles and Clinical Practice,* ed. 2, Eds., RW Colman, J Hirsh and EW Salzman, pp. 1048–1060. Philadelphia: JB. Lippincott.
85. Pegels, JG, et al. 1982. Pseudothrombocytopenia: An immunologic study on platelet antibodies dependent on ethylenediaminetetraacetate. *Blood* 59:157–161.
86. Bowie, EJW, and Owen, CA, Jr. 1977. Hemostatic failure in clinical medicine. *Semin Hematol* 14:341–364.
87. Oberman, HA. 1986. Indications and monitoring of use of fresh frozen plasma as a hemostatic agent. *Curr Stud Hematol Blood Transf,* 53:125–132.
88. Ness, M, and Perkins, HA. 1979. Cryoprecipitate as a reliable source of fibrinogen replacement. *JAMA* 241:6P, 1690–1852.
89. Breen, FA, Jr, and Tullis, JL. 1969. Prothrombin concentrates in treatment of Christmas disease and allied disorders. *JAMA* 208:1848.
90. Hoag, MS, et al. 1969. Treatment of hemophilia B with a new clotting-factor concentrate. *N Engl J Med* 280: 581–586.
91. O'Leary, DS, Ruymann, FB, and Conrad ME. 1971. Therapeutic approaches to factor X deficiency with emphasis on the use of a new clotting-factor concentrate (Konyne). *J Lab Clin Med* 77:23–32.
92. Hellerstein, LJ, and Deykin, DL. 1971. Hepatitis after Konyne administration. *N Engl J Med* 284:1039–1040.
93. Blatt, PM, et al. 1974. Thrombogenic materials in prothrombin complex concentrates. *Ann Intern Med* 81: 766–770.
94. Blatt, PM, et al. 1984. Failure of activated prothrombin complex concentrates in a hemophiliac with an anti-factor VIII antibody. *JAMA* 251:67.
95. Cedarbaum, AI, Blatt, PM, and Roberts, HR. 1976. Intravascular coagulation with the use of human prothrombin complex concentrates. *Ann Intern Med* 84:683–687.
96. Lusher, JM, et al. 1980. Efficacy of prothrombin-complex concentrates in hemophiliacs with antibodies to factor VIII: A multicenter therapeutic trial. *N Engl J Med* 303:421–425.
97. Lusher, JM, et al. 1983. Autoplex versus Proplex: A controlled, double-blind study of effectiveness in acute hemarthrosis in hemophiliacs with inhibitors to factor VIII. *Blood* 62:1135–1138.
98. Fuerth, JH, and Mahrer, P. 1981. Myocardial infarction after factor IX therapy. *JAMA* 245:1455–1456.
99. Sjamsoedin, LJ, et al. 1981. The effect of activated prothrombin complex concentrate (FEIBA) on joint and muscle bleeding in patients with hemophilia A and antibodies to factor VIII: A double-blind clinical trial. *N Engl J Med* 305:717–721.
100. Holmberg, L, et al. 1983. Platelet aggregation induced by 1-desamino-8-d-arginine vasopressin (DDAVP) in type IIB von Willebrand's disease. *N Engl J Med* 309: 816–821.
101. Takahashi, H, et al. 1984. Letter: Platelet aggregation induced by DDAVP in platelet-type von Willebrand's disease. *N Engl J Med* 310:722–723.
102. Kobrinsky, NL, et al. 1984. Shortening of bleeding time by 1-deamino-8-d-arginine vasopressin in various bleeding disorders. *Lancet* 2:1145–1148.
103. Grant, PJ, et al. 1986. Intra-operative activation of coagulation—a stimulus to thrombosis mediated by vasopressin? *Thromb Haemost* 55:104–107.
104. Melissari, E, et al. 1986. The influence of DDAVP infusion on the coagulation and fibrinolytic response to surgery. *Thromb Haemost* 55:54–57.
105. Kentro, TB, Lottenberg, R and Kitchens, CS. 1987. Clinical efficacy of desmopressin acetate for hemostatic control in patients with primary platelet disorders undergoing surgery. *Am J Hematol* 24:215–219.
106. McNicol, GP, et al. 1961. The use of epsilon aminocaproic acid, a potent inhibitor of fibrinolytic activity, in the management of postoperative hematuria. *J Urol* 86: 829–837.
107. Naeye, RL. 1962. Thrombotic state after a hemorrhagic diathesis, a possible complication of therapy with epsilon-aminocaproic acid. *Blood* 19:694–701.
108. Reid, WO, et al. 1964. The use of epsilon aminocaproic acid in the management of dental extractions in the hemophiliac. *Am J Med Sci* 248:184–188.
109. Strauss, HS, Kevy, SV, and Diamond, LK. 1965. Ineffectiveness of prophylactic epsilon aminocaproic acid in severe hemophilia. *N Engl J Med* 273:301–304.
110. Bergin, JJ. 1966. The complications of therapy with epsilon-aminocaproic acid. *Med Clin North Am* 50: 1669–1678.
111. Mullan, S, and Dawley, JF. 1968. Antifibrinolytic therapy for intracranial aneurysms. *J Neurosurg* 28: 21–23.
112. van Itterbeek, H, Vermylen, J, and Verstraete, M. 1968. High obstruction of urine flow as a complication of the treatment with fibrinolysis inhibitors of haematuria in haemophiliacs. *Acta Haematol* 39:237–242.
113. Ratnoff, OD. 1969. Editorial: Epsilon aminocaproic acid—a dangerous weapon. *N Engl J Med* 280: 1124–1125.
114. Walsh, PN, et al. 1971. Epsilon-aminocaproic acid therapy for dental extractions in haemophilia and Christmas disease: A double-blind controlled trial. *Br J Haematol* 20:463–475.
115. Gralnick, HR, and Greipp, P. 1971. Thrombosis with epsilon aminocaproic acid therapy. *Am J Clin Pathol* 56: 151–154.
116. Jaques, LB. 1973. Protamine-antagonist to heparin. *Can Med Assoc J* 108:1291–1297.
117. Smith, RB, Riach, P, and Kaufman, JJ. 1984. Epsilon aminocaproic acid and the control of post-prostatectomy bleeding: A prospective double-blind study. *J Urol* 131: 1093–1095.
118. Schwartz, BS, et al. 1986. Epsilon-aminocaproic acid in the treatment of patients with acute promyelocytic leukemia and acquired alpha-2-plasmin inhibitor deficiency. *Ann Intern Med* 105:873–877.
119. Green, D. 1971. Suppression of an antibody to factor VIII by a combination of factor VIII and cyclophosphamide. *Blood* 37:381–387.
120. Vera, JC, et al. 1975. Acquired circulating anticoagulant

to factor VIII: Response to high doses of cryoprecipitate and immunosuppressive therapy. *JAMA* 232:1038–1039.

121. Spero, JA, Lewis, JH, and Hasiba, U. 1981. Corticosteroid therapy for acquired factor VIII: C inhibitors. *Br J Haematol* 48:635–642.
122. Cohen, P, and Gardner, FH. 1961. The thrombocytopenic effect of sustained high-dose prednisone therapy in thrombocytopenic purpura. *N Engl J Med* 265:611–617.
123. Bouroncle, BA, and Doan, CA. 1969. Treatment of refractory idiopathic thrombocytopenic purpura. *JAMA* 207:2049–2052.
124. Finch, SC, et al. 1974. Immunosuppressive therapy of chronic idiopathic thrombocytopenic purpura. *Am J Med* 56:4–12.
125. Nord, E, et al. 1976. Sclerosing reticulum cell sarcoma following prolonged treatment with azathioprine for idiopathic thrombocytopenic purpura. *Scand J Haematol* 17:321–325.
126. Mannucci, PM, et al. 1983. Deamino-8-d-arginine vasopressin shortens the bleeding time in uremia. *N Engl J Med* 308:8–12.
127. Vicente, V, et al. 1984. DDAVP in uremia. *Nephron* 36:145–146.
128. Liu, YK, Kosfeld, RE, Marcum, SG. 1984. Treatment of uraemic bleeding with conjugated oestrogen. *Lancet* 2:887–889.
129. Di Minno, G, et al. 1985. Platelet dysfunction in uremia. *Am J Med* 79:552–559.
130. Salzman, EW, et al. 1986. Treatment with desmopressin acetate to reduce blood loss after cardiac surgery *N Engl J Med* 314:1402–1406.
131. Livio, M, et al. 1986. Conjugated estrogens for the management of bleeding associated with renal failure. *N Engl J Med* 315:731–735.
132. Brown, CH, III, et al. 1975. Glanzmann's thrombasthenia: Assessment of the response to platelet transfusions. *Transfusion* 15:124–131.
133. Rapaport, S. 1983. Preoperative hemostatic evaluation: Which tests, if any? *Blood* 61:229–231.
134. Bowie, EJW, and Owen, CA. 1980. The significance of abnormal preoperative hemostatic tests. *Prog Hemost Thromb* 5:179–209.
135. Burns, ER, et al. 1986. The preoperative bleeding time as a predicator of postoperative hemorrhage after cardiopulmonary bypass. *J Thor Cardiovas Surg* 92: 310–312.
136. Suchman, AL, and Mushlin, AI. 1986. How well does the activated partial thromboplastin time predict postoperative hemorrhage? *JAMA* 256:750–753.
137. Suchman, AL and Griner, PF. 1986. Diagnostic uses of the activated thromboplastin time and prothrombin time. *Ann Intern Med* 104:810–816.

12

Neurologic Changes in the Elderly

Janice E. Knoefel and Martin L. Albert

All neurologic systems are affected by aging: intellectual, sensorimotor, perceptual, and autonomic. This is of both theoretical and practical interest. On the theoretical level, in attempting to understand the nature of aging, one seeks to answer fundamental questions of life and death. On a more practical level, the geriatric neurologist seeks to help the ailing elderly, for example by answering the puzzled student's question regarding a 75-year-old patient with Alzheimer's disease, "But how does this differ from the normal changes of old age?"

This chapter reviews what is known about normal, age-related changes of the nervous system. For discussion purposes, the neurologic functions have been grouped into cognitive, sensory-perceptual, and motor, and will be discussed in that order.

General Considerations

Studies of human aging are frought with methodological difficulties. There is considerable heterogeneity among elderly populations and varying appreciation of what may be called normal, with marked differences among cultures. For example, in some regions of the world, it is desirable and acceptable to exaggerate one's age (1). This contrasts with our own youth-oriented society, where age tends to be revised downwards in an attempt to cling to fading youthfulness.

Selection of experimental design remains a major, unresolved problem in human aging studies. The relative merits and validity of cross-sectional and longitudinal studies are much debated (2). As a general rule, cross-sectional studies tend to maximize age-related changes in testing, while longitudinal designs tend to minimize such changes. Differences among the age groups (cohort effects) are seen in areas of nutrition, education, health care, vocation, and avocation. These factors alone may account for a significant portion of the decline with age seen on tests of cognitive and motor skills.

Longitudinal studies, on the other hand, may be biased toward extraordinarily healthy and skilled individuals. Selection of highly motivated, healthy subjects (volunteers to be tested in their remarkably preserved abilities), dropout of less motivated or ill subjects, and death may influence the outcome and prevent generalization to the larger, but less extraordinary population.

Cognitive Changes in Normal Aging

This section reviews key changes in attention, memory, language, and intellect. Many authors have discussed methodological problems in evaluating cognitive changes in the elderly (3). The authors provide here their own analysis of cognitive function in normal aging and mention areas of controversy in passing.

Attention

Attention may be defined clinically as the ability to focus mental energy on a specific stimulus, while effectively

This work was supported in part by the National Institutes of Health (NS-06209), the VA Medical Research Service, and the Seidel Fund for Research on Dementia.

screening out distractions from peripheral stimuli. Vigilance is sustained attention. Changing mental set (shifting set) includes the concept of refocusing attention from one stimulus to another. Divided attention allows attention to be focused on competing stimuli simultaneously.

Attention may be tested with a range of bedside or laboratory tests: digit span (the immediate repetition of numbers) forward and backward (4, 5); continuous performance tasks (auditory recognition of a recurring stimulus letter in a random series of letters) (6); trail making tests (graphomotor sequencing of letters, numbers, or both in a random array) (7); Paced Auditory Serial Addition Test (sequential addition of a random series of digits presented orally at regular intervals) (8); cancellation tasks (identification of recurring stimulus in visually presented random array of letters) (9); symbol digit substitution tasks of the Wechsler Adult Intelligence Scale (WAIS) (visual matching of a series of symbols with numbers) (5); and so forth. These tasks have been validated and are commonly used in neuropsychologic test batteries and in the basic clinical examination of neurologists, psychiatrists, and geriatricians.

Another test, serial subtraction of sevens from one hundred, is often used by clinicians but lacks statistical support of its validity (10). Observations of distractibility, inattention, and perseveration are also recorded at bedside and under test conditions.

Simple tests of attention are performed equally well by old and young alike. Tasks of sustained attention and concentration are not performed as well in old as in young groups of subjects (5). Performance on timed tasks of attention show even greater deficits. The digit symbol substitution tests shows an age effect in both cross-sectional (5) and longitudinal studies (11). The trail-making test also demonstrates significant age-related decline in time-to-performance criteria. In addition to impaired performance on tasks of sustained attention, elderly people also show impairment on tests of divided attention.

In summary, the elderly show no decrement on tasks of simple attention; however, tasks of sustained and divided attention reveal significant decreases in performance with age. This effect is compounded by timed performance.

Intact attention and concentration are prerequisites for all aspects of memory function and coherent cognitive integration. The elderly person with a decrement in sustained or divided attention may not capture all necessary details in everyday exchanges of information. Similarly, the elderly person is not as facile in shifting from one important idea to another. Attentional slowing and an increased need for additional time to register information predispose the elderly to misunderstood instructions.

Memory

Complaints of memory loss are so common in the elderly that it has become the standard belief that memory impairment is the principal cognitive problem of normal aging. This belief may be unwarranted. Memory is mildly impaired with normal aging, but not nearly as much as commonly believed. Other cognitive deficits may interact with mild memory problems, making the memory impairment of old age seem worse than it really is.

Memory is not a single, unitary cognitive function. Memory involves multiple sequential and parallel processes that are mutually interdependent. To understand memory, one must test not only each of these independent processes, but also the interactions.

Recent memory can be tested by questions of orientation regarding the year, month, day of the week, time, and place. A test for recent memory is also a test of new learning ability. For example, the patient may be asked to recall three unrelated words presented a few minutes previously. Healthy individuals at any age can be expected to recall all three words at 5 minutes and again at 10 minutes. Objects may be hidden in different locations about the room for later recall to test visual memory. Recall of distant events, personal and historical, can be used at the bedside to evaluate remote memory.

Bedside testing of the elderly is valuable for detecting qualitative abnormalities, while quantitative changes are the province of the neuropsychologist and psychologist. Commonly employed formal measurements to assess recent memory and new learning include: Rey Auditory Verbal Learning Test (a 15-word list is presented for immediate recall for five trials, then is requested as free recall at a later time, followed by recognition conditions) (12); Wechsler Memory Scale combining the subtests of associative learning (word pairs), logical memory, and visual reproduction (memory for designs) (13); Benton Visual Retention Test (free recall and recognition for designs) (14). Tests of remote memory include Wechsler Memory Scale subtests (personal and current information); the test of Famous Faces (visual memory for pictures of famous people in different epochs) (15); the information and vocabulary subtest of WAIS.

Recent memory tasks of orientation are performed equally well in old and young people. Learning and recall of short lists of words and location of hidden objects is similarly well performed by older groups. The differences in recent memory seen with age are demonstrated with: (*a*) a longer, more complex body of information to be learned; and (*b*) information of little logical associative value. The Auditory Verbal Learning Test readily shows a significant decrease in its standard scores for both highly educated and poorly educated groups of old people (12). This same effect is seen with designs (16).

Material of little logical associative value is more difficult for most old people to learn and recall. The Wechsler Memory Scale subtests of associative learning and visual reproduction show significant decremental effects with age. The negative age effect upon learning is reduced when logical word association is possible (17). Conversely, when nonsense items are presented for learning and recall, the age effect is worsened (18). Incidental learning (recall of information not intentionally learned) is diminished in old as compared to young groups of subjects (19).

Are age-related changes in memory preferential for modality of testing? The effects described above (i.e., slight loss with material of logical associative value, greater loss with complex and longer material and with incidental, rather than intentional learning) are seen with both verbal and visual tests. It does not appear that the deterioration of learning and short term memory with age is necessarily less for verbal than for visual material.

Remote memory is retained in normal healthy aging. The information and vocabulary subtests of the WAIS show little change with age. Semantic memory is tested by the vocabulary test; information items test general knowledge learned years ago, generally through education. Although older subjects take longer to learn, once the material is learned, it is recalled equally well.

In summary, the elderly show no deterioration in immediate memory, and in recent memory for short lists and logically associated material. Likewise, no deterioration is evident in remote memory for information, semantics, and overlearned material. Age-related impairments are seen in learning and recent memory for longer, more complex, and logically unassociated material. Capacity for incidental memory is lessened for both verbal and visual material in older subjects.

The elderly individual with these typical age-related changes in memory and learning may be disrupted in everyday functioning. Difficulty in learning complex material and long lists (e.g., shopping) may affect occupational and daily routine activities. Nonsense words (foreign languages) and logically unassociated facts will be harder to master. Changes in incidental memory ("Where did I put my glasses when I finished the newspaper?") will show up with irritating regularity. This usually leads the elderly to rely more heavily on reminders (written lists for shopping) and on routines (glasses always in the same place). These difficulties may also be expressed as an unwillingness to attempt new tasks or ways, i.e., the "inflexibility" of the aged. The pace at work may be slow, and efficiency in work may drop, as the elderly take longer to master new tasks (e.g., more rehearsals for a sales presentation).

On the other hand, performance of tasks based on remote memory, discussion of information already learned, and attention to the tasks at hand will be competitive or superior to that of a younger individual. ("They had to hire two people to do my job after I retired.")

Language

Communication, written and spoken, verbal and nonverbal, is a crucial cognitive function in everyday life. Language can be defined as the ability to communicate through the use of auditory (oral) and visual (written or gestural) symbols (20). Language incorporates the attendant abilities of speech (formation of oral language), comprehension of spoken language, repetition of spoken language, naming (assigning a symbolic label stored in memory to an object or idea), reading (comprehension of written language), writing (forming graphic, visual symbols), comprehension of prosody (interpretation of emotional tone, inflection, rhythm, and melody in speech), discourse (continuous communication), and comprehension of pragmatics (the social context of communication). Each of these aspects of language function can be affected differently in normal aging.

Bedside testing of language probes the major functional areas of language (4). Detailed evaluation of language in normal aging is a relatively new specialty (21). However, excellent language batteries have been developed for the testing of aphasic language disturbances. Among these are the Boston Diagnostic Aphasia Examination (22) and others (23–27).

Language functions are also tested as part of standardized intelligence batteries. WAIS subtests of comprehension, information, similarities, and vocabulary measure verbal ability, memory, general knowledge, and verbal concept formation. Verbal fluency is well assessed with the Controlled Word Association Test (28). The subject is asked to generate orally as many words as possible beginning with a certain letter within a given time period.

In the absence of disease, the elderly perform as well as younger subjects on bedside tests of language. Errors, such as paraphasic substitutions, neologisms, and misinterpretation of commands, should be viewed with concern, regardless of the age of the subject.

It has generally been held that verbal behavior is preserved into old age. The initial 1955 standardization of the WAIS shows a drop of less than one standard deviation in the score of the verbal subtests across ages 25 to 74. This cross-sectional study was felt to reflect major cohort differences in education rather than a true age effect (29).

Longitudinal studies show that the language functions of vocabulary, information, and comprehension do not change until well past age 70 (30, 31). These studies have their critics as well; longitudinal studies are weighted with healthy, highly motivated subjects who continue in the study well past the time when unhealthy subjects have dropped out. The apparent preservation of verbal skills has prompted psychologists to label verbal functions as part of "crystallized intelligence" to signal their relative stability, in contrast to "fluid intelligence," which indicates functions that deteriorate at a younger age (32).

However, it is not at all clear that verbal skills are uniformly as well preserved into old age as is generally claimed. The Communicative Abilities in Daily Living Test shows differences in functional communication for normal controls over 75 years of age (33). Verbal fluency shows a significant decrease with age, although the decrease is not as great with higher educational levels.

Older adults often complain of difficulty finding an intended word or proper name. This difficulty has been explored in subjects aged 70 and above (34) and recently confirmed (21). This latter study showed a significant decrease in correct answers from ages 30 to 79. The most common errors for the elderly groups were circumlocutions, unnecessary comments, and perceptual errors. Cues, both semantic and phonologic, were equally facilitative in all age groups. This study suggests that the elderly have difficulty retrieving words from an intact lexicon. These findings may explain, in part, the commonly observed loquacity in older people. Tasks designed to allow the elderly to define or explain rather than retrieve target words demonstrate that elderly, more often than younger subjects, give superior explanations, but not synonyms (35). These observations also help explain the tendency toward loquacity.

Comprehension at the one-word level is unchanged in the elderly. Stimuli at the sentence and longer level show decrements with age (36). This is true for older adults regardless of educational attainment.

Discourse in the elderly is perceived to be tangential and circumlocutory, often called "long-winded". Qualitative studies of discourse (both written and oral) find that older groups use more paraphrasing, full sentences, indefinite terms, comments, and questions (37).

In summary, although verbal subtests of the WAIS show little, if any, decrement until the mid to late seventies in the absence of disease, major qualitative changes are nevertheless seen in language with normal aging. Decrements are observed on tests of naming and in comprehension of complex material. The elderly tend to have more elaborate and longer discourse styles. Retrieval of words from an intact lexicon is impaired. Practically speaking, communication remains functional throughout the life span. Elderly people cannot always find the word they want and tend to communicate in a descriptive and circumlocutory fashion. If the audience is patient and the conversation is slowed down, the elderly understand what is being communicated.

Higher Cognitive Functions

Attention, memory, and language are building blocks, basic processes upon which other more complex intellectual functions are founded. Sensory-perceptual abilities are also fundamental to higher order cognition and will be discussed in the next section. For want of a better term, these complex intellectual functions will be called the higher cognitive functions; abstract thinking, concept formation, generalization, mathematical computations, problem solving, and hypothesis testing are included. These abilities are complex functions dependent upon interactions and synthesis of basic neuropsychological processes. A decline or change in any basic process will produce a concomitant change in higher cognitive functions (38).

Bedside testing of higher cognitive functions includes the interpretation of idioms and simple and complex proverbs, and elucidation of similarities and differences between objects. These tests differ from other cognitive tests in that the score for each item depends in large measure on the examiner's subjective assessment of the response in terms of relevancy, accuracy, and complexity.

Neuropsychologic tests attempt to quantify cognitive functions using much the same testing format in a standardized fashion. Proverbs Test (39) and Similarities subtest of WAIS (29) are examples of verbal abstraction tests. Nonverbal concept formation may be tested by the Wisconsin Card Sorting Test (40).

Interpretation of idioms and simple proverbs should be abstract, regardless of age, educational level, and occupation (6). More complex proverb interpretation will be influenced by education level, general intelligence, and cultural and occupational status, but not by age.

The Similarities subtest of the WAIS is considered a "Don't Hold" test in reference to age effects, showing a significant decrease beyond 70 years of age (5). This suggests a change in the ability to generate, generalize, compare, and contrast verbal concepts. The same is true for nonverbal concept formation, as measured by the Wisconsin Card Sorting Test. This test measures the ability to change, evaluate, and formulate strategies nonverbally. The elderly were found to be less efficient, making more errors and needing more trials for correct completion of the test. Other tests of problem solving also show age-related decrements (41–43).

"Mental flexibility" refers to the ability to adapt to new situations, solve novel problems, and change mental set (44). A decrement in this cognitive capacity, which also reflects impaired conceptualization, is found as a general trait within the intellectual performance failures of old age (45).

In summary, tests of abstract thinking should not be affected by age, but will be affected by general intelligence level, education level, and occupational status. More difficult tests of concept formation and manipulation of acquired knowledge (WAIS Similarities Subtest, Wisconsin Card Sort) show age-dependent decrements in verbal and nonverbal capacities. Impairments in related measures of mental flexibility, problem solving, and changing mental set are also found in groups of elderly people in a laboratory setting. This set of differences, taken together, has evolved into a general belief that the elderly are deficient in higher cognitive processes, relative to younger people. However, this general belief may be erroneous.

Concept formation and problem solving form the basis for much of the intellectual workload in occupational and daily living activities. If capabilities for concept formation are reduced among the elderly, that may account for the observed peak in creative potential usually described between the ages of 30 and 40 for most individuals (earlier with physical sciences, later for literature and humanities). Rabbitt (41) has observed that not much original work is accomplished beyond the 5th decade.

Unfortunately, laboratory investigations of conceptualization do not always seem to relate directly to real-life problems, which elderly people are often able to solve adequately. Elderly people tend to be more cautious than younger people in all endeavors (46). This cautiousness, together with reduced speed of information processing and a slight tendency to concreteness of thought, produces low scores on laboratory tests of cognitive functioning. It is not at all clear, however, that elderly people have less capacity for functioning than younger people in real-life situations. Indeed, there is some evidence that older people, with accumulated experiences to aid them, may actually be better than younger people in solving real-life problems.

Sensory-Perceptual Changes in Normal Aging

Reception, transmission, perception, and interpretation of multimodality sensory information are complex processes requiring the cooperation and interdependence of both the peripheral and central nervous system. If incoming information is missing, contradictory, or erroneous, then the individual may commit errors based on insufficient data. Assessment of the state of sensory-perceptual mechanisms in the elderly is essential to the assessment of cognitive functions. The sensory systems to be dealt with in this section are visual, auditory, and somatosensory.

Visual Perception

Ours is a visual world, and individuals of any age with impairment of any of the visual functions are at a significant disadvantage. Age-dependent changes may occur in ocular structures, visual pathways, and cerebral cortical regions responsible for such functions as spatial resolution, perception of depth, color vision, and temporal mediation (47). Neuropsychologic processes of visuospatial and visuoconstructive tasks are dependent upon these basic visual functions.

Assessment of visual functions at the bedside includes charting of visual acuity, peripheral field of vision and color vision, and the direct viewing of the ocular apparatus, retina, and optic nerve (48). Visuoverbal tasks of reading and writing are described in the section on language. Visuospatial functioning may be tested through the use of visuoconstructive tasks. Constructional tasks include copy of two- and three-dimensional line drawings and free hand line drawings of objects to command (e.g., clock, house). Observations in real-life situations also provide information on visuospatial skills: finding the way around the hospital ward, dressing, and navigating the city streets. Neurophysiologic testing with averaged evoked potentials recorded from the scalp can be used to provide measurements of the locations and speed of visual events in the brain.

Neuropsychologic testing of visuoperceptual functions overlap inevitably and consistently with cognitive memory tasks (44). WAIS performance subtests include: Block Design (construction of replica of printed design using colored cubes); Object Assembly (cut-up figures of familiar objects); Picture Arrangement (arrangement of pictures in a series to tell a logical study); and Digit Symbol (substitution of symbols for digits). These are tests of visual recognition, visuospatial organization, visual conceptualization, and visuomotor performance.

Tests which require no physical manipulation of test materials are also used. Hooper Visual Organization Test (49) is a mental assembly task based on cut-up and disorganized line drawings on an object. The influence of visual interference can be assessed by figure ground tests, such as hidden figures (50), and hidden words (9). Visual tracking can be assessed by Rey's Targeted Lines (12).

Visual acuity tested with corrective lenses and ample light (to ensure adequate black-white contrast) should be no worse than 20/30 on the near card. Peripheral visual fields show a consistent constriction, starting at about age 40 and accelerating after age 50. Whether a consequence of reduction in pupillary size (i.e., senile miosis) (51) or of retinal ischemia (52), the constriction is symmetrical bilaterally and affects the temporal field of each eye to a greater degree. Referral for an ophthalmic examination should be made for visual acuity deficits unable to be corrected by eyeglasses, for asymmetrical constriction or loss of peripheral vision, and for retinal or optic nerve alterations. Visual evoked potentials in the elderly characteristically show an increase in both the latency and amplitude of the last components and is felt to be reflective of slowed higher order visual processing (53).

Simple visuoconstructive tasks, such as copying words and designs, should still be executed accurately, albeit more slowly, by the older individual. These examinations likewise serve as a good screening battery for serious dysfunction. Impairment in these areas should prompt more detailed, formal testing.

The "classical aging pattern" detected in the WAIS is that of preserved verbal skills in the face of deteriorating performance skills. The WAIS performance subtests are timed tasks, requiring motor responses. Block Design, Picture Completion, Picture Arrangement, and Object Assembly show a modest decrement with age. Digit-Symbol subtest, with its major attentional input, shows an even greater decrement. The decline in scores on the WAIS performance subtests remains even with the element of speed of response removed (54). Other visuospatial tests also consistently show age-related impairments.

The highest rate of decline is seen with test procedures that depend upon two or more cognitive processes that are vulnerable to the effects of age. For example, the digit symbol substitution subtest of the WAIS tests attention, incidental learning, visuomotor coordination, and speed of response. Scores on this test require the largest age correction of all the WAIS subtests. Benton Visual Retention Test is dependent upon visual attention, visual memory, spatial organization, and visuomotor ability (14) and is quite sensitive to age (55).

Cross-sectional studies showing clear differences between young and old on visuospatial tests suggest impairment of right parietal function. However, elderly people have no difficulty with other tests supposedly testing right parietal activity (e.g., drawing familiar objects, localizing places on maps). Thus, it would be a mistake to conclude that the right parietal region undergoes a process of preferential aging. These seemingly contradictory findings demand a more comprehensive theory of neurologic aging.

In summary, neuropsychologic techniques show age-related decrements in performance for the majority of visuospatial, visuoconstructive, visual recognition and scanning, visual conceptualization, and visuomotor abilities. Performance in visuospatial assessment tasks containing an element that tests other age-sensitive cognitive abilities shows an even greater decline with age.

Although much is known about age-related decrements in visual and spatial functioning in test situations, the resulting translation to everyday life is not clear-cut. Performance of elderly people on visuomotor tasks, such as driving and walking, is carried out more slowly, but apparently with no less skill under ordinary conditions. The capacity to adapt to different physical surroundings and the ability to use unfamiliar tools and objects are nevertheless reduced.

Auditory Perception

As with the visual system, the auditory system shows age-related decline in functions. Hearing shows decrements in both its sensory and perceptual portions. The impact upon verbal and nonverbal communication can be profound.

Testing for auditory function at the bedside is by both observation and elicitation. Observations of actions of an individual turning toward a sound, lip reading, or reacting to conversation over background noise (repeating questions, misunderstanding statements) is of clinical use. Quiet conversation in a soft voice can allow assessment of hearing capability in practical terms. The so-called "noise test" (distance from each ear the patient is able to hear the examiner's whispered voice) is more a qualitative (hearing impaired) than a quantitative (degree of impairment) clinical assessment (48). For an accurate and qualitative test, a referral should be made to an audiologist for an audiogram to assess auditory acuity and speech sound discrimination.

Once integrity of the peripheral auditory system is established, further testing can be done. Clinical bedside testing of higher auditory functions for the most part consists of language subtests (auditory comprehension of one-, two- and three-step commands; repetition of increasingly long and complex phrases and sentences) and recognition of nonverbal sounds (bell ringing, hand clapping). Tests of expressive and receptive prosody are now included in many testing batteries.

Neuropsychologic assessment of auditory perceptual function is measured in both verbal and nonverbal conditions. Verbal measures of language, memory, and problem solving present the opportunity for the individual to display adequate auditory comprehension and processing. When impairment in auditory processing is suspected, the examiner should compare the impaired auditory performance with that of a similar task presented visually (44). Nonverbal auditory perception is infrequently assessed routinely. Music recognition, rhythms, and meaningful sounds (traffic, door slamming) can be tested both informally and formally (56, 57).

Bedside tests of auditory acuity should reveal normal results, even though age-related changes at every level of the auditory sensory apparatus have been described (58). Referral for formal testing and evaluation for a prosthesis should be made if bedside testing shows a decrement in hearing. Presbycusis is one of the major sensory changes associated with aging. With estimates of up to 75% of the population between the ages of 75 and 79 having hearing problems (59), it is difficult to say that hearing loss is not a significant part of aging. Hinchcliffe (60) describes the findings in presbycusis as follows: impairment of pure tone thresholds, particularly in higher frequency ranges; impairment of frequency discrimination; impairment of auditory temporal discrimination and sound localization ability; impairment of speech discrimination ability; and decreased ability to understand distorted speech.

Clinically applicable tests of hearing impairment include speech reception thresholds, which are progressively impaired after age 50 (61), and sound discrimination. This latter test is especially important, in that it evaluates functions necessary for day-to-day verbal communication. In this test, speech is presented to the subject at various intensities, and the correct number of words/sentences is measured. Most elderly persons with presbycusis require an elevation of speech sound threshold of 5 to 10 decibels for intelligibility (62). Speech intelligibility has also been measured under adverse listening conditions (e.g., background noise) and is found to be even further impaired in the elderly (63). This test again simulates a real-life situation and corresponds to a frequent complaint of hearing-impaired elderly, that of worsening speech perception in noisy surroundings.

Considerable research has looked at auditory perceptual processes in relation to comprehension in the elderly. Much of what we hear in everyday communication is ambiguous and must be processed into a meaningful message. Some of the processing mechanisms involve linguistic and contextual devices (semantic, syntactic, phonologic, and metalinguistic) (64, 65). Some involve attentional and memory mechanisms and are dependent on processing speed. All of these processing mechanisms seem to be impaired in the elderly to varying degrees. The result is a reduction of auditory comprehension (58).

Auditory perceptual function is impaired in the majority of elderly people. This reduced capacity is due to primary sensory loss in hearing coupled with impaired speech sound discrimination and speech reception thresholds. These difficulties in the peripheral auditory apparatus are compounded by age-sensitive vulnerabilities in central mechanisms linked to auditory processing, including memory for complex material, processing speed, and accessing lexical items in long-term memory stores. Impaired auditory comprehension is exaggerated in settings with increased background noise.

Given what we know about auditory processing in the elderly, we can make specific recommendations for manipulating the environment and improving communication for elders and their families. Quiet background conditions, clear and well-enunciated speech, and an environment free of distraction will foster optimal communication.

Somatosensory Perception

Somatosensory information is the sum total of sensation from the skin and viscera; kinesthesis is information of movement coming from the muscles and joints. These senses are important in all tasks of mobility and ambulation, for homeostasis, and for overall well-being. They have been independently studied in the elderly.

Bedside testing of peripheral sensation has generally been considered to be modality specific; pain, temperature, touch, vibration, and kinesthesis are tested using specific techniques (48). Each limb, both proximal and distal, is tested, as well as trunk, face, and neck. Cortical contributions are made to perception of complex sensory signals through integration, interpretation, recognition and comparison to previous somatosensory memories. The so-called "cortical" sensory functions are tested individually, e.g., graphesthesia, stereognosis, two-point discrimination, sensory extinction, sensory inattention.

Somatosensory functions may be tested in neuropsychologic test batteries with tasks such as finger agnosia (66), stereognosis for objects and textures (67), and graphesthesia for numbers and letters (12). These tests have been insufficiently applied to elderly populations.

In the elderly, there is a loss of receptors in the skin of heavily myelinated nerve fibers and of neurons in the spinal cord and parietal cortex. The largest and longest nerve fibers of the posterior columns, subserving vibration and position in the distal lower extremities, seem the most affected. Sensory peripheral nerve conduction slows with age (68). This slowing is seen in the bedside neurologic examination as a diminution of ankle jerks. There is loss of vibratory sensation in lower extremities of up to 60% and in upper extremities of up to 40% (69). Little change in touch sensation is found in the elderly, even up to age 75.

In the absence of disease-induced parietal lobe dysfunction, the elderly perform as well as younger groups in tests of finger agnosia. However, they perform consistently less well in tests of two-point discrimination (70), stereognosis (71), and graphesthesia (12). The explanation for these sensory decrements is thought to be the combined effect of peripheral sensory blunting and central processing impairments (72). Importantly, kinesthetic capabilities in normal elderly are found to be impaired to both passive and active movement; however, more study is needed on this issue.

Deficits in peripheral sensation among normal elderly are seen, most clearly in reduced vibratory sensation and diminished deep tendon reflex responses in the lower extremities. Mild decrement in cortical sensory findings are also seen.

The somatosensory system is yet another neural network that displays deficiencies at several levels in the elderly. Slight but real reductions in sensory function interfere with activities, such as ambulation and skilled motor movements, as well as with occupational skills that are dependent on these neurosensory functions.

Motor Changes in Normal Aging

A motor act is required for all behavior to be effected. From the simplest of reflex reactions to the most complex of problem-solving tasks, a motor performance ultimately forms the basis upon which other cognitive and perceptual processes are judged. Thus, a change in motor performance can be expected to have broad implications and wide-ranging effects. Motor performance is significantly affected in normal aging.

Motor testing individually addresses several levels of motor functioning. Muscular strength, tone, tendon stretch reflexes, bulk of musculature, coordination, rapid volitional movements, postural and righting reflexes, skilled motor acts, and gait are all evaluated. The usual criteria for testing, however, are designed to screen for gross differences in motor performance usually seen with pathologic conditions, and not the subtle differences found with age-related decrement. Hence, results of motor system examinations of aged individuals are usually interpreted in relation to various human pathologic entities. This approach is not necessarily the most useful for understanding changes in motor performance with normal aging.

Neuropsychologic techniques may sample motor performance in such timed tasks as the Performance Scale subtests of the WAIS. Speed of response is tested by reaction time tests, among others. Free drawing tasks also measure motor skills. Tests designed to assess manual dexterity include the Finger Tapping Test (73) (number of taps per 10-second trial alternating hands) and the Purdue Pegboard Test (74) (placement of pegs in the pegboard with individual, then both hands, under timed conditions).

Sparse data are available from a handful of cross-sectional studies that have examined motor parameters as a function of age (69); there are no comparable longitudinal studies. A moderate decrement, up to 60%, of muscular strength (leg flexion, foot dorsiflexion) and a lesser decrement, up to 40%, in manual dexterity (manipulating small objects, finger dexterity, zipping garments) was seen at age 80 as compared to age 20. Changes in muscular tone with age have not been studied systematically; increased tone of the lower extremities in a mildly spastic pattern may be seen (75). Evidence of frank spasticity or cogwheel rigidity suggests an underlying pathologic condition.

Speed of skilled motor acts, simple or choice reaction time, and foot or hand tapping have consistently been shown to decrease with age (76). The sum total of all decrements is a slowing of activities. Nonetheless, elderly individuals remain able to improve performance with practice to a degree equivalent to that of the younger comparison group (77). This principle, the so-called "practice effect," is the theoretical basis for geriatric exercise groups and rehabilitation aimed at improved neuromuscular conditioning.

Normal gait depends not only on competent motor abilities. Somatosensory and kinesthetic sensory systems have major roles to play in balance, mobility, and coordination in the upright position. We have already examined the effects of age-related decrements in sensory function. For control of gait, these sensory changes in the elderly are compounded by decrements in motor performance. Gait, even in the healthy elderly person, is thus impaired. As stated by M. Malcolm Cowley (78) writing at age 80, "Age is not different from earlier life, as long as you are sitting down."

Age-related changes cause the gait to assume a characteristic pattern. Posture in the upright position is slightly flexed; forward progress is made more slowly; length of stride shortens; clearance of the foot and heel from the ground decreases; extra steps are taken in turning; side-to-side sway is slightly increased. In its extreme form, this gait resembles that of Parkinson's disease without the tremor and festination. Although the gait of elderly people is changed to a significant degree, full activities are possible. Falling or extreme slowness are indicative of pathologic states, not simply normal aging.

Neurophysiologic studies show slowing in both peripheral and central components of motor activity. With aging, nerve conduction velocities slow in motor and sensory peripheral nerves, but to only a mild degree (79). A greater degree of decrease in speed of the central component of motor processing accounts for the majority of slowing seen in motor acts. This reduction in speed of processing centrally is demonstrated by comparison of reaction time utilizing efferents of varying distance of peripheral nerve conduction. Birren and Botwinick (80) found no difference in reaction time of jaw, finger, or foot in response to an auditory signal. Central slowing is also demonstrated by the greater magnitude of age-related decrements in complex motor tasks. For example, the usual difference between simple and choice reaction times is exaggerated with older age groups (81).

Age-related decrements are also seen with standardized tests of manual dexterity and speed. For example, the Purdue test utilizes a separate set of cut-off scores, up to 30% slower for those aged 60 and above (82).

In summary, age-related slowing in all aspects of motor performance has been documented. Relative performance deteriorates more when motor skills are combined with other skills known to be vulnerable to aging. Hence, the complex, integrated sensory-motor task of ambulation is affected to a greater degree than simple reaction time. Tasks of greater complexity, which utilize greater cognitive processing and interpretation (e.g., choice versus simple reaction time), show a greater decline in the elderly than simple perceptual or motor tasks. Of note, however, is the positive practice effect for motor tasks which is equal in elderly and young groups.

Although society expects a functional decline in the aged, all motor activities, albeit slower, should be maintained throughout the life span in the absence of disease. The optimal performance of motor acts requires practice and good physical conditioning. Thus, if one's definition of being old is "when he can't stand on one leg and has trouble pulling on his pants" (78), then one can postpone growing old by practicing putting on one's pants a leg at a time while standing.

Conclusions

A neurologic scorecard, balancing the debits and credits of aging, is shown in Table 12-1. The table summarizes

Table 12-1. Neurologic/neurobehavioral functions in aging

Function	Decline	No change
Cognitive		
Attention	Divided attention Sustained attention	Simple attention
Memory	Short-term memory: lengthy information unassociated material Incidental learning: verbal visual	Immediate memory Short-term memory: brief information associated material Remote memory: information semantics over-learned material
Language	Comprehension: complex material Active naming	Elaborate narratives Vocabulary Functional communication
Conceptualization	Concept formation: novel information complex concepts Problem solving: novel and complex Changing mental set	Concept formation: idioms and proverbs Problem solving: real-life
Sensory		
Visual	Visual recognition and scanning Visuoconstructive Visuomotor	Visual acuity Visuospatial tasks in real life
Auditory	Primary sensory loss Speech discrimination Auditory processing	Comprehension in quiet surroundings
Somatosensory	Peripheral vibratory sensation Cortical sensory abilities	Finger gnosis
Motor	Choice reaction time Complex sensorimotor tasks	Simple reaction time Practice effect

important changes of neurologic and neurobehavioral functioning with age. These changes are generalizations from statistical studies of large groups. To understand how these changes affect individuals, factors such as general intelligence, education, occupation, activity, nutrition, avocations, personality, and social support must be taken into account. An individual, free of disease, should be able to maintain an active, independent life through the years.

This optimistic picture of aging is often complicated, however, in individuals of advanced age by significant loss of primary sensory functions. Visual and auditory disturbances are present more often than not, even in healthy aging. These losses of primary sensation, coupled with a mild reduction of perceptual and motor speed, seriously compound subtle, age-related decrements in sensory processing and perceptual functions, which in turn, exaggerate otherwise mild declines in attention, short-term memory, incidental learning, verbal communication, and complex problem-solving. These authors conclude that early intervention to optimize sensory functions is one of the keys to successful, healthy aging.

Another positive factor the authors wish to emphasize for healthy aging is the preserved practice effect observed in motor tasks. As individuals age, physiologic reserves decrease, and the line between healthy functioning and impairment narrows. By maintaining optimal neuromuscular conditioning, in the absence of disease, performance of day-to-day activities may be maintained and potentially enhanced.

Table 12-2. Recommendations for enhanced care of elderly

Cognitive	
Attention:	Use of attention-getting signals Screen out distractions
Memory:	Keep new information brief and relevant Use logical relationships Tie new information to old knowledge Use repetition for learning Write down information State the important information to be learned
Language:	Expect elaborate narratives Ask close-ended questions when necessary Allow adequate time for communication Speak in concrete terms
Problem solving:	Anticipate problems Rehearse with elderly what to do Encourage to summon assistance readily
Sensory	
Visual:	Use eyeglasses Orientation materials within visual field
Auditory:	Use hearing aids Adequate verbal communication
Somatosensory:	Maximize somatosensory input Caregiver contact
Motor	
Pre-op:	Optimize cardiovascular conditioning Optimize musculoskeletal conditioning
Post-op:	Early mobilization

Implications for Care of the Elderly Surgical Patient

Upon consideration of the previous discussion of changes in nervous system function with age, several concrete suggestions can be made to enhance care of the elderly individual. Table 12-2 summarizes the recommendations for patient care, based upon the known changes in the aging nervous system.

To improve communication with the elderly, attention-getting and maintaining signals (close face-to-face discussion, touching the patient, abundant use of gestures and facial/voice expression) are needed. Screening out distractions (draw the curtains, close doors, turn off TV or radio, provide one to one interaction) are helpful. The older individual remembers brief and relevant new information the best. Keep instructions and information brief, logical, and organized. Try to tie together new information with what the individual already knows ("Now you remember that President Reagan had a cancer in his bowel," etc.). Don't use new medical terms or abbreviations without knowing if the patient clearly understands them. Ask the patient what he or she already understands ("Mrs. Jones, now what did the nurse tell you about the colostomy bag?"). Use pre-existing knowledge to build on. Write down or give printed information for further review to the patient and family. Plainly state what is to be remembered, and what is important ("You must remember to take the pills the night before the test.").

In eliciting information from the elderly, expect lengthy and elaborate descriptions, which may be tangential. Allow enough time to obtain a good narrative history. Then, ask focused questions which can be answered by a yes or no. Don't overuse slang, abstract sayings, and metaphors.

Problem solving in new situations and novel surroundings, and with unfamiliar equipment can be quite difficult. Explain what problems may arise and what to do about them. Tell the individual when to summon assistance ("If the needle in your arm hurts or swells up, tell the nurse about it.").

Sensory functions should always be optimized. Eyeglasses and hearing aids must be available, in working order, and in use as soon as possible after all procedures. The amount of orienting information that is denied to the sensory-deprived individual is not to be underestimated. This is especially important if one mode of sensory input is severely disordered and not amenable to improvement (e.g., flotation mattress for treatment of decubitus ulcers may disorient totally an elderly deaf patient who is not using his or her eyeglasses consistently).

Exercises to condition cardiovascular and musculoskeletal systems should be undertaken in advance of procedures, whenever it is safe and feasible. Nonweight bearing exercises and gentle stretching for flexibility should be recommended, as much as stopping cigarettes and reducing weight. Early mobilization is also well recommended for this age group. The bed is a dangerous place for the elderly, and surgical procedures only add stress.

References

1. Mazess, RG, and Forman, SHL. 1979. Longevity and age exaggeration in Vilcabamba, Ecuador. *J Gerontol* 34:94.
2. Nesselroade, JR, and Labouvie, EW. 1985. Experimental design in research on aging. In *Handbook of the Psychology of Aging,* ed. 2, Eds., JE Birren and KW Schaie. New York: Van Nostrand Reinhold.
3. Schaie, KW, and Hertzog, C. 1985. Measurement in the psychology of adulthood and aging. In *Handbook of the Psychology of Aging,* ed 2, Eds., JE Birren and KW Schaie. New York: Van Nostrand Reinhold.
4. Strub, RL, and Black, FW. 1977. *The Mental Status Examination in Neurology.* Philadelphia: F.A. Davis Company.
5. Wechsler, D. 1958. *The Measurement and Appraisal of Adult Intelligence,* ed. 4. Baltimore: Williams & Wilkins.
6. Cummings, JL. 1985. *Clinical Neuropsychiatry.* Orlando: Grune & Stratton.
7. Army Individual Test, *Manual of Directions and Scoring.* 1944. Washington, DC: War Department, Adjutant General's Office.
8. Gronwall, D, and Wrightson, P. 1974. Delayed recovery of intellectual function after minor head injury. *Lancet* 2(1):605.
9. Talland, GA. 1965. *Deranged Memory.* New York: Academic Press.
10. Smith, A. 1967. The serial sevens subtraction test. *Arch Neurol* 17:78.
11. Granick, S. 1971. Psychological test functioning. In *Human Aging II,* Eds., S Granick and RD Patterson. Rockville, Maryland: U.S. Dept. of Health, Education and Welfare, Publication 71–9037.
12. Rey, A. 1964. *L'examen clinique en psychologie.* Paris: Presses Universitaires de France.
13. Wechsler, D. 1945. A standardized memory scale for clinical use. *J Psychol* 19:87.
14. Benton, AL. 1963. *The Revised Visual Retention Test.* New York: Psychological Corporation.
15. Albert, MS, Butters, N, and Levin, J. 1979. Temporal gradients in the retrograde amnesia of patients with alcoholic Korsakoff's disease. *Arch Neurol* 36:211.
16. Davies, AD. 1967. Age and the memory-for-designs test. *Br J Soc Clin Psychol* 6:228.
17. Hultsch, DF. 1975. Adult age differences in retrieval: Trace-dependent and cue-dependent forgetting. *Develop Psychol* 11:197.
18. Gilbert, JG. 1941. Memory loss in senescence. *J Abnorm Soc Psychol* 36:73.
19. Eysenck, MW. 1974. Age differences in incidental learning. *Develop Psychol* 10:936.
20. Benson, DF. 1979. *Aphasia, Alexia and Agraphia.* New York: Churchill Livingstone.
21. Sandson, J, Obler, LK, and Albert, ML. 1987. Language changes in healthy aging and dementia. In *Advances in Applied Psycholinguistics,* Ed., S. Rosenberg. New York: Cambridge University Press.
22. Goodglass, H, and Kaplan, E. 1972. *The Assessment of Aphasia and Related Disorders.* Philadelphia: Lea & Febiger.
23. Porch, B. 1967. *Porch Index of Communicative Ability.* Palo, Alto, CA: Consulting Psychologists.
24. Spreen, O, and Benton, A. 1960. *Neurosensory Center Comprehensive Examination for Aphasia.* Victoria, British Columbia, Canada: Neuropsychology Laboratory, University of Victoria.
25. Kertesz, A. 1982. *Western Aphasia Battery.* New York: Grune and Stratton.
26. Sarno, MT. 1969. *The Functional Communication Profile: Manual of Directions.* Monograph 42. New York: Institute of Rehabilitation Medicine, New York University Medical Center.
27. Holland, AL. 1981. *A Test for Measuring Aphasic Patients' Communicative Abilities in Daily Living.* Baltimore: University Park Press.
28. Benton, AL. 1973. The measurement of aphasic disorders. In *Aspectos patalogicos del lengae,* Ed., A. Caceres Velasquez. Lima, Peru: Centro Neuropsicologier.
29. Wechsler, DL. 1955. *Wechsler Adult Intelligence Scale Manual.* New York: Psychological Corporation.
30. Owens, WA. 1966. Age and mental abilities: A second adult followup. *J Educ Psychol* 57:311.
31. Eisdorfer, C, and Wilker, F. 1973. Intellectual changes with advancing age. In *Intellectual Functioning in Adults,* Eds., LF Jarvik, C Eisdorfer, and JE Blum. New York: Springer Publishing.
32. Cattell, RB. 1971. *Abilities: Their structure, growth and action.* Boston: Houghton-Mifflin.
33. Holland, AL. 1980. Working with the aging aphasic patient: Some clinical implications. In *Language and Communication in the Elderly,* Eds., LK Obler and ML Albert. Lexington, MA: DC Heath and Company.
34. Goodglass, H. 1980. Naming disorders in aphasia and aging. In *Language and Communication in the Elderly,* Eds., LK Obler and ML Albert. Lexington, MA: DC Heath and Company.
35. Botwinick, J, and Storandt, M. 1974. *Memory, Related Functions and Age.* Springfield, IL: Charles C Thomas.
36. Cohen, G. 1979. Language comprehension in old age. *Cogn Psychol* 11:412.

37. Obler, LK. 1980. Narrative discourse style in the elderly. In *Language and Communication in the Elderly.* Eds., LK Obler and ML Albert. Lexington, MA: DC Heath and Company.
38. Reese, HW, and Rodenheaver, RD. 1985. Problem solving and complex decision making. In *Handbook of the Psychology of Aging,* ed. 2, Eds., JE Birren and KW Schaie. New York: Van Nostrand Reinhold.
39. Gorham, DR. 1956. A proverbs test for clinical and experimental use. *Psychol Rep* Monograph suppl., no. 1.
40. Berg, EA. 1948. A simple objective technique for measuring flexibility in thinking. *J Gen Psychol* 39:15.
41. Rabbitt, P. 1977. Changes in problem solving ability in old age. In *Handbook of the Psychology of Aging,* Eds., JE Birren and KW Schaie. New York: Van Nostrand Reinhold.
42. Bigler, ED, Steinman, DR, and Newton JS. 1981. Clinical assessment of cognitive deficit in neurologic disorders: Effects of age and degenerative disease. *Clin Neuropsychol* 3:5.
43. Arenberg, D. 1968. Concept problem solving in young and old adults. *J Gerontol* 23:279.
44. Lezak, MD. 1983. *Neuropsychological Assessment.* New York: Oxford University Press.
45. Williams, M. 1970. *Brain Damage and the Mind.* Baltimore: Penguin Books.
46. Okun, MA. 1976. Adult age and cautiousness in decisions: A review of the literature. *Human Dev* 19:220.
47. Kline, DW, and Schieber, F. 1985. Vision and aging. In *Handbook of the Psychology of Aging,* ed. 2, Eds., JE Birren and KW Schaie. New York: Van Nostrand Reinhold.
48. DeJong, RN. 1979. *The Neurologic Examination,* ed. 4. Hagerstown, Maryland: Harper and Row.
49. Hooper, HE. 1958. *The Hooper Visual Organization Test Manual.* Los Angeles: Western Psychological Services.
50. Thurstone, LL. 1944. *A Factorial Study of Perception.* Chicago: University of Chicago Press.
51. Weale, RA. 1961. Retinal illumination and age. *Transactions of the Illuminating Engineering Society* 26:95.
52. Wolf, E, and Nadroski, AS. 1971. Extent of the visual field changes with age and oxygen tension. *Arch Ophthalmol* 86:637.
53. Beck, EC, Swanson, C, and Dustman, RE. 1980. Long latency components of the visually evoked potential in man: Effects of aging. *Exper Aging Res* 6:523.
54. Storandt, M. 1977. Age, ability level and method of administering and scoring the WAIS. *J Gerontol* 32:175.
55. Benton, AL, Eslinger, PJ, and Damasio, AR. 1981. Normative observations on neuropsychological test performance in old age. *J Clin Neuropsychol* 3:33.
56. Seashore, CE, Lewis, D, and Saetveit, DL. 1960. *Seashore Measures of Musical Talents.* New York: Psychological Corporation.
57. Halstead, WC. 1947. *Brain and Intelligence.* Chicago: University of Chicago Press.
58. Olsho, LW, Harkins, SW, and Lenhardt, ML. 1985. Aging and the auditory system. In *Handbook of the Psychology of Aging,* ed. 2, Eds., JE Birren and KW Schaie. New York: Van Nostrand Reinhold.
59. Butler, RA, and Lewis, ML. 1977. *Aging and Mental Health.* St. Louis, MO: Mosby.
60. Hinchcliffe, R. 1962. The anatomical locus of presbycusis. *J Speech Dis* 27:301.
61. Plomp, R, and Mimper, AM. 1979. Speech reception threshold for sentences as a function of age and noise level. *J Acoust Soc Am* 66:1333.
62. Punch, JL, and McConnell, F. 1969. The speech discrimination function of elderly adults. *J Aud Res* 9:159.
63. Bergman, M. 1971. Changes in hearing with age. *Gerontologist* 11:148.
64. Warren, RM. 1970. Perceptual restoration of missing speech sounds. *Science* 167:393.
65. Spencer, NJ, and Wollman, NL. 1980. Lexical access for phonetic ambiguities. *Lang Speech* 23:171.
66. Kinsbourne, M, and Warrington, EK. 1962. A study of finger agnosia. *Brain* 85:47.
67. Weinstein, S. 1964. Deficits concomitant with aphasia or lesions of either hemisphere. *Cortex* 1:151.
68. Dorfman, LJ, and Bosley, TM. 1979. Age-related changes in peripheral and central nerve conduction in man. *Neurology* 29:38.
69. Potvin, AR, et al. 1980. Human neurologic function and the aging process. *J Am Ger Soc* 28:1.
70. Bolton, CF, Winkleman, RK, and Dyck, PJ. 1968. A quantitative study of Meissner's corpuscles in man. *Neurology* 16:1.
71. Axelrod, S, and Cohen, LD. 1961. Senescence and embedded figure performance in vision and touch. *Percept Psychophys* 12:283.
72. Kenshalo, DR. 1977. Age changes in touch, vibration, temperature, kinesthesis and pain sensitivity. In *Handbook of the Psychology of Aging,* Eds., JE Birren and KW Schaie. New York: Van Nostrand Reinhold.
73. Goldstein, SG, Deysaack, RE, and Kleinknecht, RA. 1973. Effect of experience and amount of information on identification of cerebral impairment. *J Consu Clin Psychol* 41:30.
74. Purdue Research Foundation. 1948. *Examiner's Manual for the Purdue Pegboard.* Chicago: Science Research Associates.
75. Durso, R, and Feldman, RG. 1984. Parkinson's disease and its relationship to aging. *Neurologic Consultant* 2(4):1.
76. Salthouse, TA. 1985. Speed of behavior and its implications for cognition. In *Handbook of the Psychology of Aging,* ed. 2. Eds., JE Birren and KW Schaie. New York: Van Nostrand Reinhold.
77. Salthouse, TA, and Somberg, BL. 1982. Isolating the age deficit in speeded performance. *J Gerontol* 37:59.
78. Cowley, ML. 1976. *The View from 80.* New York: Viking Press.
79. LaFratta, CW, and Canestrari, RE. 1966. A comparison of sensory and motor nerve conduction velocities as related to age. *Arch Phys Med Rehabil* 47:286.
80. Birren, JE, and Botwinick, J. 1955. Age differences in finger, jaw and foot reaction time to auditory stimuli. *J Gerontol* 10:429.
81. Welford, AT. 1977. Motor performance. In *Handbook of the Psychology of Aging*, Eds., JE Birren and KW Schaie. New York: Van Nostrand Reinhold.
82. Vaughan, HG, Jr, and Costa, LD. 1962. Performance of patients with lateralized cerebral lesions, II: Sensory and motor test. *J Nerv Ment Dis* 134:237.

13

Psychiatric Changes in the Elderly

Donna Cohen, Gregory J. Paveza, and Philip B. Gorelick

> . . . nothing you are can stay
> But all the time you keep going
> away, away.

W.S. Merwin wrote these lines in his poem "Grandmother Watching at the Window," where he captures the elegiac awareness of mortality with an acceptance of the human condition of aging. The phenomenon of increased life expectancy has never been witnessed in the history of our world. Currently, more than 20% of our population now dies after age 80, and if present trends continue, within the next 10 to 12 years half of all deaths will occur after age 80 (1).

Death rates have declined greatly since 1900. A steep decline persisted from 1900 until about 1950 and then suddenly reached a plateau for almost a quarter of a century (1). During those years, it was erroneously assumed that Americans had achieved a maximum life expectancy of age 67, and both the Social Security and Medicare programs developed under this faulty assumption. In 1968, a sharp decline in mortality resumed and continues today. We do not know what is causing this increasing life expectancy or at what point it will slacken. However, the central health issue raised by increasing longevity is net gain of active, functional, and happy years of life versus total years of compromised health spent in pain and misery. The latest U.S data suggest that for each year of healthy active life gained in our population, about 3.5 compromised years are added (1). This means that while most of us can expect to live longer active lives, we can also expect that some portion of our late life will be accompanied by a loss of function and a reliance on others to care for us. Therefore, it is not surprising that so many people—from poets to physicians—are ambivalent about growing old.

Another form of ambivalence, uncertainty, characterizes many decisions about older persons, especially whether the very old should be surgical candidates. Little is known about the natural history of most physical and psychiatric diseases in the aged, limiting the data base for rational medical decisions about the risks of surgery (2). Preoperative, intraoperative, and postoperative decisions about older patients are also complex because many older persons have multiple coexisting and interacting comorbidities and co-disabilities; they also may live under adverse social and economic circumstances.

Accurate assessment of operative risks and benefits of surgical intervention as well as proper management of older surgical patients requires an awareness of each older person's motivation and view of his or her disorder as well as an understanding of his or her intellectual, emotional, and physical status. Where possible, a preoperative mental status examination and a psychiatric consultation are recommended for older patients. Therapy can then be focused on maximizing optimal functional effectiveness in the preoperative, intraoperative, and postoperative periods.

Time spent with older patients and their families clarifies the indications for surgery as well as the outcomes. This chapter will therefore present an overall approach to communicating with older patients during surgical contacts and will review common issues in the surgical care of patients with psychiatric and behavioral disturbances. Guidelines for family interviews are discussed since helping patients and family understand what can be expected before, during, and after an operation maximizes successful convalescence.

An Approach to Caring for Older Patients

Effective health care for all patients, young and old, transcends the diagnosis and treatment of specific conditions. Caring also involves an awareness of the needs of patients as individuals who are reacting and adapting to symptoms, a disease or a disability, as well as communicating effectively with them about their life-style and health care. Communication skills have always been integral to patient contact—history taking, the physical examination, prescription writing, patient counseling, and psychotherapy. Communication skills are even more essential today not only because of the increasingly complex legal relationships between patients and physicians, but because older patients with multiple co-morbidities and disabilities make the evaluation for surgery complex.

An interactive, respectful, and trusting partnership between physicians and patients is essential for effective health care. However, the majority of older patients report difficulty communicating with their physicians (3). Medical interviews with older persons are a challenge. Older adults bring a lifetime of experiences and a rich history of interpersonal and intergenerational relationships to the physician's office which need to be understood in the context of presenting problems and symptomatology. Furthermore, older persons are often accompanied by family members who have requested the appointment on behalf of the individual or have pressured their relative to see a doctor. This puts the physician in the complex and sometimes difficult position of establishing a relationship with an older patient in which the patient's autonomy is respected while simultaneously promoting a therapeutic family relationship.

Interviewing older patients is a complex experience precisely because of the person's age. There are major differences in the life experiences, motivations, and capabilities of older as compared to younger adults. The heterogeneity in the older population over the entire range of biopsychosocial variables is greater than in any other age group. Moreover, the life experiences of older patients often surpass those of a younger physician. In some instances, this may limit the latter's ability to understand older patients despite clinical training. Finally, frail older persons and the very old with multiple chronic illnesses in hospitals and long-term care institutions may require professionals to adopt less formal and more personalized approaches to medical examinations and interviews.

Medical interviews flow easily with many older persons who are in good physical and mental health. Patients often become ready participants in the process with little inhibition, and a certain wisdom in the patient may even help the physician to enhance his or her understanding of the resiliency and endurance of older patients. However, at the other end of the spectrum are the difficulties associated with severely disabled and frail hospital and nursing home patients, who challenge the physician's ability to establish a relationship in order to understand the patient's needs and desires, diagnose existing disease, identify excess disability amendable to therapy, and in general care for the human being.

The success of medical interviews depends upon the quality of the relationship that develops between the physician and the older patient. The initial phase of interviewing should focus on understanding what is required to foster the optimum relationship to help the patient. Older people have had a lifetime of dealing with others, and many are adept at "sizing up" new people, while others are not. But all older persons experience a process of transference with the physician. The patient, to a greater or lesser extent, experiences the physician as a physician, but he or she will also respond with emotions appropriate to another relationship important to them. It is not uncommon for older patients to react to physicians in ways that developed in relation to a parent, a younger sibling, or an aunt or uncle. The severely cognitively impaired patient may react to the physician as a long dead parent or relative, whereas a retired business executive with mild cognitive impairment may experience a physician as a subordinate and behave in ways that are inappropriate in a physician's office but were appropriate in the working environment.

Many discussions with older patients flounder at the start when physicians fail to understand the powerful misidentification that may occur. Moreover, discussions that begin well may collapse at a later time as the unconscious misidentification process changes the patient's ability to maintain trust and confidence in the physician.

These same unconscious mechanisms are operating in physicians. It is easy to experience an older patient as an older relative or an image of what the physician will ultimately become. It is not uncommon to feel uncomfortable around older patients who are very sick and impaired. The smell of feces, urine, foul breath, and other body odors are often barriers to spending sufficient time with patients to conduct an adequate examination, which affects the diagnostic accuracy and the efficacy of treatment and rehabilitation.

Physician reactions are often helpful to understand the patient. Older patients frequently arouse anger in physicians during an examination with belligerent or irritating behaviors that are often a projection of the patient's anger about being sick and dependent. Becoming old and frail or old and sick is often frightening and upsetting. Having a chronic illness changes a person's life as the illness becomes part of an individual's identity. Pain often accompanies illness and medical procedures, and it is common for patients not only to be angry with the pain and deterioration but also to be upset with relatives, doctors, and nurses who may not understand these feelings or who appear indifferent.

There is perhaps no greater fear among older persons than that of ongoing dependency on others. Many older patients experience health or social crises as personal events and think about the future in terms of their own individual resources. For many the desire for independence is a powerful force, and adjustment to illness is a battle. Other persons may adjust more easily. What is important to understand are the perceptions of older persons and how a medical episode or health "catastrophe" fits with their perceptions of themselves and their ability to manage.

The physician's behavior with older patients decisively influences the quality of the relationship and participation in health care procedures. It is essential to foster a sense of comfort and trust as a prerequisite to an adequate flow of medical and personal information from the older patient. This can be quite difficult especially when sick older patients are unaware of the reason for a physician visit, which is often the case in hospitals and nursing homes where physical infirmity and pain interfere with comprehension. In more intact patients, physicians will often encounter a suspiciousness that effectively blocks the flow of discussion. This suspiciousness occasionally develops as an appropriate response to traumas experienced in other relationships, including poor physician relationships in the past. It may also be the result of a florid paranoid condition with delusions or vivid visual and auditory hallucinations that require a psychiatric consultation.

Older patients are often exquisitely sensitive to the slightest emotional nuances. This sensitivity may relate to a fear of rejection often experienced by older patients who feel their age is a barrier to being perceived as a worthwhile and desirable person. It is particularly important to avoid comments which may be perceived as intrusive, critical, or overly familiar. Older patients often express a sense of being "locked in" and isolated from the real world as well as feelings of abandonment and decreased self-esteem, making it even more critical to approach patients with a genuine sense of acceptance. Older persons are frequently sensitive to artificial involvement. Nonverbal communication readily conveys whether a physician empathizes with the predicament, is available, and truly wants to be helpful.

This honest, comfortable, and forthright attitude is particularly important for those with Alzheimer's disease or a related disorder. It is essential to understand the patient's use of language and enter into an interactive pattern as much as possible (4). In its simplest form, this often means using short phrases and simple direct questions, giving the person time to answer, inserting words when necessary, repeating questions slowly, maintaining eye contact, and generally letting the individual know you care about his or her answers. This ability requires considerable practice, but once acquired, fosters communication with many cognitively impaired older patients who were once thought impenetrable.

Sensory acuity is fundamental to successful medical interviews since the ability to see, hear, feel, and touch affects effective communication. Older patients with impaired hearing will often attempt to cover up deficits out of a sense of embarrassment. If the person does not use a hearing aid, speak face-to-face to maximize lip reading. Where hearing loss is serious, it is possible to conduct a successful interview by writing out the questions for the individual to read and answer. Some physicians place their stethoscope in the patient's ears and speak loudly into the diaphragm to amplify their voice.

Fatigue, particularly in very frail and sick patients, is one of the greatest barriers to understanding a person's needs, problems, and preferences. Short interviews spaced over time often elicit material from the most inaccessible patient in a hospital or nursing home. As much as possible, patients should be interviewed privately to convey a sense of intimacy and respect. Even in crowded hospital or nursing home wards, it is appropriate to pull the curtain around the patient's bed to symbolically communicate this sense of privacy.

As is true for most patients, older persons are often anxious about talking to a doctor. Fortunately, this anxiety usually diminishes as a history is being developed. Physicians must take the initiative to deliberately structure their questions and be clear about why it is important to talk about a specific condition or symptom. Initial questions should be cast broadly in terms that reduce anxiety and stimulate a flow of information. For example, "How can I help you?" or "What has brought you to see me?" An optimistic tone may also help reduce anxiety. If patients do not relax, question the patient more directly about his or her anxiety.

The initial phase of history taking should focus on understanding the chief complaints or distress experienced. Paradoxically, some lucid older patients have little if any insight into their problems, while those with mild to moderate dementia may be able to explain difficulties with disarming clarity. A man in his mid-70s with profound memory loss of at least 6 years duration was seen in the hospital after a car accident in which he sustained multiple broken bones (5). He talked about his feelings of sadness and frustration about his memory problems. In spite of aphasia, he conveyed his deep frustration and sense of inadequacy. He expressed a desire to die from his injuries so that he would not be a burden to his wife in the later stages of dementia. The surgeon requested psychiatric consultation, and during brief supportive psychotherapy the patient was relieved to share his feelings, which had been hidden from his wife and family.

It is essential to develop at least a preliminary understanding of the patient's thoughts, fears, and beliefs about presenting symptoms and conditions. Psychiatric consultation was requested for an older woman because of constant screaming on the ward. She was suffering from a mild anoxic encephalopathy following cardiac bypass surgery. During the interview, she was calm and agreeable, but when questioned about her screaming she stated that she became fearful at night when the doctors were gone, and she was particularly fearful when the nurses were no longer present. The presence of a private duty nurse for several days eliminated the screaming.

Understanding a patient's major complaints is only the prologue to discerning the history of an illness, and many older patients are able to adequately describe the development of their symptoms. A 70-year-old patient was seen in the hospital following a successful course of electroshock treatments for a psychotic depression (5). Approximately 1 year earlier, she had been hospitalized following an automobile accident in which her cervical spine was fractured. Shortly before the onset of the psychotic depression, an orthopedist had told her she might need surgery and traction for several months because her vertebra had not knitted together properly. The psychotic symptoms developed around the fears of being in traction, which reminded her of experiences 40 years earlier in a concentration camp.

If physicians are tactful, patient, and flexible, many older patients will discuss life issues relevant to their current situation and medical status. Nonverbal cues of patience and understanding (e.g., sitting down and trying to convey a sense of having the time to spend talking regardless of a hectic schedule) may permit even delusional patients to reveal personal thoughts. For example, a lady with terminal breast cancer was seen by a psychiatrist at the request of nursing home staff who were concerned about what they believed was a depression (5). As the lady spoke, she made vague references to a staff member who was abusing her. Eventually, she revealed a delusional system in which she perceived a plot to extract money from her by the entire nursing staff. What was seen by the staff as depression was actually a paranoid fear of them.

As the medical history evolves, the physician must begin to formulate hypotheses about the patient and his or her medical needs. How has the patient adapted to old age and his or her injury or medical problems? Are there unusual problems or symptoms? What resources does the patient have to deal with his or her illness, injury, or circumstances? The answers to these questions provide the basis for developing diagnostic and treatment strategies that will not only deal with the medical-surgical situation but also engage the older person in his or her recovery.

Interviewing About the Relevant Past

Many older persons have a great need to share their memories as well as their present circumstances, and the physician is usually exposed to the patient's seemingly unending life history, regardless of firm attempts to structure the interview. Advancing age in the face of illness, impending surgery, or disability is frequently a time of heightened psychologic investment in the resolution of present and past conflicts. To the casual observer, the intensity of these processes are not always discernible, and they are often confusing if not frustrating.

When patients face life-threatening situations, it is often appropriate to probe into the patient's thoughts about life and death. One patient with pancreatic cancer, seen for evaluation of a recent onset of severe depression, described a difficult past, which consisted of early widowhood and the birth of a child profoundly crippled with cerebral palsy (5). The symptoms of depression developed shortly after her 65th birthday, and when questioned about a possible linkage, she insisted that she was now old and would soon die. She felt cheated and angry because she had never really lived.

Some older patients almost seem to court or welcome death. It is important to establish how much the individual worries about death and illness as well as what personal resources are present to deal with these realities. Indeed, behavior may be more important than words. A 99-year-old woman whose mental status was remarkably intact was seen in a nursing home shortly after a mild stroke (5). She had formerly been independent, making trips alone to Florida to spend winters in her trailer. She spoke freely about not fearing death yet expressed a desire to die. The nursing home staff reported, however, that she demanded constant attention from them, as well as her family and the rehabilitation staff. As she gradually improved it was clear that she, in fact, did not wish to die.

A patient's history is important because of the insights it can reveal about the present. Sometimes even in the most difficult interviews the importance of the past can be profound. A 70-year-old patient with terminal breast cancer was seen in the intensive care unit of a hospital. The consultation request stated that the patient was expecting to die momentarily but seemed to be lingering as if she were fighting death. The referring oncologist wanted advice on how to deal with the patient's constant piercing screams. When interviewed the patient was weak, jaundiced, and barely audible. After some time, she revealed that as a young secretary many years before she had had an abortion. As her cancer worsened she became intensely religious, returning to her earlier Catholic faith. She stated that her screaming was out of fear of the punishment she might receive after death for the abortion. She accepted the interviewer's suggestion to speak with a priest and died peacefully the day following that visit.

An older person's attitudes and perceptions about his or her strengths and weaknesses reveal a great deal about coping styles during illness. A wealthy client with a profound dementia of 10 years duration still had good social skills, which allowed him to relate to old acquaintances (5). He insisted that his family be silent about his memory problem because "he would be ruined if the word got out." Everyone knew about his disorder, but as one relative stated, family and friends treated him like "the emperor with no clothes." Everyone feared he would become deeply depressed if he felt he was no longer valued for his prowess. A solid appreciation of the way individuals view themselves provides important insights and a basis for providing meaningful health care.

Interviewing Family

Interviews with the individual's family are often helpful, but these must be carefully structured because the relationship between older persons and their families is extraordinarily complex. As described by Boszormeyi-Nagy and Spark (6) there are powerful loyalties within families which bind them across and within the generations. This is often a positive and beneficial affiliation, but at other times emotional forces can be negative and destructive.

Many puzzling behaviors of older patients may be unraveled by skillful interviews with family members. For example, a 79-year-old nursing home patient, alert but with severe arteriosclerotic heart disease, periodically developed congestive heart failure. He had been a resident in the home for approximately 6 months when first seen. He had been married for 50 years in what was described as an ambivalent relationship. The wife, who herself had serious heart disease, lived alone at the time. During a joint interview with the couple, it emerged that the episodes of heart failure developed whenever the wife left town to visit their daughter. Subsequent discussions with the patient led to a decrease in the frequency of cardiac crises when he was better able to anticipate and cope with the anxiety of separation.

Physician interviews with families must elicit several types of data. It is important to be sensitive to the authority the older patient may still exert in the family system since this provides a handle on how to respond to family members who appear to want to control the medical encounter and their relative's illness. Does the patient still maintain leadership and power or is he or she becoming infantilized by family members? If a spouse is alive, what is the status of the marital relationship as well as the spouse's health? Is the family affectionate or hostile in interactions with the patient as well as one another? Is there legitimate family conflict because of excessive demands by the patient or unusual and inappropriate family behaviors in caregiving tasks?

Probing into the pattern of family relationships provides clues about loyalty across generations, and the ability as well as capacity of family members to be involved in a supportive way in a relative's care, even when there has been a history of indifference or hostility. An older woman with chronic leukemia was interviewed jointly with her daughter, who admitted that she had always been angry with her mother for not meeting her needs (5). Although she had been alienated from her mother and had not spoken to her for 7 years, the daughter stated that she now felt it was her duty to care for the mother as repayment for her very existence. When her mother died a year later, the daughter told the staff that she had found her mother again.

Older patients must be carefully prepared prior to family members being interviewed, even when relatives accompany them on an office visit. Such preparation is necessary in order to ensure that the older person understands why the family is being interviewed and to allay any fears that the family is being brought in to make plans about the aged person's care. It is important that the older patient be permitted to remain in a relationship with the doctor in which the older patient perceives that he or she and the doctor are making decisions about his or her life. The essential element needed in working with older patients is their trust, which may be lost if they do not consent to and understand the reason for family members being brought into discussions about their health care. If the patient objects, family discussions might be postponed until the individual is less threatened, if the medical situation permits.

With many older persons, even those who come to a physician appointment alone, a joint meeting with the family is sometimes indicated; depending on the medical situation, separate interviews are also useful. It is important not to ask questions in a manner that heightens guilty feelings in family members. Relatives are often guarded in their willingness to share information, and they may quickly become defensive. It is important to keep the discussions centered around the needs of the older patient as much as possible. If interviews are held separately the physician must not share information with the family that the patient considers confidential.

Interviewing and history taking are essential first

steps in caring for older patients, even for surgeons who often rely upon the internist or family physician to carry out their evaluations. They must be done carefully, thoughtfully, systematically, and with the highest respect for the autonomy, dignity, and complexity of the individual and often the family. Family members should be included as informants when individuals are mentally impaired or incapacitated, but even then patients should be participants in this process. The determination of surgical risks as a balance between the results of surgical therapy versus no surgery as well as effective management may rest upon the information extracted from family interviews.

Discussing surgical procedures with patients and families will help prepare them for the acute decline in physical and mental functioning that frequently follows surgery. Delirium and acute psychiatric conditions may occur in 25% or more of patients in surgical intensive care units (7). Patients and families need to be prepared for this common and reversible deterioration. If understood, inappropriate institutionalization by upset relatives can be avoided (8).

The Challenge of Surgical Decisions When Older Patients Have Psychiatric Problems

Older patients with psychiatric conditions require special attention when elective and major surgery is being considered. Psychiatric consultation is often valuable not only to assess the relative risks and benefits of surgery but to develop effective strategies for preoperative and postoperative care. Other health professionals such as nurses, psychologists, and social workers provide important pre- and postoperative services, helping patients adjust to the hospital environment as well as make a smooth transition home or to a nursing home. Behavioral strategies during convalescence are far more effective than psychotropic medications that often make the patient worse and delay recovery.

Surgical decision making should be based on a collaborative relationship between the patient and the physician as well as family members and other health professionals when appropriate. Whenever possible, the authority to accept or reject diagnostic and treatment procedures, including surgery, rests with the patient, who may choose to delegate authority to someone else. Hospitals should have institutional procedures to protect the rights of older surgical patients who are cognitively and/or emotionally impaired to the extent that their ability to make an informed voluntary decision is questioned (8). Likewise, hospitals should have procedures to clarify circumstances under which the patient's authority may be limited and where other parties, including the courts, may substitute judgment. Only when a patient's capacity to make decisions is definitely impaired and potentially dangerous should the patient's right for decision making be transferred to others.

The right to accept or refuse surgical procedures presumes that an older patient is capable of talking with the physician, understanding treatment alternatives, and evaluating potential risks and benefits. When older persons are seriously impaired emotionally and cognitively, it is appropriate to question the patient's ability to participate in a process of informed consent and evaluate the patient's mental status. It is essential to emphasize that even patients with cognitive disorders are capable of understanding their options when information is presented to them in simple language and there is a basis for trust and understanding between these patients and their physicians. It is also advisable and useful that information be shared with the patient's family.

Discussions between patient, family, and physician are valuable in ensuring that patients understand surgical information presented to them and treatment choices available. Even in cases where patients have chosen to delegate decisions to family members or a physician, a discussion with the patient about the implications of treatment is recommended. There are clearly some emergencies where obtaining voluntary informed consent is impossible. In these cases, the patient's consent to surgery chosen by a physician may be legally supported by the circumstances surrounding the provision of such care.

The right to choose surgery includes the right to refuse it or to select an alternative treatment. If a patient refuses all forms of treatment, a written refusal is recommended to protect the hospital and physicians. This decision should also be documented in the patient's chart. If the patient chooses a treatment course unacceptable to the attending physician, the latter may withdraw as long as this does not constitute legal abandonment. If a qualified alternative physician is willing to comply with a patient's preferences, transfer to the care of such a person should be offered to the patient. If no physician or qualified health care professional is willing to undertake the patient's choice of treatment, hospitals should have policies relative to the care of such patients. Hospitals should also have policies to clarify and deal with situations where the treatment course is unacceptable to the mission of the institution. Laws regarding the rights of patients or someone on the patient's behalf to refuse treatment differ across states.

In surgical situations, decision making is best defined as the patient's ability to understand the treatment options and their effect on him or her. Only when the patient's capacity to make decisions is definitely impaired and the impact of a bad decision is potentially serious should his or her right and responsibility be transferred to others. When there is doubt about a patient's ability for adequate decision making, the physician should assess this capacity in consultation with family, friends, and other health care professionals. Hospitals and nursing homes should have appropriate policies for this assessment and identified methods to ensure that physicians conduct them when necessary. There should also be procedures for family, friends, and other health care professionals to question a patient's capacity to make decisions.

The following case anecdote illustrates some of the important issues regarding the legal protection of patient rights in the absence of a previously diagnosed dementia or psychiatric condition (9). The case is the matter of Bertha Harris (*Harris,* 477, A.2d 724 (D.C. 1984)), which was eventually referred to the D.C. Superior Court in 1984 (*In the Matter of Bertha Harris,* Misc. No. 126-84 (D.C. Superior Ct., June 4, 1984)). Bertha Harris, 73 years old, had both diabetes and circulatory problems when she was transferred from a nursing home to the hospital for surgery. Ms. Harris had been told that gangrene in her foot would probably spread, and she consented to amputation of her left leg above the knee. Her sister and niece (who was a court–appointed conservator of Ms. Harris's estate) also consented to the operation.

Several weeks later, physicians observed a black patch on her right foot and recommended that the right leg also be amputated. Ms. Harris refused, and when the physician could not persuade Ms. Harris, her sister, or niece to consent to the second amputation, the hospital requested the court to declare Bertha Harris incompetent and authorize the surgery.

The court ruled that a ruling of incompetency required convincing evidence that Bertha Harris lacked the capacity to make the decision about a second amputation. The court also ruled that Ms. Harris had the right to be examined by a psychiatrist and physician of her own choosing. Following further hearings the court found that Bertha Harris understood the consequences of not amputating her second leg. The court recognized that there was evidence that Ms. Harris did display confusion and some memory difficulties, but that this did not affect her ability to make a treatment decision about her leg. Ms. Harris was competent to decline treatment and there was no basis for the court to interfere with her decision.

The case of Bertha Harris illustrates accepted methods of dealing with health care decisions when patient competence is questioned. The hospital obtained the consent of appropriate family members in addition to the patient before the first amputation. When the patient and family members refused permission to amputate the second leg, the hospital approached the court to determine whether she was capable of making such a decision and to authorize surgery if it concluded that Bertha Harris was not competent to make her own decision about the second amputation.

Competent adult patients have the right to make decisions even if they are inconsistent with the judgment of their physicians. Bertha Harris's physician did not question her competence when she agreed to the first amputation, only after she refused to have the second amputation. The court ruled that she had the right to make a decision contrary to her doctors', as long as she understood the nature and consequences of that decision.

Assessing decision making in patients with cognitive impairments requires careful sensitive interviews, usually over several time periods. Bertha Harris performed poorly on a mental status examination, but she also had difficulty understanding the foreign-born psychiatrist who testified that Ms. Harris was incompetent because she had problems processing what was said to her. However, Ms. Harris clearly demonstrated that she understood the doctors wanted to amputate her second leg and that they thought she would die within weeks if this surgery were not performed. Questioning by another physician revealed that Bertha Harris's poor performance on the mental status examination was a function of her fears and anxiety, not a brain disorder that impaired competent judgment. Physicians evaluating an older patient's cognitive status should speak fluently and clearly using language understood by the patient, and have appropriate training and experience in geriatric psychiatry, neurology, medicine, or psychology.

Summary

Using illustrative case anecdotes, this chapter reviews guidelines for effective communication with older persons during surgical contacts. Most of the relevant information about surgical risks is derived from the patient's history, a process often problematic for physicians, older patients, and families. Time spent with older patients and family members will help clarify unusual symptomatology, identify ways to ameliorate risk factors, and prepare them for a delayed convalescence.

References

1. Brody, JA. 1987. The best of times, The worst of times: Aging and dependency in the 21st century. In *Ethical Dimensions of Geriatric Care,* Eds., SF Spicker, SR Ingman, and IR Lawson. New York: D. Reidel.
2. Weksler, MD. 1985. The evaluation of the elderly patient for

surgery. In *Practical Geriatric Medicine,* Eds., AN Exton-Smith and ME Weksler. New York: Churchill Livingstone.
3. American Association for Retired Persons. 1984. *Truth About Aging: Guidelines for Accurate Communications.* Washington, DC: AARP.
4. Cohen, D, and Eisdorfer, C. 1986. *The Loss of Self: A Family Resource for Alzheimer's Disease and Related Disorders.* New York: WW Norton.
5. Cohen, D, and Speken, R. 1985. Interviewing older adults. In *Effective Interviewing,* Ed., A Tolor. Springfield, IL: Charles C Thomas.
6. Boszormeyi-Nagy, I, and Spark, GM. 1973. *Invisible Loyalties: Reciprocity in Intergenerational Family Therapy.* Hagerstown, MD: Harper & Row.
7. Heller, SS, et al. 1970. Psychiatric complication of open-heart surgery. *N Engl J Med* 203:1015–1020.
8. Levilan, SJ, and Kornfeld, DS. 1981. Clinical and cost benefits of liaison psychiatry. *Am J Psychiat* 138:790–793.
9. American Association of Retired Persons. 1986. *A Matter of Choice: Planning Ahead for Health Care Decisions.* Washington, DC: AARP.

14

Immunologic Changes in the Elderly

Douglas C. Powers, James E. Nagel, and William H. Adler

Declining immune function has long been recognized as a correlate of advancing age. Immune factors are even postulated as the primary determinants of biologic senescence (1). Although the immunologic theory of aging remains unproven, there is no question that many diseases of the elderly are associated with alterations of immune function. This chapter briefly describes the organization and cellular components of the immune system, and then summarizes current knowledge about age-related changes. A brief discussion of clinical considerations relating to these changes follows.

General Organization

Major structures of the immune system include the spleen, thymus, bone marrow, lymph nodes, the cellular elements of the blood, and the gut- and lung-associated lymphoid tissues (Fig. 14-1). In general, the distribution and histologic structure of these lymphoreticular organs provides for the efficient exposure of foreign immunogens to the various cells involved in the immune response. All of the solid lymphoid organs, such as the spleen, thymus, and lymph nodes, contain large numbers of lymphocytes as well as other immunocompetent accessory cells (Table 14-1). Of the various cell types that participate in an immune response, lymphocytes are by far the most numerous and important. Lymphocytes have receptors on their surface that enable them to recognize "self" as well as to respond to various foreign or "nonself" substances or cells. Lymphocytes are divided into two major categories, the T and B lymphocytes. The B refers to the bursa of Fabricius of birds or the bone marrow of mammals and the T refers to the thymus. The B lymphocytes, the progenitors of antibody-forming cells, undergo partial maturation in the bone marrow. The T lymphocytes, which are the effectors of cellular immunity as well as regulators of various immune functions, derive from the thymus. The T and B lymphocytes are not homogenous and include various functional subpopulations of cells.

A third type of lymphoid effector cell is the natural killer (NK) cell. These cells, which have a large granular morphology and appear to be lymphocytes, play an important role in host defense. They are capable of recognizing, without the need for prior immunologic sensitization, and lysing cells that have been altered by neoplastic transformation or viral infection.

The most important nonlymphoid effector cells are the monocyte and macrophage. Along with polymorphonuclear cells, monocytes are responsible for antibody-dependent cell-mediated cytotoxicity (ADCC), another type of cytolytic reaction mediated through cells with surface receptors for the Fc portion of immunoglobulin. Macrophages and other accessory cells of the reticuloendothelial system (RES) also participate in the immune response by presenting antigens to immunocompetent lymphocytes, by phagocytizing immune complexes and tissue debris, and by regulating lymphocyte activity through the production of soluble mediators, such as interleukin-1 and prostaglandins.

Age-Related Changes in Immune Function

On a very basic level, the senescence of the immune system might be inferred from anatomic changes of the lym-

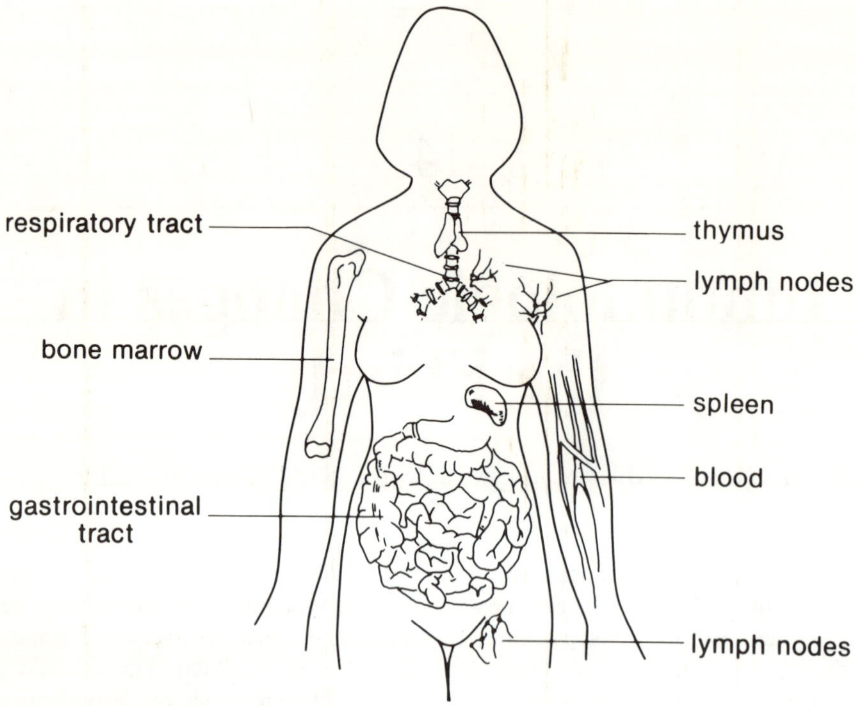

Figure 14-1. Anatomic organization of the immune system.

phoreticular network that accompany aging (2). Over time, virtually all of the solid lymphoid organs undergo a progressive reduction of both volume and mass. This decrease in size is paralleled by morphologic changes, which include blurring of histologic architecture, alterations in the numbers of cells, and fatty infiltration. The most striking example of the impact of aging on an organ involves the thymus, which begins to involute at puberty. This process continues through adult life until the thymus is replaced with fat by the 6th to 7th decade. The germinal centers are reduced in number and become fibrotic or calcified.

A great deal has been learned in recent years about age-related changes of immune function that occur at the cellular level. A number of these are summarized in Table 14-2. For purposes of discussion, we will consider each of the various cell types involved in the immune response separately, realizing that such a division is somewhat artificial due to the close interactions the cells have with each other.

T Lymphocytes and Cell-Mediated Immunity

Longitudinal studies of healthy adults have shown that total numbers of peripheral blood lymphocytes do not change significantly with advancing age (3). Interestingly, there appears to be a correlation between depressed lymphocyte counts and subsequent mortality (4). Although the physiologic basis for this correlation remains unknown, similar factors may account for the observed association in surgical patients between preoperative lymphopenia and postoperative mortality (5). An age-related

Table 14-1. Functions of immunocompetent cells

T Lymphocytes	B Lymphocytes	Natural killer (NK) cells	Monocytes/macrophages
Cell-mediated immunity Delayed hypersensitivity Helper and suppressor cell activity Soluble mediator production (i.e., IL-2)	Immunoglobulin and specific antibody production	"Immune surveillance" Lysis of neoplastic and viral-infected cells	Antigen recognition and presentation to lymphocytes Phagocytosis of tissue debris and bacteria Participation in ADCC Regulation of lymphocyte activity Soluble mediator production (i.e., IL-1)

Table 14-2. Age-related changes of immune function

1. Decreased numbers and proportion of peripheral blood T cells
2. Decreased T cell proliferative response to mitogenic and antigenic stimulation
3. Decreased T cell proliferative response to irradiated allogeneic lymphocytes
4. Decreased T cell-mediated cytotoxicity
5. Increased numbers of autorosette-forming T cells
6. Decreased in vivo delayed hypersensitivity
7. Decreased T cell production of and response to IL-2
8. Increased responsiveness of suppressor T cells to PGE_2
9. Increased proportion of individuals with B cells not responsive to mitogenic or antigenic stimulation
10. Decreased levels of specific antibody
11. Decreased heterogeneity of the antibody response
12. Decreased antigen-avidity of antibody
13. Increased frequency of monoclonal gammopathy
14. Increased levels of immunoglobulin among the very old
15. Increased prevalence of autoimmune antibodies
16. Increased numbers of peripheral blood NK cells
17. Increased suppression of lymphocytes by macrophages
18. Decreased T cell IL-2 receptor expression
19. Decreased transcription of mRNA for IL-2 and IL-2 receptor

decline is demonstrable for both the absolute number and relative proportion of peripheral blood T lymphocytes (6). The data is less consistent for specific T cell subsets, since numbers of both helper and suppressor cells have been reported to increase, decrease, and remain the same (6–8). Even though the differences in T cell numbers between young and old subjects reach statistical significance, most researchers do not believe they are of sufficient magnitude to account for observed differences in T cell immune function.

Several parameters of in vitro T lymphocyte functional activity can be assayed. Proliferative responses of peripheral T cells from elderly subjects to nonspecific mitogens, including phytohemagglutinin, concanavalin A, and pokeweed lectin, are diminished when compared to young controls (9, 10), as are responses to specific recall antigens, such as streptokinase-streptodornase (SKSD), tetanus toxoid, and purified protein derivative of tuberculin (PPD) (11). An age-related decline of T cell-mediated cytotoxicity has been demonstrated in both xenogenic and allogenic assays using murine and human target cell lines, respectively (12, 13). Although some investigators have reported conflicting data (14), the proliferation of T cells in the presence of irradiated allogenic lymphocytes, known as the one-way mixed lymphocyte reaction, is also diminished in the elderly (9). Yet another in vitro assay involves the response of T cells cocultured with irradiated autologous non-T lymphocytes (the autologous mixed lymphocyte reaction), and has been shown to be enhanced in elderly females, but comparably lower in both young adults and elderly males (15). A subset of T lymphocytes is capable of forming rosettes with autologous erythrocytes, and the proportion of these autorosette-forming cells in the peripheral blood has been shown to increase with age, more so in females than males (16). It is believed that autorosette-forming cells and responder T cells involved in the autologous mixed lymphocyte reaction are either the same or represent two overlapping cell populations.

In vivo correlates of T cell function include cutaneous delayed hypersensitivity responses to skin test antigens, lymphocyte transfer reactions, graft rejection, and graft-versus-host disease. Many authors have reported an increased prevalence of total or relative anergy among aged populations, but the subjects studied have frequently been uncharacterized or affected by illnesses or conditions known to impair the cutaneous immune response. At least 90% of healthy young adults will have one or more positive responses to antigens from *Candida,* mumps, trichophyton, tetanus, or streptokinase-streptodornase (SK SD), but it is unclear whether this degree of reactivity is to be expected in the healthy elderly (17). The lymphocyte transfer reaction occurs following the intracutaneous injection of viable allogenic lymphocytes and may be thought of as an in vivo one-way mixed lymphocyte reaction. Measurable responses to the lymphocyte transfer assay are decreased in older recipients relative to younger controls (18). Age-associated changes in transplantation immunology have been characterized more extensively in animal models than in humans, and as might be expected, very little data is available regarding the truly elderly. It has long been known that aged mice have a prolonged survival of homologous skin grafts (19). Renal allograft survival in humans declines with advancing recipient age, but this probably has as much or more to do with nonimmune factors.

The senescence of T lymphocyte function is thought to arise through several mechanisms, which include factors both intrinsic and extrinsic to the cells. Lymphocyte preparations from elderly humans contain smaller numbers of mitogen or antigen responsive cells when compared to young controls (20, 21). Moreover, there is an impaired capacity of responding cells from old individuals to undergo clonal expansion, demonstrated by the fact that they have fewer subsequent cell divisions and may take longer to do so (22, 23). Studies using mice have shown that there is an age-related decline in the frequency of T cell precursors capable of carrying out various responses to both antigen-specific and nonspecific stimuli

(24). In addition to proliferative responses, both lymphokine production and cytotoxicity were assayed. The actual performance of effector T cells involved in these responses was comparable between young and old mice. Overall, the data suggests that diminished T lymphocyte activity in the elderly occurs because there is an increased proportion of nonresponding cells rather than a uniformly impaired response among all cells.

Various other age-related changes of intrinsic T cell properties have been described, including decreased levels of intracellular enzymatic activity and protein synthesis, increased variability and mutation frequency of DNA content, impaired calcium uptake following mitogenic stimulation, and alterations of cell membrane components. Intensive research efforts have recently been focused on a group of membrane phospholipids, the polyphosphoinositides, and their effects on transmembrane signaling. Recent biochemical studies suggest that an intermediary step between antigen or mitogen binding and cell activation is the hydrolysis of phosphoinositol 4,5-biphosphate to produce 1,2-diacylglycerol and inositol triphosphate (25, 26). These intermediate products respectively activate protein kinase C and mobilize intracellular calcium, which are closely linked with cell membrane interleukin-2 receptor (IL-2R) expression and IL-2 secretion. Both events are essential to lymphocyte proliferation.

Several extrinsic factors can be implicated in the age-related decline of T lymphocyte function. The thymus gland has a critical role, not only because it serves as a site of T lymphocyte maturation but also because it secretes a number of hormones that promote T cell differentiation. It seems logical, then, that thymic involution would somehow contribute to the waning of cell-mediated immunity, and available evidence seems to support this conclusion. Morphologic changes of the aging thymus are correlated with depressed serum levels of thymic factors and appear to precede the onset of demonstrable immunodeficiency (27). It has also been shown in animal models when thymus grafts are transplanted into thymectomized, irradiated, and marrow-reconstituted hosts that the degree of subsequent T cell immunocompetence declines with advancing donor age (28).

Effector T cell function is exquisitely regulated by complex interactions with a variety of other cells, including both lymphocytes and monocytes. It was mentioned earlier that there is no consistent evidence of an age-related change in the relative proportions of T helper and suppressor subsets. On the other hand, qualitative changes in the functions of these subsets, including both decreased helper and increased suppressor activity, have been clearly demonstrated in animal models (29). The situation is less certain for humans, but evidence available thus far suggests similar changes with aging. Immunoregulatory interactions between lymphocytes are thought to be mediated in part by soluble lymphokines. Of these, the most extensively investigated has been interleukin-2 (IL-2; formerly T cell growth factor, TCGF), which is secreted primarily by helper T cells and has been shown to modulate various T cell activities, including antigen-specific proliferative responses, cell-mediated cytotoxicity, and suppressor cell function. Both the production of and response to IL-2 by human lymphocytes have been shown to be depressed among the elderly (30). The diminished response in particular may be related to the fact that activated lymphocytes from older individuals express fewer IL-2 receptors. Recently, cDNA probes to IL-2 and IL-2R have demonstrated that the induction of mRNAs for both genes is decreased in cells from elderly humans (31). Much of the research involving suppressor cell activity in humans has been concerned with the role of prostaglandins. It appears that prostaglandin E_2 (PGE_2) exerts a suppressive effect on immune function and that suppressor cells from the elderly are hyperresponsive to the effects of PGE_2 (32).

B Lymphocytes, Immunoglobulins, and Humoral Immunity

Absolute numbers of B lymphocytes in the peripheral blood do not change significantly with age (33). Peripheral blood counts may not accurately reflect the true number and distribution of B cells within lymphoid tissues, but this issue has not been systematically studied in elderly humans. Aged mice are known to have an increased proportion of immunoglobulin-secreting cells in the spleen, marrow, and lymph nodes but diminished numbers in Peyer's patches (34).

Numerous studies have demonstrated an age-related decline of B cell function. This has been shown to hold true for both nonspecific (polyclonal) and antigen-specific humoral immune responses. Nonspecific activation of B lymphocytes in vitro by pokeweed mitogen has been indirectly measured by a number of assays: enumeration of the numbers of immunoglobulin-secreting cells, [^{3}H]thymidine incorporation, and total immunoglobulin production. Mean levels of all of these indices are diminished with peripheral blood lymphocytes from aged subjects (8, 35, 36). A large proportion of the elderly have nonspecific B cell responses that are comparable to young controls, but there is a substantial increase in the frequency of nonresponders over the age of 55, and it is this subset that skews the mean downward for the entire group (37). It appears, then, that age-associated alterations in B lymphocyte function may not affect the population uniformly.

It is important to note that pokeweed mitogen is able

to activate B lymphocytes only in the presence of T cells and monocytes, and so the aforementioned studies could be interpreted as showing that impaired B cell function is partly or wholly attributable to defective interactions with other types of cells. The degree to which measurable deficiencies of B lymphocyte function are due to intrinsic properties of these cells versus altered T cell regulation is a central question addressed by recent research. In studies using cocultures of T and B cells from both responders and nonresponders to pokeweed mitogen, it has been shown that nonresponder B cells can be "driven" to produce significantly more immunoglobulin in the presence of activated helper T cells from responders (38). On the other hand, the fact that the proliferative response of B lymphocytes from aged donors in coculture with T cells from young responders or in assays using a putative T cell independent polyclonal activator was less than that of cells from young donors, has been purported as evidence of an intrinsic B cell defect (39, 40).

Antigen-specific activation of human B lymphocytes in vitro, which is assayed by enumeration of the numbers of specific antibody-secreting cells, has been shown to diminish with age (35). The deficiency appears to be more marked for primary than for secondary humoral immune responses (41). As with polyclonal activation, the variability of an antigen-specific response is greater among the elderly, with a significant subset of very poor responders. Specific antibodies in a given individual are normally found to be heterogenous in terms of their antigen avidity. Antibody secreted in vitro by B cells from aged mice is less heterogenous than in young mice, due mainly to the loss of the high avidity fraction (42). In short, there are quantitative and qualitative changes in which the B cells make less antibody, and that which is produced is less able to bind antigen.

Humoral immunity can be assayed by measurement of pre- and postimmunization specific antibody titers to known antigens. In fact, vaccination is the most important clinical application of the specific immune response. It is currently recommended by the Centers for Disease Control (CDC) and the American College of Physicians that persons aged 65 or older receive influenza vaccine annually, booster tetanus toxoid every 10 years, and pneumococcal polysaccharide vaccine once. A primary series of tetanus immunizations should be administered to all individuals who have never received one. Along this line, it should be recalled that not until the 1940s were routine immunizations given to infants and children, and therefore many older persons may never have received a primary series of vaccinations. Studies comparing serum antibody responses following influenza vaccination of healthy elderly versus young adults have yielded conflicting data (43, 44). Elderly subjects often have higher preexisting antibody titers that may attenuate their response to influenza vaccine. Specific antibody responses to both tetanus toxoid and certain serotypes of pneumococcus are less vigorous and persist for shorter periods in the elderly than in young adults (45, 46). The depressed anti-tetanus responses can be attributed to both lower numbers of antibody-secreting precursors and impaired helper T cell signals (47). Data about the actual clinical efficacy of vaccination among the elderly is relatively limited. In at least one study, the use of pneumococcal vaccine has not been shown to have an impact on the incidence or mortality rate of pneumococcal pneumonia among institutionalized geriatric patients (48). It may be that those individuals who are most at risk for developing infectious complications from immunosuppression are the least capable of mounting specific responses following vaccination. Another recent study has found that the individuals most likely to develop pneumococcal pneumonitis have been hospitalized for other medical problems in the preceding 5 years (49). This has led to the suggestion that at-risk hospitalized patients should be immunized prior to hospital discharge. Vaccines may be more efficacious in the elderly if they are administered to individuals in their fifties and sixties, when there is little significant impairment of the immune response. Later in life, a reimmunization procedure would then provide a secondary response, which usually is less impaired than a primary response.

Serum levels of total immunoglobulin and of the major immunoglobulin subclasses (IgG, IgA and IgM) do not undergo major changes through the 6th decade, but levels of IgG and IgA are significantly increased in individuals beyond the 7th decade (50). In addition, plasma cell dyscrasias manifested as benign and malignant forms of monoclonal gammopathy are not uncommon by the age of 40 (approximately 0.5% of the population) and increase in prevalence thereafter. The elderly also have a threefold to fivefold increased frequency of serum autoantibodies, particularly rheumatoid factor and antinuclear antibodies (51). There is no definite correlation between the presence of autoantibodies in the elderly and clinically evident autoimmune disease or general health status, nor is there a striking difference between females and males in the prevalence of autoantibodies, as is the case among younger patients. Possible explanations for the increased incidence of autoantibodies with advancing age include a decreased ability to recognize self-antigens as such, the deregulation of corresponding B cell clones, perhaps again because of abnormal interactions with T cells, and alterations of self-antigens by viruses.

Mucosal immunity is thought to be an important first-line defense against pathogens in the respiratory, gastrointestinal, and urogenital tracts, but very limited data is available concerning age-related alterations in this branch of the immune network. This is in part because detailed knowledge about many aspects of the "normal" mucosal immune response is lacking, and so models to study the effects of aging have yet to be developed. Elderly subjects have higher total concentrations of secretory IgA in their saliva than younger controls (52). Concentrations of IgA in nasal washings have been reported to diminish with age, but the patients chosen for study had chronic respiratory disease (53). Virtually nothing is known about S-IgA levels in the intestinal secretions of humans, but there appears to be a slight age-related decline in mice (54). Local antibody responses measured in nasal washings are lower in elderly volunteers than in children following both parenteral and intranasal immunization using inactivated influenza virus vaccine (55). Possible age-related changes in the processing of foreign antigens presented to mucosal surfaces, migration of lymphocytes between secretory sites, and the role of cell-mediated immunity within the mucosal network have yet to be delineated.

Several parameters of immediate hypersensitivity are known to change with age. Serum IgE levels in atopic patients are decreased among older individuals, as are skin test responses and RAST scores to a number of common inhalant antigens (56). Changes in immediate skin test reactivity may be partly due to non-immune factors, such as degranulation kinetics of mast cells from old people. However, there does appear to be an age-related decline in clinically apparent allergic reactions except in those that are secondary to drugs or related to lymphomas.

Natural Killer Cells and Antibody-Dependent Cell-Mediated Cytotoxicity

There is a striking increase in the number of peripheral blood NK cells among healthy elderly subjects (57). It is uncertain whether this change is an expected correlate of normal aging, a homeostatic response to increased demands on host defenses, or a positive selection factor for survival that is apparent only because individuals having a lower number of NK cells tend to die at a younger age.

Although there is agreement that the activity of splenic NK cells declines in aging rats and mice, the data from humans using peripheral blood NK cells is much less consistent (58). The in vitro cytotoxic potential of human NK cells has been reported to increase, decrease, and remain unchanged with advancing age. Differences in the target cells employed for these assays may account for the variation of results. Clearly, further work is needed to clarify the effect of aging on NK cell function.

As mentioned earlier, ADCC reactions are carried out by cells bearing receptors for the Fc portion of immunoglobulin. Surface marker analysis has demonstrated a considerable overlap in the populations of cells that mediate ADCC and NK functions (59). Not surprisingly, age-related changes observed in ADCC activity have tended to parallel the changes reported by the same investigators for NK function and have ranged from increased to decreased levels (58). Researchers who have shown a decline in ADCC among the elderly have correlated it with diminished acid phosphatase activity in peripheral blood lymphocytes from the same subjects, and speculate that this enzyme may be an important mediator of cytolysis, which is impaired with advancing age.

Reticuloendothelial Cells

The RES contains both wandering and fixed cells. The former group includes monocytes and tissue macrophages, whereas the latter is comprised of specialized endothelial and reticular cells sharing one or more accessory functions: phagocytosis, antigen processing and presentation, monokine production, and ADCC reactions. In general, age-related changes are less striking for RES activity than for lymphocytes. The clearance capacity of the human RES for intravenously injected colloid substances declines by about 15% between 30 and 80 years of age, although it is uncertain whether this change is due to decreases in effector cell numbers and/or function, opsonin levels, or blood circulatory capacity (60). In vitro studies of macrophage phagocytic capacity have failed to demonstrate any difference between cells from young and elderly subjects (61).

The evidence has been variable regarding age-related changes of the role of macrophages in the immune response. On the one hand, macrophages from aging mice retain full capacity for both antigen processing and participation in lymphocyte mitogenic activation (62, 63). On the other hand, the production of and response to certain monokines appears to be altered during senescence. Interleukin-1 (IL-1) functions primarily by potentiating the activation of helper T cells, whereas PGE_2 stimulates suppressor cells. Macrophages from old mice synthesize less IL-1 but more PGE_2 than cells from younger controls (64, 65). In addition, as mentioned earlier, suppressor cells from elderly humans are hyper-responsive to PGE_2. It appears, then, that macrophages from old donors have enhanced suppressor effects on the immune response. Interestingly, in vitro monocyte-induced suppression of antibody responses by peripheral blood lymphocytes from elderly subjects can be abolished with the addition of non-steroidal anti-inflammatory drugs, presumably by blocking PGE_2 synthesis (32).

Clinical Implications of Immunosenescence

Two types of disease that are common among the elderly and thought to be related to immunologic decline are infection and malignancy. Infectious illnesses have a strikingly increased incidence and related mortality among geriatric populations (66). Frequent sites of infection include the respiratory and urinary tracts, soft tissues, and the abdominal cavity. Endocarditis is more common in the elderly, as is bacteremia from unidentified sources. The range of pathogens varies somewhat from that seen in younger patients, particularly due to the increased rate of gram-negative bacterial colonization and sepsis among the aged. Infections with *Mycobacterium tuberculosis* and herpes zoster are most commonly encountered in the elderly. Although tetanus is a completely preventable disease and cases are rare, it has become a geriatric illness, with a mortality rate approaching 80% among the elderly.

The management of infectious diseases in older patients is further complicated by the fact that the clinical presentation is frequently less clear than in younger people. Symptoms and signs that are commonly sought for purposes of diagnosis, such as fever, chills, urinary irritation, productive cough, etc., are often unimpressive or not present at all among the elderly. Subtle changes of mentation, function, or metabolic status are at times the only indication of underlying sepsis. Prudent management of geriatric patients requires a high index of suspicion for infection and the empiric early use of broad-spectrum antibiotics in those cases where sepsis is considered.

The increasing incidence of malignancy with advancing age may be related in part to a decline of "tumor surveillance" by immune and nonimmune mechanisms. Senescent animals have been shown to have a diminished in vivo cytotoxic response to transplanted neoplastic cells (19), but evidence of similar changes in humans is obviously circumstantial. As mentioned earlier, peripheral blood NK cells increase in number with age and appear to have functional abilities similar to those of young persons. Thus, the relationship of NK cells to neoplastic processes within the host remains uncertain.

Conclusion

Diverse changes of immune activity occur with aging, and are apparent at the organ, cellular, and subcellular levels. A few important generalizations may be made. First, age-related alterations are better documented and more profound for immunocompetent lymphocytes than for nonspecific accessory cells. Second, changes in T cell activity may be more important than, and largely responsible for, changes in B cell activity. Third, alterations in lymphocyte activity are more qualitative (i.e., involving cell function) than quantitative (i.e., involving cell numbers or immunoglobulin levels). It is hoped that by advancing our understanding of the relationship between immune deficiency and medical illness, as well as of potential methods for correcting these deficiencies, the care of our growing elderly population will continue to improve.

References

1. Walford, RL. 1969. *The Immunologic Theory of Aging*. Copenhagen: Munksgaard.
2. Adler, WH, Jones, KH, and Nariuchi, H. 1977. Aging and immune function. In *Recent Advances in Clinical Immunology,* vol 1, Ed., RA Thompson. Edinburgh: Churchill Livingstone.
3. Sparrow, D, Silbert, JE, and Rowe, JW. 1980. The influence of age on peripheral lymphocyte count in men: A cross-sectional and longitudinal study. *J Gerontol* 35:163–166.
4. Bender, BS, et al. 1986. Absolute peripheral blood lymphocyte count and subsequent mortality of elderly men: The Baltimore longitudinal study of aging. *J Am Geriatr Soc* 34:649–654.
5. Grossbard, LJ, et al. 1984. Lymphocytopenia in the surgical intensive care unit patient. *Am Surgeon* 50:209–212.
6. Nagel, JE, et al. 1983. Monoclonal antibody analysis of T-lymphocyte subsets in young and aged adults. *Immunol Comm* 12:223–237.
7. Moody, CE, et al. 1981. Lymphocyte transformation induced by autologous cells. XI. The effect of age on the autologous mixed lymphocyte reaction. *Immunology* 44: 431–438.
8. Mascart-Lemone, F, et al. 1982. Characterization of immunoregulatory T lymphocytes during aging by monoclonal antibodies. *Clin Exp Immunol* 48:148–154.
9. Weksler, ME, and Hutteroth, TH. 1974. Impaired lymphocyte function in aged humans. *J Clin Invest* 53:99–104.
10. Birnbaum, G, and Swick, L. 1981. Human suppressor lymphocytes. II. Changes in concanavalin A inducible suppressor cells with age. *J Gerontol* 36:410–415.
11. Sohnle, PG, et al. 1980. Failure of lymphokine-producing lymphocytes from aged humans to undergo activation by recall antigens. *J Immunol* 124:2169–2174.
12. Becker, MJ, et al. 1979. Cell-mediated cytotoxicity in humans: Age-related decline as measured by a xenogeneic assay. *Clin Immunol Immunopathol* 14:204–210.
13. Kishimoto, S, et al. 1978. Age-related changes in the subsets and functions of human T lymphocytes. *J Immunol* 121:1773–1780.
14. Charpentier, B, et al. 1981. Immunological studies in human aging. I. In vitro functions of T cells and polymorphs. *J Clin Lab Immunol* 5:87–93.
15. Fournier, C, and Charreire, J. 1981. Autologous mixed lymphocyte reaction in man. I. Relationship with age and sex. *Cell Immunol* 60:212–219.

16. Fournier, C, and Charreire, J. 1977. Increase in autologous erythrocyte binding by T cells with aging in man. *Clin Exp Immunol* 29:468–473.
17. Goodwin, JS, Searles, RP, and Tung, KS. 1982. Immunological responses of healthy elderly population. *Clin Exp Immunol* 48:403–410.
18. Andersen, E. 1972. The influence of age on transplantation immunity. Reactivity to normal lymphocyte transfer at different ages. *Scand J Haematol* 9:621–624.
19. Teller, MN, et al. 1954. Aging and cancerigenesis. I. Immunity to tumor and skin grafts. *J Natl Cancer Inst* 33:649–656.
20. Inkeles, B, et al. 1977. Immunological studies of aging. III. Cytokinetic basis for the impaired response of lymphocytes from aged humans to plant lectins. *J Exp Med* 145: 1176–1187.
21. Sohnle, PG, Collins-Lech, C, and Huhta, K. 1982. Age-related effects on the number of human lymphocytes in culture initially responding to an antigenic stimulus. *Clin Exp Immunol* 47:138–146.
22. Hefton, JM, et al. 1980. Immunologic studies of aging. V. Impaired proliferation of PHA responsive human lymphocytes in culture. *J Immunol* 125:1007–1010.
23. Tice, RR, et al. 1979. Cytokinetic analysis of the impaired proliferative response of peripheral lymphocytes from aged humans to phytohemagglutinin. *J Exp Med* 149: 1029–1041.
24. Miller, RA. 1984. Age-associated decline in precursor frequency for different T cell-mediated reactions, with preservation of helper or cytotoxic effect per precursor cell. *J Immunol* 132:63–68.
25. Isakov, N, Scholz, W, and Altman, A. 1986. Signal transduction and intracellular events in T-lymphocyte activation. *Immunol Today* 7:271–277.
26. Dröge, W. 1986. Protein kinase C in T-cell regulation. *Immunol Today* 7:340–343.
27. Bach, JF, et al. 1975. Isolation, biochemical characteristics, and biological activity of a circulating thymic hormone in the mouse and in the human. *Ann NY Acad Sci* 248:186–210.
28. Hirokawa, K, and Makinodan, T. 1975. Thymic involution: Effect on T cell differentiation. *J Immunol* 114:1659–1664.
29. Liu, JJ, Segre, M, and Segre, D. 1982. Changes in suppressor, helper, and B cell functions in aging mice. *Cell Immunol* 66:372–382.
30. Gillis, S, et al. 1981. Immunological studies of aging. Decreased production of and response to T cell growth factor by lymphocytes from aged humans. *J Clin Invest* 67:937–942.
31. Nagel, JE, et al. 1988. Decreased proliferation, interleukin 2 synthesis and interleukin 2 receptor expression are accompanied by decreased mRNA expression in phytohemagglutinin-stimulated cells from elderly donors. *J Clin Invest* 81:1096-1102.
32. Delfraissy, JF, et al. 1982. Abolished in vitro antibody response in elderly: Exclusive involvement of prostaglandin-induced T suppressor cells. *Clin Immunol Immunopathol* 24:377–385.
33. Jamil, NA, and Millard, RE. 1981. Studies of T, B, and 'null' blood lymphocytes in normal persons of different age groups. *Gerontology* 27:79–84.
34. Benner, R, et al. 1981. Frequencies of background immunoglobulin-secreting cells in mice as a function of organ, age, and immune status. *Immunobiology* 158:225–238.
35. Pahwa, SG, Pahwa, RN, and Good, RA. 1981. Decreased in vitro humoral immune responses in aged humans. *J Clin Invest* 67:1094–1102.
36. Ceuppens, JL, and Goodwin, JS. 1982. Regulation of immunoglobulin production in pokeweed mitogen stimulated cultures of lymphocytes from young and old adults. *J Immunol* 128:2429–2434.
37. Nagel, JE, Chrest, FJ, and Adler, WH. 1981. Human B cell function in normal individuals of various ages. I. In vitro enumeration of pokeweed-induced peripheral blood lymphocyte immunoglobulin-synthesizing cells and the comparison of the results with numbers of peripheral B and T cells, mitogen responses, and levels of serum immunoglobulins. *Clin Exp Immunol* 44:646–654.
38. Chrest, FJ, et al. 1983. Human B cell function in responder and non-responder individuals. II. The role of T helper cells in promoting the PMW-induced B cell production of immunoprotein. *Clin Exp Immunol* 53:465–472.
39. Antel, JP, et al. 1983. Mechanisms responsible for reduced in vitro immunoglobulin secretion in aged humans. *Mech Ageing Dev* 23:11–19.
40. Wrabetz, LG, et al. 1982. Age-related changes in in vitro immunoglobulin secretion: Comparison of responses to T-dependent and T-independent polyclonal activators. *Cell Immunol* 74:398–403.
41. Makinodan, T and Peterson, WJ. 1962. Relative antibody-forming capacity of spleen cells as a function of age. *Proc Natl Acad Sci USA* 48:234–238.
42. Goidl, EA, Innes, JB, and Weksler, ME. 1976. Immunological studies of aging. II. Loss of IgG and high avidity plaque-forming cells and increased suppressor cell activity in aging mice. *J Exp Med* 144:1037–1048.
43. Feery, BJ, et al. 1979. Antibody responses to influenza vaccines containing A/USSR/90/77. *Aust J Exp Biol Med Sci* 57:335–344.
44. Ershler, WB, Moore, AL, and Solinski, MA. 1985. Specific antibody synthesis *in vitro*. III. Correlation of *in vivo* and *in vitro* antibody response to influenza immunization in young and old subjects. *J Clin Lab Immunol* 16:63–67.
45. Kishimoto, S, et al. 1980. Age-related decline in the in vitro and in vivo syntheses of antitetanus toxoid antibody in humans. *J Immunol* 125:2347–2352.
46. Landesman, SH, and Schiffman, G. 1981. Assessment of the antibody response to pneumococcal vaccine in high-risk populations. *Rev Infect Dis* 3 Suppl: S184–S196.
47. Kishimoto, S, et al. 1982. Age-related decrease in frequencies of B-cell precursors and specific helper T cells involved in the IgG anti-tetanus toxoid antibody production in humans. *Clin Immunol Immunopathol* 25:1–10.
48. Bentley, DW, et al. 1981. Pneumococcal vaccine in the institutionalized elderly: design of a nonrandomized trial and preliminary results. *Rev Infect Dis* 3 Suppl: S71–S81.
49. Fedson, DS, and Baldwin, JA. 1982. Previous hospital care as a risk factor for pneumonia. Implications for immunization with pneumococcal vaccine. *JAMA* 248:1989–1995.
50. Proust, JJ, et al. 1989. Developmental biology, senescence, and natural immunity. In *Natural Immunity*, Ed., D Nelson. Marnickville, NSW, Australia: Harcourt Brace Jovanovich.
51. Hallgren, HM, et al. 1973. Lymphocyte phytohemag-

glutinin responsiveness, immunoglobulins, and auto-antibodies in aging humans. *J Immunol* 111:1101–1107.

52. Finkelstein, MS, Tanner, M, and Freedman, ML. 1984. Salivary and serum IgA levels in a geriatric outpatient population. *J Clin Immunol* 4:85–91.
53. Alfrod, R. 1986. Effects of chronic bronchopulmonary disease and aging on human nasal secretion IgA concentrations. *J Immunol* 101:984–988.
54. Kawanishi, H, and Kiely, J. 1985. Effect of aging on murine gut-associated lymphoid tissue. *Gastroenterology* 88:1440.
55. Fulk, RV, et al. 1970. Antibody responses in serum and nasal secretions according to age of recipient and method of administration of A2/Hong Kong/68 inactivated influenza virus vaccine. *J Immunol* 104:8–13.
56. Stoy, PJ, et al. 1981. Aging and serum immunoglobulin E levels, immediate skin tests, and RAST. *J Allergy Clin Immunol* 68:421–426.
57. Ligthart, GJ, et al. 1986. The expanded null set compartment in aging: Increase in the number of natural killer cells and changes in T-cell and NK-cell subsets in human blood. *Immunology* 59:353–357.
58. Bender, BS. 1987. Natural killer cells in senescence: Analysis of phenotypes and function. In *Review of Biological Research in Aging,* Ed., M Rothstein, vol 4. New York: Alan R. Liss.
59. Wahlin, B, and Perlmann, P. 1983. Characterization of human K cells by surface antigens and morphology at the single cell level. *J Immunol* 131:2340–2347.
60. Brouwer, A, and Knook, DL. 1983. The reticuloendothelial system and aging: A review. *Mech Ageing Dev* 21:205–228.
61. Gardner, ID, Lim, ST, and Lawton, JW. 1981. Monocyte function in ageing humans. *Mech Ageing Dev* 16:233–238.
62. Heidrick, ML, and Makinodan, T. 1973. Presence of impairment of humoral immunity in nonadherent spleen cells of old mice. *J Immunol* 111:1502–1506.
63. Callard, RE. 1978. Immune function in aged mice. III. Role of macrophages and effect of 2-mercaptoethanol in the response of spleen cells from old mice to phytohemagglutinin, lipopolysaccharide and allogeneic cells. *Eur J Immunol* 8:697–705.
64. Bruley-Rosset, M, and Vergnon, I. 1984. Interleukin-1 synthesis and activity in aged mice. *Mech Ageing Dev* 24:247–264.
65. Rosenstein, MM, and Strausser, HR. 1980. Macrophage induced T cell mitogen suppression with age. *J Reticuloendothel Soc* 27:159–166.
66. Berk, SL, and Smith, JK. 1983. Infectious diseases in the elderly. *Med Clin North Am* 67:273–293.

15

Infectious Disease in the Elderly

Gary Victor and Marsha Fretwell

Infection is both a common indication for surgery and an occasional associated outcome of surgery. In both cases, the ability to mount an effective immunologic response to an infection and the ability to heal wounds are critical in achieving the optimal outcome for any given surgical procedure.

This chapter first discusses the central role of adequate nutrition in immune function and wound healing and the associated disease factors that predispose older surgical patients to infection. Common presentations are then described as well as the appropriate management of those infections that frequently present as indications for surgery or become unwanted consequences of surgery.

Nutrition

Recently, there has been increased interest in the interaction of nutritional intake with the processes of aging in various organ systems (1–3). Many factors, both physical and psychologic, influence the nutritional status of the elderly surgical population. Physical factors include diminished taste and smell, poor dentition, and difficulty feeding or swallowing. Psychologic factors include social isolation, bereavement, and depression. The single most common cause of weight loss in the elderly is decreased oral intake of food (4). Underlying diseases and their required medications can also account for impaired utilization of food. Such diseases include achlorhydria, diabetic gastroparesis, chronic pulmonary disease, and pancreatic insufficiency.

The effects of malnutrition are complex because they include both a delay in effective healing of surgical wounds and alterations in specific host defense mechanisms such as (*a*) an associated decrease and function of circulating T lymphocytes; (*b*) normal or increased number of circulatory B lymphocytes, which are characterized by depressed primary antibody responses; (*c*) impaired intracellular killing of organisms by neutrophils; and (*d*) a decrease in both classic and alternate complement pathway components (5). Thus the risk of a wound infection or other nosocomial infection is increased. Obtaining an albumin level prior to surgery and using various forms of supplemental nutrition prophylactically will maximize nutritional status in the elderly surgical patient, thereby avoiding these complications of surgical and medical therapy.

Alterations in Host Defense Mechanisms

Nonspecific Defense Factors

Dermal, respiratory, gastrointestinal, and urinary epithelium are important first-line defenses against infectious agents and are all subject to age-related changes. In the skin, there is thinning of the epidermis, slowing of cell replacement in the stratum corneum, decreased output of exocrine and apocrine glands and diminished blood flow, all of which may contribute to an increased incidence of skin and soft-tissue infections as well as an additional delay in wound healing (6–9).

In the lung, a reduction in the overall tone of airways results from a loss of elastic tissue surrounding the alveoli, an increase in the chest diameter, and a weakening of the respiratory muscles. These factors lead to an increased tendency toward atelectasis of the lower airways, impairment of the ability to mobilize secretions, and a greater incidence of microbial colonization of the tracheobronchial system (10). Thus, older individuals have an increased risk of respiratory tract infection.

Similar changes occur in the gastrointestinal tract (11). There is decreased production of saliva and a consequent reduction in its antibacterial components. Alterations in esophageal and gastric motility and achlorhydria increase with age (12), leading to an increased risk of aspiration and the probability of becoming infected with certain enteric gram negative bacilli (13).

In females, there is a decline in the efficiency of bladder function, possibly as a result of loss of elastic properties of the tissues. Consequently, residual urines of greater than 100 cc are common and may predispose to bacteriuria. In males, prostatic hypertrophy can lead to outflow obstruction and hence a similar reduction in the efficiency of bladder emptying.

Other predisposing factors for the development of urinary tract infections have been reviewed (14, 15) and include the following:

1. Urinary obstruction, stasis, reflux
2. Age
3. B or AB blood type
4. Hyperosmolality of the renal medulla, which inhibits mobilization of granulocytes into the injured medulla and decreases their ability to phagocytose bacteria
5. Differences in bladder and kidney host cell receptor sites for uropathic bacteria
6. Possible increased receptivity of uroepithelial, periurethral, and vaginal cells for uropathic coliforms in some patients with recurrent urinary tract infections
7. Immunologic mechanisms related to persistence of bacterial antigen and to cross-reactivity between Tamm-Horsfall protein and gram-negative bacteria. Other factors that have been implicated include bladder wall ischemia caused by distension, fecal incontinence, urinary tract abnormalities, and instrumentation of the urinary tract.

Fever in Older Surgical Patients

The substance found to cause fever was initially described in 1948 by Beeson (16) and subsequently named endogenous pyrogen (17). It is a product of bacterial cells, principally mononuclear phagocytes. The mechanism of fever is complex and is the result of the following sequence of events (18): (*a*) macrophage or monocyte recognition of a neoantigen and phagocytosis; (*b*) release of interleukin I; (*c*) circulation of interleukin I to the interior hypothalamus; (*d*) abrupt increase in the synthesis of the cyclic endoperoxides, including prostaglandin E as stimulated by the presence of interleukin I in the hypothalamus; (*e*) elevation of prostaglandin E2 levels, which raise the hypothalamic thermostat, initiating mechanisms of heat conservation to re-establish homeostasis; and (*f*) heat conservation mechanisms, vasoconstriction, and muscle shivering, which increase core temperature until the hypothalamic set point is reached.

Fever has both theoretic and practical implications when considering infections in older patients. Theoretically, certain animals including reptiles, amphibians, and fish do benefit from elevated body temperatures, and *Neisseria gonorrhea* and *Treponema pallidum* are quite sensitive to heat and can be killed by inducing fever in experimental animals (19). Unfortunately, natural infection does not result in body temperatures high enough to kill these organisms.

Practically speaking, a fever is an early indication of the presence of an infection. Failure to mount a fever might conceivably lead to a delay in diagnosis of the infection and the need for surgical intervention. Controversy exists as to the ability of elderly patients to mount a febrile response (20, 21). Recently, it has been observed that most older patients do exhibit some type of febrile response (22). A diminished febrile response may not necessarily be related to old age but may be due to malnutrition and decreased leukocyte production rather than to chronological age (3). Other possibilities include a latency between the introduction of the stimulus and production of interleukin I, a defect in the hypothalamus which impairs its ability to respond to interleukin I, or an alteration in other mechanisms of thermoregulation.

Management of the febrile patient includes treatment of the underlying disorder (which should include antibiotic therapy if infection is suspected) as well as other conservative measures, including hydration, nutrition, and oxygenation. Only if cardiac, respiratory, or neurologic deterioration ensues, are antipyretics indicated. Theoretically, any defect leading to a diminished febrile response may lead to increased susceptibility to infection and hence to increased morbidity and mortality.

Specific Immune Responses

B Cell Function

There is no doubt that aging alone does have an effect on the immune response. Whether this single effect translates into meaningful reduction in overall host defense is less clear. The first alteration noted in humans was a distinct age-related reduction in serum isoagglutinins in normal individuals (23, 24).

Significantly lower concentrations of IgM have also been found in older individuals when compared with younger control groups, although the concentrations could be considered within normal limits (25).

Significantly decreased levels of IgG were found in a group of very old individuals, and these did appear to correlate with an increased mortality (26). In these individuals, the initial levels of the IgG determined approximately 8 years prior to death were normal. Humoral immune response or antibody production can also be detected by response to vaccines and, although the elderly are capable of humoral responses, they may not be able to mount a response comparable to that of younger individuals (27, 28).

Low IgM and IgA levels in *some* older people have been associated with decreased responses to pneumococcal capsular polysaccharide vaccine (29).

Cell-Mediated Immunity

T cell numbers. The most striking immune system abnormalities are in the T cell population. Although normal aging appears to be associated with qualitative changes in the T lymphocytes circulating in the peripheral blood, again, it is unclear if this contributes to an increased mortality rate (30, 31). Age-related reductions in T cell helper activity, increases in T cell suppressor activity, and the reduced ability of B cells to produce normal heterogeneous high affinity antibodies in response to an antigen all appear to have their origins in the involution of the thymus gland (24).

Recent evidence has shown that lymphopenia induced by acute bacterial infections in the elderly population may well be a sign of prognostic significance (32). Additionally, a second group of investigators has noted a correlation between the absolute peripheral blood lymphocyte count and mortality in elderly men in the three years before their death (33). These associations were not considered causal, suggesting that other factors may also cause this diminution in the lymphocyte count.

T cell function. Another manifestation of a reduction in T cell activity is found in the decreasing number of positive skin tests in those over 60 years of age. In one study, this hyporesponsiveness to tests for delayed hypersensitivity could be correlated with increased mortality over a two-year period (34). The elderly also show a decreased ability to be sensitized to dinitrochlorobenzene (35).

Mitogen testing has revealed decreased responses in both aged animals and humans (36, 37). However, other studies have demonstrated no significant differences (38). Despite all evidence to date, no consistent defect in the immunologic system has been found that can explain why the elderly appear to be at an increased risk for infection (37).

Wound Healing

Wound healing involves a complex interaction of inflammatory cells, including lymphocytes, macrophages, granulocytes, tissue complement, and other proteins (39). If nutrition is impaired, various aspects of wound healing are affected. The early effects of malnutrition alter this inflammatory and immune response. Later effects include disorders of fibroblast function, collagen synthesis, and neovascularization. The role of vitamins A and C has been well documented. Trace elements, in particular zinc, have been shown to be of significance in wound healing (40).

As previously noted, the effects of aging on the skin include epidermal thinning, loss of connective tissue, and diminished blood flow, all of which increase the risk for injury, breakdown, and subsequent infection of thin lax skin. The overall result of any impairment in the process of wound healing is an increased risk of infection to the wound, surrounding skin, and contiguous structures.

It is not difficult to understand why wounds in the elderly not only heal slowly but are at increased risk for infection.

Predisposing Factors in the Aged

Chronic Disease Associated with Aging

Hyperglycemia or diabetes mellitus has been shown to be associated with defects in polymorphonuclear leukocyte chemotaxis as well as phagocytosis (41). The accompanying microvascular changes enhance the risk of skin and soft-tissue infection. Advancing renal insufficiency can also reduce immune competency. The incidence of bacteriuria in women with diabetes is twice as high as that in other women, but this may be due in part to the frequency of catheterization (42, 43). Diabetic patients have been reported to have increased susceptibility not only to urinary tract infections but to septic arthritis as well (24). Because of the incidence of hyperosmolar coma and its attendant decrease in level of consciousness, it is not unexpected that aspiration pneumonia and skin trauma occur with increased frequency in this group of patients.

Arteriosclerosis is the most common of the degenerative diseases in developed countries. As a result of reduction in blood flow, organs are subjected to diminished blood supply and the risk of ischemic damage and necrosis.

When this occurs in limbs, in particular lower extremities, soft-tissue infection ensues quickly. As a result of diminished blood flow, healing is delayed and underlying structures including bone are at increased risk as well.

Arteriosclerotic changes occur in all blood vessels, including the cerebral vessels and major arteries. Cerebral vascular accidents with their attendant sequelae increase the risk of infection in the elderly population. Similarly, arteriosclerotic plaques can lead to foci of endovascular infection in this population as well.

Hematologic disorders predispose patients to infection in several ways, including intrinsic host immune deficits secondary to these diseases, neoplastic disruption of normal tissue barriers, and exogenous immunosuppressive therapy (44).

Chronic pulmonary disease in the elderly compromises an already altered respiratory tract and the host defense mechanisms as described earlier. With repeated episodes of exacerbated bronchitis, more damage occurs to a compromised airway, and the patient is also subjected to increasingly serious infections.

Prostatic disease in the form of benign prostatic hypertrophy, prostatitis, carcinoma, or calculi can lead to prostate enlargement and subsequent prostatic obstruction. This can lead to bacteriuria in men, particularly those over 50. Acute bacterial prostatitis is not usually a problem in older men. On the other hand, chronic prostatitis is a more difficult problem to manage because of the difficulty in ascertaining a microbiologic diagnosis and also poor penetration of the prostate with antibiotics. However, the new quinoline antibiotics have better penetration into the prostate and may offer a therapeutic modality for this problem (45).

Culture Methodology

Proper specimen collection is of utmost importance in allowing the microbiology laboratory to isolate and identify microorganisms and determine their susceptibility to antimicrobial agents. The guidelines for microbiologic specimen collection and transport have been documented elsewhere (46, 47).

Pleural fluid should be sent not only for gram stain and culture and sensitivity, but the syringe should be capped and transported to the lab to try to isolate anaerobic organisms as well. An acid-fast bacilli (AFB) smear and culture should be obtained. If *Legionella* is suspected, then both culture and direct fluorescent staining can be ordered.

In intra-abdominal infections, anaerobic organisms often play a significant role. Measures should be taken to ensure isolation of these organisms as well as routine aerobic organisms. If granulomatous lesions are found, the material should be cultured for mycobacteria, fungi, and *Brucella* as well.

Soft-tissue infections are usually caused by bacteria, but some are also due to fungi, and care must be taken to obtain specimens in a proper fashion. The most useful method is with a sterile syringe and needle as opposed to a swab. Irrigation of the lesion with bacteriostatic saline is sometimes necessary (46). Soft-tissue lesions are often indicators of deep-seated infections (i.e., bone), and it is sometimes important to obtain a specimen of bone to better guide the antimicrobial therapy. Bone biopsy once obtained should be collected and sent to the laboratory for aerobic and anaerobic cultures as well as other special cultures if indicated, including fungi and mycobacteria.

Infections as an Indicator for Surgery

Cholecystitis

The incidence of cholelithiasis increases with age, occurring in 10% of women and 20% of men aged 55 to 64 years and 30% of all those over 80 years (48). Obstruction of the cystic duct results in cholecystitis. Approximately 3% to 5% of cases of acute cholecystitis occur in the absence of gallstones, usually in critically ill patients.

Symptoms of biliary tract infection include right upper quadrant pain, usually colicky, associated with nausea, vomiting, chills, and fever. Laboratory data usually reveal leukocytosis, hyperbilirubinemia, and elevated transaminases and alkaline phosphatase. Radiologic tests to assist in diagnosis include ultrasound and HIDA scan. Microbiological flora causing infections include *Escherichia coli*, *Klebsiella*, and Group D *Streptococcus* (49–51). Because anaerobic organisms have been found to be an important pathogen in biliary disease (52), therapy is directed toward these organisms. Antimicrobial therapy consists of an extended spectrum penicillin and aminoglycosides as well as an anti-anaerobic drug.

Diverticulitis

Diverticular formation in the colon relates to two factors: increased intraluminal pressure and weakness in the intestinal wall (53). Diverticulitis develops in approximately 15% to 25% of individuals over 70 years. The mortality rate for diverticulitis may be as high as 12% (54).

The clinical manifestations include abdominal pain (usually left lower quadrant), alteration in bowel habits, fever, and leukocytosis. This should be differentiated from ischemic colitis and inflammatory bowel disease. Diagnosis is usually confirmed by radiologic investigation with water-soluble media (55).

Sigmoidoscopy is of limited value because of the angulation and fixation of the bowel, which does not permit adequate visualization of the affected segments. Endoscopy is performed principally to rule out other disease conditions (i.e., carcinoma, inflammatory bowel disease). Once the diagnosis has been made, treatment depends on the severity of the illness. Treatment for mild symptoms includes making the patient NPO and, once symptoms improve, a high fiber diet. Patients with abdominal tenderness, fever, and leukocytosis are hospitalized and treated with intravenous fluids for rehydration, nasogastric suctioning, and antibiotic therapy. Antibiotic therapy is empiric, and a regimen to cover bowel flora (i.e., gram-negative aerobic bacilli and anaerobic organisms) should be chosen (56). A broad-spectrum penicillin in combination with an aminoglycoside as well as clindamycin or metronidazole should be used. Complications that can arise from an episode of diverticulitis and warrant surgical intervention include fistula formation, bowel obstruction, peritonitis, and macroperforation with pericolic abscess.

Appendicitis

Although this disease is associated with a younger age group, the mortality rate from appendicitis varies from 2% to 14% (57–60). The classic presentation of acute appendicitis is periumbilical pain that subsequently localizes to the right lower quadrant with associated peritoneal signs. This pattern does not occur as frequently in the older patient. However, most patients will complain of abdominal pain of some type during the course of appendicitis (57–60). As with other illnesses in this population, nonspecific symptoms including confusion, anorexia, and incontinence may be presenting features of acute appendicitis. Because of the atypical presentation in the elderly, delays in diagnosis occur. Norman and Yoshikawa (61) have proposed other factors contributing to the delay in diagnosis which include:

1. Failure of patients to seek medical attention
2. Failure of physicians to consider the diagnosis for elderly patients
3. Atypical clinical presentation or findings
4. Excessive laboratory and radiographic studies
5. Reluctance to operate on elderly patients

The rate of perforation is significantly higher in the elderly population (62), and the reason for this is unclear although anatomic changes that occur with aging, including thinning of the mucosa and loss of lymphoid tissue, may potentially contribute to the risk of perforation. As suggested by Norman and Yoshikawa (61), the diagnosis of acute appendicitis should be considered in the differential diagnosis of the elderly patient in whom prior appendectomy has not been performed, who has unexplained abdominal pain of recent onset, or who manifests evidence of an acute confusional state or signs of infection.

Once the diagnosis is considered, empiric antibiotic therapy should be instituted after blood cultures have been obtained. An antimicrobial regimen should be chosen to include coverage for both aerobic and anaerobic bacteria (63). A beta-lactam antibiotic alone or in combination with an anti-anaerobic drug and an aminoglycoside may well be warranted depending on the clinical status of the patient.

Pyogenic Liver Abscess

This infection occurs most often now as a disease of the elderly with biliary sepsis, diverticulitis, or bowel carcinoma with perforation. Some authors have shown that 33% to 56% of patients with pyogenic liver abscess are over 60 years of age (64, 65). Unfortunately, there is a significant mortality rate in this age group, especially in those with multiple abscesses, underlying malignancy, and delay in diagnosis.

The bacteriology of this disease principally involves enteric bacteria. A significant proportion of the abscesses are polymicrobial, with anaerobes playing an important role (64, 65). Clinical features include fever, chills, and nonspecific gastrointestinal symptoms. Computed tomographic (CT) scan appears to be the most accurate diagnostic technique (66).

Percutaneous drainage should be the initial drainage procedure in most patients, in combination with antibiotic therapy (67, 68). The choice of antibiotic therapy should be similar to that of diverticulitis, and alterations should be made based on microbial studies. The duration of antimicrobial therapy is usually prolonged (5).

Fasciitis

Inflammation of the fascial planes may present an area of localized pain with minimal swelling and usually no obvious break in the skin surface (69). Over time, the involved skin becomes indurated, with erythema, blisters, and bullae (70). The patient is usually systemically ill with fever and altered mental status, but with the geriatric population, some of these manifestations may be blunted. Individuals with diabetes mellitus and peripheral vascular disease seem to be at increased risk for this disease (56). β-Hemolytic *streptococci* and *Staphylococcus aureus* account for a majority of cases, however gram-negative bacteria have been associated with this entity as well.

Once the diagnosis is confirmed (70), most authorities agree that an aggressive approach (71, 72) is warranted to treat this potentially life-threatening emergency. Antibiotic therapy is initiated with an antistaphylococcal penicillin, broad-spectrum penicillin, aminoglycoside, and an anti-anaerobic agent. Therapy is modified as culture results are obtained.

Empyema

Empyema exists when there is accumulation of purulent material in the pleural space resulting from direct spread of a pulmonary infection such as pneumonia or a lung abscess. Transdiaphragmatic spread from a subdiaphragmatic focus has also been implicated in the pathogenesis of this infection (73).

The bacteriology of this infection has changed over time (74, 75). *Staphylococcus aureus* is the most common cause of empyema, followed in frequency by various gram-negative bacilli. Anaerobic organisms may also be significant pathogens in this disease.

The patient may present with fever, dyspnea, chest pain, and cough. These symptoms, however, may well be lacking in the geriatric patient. Physical findings are consistent with those of pleural effusion (i.e., dullness to percussion with decrease in available breath sounds). Radiologically, there will be evidence of pleural effusion; if it does not change location with a change in posture of the patient, it may be loculated. This can be confirmed with ultrasound or CT scan. Once the presence of fluid has been confirmed by these ancillary methods, sampling of the pleural space is imperative. Thoracentesis usually reveals an exudate with its characteristic findings: protein levels > 3.0 g/100 ml and LDH > 550 units (76). Gram stain of the pleural fluid will often be positive and indicative of the underlying organism. Appropriate cultures, both aerobic and anaerobic, are indicated.

Therapy for empyema involves both antibiotic therapy and adequate drainage of the effusion. Antibiotic therapy is based upon the causative organism and is usually prolonged (3 weeks or longer). Drainage of the pleural space is achieved via a thoracostomy tube or repetitive thoracentesis. If the fluid becomes loculated, then surgical drainage is usually required.

Infections as Unwanted Consequences of Surgery

Nosocomial Pneumonia

Pneumonias acquired by patients while in the hospital result from a complex mixture of factors. Colonization of the pharynx by gram-negative bacteria is thought to be a prerequisite for such infections (77). The leading hypothesis for these pneumonias suggests that patients aspirate these potential gram-negative pathogens, which have colonized in the oropharynx. Factors predisposing to aspiration include constipation or impaction, seizure disorder, stroke, muscle weakness, impaired cognition, lack of coordination, and medications (78). Intubation of the respiratory tract not only allows a breach of the natural host defenses, but also promotes retrograde pharyngeal colonization by organisms in the stomach (79), thus increasing the possibility of nosocomial pneumonia. Driks et al. (80) have shown that intubated patients have less morbidity and mortality from nosocomial pneumonia if they are not treated with histamine type 2 (H-2) antagonists drugs, which diminish the natural gastric acid barrier.

The clinical presentation in this age group is often misleading and may be subtle. Change in mental status, weakness, and anorexia may be the initial manifestation of pneumonia.

Hypothermia, hypotension, hyperventilation, leukopenia, thrombocytopenia, oliguria, and jaundice occur, but usually late in the course of infection and are associated with a poor prognosis (81).

Gram stain of the sputum remains the single most useful test to establish the diagnosis. It is important to obtain a sputum free of oropharyngeal contamination, but this is sometimes difficult in the debilitated patient. One must always consider the possibility of underlying primary or metastatic disease. Bacterial pathogens, which are more likely to cause pneumonia in the elderly, include *Escherichia coli, Klebsiella, Enterobacteriaceae, Hemophilus influenza,* and anaerobic organisms. Although *Legionella pneumophila* is more likely to be acquired outside the hospital environment, it should be considered as a diagnosis if the clinical presentation is compatible.

Therapy of pneumonia consists of supportive measures such as respiratory support, metabolic support (including electrolyte, fluid, and nutritional balance), treatment of underlying medical conditions, and specific treatment with antibiotic therapy.

Therapeutic decisions should be supported by gram stain of a well-collected specimen or if available by documentation of the susceptibility of the most common hospital acquired organisms in your local environment. Broad-spectrum penicillins, i.e., mezlocillin in combination with an aminoglycoside for *Pseudomonas* coverage, is an adequate first choice. For less virulent organisms second or third generation cephalosporins may be quite adequate. Erythromycin is the drug of choice for *Legionella pneumophila*.

Nosocomial Urinary Tract Infection

There is a high prevalence of bacteriuria in populations of older individuals and prevalence continues to increase with advancing age (82). For instance, epidemiologic studies have shown that approximately 20% of women and 2% to 3% of men 65 to 70 years of age have bacteriuria as compared with 23% to 50% of women and 20% of men over 80 years of age (82, 83).

Most older patients with significant bacteriuria are asymptomatic (84). Studies have shown that symptoms related to the urinary tract ranged from 2.6% to 18%. Six percent had flank tenderness, and most had systemic complaints, consisting of anorexia, malaise, nausea, altered mental state, lethargy, and confusion (85). Even when these patients have symptoms, they are often vague and difficult to interpret. Bacteriuria has been associated with an increased mortality rate (38). Whether the mortality is directly related to bacteriuria alone or from factors that increase both bacteriuria and mortality is not well defined. Recent evidence suggests that underlying diseases associated with bacteriuria may account for the increase in mortality (86). Using antibody coating of bacteria as a marker for upper tract infection, Nicolle et al. (87) recently showed that 67% of the infections in older women were localized to the kidney, whereas 33% were in the bladder. Further approaches localizing urinary infection will undoubtedly assist physicians in their management.

The indwelling urinary catheter has been the most common predisposing factor in fatal gram negative sepsis in hospitals (54). Of 100 consecutive episodes of bacteremia, the most common source for bacteremia was the urinary tract (85).

The diagnosis is usually made from the urinalysis of a midstream clean catch specimen (if possible) with gram stain of the sediment and urine culture and sensitivity. A sterile catheterized specimen can be processed as above. The most likely organisms causing bacteriuria include *Escherichia coli, Proteus mirabilis, Klebsiella pneumoniae*, and *Enterococcus* (86, 88).

Treatment of bacteriuria is still controversial. Nicolle et al. (88) investigated the effect of therapy and found that although single-dose antibiotic therapy was effective in sterilizing the urine for short periods of time, there was recurrence of infection. Also of interest was that treatment had no effect on mortality. When therapy is indicated, antimicrobial agents that are excreted in the urinary tract should be chosen, thereby achieving high urine concentrations and decreased likelihood of adverse systemic effects. β-lactam antibiotics are usually the safest choices. The duration of therapy is usually 7 to 14 days. In the case of underlying urinary tract abnormality, however, a longer duration of therapy is warranted. If the Foley catheter can be removed, this may allow the normal host defense mechanisms to clear the infection. Another group of antimicrobial agents, the quinolines, are an alternative in the management of most gram-negative bacilli and some gram-positive cocci (including some species of *streptococci*), but they have no activity against anaerobic organisms (38, 89).

Perinephric abscess occurs as a complication of urinary tract infection (90), usually secondary to an obstruction or even bacteremia. The likely organisms include gram-negative bacilli. Clinical symptoms include fever, flank pain, and abdominal pain. A mass may be detected by palpation but is not a consistent finding. Ultrasonography and computed tomography can assist in the diagnosis. In some instances, percutaneous drainage has obviated the need for surgical drainage (91).

Antibiotic therapy directed against organisms isolated from urine or blood should be started once the diagnosis has been made. Alterations in the regimen can then be made once appropriate culture results have been obtained.

Cellulitis

The skin acts as an important barrier to microbial attachment and subsequent tissue invasion. Age-related changes can affect organs and organ systems. As discussed earlier, the skin undergoes changes that can lead to secondary invasion from bacteria. Patients who are at risk of developing cellulitis include diabetic patients and those who have undergone venous stripping (92) or bypass grafting (92, 93). Poor hygiene and maceration are predisposing factors as well. The most likely organisms involved in these infections are the usual skin flora, including *Staphylococcus aureus* and Group A *Streptococcus*. Antibiotic therapy with a first generation cephalosporin or anti-staphylococcal penicillin is usually warranted. Therapy should also include measures to prevent further skin maceration and antifungal agents if dermatophytosis infections are present.

Pressure Sores

Pressure sores are a constant threat to the debilitated patient. Critical factors leading to their formation include immobility of the patient in bed or sitting (for more than 2 hours), poor protein nutrition, and shearing forces on the skin (94). Prevention by strict attention to nutrition and frequent shifting of the patient's weight is within the standards of good medical and nursing care. When sores do occur, secondary infection is relatively common with gram-negative bacilli and anaerobes. It is important not only to treat these lesions adequately but to rule out underlying infection. Sugarman (95, 96) reviewed this topic and found that a significant number of patients with poorly healing sores had evidence of osteomyelitis. An aggressive approach to these lesions is warranted, including debridement, radiologic studies, bone biopsy, and antibiotic therapy (97).

Reactivated Tuberculosis

The most common clinical form of tuberculosis (TB) seen in older patients is reactivation. Although reactivation often occurs within a few years of the initial infection or at times of altered host resistance, it can occur many decades after the initial infection. Tuberculosis should be considered in every older surgical patient who has a "failure-to-thrive" syndrome either preceding or following surgery. Chest x-ray may be helpful in the diagnosis. The clinical features of presentation may well be atypical in the elderly. Symptoms may often be quite insidious. In other cases, systemic symptoms may be prominent, including anorexia, weight loss, and night sweats (98).

In patients with proven TB who are given a skin test (properly performed), there seems to be little aged-related loss in the size of the measured reactions to purified protein derivative (PPD). There is a slowly progressive increase with age in the number of totally nonreactive patients (anergy) to nearly 20% in those over 80 years old. The so-called booster effect, where a supermaximal antigenic stimulus must be applied more than once to elicit a positive PPD, appears to be more common in older patients (24). The diagnosis of pulmonary tuberculosis can be confirmed by examination of the sputum in most patients. Other diagnostic tests may be necessary.

Treatment of tuberculosis in the elderly is generally similar to that in younger patients. Toxicities from antituberculosis medications pose the greatest problems to the elderly, and for this reason, streptomycin should usually be avoided as this drug can cause ototoxicity as well as vestibular toxicity (99). Isoniazid (INH) prophylaxis is recommended for those older than age 35 with recent conversion and impairment of the immune system.

Tuberculosis remains a significant problem in the 1980s. Although this disease has shown significant decline over the years, recent data from the Centers for Disease Control reveal an increase of 2.6% in the number of reported cases (100). Although the largest increase occurred in the 25 to 44 year age group, the incidence rate was highest in the over 65 age group. Stead (101) and colleagues have shown that there is a 3.5% skin test conversion rate in nursing home patients even in the absence of known exposure. This is not surprising as these people have lived through an era when the risk of being infected with *Mycobacterium* was much higher than it is today (24).

References

1. Elahi, VK, et al. 1983. A longitudinal study of nutritional intake in men. *J Gerontol* 38:162–180.
2. Lipschitz, DA, and Udupa, KB. 1986. Age and the hematopoietic system. *J Am Ger Soc* 34:448–454.
3. Kaufman, CA, et al. 1983. Aging and nutrition. Effects on leukocytic pyrogen production by monocytes. *Clin Res* 31:773A.
4. Morley, JE, et al. 1986. Nutrition and the elderly. *J Am Geriatr Soc* 34:823–832.
5. Rubin, RH, and Cosimi, AB. 1988. Infection in the immunocompromised host. In *Surgical Infectious Diseases*, Eds., RH Howard and RL Simmons, pp. 849–851. Norwalk: Appleton and Lange.
6. Selmanowitz, VJ, et al. 1977. Aging of the skin and its appendages. In *Handbook of the Biology of Aging*, Eds., CE Finch and L Mayflick, p. 496. New York: Van Nostrand Reinhold.
7. Gilchrest, BA. 1979. Some gerontologic considerations in the practice of dermatology. *Arch Dermol* 115:1343.
8. Gilchrest, BA. 1982. Age-associated changes in the skin. *J Am Geriatr Soc* 30:139–143.
9. Yoshikawa, TT. 1983. Geriatric infectious diseases: An emerging problem. *J Am Geriatr Soc* 31:34–39.
10. Levitsky, MG. 1984. Effects of Aging on the Respiratory System. *Physiologist* 27(2); 102.
11. Gorbach, SL, et al. 1967. Studies of intestinal microflora: Effects of diet, age and periodic sampling on numbers of fecal microorganisms in man. *Gastroenterology* 53: 845–855.
12. Weinstein, L, and Dalton, AC. 1968. Host determinants of response to antimicrobial agents. *N Engl J Med* 279:467–473.
13. Valenti, WM, Trudell, RG, and Beverly, DW. 1987. Factors predisposing to oropharyngeal colonization with gram negative bacilli in the aged. *N Engl J Med* 298:1108–1111.
14. Andriole, VT. 1987. Urinary tract infections: Recent developments. *J Infect Dis* 156:865–869.
15. Zweig, S. 1987. Urinary tract infections in the elderly. *Am Fam Phys* 35(5) 123.
16. Beeson, PB. 1948. Temperature-elevating effect of a substance obtained from polymorphonuclear leukocytes. *J Clin Invest* 27:524.
17. Atkens, E, and Wood, WB, Jr. 1955. Studies in the pathogenesis of fever. The presence of transferable pyrogen in the blood stream following injecting of the typhoid vaccine. *J Exp Med* 101:519.
18. Dinarello, CA, et al. 1984. Interleukin I and pathogenesis of acute phase response. *N Engl J Med* 311: 1413–1419.
19. Mackowiak, PA. 1981. Direct effects of hyperthermia on pathogenic microorganisms: Teleologic implications with regard to fever. *Rev Infect Dis* 3:508.
20. Gleckman, R, and Hibert, D. 1982. Afebrile bacteremia: A phenomenon in geriatric patients. *JAMA* 248: 1478–1481.
21. Finklestein, MS, et al. 1983. Pneumococcal bacteremia in adults: Age dependent differences in presentation and in outcome. *J Am Geriatr Soc* 31:19–27.
22. Berman, P, Hogan, DB, and Fox, RA. 1987. The atypical

presentation of infection in old age. *Age Aging* 16:210–207.
23. Thomson, O, and Kettek, K. 1929. Die Storke der menschlichen Isoagulinine and ent sprechen-den Blut korperchenzezeptoren in verschiedonen Leb-ensoltem. *Z Immunitaetsforsh* 63:67.
24. Fretwell, M, and Lipsky, BA. 1985. Infectious agents: The compromised host. In *Principles of Geriatric Medicine*, Eds., R Andres et al. New York: McGraw/Hill.
25. Phair, JP. 1979. Aging and infection: A review. *J Chron Dis* 32:535.
26. Buckley, CE, Buckley, EG, and Dorsey, FC. 1974. Longitudinal changes in serum immuno-globulin levels in older humans. *Fed Pract* 33:2036–2039.
27. Cate, TR, et al. 1977. Clinical trials of bivalent influenza A/New Jersey/ 76-A/Victoria/75 vaccines in the elderly. *J Infect Dis* 136(suppl):518–525.
28. Scheider, EL. 1983. Infectious diseases in the elderly. *Ann Intern Med* 98:395.
29. Ammann, AJ, et al. 1980. The antibody responses to pneumococcal capsular polysaccharides in aged individuals. *Proc Soc Exp Med* 164:312–316.
30. Green, GM, et al. 1977. Defense mechanisms of the respiratory membrane. *Am Rev Resp Dis* 115:479–514.
31. Waldorf, DS, et al. 1968., Impaired delayed hypersensitivity in an aging population. *JAMA* 203:831.
32. Proust, J, et al. 1985. Lymphopenia induced acute bacterial infections in the elderly: A sign of age related immune dysfunction of major prognostic significance. *Gerontology* 31:178–185.
33. Bender, BS, et al. 1986. Absolute peripheral blood lymphocyte count and subsequent mortality of elderly men. *J Am Geriatr Soc* 34:649–654.
34. Roberts-Thomson, IC, et al. 1974. Aging immune responses and mortality. *Lancet* 2:368–370.
35. Portano, JK, et al. 1978. Population immunology age and immune cell parameters. *Clin Immunol Immunopathol* 11:339.
36. Goodwin, JS, et al. 1982. Immunological responses of a healthy elderly population. *Clin Exp Immunol* 48: 403–410.
37. Felser, JM, and Raff, MJ. 1983. Infectious diseases and aging: Immunologic perspectives. *J Am Geriatr Soc* 31: 802–807.
38. Platt, R, et al. 1982. Mortality associated with nosocomial urinary tract infection. *N Engl J Med* 307: 637–642.
39. Marchese, V. 1985. Inflammation and healing. In *Anderson's Pathology*, Ed., JM Kissane, p. 47. St. Louis: CV Mosby.
40. Wolman, SL, et al. 1979. Zinc in total parenteral nutrition: Requirements and metabolic effects. *Gastroenterology* 76:458.
41. Mofenaar, D, et al. 1976. Leukocyte chemotaxis in diabetic patients and their nondiabetic first degree relatives. *Diabetes* 25:880(suppl).
42. Veilsgaard, R. 1973. Studies on urinary infections in diabetes mellitus. Significant bacteriuria in pregnancy in relation to age and onset, duration of diabetes, angiopathy and urological symptoms. *Acta Med Scand* 193:343.
43. Forland, M, Thomas, V, and Shelokov, A. 1977. Urinary tract infections in patients with diabetes mellitus: Studies on antibody coating of bacteria. *JAMA* 238:1924–1926.
44. Mayer, K, and Opal, SM. 1987. Antibacterial therapy in patients with malignancies. *Cancer Metastasis Rev* 5:271.
45. Percival, A. (ed). 1986. Quinolines: 1986. Their future in Clinical Practice. London: Royal Society of Medicine Services.
46. Washington, JA, III. 1985. Bacteria, fungi and parasites. In *Principles & Practice of Infectious Disease*, Ed., G Mandell, pp. 110–111. New York: Wiley.
47. Lennette, EH (Ed). 1985. *Manual of Clinical Microbiology*. Washington DC: Society for Microbiology.
48. Maasden, CF, and Anuras, S. 1981. Are you overlooking GI infections in your elderly patients? *Geriatrics* 36:127.
49. Chetlin, SH, and Elliot, DW. 1971. Biliary bacteremia. *Arch Surg* 102:303–307.
50. Mason, GR. 1968. Bacteriology and antibiotic selection in biliary tract surgery. *Arch Surg* 97:533.
51. Saek, RP, et al. 1975. Spectrum of cholangitis. *Am J Surg* 130:143.
52. England, DM, and Rosenblatt, JE. 1977. Anaerobes in human biliary tracts. *J Clin Microbiol* 6:494–498.
53. Burakoff, R. 1986. An updated look at diverticulitis. *Geriatrics* 36:83–91.
54. Kyle, J. 1968. Prognosis in diverticulitis. *JR Coll Surg Edinb* 13:136.
55. Cello, JP. 1981. Diverticular disease of the colon. *West J Med* 134:515–523.
56. Cohn, J, Jr, and Bornside, GH. 1984. Infections. In *Principles of Surgery*, Ed., SI Schwartz, pp. 205–208. New York: McGraw Hill.
57. Albano, WA, Zielinski, CM, and Organ CH. 1975. Is appendicitis in the aged really different? *Geriatrics* 30: 81–88.
58. Owens, BJ, and Hamet HF. 1978. Appendicitis in the elderly. *Ann Surg* 187:392.
59. Peltokallio, P, and Jauhiaunen, K. 1970. Acute appendicitis in the aged patient. *Arch Surg* 100:140.
60. Yusuf, MF, and Dunn, E. 1979. Appendicitis in the elderly—learn to discern the untypical picture. *Geriatrics* 34:73.
61. Norman, DC and Yoshikawa, TT. 1983. Intra-abdominal infections in the elderly. *J Am Ger Soc* 31:677–684.
62. Lewis, FR, et al. 1975. Appendicitis: A critical review of diagnosis and treatment in 1000 cases. *Arch Surg* 110:677.
63. Berne, TV, et al. 1982. Antibiotic management of surgically treated gangrenous or perforated appendicitis. Comparison of gentamycin and clindamycin versus cefamandole versus cefoperazone. *Am J Surg* 144:8–13.
64. de la Maza, LM, Naceim, F, and Berman, LD. 1974. The changing etiology of liver abscess. *JAMA* 227:161–163.
65. Rubin, RH, et al. 1975. Hepatic abscess changes in clinical, bacteriologic and therapeutic aspects. *Am J Med* 57:601.
66. McDonald, MI. 1984. Single and multiple pyogenic liver abscess, natural history, diagnosis and treatment with emphasis on percutaneous drainage. *Medicine* 63:291.
67. Bertel, CK, Van Heerden, JA, and Sheedy, PF. 1986. Treatment of pyogenic hepatic abscesses, surgical vs. percutaneous drainage. *Arch Surg* 121:554–558.
68. Gerzol, SG, et al. 1985. Intrahepatic pyogenic abscesses treatment by percutaneous drainage. *Am J Surg* 149:487.

69. Janevicius, RV, Hann, SE, and Batt, MD. 1982. Necrotizing fasciitis. *Surg Gynecol Obstet* 154:97–102.
70. Ahrenholz, DA. 1988. Necrotizing soft-tissue infections. *Surg Clin North Am* 68:199–214.
71. Dellinger, EP. 1981. Severe necrotizing soft tissue infections. Multiple disease entities requiring a common approach. *JAMA* 246:1717–1721.
72. Frieschlag, JA, et al. 1985. Treatment of necrotizing soft tissue infections: The need for a new approach. *Am J Surg* 149:757.
73. Quinn, E. 1985. Pleural effusion and empyema. In *Principles and Practices of Infectious Disease*, Ed., G Mandell, p. 404.
74. Ukese, WC, et al. 1973. Empyema of the thorax then and now: A study of 122 cases over four decades. *Arch Intern Med* 131:156.
75. Finland, M, and Barnes, MW. 1978. Changing ecology of acute bacterial empyema; Occurrence and mortality at Boston City Hospital during 12 selected years from 1935–72. *J Infect Dis* 137:274–291.
76. Chandrasekhar, AJ, et al. 1969. Pleural fluid lactic acid dehydrogenase activity and protein content: Value in diagnosis. *Arch Intern Med* 123:48–50.
77. Johanson, WG, et al. 1972. Nosocomial respiratory tract infections with gram-negative bacilli. The significance of colonization of the respiratory tract. *Ann Intern Med* 701–706.
78. Esposito, AL. 1983. Bacterial pneumonia in the elderly in respiratory infections. In *Diagnosis and Management*, Ed., J Pennington, pp. 159–169. New York: Raven Press.
79. Atherton, ST, and White, DJ. 1982. Stomach as source of bacteria colonizing respiratory tract during artificial respiration. *Lancet* 1:242–245.
80. Driks, MR, et al. 1987. Nosocomial pneumonia in intubated patients given sucralfate as compared with antacids or histamine Type 2 Blockers. *N Engl J Med* 317: 1376–1382.
81. Kerzner, LG, et al. 1983. Presentation of disease in the elderly. In *Primary Care Geriatrics: A Case-based Learning Program*, Ed., RJ Hom, Module 10. Littleton, MA: Wright-PSG.
82. Brocklehurst, JC, et al. 1968. The prevalence and symptomology of urinary infection in an aged population. *Gerontol Clin* 10:242–253.
83. Sourander, LB. 1966. Urinary tract infection in the aged—an epidemiological study. *Ann Med Intern* 55 (suppl 45) 7.
84. Boscia, JA, et al. 1986. Lack of association between bacteriuria and symptoms in the elderly. *Am J Med* 81: 979–982.
85. Esposito, AL. 1980. Community-acquired bacteremia in the elderly: Analysis of one hundred consecutive episodes. *J Am Geriatr Soc* 28:315.
86. Nordenstam, GR, et al. 1986. Bacteriuria and mortality in an elderly population. *N Engl J Med* 314:1152–1156.
87. Nicolle, LE, et al. 1988. Localization of urinary tract infection in elderly institutionalized women with asymptomatic bacteriuria. *J Infect Dis* 157:65.
88. Nicolle, LE, et al. 1983. Bacteriuria in elderly institutionalized men. *N Engl J Med* 309:1420–1425.
89. *Medical Letter*. 1988. 30:11.
90. Thaley, JD, Jones, SR, and Sanford, JP. 1974. Perinephric abscess. *Medicine* 53:441–451.
91. Costello, AJ, Blandy, JP, and Hately, W. 1983. Percutaneous aspiration of renal cortical abscess. *Urology* 21:201–204.
92. Baddour, LM, and Bisno, AL. 1984. Recurrent cellulitis after coronary bypass surgery. *JAMA* 251:1049–1052.
93. Baddour, LM, and Bisno, AL. 1985. Recurrent cellulitis after saphenous venectomy for coronary bypass surgery. *Ann Intern Med* 79:155–159.
94. Reuler, JB, and Cooney, TG. 1981. The pressure sore: Pathophysiology and principles of management. *Ann Intern Med* 94:661.
95. Sugarman, B, et al. 1983. Osteomyelitis beneath pressure sores. *Arch Intern Med* 143:683–688.
96. Sugarman, B. 1987. Pressure sores and underlying bone infection. *Arch Intern Med* 147:553–555.
97. Sugarman, B. 1985. Infection and pressure sores. *Arch Phys Med Rehab* 66:177.
98. Simon, M. 1986. Mycobacteria. In *Scientific American Medicine* Vol 2 VIII: 1. Eds., E Rubenstein and DD Federman. New York: Scientific Am Inc.
99. Kopanoff, DE, et al. 1978. Isoniazid-related hepatitis: A US Public Health Service Cooperative Surveillance Study. *Am Rev Resp Dis* 117:991.
100. Tuberculosis, Final Data—United States, 1986. *MMWR*, Jan 1988; 36:50–51.
101. Stead, W, et al. 1985. Tuberculosis as an endemic and nosocomial infection among the elderly in nursing homes. *N Engl J Med* 312:1483–1487.

16

Neoplastic Disease in the Elderly

Frederick F. Holmes

One-eighth of the population of the United States is over age 65, and this small portion suffers one-half of all cancers diagnosed. Shortly after the year 2,000, it is likely that one-fifth of the United States population will be over 65. If cancer incidence patterns remain the same, this demographic change alone will increase the number of cancers in America by about 30% and the number of cancers in the elderly by about 60%. It is believed by some that life expectancy is close to the maximum in the western world (1). Others believe that substantial further improvement is possible.

Epidemiology

No other single factor is as important in cancer incidence as is age. For example, prostate cancer, the quintessential cancer of old men, increases in incidence from 1 in 100,000 for 40-year-old men to nearly 1,000 in 100,000 for 80-year-old men. This is an increase of four orders of magnitude in four decades, a logarithmic increase. The increase in incidence with aging for all cancers combined is shown in Table 16-1 with data derived from the Survival, Epidemiology, and End-Results program of the National Cancer Institute (2). Between ages 40 and 80, there is an increase of about one order of magnitude for all cancers combined. Breast and cervical cancer account for most of the excess of female cases in middle age and then prostate and lung cancer account for most of the excess of male cases in old age, with men over 70 just about twice as likely to have cancer as women of that age. Cancer incidence data beyond age 85 are not generally available, but there is some evidence that incidence may decrease in the nineties (3). The autopsy is the final arbiter of human disease. A classic autopsy study of 3,535 patients over 65 years of age found 23.9% of females to have cancer and 40.3% of males. Previously undiagnosed cancers increased from 20.7% in those aged 66 to 75 to 36.2% in those over age 85. Cancer prevalence stayed the same with age for females but increased in males. The percentage of cancers with metastases decreased from 59.5% in the 66 to 75 age group to 46.9% in those over 85 (4). It has been suggested that the autopsy can be used as an epidemiologic resource (5). Such study might be quite useful in the better understanding of the natural history of cancer in the elderly.

It is assumed by the general public that improvement in cancer treatment has steadily increased cure and survival rates in recent decades. In 1975, a review of survival trends over four decades showed improved 5-year survival rates for cancer of most sites between 1940 and 1970, including colon, rectum, lung, and stomach (6). This is important to the elderly because they suffer the common cancers and are less likely to have the kinds of cancer in which the most spectacular gains have been made, such as Hodgkin's disease. However, survival rates may not have improved much at all, when calculated by stage, if one ascribes to Feinstein's thesis that apparent improved survival in recent decades in some kinds of cancer is in fact due to earlier diagnosis (7). However, this can also be seen as a clear indication that some kinds of cancer are now being diagnosed at an earlier stage than in previous decades.

Unfortunately, the elderly may not have benefited from this trend of earlier diagnosis. There is good evidence that stage at diagnosis increases directly with age

Table 16-1. Cancer incidence in the United States by age for males, females, and both sexes combined expressed as cases per 100,000 population per year

Age group	Males	Females	Both sexes
0–4	19	15	17
5–9	11	8	10
10–14	11	11	11
15–19	17	18	18
20–24	28	31	30
25–29	39	56	47
30–34	51	93	72
35–39	75	148	112
40–44	131	251	192
45–49	248	407	329
50–54	429	562	497
55–59	719	777	749
60–64	1,137	938	1,033
65–69	1,660	1,114	1,361
70–74	2,266	1,259	1,686
75–79	2,847	1,507	2,029
80–84	3,206	1,629	2,195
85+	3,381	1,795	2,308

Source: Young et al. (2).

for most common cancers (8). They found this true for cancers primary to bladder, breast, cervix, kidney, ovary, stomach, and endometrium. Interestingly, there was only a slight trend with colorectal cancer and a highly significant inverse relationship for lung cancer. This work was largely confirmed by Goodwin et al. in 1986 (9). In a very controversial paper, little change in cancer mortality rates in America since 1950 was equated with little progress in cancer treatment (10). In fact, even in a flurry of letters denouncing the study, two showed that while cancer mortality rates in the young and middle aged have decreased in recent decades, rates have substantially increased in the elderly in America (11, 12). Thus, one might conclude that cancer is a very large health problem for the elderly and that the magnitude of this problem grows year by year.

Carcinogenesis

Why does cancer incidence increase with age? There is no simple single answer to this question. Rearrangements of genomes accompanying cellular aging and age-dependent alterations in immune function and host defense are surely two important factors in this phenomenon (13). To this must be added age-related hyperplasias (14) and the obvious fact that the longer we live, the longer we are exposed to environmental carcinogens. Finally, speculation must focus on the oncogenes, which are in fact common genes widely distributed in living matter. Many of these are responsible for the production of cellular growth factors and their roles in the progression of normal cell to lethal cancer cell are rapidly becoming more clear (15, 16). It is accepted that most cancers have a chromosomal defect. Trisomy, chromosome band deletions, and translocations are easily demonstrated in cancers in animals and man. Trisomies provide extra gene dosage, translocations could place an oncogene next to an activating DNA sequence, and deletions could eliminate oncogene repressors (17). Of course the longer we live, the greater the likelihood of damage to and mutation of our DNA.

To acquire an appreciation of the complexities of carcinogenesis and aging, one must consult the animal literature. In mice, aging was found to increase susceptibility of mouse skin to a chemical carcinogen independent of the general immune status of the animals (18). Again in mice, DNA repair mechanisms seem to deteriorate with aging (19). In a study of mice given diethylnitrosamine in their drinking water, it was found that age at beginning of treatment had little effect on incidence or distribution of tumors among various organs but that old mice survived less long with their tumors than young mice (20). In Russia, V.N. Anisimov has conducted extensive studies of carcinogenesis in aged rodents. He found rat mammary gland epithelium, ovarian tissue, and thyroid tissue to be less sensitive to x-ray carcinogenesis with increasing age and concluded that it was related to age-related decrease in proliferative activity of these tissues (21). With respect to chemical carcinogenesis, he concluded that age does have a modifying effect on chemical carcinogenesis, but the effect can be either stimulating or inhibitory, depending on the carcinogen, the species of animal, the particular target tissue, and other factors (22, 23). Among the other factors, he identified polypeptides from thymus, pineal, and anterior hypothalamus which he has studied (24). In an ingenious experiment comparing development of prostatic carcinoma in two quite different strains of aged male rats, one investigator concluded that alterations of the testosterone:estrogen ratio might be an important host factor influencing carcinogenesis, but he was unable to induce precocious development of microscopic prostate cancer by exogenous testosterone treatment of one strain of rats, and invoked other unidentified factors as being important (25). Finally, on the basis of work with mice, British investigators have concluded that no intrinsic effects of aging whatever need be postulated to explain the vast increases in old age of the incidence rates of human cancers, just duration of exposure to carcinogens alone (26).

Obviously, it is impossible to study carcinogenesis in humans other than by inference from incidence statistics. The vast amount of research linking lung cancer with cigarette smoking could be cited as demonstrating that for a given chemical carcinogen, some humans are susceptible and some are not, and that for those who are susceptible, dose and length of exposure are both important. In regard to radiation carcinogenesis, perhaps everyone is susceptible with dose and latency being important factors. In humans, it would appear that old lymphocytes in cell culture express more damage from radiation than young lymphocytes and repair damaged DNA less well (27, 28). Setlow suggests that compromised ability to repair DNA as a consequence of aging may be a result of the turning off of parts of the repair system at early ages in the development of some animals (29). At this point, some mention must be made about nutrition because of its continuing fascination for both the scientific and lay communities with respect to cause and prevention of cancer. It can be succinctly stated that cause and effect data in humans are lacking. Vitamins A, C, and E may be chemopreventives, but their utility is unproven in human prospective intervention studies (30). The entire matter was beautifully summarized by Ames who describes food as containing countless carcinogens and anticarcinogens, making research on diet and cancer in humans very difficult indeed (31).

Clinical Perspectives

The age of the patient at the time of diagnosis of cancer has some importance, but when treatment decisions must be made, the general condition of the patient and the status of concurrent diseases are of much greater importance. It is well established that the proportion of cancer cases receiving potentially curative therapy declines with age and the presumption is that the presence of other diseases is the major influence in initial treatment decisions (32). However, the role of concurrent disease affecting treatment decisions has been brought into question, and some wonder if older cancer patients may be denied appropriate therapy on the basis of age alone (33). After the general condition of the patient, the most important considerations are the site of the primary lesion and the stage at the time of diagnosis. To provide a framework for understanding the relationships between age, site, and stage, data are presented in tables by site from an analysis of 61,654 patients aged 60 to 99, diagnosed with cancer in Kansas hospitals between 1975 and 1984. Survival data are also presented for these patients by stage and age in the tables. These are observed survival rates at 5 years calculated by an actuarial method (34). Each table has corresponding survival rates for the general population, so relative survival rates may be appreciated. Survival data for the general population are derived from USA published life tables (35). A note of caution must be sounded here. Data used to calculate life tables for the elderly in America are weak, and the numbers shown should be regarded as the best approximations possible and not as absolutes. (The author thanks his colleague, Dr. Khatab Hassanein, for doing his best with these weak data in estimating expected survival in the oldest age ranges.) Of these 61,654 patients, 38% were aged 60 to 69, 39% were 70 to 79, 20% were 80 to 89, and 3% were 90 to 99 at the time of diagnosis.

Breast

The most common cancer in older women arises in the breast. Incidence increases progressively to age 85 and then may decline slightly (2, 3). The histologic pattern changes with age, with inflammatory and medullary carcinoma being less common and colloid carcinoma being more common in older women (36). Perhaps of more importance is the fact that both the percentage of patients with estrogen-receptor positive tumors and the concentration of estrogen-receptor protein in those tumors increases with age (37, 38). Histology and the presence or absence of estrogen-receptor protein are important factors in treatment choice as well as in prognosis. While the general medical condition of the patient might alter treatment decisions, it is felt that the older woman should be accorded the same treatment as the younger woman, at least with respect to surgery (39).

Table 16-2 shows the percentage distributions of 6,677 breast cancer patients by age and stage. Just about half are locally confined for patients in their 60s, 70s, and 80s, with the percentage of local lesions declining during the 90s. Disease regionally spread at the time of diagnosis declines from 36% for women in their 60s to 26% for those in their 90s. The percentage distantly spread at the time of diagnosis is constant at 8% for all ages, but the percentage of those who were not staged increases from 7% in the 60s to 24% in the 90s. This latter trend will be noted for most sites and the reason or reasons cannot be determined from the data available.

All else being equal, most authors feel that age at

Table 16-2. Distribution of percentages of 6,677 female breast cancer patients by stage and age at diagnosis, Kansas 1975–1984

	Stage			
Age group (number)	Local	Regional	Distant	Not staged
60–69 (2,769)	49	36	8	7
70–79 (2,457)	51	34	8	8
80–89 (1,247)	54	34	8	8
90–99 (204)	41	26	8	24

diagnosis should not be an important consideration in treatment choices for breast cancer patients and end results will be determined by factors other than age, particularly with regard to surgery (40–43). Because of the greater percentage of estrogen-receptor-positive tumors among older women, tamoxifen appears to be more useful in this group of patients. A group of Scottish surgeons even suggests using tamoxifen as initial sole therapy for localized breast cancer in older women (44). There is lack of agreement about the use of adjuvant chemotherapy in older women with positive axillary lymph nodes removed at the time of surgery. Available data indicate that fewer older than younger women receive adjuvant chemotherapy (36).

Because breast cancer is a capricious disease, it has been difficult to determine the effect of age at diagnosis on subsequent survival. Recurrence decades after treatment with curative intent is not uncommon (45). Long survival with disease metastatic only to the skeleton is also not uncommon (46). It has been thought that older women have better relative survival rates than younger women with breast cancer (47). However, the weight of the evidence suggests that older women have lower relative survival rates than younger women (48–52). There is a subset of older women with locally confined breast cancer who are either easily cured or who have very indolent disease. Their survival is exceptionally good, and it may even be possible to speak of cure of breast cancer in this group (53, 54).

Table 16-3 shows 5-year survival of 6,677 older women with breast cancer by stage and age at diagnosis with expected survival for that age population for comparison. At all ages, survival decreased with increasing extent of disease at the time of diagnosis, as would be expected. Applying the correction of expected survival for the four decades, it appears that women in their seventies do as well at 5 years as women in their sixties but that there is a decrement in relative survival for the oldest two groups.

With regard to improvement in survival in breast cancer in the past four decades, it is important to know that survival in women over age 75 with locally confined disease is very close to that of the age-matched female population at large. Survival in disease regionally spread has not improved significantly in the past several decades. In disease distantly spread at the time of diagnosis, a highly significant increase in survival was noted for women treated during the 1970s when compared to those treated during the 1950s and 1960s, suggesting that multiagent chemotherapy is effective in improving survival rates in advanced disease (53).

Table 16-3. Percentages of 5-year survival for 6,677 female patients with breast cancer by stage and age at diagnosis, compared with expected survival for the general female population, Kansas 1975–1984

	Survival			
		Observed		
Age group (number)	Expected	Local	Regional	Distant
60–69 (2,769)	92	79	59	16
70–79 (2,457)	83	74	54	20
80–89 (1,247)	62	56	40	26
90–99 (204)	39	27	32	10

Prostate

The most common cancer in older men arises in the prostate gland. Incidence increases steadily with age until at least 90, and there is some question whether it stays the same or decreases slightly after that advanced age (2, 3). Prostate carcinoma is often found at rectal examination in older men when they have no symptoms of the disease. At the other extreme is the man who consults his physician for arthritis, which is found to be painful bony metastases from undetected, and perhaps not even symptomatic, primary prostate carcinoma. As many as 40% of men in their 70s may have occult prostate carcinoma, as suggested by autopsy studies, and the percentage is probably even higher in men in their 80s and 90s (55). Given the natural history of this disease, in some patients very indolent and in others very aggressive, one author suggests that screening and early diagnosis are not worthwhile (56). A recent study has demonstrated the presence of a ras oncogene protein in a high percentage of prostate carcinomas, particularly those of high histologic grade (57). There is a strong correlation between likelihood of metastases and both histologic grade and size of the primary tumor (58).

Table 16-4 shows the distribution by stage and age for 8,157 older men with prostate cancer. Just about two-thirds of cases are diagnosed during the 60s, 70s, and 80s, when the disease is apparently locally confined. This declines to 57% for those in their 90s. The percentage of regionally spread disease actually decreases with age and that distantly spread at the time of diagnosis increases slightly. Unstaged disease constitutes just about 10% until the 90s when it increases to 16%.

There are two landmarks in the history of prostate cancer treatment. In 1941, castration and estrogen administration were described as effective treatment for metastatic prostate carcinoma (59). This therapy was quickly adopted even for carcinoma of lesser magnitude, and this

Table 16-4. Distribution of percentages of 8,157 male prostate cancer patients by stage and age at diagnosis, Kansas 1975–1984

	Stage			
Age group (number)	Local	Regional	Distant	Not staged
60–69 (2,290)	63	12	15	11
70–79 (3,519)	66	10	14	10
80–89 (2,059)	63	9	17	12
90–99 (289)	57	8	19	16

therapy was largely unchallenged until the results of the large cooperative Veterans Administration study were published in 1967 (60). It was found that treatment did not substantially alter survival and that use of estrogens was associated with increased mortality from cardiovascular disease. Estrogen doses were markedly decreased after this study, but a recent Swedish study comparing castration with estrogen administration showed that estrogens given even in the lowest recommended dosage increased morbidity from cardiovascular disease in men over age 75, even in those with little or no evidence of pre-existing cardiovascular disease (61). However, estrogens may disappear into history as gonadotropin-releasing hormone analogs come into their own. They are clearly equal to diethylstilbestrol in suppressing pituitary release of FSH and LH and subsequent testicular elaboration of steroid hormones, without increasing cardiovascular morbidity or mortality. They exert comparable effects on the prostate carcinoma itself (62).

With respect to treatment of prostate carcinoma, there are several important questions. Is it possible to cure locally confined prostate carcinoma by radical surgery with acceptable morbidity and mortality rates? Most people think not. If the disease cannot be cured, then what are the best methods of controlling it in older men whose life expectancy is usually measured in years rather than decades? Chemotherapy with existing agents has proved worthless (63). Radiation therapy in various modes has proved efficacious for management even in the very elderly (64). Thus, prospective controlled studies will be necessary to identify the best ways to manage men with aggressive disease as well as men with indolent disease. Several such studies have been suggested or are underway (65, 66). Until the answer is clear, it is probably best to be conservative and to be cognizant of the survival of men of different ages with this disease at different stages as compared to survival of the male population generally.

Table 16-5 shows percentages of 5-year survival for 8,157 older men distributed by age and stage. When compared with expected survival for the male population generally, the excess mortality for locally confined prostate cancer is not great and that for disease regionally spread at diagnosis, not much more. Disease distantly metastatic at the time of diagnosis extracts considerable excess mortality at any age, however. When survival data are reviewed for the past several decades, a highly significant increase in survival was noted after the 1960s, particularly for men over age 75, suggesting that reduction of estrogen doses correspondingly reduced cardiovascular mortality in these very vulnerable elderly men (53).

Table 16-5. Percentages of 5-year survival for 8,157 male patients with prostate cancer by stage and age at diagnosis, compared with expected survival for the general male population, Kansas 1975–1984

	Survival			
		Observed		
Age group (number)	Expected	Local	Regional	Distant
60–69 (2,290)	85	70	62	30
70–79 (3,519)	72	62	51	22
80–89 (2,059)	51	37	41	15
90–99 (289)	28	24	—	0

Lung

Cancer primary to the bronchus is a major cause of mortality in the western world. Until recently, it was considered a disease of men, but in the past decade its incidence has increased in women, probably the result of increased cigarette smoking in women. After decades of steadily increasing incidence in men, the incidence in the United States leveled out in the late 1970s and has actually declined in the 1980s, perhaps a consequence of decreased cigarette smoking in men (67). Quite apart from this salutary phenomenon is the fact that lung cancer incidence declines after about age 75, making it less common in the elderly (2). The reason or reasons for this are unclear. Another curious fact about the natural history of lung cancer is that it is much more likely to be diagnosed at an early stage in the elderly as compared to those who are younger. This makes it unique among the common cancers (8, 68). One of the reasons for this is the decreased incidence of small-cell carcinoma with age and the relative increase in the proportion of the squamous-cell histology (69).

Unfortunately, most lung cancers are incurable at the time of diagnosis. Screening programs based on frequent chest x-rays and sputum cytologies in men at high risk of developing lung cancer have proven to be of very limited utility (70, 71). They might be more useful in the elderly but have not been tested specifically in this group. So, at present, lung cancer patients are diagnosed because of symptoms or have a mass lesion discovered on a chest x-ray taken for another reason.

Table 16-6 shows the distribution by stage and age of 8,805 lung cancer patients from Kansas. The percentage of local lesions increases and that of regional and distant lesions decreases with increasing age. However, there is also an increase of lesions not staged at all from 15% in the 60s to 49% in the 90s. The reason for this increase of unstaged patients is unknown, but it is likely that concurrent disabling disease plays a major part, most notably heart and other lung disease.

In that cure of lung cancer is largely in the hands of the surgeon, one might hope that the increased percentage of locally confined lesions in older patients could be exploited for a greater cure rate. All else being equal, it is known that elderly patients tolerate thoracotomy quite well and age, per se, is not a contraindication to thoracotomy (72). The results of major pulmonary resection for bronchogenic carcinoma in elderly patients are comparable to those in younger patients. One series reported a 30% 5-year survival rate in patients over 70 years of age (73). Radiotherapy has proven very useful in control of lung cancer of all of the common histologies, and some believe that it may occasionally be curative (74). Chemotherapy is essentially worthless in squamous, adenocarcinoma, and large-cell histologies. It remains the treatment of choice, combined with radiotherapy, for small-cell carcinoma, with dramatic improvement in survival time and occasional cures well documented, even in elderly patients (75, 76).

Table 16-7 shows 5-year survival in 8,805 lung cancer patients seen in Kansas in the past decade. As is apparent, the survival rate is not improved with age despite the increased percentage of early lesions documented in Table 16-6. It may be that concurrent disease in this elderly population exacts considerable mortality in those who might otherwise be cured of their cancers. In any event, the record of long survival and cure in lung cancer remains poor at any age. There has been little improvement in survival in the past four decades (53). It would seem that the management of the elderly lung cancer patient is not different from one of lesser age, in that the chance of cure rests with a locally confined lesion in a patient who can tolerate major pulmonary resection. Otherwise, the goal of treatment must be control, with radiotherapy playing a major part and chemotherapy useful only for small-cell carcinoma.

Table 16-6. Distribution of percentages of 8,805 lung cancer patients by stage and age at diagnosis, Kansas 1975–1984

	Stage			
Age group (number)	Local	Regional	Distant	Not staged
60–69 (4,360)	27	25	33	15
70–79 (3,365)	29	21	28	21
80–89 (988)	30	15	23	32
90–99 (92)	21	10	21	49

Table 16-7. Percentages of 5-year survival for 8,805 patients with lung cancer by stage and age at diagnosis, compared with expected survival for the general population, Kansas 1975–1984

	Survival			
		Observed		
Age group (number)	Expected	Local	Regional	Distant
60–69 (4,360)	89	29	14	2
70–79 (3,365)	78	15	7	1
80–89 (988)	58	6	3	2
90–99 (92)	35	—	—	—

Colorectum

The most commonly occurring cancer of the elderly arises in the large intestine, either the colon itself or the rectum. Incidence increases steadily into the oldest age groups (2). While diet and polyps may be important considerations with respect to etiology of colorectal cancer, the actual cause or causes are unknown. Several recent studies have suggested that what causes cancer in the cecum may not be the same as what causes cancer in the rectum, because there has been a trend toward less cancer in the distal colorectum and more in the proximal colon in recent decades (77). Part of this trend is related to a decreased left, unchanged transverse, and increased right occurrence of colorectal cancer with increasing age, statistically significant for women but not for men, in 948 Kansans studied (78). Beyond the implications for incidence and etiology, these findings mean that fewer colorectal cancers are within reach of the examining finger, the rigid proctoscope, or even the flexible sigmoidoscope. Colonoscopy and the colon x-ray assume greater importance in light of these findings. There is now general agreement that removing all colorectal polyps decreases the chance of subsequent colorectal cancer (79, 80). This becomes an important strategy at any age since the possibility that most colorectal polyps and cancers may be related to an inherited autosomal dominant gene for susceptibility was recently demonstrated (81).

Table 16-8 shows that the distribution by stage of colorectal cancers remains just about the same from the 60s to the 90s, with about 35% being confined to the bowel itself, about 40% being regionally spread, and about 15% being distantly spread at the time of diagnosis. Unfortunately Duke's staging cannot be presented because it was available for only a minority of these 9,695 cases.

Curative treatment of this common disease is totally in the hands of the surgeon. Five-year survival usually means cure, but long survival with disease or late recurrence is by no means uncommon. Table 16-9 shows relative 5-year survival to be much the same in the four age groups, which is salutary indeed. Survival is fair in regionally spread disease and largely independent of age even in the older patients in this series. Survival in disease distantly spread at diagnosis is, of course, uniformly poor. Radiotherapy and chemotherapy do not have a large role in colorectal cancer. Surgical adjuvant chemotherapy was not useful in colon cancer in a prospective randomized study, but radiation and chemotherapy were useful after potentially curative rectal cancer surgery (82, 83). More recent analysis of the rectal cancer data suggests considerable benefit from combined radiotherapy and chemotherapy for patients who have tumor penetrating into perirectal fat or in regional lymph nodes (84). Conservative and effective palliative therapy of rectal cancer in debilitated elderly patients has received considerable attention in recent years, and irradiation, even by intrarectal application, has proven useful, perhaps occasionally curative (85, 86).

Stomach

The incidence of gastric cancer varies widely around the world, and environmental factors, presumably dietary influences, must play a large role in gastric carcinogenesis. It is generally agreed that the incidence of gastric cancer has declined markedly in the past five decades in most of the western world. However, there is genuine concern that lack of histologic confirmation in former times may have inflated the incidence rate. Indeed in a necropsy study in Norway, the incidence of this disease was found not to have changed from 1955 to 1980 (87). In any event, the incidence increases steadily with age into the oldest age groups (2). The disease is sufficiently uncommon in the young and middle-aged populations that stomach cancer can be considered a disease of old age.

Usually vague symptoms bring the patient to the doctor's attention; weight loss, poorly localized abdominal pain, tiredness from anemia, and the like. The disease has not been common enough in the western world to prompt interest in screening for early lesions as in Japan where incidence is relatively high. Table 16-10 shows the distribution of stage by age for 1,143 cases in Kansas. Just about one-fifth of cases are locally confined by clinical or operative estimation, regardless of age, and slightly more than one-third are regionally spread. However, review of the 5-year survival data in Table 16-11 shows that survival

Table 16-8. Distribution of percentages of 9,695 colorectal cancer patients by stage and age at diagnosis, Kansas 1975–1984

	Stage			
Age group (number)	Local	Regional	Distant	Not staged
60–69 (3,058)	34	42	16	8
70–79 (3,938)	35	41	15	9
80–89 (2,324)	36	39	13	11
90–99 (375)	29	42	12	18

Table 16-9. Percentages of 5-year survival for 9,695 patients with colorectal cancer by stage and age at diagnosis, compared with expected survival for the general population, Kansas 1975–1984

	Survival			
		Observed		
Age group (number)	Expected	Local	Regional	Distant
60–69 (3,058)	89	66	42	3
70–79 (3,938)	78	56	38	7
80–89 (2,324)	58	42	27	4
90–99 (375)	35	22	20	0

Table 16-10. Distribution of percentages of 1,143 stomach cancer patients by stage and age at diagnosis, Kansas 1975–1984

	Stage			
Age group (number)	Local	Regional	Distant	Not staged
60–69 (351)	22	37	28	13
70–79 (456)	20	43	22	14
80–89 (281)	20	35	20	25
90–99 (55)	22	35	7	36

Table 16-11. Percentages of 5-year survival for 1,143 patients with stomach cancer by stage and age at diagnosis, compared with expected survival for the general population, Kansas 1975–1984

	Survival				
		Observed			
Age group (number)	Expected	All	Local	Regional	Distant
60–69 (351)	89	20	47	12	6
70–79 (456)	78	10	24	8	—
80–89 (281)	58	9	22	12	0
90–99 (55)	35	10	—	—	—

for disease thought to be locally confined is poor, implying that staging of this disease is wrong at least half of the time. Survival for regionally spread disease is very poor, and for distantly spread disease essentially zero at 5 years. There may be some distortion of the survival data by cases of gastric lymphoma, which have a much better prognosis than carcinoma. Radiotherapy and multi-agent chemotherapy have some place in palliation, but their effect is small (53, 88).

Esophagus

In the United States, the incidence of esophageal cancer increases directly with age into the 80s but may decline somewhat in the 90s; the disease is about twice as common in males as in females (2, 3). However, in other parts of the world, notably Linxian County in Henan Province in the People's Republic of China, the disease is extremely common and just about equally common in the two sexes (89). Rather like that for lung cancer in the United States, the incidence in China declines in old age, implying a powerful carcinogen of spent force by the time a population is elderly. Extensive epidemiologic research in Henan Province has yet to identify this carcinogen, though there are many fascinating leads. In the United States, esophageal cancer has been associated with cigarette smoking and alcohol use, particularly in concert.

Comparison of Table 16-12 with Table 16-13 shows that, although the percentage of cancers which are locally confined increases from about one-third to one-half with increasing age, survival is very poor. Almost all of these tumors are of squamous origin, though adenocarcinoma does occur in the lower third. This cancer kills its victim by local and regional spread; the patient dies of starvation. Early lesions can be surgically cured. In Henan Province in China screening programs using an inflated balloon and exfoliative cytology have identified such early lesions (90). The author observed extensive esophageal resections done by experienced thoracic surgeons in Zhengzhou, Henan, completed in less than two hours without blood transfusion. Chemotherapy is of no benefit and radiotherapy of some use in the United States (91). Palliative esophageal dilatation and intubation may be particularly useful in the older patient (92).

Table 16-12. Distribution of percentages of 520 esophagus cancer patients by stage and age at diagnosis, Kansas 1975–1984

	Stage			
Age group (number)	Local	Regional	Distant	Not staged
60–69 (251)	37	23	18	23
70–79 (169)	39	21	15	25
80–89 (88)	40	15	17	28
90–99 (12)	50	0	8	42

Pancreas

Few diseases are as hopeless as adenocarcinoma of the pancreas. The incidence of this disease increases steadily with age into the oldest age groups with the male-to-female ratio being about 3:2 (2). Three-fourths of patients are over age 59, so this is essentially a disease of old age (93). It is thought that incidence has increased in recent years in the United States, but one must wonder if this might be the obverse of the decrease in stomach cancer during the same period. In reviewing data on 1,500 Kansans with this disease, it is obvious that stage has no meaning and that survival is abysmal. The surgeon can

Table 16-13. Percentages of 5-year survival for 520 patients with esophagus cancer by stage and age at diagnosis, compared with expected survival for the general population, Kansas 1975–1984

	Survival				
		Observed			
Age group (number)	Expected	All	Local	Regional	Distant
60–69 (251)	89	10	15	11	0
70–79 (169)	78	12	14	—	—
80–89 (88)	58	0	0	—	—
90–99 (12)	35	—	—	—	—

improve quality of life and perhaps increase survival slightly by biliary diversion in the face of obstructive jaundice. Radiotherapy seems to be of some benefit for palliation, but chemotherapy is essentially worthless. Cure, except for the occasional unusual endocrine tumor, is very rare.

Bladder

Cancer of the bladder is a disease of old men although not as common as prostate cancer. The incidence doubles every 10 years from age 50 to age 80 in men; it is only about one-fifth as common in women but still increases in incidence into the oldest ages. Bladder cancer is the first neoplasm for which a major cause was identified, when Rehn described the link with aniline dyes in Germany (94). Beyond this there is a strong association with cigarette smoking (95). Hematuria is perhaps the most common presenting symptom, but minor urinary discomfort may be the only early symptom of this disease.

Table 16-14 shows the stage distribution by age in 3,331 patients. Just about three-fourths of cases are locally confined at the time of diagnosis, although this declines to two-thirds in the 90s. Consistently, 3% of patients are diagnosed when the disease is widespread, and those not staged increase from 7% to 16% between the 60s and the 90s. Table 16-15 shows that survival is quite good for those with locally confined disease with an excess mortality at 5 years of only about 20%. Even those with regionally spread disease have substantial survival at 5 years. However, it must be recognized that survival beyond 5 years with disease present is fairly common. Thus, bladder cancer becomes a chronic disease for some, perhaps particularly for older people. Combined modality therapy has been the standard for many years, even in the elderly (96). Chemotherapy is of little use in this disease and, in the elderly, is likely to cause considerable harm. Survival in local and regional stages has improved in the last three decades but not very much (53).

Table 16-14. Distribution of percentages of 3,331 bladder cancer patients by stage and age at diagnosis, Kansas 1975–1984

	Stage			
Age group (number)	Local	Regional	Distant	Not staged
60–69 (1,073)	78	13	3	7
70–79 (1,388)	74	15	3	8
80–89 (743)	71	16	3	10
90–99 (127)	67	17	1	16

Table 16-15. Percentages of 5-year survival for 3,331 patients with bladder cancer by stage and age at diagnosis, compared with expected survival for the general population, Kansas 1975–1984

	Survival			
		Observed		
Age group (number)	Expected	Local	Regional	Distant
60–69 (1,073)	89	68	33	13
70–79 (1,388)	78	57	30	22
80–89 (743)	58	39	15	—
90–99 (127)	35	24	—	—

Ovary

Cancer of the ovary is responsible for as many deaths as all of the other gynecologic cancers combined and is the fifth leading cause of cancer death among American women. The incidence of ovarian cancer increases steadily into the oldest age groups (2). The histology of ovarian cancer is varied, but nearly 90% are of the common epithelial type. Causes are unknown, but familial factors, previous use of talc on sanitary napkins, and no or low parity have significant associations with ovarian cancer (97). The greatest tragedy about ovarian cancer is the fact that the minority of cases are diagnosed at an early stage. At present the only screening test is a pelvic examination. Despite the increasing incidence of this disease with age, there is a decrease in frequency of pelvic examinations as women proceed beyond menopause. Real-time ultrasonography for determination of ovarian morphology and volume holds promise as a screening test (98).

Table 16-16 shows the distribution of stage by age for 1,092 patients. The proportion that is distantly spread at the time of diagnosis increases from about 50% to 60%

Table 16-16. Distribution of percentages of 1,092 female patients with ovary cancer by stage and age at diagnosis, Kansas 1975–1984

	Stage			
Age group (number)	Local	Regional	Distant	Not staged
60–69 (514)	20	23	51	7
70–79 (370)	19	21	51	9
80–89 (186)	19	22	48	10
90–99 (22)	9	18	59	14

from the 60s to the 90s. Probably the only curable disease is that which is locally confined, and local cancer decreases from 20% to 9% over the same age range. Disease that has not been staged doubles.

Table 16-17 shows 5-year survival for these patients by stage and age. As survival past 5 years with disease present is uncommon, 5-year survival may be nearly synonymous with cure. In locally confined disease, nearly two-thirds are cured by surgery in the 60s. This falls to one-half during the 70s and to one-third during the 80s. Even in regionally spread and distantly spread disease, there are substantial percentages of patients alive at 5 years. This corresponds with the observation that survival in this disease has increased quite significantly in recent decades (53). There seems little doubt that chemotherapy and perhaps more imaginative strategies of radiotherapy have contributed to this (99, 100).

Endometrium

During the last several decades, the incidence of endometrial cancer has changed, with an increase after menopause. This is generally attributed to the increase in use of estrogens unopposed by progestins in women after menopause (101, 102). It must be recognized that endometrial cancer is not uncommon in old age and any postmenopausal woman with vaginal bleeding should be assumed to have endometrial cancer until it is ruled out. The only screening test, at any age, is the periodic pelvic examination. Certainly this should be mandatory for women who have received estrogens after menopause, as their risk of endometrial cancer continues for a decade or more after they have stopped taking supplemental estrogens (103).

As is shown in Table 16-18, most endometrial cancers are diagnosed when the disease is locally confined, but this proportion declines from about three-fourths in the 60s to about one-half in the 90s. Disease distantly spread at the time of diagnosis is uncommon; the percentage of patients not staged rises from one-tenth in the 60s to about one-fourth in the 90s. Scrutiny of Table 16-19 shows that 5-year survival in locally confined disease is quite good, even through the 80s. This suggests that for many women this disease may not be very aggressive. Even in regionally spread disease, 5-year survival is substantial. The possibility for salvage after failure of initial therapy is real in distinction to many of the common kinds of cancer (104).

Table 16-18. Distribution of percentages of 2,401 female patients with endometrial cancer by stage and age at diagnosis, Kansas 1975–1984

	Stage			
Age group (number)	Local	Regional	Distant	Not staged
60–69 (1,256)	74	12	3	11
70–79 (819)	69	14	5	12
80–89 (282)	60	16	7	17
90–99 (44)	57	11	5	27

Cervix

The incidence of invasive cancer of the uterine cervix increases steadily into old age. An 80-year-old woman is four times more likely to have invasive cervical cancer than a 30-year-old woman, despite the fact that the peak incidence of carcinoma of the cervix in situ occurs at age 30 (2). This interesting paradox is not widely appreciated. The evidence that cervical carcinoma is directly related to wart virus infection is mounting, particularly that suf-

Table 16-17. Percentages of 5-year survival for 1,092 female patients with ovary cancer by stage and age at diagnosis, compared with expected survival for the general female population, Kansas 1975–1984

	Survival				
		Observed			
Age group (number)	Expected	All	Local	Regional	Distant
60–69 (514)	92	29	62	28	14
70–79 (370)	83	18	48	17	6
80–89 (186)	62	15	36	17	8
90–99 (22)	39	—	—	—	—

Table 16-19. Percentages of 5-year survival for 2,401 female patients with endometrial cancer by stage and age at diagnosis, compared with expected survival for the general female population, Kansas 1975–1984

	Survival				
		Observed			
Age group (number)	Expected	All	Local	Regional	Distant
60–69 (1,256)	92	76	82	48	6
70–79 (819)	83	62	69	53	8
80–89 (282)	62	40	51	20	—
90–99 (44)	39	0	0	—	—

fered by younger and middle-aged women (105–107). A strong case can be made for regular pelvic examinations and Papanicolaou smears for older women regardless of their previous history of screening or gynecologic disease (108, 109). There is a disquieting note in that one small study found that 4 of 50 postmenopausal women had cervical carcinoma in situ in face of normal cervical cytology (110). There may yet be much to learn about the natural history of cervical cancer in older women.

Table 16-20 shows the distribution of stage by age of cervical cancer for older women with the in situ stage included. As a percentage of the whole, the fraction of in situ cancer decreases rapidly with increasing age. Other locally confined disease decreases from about 40% to about 30% with aging. As is obvious, there is a strong trend toward increasing stage with increasing age in this particular disease. Table 16-21 shows survival for in situ stage to be essentially that of the general female population, with quite good survival for local and regional disease. There were not enough patients to analyze survival for disease distantly spread at the time of diagnosis.

Both surgery and radiotherapy play a part in the treatment of this disease at any age, and the results of treatment are as good in older women as in younger ones according to one study (111). This author's data would generally support this. Chemotherapy as presently applied is of little use in this disease.

Melanoma

The incidence of melanoma of the skin increases steadily to the 80s and is slightly more common in older men than in older women, a contrast to the incidence pattern of younger people (2). The relationship to sex hormones has been considered, and this may be a factor in the age differential in incidence as well as spread of disease and survival (112, 113). There is a strong association of incidence both with being fair-skinned and with sun exposure (114).

Table 16-20. Distribution of percentages of 825 female patients with cervical cancer by stage and age at diagnosis, Kansas 1975–1984

	Stage				
Age group (number)	In situ	Local	Regional	Distant	Not staged
60–69 (402)	29	38	21	6	6
70–79 (286)	22	31	29	8	9
80–89 (123)	15	33	27	9	16
90–99 (14)	0	29	50	14	7

Table 16-21. Percentages of 5-year survival for 825 female patients with cervical cancer by stage and age at diagnosis, compared with expected survival for the general female population, Kansas 1975–1984

	Survival				
		Observed			
Age group (number)	Expected	In situ	Local	Regional	Distant
60–69 (402)	92	92	72	59	—
70–79 (286)	83	93	58	44	—
80–89 (123)	62	—	46	21	—
90–99 (14)	39	—	—	—	—

This disease is capricious and unpredictable. Animal studies have shown a difference in metastatic potential when young mice are compared to old (115).

Table 16-22 shows the distribution of 805 older patients with melanoma of the skin by age and stage. Unfortunately, data on the thickness of the primary lesions were unavailable for most of these patients. However, it can be noted that two-thirds or more of these lesions appear to be locally confined at the time of diagnosis and original treatment, but with a suggestion of increasing stage with increasing age. This is an interesting contrast to the relative improvement of 5-year survival with increasing age for all melanomas and for the local and regional stages as shown (Table 16-23). One might wonder if host factors are not very important in the prognosis of this disease.

Hematologic Malignancies

Though the surgeon plays a minor part in the initial treatment of this large family of cancers, the surgeon is nonetheless often involved in the care of these patients because they are prone to have complications requiring surgical intervention.

Table 16-22. Distribution of percentages of 805 patients with melanoma by stage and age at diagnosis, Kansas 1975–1984

	Stage			
Age group (number)	Local	Regional	Distant	Not staged
60–69 (350)	69	8	10	13
70–79 (287)	73	9	6	12
80–89 (151)	59	12	8	19
90–99 (17)	65	12	18	6

Table 16-23. Percentages of 5-year survival for 805 patients with melanoma by stage and age at diagnosis, compared with expected survival for the general population, Kansas 1975–1984

	Survival				
		Observed			
Age group (number)	Expected	All	Local	Regional	Distant
60–69 (350)	89	60	68	56	22
70–79 (287)	78	50	58	32	—
80–89 (151)	58	41	50	—	—
90–99 (17)	35	—	—	—	—

The incidence of the acute and chronic leukemias, lymphoma, Hodgkin's disease, and multiple myeloma all increase progressively into old age. Chemotherapy is the mainstay of treatment for these diseases, although radiotherapy plays an important part.

In general, there has been little improvement in survival in the leukemias in the elderly, either acute or chronic, in recent decades. This is in contrast to the improvements noted in children and younger adults. Older patients do very poorly with bone marrow transplants. Because of the markedly diminished chance of altering the course of the disease in the various leukemias, aggressive chemotherapy seems less appropriate in older people. However, some believe that age per se is not an important factor in predisposition to toxicity from cancer chemotherapy (116). The quintessential leukemia of old age is chronic lymphocytic leukemia. It is likely to be a very indolent disease and likely to be present in older patients having elective surgical procedures unrelated to the leukemia. If clotting factors, including platelets, are normal and if careful attention is paid to the possibility of postoperative infection, these patients should be good surgical candidates. Incidental surgery in the older patient with acute leukemia will be associated with increased morbidity and mortality.

Chemotherapy has improved the lot of the older patient with lymphoma or Hodgkin's disease, and age is not an important limiting factor in chemotherapy in these diseases. Improvement in survival in multiple myeloma in recent decades has been at least as good in the elderly as in younger patients (53, 117, 118). Morbidity and mortality associated with incidental surgery in these patients would be related to whether or not they were in remission.

Other Malignancies

Primary brain tumors in the elderly are of interest for several reasons. The actual incidence of the various gliomas declines after the 70s. There is a cohort effect underlying all of this (119). The reason or reasons for this decreased incidence are unknown, but one could speculate about the spent force of environmental carcinogens. Because intracranial disease is very common in the elderly—stroke, subdural hematoma, and metastatic malignancy—it is important to identify meningiomas, which may be cured, and gliomas, which may be palliated, even in the elderly.

The various head and neck malignancies constitute a collection of kinds of cancer that generally increase in incidence with increasing age or plateau after the 70s. At the present time, those related to smoking are much more common in males than in females, even in old age. Cancer of the thyroid gland is more common in elderly women than in elderly men. Stage distributions and 5-year survival vary widely from lip and larynx to the pharynx.

Finally, mention must be made of cancer of unknown primary site. The incidence increases with age. Surprisingly, length of survival after diagnosis has improved significantly in recent decades (53).

Conclusion

Cancer and aging seem inextricably linked, quite probably at the level of DNA itself. In recent years the understanding of the molecular biology of cancer has been rapidly improved, whereas there is little understanding of the mechanisms of aging in this context. The interaction is very important because cancer incidence increases as physical vigor decreases in humans. Surgeons and physicians who treat the elderly with cancer are well advised to keep in focus the finitude of human life and the natural history of the various kinds of cancer in their patients. With these data at hand, the surgeon and the physician can balance benefit and risk and provide the best treatment for each elderly patient with due consideration both to functional status and life expectancy.

References

1. Fries, JF, and Crapo, LM. 1981. Vitality and Aging: Implications of the Rectangular Curve. San Francisco: W.H. Freeman and Company.
2. Young, Jr, J, Percy, C, and Asire, A. 1981. Surveillance, Epidemiology, and End-Results: Incidence and Mortality Data, 1973–1977. NIH Publication No. 81-2330, Bethesda, MD: National Cancer Institute.
3. Lew, EA. 1978. Cancer in old age. *Ca* 28:2–6.
4. Suen, KC, Lau, LL, and Yermakov, V. 1974. Cancer and old age: An autopsy study of 3,535 patients over 65 years old. *Cancer* 33:1164–1168.
5. McFarlane, MJ, Feinstein, AR, and Wells, CK. 1985.

The "Epidemiologic Necropsy," unexpected detections, and the changing rates of lung cancer. *Clin Res* 33:260A.

6. Cutler, SJ, Myers, MH, and Green, SB. 1975. Trends in survival rates of patients with cancer. *N Engl J Med* 293: 122–124.
7. Feinstein, AR, Sosin, DM, and Wells, CK. 1985. The Will Rogers' Phenomenon: Stage migration and new diagnostic techniques as a source of misleading statistics for survival in cancer. *N Engl J Med* 312:1604–1608.
8. Holmes, FF, and Hearne, EM. 1981. Cancer stage-to-age relationships: Implications for cancer screening in the elderly *J Am Geriatr Soc* 29:55–57.
9. Goodwin, JS, et al. 1986. Stage at diagnosis of cancer varies with the age of the patient. *J Am Geriatr Soc* 34: 20–26.
10. Bailar, JC, and Smith, EM. 1986. Progress against cancer? *N Engl J Med* 314:1226–1232.
11. del Junco, DJ, and Annegers, JF. 1986. Progress against cancer? (letter in response) *N Engl J Med* 315:964–965.
12. Mann, DA. 1986. Progress against cancer? (letter in response). *N Engl J Med* 315:966.
13. Lipschitz, DA, et al. 1985. Cancer in the elderly: Basic science and clinical aspects. *Ann Intern Med* 102: 218–228.
14. Martin, GM. 1979. Proliferative homeostasis and its age-related aberrations. *Mech Ageing Dev* 9:385–391.
15. Hamlyn, P, and Sikora, K. 1983. Oncogenes. *Lancet* 2: 326–330.
16. Robertson, M. 1983. Oncogenes and multistep carcinogenesis. *Br Med J* 287:1084–1086.
17. Yunis, JJ. 1983. The chromosomal basis of human neoplasia. *Science* 221:227–236.
18. Ebbesen, P. 1974. Aging increases susceptibility of mouse skin to DMBA carcinogenesis independent of general immune status. *Science* 183:217–218.
19. Ishikawa, T, and Sakurai, J. 1986. In vivo studies on age dependency of DNA repair with age in mouse skin. *Cancer Res* 46:1344–1348.
20. Clapp, NK, et al. 1981. Temporal advancement of diethylnitrosamine carcinogenesis in aging mice. *J Gerontol* 36:158–163.
21. Anisimov, VN and Prokudina, EA. 1986. Carcinogenesis and aging—VII. Carcinogenic effect of single total-body x-ray irradiation in young and old female rats. *Exp Pathol* 29:165–171.
22. Anisimov, VN, and Turusov, VS. 1981. Modifying effect of aging on chemical carcinogenesis: A review. *Mech Ageing Dev* 15:399–414.
23. Anisimov, VN. 1982. Carcinogenesis and aging—III. The role of age in initiation and promotion of carcinogenesis. *Exp Pathol* 22:131–147.
24. Anisimov, VN, Khavinson, VK, and Morozov, VG. 1982. Carcinogenesis and aging—IV. Effect of low-molecular-weight factors of thymus, pineal gland, and anterior hypothalamus on immunity, tumor incidence and life span of C3H/Sn mice. *Mech Ageing Dev* 19: 245–258.
25. Isaacs, JT. 1984. The aging ACI/Seg versus Copoenhagen male rat as à model system for the study of prostatic carcinogenesis. *Cancer Res* 44:5785–5796.
26. Peto, R, et al. 1975. Cancer and ageing in mice and men. *Br J Cancer* 32:411–426.
27. Dutkowski, RT, et al. 1985. Increased chromosomal instability in lymphocytes from elderly humans. *Mutat Res* 149:505–512.
28. Staiano-Coico, L, et al. 1983. Increased sensitivity of lymphocytes from people over 65 to cell cycle arrest and chromosomal damage. *Science* 219:1335–1337.
29. Setlow, RB. 1978. Repair deficient human disorders and cancer. *Nature* 271:713–717.
30. Holmes, FF. 1985. Vitamins and Cancer. In *Pathophysiological Aspects of Cancer Epidemiology,* Eds., G Mathe and P Reizenstein. Oxford: Pergamon Press.
31. Ames, BN. 1983. Dietary carcinogens and anticarcinogens: Oxygen radicals and degenerative disease. *Science* 221:1256–1264.
32. Samet, J, et al. 1986. Choice of cancer therapy varies with age of patient. *JAMA* 255:3385–3390.
33. Mor, V, et al. 1985. Relationship between age at diagnosis and treatments received by cancer patients. *J Am Geriatr Soc* 33:585–589.
34. Berkson, J, and Gage, RP. 1950. Calculation of survival rates for cancer. *Proc Staff Meet Mayo Clinic* 25: 270–286.
35. National Center for Health Statistics. 1985. Vital Statistics of the United States, 1982, vol. II, sec. 6, Life Tables. DHHS Pub. No. (PHS) 85-1104. Washington, DC: Public Health Service, U.S. Government Printing Office.
36. Allen, C, et al. 1986. Breast cancer in the elderly: Current patterns of care *J Am Geriatr Soc* 34:637–642.
37. McCarty Jr, KS, et al. 1983. Relationship of age and menopausal status to estrogen receptor content in primary carcinoma of the breast. *Ann Surg* 197:123–127.
38. Elwood, JM, and Godolphin, W. 1980. Oestrogen receptors in breast tumours: associations with age, menopausal status, and epidemiological and clinical features in 735 patients. *Br J Cancer* 42:635–644.
39. Davis, SJ, et al. 1985. Characteristics of breast cancer in women over 80 years of age. *Am J Surg* 150:655–658.
40. Kesseler, HJ, and Seton, JZ. 1978. The treatment of operable breast cancer in the elderly female. *Am J Surg* 135: 664–666.
41. Hunt, KE, Fry, DE, and Bland, KI. 1980. Breast carcinoma in the elderly patient: An assessment of operative risk, morbidity and mortality. *Am J Surg* 140:339–342.
42. Devitt, JE. 1970. The influence of age on the behaviour of carcinoma of the breast. *Can Med Assoc J* 103: 923–926.
43. Cortese, AF, and Cornell, GN. 1975. Radical mastectomy in the aged female. *J Am Geriatr Soc* 23:337–342.
44. Preece, PE, et al. 1982. Tamoxifen as initial sole treatment of localised breast cancer in elderly women: A pilot study. *Br Med J* 284:869–870.
45. Sutton, M. 1960. Late recurrence of carcinoma of the breast. *Br Med J* 1:1132–1134.
46. Sherry, MM, et al. 1986. Metastatic breast cancer confined to the skeletal system: An indolent disease. *Am J Med* 81:381–386.
47. Herbsman, H, et al. 1981. Survival following breast cancer surgery in the elderly. *Cancer* 47:2358–2363.
48. Adami, HO, et al. 1985. Age as a prognostic factor in breast cancer. *Cancer* 56:898–902.
49. Adami, HO, et al. 1986. The relation between survival and age at diagnosis in breast cancer. *N Engl J Med* 315: 559–563.
50. Mueller, CB, Ames, F, and Anderson, GD. 1978. Breast

cancer in 3,558 women: Age as a significant determinant in the rate of dying and causes of death. *Surgery* 83: 123–132.
51. Rosen, PP, Lesser, ML, and Kinne, DW. 1985. Breast carcinoma at the extremes of age: A comparison of patients younger than 35 years and older than 75 years. *J Surg Oncol* 28:90–96.
52. Schottenfeld, D, and Robbins, GF. 1971. Breast cancer in elderly women. *Geriatrics* 26:121–131.
53. Holmes, FF. 1983. Aging and Cancer. Recent Results in Cancer Research, vol 87. Berlin: Springer-Verlag.
54. Langlands, AO, et al. 1979. Long-term survival of patients with breast cancer: A study of the curability of the disease. *Br Med J* 2:1247–1251.
55. Rich, AR. 1979. On the frequency of occurrence of occult carcinoma of the prostate. *Ca* 29:115–119.
56. Meyers, FJ. 1986. Tumor biology in explanation of the failure of screening for cancer and in determination of future strategies. *Am J Med* 80:911–916.
57. Viola, MV, et al. 1986. Expression of *ras* oncogene p21 in prostate cancer. *N Engl J Med* 314:133–137.
58. McNeal, JE, et al. 1986. Patterns of progression in prostate cancer. *Lancet* 1:60–63.
59. Huggins, C, and Hodges, CV. 1941. The effect of castration, of estrogen, and of androgen injection on serum phosphatases in metastatic carcinoma of the prostate. *Cancer Res* 1:293–297.
60. Arduino, LJ, and Bailar, JC, The Veterans Administration Cooperative Urological Research Group. 1967. Carcinoma of the prostate: Treatment comparisons. *J Urol* 98:516–522.
61. Henriksson, P, and Edhag, O. 1986. Orchidectomy versus oestrogen for prostatic cancer: Cardiovascular effects. *Br Med J* 293:413–415.
62. Garnick, MB, Glode, LM, and The Leuprolide Study Group. 1984. Leuprolide versus diethylstilbestrol for metastatic prostate cancer. *N Engl J Med* 311:1281–1286.
63. Torti, FM, and Carter, SK. 1980. The chemotherapy of prostatic adenocarcinoma. *Ann Intern Med* 92:681–689.
64. Green, N, Bodner, H, and Broth, E. 1985. Prostate cancer: Experience with definitive irradiation in the aged. *Urology* 25:228–232.
65. Kirk, D. 1985. Prostatic carcinoma. *Br Med J* 290: 875–876.
66. Torti, FM. 1984. Hormonal therapy for prostate cancer. *N Engl J Med* 311:1313–1314.
67. Horm, JW, and Kessler, LG. 1986. Falling rates of lung cancer in men in the United States. *Lancet* 1:425–426.
68. Ershler, WB, Socinski, MA, and Greene, CJ. 1983. Bronchogenic cancer, metastases, and aging. *J Am Geriatr Soc* 31:673–676.
69. Teeter, SM, Holmes, FF, and McFarlane, MJ. 1987. Lung carcinoma in the elderly: The influence of histology on the inverse relationship of stage to age. *Cancer* 60: 1331–1336.
70. Woolner, LB, et al. 1981. Mayo lung project: Evaluation of lung cancer screening through December 1979. *Mayo Clin Proc* 56:544–555.
71. Grant, IW. 1982. Screening for lung cancer. *Br Med J* 284:1209–1210.
72. Wellington, JL, and Lynn, RB. 1966. Thoracic surgery in the elderly. *Canad Med Assoc J* 95:252–256.
73. Kirsh, MM, et al. 1976. Major pulmonary resection for bronchogenic carcinoma in the elderly. *Ann Thorac Surg* 22:369–373.
74. Cox, JD, Komaki, R, and Eierst, DR. 1980. Irradiation for inoperable carcinoma of the lung and high performance status. *JAMA* 244:1931–1933.
75. Livingston, RB, et al. 1984. Long-term survival and toxicity in small cell lung cancer. *Am J Med* 77:415–417.
76. Clamon, GH, Audeh, MW, and Pinnick, S. 1982. Small cell lung carcinoma in the elderly. *J Am Geriatr Soc* 30: 299–302.
77. Rhodes, JB, Holmes, FF, and Clark, GM. 1977. Changing distribution of primary cancers in the large bowel. *JAMA* 238:1641–1643.
78. Butcher, D, et al. 1985. Female gender is a major determinant of changing subsite distribution of colorectal cancer with age. *Cancer* 56:714–716.
79. Gilbertsen, VA, and Nelms, JM. 1978. The prevention of invasive cancer of the rectum. *Cancer* 41:1137–1139.
80. Lotfi, AM, et al. 1986. Colorectal polyps and the risk of subsequent carcinoma. *Mayo Clin Proc* 61:337–343.
81. Burt, RW, et al. 1985. Dominant inheritance of adenomatous colonic polyps and colorectal cancer. *N Engl J Med* 312:1540–1544.
82. Gastrointestinal Tumor Study Group. 1984. Adjuvant therapy of colon cancer—results of a prospectively randomized trial. *N Engl J Med* 310:737–743.
83. Gastrointestinal Tumor Study Group. 1985. Prolongation of the disease-free interval in surgically treated rectal carcinoma. *N Engl J Med* 312:1465–1472.
84. Douglass, HO, and Moertel, CG. 1986. The Gastrointestinal Tumor Study Group: Survival after postoperative combination treatment of rectal cancer. *N Engl J Med* 315:1294–1295.
85. Kligerman, MM. 1975. Irradiation of the primary lesion of the rectum and rectosigmoid. *JAMA* 231:1381–1384.
86. Papillon, J. 1975. Resectable rectal cancers, treatment by curative endocavitary irradiation. *JAMA* 231:1385–1387.
87. Maartmann-Moe, H, and Hartveit, F. 1985. On the reputed decline in gastric carcinoma: Necropsy study from western Norway. *Br Med J* 290:103–105.
88. MacDonald, JS, et al. 1980. 5-Fluorouracil, doxorubicin, and mitomycin (FAM) combination chemotherapy for advanced gastric cancer. *Ann Intern Med* 93: 533–536.
89. Yang, CS. 1980. Research on esophageal cancer in China: A review. *Cancer Res* 40:2633–2644.
90. Guo, JH, and Wu, YK. 1984. Carcinoma of the esophagus and gastric cardia. Berlin-Heidelberg: Springer-Verlag.
91. Lowe, WC. 1972. Survival with carcinoma of the esophagus. *Ann Intern Med* 77:915–918.
92. Heit, HA, Johnson, LF, Siegel, SR, et al. 1978. Palliative dilation for dysphagia in esophageal carcinoma. *Ann Intern Med* 89:629–631.
93. Maruchi, N, et al. 1979. Cancer of the pancreas in Olmstead County, Minnesota, 1935–1974. *Mayo Clin Proc* 54:245–249.
94. Rehn, L. 1895. Blasengaschwultste bei Anilinarbeitern. *Arch Clin Chir* 50:588.
95. Cobb, BG, and Ansell, JS. 1965. Cigarette smoking and cancer of the bladder. *JAMA* 193:329–332.

96. DeWeerd, JH, and Colby Jr, MY. 1967. Bladder carcinoma: Combined radiotherapy and surgical treatment. *JAMA* 199:109–111.
97. Richardson, GS, et al. 1985. Common epithelial cancer of the ovary. *N Engl J Med* 312:415–424.
98. Campbell, S, et al. 1982. Real-time ultrasonography for determination of ovarian morphology and volume: A possible early screening test for ovarian cancer? *Lancet* 1:425–426.
99. Young, RC, et al. 1978. Advanced ovarian adenocarcinoma: a prospective clinical trial of melphalan (L-PAM) versus combination chemotherapy. *N Engl J Med* 299: 1261–1266.
100. Katz, ME, et al. 1981. Epithelial carcinoma of the ovary: Current strategies. *Ann Intern Med* 95:98–111.
101. Weiss, NS, Szekely, DR, and Austin, DF. 1976. Increasing incidence of endometrial cancer in the United States. *N Engl J Med* 294:1259–1262.
102. Weiss, NS, et al. 1979. Endometrial cancer in relation to patterns of menopausal estrogen use. *JAMA* 242: 261–264.
103. Shapiro, S, et al. 1985. Risk of localized and widespread endometrial cancer in relation to recent and discontinued use of conjugated estrogens. *N Engl J Med* 313: 969–972.
104. Yoonessi, M, Anderson, DG, and Morley, GW. 1979. Endometrial carcinoma: Causes of death and sites of treatment failure. *Cancer* 43:1944–1950.
105. Campion, MJ, et al. 1985. Increased risk of cervical neoplasia in consorts of men with penile condylomata acuminata. *Lancet* 1:943–946.
106. Mitchell, H, Drake, M, and Medley, G. 1986. Prospective evaluation of risk of cervical cancer after cytological evidence of human papilloma virus infection. *Lancet* 1: 573–575.
107. Wickenden, C, et al. 1985. Screening for wart virus infection in normal and abnormal cervices by DNA hybridization of cervical scrapes. *Lancet* 1:65–67.
108. Mandelblatt, J, Gopaul, I, and Wistreich, M. 1986. Gynecologic care of elderly women: Another look at Papanicolaou smear testing. *JAMA* 256:367–371.
109. Riesenberg, DE. 1986. The Papanicolaou test in elderly women. *JAMA* 256:393.
110. Roberts, AD, Denholm, RB, and Cordiner, JW. 1985. Cervical intraepithelial neoplasia in postmenopausal women with negative cervical cytology. *Br Med J* 290: 281.
111. Lewis, DR. 1966. Management of cervical carcinoma in the elderly patient. *J Arkansas Med Soc* 63:109–111.
112. Lee, JAH, and Storer, BA. 1980. Excess of malignant melanoma in women in the British Isles. *Lancet* 2:1337–1339.
113. Rampen, FHJ, and Mulder, JH. 1980. Malignant melanoma: an androgen-dependent tumor. *Lancet* 1:562–564.
114. Elwood, JM, et al. 1982. Pigmentation and skin reaction to sun as risk factors for cutaneous melanoma: Western Canada Melanoma Study. *Br Med J* 288:99–102.
115. Hirayama, R, et al. 1984. Different metastatic modes of malignant melanoma implanted in the ear of young and old mice. *Cancer Immunol Immunother* 18:209–214.
116. Begg, CB, and Carbone, PP. 1983. Clinical trials and drug toxicity in the elderly. *Cancer* 52:1986–1992.
117. Ludwig, H, Fritz, E, and Friedl, HP. 1982. Epidemiologic and age-dependent data on multiple myeloma in Austria. *JNCI* 68:729–733.
118. Peterson, BA, et al. 1982. Effect of age on therapeutic response and survival in advanced Hodgkin's disease. *Cancer Treat Rep* 66:889–898.
119. Bharucha, NE, Raven, RH, and Schoenberg, BS. 1985. Primary malignant nervous system neoplasms: Birth cohort effect in the elderly. *Arch Neurol* 42:1061–1062.

17

Pharmacotherapeutic Considerations in the Elderly Surgical Patient

Peter P. Lamy and Thomas H. Wiser

As the number of elderly persons is increasing rapidly (1), it is important to provide principles of pharmacotherapy in the elderly patient being considered for surgical intervention. Definition of therapeutic evaluation, use of practical bedside techniques, prevention of iatrogenic disease, and guidelines for therapeutic monitoring will be discussed to assist the surgeon to best monitor preoperative and postoperative outcomes in the elderly patient as they may be affected by drugs. Patients must be approached in a systematic manner depending on their physiologic and functional status. A practical and realistic pharmacotherapeutic database and management strategy should be established only after a thorough evaluation of the patient and consultation with the primary provider, family, and/or caregiver. Once a comprehensive data base is obtained, the general goals can be specifically tailored for special medical, psychosocial, and rehabilitative problems in order to define risk factors for surgical intervention, to minimize adverse perioperative outcomes (e.g., drug interactions or drug toxicity), and to assist the patient in a quick recovery without adverse or moribund outcome.

Because pharmacotherapeutic misadventures frequently occur in the elderly patient, there are several goals of the pharmacotherapeutic evaluation: (*a*) to provide an accurate definition of the current medical regimen (including the recent past) of both prescription and over-the-counter (OTC) medications; (*b*) to document previous adverse drug reactions; (*c*) to identify potential drug interactions with commonly used pre-anesthetic medications, anesthetic, and postoperative medications; (*d*) to identify pharmacokinetic/pharmacodynamic alterations in individual elderly surgical patients; and (*e*) to provide patient information and education about anesthetic agents, pain management, and other commonly used surgical medications.

Hospitalized patients receive numerous medications (2, 3), and surgical patients receive additional medications related to operative procedures and perioperative care. Drug use among elderly patients is even higher than among the younger population, leading to a higher prevalence of adverse drug reactions as well as drug interactions (4–7). By carefully performing a comprehensive medication history, thoroughly evaluating the patient's disease(s)/and problems, and knowledgeably applying basic pharmacodynamic/therapeutic/kinetic principles, most drug-related problems in the elderly surgical patient can be avoided.

Medication History

The first step is the determination of currently prescribed and over-the-counter medications. This information must include documentation of allergies, previous drug reactions, screening for drug interactions, determination of patient's compliance behavior, and efficacy of current therapeutic regimen.

The patient's medication history is usually incorpo-

Note: Dosages given in this chapter, unless otherwise specified, are the "usual" adult dose and may have to be adjusted to meet the needs of the individual patient.

rated into the medical data base. It is important to assist the patient in responding to this survey by determining the medications the patient has taken during the previous 24-hour period, starting with awakening the day before the survey. A similar procedure is helpful for nonprescription medications and can be initiated by asking what nonprescription medications the patient has taken within the last 30 days. Requesting the patient to bring all of the current medications at the time of evaluation, in the clinic or at the hospital, may obviate patient hesitancy, poor recall, or inappropriate drug labeling. The dosing schedule, indications, efficacy, and any adverse effects should be thoroughly documented (i.e., dose, frequency, specific time of administration during the day, effectiveness of therapy, duration of therapy, and any specific problems with the therapy).

In an effort to facilitate patient recall and increase accuracy and completeness of the medication history, one can ask about specific medication use during the review of systems. For example, in questioning the patient about ear-related problems, the provider should question about the specific use of any medication for the ears. It is not uncommon for a patient to respond negatively to a global question such as, "What nonprescription medications do you use?" yet respond positively to the specific question, "Do you use ear drops or any kind of medications for your ears?" Commonly used prescription and over-the-counter medications include those medications listed in Tables 17-1 and 17-2.

The second major objective of the medication history is to document previous adverse drug reactions including allergic, idiosyncratic, and toxic reactions. One may simply ask if the patient is allergic to any medications, foods, chemicals, or insects. Because medications are commonly used in the perioperative setting (anesthetics, narcotics, nonsteroidal anti-inflammatory agents, or antibiotics to mention a few), questions about specific adverse effects, side effects, or unusual reactions to these specific medications may help to obtain a positive response or document a pertinent negative response. When a positive response is obtained, further questioning should include: What symptoms were experienced?; Did the adverse reaction improve when the drug was discontinued or when a specific antagonist was given?; Did the adverse drug reaction reappear when the drug was readministered?; Was the severity of the reaction related to an increase or decrease in the dose?; Was a similar reaction to the same or similar therapeutic agent present earlier?; and Did your physician confirm the adverse events with any tests? During the evaluation process of the elderly surgical patient, previous administration of anesthesia should be specifically documented including when, where, type of surgery, and presence of any adverse effect.

Table 17-1. Prescription and over-the-counter drugs that elderly individuals commonly take

Analgesics Headache (Bufferin, Anacin, Excedrin) Arthritis (Anacin 3, Motrin, Nuprin)
Antihypertensives (Methyldopa, Propranolol, Reserpine)
Antianxiety (Compoz, Miles Nervine, Cope, Valium)
Diuretics (Chlorthalidone, HCTZ, Furosemide)
Hypnotics (Sominex, Dalmane)
Cough, cold, allergy products (Contac, Robitussin DM, Nose sprays)
Antacid products (Maalox, Mylanta)
Laxative products (Milk of Magnesia, Chronulac)
Antidiarrheal products (Kaopectate, Pepto Bismol, Lomotil)
Asthma products (Primatene inhaler, Alupent, Aminophyllin)
Weight control products (Dexatrim, Ayds)
Stimulant products (Sleep-eze, No Doz)
Otic products (Debrox, Cerumenex)
Eye products (Murine, Visine)
Ointments, creams, powders
Injections (Insulin, B_{12})
Personal care products (douches, deodorant products, depilatories, medicated shampoos)
Home remedies (herbal teas, sweet oil)
Vitamins, minerals, nutritional supplements

Note: List of products is not meant to be all-inclusive.

The most common causes for drug-related hospital admissions are noncompliance to prescription medications (10.5%) and adverse drug reactions (7.9%) (8). Early identification of noncompliance may not only preclude a hospital admission and possible surgical procedures, but explain the patient complaint. Noncompliance to long-term medication regimens can affect morbidity and mortality and may even pose serious threats to public health in chronically infected patients. Studies in inpatient as well as outpatient settings have shown that as many as

Table 17-2. The most frequently prescribed drugs for the elderly

Drug entities for those 85 years and older	Dollar volume Pennsylvania Pace Program[a]
Hydrochlorothiazide	Tagamet[R]
Digoxin	Feldene[R]
Aspirin	Procardia[R]
Potassium products	Zantac[R]
Triamterene	Transderm-Nitro 5[R]
Vitamin B_{12}	Aldomet[R]
Papaverine	Clinoril[R]
Isosorbide dinitrate	Darvocet-N[R] 100

[a]A prescription program for poor elderly in Pennsylvania.

75% of geriatric patients make errors in their compliance to prescriptions and one-fourth of those may be potentially serious. While noncompliance can be a problem at all ages, patients over 85 years who live alone, become confused, have memory lapses, and are not coping with disease states or life situation may be particularly likely to make errors in drug therapy, both over- and under-compliance (9). Compliance rates to long-term therapy are listed in Table 17-3.

Hypertension is an excellent example of how noncompliance can be a major problem. It has been suggested that the major problem in controlling hypertension is the failure of the patient to comply with therapy over time (10). It has also been suggested that the incidence of hypertension may be as high as 50% of patients aged 55 and over (11). Further, an evaluative study of 1001 patients over the age of 40, presenting for surgical interventions at Massachusetts General Hospital in 1977, indicated that 28% were hypertensive (12). Perhaps of even greater significance is the fact that abrupt discontinuation of antihypertensive medication is associated with rebound hypertension, angina, and edema (13). Numerous other chronic diseases, including cardiac arrhythmias, asthma, angina, and epilepsy, require continued compliance and maintenance of adequate therapeutic serum concentrations for successful management. Despite the severity of these disorders, less than 50% of recommended minimum serum concentrations of anti-arrhythmic, anti-asthmatic, and anticonvulsive therapy has been documented by various compliance studies (14–16). The Center for Disease Control stated that 23% to 31% of tuberculosis patients in the United States did not complete their antituberculosis therapy (17). Therfore, it is obvious that noncompliance with medication regimens plays a significant role in therapeutic failures, drug toxicities, hospitalizations, and disease and drug morbidity and mortality.

Table 17-3. Compliance to chronic therapeutic regimens

Therapeutic regimens	Compliance rate (%)
Hypertension treatment	
1 year	94
2 years	65
3 years	34
In general	53
Antibiotic treatment (in general)	33
Tuberculosis therapy	55
Sedative/hypnotics	42
Tranquilizers (in general)	54
Tranquilizers (in schizophrenic patients)	42
Insulin injections	48
Asthmatic medications	46
Glaucoma treatment	42

Source: Adapted from Sackett and Snow (149) and Dirks and Kinsman (150).

Identification, appropriate intervention, and documentation of a drug interaction with a current medication regimen or with anesthetic agents and other medications commonly used in the perioperative circumstance are important. Almost 7% of adverse drug reactions are attributed to drug interactions (18), with fatalities due to adverse drug interactions occurring at a rate of 0.29% of hospitalized patients (3). Studies evaluating drug interactions in institutionalized elderly patients suggest a rate substantially higher, 2.7% to 23.4% (19–21). Common, well-known risk factors predisposing elderly patients to drug interaction include the following: (*a*) increased medication use; (*b*) multiple health care providers; (*c*) purchase of medications from multiple pharmacies; (*d*) altered physiology; (*e*) concurrent use of nonprescription medications; and (*f*) concurrent use of alcohol (22, 23). Because of the plethora of drugs and the potential for drug interactions, it is impossible for the health care professional to remember virtually all drug interactions. A number of computerized drug interaction systems have been reported in the literature (24, 25) and a number of references on drug interactions are also available (26–28). The possibility of drug interactions should be considered during: (*a*) initiation of any new therapy; (*b*) occurrence of a possible adverse drug reaction; (*c*) inadequate therapeutic effects; and (*d*) for all patients on multiple drug therapies and for those demonstrating laboratory abnormalities.

Adverse drug reactions are significantly more common in elderly patients for the following reasons: (*a*) signs and symptoms of adverse reactions may be different in older individuals; (*b*) temporal relationships may be prolonged for the development of an adverse drug reaction to occur; (*c*) adverse reactions may occur even after a medication has been discontinued in an older individual, and untoward reactions can suddenly develop even to a medication that has been used chronically without problems. Therapeutic misadventures are also known to increase in frequency with age as documented by the classic study by Hurwitz and Wade (29) who also identified predisposing factors to these adverse drug reactions (30). Data in Table 17-4 clearly demonstrate that the rate of adverse drug reactions increases with age. Reasons for this apparent increased susceptibility to adverse drug reactions are multifactorial, including physical, psychologic and/or socioeconomic factors. Elderly patients have multiple medical problems. Four of every 5 elderly patients have at least one chronic illness and often more, and thus, the frequency of drug use by elderly patients also increases with age (Table 17-5) (31).

Altered physiologic functions also play a significant

Table 17-4. Age and adverse reactions

Age of patients (years)	Number of given drugs	Number with reactions	Rate (%)
<60	667	42	6.3
60–69	252	27	10.7
70–79	178	38	21.3
80–89	59	11	18.6
90–99	4	0	0

Adapted from Hurwitz, N, and Wade, OL (29).

role in the development of adverse drug reactions. First, body composition changes with age, affecting drug distribution significantly. For example, total body water decreases linearly with age after age 25 in both men and women (6, 32). The ratio of lean body mass to body weight also decreases. Lean body mass may be as much as 30% less in elderly than in young persons (6). Total body fat also increases with age, proportional to total body mass (33), and may represent an average increase in total adipose tissue from 18% to 36% in men to 33% to 45% in women. These changes prolong and possibly increase the activity of lipophilic drugs (benzodiazepines, phenothiazines, barbiturates) and may have an opposite effect on water-soluble drugs such as antibiotics.

The cardiovascular system undergoes significant pathologic and physiologic changes with aging, including increased peripheral vascular resistance (resulting in redistribution of blood flow), increased atherosclerotic coronary artery disease and valvular aortic stenosis, and a decline in cardiac output. While blood flow to the muscles, brain, and coronary arteries seems to be maintained, blood flow to the kidneys, liver, and gastrointestinal tract is decreased. These changes may alter drug absorption, metabolism, and elimination. They may also adversely affect the patient's operative survival (34). It should be pointed out that cardiac output in healthy elderly patients is unchanged (35).

The effect of aging on renal function has been well documented and is easily measured by routine clinical laboratory procedures. Because many drugs are excreted by renal processes, either fully or to a significant degree, impaired renal function could result in retention of drugs and increased drug toxicity. A number of anatomic and physiologic changes are known to occur in renal function with increasing age. For example, kidney mass (weight and volume) decreases approximately 20% to 30% between the ages of 30 and 90 years, and total number of glomeruli decrease approximately 30% to 50% (4, 36–38). Renal plasma flow decreases by approximately 1.5% per year between the ages 20 to 90 years, with a resulting diminished glomerular filtration rate by about 1 ml/min / 1.73 m^2/year and an average reduction of about 30% to 46% (4, 39). Other important changes in renal function include the lessened ability to concentrate urine and conserve the sodium (and water) balance (40, 41). These changes result in a reduction in creatinine clearance. A parallel reduction in urinary creatinine excretion per 24 hours (thought to be the result of decreased muscle mass with increased age) also takes place, resulting in serum creatinine concentrations that remain constant. A decrease in creatinine clearance is much more extensive in the elderly patient before serum creatinine increases. Thus, there is a false normalcy in serum creatinine in the elderly person, even though renal function may be substantially reduced. Commonly used nomograms and formulas are highly recommended to estimate true creatinine clearance with respect to increasing age (42, 43). Alterations in dosages and schedules of commonly used therapeutic agents as developed by Bennett et al. (44) are also extremely helpful and serve as guidelines for drug usage in elderly patients.

These anatomic and physiologic changes in renal function create the need for cautious use of many therapeutic agents. Commonly prescribed agents that require adjustments in dose or dosing intervals based on renal function are seen in Table 17-6. Particularly in patients 75 years or older, substantive changes in dosing and/or intervals of administration may be required (Table 17-7).

In addition to important pharmacokinetic implications for commonly used drugs for the elderly, there is a

Table 17-5. Prescription and nonprescription drug use

	Number of prescription drugs		Number of nonprescription drugs	
Age in years	Female	Male	Female	Male
All ages	3.8	2.2	3.1	2.6
50–64	4.2	2.4	3.1	3.0
65+	5.7	4.1	3.2	3.7

Adapted from Stewart, RB, and Cluff, LE (31).

Table 17-6. Commonly prescribed therapeutic agents requiring a change in dose and/or dosing intervals as a result of altered kidney function

Allopurinol	Indomethacin
Antimicrobial agents (most antibiotics)	Lithium Meperidine
Carbamazepine	Metoclopramide
Chlorpropamide	Propoxyphene
Cimetidine	Procainamide
Digoxin	Sulindac
Disopyramide	Tolbutamide

Table 17-7. The 10 most frequently prescribed drugs for patients 75 years and older

Drugs	Alteration required with decreased renal function
Hydrochlorothiazide	Avoid use when GFR is less than 25–30 ml/min.
Digoxin	Dose alterations required when GFR is less than 50 ml/min (therapeutic drug monitoring helpful in reduced creatinine clearances).
Furosemide	No dose alteration required as the result of diminished GFR, but significant dehydration may occur as the result of inability to conserve sodium as efficiently as younger patients.
Triamterene	Avoid when GFR is less than 10 ml/min. Active metabolites have increased $T_{1/2}$ with decreased GFR.
Aspirin	Avoid when GFR is less than 10 ml/min, but may add to gastrointestinal hemorrhage associated with uremia and may decrease GFR when renal blood flow is prostaglandin-dependent.
Propranolol	No alterations required with decreased GFR but active metabolites may accumulate. Titrate to desired pharmacodynamic response and monitor for commonly encountered beta-blocking agent toxicities.
Methyldopa	Drug and metabolites accumulate with decreasing GFR. Monitor pharmacodynamic responses (blood pressures including orthostatic changes) more closely.
Potassium Supplement	Potassium tends to be retained in most diminished GFR states (exceptions always noted). Increased serum electrolyte monitoring is paramount.
Vitamin B_{12}	No dose alterations required.
Nitroglycerin	No dose alterations required in diminished GFR, but increased pharmacodynamic monitoring is prudent (blood pressure, creatinine clearance).

Adapted from Koch, H, and Smith, MC (151).

host of drugs used by the anesthesiologist and surgeon that requires similar changes in doses or dosing intervals as a result of diminished renal function in elderly patients (Table 17-8).

Impairment of renal function also mandates careful monitoring of intraoperative fluid administration and urinary output. It has been demonstrated by Rush and coworkers (45) that postoperative depression of renal function can also be determined by the site and magnitude of surgery. For example, diminished renal blood flow and concomitant glomerular filtration rate reduction may occur more often in patients undergoing an extensive abdominal operation when compared to patients undergoing lesser abdominal surgery.

In conclusion, impairment of renal function has several implications: altered pharmacodynamic and pharmacokinetic variables of commonly used drugs are likely, and the diminished capacity of the elderly to conserve water with a blunted response to sodium shifts produce altered pharmacodynamic responses in many agents. For example, diuretics increase the risk of volume depletion during common processes such as mild diarrhea and vomiting, often seen in elderly surgical patients.

The liver is responsible for drug metabolism. These metabolic processes are highly variable and are affected by numerous parameters including race, gender, genetics, environment, smoking, other drugs, nutritional status, and diseases (6). The lack of routine clinical laboratory measurements of liver function also dramatically influences how clinicians can monitor for structural and functional changes in the liver. Several variables are known. Liver weight decreases with age by about 1% per/year after the age of 40 (46). Blood flow to the liver also declines as age increases, as evidenced by delayed clearance of indocyanine green, by about 40% from age 25 to 75, which averages about 0.5% to 1% per year (47). Other studies indicate that the aging process is also associated with an age-related decline in most liver enzyme activity, reduced drug metabolism by mixed-oxidase enzyme systems, and increased susceptibility to drug-induced liver dysfunction (48–50). While it is clear that altered pharmacodynamic and pharmacokinetic changes in drug therapy are not as well documented with hepatic disease as they are with renal disease, a number of therapeutic agents commonly used during the perioperative period are affected by hepatic dysfunction (Table 17-9) (46, 47, 49–56).

It is apparent, then, that pharmacokinetic alterations of numerous therapeutic agents may play a significant role in the perioperative evaluation of all patients, particularly the elderly. Preoperative liver disease is also associated with a high rate of postoperative morbidity and mortality, whereas the clinical significance of mild liver impairment is uncertain (57). In addition, it is clear that the general pharmacodynamic response to a general anesthetic agent can be affected by reduced liver blood flow, which seems to have no clinical significance in a patient with a normal liver. Well elderly patients who tend to have lower hepatic blood flow may be more susceptible to the effects of anes-

Table 17-8. Therapeutic agents commonly used by anesthesiologists and surgeons requiring dosing adjustment in diminished GFR

Therapeutic agent and/or therapeutic classification	Dosing changes as the result of diminished renal function
Aminoglycosides Amikacin Gentamicin Tobramycin	Dosage adjustment is required and/or lengthening dosing intervals as GFR decreases; therapeutic drug monitoring is paramount in patients with diminished GFR. Nephrotoxicity common with elevated, sustained peak and/or trough serum drug concentrations.
Anesthetic Agents Halothane Enflurane Isoflurane Methoxyflurane Nitrous Oxide (N_2O)	Detrimental only during periods of hypotension. The general pharmacologic properties of general anesthetic agents include decreased cardiac output, decreased cardiac contractility, decreased total vascular resistance and hypotension; all of these pharmacologic effects also decrease GFR. The exception to this principle is nitrous oxide, which increases total peripheral vascular resistance and increases cardiac output. Methoxyflurane has also been associated with nephrotoxicity and its use should be limited.
Analgesics	
Non-narcotic analgesics	
Acetaminophen	No changes in dosage required with 4–6-hour intervals in patients with 10–50 ml/min. GFR and 8-hour intervals in patients with less than 10 ml/min.; nephrotoxic in overdose.
Aspirin	Avoid use with GFR less than 10 ml/min; nephrotoxic in overdose; may decrease GFR when renal blood flow is prostaglandin dependent; gastrointestinal bleeding tendencies increase during uremia.
NSAIDs[a]	
Ibuprofen, Indomethacin Naproxen Sulindac	Dosages are generally unchanged with decreased GFR but may produce decreased GFR when renal blood flow is prostaglandin dependent.
Narcotic analgesics and narcotic antagonists	
Butorphanol	Unchanged with diminished GFR; increased need for monitoring for sedation and respiratory depression.
Codeine	Unchanged with diminished GFR; increased need for monitoring for sedation and respiratory depression.
Fentanyl	Unchanged with diminished GFR; increased need for monitoring for sedation and respiratory depression.
Meperidine	Unchanged with diminished GFR; metabolite accumulates in renal failure resulting in seizures.
Methadone	Dosage and intervals unchanged except where GFR is less than 10 ml/min, dosage should be reduced by approximately half; $T_{1/2}$ equals approximately 22 hours during chronic therapy.
Morphine	Dosage unchanged with diminished GFR; sedation and respiratory depression may occur with increased frequency in elderly patients; recent data show that indeed some accumulation may occur with diminished renal function and chronic administration (155).
Naloxone	Dosage unchanged with diminished GFR.
Propoxyphene	Dosage unchanged until GFR less than 10 ml/min; dose should be reduced dramatically (25%) or not used at all.
Barbiturates	
Thiopental	Dosage is unchanged until GFR is less than 10 ml/min at which time dose should be reduced to 75%.
Benzodiazepines Chlordiazepoxide Diazepam Lorazepam Oxazepam	In general, benzodiazepines are metabolized by liver mechanisms (except lorazepam and oxazepam) and require no dosage adjustment with diminished GFR; increased pharmacodynamic effects are noted. Shorter acting and renally excreted drugs are preferred with dosage titration to pharmacologic effect to avoid adverse effects.
Neuromuscular blocking agents	
Atracurium	No dosage adjustments required for renal failure.
Gallamine	Drug should be avoided with GFR less than 50 ml/min.; increased neuromuscular blockade with aminoglycoside antibiotics, hypokalemia (diuretics, amphotericin B), and narcotics.
Neostigmine	Dosage adjustments not required until GFR less than 10 ml/min; intervals should be extended from 6 to 12 hours.
Pancuronium	Dosage adjustment not required until GFR less than 10 ml/min; drug should be avoided at that time because active metabolites accumulate.

(*continued*)

Table 17-8. (*continued*)

Therapeutic agent and/or therapeutic classification	Dosing changes as the result of diminished renal function
Pyridostigmine	Dosage adjustments not required in renal failure, however patients with endstage renal disease may be predisposed to drug action and develop bladder atony.
Succinylcholine	Dosage adjustment not required in renal failure; close monitoring for hyperkalemia is required in patients with endstage renal disease.
Tubocurarine	Dosage adjustment not required in renal failure.
Vecuronium	Dosage adjustment not required during renal failure.

[a]Nonsteroidal anti-inflammatory drugs.

thesia on hepatic blood flow, but clinical research has not yet tested this hypothesis. A few patients appear to have a specific hypersensitivity, "halothane hepatitis," predisposing these patients to postoperative hepatocellular dysfunction after the administration of a general anesthetic (57).

Certain "stresses" have been identified as having the potential for causing further deterioration of a previously damaged liver, including abdominal surgery, sepsis, hypotension, hypokalemia, and hypovolemia (58). Therefore, in the clinical strategic process in the evaluation of the elderly surgical patient, preoperative liver function tests are required to establish a baseline. Prevention of the predisposing "stresses" is essential.

Altered Pharmacodynamic Responses

Drug receptor response, defined as the pharmacologic response after a drug-end-organ interaction and often called tissue sensitivity, may be altered in elderly patients. There may be an exacerbated or diminished pharmacodynamic response. For example, warfarin will achieve the same degree of elevation in the prothrombin time with a lower serum concentration in elderly persons compared to younger patients (59). In elderly patients propranolol and isoproterenol produce a lesser cardiac pharmacodynamic effect when compared to younger patients (i.e., older patients seem to be resistant to isoproterenol and propranolol) (60). Numerous explanations for these altered pharmacodynamic responses include depletion of neurotransmitters, presence of disease, and physiologic and nutritional changes that occur in the normal aging process. An interesting phenomenon demonstrating this altered response pertinent to the surgical evaluation of the elderly patient is the inverse relationship between age and general anesthetic requirements. Older patients are more easily anesthetized. Gregory et al. (61) found that the minimum alveolar anesthetic concentration (MAC) decreases with advancing age from a value of 1.1% in the neonate to 0.64% in the patient over 70 years of age (61). Other drugs pertinent to surgery and anesthesia that exhibit altered responses in elderly patients are the muscle relaxants and analgesics. Neuromuscular blockade is more intense and prolonged, and reversal by antagonists is more difficult with advancing age (62, 63). It has been suggested that the neuromuscular junction is more sensitive to these agents and clearance is diminished. Reversal of the action of these agents should be accomplished with short-acting agents, such as edrophonium chloride, which may also have a longer duration and more pronounced effect in the elderly. Elderly patients are also known to have increased sensitivity to narcotics and analgesics. It is difficult to differentiate between pharmacokinetic and pharmacodynamic influences responsible for increased central nervous system sensitivity. Kaiko (64) demonstrated that morphine is approximately twice as effective in the elderly as compared to young persons. Other agents with increased pharmacodynamic responses in elderly patients are listed in Table 17-10. Because elderly patients may demonstrate increased sensitivity to numerous therapeutic agents, careful clinical monitoring of efficacy and toxicity concomitant with therapeutic drug monitoring (use of plasma drug concentrations) is required to obtain the specific therapeutic goal(s) and prevent adverse effects.

Pulmonary Alterations

Numerous changes occur in pulmonary function with age, including increased chest wall rigidity, narrowing of the airway, loss of elastic recoil, reduced alveolar surface area, and decreased diaphragmatic excursion. These changes combine to reduce pulmonary function oxygenation and thus increase the risk for respiratory failure (65, 66). A thorough evaluation, coordinated with the internist/family physician, surgeon, anesthesiologist, and allied health professionals from nursing, pharmacy, and dietary will serve to decrease the likelihood of untoward events (including pharmacologic misadventures) in the perioperative period.

Table 17-9. Commonly used perioperative medications affected by hepatic dysfunction

Drug	Comments
Acetaminophen	Reduced clearance may occur in the presence of hepatitis.
Alprazolam	Increased plasma protein binding, decreased clearance, and increased half-life in the presence of cirrhosis and aging.
Amikacin	No apparent changes occur in liver disease.
Atracurium	No apparent changes occur in liver disease.
Carbamazepine	Few data available on the effects of various liver disease states, however, because the drug is almost completely metabolized by the liver its clearance may be decreased in liver disease.
Carbenicillin	Half-life is significantly increased in oliguric patients with concomitant liver disease.
Cefoperazone	Hepatitis decreases hepatic clearance without change in volume of distribution and serum half-life; cirrhosis has no effect on clearance but increases volume of distribution and serum half-life.
Cefotaxime	Has been associated with drug-induced hepatic disease; no change in serum half-life noted during hepatitis.
Chloramphenicol	Cirrhosis decreases plasma protein binding, decreases clearance, increases serum half-life without apparent changes in volume of distribution.
Chlordiazepoxide	Cirrhosis decreases plasma protein binding, clearance, and increases serum half-life and volume of distribution.
Chlorpromazine	Cirrhosis causes no apparent changes in pharmacokinetic variables.
Cimetidine	Cirrhosis causes no apparent changes in pharmacokinetic variables.
Desmethyldiazepam	An active metabolite of diazepam; clearance is decreased in hepatitis and cirrhosis with no changes in volume of distribution and increased serum half-life.
Diazepam	Plasma protein binding and clearance are decreased in cirrhosis and hepatitis, whereas volume of distribution and serum half-life are increased.
Diphenhydramine	Plasma protein binding is decreased in the presence of cirrhosis whereas clearance and volume of distribution are unchanged; serum half-life is increased.
Erythromycin	Serum half-life increased in the presence of cirrhosis.
Furosemide	Volume of distribution and serum half-life are increased in the presence of cirrhosis, whereas clearance is unchanged and plasma protein binding is decreased.
Hexobarbital	Serum half-life is increased in the presence of cirrhosis; volume of distribution and protein binding are unchanged; clearance is decreased.
Isoniazid	Serum half-life is increased in the presence of cirrhosis.
Isosorbide dinitrate	Clearance is decreased in the presence of cirrhosis.
Labetalol	Clearance and serum half-life is unchanged in the presence of cirrhosis; oral bioavailability is increased.
Lidocaine	Clearance is decreased in the presence of cirrhosis; volume of distribution and serum half-life are increased.
Lorazepam	Volume of distribution and serum half-life are increased in the presence of cirrhosis; clearance is unchanged and protein binding is decreased.
Meperidine	Volume of distribution and serum half-life are increased in the presence of cirrhosis; clearance and plasma protein binding are decreased.
Metoprolol	Serum half-life and oral bioavailability are increased in the presence of cirrhosis.
Metronidazole	Clearance is decreased in the presence of cirrhosis.
Morphine	Plasma protein binding is decreased in the presence of cirrhosis, whereas clearance, volume of distribution, and serum half-life are unchanged.
Nafcillin	Significant increase in serum half-life noted in extrahepatic biliary obstruction; half-life unchanged in the presence of unobstructed cirrhosis; cirrhosis also decreases volume of distribution and clearance but increases the percent of urinary excretion.
Naproxen	Plasma protein binding and volume of distribution are increased in the presence of cirrhosis along with a decrease in the clearance of unbound drug suggesting a dosage decrease in the presence of cirrhosis.
Oxazepam	No apparent pharmacokinetic variable changes in the presence of cirrhosis.
Phenobarbital	Serum half-life increases in the presence of cirrhosis (also with aging) with no apparent changes in urinary excretion percentage.

(*continued*)

Table 17-9. *(continued)*

Drug	Comments
Phenytoin	Decreased plasma protein binding in the presence of hepatitis and cirrhosis.
Prednisolone	No pharmacokinetic changes in the presence of hepatitis.
Prednisone	No pharmacokinetic changes in the presence of hepatitis.
Propranolol	Serum half-life and volume of distribution are increased in the presence of hepatitis; clearance decreases.
Quinidine	Cirrhosis increases serum half-life and volume of distribution and decreases plasma protein binding with no apparent change in clearance.
Ranitidine	Serum half-life increases in the presence of cirrhosis with no changes in volume of distribution and increases noted in oral bioavailability.
Theophylline	Cirrhosis and hepatitis increase serum half-life, volume of distribution clearance, and plasma protein binding.
Thiopental	Increased serum half-life, decreased plasma protein binding, and no change in clearance in patients with cirrhosis.
Tubocurarine	No apparent changes in pharmacokinetic variables occur as a result of cirrhosis.
Verapamil	Serum half-life, volume of distribution, and plasma protein binding are increased in the presence of cirrhosis, whereas clearance is decreased.

Adverse Drug Reactions (ADRs)

Definition/Classifications

A major goal of the medication history is to document previous adverse drug reactions including allergic, idiosyncratic, and toxic reactions. To adequately assess and document adverse drug reactions, clarification of definitions and classifications is necessary.

An adverse drug reaction can be defined as any noxious, unintended, and undesired effect of a drug after administration for prophylaxis, diagnosis, or therapy (67). The clinical manifestations of an ADR may be any abnormal sign or symptom, an abnormal laboratory test, or a combination of both. This definition excludes therapeutic failures, overdoses (intentional or accidental), and drug abuse.

An adverse drug reaction may be classified into three categories: (*a*) hypersensitivity reactions; (*b*) idiosyncratic reactions, or (*c*) predictable reactions (extensions of the pharmacologic effect or toxic reaction).

Table 17-10. Therapeutic agents demonstrating increased pharmacodynamic responses in elderly patients

- Antihypertensives
- Antipsychotics, e.g.,
  - Chlorpromazine
  - Thioridazine
- Barbiturates
- Benzodiazepines
- Digoxin
- Heparin
- Narcotic analgesics
- Warfarin

Hypersensitivity Reactions

Hypersensitivity reactions are allergic phenomena mediated immunologically. There are many different manifestations of drug hypersensitivity. They rarely are diagnostic or unique to any specific drug or allergic reaction; all allergic clinical manifestations can be evoked by antigens other than drugs. Allergic responses, regardless of the etiology, have several distinctive characteristic features: (*a*) there is no correlation with known pharmacodynamic characteristics of the suspected agent, unlike a toxic reaction; (*b*) there is no dose response relationship; (*c*) numerous associated symptoms often coexist, including rash, angioedema, anaphylaxis, asthma, or even a serum sickness-like syndrome; (*d*) clinical manifestations do not occur on primary exposure; (*e*) clinical manifestations disappear with cessation of therapy and reappear after administration of therapy, and (*f*) responses usually occur in only a small number of persons receiving the suspected offending agent. Because of the heterogeneity of hypersensitivity reactions, classification is useful not only in providing insight into the pathogenesis, but also for allowing appropriate therapeutic intervention.

Type I hypersensitivity reactions occur in a small number of surgical patients with a frequency of about 1 in 5000 due to anesthetic agents (68). Clinical features of Type I hypersensitivity reactions include urticaria, asthma (shortness of breath, wheezing, stridor), angioedema, anaphylaxis, flushing, itching, hypotension, nausea, vomiting, or diarrhea with/without abdominal pain, and occasionally convulsions, coma, and urinary incontinence. Anaphylaxis is thought to be secondary to a rapid, massive release of mediators such as histamine, kinins, and SRS-A (slow reacting substance of anaphylaxis). A sensitized individual will release these mediators when the antibody (usually from the IgE class), is fixed on the cell surface in the presence of the antigen, resulting in a sudden release of the mediators. These rare reactions are important, since a large proportion of these reactions can lead to death, with drug allergies being the most common cause (69). Certain drugs, such as morphine, meperidine, or radiocontrast dyes, cause physical degranulation of mast cells and histamine release without IgE involvement. The end result, however, is similar to anaphylaxis and is referred to as an anaphylactoid reaction (70).

Type II hypersensitivity reactions occur when an antibody reacts with antigenic components of a cell or tissue or an antigen that has become intimately coupled to cells or tissues. These antibodies (IgM or IgG) are cytotoxic. This least common category of drug hypersensitivity reaction is best exemplified by the Coombs' test, i.e., positive autoimmune hemolytic anemia, occurring secondary to the administration of methyldopa. Mismatching of blood products or plasma transfusions can also result in Type II hypersensitivity reactions. In the latter example, the antigen binds to the red blood cell surface, and the antibodies react to activate complement and destroy the red blood cells.

Type III hypersensitivity reactions are also referred to as Arthus reactions and are mediated by IgG, IgM, and complement. Common examples include the immune complex reaction, which occurs when IgG reacts with tissue and causes destruction, as exemplified by serum sickness commonly reported with penicillin, aspirin, and sulfa drugs. The serum sickness usually develops in about 1 to 2 weeks after the initiation of therapy and is commonly characterized by the following clinical features: fever, arthralgias, urticaria, and lymphadenopathy. Treatment of such reactions includes early recognition, discontinuation of the offending agents, antihistamines (for itching), analgesics (for pain), and antipyretics (for fever).

Type IV hypersensitivity reactions are also commonly referred to as cell-mediated, delayed, or tuberculin-type hypersensitivity reactions. These reactions are produced by sensitized T-cells. Lymphocytes (or macrophages), after contact with an antigen, produce an inflammatory reaction that results in direct cytotoxicity or the release of lymphokines with a subsequent influx of neutrophils in macrophages. Type IV hypersensitivity reactions differ from other immune reactions in that they are mediated by sensitized lymphocytes and not antibodies. Allergic contact dermatitis from the topical use of medications is a common and important example of this type of reaction. Another important and interesting aspect of this reaction is exemplified by the patient with a known contact dermatitis who subsequently receives the specific offending agent systemically and has a generalized reaction with a more pronounced reaction over the area previously affected. Type IV reactions can be manifested in various responses, including eczema, pruritus, or erythema, and form a papillar eruption which, in turn, can be followed by edema and vesiculation and progress to bullae and other severe reactions (71). The histologic characterization of these lesions include infiltration of lymphocytes, basophils, and eosinophils. Chronic exposure to known offending agents may result in lichenification acanthosis. Drugs commonly associated with conditions related to contact dermatitis include local anesthetics, topical antihistamines, topical antibiotics, cosmetic creams containing paraben esters, and even corticosteroid creams.

Drug Fever

Drug fever is thought to be due to a number of different mechanisms in addition to hypersensitivity, including: (*a*) release of bacterial pyrogens, (*b*) contamination of drugs with exogenous pyrogens, (*c*) release of endogenous pyrogens from sterile inflammatory lesions at the site of an intramuscular injection, (*d*) increased tissue metabolism, (*e*) peripheral vasoconstriction with reduced heat loss, (*f*) central effects, and (*g*) hormonal effects (71). However, as many as 25% of drug fevers may be hypersensitivity related (72) including the following commonly encountered perioperative medications: ketamine, methoxyflurane, thiopental, halothane, D-tubocurarine, and scopolamine (72). It should be noted, however, that drug fever has not been reported secondary to cross sensitization between anesthetics (73).

To make the issue more confusing, elderly patients tend to maintain lower body temperatures without appearing ill or feeling cold (22). Also, elderly patients with infections or allergic responses present with more general symptomatology than younger patients, including confusion, anorexia, lethargy, rapid respiratory rate, or tachycardia and, less reliably, a high-grade fever (74). In fact, classic signs and symptoms of a focal infection are often missing, and the rule of thumb is to suspect infection or allergy in any elderly patient with a low-grade fever and multiple, nonspecific complaints.

When febrile responses are noted, it may be the direct effect of pharmacologic intervention. For example, phenothiazines and other agents causing dopamine blockade interfere with hypothalamic thermal regulation by inhibiting normal compensatory cooling mechanisms (75). In addition, the anticholinergic effect of many medications may prevent heat loss by CNS-induced anhydrosis, and vasoconstrictors such as epinephrine, may increase temperature by peripheral mechanisms (75). Rarely, general anesthetics cause a malignant hyperthermic response in genetically susceptible individuals. The clinical manifestations of this reaction include a rapid increase in body temperature with a concomitant increase in oxygen consumption and carbon dioxide production with possible death. Early recognition by frequent temperature monitoring and treatment with dantrolene sodium and supportive measures are generally recommended for early detection and prevention of mortality (76).

Idiosyncratic Reactions

Idiosyncratic reactions are rare effects unrelated to the pharmacology of the specific offending agent and differ from hypersensitivity reactions by failure to demonstrate an immunologic basis of the adverse effect.

Idiosyncratic reactions are unpredictable and often are difficult to distinguish from hypersensitivity reactions, as exemplified by the halothane-induced hepatitis syndrome. Halothane hepatitis is heralded by the onset of fever accompanied by anorexia, nausea, and vomiting 2 to 5 days after anesthesia. Biochemical and histologic abnormalities indicative of hepatitis are characteristically found, and mortality is significant, as high as 50%. Eosinophilia only rarely accompanies the syndrome, and the syndrome seems to be unrelated to mild elevations in serum transaminases, which occur in about 20% of patients receiving halothane. The hepatitis syndrome may occur between 1 in 6,000 and 1 in 22,000 exposures. The mechanism of hepatitis is further confounded by the fact that one of halothane's main metabolites, trifluoro acetic acid, has been shown to be antigenic in animal studies (48).

Predictable Reactions

Most adverse drug reactions are direct extensions of the pharmacologic effect of any therapeutic agent. For example, dry mouth with antidepressants, sedation with phenobarbital, postural and/or exercised-induced hypotension with an adrenergic blocking agent, such as guanethidine, are predictable events and result from an exaggerated pharmacologic effect. Well-known examples seen perioperatively are the prolongation of bleeding time up to twice normal by inhibition of platelet aggregation with less than 1 aspirin tablet (77), and prolonged apnea secondary to neuromuscular blocking agents such as d-tubocurarine, pancuronium, or succinylcholine.

Probability of Adverse Drug Reaction

Adverse drug reactions are categorized into definite, probable, possible, conditional, or doubtful probability using the following definitions (78–80).

A definite adverse drug reaction meets the following criteria: 1) follows a close temporal relationship to the administration of the drug or occurs in the presence of a documented drug level in body fluids or tissues, 2) follows the known adverse drug response patterns to the suspected etiologic agent, 3) improves on discontinuation of the suspected agent (dechallenge) and 4) reappears upon reexposure (rechallenge), and 5) the reaction is not compatible with the known characteristic of the patient's disease(s).

A probable adverse drug reaction meets the following criteria: 1) follows a reasonable temporal sequence with respect to drug administration, 2) demonstrates a known adverse drug reaction response pattern of the suspected drug, 3) improves with dechallenge, 4) is not compatible with the known characteristics of the patient's disease(s).

A possible adverse drug reaction meets the following criteria: 1) demonstrates a reasonable temporal sequence with respect to drug administration, 2) follows a known adverse drug reaction response pattern of the suspected etiologic agent, 3) may have been compatible with the patient disease(s) or other medications patient was taking concomitantly (or recently discontinued).

A conditional adverse drug reaction meets the following criteria: 1) follows a reasonable temporal sequence with respect to the administration of the suspected etiologic agent, 2) may not follow a known adverse drug reaction response pattern, and 3) cannot be ruled out by the known characteristic of the patient clinical status. (The purpose of this category is to prevent the loss of a previously unsuspected reaction and serve as a basis to help identify new adverse drug reactions.)

A doubtful adverse drug reaction does not meet any of the previously mentioned criteria.

Many adverse drug reactions are categorized as probable or possible because rechallenge is not commonly performed for obvious reasons.

Adverse Drug Reactions to Specific Perioperative Medications

Narcotic analgesics and sedatives/tranquilizers are often administered before surgery to reduce the intensity and/or severity of pain anxiety, to facilitate a smooth induction of anesthesia, and to allow reduced dosage of general anesthetic agents. Although a degree of respiratory depression occurs in most patients, treatment is not required until significant clinical symptomatology or abnormal arterial blood gases are obtained.

Morphine is a potent narcotic analgesic used to relieve severe, acute pain. It is the standard for opioid analgesics and antagonists. It is used in the preoperative stages for its sedative properties and as a supplement to anesthetic analgesia. Most adverse drug reactions related to morphine are extensions of its pharmacologic effect, such as hypotension through histamine-induced arterial dilatation, depression of respiration due to decreased carbon dioxide responsiveness of the medulla, pupillary constriction, and nausea/vomiting most likely secondary to a direct effect on the central nervous system (70). A serious adverse effect of morphine is respiratory depression. This may require use of resuscitative equipment, oxygen therapy, or possibly an opiate antagonist such as naloxone, throughout the operation and into the postoperative phase. Because morphine induces smooth muscle hypertonicity, difficult urination may subsequently develop and require catheterization, especially in elderly patients. The urinary retention may persist for 10 to 20 hours postadministration and is more commonly associated with epidural or intrathecal administration. Administration of low-dose naloxone (0.2 mg) is usually adequate to reverse the urinary retention abnormality. Hypersensitivity reactions to morphine include skin rashes with wheal and flair-type reactions proximal to the site of intravenous injection. Presumably, this is caused by a direct histamine release mechanism and is not immunologically mediated. An interesting explanation for prolonged or delayed adverse reactions to morphine in elderly patients is the observation that analgesia lags behind plasma morphine levels, implying that brain morphine concentrations may be delayed. They may be reduced at a slower rate than plasma levels.

Other major disadvantages of systemic morphine administration include: (*a*) nausea and vomiting, which can be severe and prolonged; (*b*) drowsiness, preventing early ambulation; and (*c*) reduced gastrointestinal motility (81).

Meperidine (Demerol[R]) is another commonly used narcotic analgesic with a very similar adverse drug reaction profile and pharmacologic actions similar to morphine. It requires dosages 10 times those of morphine for equianalgesic effects. Meperidine depresses the respiratory center but appears to produce less nausea and vomiting than morphine, as well as less reduction in blood pressure, but is more often associated with tachycardia. A variety of CNS excitation effects have been reported, including tremors, muscle twitching, myoclonus and seizures, presumably due to normeperidine, the metabolite of meperidine. Normeperidine accumulates when high doses of meperidine are used and also in renal dysfunction. Therefore, close and careful monitoring is required when meperidine is used in elderly patients (82). Meperidine is commonly used in combination with promethazine (Phenergan[R]), or hydroxyzine (Vistaril[R]) to provide increased sedation. When meperidine is used with a phenothiazine or a related drug, its dosage should be reduced by 25% to 50% to reduce respiratory depression and prevent prolonged serum half-life (83, 84).

Short- and intermediate-acting barbiturates (pentobarbital/secobarbital) produce sedation and hypnosis without analgesia and may, in fact, possess some anti-analgesic activity, thus increasing the requirements for anesthetic agents intraoperatively. The serum half-life for pentobarbital and secobarbital, respectively, are 21 to 42 hours and 19 to 34 hours (85). The most significant adverse drug reaction to the short-intermediate-acting barbiturates is depression of the respiratory drive. There is little effect on cardiovascular functions. These agents may be used alone and/or in combination with narcotics and/or anticholinergics. When used as a pre-anesthetic medication, the dosage is usually 1 to 4 mg/kg IM up to a total dose of 200 mg with careful monitoring of respiration and pain.

Benzodiazepines, most commonly diazepam, chlordiazepoxide, and lorazepam, have been used in combination with other premedication/anesthesia for relief of anxiety and tension. Of equal efficacy are the barbiturates; they cause less respiratory depression and hypotension. Parenteral benzodiazepines induce light anesthesia and anterograde amnesia, which is of obvious benefit. Rapid intravenous administration of diazepam, however, has been associated with hypotension, probably secondary to its diluent, 40% propylene glycol (86, 87). Intramuscular administration of diazepam and chlordiazepoxide is associated with considerable pain, erratic absorption, and unreliable clinical effects, whereas kinetic and clinical trials of lorazepam suggest that it will offer less pain and reliable absorption and therapeutic effect (87). A new parenteral benzodiazepine, midazolam (Versed[R]), is used intravenously for sedation for short diagnostic or endoscopic procedures, sedation before general anesthesia, induction of general anesthesia, and as a hypnotic drug in balanced anesthesia regimens. Clinical studies demonstrate that midazolam is 3 to 4 times as potent as diazepam and is rapidly metabolized in the liver by microsomal oxidation with an elimination half-life ranging from 1 to 4 hours (88). Its adverse drug reaction profile demonstrates respiratory depression and apnea, particularly in patients with preexisting lung disease but with no greater frequency than with other benzodiazepines. Its main advantage is the short serum half-life and duration of action. It will likely replace other benzodiazepines for perioperative use because of the faster onset of action, shorter duration of action, and lesser tissue irritation (89). A comparison of the pharmacokinetic and pharmacodynamic properties of injectable benzodiazepines is shown in Table 17-11.

Anticholinergic agents are used primarily as anti-sialagogues. They decrease oral, tracheal, and bronchial secretions, which minimizes bronchospasm and laryngospasm associated with general anesthetic agents. Caution is warranted in patients with chronic bronchitis or other diseases where inspissation of mucus may result in obstruction of small airways, predisposing patients to respiratory embarrassment. Among the most commonly used anticholinergic agents are atropine (0.4 to 0.6 mg IM), scopolamine (0.3 to 0.4 mg IM), and glycopyrrolate

Table 17-11. Pharmacokinetic/pharmacodynamic considerations of injectable benzodiazepines

Drug	Half-life (hours)	Common dosage units	Major active metabolites (half-life/hours)
Diazepam (Valium[R])	20–50	5 mg/ml	Desmethyldiazepam (30–200) 3-Hydroxydiazepam (5–20) Oxazepam (3–21)
Chlordiazepoxide (Librium[R])	5–30	100 mg/unit	Demoxepam (14–95) Desmethylchlordiazepoxide (18) Desmethyldiazepam (30–200) Oxazepam (3–21)
Lorazepam (Ativan[R])	10–20	2 mg/ml 4 mg/ml	None
Midazolam (Versed[R])	1–4	10 mg/ml	None

(Robinul[R], 0.2 to 0.3 mg IM/IV). When succinylcholine is used, atropine is recommended to reduce both vagal effect and secretory stimulation, although atropine is contraindicated in glaucoma. Scopolamine has sedative properties but has been associated with emotional lability and/or thought dissociation in elderly patients, reversible with 1 to 2 mg of intravenous physostigmine. Glycopyrrolate is a synthetic anticholinergic with little pharmacokinetic information available on its use. It is a quaternary ammonium antimuscarinic that is completely ionized. Because of poor lipid solubility, it does not readily cross the blood-brain barrier and may cause fewer CNS side effects than scopolamine or atropine. In addition, it reduces gastric secretions and acidity (90).

Adverse Reactions to General Anesthetics

The overall surgical death rate in elderly has declined steadily in recent years ranging from 30% to 40% in older studies to 5% to 10% in more recent studies including patients over the age of 80 (91). Still, perioperative mortality in elderly patients is four times greater in patients with coexisting diseases and 20 times greater in elderly requiring emergency surgery (92). In general, though, elderly patients are not at significantly greater risk of perioperative morbidity or mortality (92). The causes of geriatric postoperative death include problems with the cardiovascular, pulmonary, and renal systems. Specific causes of postoperative mortality in patients over the age of 70 have been summarized as follows (93): pneumonia (13% to 38%), pulmonary embolism (3% to 14%), mild myocardial infarction and heart failure (12% to 32%), sepsis and primary surgical disease (9% to 43%), stroke (2% to 9%), and renal failure (3% to 8%). These reinforce the need for a thorough preoperative evaluation of the cardiovascular system, respiratory system, renal function, and nutritional status in elderly patients.

One of the major risk factors involved in surgical procedures is the use of a general anesthetic. It must provide the most efficacious anesthesia and prevent the development of toxicity. Much debate exists about whether elderly patients should receive regional or general anesthesia for operations such as vascular surgery, hip replacement, or transurethral prostatectomy. In general, outcomes are determined by the status of the pre-existing cardiopulmonary sytem. Normalcy implies better outcomes. Regional anesthetics cause less respiratory depression but may induce an equally high incidence of hypotension as others. Inadequate doses of regional anesthetics may lead to pain with subsequent tachycardia and hypertension, with ensuing myocardial ischemia. In the uncooperative or anxious patient, increased sedation may be required, which may result in cardiopulmonary depression. General anesthesia allows for significantly greater airway control and monitoring as well as muscle relaxation. It has been suggested that pharmacologic stabilization of vital signs can be provided more effectively by use of these agents (94). Nevertheless, depression of myocardial function with its associated reduced blood flow to the central nervous system, coronary arteries, liver, and kidneys must be closely monitored to prevent hypotension and reflex tachycardia, postoperative renal failure, dehydration (or fluid overload), hypothermia, and hypoxia.

The ideal inhalational general anesthetic agent should have the following characteristics: (*a*) rapid and pleasant induction of and recovery from anesthesia; (*b*) rapid changes in the depths of anesthesia; (*c*) adequate relaxation of skeletal muscles; (*d*) a wide margin of safety; and (*e*) absence of toxic or other adverse effects. Because of the availability of multiple short-acting analgesics and muscle relaxants, the primary determinants for general anesthetic use are the margin of safety and a low incidence of adverse effects. The agents most widely used include halothane, nitrous oxide, enflurane, isoflurane, and methoxyflurane (least used). Table 17-12 lists their basic pharmacologic properties and possible adverse effects.

Hypotension

As noted in Table 17-12, hypotension occurs with many inhalational anesthetic agents. It is the result of decreased intravascular volume, decreased total peripheral vascular resistance, and/or decreased cardiac output. If hypotension occurs, volume expansion and/or vasopressor agents are primary interventions. Volume expansion is usually performed with either colloids (albumin or hetastarch) or crystalloids (normal saline or 5% dextrose). Both have similar hemodynamic influence and selection of one as opposed to the other is controversial (95). Other methods used to increase blood pressure depend on the etiology of the hypotension. They include positive inotropic drugs, antiarrhythmic drugs, and cardiac pacing or vagolytic drugs, such as atracurium, metocurine, and d-tubocurarine. The primary intervention for arterial hypotension is prevention, that is, choosing the anesthetic agent that will not worsen hypotension. It is necessary to carefully and systematically monitor blood pressure, pulse, respiration, and electrocardiograms. Other instruments recommended for facilitating and allowing hemodynamic monitoring and fluid management include central venous pressure catheters, pulmonary artery catheters, and radial artery lines, when appropriate. Cautious and judicious use of preoperative medications that are known to interfere with blood pressure control, such as narcotics, barbiturates, butyrophenones, phenothiazines, antidepressants, and diuretics is necessary. Their use must be carefully evaluated prior to the induction of anesthesia.

Hypertension

Hypertension is the most frequent illness in elderly patients undergoing surgey (96). In that study of 1000 patients, the rate of postoperative complications was 36.4%, with increased hypertension and ECG changes being the most common. The most common cause of hypertension during anesthetic procedures is uncontrolled preexisting hypertension (97). A primary goal in the evaluation of hypertension, and its relationship to surgical procedures and anesthesia, is to assure that the cause of hypertension is not iatrogenic (e.g., due to the overuse of vasopressor agents such as dopamine, epinephrine, ephedrine, and phenylephrine). Excessive use of vagolytic drugs, such as pancuronium and gallamine, ketamine or inhalation general anesthetics that cause sympathetic stimulation, transfusions, or a full bladder, are all known etiologies for increased blood pressure in anesthetized patients. Special commentaries regarding neuromuscular blocking drugs (such as gallamine and pancuronium) and their use in el-

Table 17-12. Pharmacologic properties of inhalation anesthetic agents and their possible adverse effects

Agent	Comments
Halothane	*Cardiovascular effects*
	Hypotension[a]
	↓ cardiac output[a]
	Bradycardia[a]
	↓ cardiac contractility[a]
	Ectopic atrial and ventricular contractions
	Tachyarrhythmias
	↓ (mild) total peripheral vascular resistance
	Heart sensitization to catecholamines
	Dose dependent
	Respiratory effects
	↑ Respiratory rate (shallow)
	↓ Minute volume
	↑ $PaCO_2$
	↓ Ventilatory response to CO_2
	Bronchodilator
	CNS effects
	Slow wave, high amplitude (EEG changes)
	↑ Cerebral blood flow (unless severe hypotension)
	↓ Mental function (several hours postop)
	Miscellaneous effects
	↑ Action of skeletal muscle relaxants, e.g., pancuronium
	Malignant hyperpyrexia (rapid body temperature and CO_2)
	Uterine muscle relaxation
	↓ Renal blood flow and glomerular filtration rate
	Postop nausea/vomiting
	Halothane hepatitis
	Good choice in COPD patients. Avoid in presence of intracranial pressure.
Enflurane	*Cardiovascular effects*
	Hypotension
	↓ Cardiac output
	Tachycardia
	↓ Cardiac contractility[b]
	Arrhythmias (same as halothane)
	↓ Total peripheral vascular resistance
	Heart sensitization to catecholamines[b]
	Respiratory effects
	↑ Respiratory rate
	↑ $PaCO_2$
	↑ Ventilatory response to CO_2[c]
	↓ Response to hypoxia[c]
	↑ Coughing/secretion production
	CNS effects
	Tonic-clonic muscle activity (high voltage, fast frequency, EEG changes)
	↑ Cerebral blood flow (unless severe hypotension exists)

(*continued*)

Table 17-12. *(continued)*

Agent	Comments
	Jerking/twitching of jaw, face, neck and limbs Avoid in patients with seizures *Miscellaneous effects* Uterine muscle relaxation ↓ Renal blood flow and glomerular filtration rate Postoperative nausea/vomiting (3%–15%) **Avoid in seizure patients and in patients with renal disease**
Isoflurane	*Cardiovascular effects* Hypotension Cardiac output maintained Tachycardia Absent negative inotropic effect[c, d] ↓ Total peripheral vascular resistance Does not sensitize heart to catecholamines *Respiratory effects* ↓ Respiratory rate ↓ Tidal volume Respiratory depression with premedication with opioids Bronchodilation Coughing/secretion and laryngospasm[e] *CNS effects* EEG changes similar to halothane ↑ Cerebral blood flow ↑ Intracranial pressure *Miscellaneous effects* Potentiates muscle relaxants 3-fold greater than halothane Uterine muscle relaxation comparable to halothane ↓ Renal blood flow and glomerular filtration rate Postop nausea/vomiting
Methoxyflurane	*Cardiovascular effects* Hypotension ↓ Cardiac output Bradycardia ↓ Cardiac contractility Sinus bradycardia responsive to atropine A-V nodal rhythms No change in total peripheral vascular resistance *Respiratory effects* See halothane *CNS effects* See halothane *Miscellaneous effects* Additive action to competitive neuromuscular blocking agents Useful in obstetric procedures (no uterine relaxation)

(continued)

Table 17-12. *(continued)*

Agent	Comments
	↓ Renal blood flow and glomerular filtration rate Postop high output renal failure characterized by inability to concentrate urine, dehydration, hypernatremia, and azotemia—20% mortality Postop nausea/vomiting Hepatic necrosis
Nitrous oxide (N_2O) (adjuvant in most procedures)	*Cardiovascular effects* Hypertension ↑ Cardiac output ↑ Total peripheral vascular resistance *Respiratory effects* ↓ (slight) ventilatory response to CO_2 *CNS effects* No ADRs Cerebral blood flow is unchanged *Miscellaneous effects* Postop nausea/vomiting (15%)

[a]Dose-dependent

[b]Less frequent than in equipotent doses of halothane

[c]May have a wider margin of safety than halothane.

[d]May have a wider margin of safety than enflurane.

[e]Incidence is reduced with premedication and thiopental.

derly surgical patients is addressed in more detail later. Severe hypertension that develops in the perioperative period can be treated with direct vasodilators, such as nitroprusside or nitroglycerin, alpha-adrenergic blockers, such as phentolamine or droperidol, or beta-adrenergic blockers or ganglionic blockers, such as propranolol or trimethaphan, respectively.

Bradycardia

Bradycardia is a common problem during anesthesia. It is most often related to intrinsic heart disease. Preventive considerations include preoperative medications that slow the heart (e.g., succinylcholine, anticholinesterases such as neostigmine or edrophonium, propranolol, digoxin or narcotics). Common patient-related variables associated with bradycardia include increased intracranial pressure, hypoxia, and/or hypercapnia. Treatment of bradycardia includes: (*a*) cardiac pacing in patients with intrinsic heart disease, (*b*) atropine for bradycardia due to vagotonic drugs, and (*c*) vagolytic drugs.

Sinus Tachycardia

Sinus tachycardia usually represents a normal physiologic reflex response to hypotension or hypovolemia. In the absence of pheochromocytoma, thyrotoxicosis, fever, malignant hyperthermia, hypoxia, hypercapnia, mild myocardial infarction, or pulmonary embolism, there should be consideration towards a medication-induced phenomenon, and the use of drugs, such as pancuronium, gallamine, isoproterenol, epinephrine, or atropine, must be investigated.

Atrial Arrhythmias

New-onset atrial fibrillation with a rapid ventricular response is seen in patients with intrinsic heart disease, hyperthyroidism, prior surgery involving the pericardium, or excessive adrenergic or vagolytic stimulation. The heart rate may be slowed or even converted by the intravenous use of digoxin; other useful medications include propranolol or verapamil. Cardioversion may also be employed. Atrial flutter may be due to hypercapnia or hypoxia. Treatment depends on the etiology and may simply be to increase ventilation and to supply sufficient quantities of oxygen. Lidocaine may be given if ischemic heart disease is considered to be the etiology, and propranolol is given and carefully titrated if the arrhythmias are secondary to sympathetic stimulation.

Hypercapnea

Hypercapnea, elevated PCO_2, is due to increased production of carbon dioxide or inadequate ventilation. Under the assumption that the CNS causes for inadequate ventilation have been excluded, hypercapnea may be due to inadequate squeezing of the reservoir bag or low ventilation settings. Other variables to consider are partial or complete airway obstruction, increased anatomic dead space (e.g., owing to a mass lung lesion), increased physiologic dead space (e.g., due to a pulmonary embolism, sepsis, and increased CO_2 production), or malignant hyperthermia.

High glucose levels of total parenteral nutrition can also increase CO_2 production (98). Hypercapnea also causes hypertension and tachycardia and, if severe, cardiac arrhythmias. Thus, prevention and early treatment is very important.

Hypoxia

Hypoxia during the anesthetic procedure may be due to a malfunctioning oxygen supply, airway obstruction, or ventilation/perfusion problems (e.g., atelectasis, pneumonia, pulmonary edema, or interstitial pulmonary parenchymal disease). Anemia will diminish oxygen transport from the lungs to the tissues and also can be detrimental in disorders associated with hypoxia. Unquestionably, structural alterations of the aging lungs render elderly patients at increased risk for developing perioperative respiratory complications. In addition, PO_2 falls with the normal aging process; the decrease is steeper when the patient is supine (the most common position postoperatively). Certain surgical procedures (upper abdominal and thoracic incisions) have a more dramatic effect on respiratory function by decreasing vital capacity and functional residual capacity. In addition, pain may cause a reflex muscular splinting leading to hypoxia. Finally, residual anesthetic and narcotic medications may remain in the system of elderly patients through delayed elimination and add to the depressed ventilatory responses, further increasing the danger of hypoxia and hypercapnea.

Hypothermia

Hypothermia is not an uncommon postoperative event and is more pronounced and prolonged in the elderly than in younger patients (99). Because of reduced cardiac and pulmonary reserve, the elderly may develop cardiovascular problems during rewarming, for shivering postoperatively will lead to increased oxygen consumption. Elder patients with hypertension and/or increased peripheral vascular resistance may exhibit arrhythmias or even congestive heart failure. In addition, the lowered body temperature allows for increased tissue solubility of the inhaled anesthetic gas. Arousal from general anesthesia may, therefore, be delayed. The best form of treatment of hypothermia is prevention. This includes judicious use of warming blankets, anesthetic gas humidifiers, and maintenance of the operating room at the warmest possible temperature.

Postoperative Nausea and Vomiting

Postoperative nausea and vomiting is a common occurrence, its incidence ranging from 3% to 30%, depending upon numerous patient-related variables, the type of surgical operation, and the type of anesthetic used (48, 100). Drug-induced nausea and vomiting occur from the drug's action on the vomiting center receptors in the medulla and/or the floor of the fourth ventricle (the chemoreceptor trigger zone), as well as numerous other well-defined reflex arcs (101).

It is difficult to predict postoperative nausea and vomiting. Numerous patient-related variables predispose patients to a higher incidence of postoperative nausea and vomiting including age, sex, body habitus, history of motion sickness, history of postanesthetic nausea and vomiting, preanesthetic medications, the anesthetic agent itself, duration of anesthesia, and the site of surgical procedures. Women are 2 to 4 times more susceptible to nausea and vomiting than men. Obese patients have a higher incidence of nausea and vomiting than patients close to their ideal body weight, presumably due to the prolonged release of large amounts of anesthetic stored in the larger fat compartment. Diseases highly associated with nausea and vomiting include renal failure or intestinal obstruction; patients with these diseases are three times more likely to have postoperative nausea and vomiting than patients without such histories. Patients who receive narcotic analgesics preoperatively are more likely to have postoperative nausea and vomiting than patients without prior narcotic drug administration. Concomitant administration of anticholinergic agents (atropine, scopolamine), barbiturates, antihistamines (hydroxyzine), phenothiazines (chlorpromazine, promethazine), and butyrophenones (droperidol) can decrease the incidence of postoperative nausea and vomiting to 5% to 10%. Unquestionably, there is also a relationship to the type of anesthetic used. For example, intravenous barbiturates cause a much lower incidence of nausea and vomiting than inhalation agents. Diethyl ether and cyclopropane have a higher incidence of emesis than halothane and enflurane, which have a higher incidence than nitrous oxide. Presumably, in a dose-response relationship, a higher incidence of postoperative nausea and vomiting occurs with a longer duration of anesthetic therapy. Finally, the site of a surgical procedure plays an instrumental role, with abdominal surgical procedures having the highest incidence of postoperative emesis, followed by ocular procedures and head and neck operations.

The treatment and prevention of postoperative nausea and vomiting is difficult because of its unpredictability. Its time course tends to be mild and transient. Intervention with medication is often unnecessary or undesirable, especially since adverse drug reactions to antiemetic drugs are often more harmful and outweigh the drug's benefit. Careful identification of predisposing factors in patient education and discussions are highly desirable. Gentle suctioning through a nasal gastric tube and correction and/or avoidance of certain other predisposing factors, such as pain, hypotension, hypoxia, and hypercapnea, can all prevent or relieve symptoms. The commonly used antiemetic drugs given after surgery are chlorpromazine or haloperidol. They may decrease postoperative sickness in 50% of patients, but the other 50% do not respond, and the response is unpredictable. Another hazard of the antiemetic agents is their synergy with general anesthetic agents in producing respiratory depression and prolonging emergence from anesthesia (102).

Hepatitis

Hepatic necrosis is a rare but serious complication associated with general anesthetic agents, especially halothane. The incidence of this syndrome is unknown but is estimated at about 1 in 10,000 anesthetic administrations with a mortality rate of 20% to 50% (48). The pathophysiologic mechanism is unknown, but numerous theories exist including hypersensitivity, liver hypoxia, activation of reactive intermediates, and recrudescence of viral hepatitis (103). The metabolism of halothane includes the formation of unstable electrophilic intermediates that covalently bind to tissue macromolecules, causing cell death. The specific cell susceptibility through this damage may be characterized by a genetic predisposition (104, 105). Most recently, there has been a suggestion that there is a familial, constitutional susceptibility factor that predisposes persons to halothane hepatitis (104). There are no specific diagnostic criteria for determining liver necrosis and no specific criteria to determine predisposition. Some patient-related variables which seem to increase the potential for halothane-induced hepatitis include obesity, female gender, age over 40 years, multiple halothane exposures within 28 days, and previous adverse reactions to halothane anesthesia, such as an unexplained postoperative fever (103, 105). Enflurane and isoflurane may also cause adverse hepatic reactions.

Adverse Reactions to Local Anesthetics

Local anesthetics have multiple uses in surgery, especially for regional anesthetic procedures. Regional anesthesia (Table 17-13) is administered in an effort to prevent the complications that often follow the general anesthesia administration, but no technique is without danger. Care must be exercised to assure that intravascular injection is not made and that tourniquets are adequately applied to prevent leaking; leaking may permit large amounts of an anesthetic agent to enter the general circulation. Most adverse reactions to local anesthetics, therefore, represent systemic reactions to an agent inappropriately absorbed into the circulation and the accompanying altered physiologic responses.

For example, central nervous system effects represent the most serious complication that can develop from systemic absorption of local anesthetic agents (i.e., generalized seizures). Because local anesthetics readily cross the blood/brain barrier, the CNS effects correlate highly with the plasma level of the specific agent. The initial effects of CNS toxicity include stimulation and restlessness, dysphoria or euphoria, lightheadedness, dizziness, and/or visual or auditory dysfunction (e.g., blurred vision and tinnitus, respectively). These signs or symptoms may be followed by drowsiness, disorientation, and even loss of consciousness, which is subsequently followed by tonic-clonic convulsions. The EEG is of little premonitory value. CNS depression is usually followed by respiratory failure and subsequent moribund effects. Because of the abrupt onset and serious consequences on the CNS system, smallest possible dosages are generally recommended. Prevention and early recognition is paramount. Patients with congestive heart failure require diminished dosage of amide-type local anesthetics (Table 17-14) because of their decreased hepatic metabolism and excretion (106). In

Table 17-13. Classification of regional anesthetic procedures

Infiltration	Inhibition of excitation of sensory nerve ending by injection directly into the tissue.
Percutaneous	Any local anesthetic may be used for this form of anesthesia. The onset of action is rapid and duration of anesthesia is directly related to each specific agent used. The addition of epinephrine will increase the duration of anesthesia 100%.
Intravenous regional anesthesia	Administration of local anesthetic agent into the veins of an extremity that has a tourniquet inflated above arterial pressure. Useful for orthopedic procedures.
Peripheral nerve block	Inhibits neural conduction in nerve fibers of the peripheral nervous system by injection of local anesthetic directly into the peripheral nerve or nerve plexuses.
Minor nerve block	Inhibition of small nerves such as the radial or ulnar nerve. Onset of analgesia is rapid and duration of anesthesia relates to specific agents used and can be prolonged by addition of epinephrine. Usually requires only a small amount of solution (1–5 ml).
Major nerve block	Inhibits conduction of large nerves such as the sciatic or femoral nerve and usually requires larger volumes (30–50 ml). The onset of analgesia tends to be slow (10–30 minutes) and usually requires concomitant use of epinephrine to prolong duration.
Central nerve block	Inhibits neural conduction in central nerve fibers, such as spinal anesthesia that is produced by injecting the local anesthesia into the lumbar subarachnoid space.

Note: This information is presented as a general review.

addition, the drug must be discontinued at the earliest sign of toxicity. The administration of oxygen by deep breathing techniques is an important precautionary measure because seizures are associated with increased cerebral oxygen consumption (107).

Cardiovascular effects to systemic concentrations of local anesthetics usually occur after CNS effects (108). The initial cardiovascular signs of toxicity are the result of the drug's direct effect on the CNS and a direct vagal constrictor action of the local anesthetic agent; these result in tachycardia and mild elevations in blood pressure. Subsequently higher levels result in a vasodilator action on arteries and a negative inotropic action on the myocardium, approximating quinidine-like action with concomitant characteristic ECG changes.

Rarely, patients will develop a hypersensitivity reaction to local anesthetics. These reactions manifest a variety of signs and symptoms of allergic responses, including dermatitis, urticaria, pruritus, bronchial spasms, and anaphylaxis (109). Interestingly, most hypersensitivity reactions occur with ester-type local anesthetics (Table 17-14), but amide-type local anesthetics contain a methylparaben preservative that has also produced hypersensitivity reactions (109). A careful allergy history must be obtained from all patients, especially atopic patients, in an effort to preclude hypersensitivity reactions. Documentation of previous allergic responses to local anesthetics, a history of eczema, rhinitis, asthma, or chronic urticarial skin disorders should be obtained. It has been suggested that elderly patients may be more susceptible to allergic problems, increasing the importance of that documentation. Intradermal skin tests have been advocated by some to identify allergic reactions, but the absence of a positive skin test does not preclude the possibility of an allergic reaction (107). This is particularly true in the case of elderly patients, who may present with a lower incidence of reaction to standard (recall) skin test antigens and difficulty in the evaluation of anergic states. Treatment of hypersensitivity reactions of the non-alpha-adrenergic-type includes oral or intravenous antihistaminic agents. Anaphylaxis should be treated immediately with vasopressor agents for hypotension, epinephrine for bronchoconstriction, and possibly aminophylline or steroids (Table 17-15).

Adverse Drug Reactions to Muscle Relaxants

Muscle relaxants are commonly used in surgery and in anesthesiology to interrupt the transmission of the nerve impulse at the skeletal neuromuscular junction. Muscle relaxants are categorized as either competitive agents (e.g., curare) or depolarizing agents (e.g., succinylcholine) (110). Commonly used neuromuscular blocking agents, their standard dosage, and miscellaneous comments are listed in Table 17-16. The most important adverse drug reactions are related to histamine release and its effect on the respiratory and cardiovascular systems (111). Respiratory failure or prolonged apnea is a serious adverse effect of the neuromuscular blocking agents (NMBA). Other causes of respiratory failure must be ruled out, such as obstructed airways, decreased PCO_2, or excessive anticholinesterase use (e.g., neostigmine or pyridostigmine). In addition, the presence of certain patient-related variables may increase the pharmacodynamic action or exacerbate complications, including the following: (*a*) increased temperature potentiates the effect

Table 17-14. Commonly used local anesthetics

Agent	Clinical use	Equivalent in vivo anesthetic concentration (%)	Onset	Duration
Amino-esters				
Procaine (Novocain[R])	Injectable	2	Slow	Moderate
Chloroprocaine (Nesacaine[R])	Injectable, Topical	2	Fast	Short
Tetracaine	Injectable	0.25	Slow	Long
Amino-amides				
Lidocaine (Xylocaine[R])	Injectable, Topical	0.1	Fast	Moderate
Mepivacaine (Carbocaine[R])	Injectable	0.1	Moderate	Moderate
Bupivacaine (Marcaine[R])	Injectable	0.25	Slow	Long
Etidocaine (Duranest[R])	Injectable	0.5	Fast	Long

Table 17-15. Common treatment modalities for hypersensitivity reactions to local anesthetic agents

Agent	Dose[a]	Mechanism of action
Epinephrine	0.2–0.3 ml (1:1000)IM	Stimulates alpha- and beta- adrenergic receptors. Potentiates adenyl cyclase activity Relaxes bronchial smooth muscle
Ephedrine	10–25 mg IV/IM Intervals of 2–5 minutes	Stimulates alpha-adrenergic receptors Increases myocardial contractility Increases bronchodilation
Diphenhydramine (Benadryl[R])	10–50 mg PO/IV	Competitive inhibition of histamine in smooth muscles
Aminophylline	250–500 mg	Inhibits phosphodiesterase with relief of bronchospasm
Hydrocortisone	100–200 mg IV/IM	Enhances the effect of epinephrine and interferes with histamine release

[a]In normal adults.

of competitive NMBA drugs; (*b*) prolonged depolarization may cause a significant loss of intracellular potassium, resulting in cardiac arrhythmias; (*c*) decreased plasma cholinesterase or latent myasthenia gravis; (*d*) reduced skeletal muscle blood flow results in delayed removal of NMBA drugs or decreased elimination of NMBA drugs, and an increased likelihood of complications. The approach to and treatment of acute respiratory embarrassment should include identification of the etiology, positive-pressure artificial respiration with oxygen, and, when appropriate, the administration of neostigmine to block the action of competitive blocking agents. The cardiovascular system is another major system affected by toxic reactions to NMBA agents; large doses of d-tubocurarine cause a large and severe fall in blood pressure. The hypotension is related to histamine-induced peripheral vasodilation and direct sympathetic ganglionic blockade that takes place in the adrenal medulla. The hypotension is further complicated by tachycardia.

Intradermal and intra-arterial administration of muscle relaxants produce a typical histamine-like wheal and flare reaction. With significant systemic levels, bronchospasm, hypotension, and excessive bronchial and salivary secretions also occur and are thought to be directly related to histamine. *d*-Tubocurarine demonstrates the greatest histamine release, followed by succinylcholine. Pancuronium and gallamine may have the least tendency for histamine release (112, 113). In elderly patients, direct ganglionic blockade results in decreased gastrointestinal tone and motility and predisposes elderly patients to postoperative complications and fecal impaction. Succinylcholine exhibits muscarinic action and must be used very cautiously in patients with glaucoma because of the pharmacodynamic increase in intraocular tension. Patients with a

Table 17-16. Commonly used neuromuscular blocking agents

Drug	Dose	Comments
	Depolarization type[a]	
Succinylcholine (Anectine)[R]	1 mg/kg IV 1.5–2.0 mg/kg IM 2.4 mg/min (continuous infusion)	Increases intraocular pressure Increases heart rate and blood pressure Increases serum potassium (0.5–0.7 mEq/L in normal persons), higher increases in patients with massive trauma, spinal cord injury, abdominal infection, burns, malignant hyperthermia. Prolonged duration of action in severe liver disease, pregnancy, chronic renal failure, hemodialysis, and starvation Little data regarding use in aged—no known problems expected (111)
Decamethonium	See miscellaneous comments	No longer marketed in the U.S. because of propensity for entering phase II block (desensitization), which renders the cholinergic receptor inactive and unresponsive to ACh.
	Nondepolarization type[b]	
D-Tubocurarine	0.3–0.4 mg/kg 0.5–0.6 mg/kg for abdominal relaxation	Need to monitor for histamine release, hypotension, and tachycardia Eliminated via kidney/bile (useful in renal disease) Duration—about 2.5 hours
Metocurine	0.2–0.4 mg/kg	50% excretion by the kidney, possibly increased plasma levels in elderly patients, with increased toxicity (111) and increased elimination, half-life (118)
Pancuronium (Pavulon)[R]	0.05–0.10 mg/kg	Potent vagolytic (tachycardia) No histamine release Excreted via kidney About 2-hour duration of action Prolonged effects noted in aged (111) and increased elimination, half-life (118)
Gallamine (Flaxedil)[R]	1.5–3.0 mg/kg	Potent vagolytic (tachycardia) Excreted by kidney (contraindicated in renal failure), increased monitoring in aged is required Histamine release No ganglionic blockade No BP/heart rate changes
Atracurium (Tracrium)[R]	0.4–0.5 mg/kg	Less histamine release Minimal cardiovascular effects Transient tachycardia Increased blood pressure occasionally No adjustment in renal failure Highly recommended for use in elderly (111, 114)
Vecuronium (Norcuron)[R]	0.08–0.1 mg/kg	No dosage change in renal patient Optimally dialyzed No histamine release Occasional cardiovascular effects

[a]Dose for normal adults.

[b]Recommended initial dose.

predisposition for hypokalemia (e.g., elderly patients on diuretics, patients with extensive soft tissue injuries, or burn patients) demonstrate increased sensitivity to NMBA because of increased potassium loss.

Specific pharmacokinetic alterations of NMBA are seen in elderly patients and specific monitoring parameters for postoperative neuromuscular function have been suggested (114–120), but the choice of an NMBA is controversial. D'Hollander et al. (121) extensively studied the clinical pharmacology of vecuronium and demonstrated prolonged recovery from neuromuscular blockade in elderly patients (> 60 years) compared to younger patients; it was found that the steady-state dose requirement of vecuronium was significantly lower in the elderly group. Decreased elimination or biotransformation was suspected as the mechanism, although plasma concentrations were not measured. Rupp et al. (122) evaluated the pharmacokinetic and pharmacodynamic variables of vecuronium in elderly patients over the age of 70 and found that plasma concentrations did not change with age to meet a defined therapeutic end point. Plasma clearance and volume of distribution decreased in elderly patients, but elimination half-life did not change, which contradicts the D'Hollander data (122). O'Hara et al. (115) specifically looked at dose response for vecuronium with respect to age and documented no age-related change in sensitivity of neuromuscular transmission at similar steady state concentrations in younger and older patients with single doses. Triggs (119), evaluating the use of NMBA in geriatric patients, recommended use of vecuronium with caution, reduced dosage, and anticipated prolongation of neuromuscular blockade.

Bedside evaluation of neuromuscular function was recently performed on 100 patients who had received a competitive NMBA during anesthesia (120). On the patient's arrival in the recovery room, neuromuscular function was tested, using common bedside techniques. After completion of the study, the authors concluded that a large number of patients have a defect in neuromuscular transmission on arrival from the recovery room, suggesting that the bedside technique for measurement of neuromuscular transmission is inadequate. Incomplete antagonism of the competitive NMBAs leaves the patient at considerable risk for toxicity and complications (e.g., postoperative respiratory failure). The author's suggestion to obviate this problem was more reliable testing of incomplete antagonism of the competitive NMBAs with the use of a peripheral nerve stimulator (120).

A final precautionary note is that numerous drug interactions exist betwen NMBAs and other agents.

Reversal of the action of these pharmacologic agents is easily achieved by using anticholinesterase drugs, which block the hydrolysis of acetylcholine, allowing it to accumulate at the neuromuscular junction (Table 17-17).

Prevention of Adverse Reaction

Adverse drug reactions are a significant consideration in the evaluation of the elderly surgical patient in the perioperative period. The incidence of ADRs has been well documented and results in increased patient mortality and morbidity, as well as increased economic consequences. Consideration for methods to obviate adverse drug reactions are threefold: (*a*) increase awareness including the specific methods of prevention, (*b*) monitor continuously for early detection, and (*c*) develop programs for surveillance and spontaneous reporting.

The primacy of increased awareness cannot be overemphasized. Spontaneous reports play a significant role in early ADR detection as demonstrated by the fact that 35 of 47 (74%) anecdotal reports of new ADRs published in four major medical journals were subsequently validated (123). Numerous reports demonstrate that agents approved for new indications can develop previously unreported ADRs, possibly related to their use in different patient populations (124–127). Therefore, all health care providers need to be alert to the possibility of adverse drug reactions when evaluating all untoward events. Prevention of adverse drug reactions starts with the evaluation of specific variables that may predispose patients to adverse drug reactions. Most ADRs are extensions of the drug's pharmacologic effect. For example, enflurane

Table 17-17. Agents used to reverse neuromuscular blockade

Drug	Dosage	Comments
Neostigmine[a] (Prostigmin)[R]	0.06 mg/kg (maximum of 5 mg)	Drug must be given *slowly* intravenously. Need prior administration of atropine or glycopyrrolate. Adverse effects include bradycardia, bronchospasm, excess salivation, sweating, hyperperistalsis, and miosis.
Pyridostigmine[a] (Mestinon)[R]	0.1–0.25 mg/kg	Fewer muscarinic adverse effects occur than with neostigmine (administer atropine or glycopyrrolate prior to administration to minimize side effects). Full recovery expected within 15–30 minutes but delayed with hypokalemia.
Atropine	0.02–0.03 mg/kg (0.6–2.0 mg)	Give immediately prior to neostigmine or pyridostigmine to reduce the muscarinic side effects.
Glycopyrrolate (Robinul)[R]	0.01 mg/kg (0.2–0.6 mg)	Give immediately prior to neostigmine or pyridostigmine to reduce the muscarinic side effects.

[a]Antagonism is readily done with no increased efficacy or superiority of one agent over another (114, 117, 152).

causes EEG changes and, therefore, must not be used in patients with convulsions. Lastly, hospital-based drug surveillance/spontaneous reporting systems not only meet JCAH accreditation standards but also serve as useful teaching tools for improved patient care. The literature is replete with numerous programs and methods (128–133).

Drug Interactions

Information on drug interactions in the elderly and their clinical significance remains incomplete despite many reviews (134). Information is even more limited with respect to drug interactions in the elderly surgical patient. However, drug interactions play a significant role in the development of adverse drug effects. This is seen with higher frequency in the elderly because of a multiplicity of causes including increased drug use, altered physiology, multiple disease states, and compliance-related problems, among others. Because most adverse drug reactions are direct extensions of the drug's pharmacologic effect, predictability, prevention, discovery, and appropriate intervention are all possible.

A drug interaction is the alteration of the effect of one drug by prior or concomitant administration of another drug. The result may be enhanced or diminished activity, associated with desirable or undesirable therapeutic outcomes. Significant interactions resulting in overt drug toxicity occur with a frequency of about 7%, excluding minor ADRs, drug-test interactions, and undetected adverse drug interactions (135–137). Drug interactions, therefore, remain a formidable concern to the primary care physician, anesthesiologist, and surgeon. Consequently, familiarity with known drug interactions will allow health care providers to minimize or possibly prevent adverse drug reactions by adjusting dosage or scheduling of the drug administration or by selecting alternative agents (26, 27, 48, 134, 136–138).

Direct Chemical or Physical Interactions

Two drugs may interact by direct chemical or physical contact, resulting in a suppressed or nullified effect. Concomitant administration of thiopental with succinylcholine or pancuronium results in a dense, white precipitate which is the inactive free base of the muscle relaxant (139).

Altered Absorption

Drugs administered by intramuscular or subcutaneous injection may demonstrate a sustained duration of action and/or reduced level of toxicity when administered with a vasoconstrictor, which decreases absorption of the drug at the site of injection. This is commonly done to extend the duration of action of local anesthetics by concomitant use of epinephrine. Another useful example is the addition of nitrous oxide to halothane and oxygen. It is believed that use of more than one inhalational anesthetic agent will quicken the alveolar uptake of halothane by the "second gas effect," but increased halothane toxicity may occur, which requires careful monitoring (140).

Altered Protein Binding

The pharmacologic effect of any drug is related to the free, unbound portion of that drug binding to the receptor site. Because many drugs bind to plasma protein, especially serum albumin, the dynamic affinity between the protein and the unbound drug is significant with regard to its pharmacologic activity and effect. Displacement of drug A from its protein binding site by drug B with greater affinity generates a higher level of free drug A, possibly resulting in increased pharmacodynamic activity of drug A and possible toxicity. In the elderly, plasma albumin levels may be decreased. Thiopental, a commonly used perioperative drug, is highly bound to plasma protein (53); with decreased serum albumin, less of the drug would be bound, and there may be increased sensitivity (increased cardiovascular depression), decreased clearance, and increased serum half-life (141, 142).

Altered Receptor Activity

Positive or negative effects may occur between an agonist and an antagonist respectively. For example, naloxone is useful in reversing respiratory, sedative, and blood pressure depression effects of opioid analgesics by direct pharmacologic antagonism. The combination of atropine and neostigmine allows accumulation of acetylcholine at the cholinergic synapse. At the skeletal muscle, however, acetylcholine competitively antagonizes muscle relaxant, while atropine competitively antagonizes acetylcholine accumulation. Therefore, bradycardia, excessive salivary excretion, and increased gastrointestinal motility are prevented (110). Another example of altered receptor activity commonly seen in the surgical arena is the increased sensitivity of myocardial tissue to catecholamines by general anesthetics, thought to be mediated by a pharmacodynamic action between the receptor and effector (143). D-tubocurarine, pancuronium, and atracurium can have increased neuromuscular blockade when aminoglycosides, such as amikacin, gentamicin, or tobramycin, are given concomitantly. This may result in prolonged respiratory depression with an extended period of apnea which may require mechanical respiratory support (110). This interaction is thought to be caused by the inhibition of acetylcholine release from the preganglionic terminals.

Altered Drug Metabolism

Another frequent mechanism for drug interactions is the acceleration or inhibition of drug metabolism. A common example illustrating this interaction is phenobarbital and halothane. Patients on chronic phenobarbital therapy have increased mixed-function oxidase system activity and, therefore, have an increased capability of metabolizing halothane which, in turn, produces increased levels of metabolites (chloride and bromide ions). These metabolites may be responsible for mood alteration and decreased intellectual function in the postoperative period after halothane administration (144).

Altered Drug Excretion

Drugs excreted primarily through the kidney may have a prolonged pharmacologic effect in patients with decreased renal function. This is exemplified by the prolonged pharmacologic effect of gallamine in elderly patients and in patients with decreased renal function, resulting in marked prolonged respiratory paralysis. This interaction is significant and requires that gallamine not be given to patients with a creatinine clearance less than 50 ml/min (44), probably a significant number of elderly patients. Another example is the fact that nitrous oxide has delayed elimination in patients with narcotic-induced ventilatory depression (145).

General Considerations

During the evaluation of every elderly surgical patient, the consideration for drug interactions and risk for drug interactions is pivotal. It must be a consideration whenever an increased pharmacodynamic response or a therapeutic misadventure occurs, and prevention is obviously the key issue. The internist, anesthesiologist, surgeon, and other health care practitioners must consider multiple types of drug interactions in each clinical situation. A summary of specific drug-drug interactions pertinent to consideration in the perioperative elderly patient evaluation is detailed in Tables 17-18 and 17-19.

Patient Education

Preoperative counseling. This is the era of consumer advocacy; people want and need information about medications, surgical procedures, time for recuperation, costs, benefits, risks, and other pertinent information. Counseling the patient must be a team effort between the anesthesiologist, surgeon, internist, nurse, and pharmacist. The patient should be informed about the following: (a) estimated time of surgery; (b) time period whereby the patient can have nothing to eat or drink prior to surgery; (c) type, route, and time of administration of premedication agents; (d) time of transportation to the operating room; (e) monitoring of instrumentation during operating room procedure (e.g., intravenous catheters, blood pressure cuffs, ECG electrodes, and other pertinent items); (f) type of anesthesia and its risks, benefits, and alternative methods; (g) reassurances about safety throughout the operation and the recovery room; and (h) pain medications during surgery as well as postoperatively.

The patient should be explicitly counseled with respect to the risk and benefit of the operative procedures, alternative opinions regarding various surgical interventions as well as prognosis, and the diagnosis should be provided to the patient as well as the postoperative treatment plans and follow-up.

The internist should serve as a consultant to the patient, offering a second opinion on either the anesthesiologist's or surgeon's recommendations. The internist should also offer his/her opinions regarding each of the items listed above and perhaps give detailed and explicit counseling regarding perioperative medications. The patients are often worried and anxious when interacting with the anesthesiologist and the surgeon, and probably remember no more than 20% to 40% of what they were told. The internist should also encourage and motivate the patient to take an active interest in the specific management and recuperation from his/her illness, surgical procedure, or therapy.

Drug information for patients. Numerous standard references are available regarding patient consultation about medications (146–148). Education regarding specific agents can differ greatly. For example, counseling regarding a chronic pain medication will have a different emphasis than an acute anesthetic inhalation procedure that only occurs one time. In general, several agent-related variables can be emphasized during a patient education session. These include: (a) drug name and strength, which includes both generic and brand names; (b) indication for use and time of administration; (c) mechanism of action in simplistic terms; (d) effect on activities of daily living; (e) storage instructions; (f) potential adverse effects, usually separated into minor versus serious adverse reactions; and (g) commonly encountered food or drug interactions (146). Using the halothane as an example, the following information illustrates a simplistic technique for patient education (148).

> Fluothane is the brand name for halothane, which is a general anesthetic used to produce loss of consciousness before entering surgery. It is given by inhalation by a specially trained physician called an anesthesiologist. In order to decide which is the best anesthetic, you should tell your anesthesiologist any of the following: 1) past allergic reactions, especially to prior general anesthetic administration; 2) family members who have had adverse effects to anesthetics such as fevers, irregular or fast heart beats, muscle

Table 17-18. Selected drug interactions with enflurane, halothane, and isoflurane

Interacting drug (examples only)	Comments/Action
Alcohol	*Preoperative:* Alcoholic patient may present with: a. Hypovolemia. Patient sensitized to action of anesthetic. Monitor volume status. b. Hypoalbuminemia. May sensitize patient to action of anesthetic. Monitor albumin status. c. Increased activity of mixed-oxidase system. May lead to increased metabolism of anesthetic, decreased effect. *Interaction effect:* Additive CNS depressant effect with anesthetic.
Antipsychotics Chlorpromazine Haloperidol Thioridazine	*Preoperative:* Continue drug to start of anesthesia. *Interaction effect:* a. Additive postural hypotension (presumably through alpha-adrenergic receptor blockade). b. Monitor BP. Treat hypotension with alpha-adrenergic agonists.
Diuretics Furosemide Thiazides	*Preoperative:* Patient may present with reduced total body potassium or overt hypovolemia. Myocardium sensitized to arrhythmias. Monitor potassium. *Interaction effect:* a. Additive hypotensive effect. b. Possible hypovolemia, which would increase sensitivity to anesthetic.
Epinephrine	*Interaction effect:* a. Dose response ventricular irritability. Especially at risk: patients with organic heart disease. b. Lower dose of epinephrine during anesthesia.
Ketamine	*Interaction effect:* a. Halothane, and, to a lesser degree, enflurane, block cardiovascular stimulating effects of drug. b. Watch for decreased cardiac output, pulse, pulse rate, and blood pressure. c. Monitor closely blood pressure and cardiac function. d. Administer pressor agents to restore cardiac stability.
Beta-adrenergic antagonist	*Preoperative:* Continue drug up to start of anesthesia. *During procedure, postoperative:* Monitor closely BP and cardiac output. Reversal with isoproterenol or dopamine during or after anesthesia. *Interaction effect:* Mild exaggeration of hypotension (especially enflurane) and possible decompensation of congestive heart failure.
Antihypertensive drugs Clonidine Captopril Guanethidine Hydralazine Methyldopa Prazosin Reserpine	*Preoperative:* a. Continue drug to start of anesthesia. b. Do not discontinue abruptly because of danger of severe rebound hypertension. *Interaction Effect:* Additive hypotension. Decreased anesthetic dose. Maintain adequate intravascular volume.
Benzodiazepines Diazepam Lorazepam	a. Additive respiratory depression. Could cause apnea during anesthesia. b. Decreased minimum alveolar concentration needed for halothane therapy. Reduce halothane dosage.
Digoxin	*Preoperative:* a. Continue drug to start of anesthesia. b. Closely monitor serum electrolytes, particularly serum potassium. *Interaction effect:* Digoxin's positive inotropic effect offsets negative inotropic effect of anesthetic. Possible additive bradycardia.
Levodopa	*Preoperative:* Continue drug to start of surgery. a. Increased sensitivity to hypotension with blood loss. b. Increased sensitivity of myocardium to halothane. c. Blood pressure lability. d. Monitor cardiovascular status closely. *Perioperative:* Avoid antipsychotic to avoid blood pressure lability.
Phenobarbital Other barbiturates	*Preoperative:* a. Chronic barbiturate use may causes induction of mixed-oxidase enzyme system. Risk of intermediate metabolite formation, hepatitis. b. Increased metabolism may require increased anesthetic dose. *Interaction effect:* Additive CNS depression

(*continued*)

Table 17-18. *(continued)*

Interacting drug (examples only)	Comments/Action
Neuromuscular blocking agents: competitive type Atracurium Gallamine Pancuronium *d*-tubocurarine	Synergistic stabilizing action on the post-junctional membranc with additive muscle relaxation.
Theophylline	*Interaction effect:* Increased cardiac arrhythmias that appear to be dose dependent and possibly synergistic with halothane. Use enflurane or isoflurane, which are less likely to produce catecholamine-induced arrhythmias.

Adapted from References 26–28, 73, 134, 143, 144, 153, 154.

spasms or tightness, or breathing problems; and 3) any OTC (nonprescription) or prescription medications. After receiving this medication, some people feel tired, drowsy, or weak for up to a few days after its administration. Alcoholic beverages and other drugs that slow down the nervous system causing drowsiness may add to the actions of the anesthetic. Although not intended, any medicine may cause untoward effects. If you notice any of the following signs or symptoms within two weeks after anesthetic administration, check with your physician as soon as possible: black or bloody vomitus, severe or unusual headache, loss of appetite, severe or unusual nausea, stomach pain, unusual urination (either increased or decreased), unusual weight loss, or yellowing of eyes or skin. Other unwanted effects that usually do not require special evaluation by your physician and diminish as the anesthetic wears off include shivering or trembling, drowsiness, headache, mood or mental changes, nausea or vomiting, nightmares or unusual dreams. If these untoward effects continue or become bothersome in any manner, do not hesitate to check with your physician.

The preceding paragraph is only one example of how to approach a patient education session. This information obviously does not take into account the level of education and/or comprehension of the patient, and each intervention must be adapted accordingly. The importance of patient education, however, must not be underestimated.

Conclusion

Age does not present an a priori reason for withholding surgical procedures from members of the rapidly aging population. However, changes in the United States health care system and new reimbursement policies have resulted in an increase in the number of surgical procedures outside the structured environment of the acute care hospital. This mandates a new approach to the elderly surgical patient.

The elderly probably present the most heterogeneous patient population. People age at different rates and organ systems of an individual age at different rates. A host of factors, including the nutritional status of the patient, demand an individualized, careful preoperative approach to the elderly patient. Primary age changes (physiologic changes with age), secondary age changes (pathophysiologic changes with age), and tertiary age changes (behavioral changes) may interact to cause altered responses to drugs. Multiple drug therapy, likely before and during hospitalization, heightens the risk to adverse drug reactions and interactions.

Thus, a careful pharmacotherapeutic evaluation is a necessity. It should provide an accurate definition of the current medical regimen, documentation of previous adverse drug reactions, identification of potential drug interactions with commonly used pre-anesthetic medications, anesthetic, and postoperative medications, identification of pharmacokinetic/pharmacodynamic alterations in the individual surgical patient, and patient information and education about anesthetic agents, pain management, and other commonly used surgical medications.

References

1. Bureau of Census, Projections of the Population of the United States by Age, Sex, and Race, 1983–2080. 1984. Current Population Report Series P 25N0857. Washington, DC: Department of Commerce.
2. Miller, RR. 1973. Drug surveillance utilizing epidemiologic methods: A report from the Boston Collaborative Drug Surveillance Program. *Am J Hosp Pharm* 30:584–592.
3. Jick, H. 1974. Drugs: Remarkably nontoxic. *N Engl J Med* 291:824–828.
4. Rowe, JW, et al. 1976. The effect of age on creatinine clearance in men: A cross-sectional and longitudinal study. *J Gerontol* 31:155–163.
5. Lamy, PP. 1982. Comparative pharmacokinetic changes and drug therapy in an older population, *J Am Geriatr Soc* 30:11 (suppl), S11–S19.

Table 17-19. Selected drug interactions with neuromuscular blocking agents

Interacting drugs (examples only)	Comments/Action
Aminoglycoside antibiotics	*Interaction effect:* a. Neuromuscular blocking effects increased (additive or synergistic). b. Prolonged respiratory depression. c. Apnea possible. *Action:* a. Parenteral calcium may be administered for severe respiratory depression. b. Anticholinesterases may be helpful. c. Mechanical respiratory support may be needed.
Alkylating agents Nitrogen mustards Cyclophosphamide Chlorambucil	*Interaction effect:* Prolonged neuromuscular blocking effect occurs with succinylcholine (inhibition of plasma cholinesterase?). *Action:* Reduced succinylcholine dosage required.
Azathioprine	*Interaction effect:* Reverses effects of non-depolarizing muscle relaxants (atracurium, gallamine, pancuronium, tubocurarine). Mechanism unknown. *Action:* May have to increase dose of non-depolarizing muscle relaxants.
Anticholinesterases Neostigmine Pyridostigmine	*Interaction effect:* a. Neuromuscular blocking effects of succinylcholine increased. b. Prolonged respiratory depression. c. Apnea possible. *Action:* Mechanical respiratory support if needed.
Clindamycin, Lincomycin	*Interaction effect:* a. Possible increase of neuromuscular blocking action of non-depolarizing muscle relaxants (additive, synergistic). b. Respiratory depression. c. Apnea possible. *Action:* a. Parenteral calcium may be administered for severe respiratory depression. b. Anticholinesterases may be helpful. c. May still need mechanical respiratory support.
Digoxin	*Interaction effect:* a. Increased digoxin toxicity. b. Exacerbation of cardiac arrhythmias may occur (enhanced sensitivity of myocardium). *Action:* Close cardiac monitoring is required.
Diuretics Thiazides Furosemide	*Interaction effect:* a. Increased neuromuscular blocking action of non-depolarizing muscle relaxants possible (due to hypokalemia?). b. Respiratory depression. c. Apnea possible. *Action:* Monitor potassium status. Prevent hypokalemia.
Spironolactone Triamterene	*Interaction effect:* Diuretic-induced hyperkalemia potentiates succinylcholine-induced hyperkalemia. *Action:* Avoid concurrent use.
Echothiophate	*Interaction effect:* a. Increased neuromuscular blocking effects of succinylcholine (depressed plasma cholinesterase enzyme activity). b. Respiratory depression. *Action:* Avoid concurrent use.

(*continued*)

Table 17-19. *(continued)*

Interacting drugs (examples only)	Comments/Action
Lithium	*Interaction effect:* a. Possibly increased neuromuscular blocking effect of non-depolarizing muscle relaxants (mechanism unknown). b. Prolonged respiratory depression. c. Additive or synergistic interaction with succinylcholine. *Action:* a. Avoid concurrent use.
Quinidine	*Interaction effect:* a. Increased neuromuscular blocking effects (additive or synergistic activity?) b. Prolonged respiratory depression c. Apnea possible. *Action:* a. Avoid concurrent use. b. May need mechanical respiratory support.
Theophylline	*Interaction effect:* a. Possibly antagonistic activity on nondepolarizing muscle relaxants (resistance to or reversal of neuromuscular blocking action?). b. Theophylline produces a dose-dependent reversal of neuromuscular blockade. c. Concomitant use may predispose patient to cardiac arrhythmias (unsubstantiated).
Trimethaphan	*Interaction effect:* a. Increased neuromuscular blocking effect. b. Increased respiratory depression. c. Apnea possible —additive effect with nonpolarizing muscle relaxants (?) —depressed plasma cholinesterase enzyme activity with succinlycholine (?). *Action:* a. Use combination with extreme caution. b. May need mechanical respiratory support.

Adapted from references: 26–28, 73, 134, 143, 144, 153, 154.

6. Lamy, PP. 1981. Drug prescribing for the elderly. *Bull NY Acad Med* 57:718.
7. Lamy, PP. 1986. The elderly and drug interactions. *J Am Geriatr Soc* 34:586.
8. McKenney, JM, and Harrison, WL. 1976. Drug related hospital admissions. *Am J Hosp Pharm* 33:792–795.
9. Black, D, et al. 1984. Medication for the elderly: a report of the Royal College of Physicians. *JR Coll Physicians Lond* 18:7–17.
10. Joint National Committee on Detection, Evaluation and treatment of High Blood Pressure. 1984. The 1984 Report of the Joint National Committee on Detection, Evaluation, and Treatment of High Blood Pressure. *Arch Intern Med* 144:1045–1057.
11. Ostfeld, AM. 1978. Elderly hypertensive patients: Epidemiologic review. *NY State J Med* 78:1125–1129.
12. Goldman, L, et al. 1977. Multi-factorial index of cardiac risk in noncardiac surgical procedures. *N Engl J Med* 297:845–850.
13. Hubbell, FA, and Weber, MA. 1980. Adverse effects of sudden withdrawal of antihypertensive medication. *Postgrad Med* 68:129–138.
14. Squire, A, et al. 1984. Long-term antiarrhythmic therapy. Problem of low blood level in patient non-compliance. *Am J Med* 77:1035–1038.
15. Witek, TJ, Schacter, EN, and Dean, NL. 1983. A review of hospital course of asthmatic children and adults. *Ann Allergy* 50:236–240.
16. Gibberd, FB, Dunne, JF, and Handley, AJ. 1970. Supervision of epileptic patients taking phenytoin. *Br Med J* 1:147–149.
17. Center for Disease Control. 1980. *CDC Morbidity and Mortality Weekly Report* 291:97–105.
18. Boston Collaborative Drug Surveillance Program. 1972. Adverse drug interactions. *JAMA* 220:1238–1239.
19. Cooper, J, et al. 1975. A Seven Nursing Home Study. Frequency of potential drug-drug interactions. *J Am Pharm Assoc* 15:247–251.
20. Armstrong, WA, Driever, CW, and Hays, RL. 1980. Analysis of drug-drug interactions in a geriatric population. *Am J Hosp Pharm* 37:385–387.
21. Laventurier, MF, et al. 1976. Drug utilization and potential drug-drug interactions. *J Am Pharm Assoc* 16: 77–81.
22. Lamy, PP. 1980. *Prescribing for the Elderly.* Littleton PSG Publishing Co.
23. Lamy, PP. 1984. Hazards of drug use in the elderly. Common sense measures to reduce them. *Postgrad Med* 77: 50–51.
24. Greenlaw, CW, and Zellers, DD. 1978. Computerized

drug-drug interactions screening system. *Am J Hosp Pharm* 35:567–570.

25. Tatro, DS, et al. 1975. On-Line drug interactions surveillance. *Am J Hosp Pharm* 32:417–420.
26. Shinn, AF, and Shrewsbury, RP, eds. 1985. *Evaluation of Drug Interactions*. St. Louis: CV Mosby Co.
27. Hansten, PD. 1985. *Drug Interactions: Clinical Significance of Drug-Drug Interactions*. Philadelphia: Lea Febiger.
28. Mangini, RJ, ed. 1985. *Drug Interaction Facts*. St. Louis: JB Lippincott Co.
29. Hurwitz, N, and Wade, OL. 1969. Intensive hospital monitoring of adverse reactions to drugs. *Br Med J* 1: 531–536.
30. Hurwitz, N. 1969. Predisposing factors in adverse reactions to drugs. *Br Med J* 1:536–539.
31. Stewart, RB, and Cluff, LE. 1971. Studies on the epidemiology of adverse drug reactions. VI. Utilization and interaction of prescription and nonprescription drugs in outpatients. *Johns Hopkins Med J* 124:319.
32. Ritschel, WA. 1983. Pharmacokinetics in the aged. In *Pharmacologic Aspects of Aging*, Eds., LA Pagliaro and AM Pagliaro. St. Louis: CV Mosby Co.
33. Novak, LP. 1982. Aging, total body potassium, fat free mass and cell mass in males and females between ages 18–85 years. *J Gerontol* 27:438–443.
34. Weisfeldt, ML, Gerstenblith, G, and Lakatta, EG. 1985. Alterations in circulatory functions. In *Principles of Geriatric Medicine*, Eds., R Andres, EL Bierman, and WR Hazzard. New York: McGraw-Hill Book Co.
35. Rodeheffer, RJ, et al. 1984. Exercise cardiac output is maintained with advancing age in healthy human subjects: Cardiac dilation and increased stroke volume compensate for a diminished heart rate. *Circulation* 69:203–213.
36. Dunnill, MS, and Halley, W. 1973. Some observations of the quantitative anatomy of the kidney. *J Pathol* 110: 113–121.
37. Moore, RA. 1931. Total number of glomeruli in the normal human kidney. *Anat Rec* 48:153.
38. Epstein, M. 1979. Effects of aging on the kidney. *Fed Proc* 38:168–172.
39. Davies, DF, and Shock, NW. 1959. Age changes in glomerular filtration rates, effective renal plasma flow and tubular excretory capacity in adult males. *J Clin Invest,* 29:496–507.
40. Rowe, JW, Shock, NW, and DeFronzo, RA. 1976. The influence of age on renal response to water deprivation in man. *Nephron* 27:270–278.
41. Epstein, M, and Hollenberg, NK. 1976. Age as a determinant of renal sodium conservation in normal man. *J Lab Clin Med* 87:411–417.
42. Kampmann, J, et al. 1974. Rapid evaluation of creatinine clearance. *Acta Med Scand* 196:517–520.
43. Cockroft, DW, and Gault, MH. 1976. Prediction of creatinine clearance from serum creatinine. *Nephron* 16: 31–41.
44. Bennett, WM, et al. 1983. Drug prescribing in renal failure: Dosing guidelines for adults. *Am J Kidney Dis* 3: 155–193.
45. Rush, BF, Fisbein, R, and Wilder, RJ. 1965. Effective operative drama upon renal function in older patients. *Ann Surg* 162:836.
46. James, OFW. 1983. Gastrointestinal and liver function in old age. *Clin Gastroenterol* 12:671–691.
47. Wood, AJ, et al. 1976. Effect of aging and cigarette smoking on antipyrine and indocyanine green elimination. *Clin Pharmacol Ther* 26:16–20.
48. Marshall, BE, and Wollman, H. 1985. General anesthetics. In *The Pharmacological Basis of Therapeutics,* Eds., AG Gilman, LS Goodman, TW Rall, et al. New York: MacMillan Publishing Co.
49. O'Malley, K, et al. 1971. Effects of age and sex on human drug metabolism. *Br Med J* 3:607–609.
50. Salem, SAM, et al. 1978. Reduced induction of drug metabolism in the elderly. *Age Ageing* 7:68–73.
51. Rowe, JW, and Besdine, RW, eds. 1982. *Health and Disease in Old Age*. Boston: Little, Brown & Co.
52. Lamy, PP. 1986. Geriatric drug therapy. *Am Fam Phys* 34(6):119–122.
53. Benet, LZ, and Sheiner, LB. 1985. Design and optimization of dosage regimen: pharmacokinetic data (Appendix II). In *The Pharmacological Basis of Therapeutics,* Eds., AG Gilman, LS Goodman, TW Rall, et al. New York: MacMillan Publishing Co.
54. Cho-Ming, L, and Vestal, RE. 1986. The effects of age of hepatic drug metabolism. In *Drug Studies in the Elderly: Methodological Concerns,* Eds., NR Cutler and PK Narang. New York: Plenum Medical Book Co.
55. Shepherd, AMM. 1986. Physiological changes with aging: Relevance to drug study design. In *Drug Studies in the Elderly: Methodological Concerns,* Eds., NR Cutler and PK Narang. New York: Plenum Medical Book Co.
56. Pucino, F, et al. 1985. Pharmacogeriatrics. *Pharmacotherapy* 5:314–326.
57. Brown, BR, ed. 1981. *Anesthesia and the Patient With Liver Disease*. Philadelphia: FA Davis Co.
58. Norton, LW. 1981. Postoperative jaundice. In *Anesthesia and the Patient With Liver Disease,* Ed., BR Brown. Philadelphia: FA Davis Co.
59. Shepherd, AM, et al. 1979. Age as a determinant of sensitivity to warfarin. *Br J Clin Pharmacol* 4:315–320.
60. Vestal, RE, Wood, AJ, and Shand, DG. 1979. Reduced beta-adrenoreceptor sensitivity in the elderly. *Clin Pharmacol Ther* 4:315–320.
61. Gregory, G, Eger, E, and Munson, E. 1969. The relationship between age and halothane requirement. *Anesthesia* 30:488.
62. Lippmann, M, and Rogoff, R. 1974. A clinical evaluation of pyridostigmine bromide in the reversal of pancuronium. *Anesthes Analg* 53:20–22.
63. Baraka, A. 1977. Irreversible curarization. *Intens Care* 5:244.
64. Kaiko, R. 1980. Age and morphine analgesia in cancer patients with postoperative pain. *Clin Pharmacol Ther* 28:823.
65. Culver, BH, and Butler, J. 1985. Alterations in pulmonary functions. In *Principles of Geriatric Medicine,* Eds., R Andres, EL Bierman, and WR Hazzard. New York: McGraw-Hill Book Co.
66. Hewlett, MA. 1975. Postoperative pulmonary functions. *Br J Anaesth* 24:102–107.
67. Naranjo, CA, et al. 1981. A method for estimating the probability of adverse drug reactions. *Clin Pharmacol Ther* 30:239–245.

68. Fisher, M. 1975. Severe histamine mediated reactions to intravenous drugs used in anesthesia. *Anesth Intens Care* 3:180–197.
69. Matthews, KP. 1984. Clinical spectrum of allergic and pseudoallergic drug reaction. *J Allergy Clin Immunol* 74: 558–566.
70. Jaffe, JH, and Martin, WR. 1985. Opioid analgesics and antagonists. In *The Pharmacological Basis of Therapeutics,* Eds., AG Gilman, LS Goodman, TW Rall, et al. New York: MacMillan Publishing Co.
71. Kaplan, AP. 1984. Drug-induced skin disease. *J Allergy Clin Immunol* 74:573–579.
72. Martin, DW, Siegel, RC, and Smith, LH. 1978. Drug fever. *West J Med* 129:321–326.
73. Pascewski BM, and Gerbino PP. 1982. Drug reaction and interreactions in the surgical patient. In *Medical Care of the Surgical Patient: A Problem Oriented Approach to Management,* pp. 536–567. Eds., E Abrutyn, PC Atkins, MF Attie, et al. Philadelphia: JB Lippincott Co.
74. Garibaldi, RA, and Nurse, BA. 1986. Infections in the elderly. *Am J Med* 81 (Suppl 1A):53–58.
75. Hansten, PD, and Horn, JR. 1985. Heat stroke due to drug combinations. *Drug Interactions Newsletter* 5: 523–524.
76. Gronert, GA. 1980. Malignant hyperthermia. *Anesthesiology* 53:395–423.
77. Bick, RL, Adams, T, and Schmalhorse, WR. 1976. Bleeding times, platelet adhesions and aspirin. *Am J Clin Pathol* 65:69–72.
78. Karch, FE, and Lasagna, L. 1975. Adverse drug reactions: A critical review. *JAMA* 234:1236–1241.
79. Karch, FE, and Lasagna, L. 1977. Toward the operational identification of adverse drug reactions. *Clin Pharmacol Ther* 21:247–254.
80. Kramer, MS, et al. 1979. An algorithm for operational assessment of adverse drug reactions: I background, description, and instructions for use. *JAMA* 242: 623–632.
81. Scott, DB. 1982. Postoperative pain relief. *Regional Anesth* (suppl) 7:S110–S113.
82. Kaiko, RF, et al. 1983. Central nervous system excitatory effects of meperidine in cancer patients. *Ann Neurol* 13: 180–185.
83. McGee, JL, and Alexander, MR. 1979. Phenothiazine analgesia—fact or fantasy? *Am J Hosp Pharm* 36: 633–640.
84. Demerol, Product Information. 1986. New York: Winthrop Laboratory.
85. Breimer, DD. 1977. Clinical pharmacokinetics of hypnotics. *Clin Pharmacokinet* 2:93–109.
86. Bell, DS. 1969. Dangers of treatment of status epilepticus with diazepam. *Br Med J* 1:159–161.
87. Greenblatt, DJ, et al. 1979. Pharmacokinetics and bioavailability of intravenous, intramuscular, and oral lorazepam in humans. *J Pharm Sci* 68:57–63.
88. Reves, VG, et al. 1985. *Midazolam.* Pharmacology and uses. *Anesthesiology* 62:310–324.
89. Abramowicz, M., ed. 1986. *Midazolam. Med Lett Drug Ther* 28:73–74.
90. Weiner, N. 1985. Atropine, scopolamine, and related antimuscarinic drugs: In *The Pharmacological Basis of Therapeutics,* Eds., AG Gilman, LS Goodman, TW Rall, et al. New York: MacMillan Publishing Co.
91. Gibson, JR, Mendenhall, MK, and Axel, NJ. 1985. Geriatric anesthesia: Minimizing the risk. *Geriatr Clin N Am* 1:313–321.
92. Johnson, JC. 1983. The medical evaluation and management of the elderly surgical patient. *J Am Geriatr Soc* 31:621–625.
93. Stein, JM, and Hedley-Whyte J. 1986. Anesthesiology. In *The Practice of Geriatrics,* Eds., E Calkins, PJ Davis, and AB Ford. Philadelphia: WB Saunders Co.
94. Saunders, RJ. 1982. Anesthesia in the geriatric patient. *Otolaryngol Clin N. Am,* 15:395–403.
95. Ross, AD, and Angaran, DM. 1984. Colloids vs crystalloids: A continuing controversy. *Drug Intell Clin Pharm* 18:202–212.
96. Stephen, CR. 1984. The risk of anesthesia and surgery in the geriatric patient. In *Anesthesia and the Geriatric Patient,* Ed., SE Krechel. New York: Grune & Stratton.
97. Martin, DE, and Kammerer, WS. 1983. The hypertensive surgical patient: Controversy in management. *Surg Clin N Am* 63:1017–1033.
98. Askanazi, J, et al. 1980. Respiratory changes induced by large glucose loads of total parenteral nutrition. *JAMA* 243:1444–1447.
99. Vaughn, MS, Vaughn, RW, and Cork, RC. 1981. Postoperative hypothermia in adults: Relationship of age, anesthesia, and shivering to rewarming. *Anesth Analg* 60: 746–751.
100. Swenson, EJ, and Orkin, FK. 1983. Postoperative nausea and vomiting. In *Complications in Anesthesiology,* Eds., FK Orkin and LH Cooperman. Philadelphia: JB Lippincott Co.
101. Guyton, AC. 1986. Physiology of gastrointestinal disorders. In *Textbook of Medical Physiology.* Philadelphia: WB Saunders Co.
102. Mull, TD, and Smith, TC. 1974. Comparison of the ventilatory effects of two antiemetics, benzquinamide and prochlorperazine. *Anesthesiology* 40:581–587.
103. Touloukian, J, and Kaplowitz, N. 1981. Halothane-induced hepatic disease. *Semin Liver Dis* 1:134–142.
104. Farrell, G, Prendergast, D, and Murray, M. 1985. Halothane hepatitis: Detection of constitutional susceptibility factor. *N Engl J Med* 313:1310–1314.
105. Hoft, RH, et al. 1981. Halothane hepatitis in three pairs of closely related women. *N Engl J Med* 304:1023–1024.
106. Zito, RA, and Reid, PR. 1978. Lidocaine kinetics predicted by indocyanine green clearance. *N Engl J Med* 298:1160–1163.
107. Raj, PP, and Winnie, P. 1983. Immediate reactions to local anesthetics. In *Complication in Anesthesiology,* Eds., FK Orkin and LH Cooperman. Philadelphia: JB Lippincott Co.
108. Scott, DB. 1981. Toxicity caused by local anesthetic drugs. *Br J Anesth* 53:553–554.
109. Ritchie, JM, and Greene, NM. 1985. Local anesthetics. In *The Pharmacological Basis of Therapeutics,* Eds., AG Gilman, LS Goodman, TW Rall, et al. New York: MacMillan Publishing Co.
110. Taylor, P. 1985. Neuromuscular blocking agents. In *The Pharmacological Basis of Therapeutics,* Eds., AG Gilman, LS Goodman, TW Rall, et al. New York: MacMillan Publishing Co.
111. Feldman, S. 1984. Neuromuscular blocking drugs. In *A Practice of Anesthesia,* Eds., HC Churchill-Davidson

and WD Wylie. Chicago: Yearbook Medical Publishers, Inc.

112. Bowman, WC. 1980. Pre- and postjunctional cholinoreceptors at the neuromuscular junction. *Anesth Analg* 59:935–943.
113. Ertama, PM. 1982. Histamine liberation in surgical patients following administration of neuromuscular blocking drugs. *Ann Clin Res* 14:27–31.
114. Miller, RD, et al. 1984. Clinical pharmacology of vecuronium and atracurium. *Anesthesiology* 61:444–453.
115. O'Hara, DA, Fragen, RJ, and Shanks, CA. 1985. The effects of age on the dose-response curve for vecuronium in adults. *Anesthesiology* 63:542–544.
116. Shanks, CA. 1986. Pharmacokinetics of nondepolarizing neuromuscular relaxants applied to calculation of bolus and infusion dosage regimens. *Anesthesiology* 64: 72–86.
117. Miller, RD. 1984. Vecuronium: A new depolarizing neuro-muscular-blocking agent: clinical pharmacology, pharmacokinetics, cardiovascular effects and use in special clinical conditions. *Pharmacotherapy* 4:238–247.
118. Sohn, YJ, et al. 1986. Comparative pharmacokinetics and dynamics of vecuronium and pancuronium in anesthetized patients. Anesth Analg 65:233–239.
119. Triggs, EJ. 1986. Special considerations in the use of neuromuscular functions. *Anaesth Intens Care* 14:41–45.
120. Beemer, GH, and Rozental, P. 1986. Postoperative neuro-muscular functions. *Anaesth Intens Care* 14: 41–45.
121. d'Hollander, A, et al. 1982. Age-dependent dose-response relationship of ORG NC 45 in anaesthetized patients. *Br J Anaesth* 54:653–657.
122. Rupp, SM, et al. 1983. Pharmacokinetics and pharmacodynamics of vecuronium in the elderly. *Anesthesiology* 59:A270.
123. Venning, G. 1982. Validity of anecdotal reports of suspected adverse drug reactions. *Br Med J* 284:249–252.
124. Riegelman, RR. 1981. What to do until the FDA arrives. *Drug Therapy* 70:103–108.
125. Slone, P, Shapiro, S, and Miettinen, OS. 1979. Drug evaluation after marketing. *Ann Intern Med* 90:257–261.
126. Temple, RJ, Jones, JR, and Crout, JR. 1979. Adverse reactions of newly marketed drugs. *N Engl J Med* 300:1046–1047.
127. Vessell, ES. 1980. Why are toxic reactions to drugs so often undetected initially? *N Engl J Med* 302: 1027–1029.
128. Avorn, J, and Soumerai, SB. 1983. Improving drug-therapy decisions through educational outreach. *N Engl J Med* 308:1457–1463.
129. Spriet, A, et al. 1977. Methodology and results of a survey of adverse reactions to a drug in private practice. *Eur J Clin Pharmacol* 11:181–192.
130. Hulse, RK, et al. 1976. Computerized medication monitoring system. *Am J Hosp Pharm* 33:1061–1064.
131. Jacinto, M, and Kleinmann, K. 1983. Hospital pharmacy program for reporting adverse drug reactions. *Am J Hosp Pharm* 40:444–445.
132. Nelson, R. and Shane, R. 1983. Developing an adverse drug reaction reporting system. *Am J Hosp Pharm* 40: 445–446.
133. Powell, S, et al. 1982. Pharmacy-based adverse drug reaction surveillance program. *Am J Hosp Pharm* 39: 1963–1964.
134. Lamy, PP. 1986. Drug interactions in the elderly. In *Liver, Drugs and Aging,* Eds., CFA van Benzooijen, F Miglio, and DL Knook. Rijswik (The Netherlands): Eurage.
135. Tatro, DS, Moore, TN, and Cohen, SN. 1979. Computer-based system for adverse drug reaction, detection and prevention. *Am J Hosp Pharm* 36:198–201.
136. Friedman, RB, Young, DS, and Beatty, ES. 1978. Automated monitoring of drug-test interactions. *Clin Pharmacol Ther* 24:16–21.
137. Stewart, RB. 1977. Study of drug interactions. In *Drug Monitoring: A Requirement for Responsible Drug Use.* Eds., RB Stewart, LE Cluff, and JR Philp. Baltimore: Williams & Wilkins Co.
138. Hull, CJ. 1979. Pharmacokinetics and pharmacodynamics. *Br J Anaesth* 51:579–594.
139. Kramer, W, Inglott, A, and Cluxton, R. 1971. Physical and chemical incompatibilities of drugs for IV administration. *Drug Intell Clin Pharm* 5:211–228.
140. Stoelting, R, and Eger, E. 1983. An additional explanation for the second gas effect. *Anesthesiology* 30: 273–277.
141. Burch, PG, and Stanski, DR. 1983. The role of metabolism in protein binding in thiopental anesthesia. *Anesthesiology* 58:146–152.
142. Pandele, G, et al. 1983. Thiopental pharmacokinetics in patients with cirrhosis. *Anesthesiology* 59:123–126.
143. Murad, F, and Gilman, AG. 1985. Drug interactions. In *The Pharmacological Basis of Therapeutics,* Eds., AG Gilman, LS Goodman, TW Rall, et al. New York: MacMillan Publishing Co.
144. Smith, RB. 1981. Drug interactions and drug reactions. *Otolaryngol Clin N Am* 14:615–621.
145. Ngai, SH. 1980. Current concepts in anesthesiology: effect of anesthetic on various organs. *N Engl J Med* 302:564–566.
146. Rudd, CC. 1983. Teaching and counselling patients about drugs. In *Basic Skills in Clinical Pharmacy Practice,* Ed., DR Max. Chapel Hill, NC: Health Sciences Consortium, Inc.
147. Consumer Drug Digest, American Society of Hospital Pharmacists. 1982. New York: Facts on File.
148. United States Pharmacopoeial Convention, Inc; 1985. Advice for the patient, Volume II, ed. 5. Easton, PA: Mack Printing Co, USP DI.
149. Sackett, DL, and Snow, JC. 1979. The magnitude of compliance and noncompliance. In *Compliance in Health Care,* Eds., RB Haynes, DW Taylor, and DK Sackett. Baltimore: Johns Hopkins University Press.
150. Dirks, JF, and Kinsman, RA. 1982. Nondichotomous patterns of medication usage: The yes-no fallacy. *Clin Pharmacol Ther* 31:413–417.
151. Koch, H, and Smith, MC. 1985. Office based ambulatory care for patients 75 years and over: National Ambulatory Medical Care Survey, 1980–1981. *Advancedata* 110:1–4.
152. Hartvig, P, Wiklund, L, and Lindstrom, B. 1986. Pharmacokinetics of physostigmine after intravenous, intramuscular, and subcutaneous administration in surgical patients. *Acta Anaesthesiol Scand* 30:177–182.
153. Rizack, MS, and Hillman, CD. 1985. *The Medical Letter*

Handbook of Adverse Drug Interactions. New York: The Medical Letter, Inc.

154. Eltherington, LG. 1983. Complications of prior drug therapy. In *Complications in Anesthesiology,* Eds., FK Orkin and LH Cooperman. Philadelphia: JB Lippincott Co.

155. Ball, M, et al. 1985. Renal failure and use of morphine in intensive care. *Lancet* 2:784–786.

18

Nutritional Changes in the Elderly

Kenneth J. Storch and George L. Blackburn

While Americans aged 65 and over account for less than 12% of the U.S. population (1), 30% of our national health care costs (2) are expended on their care. In addition, senior citizens comprise the fastest growing segment of our population (1). Much of the extra health care allotted to the elderly relates to chronic diseases, yet impaired nutrition also plays a key role in declining health associated with aging. Estimates of malnutrition among hospitalized or institutionalized elderly patients vary from 19% to 85%, depending on the population and the criteria used (3). The contribution of poor nutritional status to increased morbidity and mortality among hospitalized patients must be curtailed, particularly since malnutrition is often iatrogenic. Increased attention to the nutritional status of our aging population could alleviate the national health care crisis as well as promote individual health and well-being.

The elderly must be treated as a distinct group when assessing nutritional status. However, of all age groups, they are the most heterogeneous. Differences in genetic endowment and environmental influences (e.g., cigarette smoking, alcohol consumption, overeating, sedentary lifestyle) exert significant individual effects over the course of decades (4). The influx of refugees who have survived famines and periods of starvation in their native lands will, as they age, constitute a group of Americans who may have an exaggerated loss of lean tissue and special nutritional vulnerabilities. Functional changes associated with aging vary from minimal deterioration in certain individuals to profound changes in less fortunate ones. It is important to realize that within each patient, the effects of aging vary at all levels, from organ systems down to organelles.

The surgeon should be aware of these nutritionally relevant effects of aging, including alterations in body composition, digestive and absorptive functions of the gastrointestinal tract, and requirements for macro- and micronutrients. Drug-nutrient interactions are also important in the elderly population. Understanding the relationship between malnutrition and pathophysiology facilitates rational nutritional evaluation and provides an effective approach to optimize wound healing, recovery, and long-term health.

Factors Predisposing to Poor Nutrition Among the Elderly

Numerous functional changes associated with chronologic aging impact on the patient's nutritional status. Appetite and the sense of taste are frequently affected by the psychological and physiologic changes of aging (5, 6), and such limitations may also impair the ability to obtain or prepare appropriate meals. The increased prevalence of chronic diseases may affect the efficiency with which nutrients are utilized, as in diabetes and renal and hepatic dysfunction. For this reason, nutrient requirements for the aged individual may be altered, both absolutely and relative to each other. Surveillance of high-risk patients should emphasize physical examinations assessing appetite, eating habits, and physical impairment.

Several widely observed consequences of aging can lead to poor food intake and subsequent poor nutrition among the elderly. Poor dental status and reduced salivation may result in changing food selections to those most easily chewed and swallowed; when dysphagia is severe, many classes of foods may be eliminated. The diminished senses of taste and smell may lessen interest in eating, reducing overall intake, so that only familiar or favorite foods that may be high in calories but low in nutrients are eaten. Zinc depletion may also affect appetite. While a four to six ounce serving of milk taken with a meal is rarely a problem, the perception that certain foods cause functional symptoms (i.e., the association of dairy products with bloating or flatulence) may lessen intake of these foods. The food and symptoms may be temporally but not causally related, since the symptom may result from normal physiologic change like the slowing of gastric emptying or other motility disorders.

Psychosocial factors can also contribute to poor intake. Decreased interest in food may be a consequence of organic brain disease as well as depression, social isolation, and grief after the loss of a spouse. Immobility may limit food shopping. Decreased vision or cognitive function may impair ability to cook, with consequent reliance on pre-prepared or packaged food, which may not provide an appropriate variety of nutrients. Even when congregate meals are available, the elderly person may find it difficult to travel to the program site, or the foods provided may be unacceptable due to ethnic or personal preferences.

The practitioner must be aware of these factors, both to understand the nutritional status of the newly admitted patient and to make appropriate discharge plans. The malnourished patient who is nutritionally rehabilitated while in the hospital will not maintain a well-nourished state unless the living conditions are supportive.

The Digestive Tract in Aging

The gastrointestinal (GI) tract is among the most metabolically active tissues in the body, undergoing rapid turnover. Deteriorated digestive and absorptive function is potentially serious due to the pivotal role in nutritional homeostasis. Studies have associated aging with physiologic changes of each segment of the GI tract.

Oral Cavity

It is difficult to excuse the health care professional for permitting semistarvation due to poorly fitting or missing dental fixtures. Decreased salivary function (7) can impair mastication of solid food, both directly and through disease of the gingivae and dentition (8, 9); however, the decrease in salivary amylase associated with aging does not measurably affect the ability to digest starch (10). Difficulty in swallowing, a frequent complaint among the elderly, may be related to reduced saliva secretion, although chronic disease may also contribute to dysphagia (11), and treatable pathology should be sought.

Esophagus

Peristalsis of the esophagus may become irregular or may not occur, though the relation between this and dysphagia is not always clear (11, 12). Hiatal hernia, lower esophageal sphincter dysfunction, and gastroesophageal reflux are more common. When meals are taken in a supine position, slower esophageal emptying and lower esophageal sphincter incompetence leads to an increased risk of aspiration and pneumonia. As a result, the diet must frequently be given in six small feedings.

Stomach

Gastric juice secretion is decreased, both in volume and in hydrochloric acid concentration, due to a decreased number of parietal cells and a decreased secretory capacity of the remaining cells (13). Loss of parietal cells in gastric mucosal atrophy can lower secretion of intrinsic factor and produce a subsequent vitamin B_{12} malabsorption and deficiency. Pepsin, but not trypsin, secretion is diminished, although the effect on protein digestion and absorption is unknown (10). Gastric emptying may be slower on average than that in younger persons (14).

Pancreas

The concentration of pancreatic lipase diminishes with age, averaging 20% less than that of younger controls (15). The amount of pancreatic juice produced, however, and the concentration of pancreatic amylase do not appear to change (16).

Liver

The flow of bile does not normally change with age, although gallbladder disease does become more common. The fraction of patients aged 70 or older, who were either undergoing gallbladder surgery or known to carry gallstones, has been found to exceed one in three (17). Gallbladder disease is a factor in the increased prevalence of fat intolerance, as discussed below.

Small Intestine

The surface area of the small intestine decreases with advancing age. Mucosal atrophy involves a lower ratio of villus surface area to volume, with a decrease in height and a slight increase in width. In the presence of concurrent chronic diseases, this effect may be pronounced with a corresponding decline in absorptive capacity (18, 19). Small intestinal diverticula are more likely to be colonized by atypical bacteria in the elderly than are those of younger persons. This may be related to decreased gastric acid, combined with ingestion of anaerobes from respiratory or oral sites and stasis of intradiverticular contents

(20). The deconjugated bile salts from bacterial action may result in malabsorptive states (20).

Large Intestine

With increasing age, the large bowel mucosa atrophies and is partially replaced with smooth muscle and connective tissue (21). As in the small intestine, diverticula become more common. Estimates of diverticular disease increase from 5% of persons at age 40, to 50% by age 90 (22).

Constipation is more frequently a problem, but the role of aging per se may be minor compared to other factors, such as decreased activity, chronic illness, and dietary changes (14).

GI Absorption

Impaired D-xylose absorption tests in the elderly (23), particularly after age 80 (24), imply reduced absorptive capacity at the mucosal surface. However, this may also reflect other factors, such as delayed gastric emptying. Decreased galactose absorption has also been documented in the elderly (25). Data on absorption of disaccharides and digestible polysaccharides (starches) are sketchier, although breath hydrogen tests reveal that one-third to two-thirds of the elderly suffer some degree of carbohydrate malabsorption (26).

While many elderly people appear to be lactose intolerant, true lactase deficiency is manifested by early adulthood and is not a normal result of aging. It has been suggested that psychological factors (e.g., the expectation that milk products will cause symptoms) are important in lactose intolerance (27).

Body Composition

Metabolic differences between the elderly and other age groups are often attributable to differences in the relative amounts of body cell mass, independent of total body weight (28). A mixed pattern is typically observed in which vital body tissue is diminished, but storage triglycerides in adipose tissue and often extracellular water are increased. On average, body weight increases with aging, but this is highly variable. Table 18-1 presents data which are considered desirable weights for the elderly. Desirable body weights are adapted from the 1959 Metropolitan Life Insurance tables and corrected for weight of clothing and height of shoes. These data reflect the average weight for medium build and have been corrected to apply to patients with shoes off (29). The Gerontology Research Center of the National Institute on Aging has established age-specific weights (Table 18-2) that apply to healthy individuals (30). Regardless of which data are used, these should only be used as a guide.

Total Body Water

Total body water (TBW), consisting of intracellular and extracellular water, is a measure of lean body mass or fat-free mass. Average TBW decreases with age from about 60% of body weight in men at age 20, to about 50% by age 60 (31). However, peripheral edema, ascites, or congestive heart failure are more likely to lead to an elevated TBW in the elderly patient due to expanded extracellular compartments (interstitial fluid, plasma, and lymph).

Body Cell Mass

Body cell mass, which decreases with age, includes non-adipose components of living tissues, such as muscle, nervous system, and visceral organ weight. Muscle mass may decrease by a factor of 50% between youth and age 70 (32). Although there is some evidence that continued activity results in less dramatic changes (33), most organs decrease in size with some exceptions, such as the prostate, lungs, and often the heart. Atrophy due to hypoplasia is generally not considered reversible.

Bone Mass

Bone mass and density reach a maximum between ages 30 and 40 in both sexes and decrease thereafter. Most women experience a greater loss than men after age 50 (34), and the presence of osteoporosis reflects markedly increased bone loss. Risk factors for postmenopausal osteoporosis include maternal history of osteoporosis, life-

Table 18-1. Desirable weights for the elderly

Height (ft/in)	Average IBW in Men (lb)	Average IBW in Women (lb)
4 9	—	100
4 10	—	103
4 11	—	106
5 0	—	109
5 1	117	112
5 2	120	116
5 3	123	120
5 4	126	124
5 5	129	128
5 6	133	132
5 7	138	136
5 8	142	140
5 9	146	144
5 10	150	148
5 11	155	—
6 0	159	—
6 1	164	—
6 2	169	—
6 3	174	—

Reprinted with permission from Simopoulos, AP. 1985. Dietary control of hypertension and obesity and body weight standards. *J Am Dietetic Assoc* 85:419 (Ref. 29).

Table 18-2. Age-specific weights

Height	Metropolitan 1983 weights for ages 25–59		Gerontology Research Center weight range for men and women by age (years)				
	Men	Women	20–29	30–39	40–49	50–59	60–69
ft-in	Pounds				Pounds		
4-10	—	100–131	84–111	92–119	99–127	107–135	115–142
4-11	—	101–134	87–115	95–123	103–131	111–139	119–147
5-0	—	103–137	90–119	98–127	106–135	114–143	123–152
5-1	123–145	105–140	93–123	101–131	110–140	118–148	127–157
5-2	125–148	108–144	96–127	105–136	113–144	122–153	131–163
5-3	127–151	111–148	99–131	108–140	117–149	126–158	135–168
5-4	129–155	114–152	102–135	112–145	121–154	130–163	140–173
5-5	131–159	117–156	106–140	115–149	125–159	134–168	144–179
5-6	133–163	120–160	109–144	119–154	129–164	138–174	148–184
5-7	135–167	123–164	112–148	122–159	133–169	143–179	153–190
5-8	137–171	126–167	116–153	126–163	137–174	147–184	158–196
5-9	139–175	129–170	119–157	130–168	141–179	151–190	162–201
5-10	141–179	132–173	122–162	134–173	145–184	156–195	167–207
5-11	144–183	135–176	126–167	137–178	149–190	160–201	172–213
6-0	147–187	—	129–171	141–183	153–195	165–207	177–219
6-1	150–192	—	133–176	145–188	157–200	169–213	182–225
6-2	153–197	—	134–181	149–194	162–206	174–219	187–232
6-3	157–202	—	141–186	153–199	166–212	179–225	192–238
6-4	—	—	144–191	157–205	171–218	184–231	197–244

Reprinted with permission from Andres, R, et al. 1985. Impact of age on weight goals. *Ann Intern Med* 103:1030–1033 (Ref. 30).

long thinness, sedentary lifestyle, and low calcium and protein intake. Chronically high protein intakes have been associated with negative calcium balance and may also have a potential role in bone disease of the aged as well. The risk of osteoporosis in later life is probably inversely related to the extent of bone accretion (mineral and protein) in the first four decades of life (35). Undoubtedly, estrogen replacement therapy will play a growing role in female metabolic support, now that the role of estrogen in bone physiology (36) and its apparent value in preventing bone fractures (37) have been demonstrated.

Adipose

The percentage of body weight as fat tends to increase with age since body cell mass and bone mass decrease. Additionally, average weight in most population groups increases through middle age and beyond, despite the decrease in body cell mass. Thus, the increase in fat is both relative and absolute (38). Lipolysis appears to be under regulation since whole body palmitate and glycerol kinetics are similar in the young and elderly, despite a doubling of the adipose tissue mass in the latter (39). Fat deposition appears to be predominantly central rather than subcutaneous, so that skin- and fatfold thicknesses, especially on the extremities, may not adequately reflect fat stores (40). Nevertheless, triceps skinfold thickness may provide a qualitative estimate of depleted or abundant fat stores (Table 18-3) (41).

At extreme ages, average weights decline, due in part to the greater mortality of the heavier individuals and in part to a decrease in caloric intake, below even the low-energy expenditure associated with aging (42).

Nutritional Assessment of the Elderly

Nutritional assessment of the elderly should be an orderly procedure, either performed following or integrated within the initial medical/surgical evaluation. The baseline assessment data profile should describe the state of nutrition and provide indications and direction for nutritional intervention. Like other forms of therapy, the initial intervention plan comprises a best, yet inexact, estimate of the patient's needs. By studying the sequential metabolic response to the nutritional intervention, the nutrition support team can optimize the anabolic effects of nutritional support, while minimizing adverse effects.

The clinical condition and level of nutrient depletion of the patient are likely to change over time. Therefore, nutritional requirements are also likely to change. Nutritional indicators are measured repeatedly to assure that the treatment remains appropriate and to judge the time point in which specialized nutritional support is no longer necessary.

Table 18-3. Triceps skinfold (TSF) and arm muscle circumference (AMC)

Test	Age 25–34.9	Age 67–74.9	Percentage of change
TSF (mm)[a]	21	24	14
AMC (cm)[a]	21.2	22.5	16

Reprinted with permission from Frisancho, AR. 1981. New norms of upper limb fat and muscle areas for assessment of nutritional status. *Am J Clin Nutr* 34:2540–2545 (Ref. 41).

[a]Fiftieth percentile values from Health and Nutrition Evaluation Survey of 1971–1974 (females).

Nutritional History

Important historical findings to focus on include:

1. *Symptoms related to body composition:* edema, recent intentional weight loss, recent unintentional weight loss (43), prolonged immobilization or limitation in physical activity; recent surgery, trauma, or sepsis
2. *Symptoms related to food intake:* difficulty eating, change in appetite, altered food intake, food allergy, food intolerance, special cultural or religious dietary needs, unusual food preferences or habits, mouth discomfort, chewing or swallowing difficulty, anorexia, nausea and vomiting, chronic illness
3. *Symptoms related to nutrient absorption:* bloating, abdominal distention, diarrhea, cramping, fistulae, prior abdominal surgery
4. *Metabolic disorders:* Type II diabetes, use of insulin, history of ketoacidosis, altered thyroid status, previous treatment for thyroid conditions, hyperlipidemia, prior or present use of corticosteroids, persistent fevers, alcohol/drug abuse, renal diseases, hepatic diseases
5. *Medical/surgical conditions:* chronicity, pharmaceutical treatments, allergies

Physical Examination

A complete physical examination is necessary for nutritional assessment. Areas of special focus include:

1. *Mental status:* Can the patient take responsibility for eating, or should oral feedings be supervised?
2. *Oral cavity:* Hypoactive gag reflex should be of concern due to the increased risk of aspiration. This applies to intragastric feedings as well as oral feedings, since some regurgitation frequently occurs in the debilitated hospitalized patient. Longitudinal furrows of the tongue are caused by reduction in tongue volume and are a reliable clinical indicator of dehydration. A dry tongue without longitudinal furrows is not a reliable index of dehydration since it is commonly the result of open-mouth breathing or hyposalivation. Atrophic glossitis (often with dryness, paresthesias, or burning) is associated with deficiencies of the B vitamins (especially B_{12} and folate) and iron as well as protein-calorie malnutrition.
3. *Skeletal muscles:* Inspection of the muscle groups provides insight into long-term physical activity levels and chronic protein-calorie malnutrition. Wasting of the skull muscles with exaggerated prominence of facial features often indicates advanced chronic semistarvation.
4. *Subcutaneous adipose deposits:* Depletion of storage triglycerides due to chronic semistarvation is often readily apparent, though peripheral edema may mask this finding.
5. *Abdomen:* Surgical scars are a clue to adhesions and prior intestinal resections. Enterocutaneous fistulae may result in significant losses of fluids and all classes of nutrients, particularly electrolytes, minerals, and proteins. Distention may suggest ileus or obstruction, making parenteral nutrition the choice intervention.
6. *Peripheral edema or ascites:* Cirrhosis or the combination of protein-calorie malnutrition and metabolic stress, leading to loss of oncotic pressure due to hypoalbuminemia, may cause peripheral edema.
7. *Evidence of hepatic disease:* Jaundice and other stigmata of liver damage should be noted.

Anthropometry

1. *Gender (male or female)*
2. *Height (cm, without shoes)*
3. *Weight (kg, in hospital gown):* Both height and weight should be measured directly, even in the nonambulatory patient. A recent weight loss of 10% is a highly significant indicator of malnutrition (44). Elderly persons may be unaware of current weight and may report their maximum height, even though height may have been lost in intervening years. Bowman and Rosenberg (45) have reported an average loss of 4.9 cm in women and 2.9 cm in men with aging.
4. *Usual body weight (UBW):* The patient or spouse can generally provide this figure. A stable lifelong weight is often a more relevant standard for the individual than a population-derived “desirable” weight.
5. *Desirable body weight (DBW):* This is derived from tables which give average weight for height by gen-

der (Tables 18-1, 18-2). Tables which take age into account should be used for aged patients (46). The body mass index (BMI), also called Quetelet Index, is a useful measure of body proportions largely independent of height. Calculated as follows, BMI = weight (kg)/height $(cm)^2$, this eliminates the need to refer to a special table of weight for height (47).

6. *Weight as %UBW*
7. *Weight as %DBW*
8. *Triceps skinfold (TSF) in mm and as percent of standard* (Table 18-3)
9. *Mid-arm circumference (MAC) in cm*
10. *Arm muscle circumference (AMC) in cm:* This quantitator of the somatic muscle protein compartment is derived from TSF and MAC. Frisancho (41) suggests the following equation for adults:

$$\text{Arm Muscle Circumference} = \frac{\text{MAC} - (3.14 \times \text{TSF})}{10}$$

Arm muscle circumference can be rated as a percentage of standards (41) applicable to older adults. As noted previously, difficulty in taking skinfold measures may particularly limit the usefulness of this parameter in the elderly.

Blood Tests

Those of nutritional relevance include:

1. *Serum electrolytes:* The physician managing nutritional treatment is in a key position to detect and participate in the treatment of disturbances in fluid, electrolyte, and acid-base homeostasis. In metabolic acidosis, one calculates the "anion gap" (Na-Cl-Bicarbonate) to screen for abnormal levels of "unmeasured" endogenous and/or exogenous anions.
2. *BUN and serum creatinine:* These aid in renal function evaluation and level of hydration and nitrogen metabolism; low BUN values may result from chronic protein inadequacy as well as advanced hepatic dysfunction and overhydration.
3. *Serum phosphorus and magnesium:* These two minerals are important components of body cell mass. Clinical deficiencies (especially hypophosphatemia) are common, yet largely preventable, and must be treated vigorously to maximize anabolism.
4. *Clotting profile, bilirubin, and liver enzymes:* These aid in evaluation of hepatic function.
5. *Hepatic secretory proteins:* All plasma protein levels are affected by various factors independent of nutritional status, and changing values must be interpreted in clinical as well as nutritional terms (48). Serum albumin has a half-life of 20 days compared to a half-life of 8 days for transferrin. When used as indices of visceral protein status (Table 18-4) (49), the former serves as a chronic index and the latter as a subacute index. Malnutrition and hypoalbuminemia predict increased risk for the development of decubitus ulcers (50, 51). Proteins such as thyroid binding prealbumin (half-life = 48 hours) and retinol binding protein (half-life = 12 hours), which are rapidly turned over, are under investigation for their acute usefulness but are generally not employed clinically.

   Serum transferrin may be calculated from total iron binding capacity (TIBC) using the following formula: Transferrin = (0.8 × TIBC) − 43. However, this relationship may be altered in certain circumstances, including iron deficiency (52).
6. *Serum cholesterol and triglyceride levels:* Serum cholesterol is a predictor for risk of atherosclerotic progression in younger age groups. In institutionalized veterans, low serum cholesterol levels (e.g., below 156 mg/dl) are found to predict short-term morbidity and mortality (53, 54). The screening of serum triglyceride levels is useful in evaluating the clearance (utilization) of intravenous lipid emulsions, although visual scanning for lipemia is adequate.
7. *Total lymphocyte count:* This crude but readily available indicator of nutritional depletion (Table 18-4) predicts a poor clinical outcome at levels below $1{,}000/mm^3$, which, in appropriate contexts, is suggestive of malnutrition.
8. *White blood cell count (WBC) differential:* shift to immature forms of the granulocyte line provides data on degree of activation of endogenous mediators of the immune response.

Table 18-4. Serum standards for nutritional assessment of the elderly

	% of Deficit		
	Mild	Moderate	Severe
Albumin (g/dl)	3.5–3.2	3.2–2.8	<2.8
Transferrin (mg/dl)	200–180	180–160	<160
TLC ($No./mm^3$)	1,800–1,500	1,500–900	<900

Reprinted with permission from Colluci, RA, Bell, SJ, and Blackburn, GL. 1987. Nutritional problems of institutionalized and free-living elderly. *Compreh Ther* 13:20–28 (Ref. 49).

24-Hour Urine Tests

The following assessments of 24-hour urine collection may help to ascertain changes in lean body mass in response to nutritional support.

1. *Daily urinary urea nitrogen excretion (UUN) in grams* (Figure 18-1): This is useful both in the calculation of nitrogen balance and estimation of degree of catabolism (net protein breakdown). Nitrogen balance may be readily calculated by assuming all nitrogen losses other than UUN add up to a total of 4 g per day (non-urea urinary nitrogen is largely creatinine, uric acid, and ammonia; GI, skin losses, and miscellaneous body fluids account for most of the rest). In clinical settings, such as protein-losing enteropathy, exceptionally severe proteinuria, peritoneal dialysis, or any other significant nitrogen losses, the 4 g per day factor becomes invalid, and direct measurements of non-UUN nitrogen losses must be quantified.

Nitrogen Balance = protein intake/6.25 − (UUN + 4)

2. *Creatinine height index:* Assuming a complete urinary collection with an insignificant contribution from dietary meat, urinary creatinine excretion indexes the size of the creatine phosphate pool, which in turn reflects muscle compartment size. This can be expressed as a percentage of standard values (Table 18-5) (55). Since muscle mass tends to decline with age, age must be factored into the table of standards (Table 18-6) (56).

Miscellaneous Tests

Fever Curve

Maximal daily temperatures are highly correlated with degree of metabolic stress from infectious and inflammatory processes.

Delayed Hypersensitivity Testing

Intradermal test panels of common antigens (e.g., mumps, candida, trichophyton, streptokinase, and tetanus toxoid) measure immune competence, specifically looking at one aspect of T cell function. Commercially available panels include multiple antigens joined by a mechanical link that allows all tests to be applied simultaneously; the skin test site is then checked 24 to 48 hours after inoculation. True induration (raised margins), at least 5 mm in diameter, indicates intact functional response to any antigen. Anergy to multiple common antigens potentially manifests protein-calorie malnutrition as

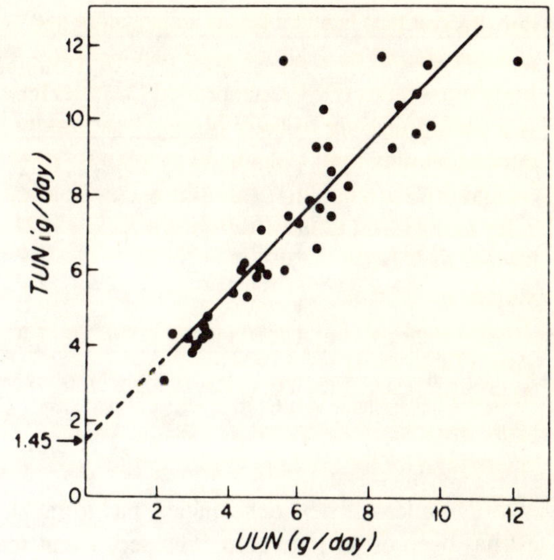

Figure 18-1. Relationship between daily total urinary nitrogen (TUN) and urinary urea nitrogen (UUN). Each patient's (n = 7) monthly UNN vs TUN is plotted for each of the 6 months. Using regression analysis of all the values ($r = 0.90, p < .01$), the line was drawn [equation: TUN (Y) = 0.99 × UNN (X) + 1.45] (74). (Reproduced with permission from Clark, NG, Rappaport, JI, DiScala, C, Lamothe, PA, and Blackburn, GL. 1988. Nutritional support of the chronically ill female at risk for elective or urgent surgery. *J Am College Nutr* 7:17–26.)

Table 18-5. Ideal urinary creatinine values

Men[a]		Women[b]	
Height (cm)	Ideal creatinine (mg)	Height (cm)	Ideal creatinine (mg)
157.5	1,288	147.3	830
160.0	1,325	149.9	861
162.6	1,359	152.4	875
165.1	1,386	154.9	900
167.6	1,426	157.5	925
170.2	1,467	160.0	949
172.7	1,513	162.6	977
175.3	1,555	165.1	1,006
177.8	1,596	167.6	1,064
180.3	1,642	170.2	1,076
182.9	1,691	172.7	1,109
185.4	1,739	175.3	1,141
188.0	1,785	177.8	1,174
190.5	1,831	180.3	1,206
193.0	1,891	182.9	1,240

Reprinted with permission from Clark, NG, and Blackburn, GL. 1983. Nutritional assessment and support of the elderly patient. *AM J IV Ther Clin Nutr* 10:14 (Ref. 55).

[a]Creatinine coefficient (men) = 23 mg/kg of ideal body weight.

[b]Creatinine coefficient (women) = 18 mg/kg of ideal body weight.

Table 18-6. Creatinine height index as a function of age

Age (yr)	*n*	Creatinine excretion (mg/24 hr)	Creatinine height index
17–24	10	1,790 + 52	10.2
25–34	73	1,862 + 31	10.6
35–44	122	1,746 + 24	10.0
45–54	152	1,689 + 18	9.6
55–64	94	1,580 + 22	9.0
65–74	68	1,409 + 25	8.0
75–84	29	1,259 + 45	7.2

Reprinted with permission from Driver, AL, and McAlvey, MT. 1980. Creatinine height index as a function of age (letter). *Am J Clin Nutr* 33:2057 (Ref. 56).

well as certain micronutrient deficiencies, including zinc. The test has been of value in predicting sepsis and mortality in the elderly (57) and in hospitalized patients (58), although not in all hands (59).

Body Composition

Accurate measurements of lean body mass (LBM), total body water, body cell mass, and percent body fat remain primarily research techniques, although the necessary technology is being validated for clinical use, while becoming more cost effective (61). The information may assist assessment of body weight data and ultimately the efficacy of nutritional support. However, present techniques which are listed below are insensitive to short-term body cell mass accretion (e.g., 1 to 3 weeks), and problems remain that complicate the interpretation of measurements performed on elderly individuals.

1. *Electrical impedance:* Because LBM conducts electrical current better than adipose tissue, electrical impedance can be used as a method to determine relative proportions of fat and lean tissue (62). This technique, also called "total body electrical conductivity" (TOBEC), is quickly and easily performed yet is reliable only if the mathematical equations are based on validation data from populations closely matching the individual patient; validation studies are actively underway.
2. *Densitometry:* The percentage by weight of bone, LBM, and fat may be determined mathematically by exploiting the differences in specific gravity of the different tissues. The technique involves weighing a subject in air and underwater, while determining the volume of water displaced at full exhalation (63). However, the increased porosity of bone with advancing age, changes in body water distribution, variability in residual lung volumes, and difficulty in performing underwater weighing in populations with reduced mobility lower the practicality of this method in the elderly.
3. *Isotopic tracer dilution:* LBM is indirectly estimated using the dilution factor measured after a stable isotope, such as ^{42}K, ^{82}Br, ^{24}Na, ^{3}H, or ^{18}O, which, following administration, is allowed to equilibrate with its total body pool or total body water (64). These measurements assume a direct relation between the size of the compartment into which the tracer distributes and lean body mass (LBM). Therefore, a calculation can be made to determine LBM. However, while LBM is estimated at 73% water, the nonfat portion of adipose tissue is 88% water. As adipose tissue increases with advancing age, isotope dilution methods overestimate the proportion of adipose tissue (61). In addition, the elderly patients may not be in fluid balance due to fluid retention or dehydration.
4. *Whole body counting:* Body potassium contains a constant percentage (~0.012%) of the radioactive isotope ^{40}K, which is assumed to comprise a fixed portion of total body water (65). However, muscle is higher in potassium (134 mEq/kg) than are other lean tissues, such as visceral organs (70 to 80 mEq/kg) or skin connective tissues (34 mEq/kg) (62). Whole body counting tends to overestimate body fat in the elderly due to muscle loss and increased connective tissue (65).

Global Appraisal of Nutritional Status

Most nutritional assessment and interpretation can be done by a dietician/nutritionist with training in nutritional support (44, 48). In conducting a global appraisal of nutritional status, two extreme patterns of macronutrient depletion can be identified.

Successful adaptation to semistarvation, or marasmus-like malnutrition, is characterized by weight loss and a decrease in other anthropometric measurements, while maintaining visceral protein levels (albumin, transferrin) and immune status.

In unsuccessful adaption to semistarvation, hypoalbuminemic or kwashiorkor-like malnutrition, visceral proteins and possibly immune function are affected. In acute cases, weight and muscle protein stores appear to be maintained. Weights may be elevated due to "third spacing" of fluid caused by decline in plasma oncotic pressure and/or increased capillary permeability due to endogenous inflammatory mediator release.

Various clinical predictors of risk for mortality and morbidity have been developed as adjuncts (66) in the assessment of nutritional depletion and metabolic stress, ranging from an "instant" technique (67) to more elaborate approaches (68, 69).

Nutritional Requirements

The Food and Nutrition Board of the National Academy of Sciences published the most recent set of recommended dietary allowances (10th edition) in late 1989. A 4-year publication delay was caused by a lack of consensus on dynamic topics, including the interactions between nutrition and aging (70).

Energy Requirements

Overall caloric requirements decrease with aging. Although the basal metabolic rate is unchanged in relation to body cell mass, the absolute rate declines as body cell mass decreases and fat mass increases. Small decreases in O_2 consumption begin as early as age 20 but are more dramatic after age 45. This translates to about a 2% decrease per decade in basal metabolic rate after age 50 (71). In addition, caloric expenditure for physical activity declines, as individuals become more sedentary. The recommended dietary allowances (RDAs) for energy intake in healthy elderly doing light work are decreased in two steps relative to young adults: by 10% between ages 50 and 75 and by a total of 20% to 25% after age 75 (72). The recommended daily intake ranges are 2,000 to 2,800 kcal (men) and 1,400 to 2,200 kcal (women) between ages 50 and 75, and 1,650 to 2,450 (men) and 1,200 to 2,000 (women) over age 75.

Basal energy expenditure (BEE) may be predicted with fair but inconsistent reliability by one of several experimentally derived algorithms. Ideally, the algorithm should be derived from a population closely resembling the patient in question. Energy needs are age related, and this should be taken into account. The most commonly employed equations were derived from the Harris-Benedict Survey (73).

Harris-Benedict Equations:

$$\text{For men: BEE} = 66 + (13.7 \times W) + (5.0 \times H) - (6.8 \times A)$$

$$\text{For women: BEE} = 655 + (9.7 \times W) + (1.8 \times H) - (4.7 \times A)$$

W is weight in kg, H is height in cm and A is age in years.

For free-living adults, the total allowance of calories includes provisions for the thermogenic effect of food (approximately 10% of the daily total) and physical activity as well as the BEE. However, clinical caloric requirements usually fall below such an estimate. Clark et al. (74) have assessed the nutritional needs of the chronically ill elderly female at risk for elective or urgent surgery. The observed mean energy requirement for weight maintenance was 98% of the calculated BEE (Fig. 18-2). While certain stresses (e.g., major burns and head trauma) show well documented large energy expenditure increases (50% to 100%) above predicted resting energy expenditure (REE), typical stresses (e.g., sepsis, uncomplicated surgery) are counterbalanced by the decrease in physical activity, keeping total caloric requirements often within 20% of predicted REE in hospitalized patients.

Resting Energy Expenditure

Indirect calorimetry is a superior method for assessing energy requirements in the individual patient, eliminating the guesswork in estimating the combined effects of body composition, nutritional status, disease processes, trauma, and clinical events on metabolic rate as predicted from nomograms (60).

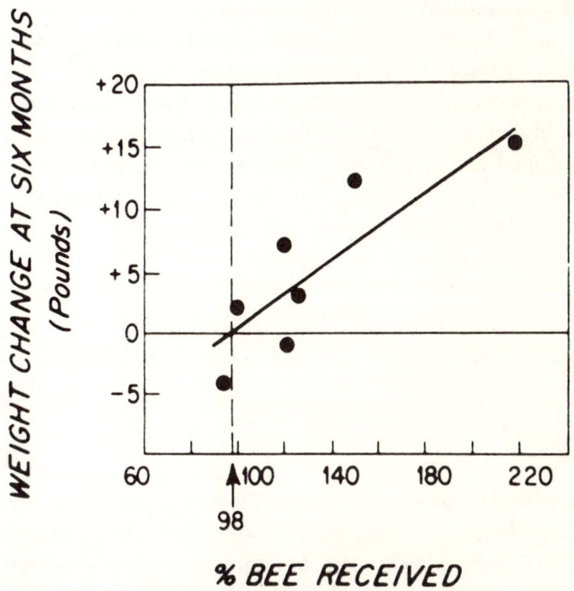

Figure 18-2. Relationship of weight change to energy intake. Each patient's ($n = 7$) weight change over the 6-month study period is indicated. Using regression analysis ($r = 0.86$, $p < .01$), the line was drawn [equation: weight change (Y) = 0.139 × BEE 8 (X) − 13.75]. As indicated, weight maintenance occurred at 98% of calculated BEE. Basal energy expenditure (BEE) = 655 + (9.6 × wt) + (1.7 × ht) − (4.7 × age) (74). (Reproduced with permission from Clark, NG, Rappaport, JI, DiScala, C, Lamothe, PA, and Blackburn, GL. 1988. Nutritional support of the chronically ill female at risk for elective or urgent surgery. *J Am College Nutr* 7:17–26.)

Protein Requirements

Unlike energy requirements, protein requirements per kilogram of lean body weight may actually rise with age. The elderly consume less protein than younger age groups on average, in part due to difficulty in chewing meat with inadequate dentition.

In various experimental models and in patients with chronic renal disease, high protein intakes have been associated with a hastening of renal function deterioration (75). Therefore, protein intake must be tailored to an adequate but not excessive level, particularly on a chronic basis.

Although the Food and Agriculture Organization/World Health Organization (FAO/WHO) recommended a minimum daily intake of 0.6 g/kg of body weight in 1973, higher intakes, 0.8 g/kg (76) or more (77), have been found necessary to maintain nitrogen equilibrium in short-term studies conducted in the United States. The U.S. RDA guidelines recommend 12% of total caloric intake for maintenance protein intake in the elderly population. In cases where repletion is necessary, temporary higher intakes of 1.2 to 1.5 g or protein per kilogram are reasonable, as long as the patient is under clinical observation, and azotemia is not excessive.

At normal levels of intake, protein appears to be as well digested and absorbed among the healthy elderly as in younger adults, despite changes in gastric secretions. At higher levels of intake (above 1.5 g/kg), however, fecal nitrogen increases (78), indicating less efficient absorption. Protein requirements may increase substantially with illness, often necessitating a 30% to 50% increase above maintenance intake. Clark et al. (74) have found that chronically ill elderly females scheduled to undergo surgery required a 30% (factorial) increase over normal protein requirements (e.g., 1.15 g/kg) (Fig. 18-3).

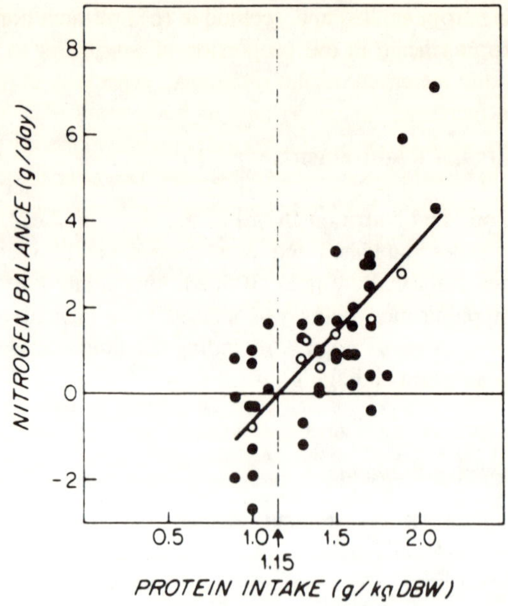

Figure 18-3. Relationship of nitrogen balance (NB) to protein intake using UUN + 4 to estimate total nitrogen loss. Each patient's (n = 7) monthly NB (g/day) vs. protein intake [g/kg desirable body weight (DBW)] is plotted. Using regression analysis of each patient's mean value for the 6-month study period (O) ($r = 0.94$, $p < .005$), the line was drawn [equation: NB (Y) = 3.55 × protein intake (X) − 4.03]. Indicated also is the minimal protein intake at which positive NB occurred (1.15 g/kg DBW) (74). (Reproduced with permission from Clark, NG, Rappaport, JI, DiScala, C, Lamothe, PA, and Blackburn, GL. 1988. Nutritional support of the chronically ill female at risk for elective or urgent surgery. *J Am College Nutr* 7:17–26.)

Lipids

Impaired GI fat absorption in the elderly appears to result from pancreatic exocrine deficiency (79). Fats are absorbed more slowly, and the absolute amount absorbed may be somewhat less. Defects in mucosal cell absorptive capacity of the small intestine cannot yet be determined (14), although experimental lipase feeding has improved fat absorption rates (80). Dietary habits may also affect fat digestion and absorption: a large amount of fat presented in a single meal may be poorly tolerated, while the same amount divided into three meals spaced throughout the day may not present problems (81). Fat intolerance can also cause flatulence, a common GI complaint in the elderly (11).

Nonprotein calories are supplied by carbohydrates and/or lipids. Calorically dense lipids (9 kcal/g compared with 4 kcal/g for carbohydrates and proteins) are required in long-term nutritional support for the provision of essential fatty acids. High carbohydrate intakes are associated with certain adverse metabolic effects, such as fatty liver and excessive bicarbonate production, which may lead to CO_2 retention. Thus "balanced" feeding regimens provide both lipid and carbohydrate calories. Novel therapeutic uses of specific types of fats are under investigation. For example, triglycerides containing omega-3 fatty acids, such as eicosapentaenoic acid (EPA) found in fish oils, may minimize the likelihood of septic shock.

Carbohydrate Intolerance

Incidence of noninsulin dependent diabetes mellitus increases with age, estimated at 16.5% of 65-year-olds and 26% of 85-year-olds (82). Even among those without overt signs of diabetes, glucose tolerance, as measured by a glucose tolerance test, may be impaired. This intolerance may be related to decreased or delayed secretion of insulin, a change in the proportion of proinsulin to insulin, and increased insulin resistance, especially in light of the increased fat percentage of body mass (32, 83). Factors, such as obesity, increased percentage of body fat, poor diet, and physical inactivity, may also contribute to observed effects, but some decrease in glucose tolerance may be a normal consequence of aging (83). When treating malnourished elderly patients, elevated blood glucose levels are more frequently seen.

Vitamins and Minerals

Important changes in vitamin and mineral nutrition among the elderly are detailed below.

Vitamin B_6

Vitamin B_6 adequacy diminishes with age due to decreased intake, absorption efficiency, and activation (84). In one study, plasma B_6 levels of unsupplemented men decreased by 0.9 mg/ml per decade after age 60 (85). The RDA for vitamin B_6 is 2.2 mg for males and 2.0 mg for females (72).

Folic Acid

Circulating levels and body pools of folate decrease with advancing age. Estimated daily requirements have recently been down-graded to 200 μg for men and 180 μg for women. Nutritional supplements can help to achieve recommended folacin intakes for older adults (72), when dietary intervention proves inadequate. Mechanisms for reduced folate nutrition include inadequate dietary intake, utilization interference from alcohol use or drug antagonism (86), and /or impaired absorption. Folate naturally occurs as a polyglutamate that must be hydrolyzed by pteroylpolyglutamate hydrolase in the mucosal cell prior to its absorption into portal blood.

Vitamin B_{12}

Among the factors contributing to declining vitamin B_{12} levels are a decreased intake of animal products (the primary source of vitamin B_{12} in human diets), decreased gastric secretion of hydrochloric acid and/or intrinsic factor, generalized malabsorption, blind loop syndrome, or even use of laxatives that increase intestinal transit time (87). The RDA for vitamin B_{12} is 2 μg for older adults (72).

Vitamin C

Ascorbic acid levels in the plasma and white cells of some elderly groups are low with occasional individuals in scorbutic ranges. This is primarily due to low dietary intake and is easily corrected by dietary changes (88). The RDA for vitamin C is 60 mg for nonsmoking adults and 100 mg for adults who smoke (72).

Vitamin D

Serum vitamin D levels are frequently lower with age due to decreased dietary intake (enriched milk is a major dietary source) and reduced exposure to direct sunlight (especially with the increased awareness of sun-exposure-related skin conditions). The efficiency of absorption and conversion to the active form also become somewhat impaired (89, 90). The RDA of vitamin D for older adults is 5 mcg (72). Vitamin D deficiency, highly prevalent among the institutionalized elderly population (91), could be a causative factor in hip fractures.

Iron

Although heme iron is apparently absorbed equally well by young and old populations, nonheme (inorganic) iron is less well absorbed by the elderly (92). This may result from decreased gastric acid secretion, since iron is better absorbed in an acid environment (93). Food choices of the elderly are also less likely to include rich sources of easily absorbed heme iron, such as meats, due to difficulty with chewing. The RDA of iron is 10 mg in adults above 50 years of age (72).

Calcium

Calcium absorption becomes less efficient with age, and the active transport system, induced by 1,25 $(OH)_2$ vitamin D, is also affected (94). Changes in vitamin D metabolism noted above contribute to poor absorption, and the elderly may decrease their intake of calcium-rich foods, further depressing calcium nutriture. The current RDA of 800 mg/day has been attacked as being too low, yet the WHO allowance (400 to 500 mg) and standards in other countries (e.g., the United Kingdom, 500 mg) are lower. While some workers have suggested that calcium intakes of 1200 mg or more per day will limit the bone loss seen in the elderly, the role of calcium intake in maintaining bone integrity has not yet been fully elucidated (34, 95), and the role of excessive protein intake in bringing about bone loss is under study. High intakes of calcium do not seem to be useful in preventing postmenopausal bone loss (36).

Zinc

Zinc deficiency is closely associated with impaired taste acuity, immune function, and wound healing. Plasma zinc levels decline slightly with age, particularly among men, but the significance of this is unclear since serum levels (and hair levels) do not adequately reflect tissue zinc status (96). Meats, fish, and poultry are primary dietary sources, providing about 40% in average diets. Vegetarian diets are low in zinc. The RDA for zinc is 15 mg for men and 12 mg for women, although impoverished or edentulous elderly frequently consume zinc below this level (7 to 13 mg in recent surveys). Due to its diverse role in health and healing, dietary evaluation of zinc intake is important, and supplementation should be prescribed if appropriate (97).

Drug-Nutrient Interactions

Roe (98) classifies drug-nutrient interactions among the elderly as falling into four distinct categories: drugs that stimulate or suppress appetite, drugs that cause alterations in nutrient digestion or absorption, drugs that alter metabolism or utilization of a nutrient, and drugs that alter excretion of a nutrient. Table 18-7 (99) summarizes drugs involved in these interactions. A few drugs or classes of drugs merit specific attention and are listed below.

Aspirin

With the recent demonstration of a prophylactic effect of aspirin against heart attacks in healthy middle-aged and older people, an increase can be expected in the number of persons who suffer iron deficiency due to GI blood loss. Aspirin may also interfere with the metabolism of folic acid and vitamin C.

Laxatives

Mineral oil type laxatives, if taken in close proximity to meals, can inhibit the absorption of fat-soluble vitamins. "Purge"-type laxatives, especially if taken frequently, can result in disturbances in electrolyte balance, although malabsorption is rare.

Antacids

Delayed gastric emptying combined with consequent postprandial discomfort, despite actual decreases in gastric acidity, may lead to frequent antacid use among the elderly. Antacids containing aluminum hydroxide bind phosphorus. When used over long periods of time, this may foster bone demineralization due to cumulative phosphate depletion (100).

Diuretics

Surveillance for excessive losses of electrolytes, including magnesium and potassium, is imperative.

Monoamine Oxidase Inhibitors

Several tyramine-containing foods must be avoided when taking a monoamine oxidase inhibitor. These include chicken and beef liver, dried fish, many pickled and preserved foods, bananas, figs, raisins, eggplant, avocados,

Table 18-7. Potential drug-nutrient interactions for some commonly used drugs

Drug	Nutrient	Potential side effect
Alcohol	Thiamin Vitamin B_6 Folate Zinc Calcium Magnesium	Deficiency Deficiency Deficiency Deficiency Deficiency Deficiency
Aluminum hydroxide	Phosphorus Calcium	Binding Deficiency
Antacids	Thiamin Calcium Iron	Decreased absorption due to altered gastrointestinal pH
Anticoagulants	Vitamin K	Deficiency
Antihistamines		Weight gain
Amphetamines		Appetite suppression Weight loss
Aspirin	Iron	Anemia
Cathartics	Calcium	Impaired gastrointestinal motility
	Potassium	Impaired gastrointestinal motility
Cholestyramine	Vitamins A, D, E, K	Deficiencies
Cimetidine	Vitamin B_{12}	Deficiency
Clofibrate	Carbohydrate Vitamin B_{12} Carotene Iron	Enzyme inactivation Decreased absorption
Colchicine	Vitamin B_{12} Carotene Magnesium	Decreased absorption due to damaged intestinal mucosa
Corticosteroids	Zinc Calcium Potassium	Damage to intestinal mucosa Gastrointestinal loss
Ethacrynic acid	Sodium	Depletion
Furosemide	Calcium Potassium Sodium	Diuretic effect Depletion
Gentamicin	Potassium Sodium	Depletion
Levodopa	Protein	Competition for absorption
Neomycin	Fat Protein Sodium Potassium Calcium Iron Vitamin B_{12}	Decreases pancreatic lipase and binds bile salts and interferes with absorption

(*continued*)

Table 18-7. (*continued*)

Drug	Nutrient	Potential side effect
Penicillamine	Zinc Vitamin B_{12} Sodium	Altered nutrient excretion
Phenobarbital	Vitamin D Folate	Impaired metabolism and utilization
Phenytoin	Vitamin D Folate	Impaired metabolism and utilization
Tetracycline	Protein Iron	Impaired uptake and utilization General malabsorption
Tricyclic antidepressants		Weight gain due to appetite stimulation

Reprinted with permission from Chernoff, R. 1987. Aging and nutrition. *Nutr Today* Mar/Apr: 4–11 (Ref. 99).

yogurt, aged cheeses, sour cream, many alcoholic beverages, coffee, cola, chocolate, yeast, soy sauce, and fava beans.

Nutritional Care of the Elderly Surgical Patient

Appropriate intervention must be instituted once the patient has been evaluated. Nutritional intervention should not only address the form of malnutrition but also consider the patient's condition(s) and dietary preferences. For the mildly affected patient, nutritious meals and snacks, supplements, or nutrient modules (meal components rich in one class of nutrient) may prove sufficient. With increasing depletion, high-calorie, high-protein supplements may be appropriate, as well as specific vitamins and minerals.

Initiation of nutritional support is rarely an emergency, and definitive treatments for serious illness should not be delayed to begin nutritional support. However, more patients suffer by far from the error of omission of nutritional management than from errors of commission.

Unless treatment is needed urgently, macronutrient pools of proteins and lipids should be restored gradually. Attempts to reverse malnutrition rapidly are fraught with danger due to complications of overfeeding (e.g., acute hypophosphatemia, hyperglycemia, hyperlipidemia, fatty liver, CO_2 retention). This is particularly evident in aged patients with impaired function of vital organ tissues (e.g., myocardium, alveoli, hepatocytes, nephrons, and endocrine and exocrine pancreas).

Acute Nutritional Intervention

In organizing the nutritional care plan, three types of initial decisions must be made: timing of the intervention, feeding routes, and dietary prescription.

Timing of Nutritional Intervention

Initiation of treatment should reflect the seriousness of the clinical situation. High-risk patients should undergo nutritional intervention as soon as possible, and elective treatments involving metabolic stress, most commonly surgery, should be delayed while repletion is underway. Patients should not become significantly malnourished in the hospital. Periods of inadequate nutrition (e.g., due to testing or procedures requiring clear liquid diets or intermittent periods of NPO status) should not be allowed to exceed 5 days without nutritional supplementation. Nutrition support should generally be instituted without delay, however, whenever such a period of suboptimal diet can be anticipated.

The process of nutritional repletion itself is stressful for the depleted or ill patient and is associated with major endocrinologic, metabolic, hemodynamic, and neurologic changes. The sudden rise in insulin and catecholamine levels can precipitate acute mineral imbalances and cardiovascular emergencies; refeeding should therefore always be performed under experienced guidance.

Overfeeding must be avoided. Excessive calories, especially in the form of carbohydrate, can produce iatrogenic pathology when the "hyper" in hyperalimentation is taken too literally. Pathophysiologic effects of overfeeding include: hypophosphatemia and hypokalemia due to imbalance between the insulin-mediated augmentation of anabolism and the provision of these obligate substrates for lean tissue accretion; hyperglycemia when the capacity of insulin-mediated glucose uptake and oxidation is overwhelmed; CO_2 retention due to excessive metabolic production of bicarbonate, beyond alveolar ventilatory capacity; "fatty liver" due to excessive hepatic triglyceride production and/or impairment of apolipoprotein synthesis; and reticuloendothelial system blockage associated with overabundant intravenous lipid emulsions or total calories.

The treatment duration for severe levels of depletion is best determined on an individual case basis. Five to 10 days of preoperative feeding are recommended for moderately depleted patients prior to nonemergent surgery. Patients requiring therapy for intervals of two or more weeks can be clinically reassessed to evaluate improvements in nutritional parameters (see "Monitoring the Course of Therapy" later in this chapter).

Feeding Routes

Optimal feeding routes should provide an appropriate balance between safety and effectiveness. The most invasive routes can be the most acutely effective, as in the extreme case of total parenteral nutrition (TPN), in which all oro-esophago-gastro-intestinal regulatory mechanisms are bypassed. Feeding via the GI tract is generally contraindicated when obstruction or perforation is suspected. In addition, pulmonary aspiration, uncontrolled diarrhea, and excessive losses of fluids and electrolytes via enterocutaneous fistulae are often indications for intravenous feedings. Nutritional repletion via the enteral route is impractical if repeated procedures that require fasting or a clear liquid diet are anticipated.

Enteral feeding tubes, either nasal or percutaneous, eliminate the need for swallowing yet are often associated with pulmonary aspiration in the elderly (101). Postpyloric tubes lower the risk of pulmonary aspiration associated with GI feeding. During abdominal surgery, one should always consider the option of placing a feeding jejunostomy if pathology is localized to the oral, esophageal, gastric, or duodenal segments of the GI tract.

Parenteral feeding requires more expertise in micronutrient management since regulation of GI nutrient absorption is bypassed. The greater flexibility and control of amino acid, mineral, and vitamin pools in parenteral nutrition proves advantageous, however, when nutrient needs are dynamic and yet fall within a narrow margin (e.g., renal and hepatic impairment).

Intravenous feeding can be life saving. Total parenteral nutrition (TPN) is usually carried out through a central vein to allow for rapid mixing and dilution of the hypertonic fluids. Patients who meet a number of criteria (Fig. 18-4) may be candidates for alimentation through a peripheral vein or peripheral parenteral nutrition (PPN). Since this requires larger volumes of solution (typically three or more liters per day), it is less widely used in elderly patients. The most common type of PPN, peripheral intravenous alimentation, employs intravenous lipid emulsions as the main caloric source to provide the highest ratio of calories per milliosmole. On a short-term basis, nondepleted patients can be given a solution of amino acids, vitamins, and minerals, while mobilizing endogenous triglycerides from adipose tissue as the chief caloric source.

Dietary Prescription

Except in routine situations, nutrition specialists should prescribe dietary intervention, and intravenous feedings are always to be monitored by an expert. Enteral feedings should be designed to provide a feeding regimen which mimics the composition of a natural diet. Complete formula diets are available when necessary. Supplemental electrolytes, minerals, and vitamins can be added when appropriate. Intragastric feedings may be administered by bolus or drip, but postpyloric feedings must maintain continuous infusion to avoid severe cramping and diarrhea.

Energy and nitrogen requirements have been reviewed earlier in this chapter. In intravenous nutrition and enteral feedings, where a profound impairment of digestive function is suspected, macronutrients are supplied as monomers in "elemental" form (e.g., monosaccharides and amino acids) instead of the predominantly polymeric form of natural foods (polysaccharides and proteins). Vitamins and minerals should be provided at RDA levels and are generally included as such in commercial enteral formulas. Individual needs, however, must always be evaluated and intakes must be tailored to the patient. Ambulation and/or physical therapy are also desirable to improve substrate utilization.

Preoperative Nutritional Care

Patients requiring elective surgery should be screened with the techniques mentioned in the "Nutritional History" and "Physical Examination" sections of this chapter. Many laboratory tests for nutritional assessment are routinely done (e.g., serum albumin, total lymphocyte count). These combined with clinical insight serve as indicators for further nutritional assessment and intervention, particularly if the patient's condition places him at nutritional risk due to interference with a normal, adequate dietary intake in the succeeding weeks or months.

The patient should be NPO for long enough to assure complete gastric emptying prior to surgery. For patients undergoing intestinal surgery, a low-fiber, low-residue diet should be prescribed for 2 to 3 days before surgery. Elemental diets (i.e., Vivonex) are low-residue but provide a full nutritional complement.

Postoperative Nutritional Care

Postoperative feeding may begin when the GI tract is functioning and bowel sounds are heard. The diet is usually begun with clear liquids, progressing to full liquids, a soft diet, and then a house diet, as the patient is able to tolerate solid foods.

When the adequacy of the patient's intake is uncertain, the physician should order "calorie counts." The dietitian will provide daily estimates of calorie and protein intake as well as any other nutrients specified. The physician should heed the nurses' and dietitians' daily notes in the patient's chart to monitor dietary progression and prescribe necessary adjustments.

The patient may require diet modification at the time

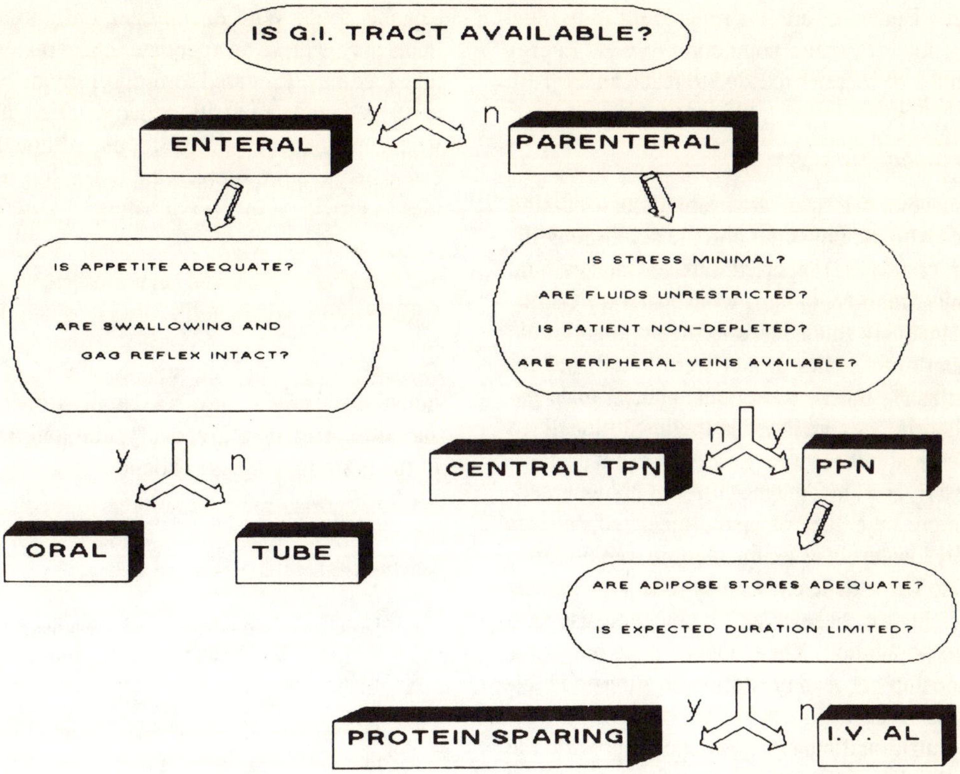

Figure 18-4. Tree diagram demonstrating choice of optimal feeding route.

of discharge. The patient must understand the diet and have access to resources for its preparation. For patients with special nutritional disorders such as diabetes, the hospital dietitian may offer educational instruction. Team conferences should involve the dietician, social worker, discharge planner, Visiting Nurse Association, and any other pertinent resources (e.g., disease-specific associations); family members should be encouraged to participate.

Trauma associated with injury, surgery, or burns and nutrients lost in malabsorption syndromes place patients in catabolic states. If conventional nutritional therapy does not restore positive nitrogen balance within 5 to 10 days, other nutritional means should be considered, such as tube feeding for patients with functioning GI tracts who are unable to ingest sufficient food.

Elemental tube-fed diets are best for patients with limited digestive and/or absorptive capacity. Depending on remaining function and tolerance, these may include sugars supplied as monosaccharides or glucose polymers and protein as free amino acids or as short polypeptides. In modular diets, differing protein, carbohydrate, and fat sources can be tailored to the patients individual needs and mixed with mineral and vitamin components. When the digestive and absorptive functions of the GI tract are seriously compromised, adequate nutrients to sustain anabolism can be provided via central venous catheter. Because this route requires surgical placement of the catheter and carries a risk of sepsis, other means of providing adequate nutrition should be evaluated thoroughly before the decision to use total parenteral nutrition is made.

Monitoring the Course of Therapy

Frequent weights and daily fluid balance determinations are integral to careful nutritional monitoring. Weight gain due to accretion of lean body mass proceeds at a rate that may only be detected by comparing weight from week to week. Weight gains of more than 1 to 2 pounds per week almost uniformly represent third space fluid retention or fat deposition. Complete 24-hour urine collections are useful to verify dietary adequacy if changes in body weight from week to week are uninterpretable, such as inconsistent fluid status. Occasional total lymphocyte counts and measurements of anthropometrics, serum protein levels, and skin tests can be useful over the long term. Another technique to verify dietary adequacy is the measurement of REE by indirect calorimetry. Routine predictors of REE based on various algorithms, such as the

Harris-Benedict Equation, are less reliable for individual estimates than for estimating population means. Energy requirement must be met or exceeded to reach anabolism.

Chronic Nutritional Management

In a recent survey of Boston area ambulatory nursing home residents who did not suffer chronic debilitating illness, Sahyoun et al. (102) reported nutrient intakes, and most biochemical markers of nutritional status were similar to a simultaneously studied free-living population. No specific nutrient deficiencies in diet were found, but intakes of vitamins B_6 and D, folate, zinc and, in male patients only, vitamin A, were lower in the institutionalized group. Biochemical indices were lower for serum protein, vitamins A and E, and zinc; magnesium was not assessed. In addition, more than 10% of institutionalized patients had abnormally low levels of serum albumin, prealbumin, and transferrin. These deficiencies may reflect the greater prevalence of chronic diseases and medication use in a long-term care population. The evidence does not prove that the relationship between institutionalization and malnutrition is causative.

Chronic nutritional management should provide the patient with a feeding regimen that is as close to a varied and "balanced" oral diet as he or she is able to assimilate safely and effectively. If eating is possible, every effort must be made to restore and preserve function of the oral cavity, including attention to dental hygiene, dental appliances, and adequate salivation. Mouth rinsing with an artificial saliva formulation can decrease the damage to oral mucosa due to xerostomia. Edentulous individuals, those with poorly fitting dentures, may benefit from a new denture fitting. Patients who have undergone mouth surgery, and those suffering oral ulcers secondary to chemotherapy or radiotherapy need an appropriately modified diet; consultation with a dietician is indicated.

Patients may be able to chew and swallow food, but if they are unable to reach their tray or unwrap or cut the food, intake will be diminished. Oral diet intake must be visually verified before assuming success. It is too common for full food trays to be returned to the kitchen unbeknownst to the physician prescribing the diet. In wards that are occasionally short of staff, a special effort is needed to ensure adequate surveillance at mealtimes.

Large gains in dietary intake may be achieved through simple measures. The physician should assure that staff, family members, or volunteers are available to assist with meals before the food has cooled and is no longer palatable. If the hospital food does not meet religious or ethnic restrictions, arrangements should be made through the dietary department for obtaining acceptable food. With encouragement and assistance, patients may achieve an adequate intake that would preclude tube feedings. Prepared formulas provide more expensive and less complete nutrition than a varied diet for a patient who can consume whole foods, although inconsistent eaters may require supplemental formula or nutrient modules to provide a margin of safety.

Conclusion

Despite the physiologic consequences of aging, nutritional management plays an equally important role in the successful treatment, recovery, and long-term well-being of the geriatric surgical patient.

References

1. US Dept of Commerce. 1987. Statistical Abstract of the U.S., ed. 10. Washington, DC: Bureau of Census.
2. Kohrs, MB. 1982. Introduction: Symposium on nutrition and aging. *Am J Clin Nutr* 36:735–736.
3. Shaver, HJ. 1980. Nutritional status of nursing home patients. *JPEN* 4:367–370.
4. Rowe, JW, and Kahn, RW. 1987. Human aging: Usual and successful. *Science* 237:143–149.
5. Arey, L, Tremaine, MJ, and Monzingo, FL. 1935. The numerical and topographical relations of taste buds to human circumvallate papillae throughout the life span. *Anat Rec* 64:9–25.
6. Glanville, EV, Kaplan, AR, and Fischer, R. 1964. Age, sex, and taste sensitivity. *J Gerontol* 19:474–478.
7. Ben-Aryeh, et al. 1984. Whole-saliva secretion rates in old and young healthy subjects. *J Dent Res* 63:1147–1148.
8. Feldman, RS, et al. 1980. Aging and mastication: changes in performance and in the swallowing threshold with natural dentition. *J Am Geriatr Soc* 28:97–103.
9. Roland, DA. 1984. Nutrition in adulthood and the later years. In *Food, Nutrition, and Diet Therapy,* Eds., MV Krause and LK Mahan. Philadelphia: WB Saunders.
10. Schlenker, ED. 1984. Nutrition in aging. *Times Mirror.* St. Louis: CV Mosby.
11. Shephard, RJ. 1986. Nutrition and the physiology of aging. In *Nutrition, Aging, and Health,* Ed., EA Young, Vol. 9 in *Contemporary Issues in Clinical Nutrition,* pp. 1–24. New York: Alan R Liss, Inc.
12. Hollis, JB, and Castell, DO. 1974. Esophageal function in elderly men: A new look at "presbyesophagus." *Ann Intern Med* 80:371–374.
13. Fikry, ME. 1965. Gastric secretory functions in the aged. *Gerontologia Clinica* 1:216–225.
14. Young, EA, and Urban, E. 1986. Aging, the aged, and the gastrointestinal tract. In *Nutrition, Aging, and Health,* Ed., EA Young, Vol. 9 in *Contemporary Issues in Clinical Nutrition,* pp. 91–131. New York: Alan R Liss, Inc.

15. Meyer, J, and Necheles, H. 1940. Studies in old age. IV. The clinical significance of salivary, gastric and pancreatic secretion in the aged. *JAMA* 115:2050–2055.
16. Rosenberg, IR, et al. 1966. The effect of age and sex upon human pancreatic secretion of fluid and bicarbonate. *Gastroenterology* 50:191–194.
17. Amberg, JR, and Zboralske, FF. 1965. Gallstones after 70. *Geriatrics* 20:539–542.
18. Warren, PM, Pepperman, MA, and Mountgomery, RD. 1978. Age changes in small intestine mucosa. *Lancet* 2:849–850.
19. Webster, SGP, and Leeming, JT. 1975. The appearance of the small bowel mucosa in old age. *Age Aging* 4:168–174.
20. Clark, ANG. 1972. Deficiency states in duodenal diverticular disease. *Age Aging* 1:14–23.
21. Yamagata, A. 1965. Histopathological studies of the colon in relation to age. *Jpn J Gastroenterol* 62:229–235.
22. Parks, TG. 1975. Natural history of diverticular disease of the colon. *Clin Gastroenterol* 4:53–69.
23. Mayersohn, M. 1982. The "xylose test" to assess gastrointestinal function in the elderly: Pharmacokinetic evaluation of the literature. *J Gerontol* 37:300–305.
24. Guth, PH. 1968. Physiologic alterations in small bowel function with age: the absorption of D-xylose. *Am J Dig Dis* 13:565–571.
25. Meyer, J, et al. 1943. Studies in old age. VII. Intestinal absorption in old age. *J Gastroenterol* 1:876–881.
26. Feibusch, JM, and Holt, PR. 1982. Impaired absorption capacity for carbohydrate in the aging human. *Dig Dis Sci* 27:1095–1100.
27. Rorick, MH, and Scrimshaw, NS. 1979. Comparative tolerances of elderly from differing ethnic backgrounds to lactose-containing and lactose-free dairy drinks: A double-blind study. *J Gerontol* 34:191–196.
28. Fukagawa, NK, et al. 1988. Glucose and amino acid metabolism in man: Differential effects of insulin. *Metabolism,* in press.
29. Simopoulos, AP. 1985. Dietary control of hypertension and obesity and body weight standards. *J Am Diet Assoc* 85:419–422.
30. Andres, R, et al. 1985. Impact of age on weight goals. *Ann Intern Med* 103:1030–1033.
31. Shock, NW, et al. 1963. Age differences in the water content of the body as related to basal oxygen consumption in males. *J Gerontol* 18:1–18.
32. Finch, C, and Hayflick, L. 1977. *Handbook of the Biology of Aging.* New York: Van Nostrand Reinhold Co.
33. Albrink, MJ, and Meigs, JW. 1971. Serum lipids, skinfold thickness, body bulk, and body weight of native Cape Verdeans, New England Cape Verdeans, and U.S. factory workers. *Am J Clin Nutr* 24:344–352.
34. Heaney, RP, et al. 1982. Calcium nutrition and bone health in the elderly. *Am J Clin Nutr* 36:986–1013.
35. Riggs, BL, and Melton, J. 1986. Involutional osteoporosis. *N Engl J Med* 314:1676–1684.
36. Riis, B, Thomsen, K, and Christiansen, C. 1987. Does calcium supplementation prevent post-menopausal bone loss? A double-blind controlled clinical study. *N Engl J Med* 316:173–177.
37. Kiel, DP, et al. 1987. Hip fracture and the use of estrogens in postmenopausal women. The Framingham Study. *N Engl J Med* 317:1169–1174.
38. Novak, LP. 1972. Aging, total body potassium, fat-free mass and cell mass in males and females between ages 18 and 85 years. *J Gerontol* 27:438–443.
39. Klein, S, et al. 1986. Palmitate and glycerol kinetics during brief starvation in normal weight young adults and elderly subjects. *J Clin Invest* 78:928–933.
40. Kohrs, MB, and Czajka-Narins, DM. 1986. Assessing the nutritional status of the elderly. In *Nutrition, Aging, and Health,* Ed., EA Young, Vol. 9 in *Contemporary Issues in Clinical Nutrition,* pp. 25–59. New York: Alan R Liss, Inc.
41. Frisancho, AR. 1981. New norms of upper limb fat and muscle areas for assessment of nutritional status. *Am J Clin Nutr* 34:2540–2545.
42. Rossman, I. 1979. The anatomy of aging. In *Clinical Geriatrics,* Ed., I Rossman, pp. 3–22. Philadelphia: JB Lippincott.
43. Marton, KI, Sox, HC, and Krupp, JR. 1981. Involuntary weight loss: Diagnostic and prognostic significance. *Ann Int Med* 95:568–574.
44. Blackburn, GL, et al. 1977. Nutritional and metabolic assessment of the hospitalized patient. *JPEN* 1:11–20.
45. Bowman, BB, and Rosenberg, IH. 1982. Assessment of the nutritional status of the elderly. *Am J Clin Nutr* 35: 1142–1151.
46. Master, AM, Lasser, RP, and Beckman, G. 1960. Tables of average weight and height of Americans aged 65 to 94 years. *JAMA* 172:658–662.
47. Thomas, AE, McKay, DA, and Cutlip, MB. 1976. Nomograph for body mass index (kg/m^2). *Am J Clin Nutr* 29:302–304.
48. Blackburn, GL, and Harvey, KB. 1982. Nutritional assessment as a routine in clinical medicine. *Postgrad Med* 71:46–63.
49. Colluci, RA, Bell, SJ, and Blackburn, GL. 1987. Nutritional problems of institutionalized and free-living elderly. *Compreh Ther* 13:20–28.
50. Pinchcofksy-Devin, GD, and Kaminski, MV. 1986. Correlation of pressure sores and nutritional status. *J Am Ger Soc* 34:435–440.
51. Holmes, R, et al. 1987. Combating pressure sores—nutritionally. *Am J Nurs* Oct:1301–1303.
52. Miller, SF, Morath, MA, and Finley, RK. 1981. Comparison of derived and actual transferrin: a potential source of error in clinical nutrition assessment. *J Trauma* 21: 548–550.
53. Rheinhardt, GF, et al. 1980. Incidence of mortality of hypoalbuminemic patients in hospitalized veterans. *JPEN* 4:357–359.
54. Rudman, D, et al. 1987. Antecedents of death in the men of a Veterans Administration nursing home. *J Am Geriatr Soc* 35:496–502.
55. Clark, NG, and Blackburn, GL. 1983. Nutritional assessment and support of the elderly patient. *Am J IV Ther Clin Nutr* 10:7–15.
56. Driver, AG, and McAlevy, MT. 1980. Creatinine height index as a function of age. *Am J Clin Nutr* 33:2057 (letter).
57. Roberts-Thompson, IC, et al. 1974. Aging, immune response and mortality. *Lancet* 2:368–370.

58. Griffin, RE, et al. 1983. Delayed cutaneous hypersensitivity testing in patients receiving nutritional support for protein-calorie malnutrition. *Clin Pharm* 2:432–435.
59. Brown, R, et al. 1982. Failure of delayed hypersensitivity skin testing to predict postoperative sepsis and mortality. *Br Med J* 284:851–857.
60. Feurer, I, and Mullen, JL. 1986. Bedside measurement of resting energy expenditure and respiratory quotient via indirect calorimetry. *Nutrition in Clinical Practice* 1: 43–49.
61. Garrow, JS. 1982. New approaches to body composition. *Am J Clin Nutr* 35:1152–1158.
62. Van Itallie, TB. 1982. Other body composition studies that could be applied. In *Assessing the Nutritional Status of the Elderly,* State of the Art Report of the Third Ross Roundtable on Medical Issues. Columbus, OH: Ross Labs.
63. Keys, A, and Brozek, J. 1953. Body fat in adult man. *Physiol Rev* 33:245–256.
64. Schoeller, DA, et al. 1980. Total body water measurement in humans with 180 and 2H labeled water. *Am J Clin Nutr* 33:2686–2693.
65. Forbes, GB, and Hursh, JB. 1963. Age and sex trends in lean body mass calculated from K^{40} measurements. *Ann NY Acad Sci* 110:255–263.
66. Baker, JP, et al. 1982. Nutritional assessment. A comparison of clinical judgement and objective measurements. *N Engl J Med* 306:969–972.
67. Seltzer, MH, et al. 1979. Instant nutritional assessment. *JPEN* 3:157–159.
68. Busby, GP, et al. 1980. Prognostic nutritional index in gastrointestinal surgery. *Am J Surg* 139:160–167.
69. Harvey, KB, et al. 1981. Biological measures for the formulation of a hospital prognostic index. *Am J Clin Nutr* 34:2013–2022.
70. Schneider, EL, et al. 1986. Recommended dietary allowance and the health of the elderly. *N Engl J Med* 314:157–160.
71. Keys, A, Taylor, HL, and Grande, F. 1973. Basal metabolism and the age of adult man. *Metabolism* 22:579–587.
72. Food and Nutrition Board. 1989. Recommended Dietary Allowances, ed. 10. Washington, DC: National Academy of Sciences.
73. Harris, JA, and Benedict, FG. 1919. Biometric studies of basal metabolism in man. Washington, DC: Carnegie Institute of Washington, Pub. No. 279.
74. Clark, NG, et al. 1988. Nutritional support of the chronically ill elderly female at risk for elective or urgent surgery. *J Am Coll Nutr* 7:17–26.
75. Brenner, BM, Meyer, TW, and Hostetter, TH. 1982. Dietary protein intake and the progressive nature of kidney disease: the role of hemodynamically mediated glomerular injury in the pathogenesis of progressive glomerular sclerosis in aging, renal ablation, and intrinsic renal disease. *N Engl J Med* 652–659.
76. Uauy, R, Scrimshaw, NS, and Young, VR. 1978. Human protein requirements: Nitrogen balance response to graded levels of egg protein in elderly men and women. *Am J Clin Nutr* 31:779–785.
77. Gersovitz, M, et al. 1982. Human protein requirements: Assessment of the adequacy of the current Recommended Dietary Allowance for dietary protein in elderly men and women. *Am J Clin Nutr* 25:6–14.
78. Werner, I, and Hambreaus, L. 1971. The digestive capacity of elderly people. *Acta Soc Med Ups* 76:239–241.
79. Webster, SGP. 1980. Gastro-intestinal function and absorption of nutrients. In *Metabolic and Nutritional Disorders in the Elderly,* Eds., AN Exton-Smith and FI Caird, pp. 86–89. Bristol: John Wright.
80. Becker, GH, Meyer, J, and Necheles, H. 1950. Fat absorption in young and old age. *Gastroenterology* 14:80–92.
81. Werner, I, and Hambreaus, L. 1972. The digestive capacity of elderly people. In *Nutrition in Old Age,* Ed., LA Carlson. Symposia Swedish Nutrition Foundation X. Stockholm: Almquest & Wiksell.
82. Bennett, PH. 1976. *Report of Work Group on Epidemiology.* National Commission on Diabetes, Vol III, Part 1. pp. 65–133. U.S. Dept. of Health, Education, and Welfare, publication (NIH) 76-1021 Washington, DC: DHEW.
83. Horowitz, DL. 1986. *Nutrition, aging, and diabetes.* In *Nutrition, Aging, and Health.* Ed., EA Young, Vol. 9 in *Contemporary Issues in Clinical Nutrition,* pp. 145–163. New York: Alan R Liss, Inc.
84. Hamfelt, A. 1964. Age variation of vitamin B_6 metabolism in man. *Clin Chim Acta* 10:48–54.
85. Rose, CS, et al. 1976. Age differences in vitamin B_6 status of 617 men. *Am J Clin Nutr* 29:847–853.
86. Rosenberg, IH, et al. 1979. Folate nutrition in the elderly. *Am J Clin Nutr* 36(Supp):2237–2243.
87. Elsborg, L, Lund, V, and Bastrup-Madsen, P. 1976. Serum vitamin B_{12} levels in the aged. *Acta Med Scand* 200:309–314.
88. Newton, HMV, et al. 1985. The cause and correction of low blood vitamin C concentrations in the elderly. *Am J Clin Nutr* 42:656–659.
89. Weisman, Y, et al. 1981. Inadequate status and impaired metabolism of vitamin D in the elderly. *Israeli Med Sci* 17:19–21.
90. Brown, WW, et al. 1986. Aging and the kidney. *Arch Int Med* 146:1790–1796.
91. Holick, MF. 1986. Vitamin D requirements for the elderly. *Clin Nutr* 5:121–129.
92. Jacobs, AM, and Owen, GM. 1969. The effect of age on iron absorption. *J Gerontol* 24:95–96.
93. Van Campen, D. 1974. Regulation of iron absorption. *Fed Proc* 33:100–105.
94. Ireland, P, and Fordtran, JS. 1973. Effect of dietary calcium and age on jejunal calcium absorption in humans studied by intestinal perfusion. *J Clin Invest* 52:5672–5681.
95. Spencer, H, et al. 1984. Calcium requirements in humans. *Clin Orthop* 184:270–280.
96. Solomons, NW. 1979. On the assessment of zinc and copper nutriture in man. *Am J Clin Nutr* 32:856–871.
97. Sandstead, HH, et al. 1982. Zinc nutriture in the elderly in relation to taste, acuity, immune response, and wound healing. *Am J Clin Nutr* 36:1046–1059.
98. Roe, DA. 1986. Drug-nutrient interactions in the elderly. *Geriatrics* 41:57–74.
99. Chernoff, R. 1987. Aging and nutrition. *Nutr Today* Mar/Apr:4–11.

100. Spencer, H, and Lender, M. 1979. Adverse effects of aluminum-containing antacids on mineral metabolism. *Gastroenterology* 76:603–606.

101. Ciocon, JO, et al. 1988. Tube feedings in elderly patients. Indications, benefits, and complications. *Arch Int Med* 148:429–433.

102. Sahyoun, NR, et al. 1988. Dietary intakes and biochemical indicators of nutritional status in an elderly institutional population. *Am J Clin Nutr* 47:524–533.

19

Response to Trauma in the Elderly

Daniel K. Lowe and Donald D. Trunkey

A quick analysis of trauma in the elderly shows it is not a common cause of death since only 2% of deaths after the age of 65 years are related to injuries. A more careful analysis, however, shows this represents over 30,000 deaths per year or 20% of the 140,000 deaths related to injury for all age groups. For those aged 75 years and older, the death rate is higher than in any other population group, including young males in the 20s. For the age group greater than 85 years, the death rate is more than 3 times that of the 20- to 30-year-old age group (1).

Not only does the elderly patient have a higher death rate from injury, but this population also has a higher hospitalization rate and emergency department usage. Overall, the elderly group consumes over 30% of the trauma medical care resources, which also impacts on cost (2). Modern reimbursement methodologies using diagnostic related groups (DRGs) show a significant disparity in reimbursements for trauma patients with an average loss for severe injury of greater than $2,000 per case (3). Additional studies of reimbursements have shown that, although patients over the age of 80 represent only a small percentage of all trauma admissions, they account for a significant reimbursement loss: approximately 17% in one study (4). More recent data from the University of California, San Francisco General Hospital, showed that over a 10-year period (1973 to 1982) people over the age of 60 years comprised 13% of the trauma admissions and 38% of all trauma deaths. The authors concluded that age greater than 40 years was associated with a higher mortality when associated with external injury (5).

The Major Trauma Outcome Study (MTOS) sponsored by the American College of Surgeons (6) has compiled a review of 33,308 traumatized patients from 91 institutions over a 3-year period (1983 to 1985). These patients represent 0.3% of all injured patients in the United States, 1% of all trauma deaths, and 2% of all in-hospital deaths. The overall mortality in this extensive review was 10%. Patients over the age of 54, however, comprised 13% of the total population examined and showed a significantly increased mortality rate. Patients over the age of 65 years comprised 8% of the study group and had a mortality rate of 17%. Epidemiologic data from these and other studies demonstrate that the injured elderly patient is a significant health care problem. *Injury in America, A Continuing Public Health Problem* (7) shows that the field of literature on injury research, epidemiology, and prevention is inadequate. Certainly this inadequacy is no more clearly seen than with a review of the literature on injury of the aged.

A review of the literature on trauma in the elderly shows that the most common mechanisms of injury are falls, motor vehicle accidents, and thermal injuries. Whereas falls or jumps comprise only 9% of all injury-related deaths, they comprise over 50% of injury deaths beyond the age of 65 years (1, 8). Motor vehicle accidents comprise 25% of injuries in the elderly compared to 50% in all age groups combined. The incidence of burns in the elderly is increased and comprises approximately 8% of injury-related mortalities. Furthermore, the mortality rate per given burn is dramatically increased over the general burn population. These three most common etiologic mechanisms of injury in the elderly describe the reduced capacity of aging to tolerate a given transfer of energy as well as a blunted response mechanism.

Falls

In the Major Trauma Outcome Study, falls comprised 14.1% of the injury etiology in 33,226 patients (6). The overall mortality incidence for this mechanism of injury was 7.8%, and the average length of hospital stay was 12 days with a 5.2 day intensive-care-unit stay. In contrast, the Harborview Medical Center reported in 1984 on 100 consecutively injured patients greater than 70 years of age (9). Falls were the mechanism of injury in 64% of this series. At the Rhode Island Hospital, in a 1986 series of 63 patients over the age of 65 years, 30 sustained falls (48%) (10). These two recently published reports show a three- to fourfold increased incidence of falls in the elderly injured population compared with the incidence of falls in the MTOS trauma population. Although different from the MTOS data on falls, these series do not show significant variation from an extensive review of the epidemiology of trauma in the elderly conducted by Hogue. This epidemiologic article on injury in the elderly showed that falls in the age group over 65 accounted for more than 75% of all of the deaths from falls (8). Additionally, falls in this elderly group accounted for more than 50% of the deaths from unintentional injury. Additionally, Hogue and others have mentioned that falls are probably under-reported as an etiologic mechanism (11). In fact, the Oregon Trauma Registry, a population-based trauma registry from a survey of all injured patients requiring hospitalization, shows that elderly patients with falls are markedly under-reported (Personal information, Oregon State Health Division).

When the elderly fall, other medical conditions, either acute or chronic, frequently are involved in the precipitating event, and these other conditions affect outcome. Fractures of the femur, wrist, and hip are the most common sites of injury from falls. Secondary sites of injury include the head and torso. When acute head injury is a part of the pattern of injury, the prognosis is worse. Oreskovich and others (9) report that the incidence of central nervous system (CNS) injury in the nonsurvivors in their traumatized elderly was twice that of the survivors (20% versus 11%).

The elderly patient is not only at risk for secondary injury; studies cited by Waller (12) describe secondary complications as well. Considerable delay in the diagnosis and treatment is implicated by a study showing that only 50% of a group of elderly and alcoholic patients sustaining an injury in a fall sought care in the 1st hour, and over 26% of the study group delayed getting care for over 6 hours. Alcohol was cited as a contributing factor to this delay. Additionally, Waller showed that overall, drinking was associated with the falls in 13% of subjects. Other potentially more damaging and lethal secondary injuries are more common because the drugged or intoxicated elderly patients are frequently unable to remove themselves from a thermal contact after a fall (12).

The elderly gait is changed because of forward stoop and stiffened lower back resulting in a more forward placed center of gravity. This results in a wider gait as well as overall increased instability. These increasing medical debilities and decreasing physical abilities create an individual increasingly susceptible to injuries secondary to falls. It is noted from epidemiologic studies that this population has a high incidence of previous and multiple falls (40%) prior to the fall resulting in serious injury (12).

Despite the serious public health problem in the elderly from falls, the incidence of death from falls in the aged has been declining since the 1950s, with a greater than 35% decline from 1970 to 1980. Perhaps this is a result of having implemented prevention measures following an increased understanding of the pathophysiology of falls in this age group.

Motor Vehicle Accidents

Motor vehicle accidents account for 25% of injury deaths in the elderly (1, 8). In the recent series described by Oreskovich and others (9) only 17% of the 100 patients had been in motor vehicle accidents; however, half of these were pedestrians hit by cars. In contrast, the recent series reported by DeMaria et al. (4) showed that 47% of injuries (30 of 63) were motor vehicle related. Differences in methodology or regional reporting of populations at risk probably account for the variations in these two studies. However, in all of these series, trauma related to motor vehicles is the second most common injury mechanism and cause of death.

Although this population tends to drive fewer miles, the accident rate is higher than that for all other age groups except males under 25 years of age. The crashes occur most frequently in the daytime with good weather conditions and have been associated with errors of judgment or perception (8). The physical attributes of aging are incompletely related to the accident rates. The visual and mental changes associated with aging alter driving habits in the elderly. They tend to avoid crowded areas, stressful situations, and night-time conditions.

Not only is the accident rate high for the elderly, but the rate and severity of injury is also high. The ability of the elderly to withstand sudden energy transferral in motor vehicle accidents has not been studied, but intuitively it appears that the elderly, as compared to the young, sustain more severe injuries related to any given insult. This pattern, based upon the combined experience of multiple trauma specialists, resulted in the addition of advanced age (> 65 years) as a comorbid triage factor (National Triage Meeting, Washington, DC, 1983).

The elderly are more susceptible to tissue damage from the usual causes of trauma. Transference of kinetic energy to the human body is reasonably well tolerated but with fragile bones and tissues as seen in the elderly both synchronous and multiple injuries are more apt to occur. The methods of kinetic energy transfer in the human body are important to understand to predict injuries. For example, a fall transfers energy from the heel along the long bones of the legs to the spine. With fragile bones multiple fractures may be seen in all these areas even when the total kinetic energy is small. Understanding of the mechanisms of injury will allow the physician to predict as well as diagnose earlier many injuries in this susceptible population.

Most surgeons appreciate that relatively minor injuries in the elderly are potentially fatal when compared to a similar injury in the younger age groups. A classic example is rib fracture. Younger patients tolerate one to three rib fractures quite well and most will not require hospitalization. In contrast, the older patient tolerates rib fractures poorly. The pain leads to hypoventilation and subsequent atelectasis. This, in turn, sets the stage for pneumonia, which has a higher mortality with advancing age. Thus, the good clinician will often admit elderly patients with what appear to be inconsequential injuries.

Thermal Injuries

Thermal injuries comprise only a small percentage (less than 8%) of deaths from injuries in the elderly, but this again is misleading. The pattern of injury from burns is frequently different in this age group compared to what is usually seen, with flames, scalds, and contact burns being most common. Any burn is more likely to result in hospitalization in an elderly patient than in a younger patient. Flame burns comprised 82% (32 of 39) of a group of patients over age 60 years who died at the Harborview Burn Center (11). In contrast, Hogue (8) cites that scalds result most frequently in hospitalization for the elderly with a thermal injury. This differs from a review of the California State Burn Registry over its first 4 years, when 327 patients were age 65 years or greater (10% of the whole) (13). The most frequent pattern of injury seen in this elderly group was flames (50%), scalds (19%), and flammable liquids (10%) (13).

Although regional differences in injury pattern must exist, all of these studies agree on the home as the site of injury in over 80%. Additionally, the authors cite greater percentage of burned surface area, longer hospital stays, and higher mortalities for the elderly. Physiologic mechanisms hypothesized to account for these findings include thinning of the skin, decreased circulation to dissipate the thermal insult, sensory deficiencies altering thermal sensitivity, a depressed immune system, and debilities limiting ability to avoid the thermal insult.

Organ System Response and Patterns to Injury

These three mechanisms (falls, motor vehicle, and burns) represent over 80% of the causes of accidental injury in the elderly. Any mechanism of injury in this age group produces varied organ system response patterns. The general theory is that the elderly human exhibits a greater extent of injury per given amount of energy in the insult as well as a reduced capacity to recover. This theory has not been scientifically examined in the laboratory. A description of what does exist in the literature regarding responses to trauma in the elderly is oriented toward individual organ systems (Table 19-1).

The most frequently injured organ system in the elderly is the musculoskeletal system. In the 100 consecutive patients over age 70 years admitted to Harborview Medical Center, 77 patients (77%) had extremity or pelvic injuries (the most frequent site of injury), and 80% had multiple system trauma (9). In contrast, Rhode Island Hospital reported on 63 elderly patients who survived a blunt trauma incident. Musculoskeletal injuries occurred in only 25 patients (40%), and overall multiple trauma was seen in 39 patients (62%) (4). Differences in methodology account for the reduced incidence of musculoskeletal trauma in the latter series, which did not include patients with isolated musculoskeletal injuries.

The Harborview series showed that musculoskeletal injury was equally present in survivors and nonsurvivors and could not be considered a factor contributing to mortality in the elderly. The quality of life following injury is a factor, however, and this series reported that 88% of the survivors did not return to independent living (9). The

Table 19-1. Aging changes affecting trauma care

System	Aging changes
Musculoskeletal	Increased bone fragility, decreased healing
Peripheral vascular	Arteriosclerotic disease, venous fragility
Cardiac	Decreased coronary perfusion, decreased myocardial reserve
Pulmonary	Decreased pulmonary reserve, chest wall fragility
Central nervous	Brain shrinkage, vascular fragility, cerebral perfusion changes

high incidence of falls and musculoskeletal injuries in this elderly group of patients must contribute to the reported overall poor prognosis for independent living. In contrast, Rhode Island Hospital reported that 89% of their elderly patients returned home after injury (4). In part, this may be attributed to the lower incidence of falls and subsequent musculoskeletal injuries seen in their group of patients.

As can be seen by the above results, the ultimate goal following a serious injury in the elderly is return to preinjury function. Musculoskeletal injury seems to be a major factor most seriously challenging this outcome. To achieve the best outcome, the principles of management as outlined by Mandelbaum and Brooker include: 1) stabilization of the fracture; 2) optimal respiratory management; 3) minimization of infection rate; 4) encouragement of union; 5) diminution of fracture disease; 6) *early* mobilization of the patient; and 7) maintenance of adequate nutrition (14).

The avoidance of complications significantly alters mortality and return of function in this fragile group of patients. Therefore, the tendency may be to avoid any aggressive, particularly operative, approach in the patient with pre-existing disease or cardiovascular instability. Paradoxically, the result is a necessarily longer hospitalization and, in the elderly particularly, a higher complication rate. Early stabilization of the fracture and mobilization of the patient result in optimization of respiratory function. Complications of the respiratory system can then be avoided, these being the most significant cause of morbidity and mortality in the elderly injured patient (15).

Although central nervous system injuries are much less frequent than musculoskeletal injuries in this age group, they have a much greater impact on recovery as well as ultimate outcome. In the Harborview series, 12 patients sustained central nervous system injuries with 3 deaths (25%), which is two times the incidence of CNS injury seen in survivors. CNS injury was seen as a significant factor in outcome, particularly when the patient required prolonged intubation (9). In the Rhode Island Hospital series, central nervous system injury was also a major factor in determining functional outcome. In this review of elderly survivors from injury, a mild to moderate central nervous system injury (Abbreviated Injury Score [AIS] 3–4) in this group resulted in more complications, longer hospital stay and less functional recovery (4).

In a series of 34 patients over age 65 years with closed head injury and acute subdural hematomas, the outcome was death in 25 patients (74%) (16). The mechanism of injury was falls in 68% (23 of the 34 patients). Aggressive neurosurgical and critical care management was given all patients, but the only patients with good recovery were those with minor injuries, a near-normal neurologic examination (Glasgow Coma Scale 13–15), and admission within 1 hour of injury (16).

The presentation of a closed head injury in the elderly can lead to confusion. The history of a blow to the head is not obtainable in a high percentage of cases. The clinical picture is frequently confusing in this elderly group because the central nervous system injury may mimic other conditions, including transient ischemic attacks (17). Thus, the elderly patient may present only with the subtle manifestations of confusion. Examination can be nonrewarding, and only computerized tomography (CT) shows the extent of injury. Additionally, the shrinkage of the brain with aging results in an increased potential for hemorrhage between the brain and the dura. An increased fragility of the veins associated with aging may also be a factor. Certainly, the elderly patient is at increased risk for a cerebral lesion with a lesser force of injury.

The elderly patient is also at risk for spinal injury because of osteoporosis and chronic bony changes with resultant stiffening of the spine. Bony spurs may impinge upon the spinal cord with even a minor force of insult and thereby damage the cord. The spinal stiffness also increases susceptibility to fracture following trivial energy transfer. Osteoporosis in the elderly adds to the tendency to fracture. This combination of stiffness, spurs, and osteoporosis requires an increased level of suspicion in the elderly for the possibility of spinal injury. The cervical spine must be evaluated by x-ray for even the most trivial of injuries in the elderly age group. In many cases additional studies are indicated, including flexion and extension films or CT scan to exclude injuries. Not only is the cervical spine at increased risk, but the thoracic and lumbar spine must be evaluated with a much higher degree of sensitivity because of an increased susceptibility for injury in this area as well.

The bony changes associated with aging similarly affect the ability of the chest wall to tolerate blunt trauma. The thoracic cage becomes brittle so that even minor forces of injury result in broken ribs. With the loss of thoracic wall integrity, there is an increased incidence of pulmonary contusion. Not only are the thoracic cage and lung at increased risk for injury from a lesser force insult than would cause damage in a younger person, but the aortic arch also has an increased susceptibility for disruption in the elderly. This is described as being secondary to a decrease in flexibility because of age-associated atherosclerosis.

The thoracic cage and its contents are not only more susceptible to injury, but also to complications leading to increased morbidity and mortality. The leading cause of death in the elderly trauma patient after the first 24 hours is adult respiratory distress syndrome (ARDS) (15). More recent studies have confirmed that respiratory complications led to increased mortality associated with injury. A fivefold increase in ARDS was seen in a series of orthopedic patients, where delay in operative repair was greater than 24 hours (18).

There are conflicting reports regarding infection as a risk factor. Increased age was not seen as a risk factor for infection in a series of 310 patients, of whom 8 were over the age of 65 years. The mean length of stay in this group of 8 patients was 40 days, however, and survival was seen in 7 patients. There was no obvious increase in infections in this group (19). In contrast, in a group of 100 patients at Harborview, thoracic injury was considered a risk factor for increased mortality in the elderly. Of the 15 nonsurvivors in this group of patients, 100% were intubated longer than 5 days, and in 80% of the fatalities, pulmonary sepsis was a significant contributing factor (9). In a series of 63 elderly survivors of major trauma, pulmonary complications were most frequent (33%) but were not seen to be related to mortality. Nine patients were intubated longer than 5 days without death, although seven developed pneumonia (4).

It is fortunate that traumatic injuries to the abdomen are less frequent in the elderly, because significant morbidity and mortality are associated with such injuries. Abdominal injuries were seen in 35% (22 of 63 patients) reported by Oreskovich and others (9). This type of injury was associated with more surgery, increased complications, and a reduction in functional recovery. Personal experience has shown that the elderly patient is at risk for a burst injury to the liver, probably because of increased liver rigidity with age. The spleen seems to have a decreased susceptibility to injury from blunt trauma, probably because of the overall tendency for a decrease in size and fragility with age. The other organs do not seem to differ in risk for blunt injury because of the aging process.

Penetrating injuries to the torso are very unusual in the elderly. Assaults are uncommon, 4% in the Seattle series, and most result in blunt trauma (9). When penetrating injuries do occur, they seem less well tolerated in this age group, particularly if accompanied by shock. This combination results in close to a 100% fatality rate.

The skin is the only other major organ system and was discussed previously in the "Mechanism of Injury" section. Burns result in 8% of accident-related deaths in the elderly. The burns seem to be deeper and more extensive because of age-associated changes. With a given percentage of burn, the mortality in the elderly is higher than that seen in younger patients.

In summary, each organ system in the elderly patient tolerates injury less well when compared to those in younger patients, and the ability to recover is reduced. Complications, primarily pulmonary, occur with a higher frequency and figure significantly in the outcome. The ability to return to preinjury function appears to be related to the injury pattern, aggressive surgical management, and avoidance of complications.

Management Principles

Strict adherence to the principles of trauma care will most likely result in a good outcome and a return to preinjury function in the elderly patient. The pattern and extent of injury can only be altered in the preinjury phase by preventive measures. Therefore, the clinician caring for the elderly trauma patient must pay attention to trauma management principles and avoid complications. Adherence to these principles is required in all three phases of injury care: prehospital, initial assessment and resuscitation, and definitive care. Any significant deviation in any phase of care increases the risk for complication and will result in an increase in mortality or a decrease in the functional outcome.

In the prehospital phase of injury care, the elderly patient presents the most significant challenge to the prehospital principle of "do no further harm." An elderly patient who is injured demands adherence to all of the principles of prehospital trauma care. Particular attention to immobilization of fractures is important in reducing bleeding. Tissue planes in the older patient are more susceptible to dissection and fail to tamponade the bleeding. Hypovolemia results and is less well tolerated. The elderly patient is more apt to have dentures or other materials in the mouth that must be removed to facilitate a patent airway. Oxygen supplementation is important in this group because of the increased incidence of vascular disease, particularly cardiac. Thermal protection should be considered as a high priority to prevent hypothermia. Frequently, the elderly patient is hypothermic because of increased heat loss secondary to diminished subcutaneous fat reserves or delay in getting medical assistance. Attention to thermal protection is increasingly important in this age group because of the attendant myocardial irritability. Electrical monitoring of the heart should be done early in the management but should not cause delay in getting the traumatized patient to a treatment facility. Attempts at stabilization in the field are not indicated for any patient with traumatic injuries. All prehospital treatments at the scene should be optimally limited to less than 10 minutes. All elderly trauma patients require admission to trauma facilities in an expeditious manner to reduce morbidity and mortality.

The prehospital team should communicate the age of the patient and mechanism of injury to the receiving trauma hospital. This advance notification will allow the trauma team to adequately prepare for assessment and resuscitation. Upon arrival, the trauma team needs to get a verbal report of the accident details and current status of the patient while the resuscitation commences. Additional details regarding past medical history, allergies, and medications need to be documented if available. Frequently, the prehospital care team has access to this information through contact with family members and can relate this to the trauma team early in the assessment and resuscitative phase.

Priorities for assessment and resuscitation are the same for the elderly patient as with any trauma patient.

A quick initial assessment of airway, breathing, and circulation should quickly allow the physician to establish priorities in the resuscitation. Airway difficulties may occur because of dentures, which should be removed. The trauma team should be alert to the possibility of cervical spine injury because of the increased fragility in the elderly patient. A protected airway should be guaranteed. All elderly trauma patients should have supplemental oxygen therapy, preferably humidified. With any question of hypothermia, the provision of warmed and humidified oxygen can be used to aid in the rewarming process. Because of the increased frailty of the thoracic cage in the elderly, a careful assessment of respiratory capabilities should be done.

Management of shock and hemorrhage in accordance with established principles of trauma patient care should next occur. Close attention to core body temperature is a must in the elderly and cannot be overemphasized. Therefore, all solutions should be warmed to 30°C prior to administration. Warming blankets at room temperature must be utilized to reduce ongoing thermal losses. Cardiac arrhythmias can occur in any hypothermic patient during resuscitation, but the elderly patient is most susceptible because of intrinsic myocardial disease.

Resuscitative measures in the elderly trauma patient should proceed according to standard protocols. Monitoring the response to treatments by physical assessment alone will frequently be misleading. Mental status may not necessarily improve because of inadequate baseline. Peripheral perfusion may be impaired as a baseline as well. Heart rate may be abnormal because of intrinsic myocardial disease or the patient may be on medication, such as a beta-adrenergic blocking agent, which may limit heart rate response to hypovolemia. More subtle physical assessments, such as tissue turgor, temperature, and pulse character, lack both sensitivity and specificity, particularly in the elderly patient.

The elderly trauma patient requires aggressive and early monitoring of the adequacy of resuscitation. Urinary output can be misleading because of the possibility of intrinsic renal disease. All elderly male patients with moderate to severe trauma should be catheterized because of the high incidence of urethral outflow problems. Catheterization under these circumstances should be done with the usual precautions in patients with pelvic fractures and the resultant potential for urethral injuries at the bladder outlet. Patients with blood at the urethral meatus, displaced or "boggy" prostates on rectal examination, or severe pelvic fractures should have retrograde urethrograms prior to catheterization.

Central venous pressure lines should be placed early in most elderly trauma patients because of the need for proper fluid management and monitoring purposes. The lines should be placed ipsilaterally to any thoracic cage injury, particularly if a tube thoracostomy has already been placed. Confirmation of the location and evaluation for pneumothorax is required. The large triple lumen venous catheters are stiff, and the fragility of veins in the elderly can lead to venous disruption. Large bore central venous lines can be utilized for fluid administration, but this should be done cautiously with cool or cold fluids or blood transfusions, because of the potential to aggravate myocardial irritability. Conversion of the central venous pressure line to a Swan-Ganz catheter will increase the ability to monitor the patient with cardiovascular compromise or chronic obstructive pulmonary disease. In the acute situation, particularly in the elderly patient, this can stimulate fibrillation and therefore should be avoided until the acidosis and hypothermia are significantly improved. The use of cardiotonic drugs in the elderly to improve myocardial performance cannot be supported with scientific evidence of benefit. The potential chronotropic action of such agents can increase the left ventricular stroke work index to high levels, which may result in myocardial failure or ischemia. Although the practice of using a low-dosage infusion of dopamine is common, the benefit is small, and the risk is large particularly if it delays volume resuscitation measures.

The initial assessment and resuscitation should proceed in an aggressive manner according to standardized protocols. The nature and severity of injury for each organ system as well as the response to the initial treatments will evolve during this time period. Plans for definitive care also require input from family or other supportive people. Knowing the baseline medical and physical activity levels becomes important in making the best clinical decision for the patient. When such knowledge is unknown or is thought to be unreliable, the clinician should assume a viable productive premorbid state and proceed with aggressive management. When the clinical situation is thought to be hopeless or the baseline function of the patient is not good, aggressive resuscitation and management may be terminated. Involvement of all pertinent family members in addition to documentation by living wills or other pieces of similar data will allow the most appropriate clinical decisions to be made.

If aggressive management is pursued, established trauma care principles should be strictly adhered to in the elderly for the best outcome. Complications of any sort in the elderly trauma patient have significant outcome consequences in terms of morbidity and mortality. The most common serious complications are pulmonary, cardiac, and septic. Close attention to prevention of these problems markedly increases the chance for a return to preinjury function.

Pulmonary complications are a common sequela of trauma management. Adult respiratory distress syndrome in the elderly patient, as defined by intubation and ventilation longer than 24 hours, carries a significant risk of mortality. Oreskovich et al. (9) showed a mortality of 100% when intubation was required for longer than 5 days in the elderly trauma patient. Many variables were involved other than just respiratory support measures, but secondary pneumonias were strongly implicated as causative. Prolonged bed rest, a high incidence of chest wall injuries, diminished upper airway protective mechanisms, and a reduction of resistance secondary to both trauma and aging all contribute to the increased incidence of pneumonia in the elderly trauma patient. Therefore, preventive and/or therapeutic measures are necessary to reduce this problem.

Measures to reduce the pulmonary complications include both overall injury treatments and specific pulmonary toilet procedures. The overall injury treatment principles to reduce pulmonary complications include aggressive and early orthopedic surgical procedures to allow patient mobilization and ambulation. Operative procedures to stabilize rib and sternal fractures may also be warranted in this high risk group to reduce complications. Pulmonary toilet measures of all kinds will reduce pneumonia in this age group. The most important consideration is the attention to detail and consideration of the elderly patient as a high-risk candidate for this problem.

The elderly patient requires a greater acuity level of nursing care. Additionally, the intensive care unit patient who is unable to get out of bed for any length of time should be considered for a rotary bed to improve pulmonary function and elimination of secretions. Daily chest x-rays, sputum gram stain, and sputum cultures on a consistent basis (every several days if the patient remains intubated) will allow early diagnosis and treatment of pneumonia should it occur. Strict attention to hand washing prior to patient contact is most important in these immunosuppressed patients at high risk for nosocomial infections.

Prevention and therapeutic interventions applied in an aggressive manner will similarly reduce cardiac complications in the elderly traumatized patient. Fluid resuscitation in patients with diminished cardiac reserve has been previously discussed. The need for invasive monitoring has been described as necessary in many of these patients. Schultz et al. (20) showed a dramatic reduction in operative mortality (29% to 3%), using routine Swan-Ganz catheterization in monitoring patients with hip fractures.

In the recovery phase the traumatized patient is particularly prone to fluid shifts, which may be poorly tolerated in the elderly. Depending on the duration of shock, the peripheral capillary beds may leak plasma; this adds to the fluid sequestration and hematoma formation directly associated with tissue damage. With stabilization of the cardiovascular system, fluid reabsorption can begin as early as 24 hours and will maximize at 72 hours. Anticipation of this fluid shift allows for optimal management, particularly in the patient with diminished cardiac reserve. The Swan-Ganz catheter measurements available during the early resuscitation phase will give several points on the patient's Starling curve. During fluid mobilization, intravenous fluid restriction may be necessary; salt restriction and prudent use of diuretics may also be required.

Improvement in the patient's overall course can lead to such optimism that the monitoring may be discontinued early, allowing a sudden unexpected deterioration in the patient. Occult fluid shifts and resultant cardiac failure may cause this deterioration. Prevention of this deterioration should occur, for the known sequelae of fluid absorption are well understood. Therefore, it is strongly recommended that elderly patients with significant peripheral fluid sequestration, as evidenced by weight gain, excess fluid requirements, and peripheral edema, be monitored by invasive catheters to properly monitor cardiac function during this vulnerable period. Consideration should be given to diuretic administration in such patients on the 2nd day through 4th day following injury. Particular attention to electrolyte balance is necessary with the use of such agents. Cardiotonic agents may occasionally become necessary as well.

As has been previously discussed, the elderly traumatized patient is susceptible to pulmonary infection. Infection is also a possibility elsewhere in the body because of the immune system suppression. Judicious use of prophylactic antibiotics is indicated in elderly patients as in other trauma patients. Careful attention should be paid to intravenous cutdown sites, and they should be treated as open, infected wounds. All intravenous lines placed in the initial resuscitation phase should be replaced in the first 24 hours because of the increased risk of infection.

A most important consideration in the management

and prevention of infections in the traumatized patient is nutrition. The enteral tract is the most appropriate means by which to return to a normal nutritional state. Parenteral hyperalimentation should also be considered for most major trauma patients. Because of the increased frailty of the elderly trauma patient, nutritional considerations are very important, and attention should be given to this early in the course of even mild to moderate injuries. As soon as gastrointestinal function returns, consideration should be given to enteral nutrition by feeding tube.

Summary

Although only 2% of deaths in the elderly are caused by injuries, this represents 20% of all trauma-related deaths. The age group over age 65 years experiences more severe injuries for a measured insult. The primary causes of injury in the elderly are falls (approximately 40% to 50%), motor vehicle accidents (20% to 30%), and pedestrian accidents (20% to 30%). Reviews of hospital care of the traumatized elderly show more serious injuries and a decreased ability to recover.

Management principles of trauma are similar in all age groups with attention to airway, breathing, and circulation in the primary survey. Special attention to previous chronic diseases should be obtained early in the management of these patients. A decreased threshold for all interventional measures is necessary for the best outcome. Early ambulation is necessary in this age group to prevent pulmonary complications and the resultant high morbidity and mortality.

Social issues complicate the hospital care in this age group. A conflict exists between the potential life-style changes, which may result from injury, and the high costs of the care to effect the outcome. These high costs are not well reimbursed by present payment mechanisms. Modern trauma care systems are collecting data on this age group to attempt to resolve some of these problems.

References

1. Baker, SP, O'Neill, B, and Karpf, RS. 1984. *The Injury Fact Book*. Lexington, MA: Lexington Books.
2. Mueller, MS, and Gibson, RN. 1976. Age difference in healthcare spending. *Soc Sec Bulletin* 36:18.
3. Schwab, CW. DRG reimbursement for trauma: The demise of the trauma center (The use of ISS grouping as an early predictor of total hospital cost). *J Trauma*, in press.
4. DeMaria, EJ, et al. 1987. Aggressive trauma care benefits in the elderly. *J Trauma* 27(11):1200.
5. Morris, JA, Jr., et al. 1986. The trauma score as a triage tool in the prehospital setting. *JAMA* 256(10):1319.
6. Champion, HR. 1986. *The Major Trauma Outcome Study.* American College of Surgeons Committee on Trauma.
7. *Injury in America, A Continuing Public Health Problem*. 1985. Washington, DC: National Academy Press.
8. Hogue, CP. 1982. Injury in late life: Part I: Epidemiology. *J Am Geriatr Soc* 30:183.
9. Oreskovich, NR, et al. 1984. Geriatric trauma: Injury patterns and outcome. *J Trauma* 24:565.
10. DeMaria, EJ, et al. Hospital costs and reimbursement in geriatric trauma patients. *J Trauma*, in press.
11. Anous, MN, and Heimbach, DM. 1986. Causes of death and predictors in burned patients more than 60 years of age. *J Trauma* 26:135.
12. Waller, JA. 1985. *Injury Control: A Guide to the Causes and Prevention of Trauma*. Lexington, MA: Lexington Books.
13. Bongard, FS, Ostrow, LB, Sacks, ST, et al. 1987. Burns in the elderly. *Am Fam Physician* 1:149.
14. Mandelbaum, ER, and Brooker, AF, Jr. 1985. Trauma to the lower extremities. In *The Management of Trauma*, ed. 4. Eds., GD Zytema, RB Rutherford, and WF Ballinger. Philadelphia: W.B. Saunders Co.
15. Trunkey, DD, et al. 1974. Management of pelvic fractures in blunt trauma injuries. *J Trauma* 14:912.
16. Howard, MA, III, Dacy, RG, Jr., and Winn, HR. 1987. *Traumatic Intracranial Hemorrhage in the Elderly.* Proceedings Am Assn of Neurologic Surgeons.
17. Russell, MA, et al. 1985. Chronic subdural hematoma mimicking transient ischemic attacks. *J Trauma* 25:1113.
18. Johnson, KD, Cadambi, A, and Seibert, GB. 1985. Incidence of adult respiratory distress syndrome in patients with multiple musculoskeletal injuries: Effect of early operative stabilization of fractures. *J Trauma* 25:375.
19. Walker, WE, et al. 1985. Patterns of infection and mortality in thoracic trauma. *Ann Surg* 201:752.
20. Schultz, RJ, et al. 1985. The role of physiologic monitoring in patients with fractures of the hip. *J Trauma* 25:309.

SECTION III
General Management of the Geriatric Surgical Patient

20

Radiologic Evaluation of the Elderly Patient

Ian Kellman and Satish Patel

Radiologic evaluation of the geriatric patient is not wholly different from that of younger individuals, if one recognizes that age-related changes associated with degenerative processes may alter the expected picture. The surgeon ordering a specific examination, as well as the technician and radiologist, must be aware of physical or mental limitations that may exist in the older patient, and understand how these factors may limit or modify the examination. In these days of Diagnosis Related Groups (DRGs) and cost containment, it is imperative that the practicing physician understand the role he or she may play in controlling the costs while assuring the patient the best in medical care.

Care of the geriatric radiology patient prior to, during, and following a study will do little to alter the radiographic picture, but may be a significant factor in the patient's well being and recovery. While many of the older patients seem to be physically fit, the rigors of some examinations may exceed the patient's ability to handle stress, resulting in further debilitation of an already ill patient. In some instances, the preparation for the examination may be as stressful to the patient as the test itself. It behooves the surgeon to keep this in mind so the cure does not end up being worse than the disease.

Failing eyesight and deficient hearing, coupled with a high level of anxiety, often result in considerable confusion on the part of the patient. It is not uncommon for an elderly patient to come for a test having no idea of what kind of examination has been ordered or why. This can usually be avoided if the ordering physician will take a few minutes to explain the test to the patient.

A better understanding of the procedure would help the surgeon recognize that a patient's physical or mental condition may not allow an adequate study without special patient preparation. It is interesting to note that many surgeons have not seen the full procedure for many of the tests they order and it would help them better understand their patients' needs if they were to spend a few hours in a radiology department during some of the more common procedures, such as barium enemas, upper gastrointestinal (GI) studies, and angiography. Knowledge of the geometry of some of the more complicated technologies, such as magnetic resonance imaging (MRI), computed tomographic (CT) scanning, and nuclear medicine, would also help the surgeon understand patient positioning problems.

Examples of some of the problems encountered by the radiologist include air contrast barium enemas ordered on patients who have just undergone hip replacement surgery, the inappropriate ordering of intravenous contrast on patients with renal failure, tests requiring patient cooperation on moribund patients, and repeated laxatives and cleansing enemas on dehydrated patients.

The use of portable studies is often abused. While this may seem to be an administrative problem, it is also a problem for the patient. Admittedly, the quality of portable studies has improved dramatically in recent years, but limitations in portable technique and patient positioning sometimes require repeat studies with both physical stress and anxiety often resulting.

In summary, recognition of an older patient's physical and mental limitations, and an understanding of the stresses encountered during some examinations, can help make the patient's visit to the radiologist a less traumatic and, in some cases, a pleasant experience.

Central Nervous System

Evaluation of the central nervous system may be crucial to determining the course of treatment in the elderly. While many patients may appear in the doctor's office or the hospital with systemic complaints, the symptoms may be somatic presentations of central nervous system disease. Confusion, lethargy, loss of memory, weakness, and many other nonspecific complaints may be due to intracranial disease. The arteriosclerotic process that is so evident in the cardiac status and peripheral vascular disease may also cause significant neurologic disease.

While a patient may present with symptoms suggesting a cerebrovascular accident (CVA), it is important to exclude other causes of intracranial disease that may be surgically treatable. A plain-film x-ray study may show bone changes hinting at an intracranial process, but technologically sophisticated modalities must be used to gain more information. In recent years, the use of magnetic resonance imaging (MRI) and computed tomography (CT) have all but replaced the nuclear brain scan, and arteriography is reserved for cases that present diagnostic confusion or require detailed knowledge of the circulatory supply. MRI applications are expanding daily and as contrast media are developed MRI will probably become as specific a test as it is now recognized to be sensitive. Because of availability, however, CT is by far the more common examination.

Recognition of cerebrovascular accidents (Fig. 20-1) and their differentiation from tumors, both metastatic and primary, can generally be accomplished with these modalities. Additionally, an unsuspected subdural hematoma is easily recognized without having to resort to arteriography. Thus, where a trauma history is not elucidated, these newer modalities enable the physician to distinguish between the surgical and nonsurgical patient.

The acute hemorrhagic lesion (Fig. 20-2) will be easily identified, and this recognition may alter the course of therapy. This refers not only to the use of anticoagulants, but also can help distinguish between the surgical and nonsurgical patient. In many instances, it may be possible to determine an approximate age of the lesion.

While carotid circulation can be evaluated in outpatients by the use of digital arteriography, preliminary ultrasound scanning is a noninvasive modality with a high degree of accuracy, especially when used with the more sophisticated doppler techniques.

Visualization of the posterior fossa, brain stem, and spinal canal contents once required invasive procedures, some of which were quite traumatic to the patient. Today, MRI can effectively delineate small lesions that previously could only be identified at surgery.

The modality selected to evaluate the spine will have to be chosen after consideration of the desired information. Plain-film radiography is the first choice as it will reveal most of the bony abnormalities associated with the degenerative process in the spine, such as disc narrowing, neural foramen encroachment, and osteoarthritis. Similarly, fractures and dislocations will usually be obvious on the plain-film study. Further evaluation of possible fractures may require tomography or CT.

Visualization of soft tissues will be limited by the presence of the bony structures, and while CT can be useful in evaluation of lumbar disc disease, the smaller spinal canal in the cervical and dorsal regions will limit the usefulness of CT in these areas. As MRI has improved in quality it has become the modality of choice in spinal evaluation, and in many instances it has replaced CT as

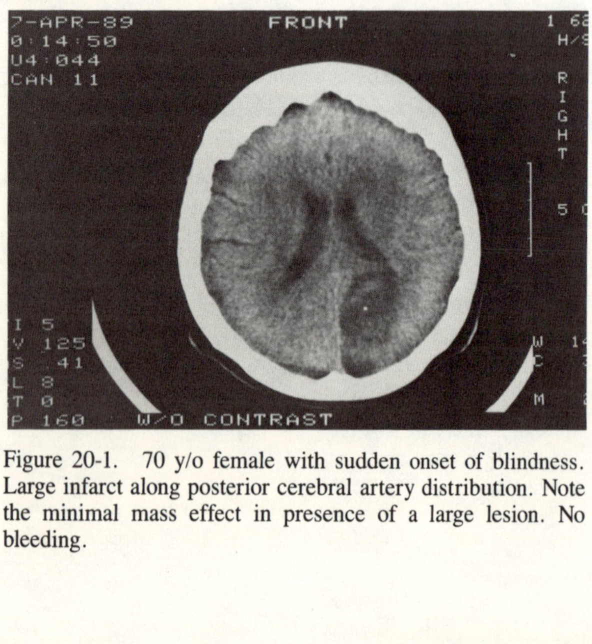

Figure 20-1. 70 y/o female with sudden onset of blindness. Large infarct along posterior cerebral artery distribution. Note the minimal mass effect in presence of a large lesion. No bleeding.

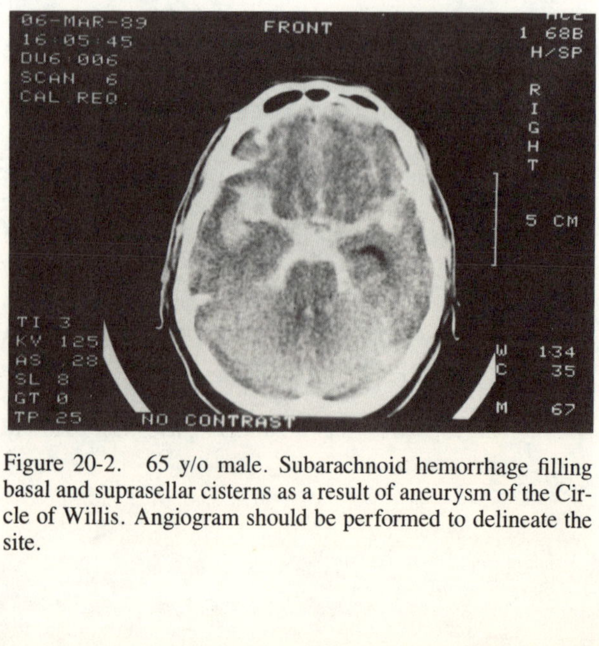

Figure 20-2. 65 y/o male. Subarachnoid hemorrhage filling basal and suprasellar cisterns as a result of aneurysm of the Circle of Willis. Angiogram should be performed to delineate the site.

well as myelography. It should be remembered, however, that MRI will not allow for optimal delineation of the bony skeleton in the spine. In this regard, CT is the examination of choice when spinal stenosis or spinal canal fracture fragments are suspected.

The Chest

The chest is a mirror of years of exposure to one's surroundings. Air, and the dust and gases within it, carry all manner of noxious agents deep within the lungs where they often remain for years. Subtle changes in the lungs are usually not appreciated on chest x-rays during the early stages of irritation. In the older patient, as a result of years of recurrent exposure, scarring from inflammation and infection, and normal changes related to tissue aging, noticeable alterations in the x-ray picture become obvious (Figs. 20-3 and 20-4).

While the chest x-ray is usually obtained for evaluation of the lungs and central cardiovascular structures, the chest is actually a complex body part with many different structures, all of which interplay to give the final "chest x-ray." When one remembers that the final radiography is a result of many overlapping shadows and soft-tissue densities, it becomes apparent that changes in the skin, muscles, bones, or any other structure may affect the appearance of the lungs. This becomes especially important in the older patient because these other structures have their own "age-related" changes that may further confuse the picture.

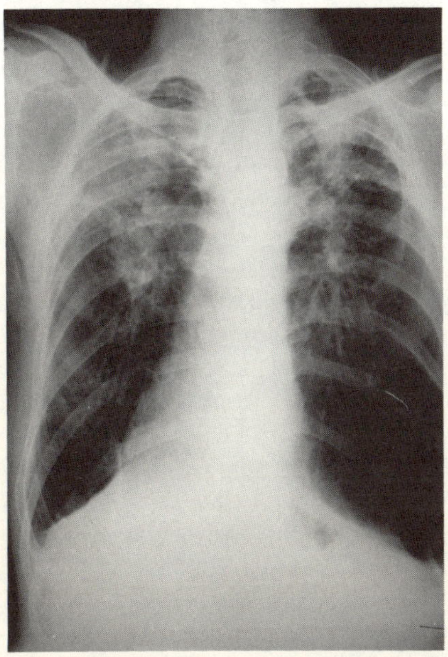

Figure 20-3. Anthracosilicosis resulting in extensive pleural and parenchymal scarring may mimic mass lesions.

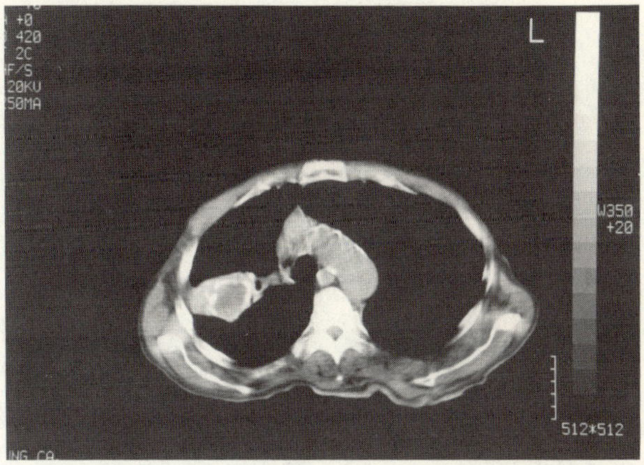

Figure 20-4. Different patient with an anthracosilicotic mass that has degenerated and is filled with fluid mimicking a carcinoma.

It is not uncommon to see a small nodule projected over a lung. The unsuspecting clinician may institute a coin lesion workup when a simple correlation of the radiograph with the physical examination would have shown a mole, verrucous tag, or possibly even a nipple to be responsible for the shadow. In our experience, the use of small BB-like markers and, in questionable cases, fluoroscopy should be sufficient to clarify the problem.

Changes in lung density do not always indicate lung disease. Alterations in the overlying skin will also affect the x-ray picture. The most common example is the postmastectomy chest in which the side that has undergone surgery will appear more lucent. Conversely, it is not uncommon for dense breast tissue to present itself as a coarsening of lung markings. It is often easy to verify this by looking at the lung bases. If the patient has taken a deep breath, and the breasts are not very large, one can see a rim of uncovered, clearer lung at the lung base. The interface may be quite striking at times.

As people get older, the skin loses its elasticity. Skin may become quite loose and the skin folds may present as areas of soft-tissue density. These may mimic pleural thickening or segmental atelectasis. Minimal skin folding that produces a faint soft-tissue interface may be confused with pneumothorax (Fig. 20-5). Careful examination of the lung and demonstration of markings beyond the edge of the "pneumothorax" should resolve this problem.

Patient positioning has a significant effect on the appearance of the chest. The chest is usually radiographed with the anterior chest against the cassette, the patient standing, and the tube 6 feet from the cassette. The patient who is weak or postsurgical may not be able to stand. Some of these patients may be able to sit erect and have a 6-foot x-ray, but others will have to be studied at shorter distances and in a supine or semi-erect position. These

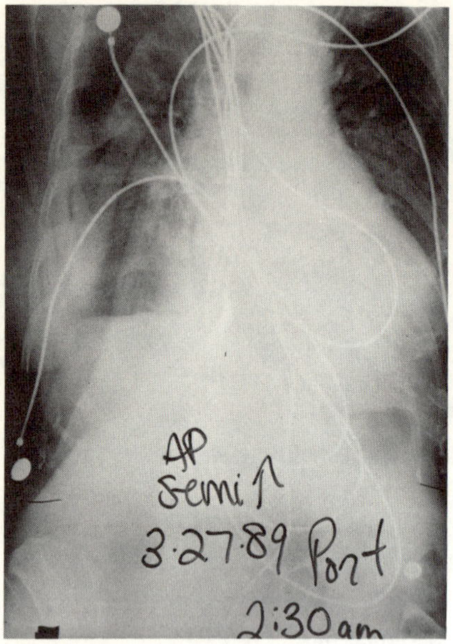

Figure 20-5. Skin fold artifacts.

studies will have to be performed with the cassette behind the patient. While some of these studies will be performed in an x-ray department, the majority will be at the bed with a portable unit. It should be noted that a modern portable x-ray unit is state-of-the-art and will produce a satisfactory study, but there may be some limitations as a result of patient size. Additionally, artifact will be introduced by the short tube to cassette distance. In this case, spatial relationships will be present that will distort the appearance of normal structures. It is therefore suggested that, when possible, the patient should be studied in the x-ray department.

The heart is an anterior structure and the least magnification results when the anterior chest is against the cassette. In the normal adult chest, heart size is considered normal when the transverse diameter of the chest is less than half the transverse diameter of the expanded lungs on an erect, posterior-to-anterior (PA) inspiratory study. The geometry of the supine anteroposterior view is such that a normal sized heart may appear enlarged. In most instances this will not pose a problem to the experienced film reader, but this may be important in serial evaluation of the patient in heart failure or with conditions such as myocarditis or pericardial effusion.

Equally important are changes in pulmonary vascular distribution with changes in patient position. In the normal chest vascular markings are most prominent in the lower lungs as a result of gravity. One of the earliest x-ray signs of heart failure is a redistribution of these markings into the upper lungs. Postural shifts in fluid volume occurring on a supine chest x-ray may obscure early changes of heart failure.

Similarly, pleural effusion normally collects in the most dependent areas of the thoracic cavity. If this fluid is free-running, it could easily layer out along the posterior chest when a patient is placed supine. The more uniform distribution may affect lung density in such a manner as to obscure the presence of the fluid. At this point it is also important to point out that fluid may sometimes distribute itself in such a manner as to conform to adjacent lung structures. Thus, fluid may present as a thickened interlobar fissure, or may mimic an area of pleural thickening. The latter is most often seen at the lung apex.

Perhaps the most important fluid distribution, because it is often the most difficult to readily identify, is the subpulmonic effusion. It is not uncommon to see a rather large effusion present in such a manner as to mimic the contour of the diaphragm. In these cases the recognition of the presence of the fluid will depend upon recognition of subtle hints such as a slight change in contour of the diaphragm when compared to earlier studies. Minimal blunting of the costophrenic recess may suggest an effusion as well. In these cases, a lateral decubitus view may provide a surprising picture of massive effusion that might otherwise have been missed completely (Fig. 20-6).

The identification of free abdominal air is a diagnostic problem of paramount importance. The recognition of air beneath the diaphragm is often the earliest indication of ruptured viscus. It must be remembered, however, that just as fluid goes to the lowest point, air goes to the highest point. Thus it is necessary to have the patient and the x-ray tube aligned in such a manner as to demonstrate this to advantage. Air may not be seen on a supine study of the chest, even when present in large quantities. The erect chest is best for the demonstration of the air (Fig. 20-7). The problem comes when a portable chest study is obtained in the semi-erect position. In order to best demonstrate the lungs, the technologist will often tilt the tube to a position perpendicular to the chest. Thus, the diaphragm is not visualized in a position advantageous to the demonstration of the air.

Rather than get involved in a discussion of the complexities of positioning, suffice it to say that fluid and free air, or air fluid levels in bowel, are best visualized when the x-ray beam is parallel to the floor and perpendicular to the body. Thus, while optimal positioning is always desired, it becomes imperative when looking for the signs of free air, free fluid, or air-fluid levels. With modern radiographic units it is now possible to perform high-quality radiography, and even fluoroscopy, at the bedside. Portable sonography is also available.

One would hope that the portable study is used with discrimination, that is, for the patient on whom a study cannot be performed in the radiology department because of patient condition or attached equipment limitations.

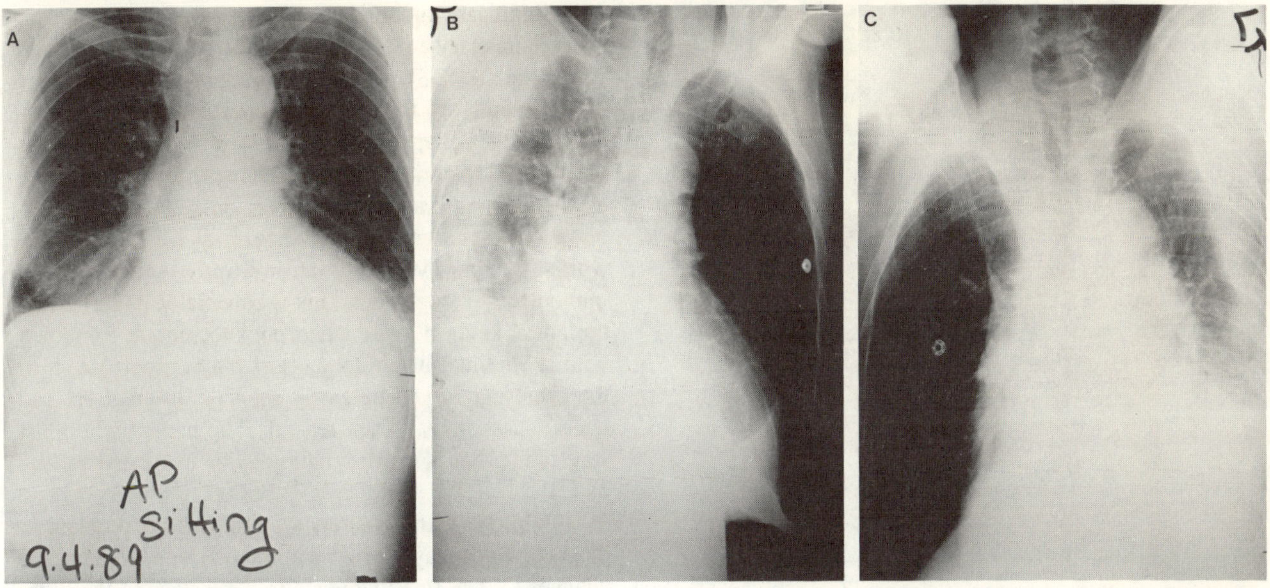

Figure 20-6, A–C. Series of chest x-rays showing development of a large bilateral pleural effusion that was not fully appreciated without the benefit of decubitus views.

Too often, the portable study is used as a convenience and needed information is not obtained.

All is not lost, however, in the debilitated patient. By a proper selection of position, the study can actually be enhanced. If the patient can be rolled up on a side, a decubitus view can be obtained. This will allow use of a horizontal beam and inclusion of the greatest surface area of the chest or abdomen, lessening the chance of missing a significant air-fluid level such as seen in an abscess or infected cyst, bowel obstruction, or even a small pneumothorax.

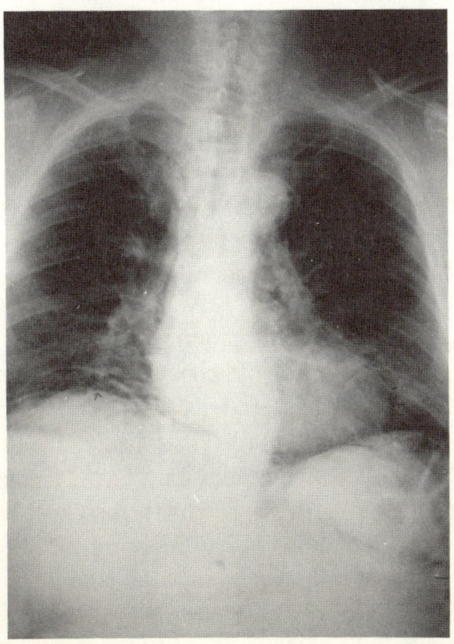

Figure 20-7. Traumatic pneumoperitoneum and pneumomediastinum. Note free air beneath right hemidiaphragm and at cardiac apex.

Changes in the configuration of the heart in the older patient are often the result of arteriosclerotic disease. It is important to have preoperative studies available for comparison in the operative patient to be certain no acute process is missed during the postsurgical period. In this age group acute heart enlargement is most likely to represent heart failure, pericardial effusion, or ventricular aneurysm. Decreased heart size, while uncommon, can be seen in severe fluid loss or Addisonian adrenal failure.

There are usually clues to past cardiac surgery in the form of opaque suture in the sternum and overlying the heart. A prosthetic valve can also be seen on a plain-film chest x-ray. The position of the valve is specific for the intracardiac location. Fluoroscopy may be used to check valve function but isotope or contrast studies that demonstrate actual blood flow are more meaningful.

More significant postoperative changes can be seen after removal of part or all of a lung. Lobectomy leaves a void that must be filled. This will cause a shift in position of normal structures. The resulting chest x-ray will usually show some degree of hyperinflation of the remaining lung in the ipsilateral thoracic cavity, and may show varying degrees of diaphragmatic elevation and mediastinal shift. The void may also fill with transudate fluid, leading to a large effusion and, on the erect x-ray, an area of abnormal density or even an air-fluid level indicating hydropneumothorax. CT will add additional information regarding tumor recurrence and adenopathy. Thoracoplasty changes are easily seen (Fig. 20-8).

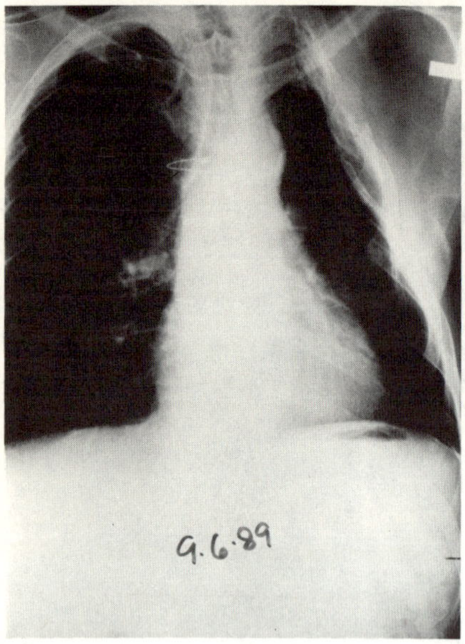

Figure 20-8. Extensive chest deformity as a result of thoracoplasty.

Thoracostomy and endotracheal tubes will be evident radiographically as will various intravascular catheters. A properly placed subclavian line may be well positioned with regard to the blood vessels, but care must be taken to be certain there is no small apical pneumothorax hidden by the clavicle. Postplacement mediastinal widening or basal shadowing may indicate intrathoracic bleeding. A feeding tube that has been passed only as far as the mid-chest may appear to be in normal position in the esophagus, but it may actually lie within the tracheobronchial tree, in an obtunded patient with no cough reflex. On rare occasions, the tube may actually pass into the lung periphery and enter the thoracic cavity. This may be an isolated finding with no pneumothorax. When there is question as to the position of a particular tube, a lateral view of the chest may help with localization.

The postpercutaneous biopsy chest is also more prone to pneumothorax. A postprocedure erect frontal view is recommended. It should be noted that small pneumothoraces are often demonstrable only on expiratory chest x-rays. If the patient has respiratory limitations, or if there are strong clinical indications of pneumothorax, but no abnormality is seen, decubitus views may provide additional information. In this instance, the pneumothorax will be evident along the margins of the nondependent lung. It should be noted that a pneumothorax may also be seen on the postbiopsy CT scan, thus obviating the need for much additional study.

Perhaps more significant than changes in the chest as a direct result of surgery are the sometimes life-threatening abnormalities that occur in the postoperative patient and manifest themselves as chest disease.

Significant among these are postoperative atelectasis, pulmonary embolism, and adult respiratory distress syndrome (ARDS). While the patient with atelectasis may present with the classical abnormal density associated with the collapse of a specific lung segment, the diagnosis may sometimes be more elusive. Mediastinal shift, diaphragmatic elevation, and loss of normal heart, mediastinum, or diaphragm borders should all be looked upon with suspicion, even when an infiltrative process is not immediately recognized. This is especially important on the portable chest x-ray when poor technique combined with suboptimal inspiratory effort may obscure areas of the chest that would be easily seen on an erect PA and lateral chest study. When feasible, the patient who must stay supine but is transportable can be evaluated further by CT.

Pulmonary embolism is a more difficult problem to diagnose for it may present with no obvious radiographic changes. When this diagnosis is suspected, in the presence of a normal chest x-ray, further evaluation by other modalities is mandatory. Ventilation-perfusion isotope lung scanning is a simple and fairly reliable examination. It does, however, require the patient's cooperation. In the noncooperative patient, or in those cases where a scan is equivocal, a pulmonary angiogram is necessary for a more definitive diagnosis.

ARDS is a serious and life-threatening process that in basic terms represents a failure of the lung's ability to function as a respiratory organ. It will present as acute respiratory distress associated with a clinical picture of severe and progressive hypoxemia refractory to oxygen therapy. Decreasing lung compliance and diffuse alveolar and interstitial infiltrate give a radiographic picture of poor inspiration and diffuse lung opacification. It starts as minimal diffuse patchy infiltration and progresses to significant consolidation. Effusion is not usually significant, if present. Life-saving therapy must be instituted at once.

Lung tumors may present as solitary or multiple lesions. It is important to distinguish between abscesses and emboli presenting as multiple nodular densities, and multiple tumors. This may not always be possible on the basis of a plain-film chest radiograph. Clinical history is of great importance, as is an old chest study for comparison. CT may not always help and, in fact, in the presence of multiple small cavitary lesions, may just add to the confusion. CT density readings may be of some help in that tumors tend to be of higher density than emboli or abscesses, but calcifications or underlying fibrotic change may just confuse the issue.

The solitary lung lesion must be carefully evaluated in the elderly patient. If this lesion was not present on recent studies, there is a good possibility that one is dealing with an inflammatory or embolic process. On the other hand, a lesion that has shown progressive growth over a period of several weeks to months, or was not present on a study taken several months previously, must, in the absence of a significant history, be considered malignant until proven otherwise. CT may be of great help in this instance, giving information not only about the nature of the lesion, but also about the presence of lymphadenopathy, pleural effusion, or additional unsuspected lesions.

The most important factor in evaluating the lesion by CT is its density number. It is generally held that a malignancy usually has density readings below 180 HU. Granulomata, on the other hand, by virtue of calcifications, will tend to have higher readings. Pneumonia or atelectasis presenting as a solitary round lesion cannot always be distinguished from neoplasm. In that case follow-up, bronchoscopy, or more invasive procedures may be required. Other criteria for malignancy include spiculated margins, eccentric and often thick-walled cavitary lesions, and eccentric calcification. The presence of fat within a lesion is more suggestive of hamartoma or adenoma. It should be noted that there have been reports of mineral oil aspiration pneumonia in patients using this material as a laxative.

Calcification is a common finding within the tissues of the chest in the elderly patient. Costal cartilage calcification and tracheobronchial tree calcification are seen with increasing frequency as the patient population ages. This is a physiologic calcification related to the aging process, and generally of no clinical significance. It is, however, important to recognize these calcifications and not see them as intrathoracic pathology.

Pleural and parenchymal calcification, on the other hand, is almost always indicative of scarring. This can be quite severe at times and may be associated with restrictive lung disease. While some patterns may indicate old granulomatous disease or old empyema, the minimal calcifications that are the more common picture are nonspecific in nature.

Vascular calcification occurs throughout the body in the elderly patient. While it may be seen in venous sites, as in pelvic phleboliths or scarred leg varicosities, it is more common to see arterial calcification. As in the abdomen, the aorta and its major branches are prone to calcification. This calcification can be used to delineate the distribution of arteriosclerosis and can be helpful in delineating aneurysms. The intracardiac valves and surrounding soft tissues can be identified; calcific density is a very common finding in the mitral annulus. Coronary artery calcification is not usually appreciated on the plain chest x-ray, yet this calcification is often recognized during fluoroscopy of the esophagus.

The skeleton of the chest wall and the external features of the chest wall, such as the musculature and skin, do not differ in the chest from those in the remainder of the body. The breast is discussed elsewhere.

A key area in the chest is the mediastinum. The site of many blood vessels, the heart, and lymphatics, as well as neural tissue, this area is often altered by disease processes elsewhere in the chest that may result in deformity and displacement of the mediastinum. Adenopathy, benign and malignant tumors, and dilated blood vessels may enlarge the mediastinum (Fig. 20-9).

For many years the esophagram and tomography were the first steps in evaluation of the mediastinum. These techniques are still useful but have been replaced for the most part by CT and, where available, MRI, which allow delineation of blood vessels and lymph nodes as well as the mediastinal contour, tracheobronchial tree, and the esophagus. Angiography can be used when additional vascular information is required. Which test is best for the patient depends on what information is sought and the reader is referred to his or her radiologist.

Skeletal System

While changes in the lung are often tempered by environmental factors, the skeletal system shows more of a "wear and tear" response to physical stresses upon the body. Constant stress from normal activities such as weight bearing, superimposition of insults from occupational and recreational activities, and the added effects of the aging process and disease, all contribute to a highly varied picture of skeletal aging. While there are many individuals who by fortune of good genetics show little deterioration of the skeletal system, it is far more common to see radiographic changes that have come to be considered "normal" in the older patient.

Underlying many of the age-related alterations in bone density and texture is the process of senile osteoporosis. While the term osteoporosis specifically refers to a process of bony atrophy with loss of the protein matrix, the term has come, through common usage, to include all processes in which there is a radiographic loss of bone density. Perhaps a more correct term would be osteopenia, as this general term includes osteomalacia, a loss of calcium, or any combination of the two.

Osteoporosis is more common in women and is related to estrogen activity and exercise during the years preceding its appearance. When it is considered that women generally have lesser bone density to start with, it is not unreasonable to expect that conditions affecting bone architecture and bone mass will have a more readily observable effect in women.

The most common presentation of senile osteoporosis is the spinal compression fracture. As the bony mass of

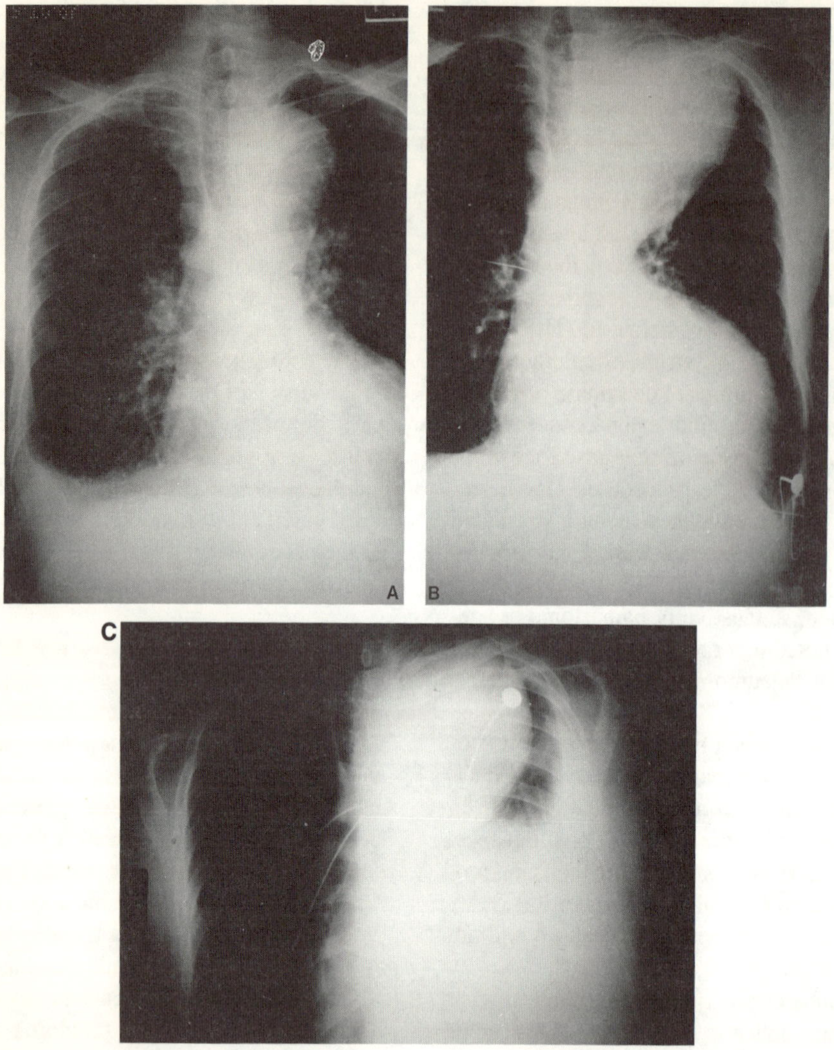

Figure 20-9, A–C. Three successive studies of a known aortic arch aneurysm. The first study preceded the other two by 2 years. There was only a 3-day interval between the last two studies. Note the large amount of free blood in the pleural space.

the vertebral body decreases, the vertebral end plate "softens" and the relatively hard intervertebral disc material encroaches upon the bony end plate and eventually protrudes through the cortex, producing the characteristic concave deformity of end plate infraction. When this process is exaggerated by weight or stress, significant end plate fractures may occur. As the vertebral bodies collapse, the forces are transmitted primarily through the anterior margin of the vertebral body resulting in "wedging." In time, this will lead to a loss of overall height of the patient, which can be further complicated by kyphosis.

The skull is another common site of changes associated with senile osteoporosis. Besides the demineralization and a somewhat grainy appearance of the calvarium, one can also see thinning of the calvarium. This often presents as thin cortices and prominent diploic vessels. Bilaterally symmetrical parietal thinning, while not common, must be differentiated from the severe demineralization characteristic of osteoporosis circumscripta of early Paget's disease. It is also important to recognize that severe demineralization of the pituitary fossa may mimic increased intrasellar pressure. As a rule, the age-related process is most severe in the posterior aspect of the floor of the fossa and in the dorsum sella. Effects of increased pressure, on the other hand, are more common in the anterior aspect of the fossa.

While the preponderance of findings are in the axial skeleton, extremities are also affected by this process. The usual picture is that of a very thin cortex, combined with decreased medullary density. These bony structures, by virtue of lesser bone mass and decreased trabecular support structures, are weakened and prone to significant fracture, even with minor trauma. This process is responsible for many fractures of the femoral neck, proximal humerus, and wrist.

Fractures are further complicated by slow healing and poor callus formation. This problem is the result of a combination of factors, which include poor blood supply, decreased physical activity, and poor nutrition, as well as osteoporosis. It is important to evaluate carefully all patients who develop fractures because metastatic disease, primary malignancy such as multiple myeloma, infection, and metabolic abnormalities, especially the renal osteodystrophies, may all result in fractures. It should be realized that the radiographic appearance of the fracture will probably not give an indication as to the etiology unless there are other pathognomonic findings in adjacent structures, such as obvious metastatic disease or classic changes of renal disease, to mention a few. When the clinical picture is equivocal, isotope bone scanning with radiography of positive findings, skeletal survey, or biopsy may be required.

In recent years, methods of quantifying osteoporosis have been developed in an attempt to predict potential risk of complications such as fractures and debility. Nuclear and CT densitometry are presently being used. These are new modalities and one should exercise some caution in making predictions of future bone loss or risk of fracture, until more experience is gained in the use of these procedures.

In some instances, it may be difficult to define a fracture line if the fracture is nondisplaced and occurs in osteoporotic bone. The clinical picture will suggest the presence of a fracture and repeated follow-up radiography or techniques such as tomography, CT, or nuclear scanning may be required to identify the fracture. Nuclear scanning will probably not be positive within the first 48 hours, but in the presence of a fracture the scan should become positive within 4 days following the injury (Fig. 20-10).

Tumors of bone in the elderly are usually metastatic. The distinction between benign and malignant tumors is easy in the presence of diffuse metastasis. The solitary lesion, however, may pose a diagnostic problem.

Sclerotic bone islands are a common solitary lesion of no clinical significance. They are especially common in the pelvis and femora. Long bones may show areas of irregular sclerosis in the ends of the marrow cavity. These are a common finding and are usually indicative of calcification in areas of fatty necrosis and bone infarcts. In some cases, an occupational history or history of pancreatic or metabolic diseases will help confirm the diagnosis.

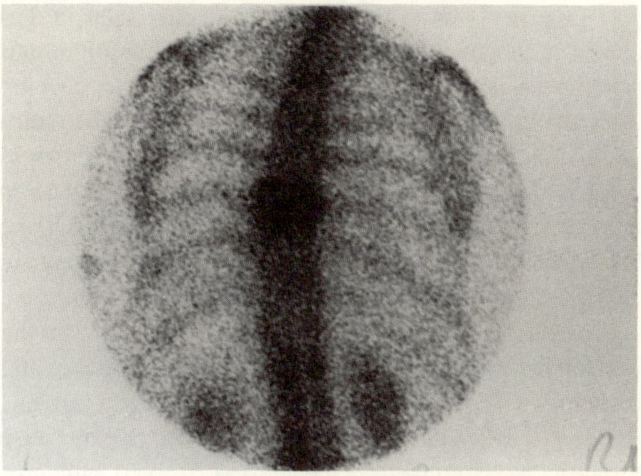

Figure 20-10. Bone scan of spine in 82 y/o female with back pain. X-ray showed osteoporosis and compression fracture of indeterminate age. Isotope concentration suggests recent, if not acute, fracture. Scan findings are nonspecific with regard to the etiology of the fracture (i.e., metastasis vs. trauma).

Solitary or diffuse sclerotic foci may be seen with some forms of metastatic disease. In the male, prostatic carcinoma is a likely diagnosis, while breast cancer may present in this manner in females. Mixed lytic and blastic lesions may be seen with any malignancy, and treatment by radiation or chemotherapy may confuse the picture. Lytic processes are usually metastatic from kidney, breast, thyroid, lung, or bowel.

While it is not always possible to distinguish benign from malignant lesions, there are some findings that may help. A soft-tissue mass in conjunction with a lytic lesion is strong evidence for a malignancy. Irregular, nonsclerotic lesion margins, periosteal reaction, and multiplicity of lesions are all suggestive of malignancy. The benign lesion tends to have well-defined, often sclerotic margins, has no associated mass, and is usually solitary. Infection may mimic tumor. Biopsy may be necessary for final diagnosis.

Avascular necrosis and osteonecrosis are common problems causing disability in the elderly. While most common in the femoral head, they may be seen in other joints. Predisposing trauma is often present but is not always clinically evident. Vascular disease, arthritis, metabolic disease, and steroid therapy may all predispose to the development of avascular necrosis. The most common picture of avascular necrosis and osteonecrosis is a flattened and irregularly sclerotic femoral head in a patient with acute onset of hip pain, or a sclerotic and deformed femoral articular surface in a patient with advanced degenerative arthritis of the knee. MRI has been shown to be a sensitive and reliable technique for the early identification of this problem. Nuclear bone scan perfusion defects can also be seen in the affected area and can be useful when MRI is not available.

Osteomyelitis in the elderly is usually seen in diabetics or in patients with cellulitis. The use of immunosuppressives can increase the propensity to develop osteomyelitis, especially in the septic patient. The radiographic picture of bone destruction and reactive changes is fairly characteristic. It should be noted that just as in other instances of bone loss, approximately 40% bone loss is required before it can be appreciated by the eye. In equivocal cases, the nuclear bone scan can be helpful.

Arthritic diseases cover a spectrum ranging from the age-related joint degeneration through inflammatory and metabolic arthritides (Fig. 20-11). In the elderly patient, the superimposition of degenerative processes may cause difficulty in distinguishing the etiology of an arthritic process. The clinical history will usually provide significant background information and allow for a proper diagnosis. Degenerative arthritis is the most common form seen in the elderly and may affect any joint. It tends to be more common in the weight-bearing joints, such as the knees and hips, and in the hands, where this may be a sequela of repeated occupational trauma.

One disease process requiring special mention is Paget's disease. This may present as either solitary or multiple lesions, and may appear lytic, blastic, or of a mixed variety. In the earliest stages, especially in the skull and distal femur, it may present as a large area of lytic disease. Over the course of the disease, there is a progression through a mixed phase to a more sclerotic phase (Fig. 20-12). In the spine and pelvis, the lytic phase may not be readily appreciated. The most common picture associated with Paget's disease of the spine and pelvis is a diffuse coarsening of bony trabeculation combined with a generalized expansion of the affected bone. The cortex is often quite thick and, in time, the bones tend to deform. In spite of the apparent increase in bone mass, the bones are actually fragile and pathologic fractures may occur. Soft-tissue mass and a change from blastic to lytic lesions are strongly suggestive of sarcomatous change. It is sometimes difficult to distinguish between severe Paget's disease and diffuse blastic metastases from prostatic carcinoma.

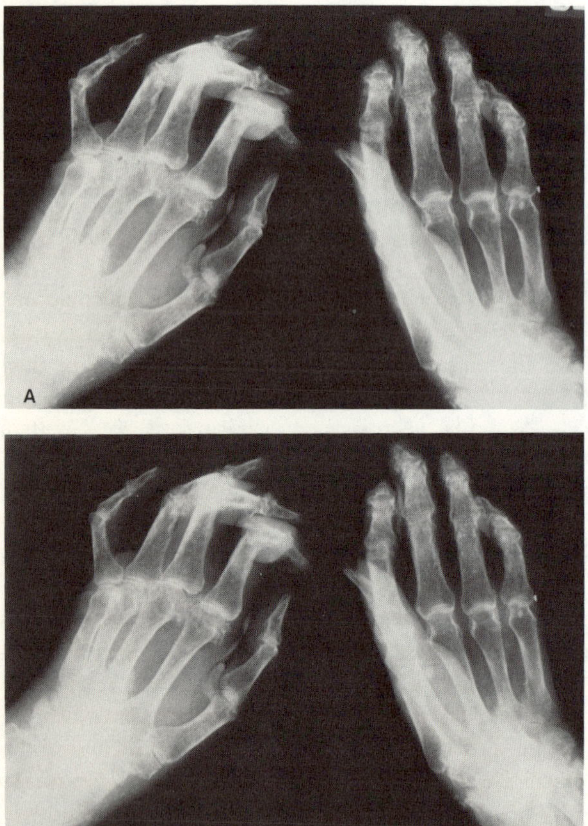

Figure 20-11, A and B. Advanced rheumatoid arthritis (two views).

Metabolic processes, especially those related to abnormal steroid production and renal disease, can cause significant changes in the skeletal system. While some of these changes, such as those seen in renal osteodystrophy, are fairly characteristic, many are nonspecific. The clinical history is very helpful in these instances.

The wide range of radiographic appearance of bony lesions often makes diagnosis on the basis of the x-ray picture alone somewhat difficult. The clinical history, results of laboratory test and, where appropriate, biopsy, and review of radiographs with a radiologist need to be combined for the best diagnostic accuracy.

Mammography

Breast cancer is a leading cause of cancer death among women, the incidence increasing with age. While a good physical examination is helpful in the detection of cancer,

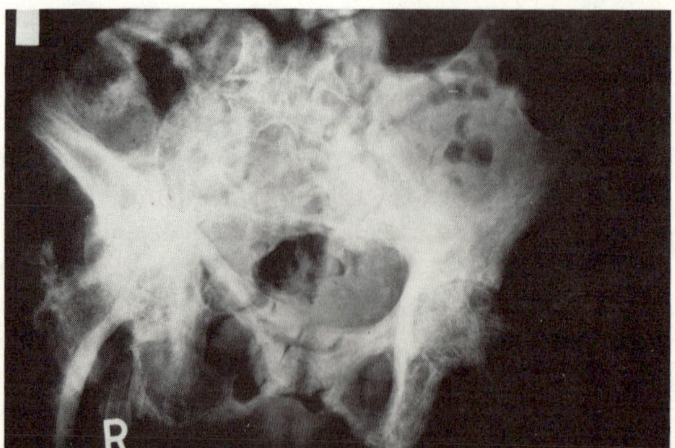

Figure 20-12. Advanced Paget's disease of the pelvis.

mammography has been shown time and again to be much more sensitive in the detection of the smaller lesion. It is unfortunate that some surgeons do not recognize the limitations of their sense of touch and do not refer their patients for mammography until a palpable lesion is discovered. This occurrence is fortunately becoming the exception rather than the rule, and with the added help of the patient with monthly self-examination, it is hoped that breast malignancy will be discovered in its earliest and curable stages.

There are many methods of breast evaluation, but as of this time only mammography has proven to be a consistent and sensitive means of early cancer detection. Whether the film-screen method or xeroradiographic method is used, is not a significant factor in the rate of detection or accuracy.

There are some technical differences between the film-screen and Xerox® methods of breast radiography that will be covered briefly. While the newest Xerox technique has a radiation dose comparable to that of the film-screen method, older units require a greater amount of radiation for the same study than the film-screen method requires. Xeroradiography needs a special unit for the electrostatic process, while film-screen studies are best done with a dedicated x-ray machine.

Which method the radiologist chooses to use is primarily a function of training and experience. Both methods use ionizing radiation and it is suggested the examination be used according to the guidelines developed by groups such as the American College of Radiology, the American College of Surgeons, and the American Cancer Society. To limit exposure in the younger patients, where there is a lower incidence of breast malignancy, and a risk of repeated exposure of the breast to radiation, mammography is discouraged in women under 30 years of age.

Ultrasound has been looked to as a nonradiation alternative to mammographic screening, but it has not yet shown the sensitivity or specificity of mammography. There is, however, a role for ultrasound in the delineation of suspected cystic lesions, and, when these lesions are poorly defined clinically, as a means of localization for aspiration. Since many of the rapidly growing lesions in the younger patients are cysts, ultrasound should be considered before mammography in the patient under 30, especially the teen or post-teen.

Preoperative localization of tumors is easily done with a fenestrated compression device. Opaque dye such as methylene blue, or a hooked wire, can be placed at the lesion to guide the surgeon. Some surgeons prefer the use of both modalities, claiming the wires tend to move in a very fatty breast. It is suggested that dye localization be performed as close to the time of surgery as possible, as the dye will rapidly diffuse into the surrounding tissues.

The postoperative breast can have a variable appearance. If surgery was minimal, it may not even be possible to identify a postoperative breast. Mastectomy, on the other hand, leaves little or no breast for examination. Most important is the need to be certain the radiologist is aware of prior surgery, as the pattern of scar tissue within a breast may mimic, or even obscure, a malignancy.

Following radiation therapy, it becomes even more difficult to evaluate the breast by mammography. Thickening of the skin, confluence of the breast markings, and even small clusters of calcification may be seen as part of the postradiation changes. These findings are easily confused with the findings in a tumor, and serial examinations may be needed to avoid unnecessary surgery.

Breast implants are a very definite limiting factor in radiographic evaluation of the breast. The surgeon must be aware of this and not be falsely secure when a clinically obvious lesion cannot be shown mammographically. More important, a small nonpalpable lesion may be obscured by the prosthesis.

Thermography and diaphanography have yet to be demonstrated to be significantly sensitive or specific as a means of breast screening.

Gynecomastia is a common problem in the older male and it has characteristic radiographic findings. Cancer does occur in the male breast, although far less frequently than in the female breast, and mammography is indicated whenever there is a suspicious breast lesion found on physical examination.

Contrast

There are two basic categories of contrast agent currently being used for radiographic examination, barium sulfate and iodinated water-soluble contrast. Air may be used with these agents for further enhancement of contrast. In the gastrointestinal tract, the majority of studies are performed using barium or a barium-air mixture. Iodinated contrast agents are usually reserved for those studies requiring injection into a blood vessel, body cavity, or the central nervous system. Here again air is sometimes used as a contrast enhancement.

There is currently much controversy in the literature as to the preferred class of water-soluble agent (i.e., high osmolar versus low osmolar) with regard to vascular and renal studies. It is not our intent to review or resolve the issues, but to give a few basic ideas for consideration. The final selection of which agent to use for your patient should be discussed with the radiologist prior to the study. Except for selected cases, low osmolar contrast is the agent of choice for intrathecal injection, while cost factors and clinical considerations do not justify the use of the newer and more expensive agents for studies such as arthrograms and fistulograms.

The major areas of controversy are intra-arterial and intravenous injection. A consensus appears to be forming that low osmolar agents are preferred in peripheral angiography and in patients with depressed renal function. Patients with heart failure or other significant compromise of the cardiovascular system would probably do well to have the newer agents. The real issue is whether or not the newer, low osmolar, and clearly more expensive agents are justified in the patient without any significant renal or cardiovascular problems. This remains to be seen and the answer will have to await further clinical studies.

It should be emphasized, however, that regardless of which form of iodinated contrast agent is being used, a few simple precautions will limit untoward results. First and foremost is a history of allergy to the contrast. Severe and sometimes life-threatening reactions can occur. If the patient has a known allergy to the contrast, its use should be weighed against both any possible benefit and the availability of alternate testing (e.g., MRI for brain). Preexisting renal dysfunction or systemic diseases with a potential for manifesting themselves in the urinary tract, such as multiple myeloma or severe diabetes, should alert the physician to a potential of disastrous renal malfunction. Perhaps the best and easiest step to take to avoid any problems following contrast injection is to maintain good patient hydration prior to as well as after the examination. There are still some physicians who instruct their patients to withhold all fluids for several hours prior to an intravenous pyelogram, thus unknowingly placing these patients at risk for renal damage.

While barium sulfate preparations are preferred for most gastrointestinal tract studies, the dangers of mediastinitis and peritonitis require use of the iodinated agents where perforation of the esophagus or an intra-abdominal viscus is suspected. On the other hand, the risk of chemical pneumonitis requires the use of barium, a relatively inert medium, where tracheobronchial aspiration is a concern.

Intestinal obstruction requires tailoring the examination according to the level of suspected obstruction. In general, a barium enema should be the first examination in suspected colon or terminal ileum obstruction. It is usually impractical to prepare this patient's colon, and a single column study is advisable to limit dilution of the agent by colonic residue.

A more proximal small-bowel lesion can be evaluated by oral contrast. Oral barium should be avoided in the presence of suspected colonic obstruction. The dehydrating function of the colon will turn ingested barium to a concrete-like mixture with serious consequences. In this instance, water-soluble agents are preferred. The more proximal bowel lesion can be evaluated with either class of agent. If a long GI tube can be advanced to a point near the suspected obstruction, water-soluble contrast or barium is usually injected through the tube and followed to the obstruction site. Where there is much dilution by retained small-bowel contents, barium is preferred.

If an extraperitoneal or walled-off perforation is suspected, as is often the case with diverticulitis, there is generally a lower risk of barium leakage complications and many radiologists will choose barium as the agent of choice.

Special attention must be given to the ostomy patient. A balloon-tipped retention catheter increases the risk of bowel wall rupture at the ostomy, or damage to an already diseased segment of bowel near the ostomy site. Devices resembling a baby bottle nipple have been developed for examination of the ostomy patient, although, with care, a catheter with no special tip can also be used. In general, if there is any question as to which contrast agent would be appropriate, direct communication with the radiologist would be best.

While evaluation of the gallbladder and biliary tree is generally performed with ultrasound, oral contrast agents are still used to opacify the gallbladder and evaluate concentration and contraction functions. Because of a high incidence of allergic reactions, and the ease with which the common duct can be evaluated on ultrasound, intravenous cholangiography has fallen into disfavor. One should leave the selection of the oral agent to the radiologist.

Gastrointestinal Tract

In addition to the common problems associated with peptic disease and hiatus hernia, the major esophageal diseases encountered in the elderly are related to swallowing, motility, and malignancy. As neuromuscular coordination deteriorates with increasing age, swallowing and esophageal peristalsis become disorganized. Movement of the soft palate and its relationship to the posterior pharyngeal wall, and properly coordinated movement of the epiglottis, are best studied by fluoroscopy. While the majority of these studies are performed with use of oral contrast agents such as barium, some examiners also use nasopharyngeal instillation of contrast.

Poor propulsion of a bolus through the esophagus as a result of the muscular dysfunction may have several results. The most obvious is difficulty with passing ingested material into the stomach. This may present as a foreign body impacted in the distal esophagus when food is not properly chewed. If this process is combined with swallowing problems, aspiration of food can occur. Once again, contrast-enhanced fluoroscopy is very useful in demonstrating the dysfunctional contractions and associated problems. Manometry may also play a role in these patients.

The distal esophagus and esophagogastric junction are a site of stricture, often related to hiatus hernia and reflux esophagitis. Malignancy is another significant factor in esophageal obstruction (Fig. 20-13). In addition to fluoroscopy, mediastinal CT can be useful in determining if a disease process within the esophagus, such as a tumor, has an extralumenal component.

The incidence of GI tract malignancy increases with age. The exact cause is uncertain but there are predisposing factors such as vitamin B_{12} deficiency, leukoplakia, polyposis, and chronic alcoholism and smoking, among others. Detection and staging is often limited by the nature of the presenting symptoms, location of the lesion, and the availability of testing methods. Both endoscopy and contrast studies play a significant role in detection of diseases in the esophagus, stomach (Fig. 20-14), and proximal duodenum, as well as the colon. The small bowel, however, is currently best examined by oral contrast. In recent years, there has been a renewed interest in the air contrast small-bowel study.

Staging of intestinal malignancy is best done with CT, although MRI and ultrasound may be helpful. These modalities will allow identification of retroperitoneal adenopathy, mesenteric nodes and tumor extension, exophytic tumor growth locally, and blood-borne spread to organs such as the liver, lungs, brain, and pelvis.

The most common intra-abdominal site of tumor spread from the bowel is the liver. Detection is easily accomplished by use of a biphasic, noncontrast CT study of the abdomen. MRI, ultrasound, and nuclear scanning

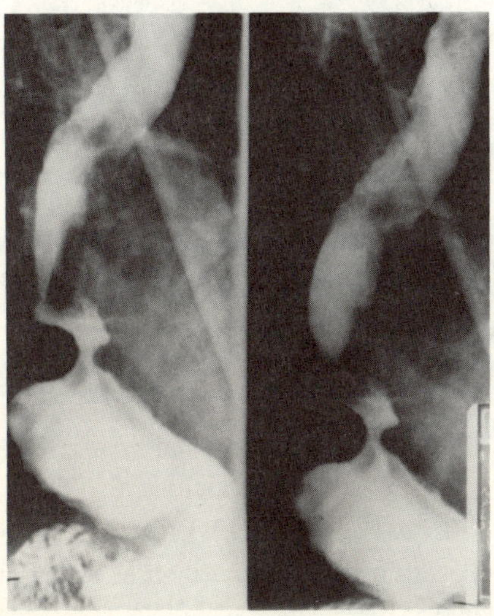

Figure 20-13. Ulcerated carcinoma of the distal esophagus.

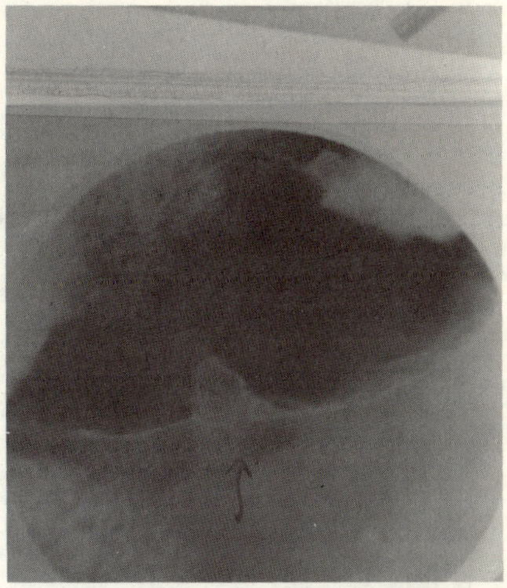

Figure 20-14. 57 y/o male with vague upper gastrointestinal complaints. Gastric carcinoma—1.5-cm nodule projecting into gastric lumen on air contrast upper GI series.

may confirm the findings, and skinny needle biopsy has a high success rate as well.

The small bowel does not have many diseases unique to the elderly. In addition to the non-age-related entities such as inflammatory bowel disease, obstruction, and metastatic disease, the elderly may also suffer from mesenteric infarcts and a motility disorder, pseudo-obstruction.

The colon also suffers from the usual problems seen at all ages, but some entities such as diverticulitis, carcinoma, infarct, and granulomatous colitis may be more frequent in the elderly (Fig. 20-15). Volvulus and megacolon, pseudomembranous enterocolitis, ischemia (Fig. 20-16) and adynamic ileus, as well as pneumoperito-

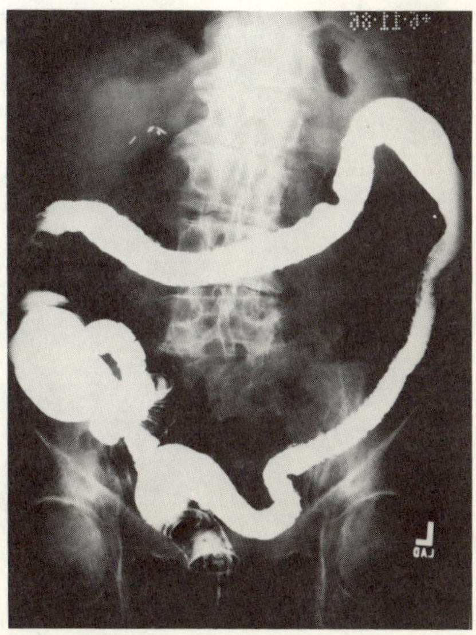

Figure 20-15. 65 y/o male with blood in stool. Inflammatory bowel disease (Granulomatous colitis).

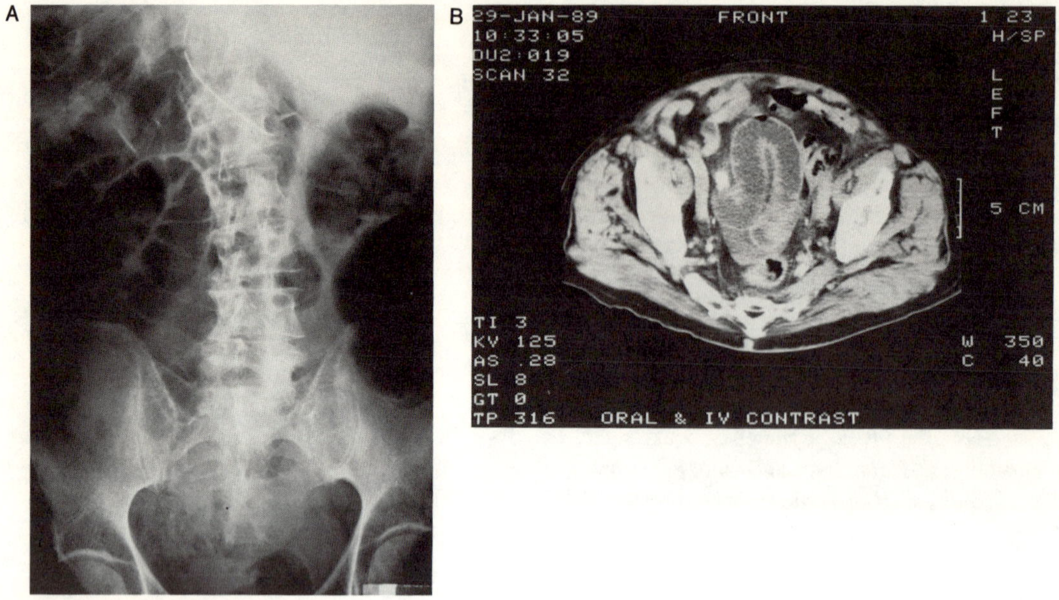

Figure 20-16, A and B. A, 76 y/o male with mesenteric infarct. Plain film of abdomen shows bowel dilatation. B, Same patient with mesenteric infarct—CT study. Note the segmental bowel dilatation with thickening of the bowel wall.

neum, may often be diagnosed without the use of contrast agents. Supine and erect or decubitus plain-film studies should be the first radiographic examination. Contrast may be used in uncertain cases. Endoscopy and angiography may be necessary.

Barium enema and CT are very useful in the diagnosis of diverticulitis and malignancy in the colon. CT has the advantage of demonstrating the extent of extralumenal disease such as abscess, mesenteric infiltration and edema, and adenopathy (Fig. 20-17).

Ultrasound is the primary method of evaluation of the biliary tree and pancreas. It allows visualization of the gallbladder walls, content, and surrounding soft tissues, as well as the intra- and extrahepatic biliary tree (Figs.

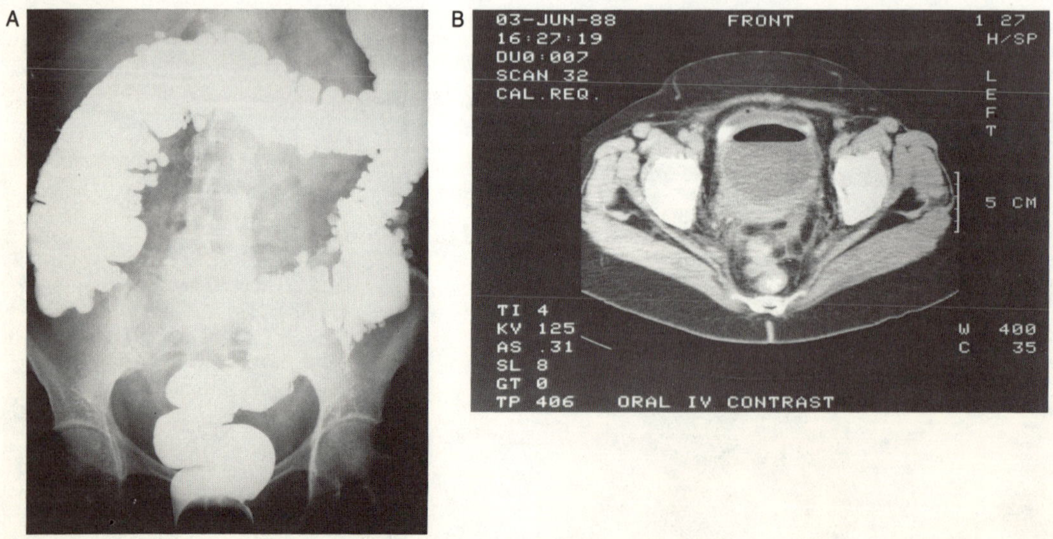

Figure 20-17, A and B. A, 62 y/o female with left lower quadrant pain. Diverticulitis with perforation of distal descending colon. B, Same patient with CT scan showing pelvic inflammation represented by thickening of fascial planes. Note how the CT scan is much better at delineating the extent of extralumenal disease.

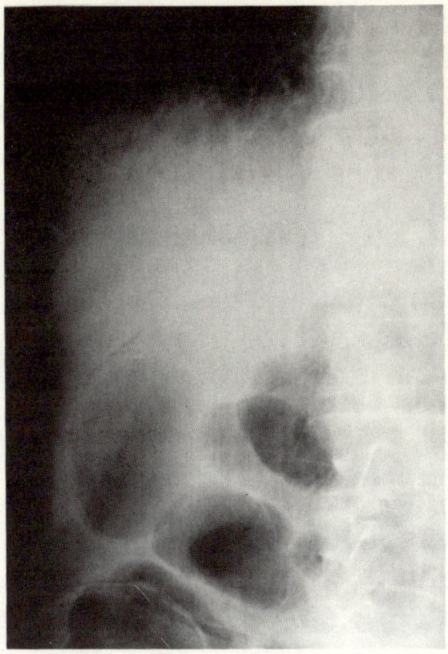

Figure 20-18. 84 y/o male with emphysematous cholecystitis. Note gas lucency outlining the dilated gallbladder. Usually seen in diabetic patients, it is a life-threatening condition requiring emergency surgery.

20-18 and 20-19). Pancreatic masses, especially cysts and pseudocysts, are readily demonstrated. The presence of bowel gas may be a limiting factor.

Biliary tract nuclear scanning with agents excreted in the bile can be very helpful in identifying biliary tract or cystic duct obstruction, or in identifying the patient with acute cholecystitis.

CT will clearly delineate the pancreas and surrounding fascial planes, tumors, cysts, pseudocysts, and phlegmon. Endoscopic retrograde cholangiopancreatography (ERCP) also plays a significant role in evaluating the biliary and pancreatic ductal systems.

Genitourinary Tract

In the elderly patient, genitourinary diseases usually center around the bladder and bladder outlet. Renal infections, obstruction, and tumors are frequently seen.

Bladder outlet obstruction is most often the result of prostatic hypertrophy (Fig. 20-20) and tumor in the male and cystocele and prolapse in the female. Physical examination is the primary means of diagnosis of these entities but the contrast urogram and cystogram can provide additional information (Fig. 20-21). As in other areas of the body, CT, MRI, and ultrasound play adjunctive roles. Prostatic tumor detection and diagnosis have been made easier with the use of ultrasound-guided needle biopsy.

CT and MRI are also helpful in revealing extension of local disease to the periprostatic area as well as local and distant metastasis. The diagnosis of female reproductive system disease, both benign and malignant, is still best done with ultrasound. Here again, CT and MRI are useful in determining extension of the disease.

Renal masses in the elderly are often simple cysts rather than tumors. Drip infusion nephrotomography has been replaced by ultrasound and CT, and these newer modalities will help in differentiating benign from malignant diseases. Percutaneous cyst aspiration and biopsy are easily performed with ultrasound or CT guidance. Angiography is not used as frequently as in the past for diagnosis, but still plays a role in preoperative determination of vascularity in large or complex tumors.

Interventional Techniques

Because of multisystem disorders and the general debilitation associated with severe illness in the elderly, many of these patients are unable to withstand the rigors of surgery.

A B

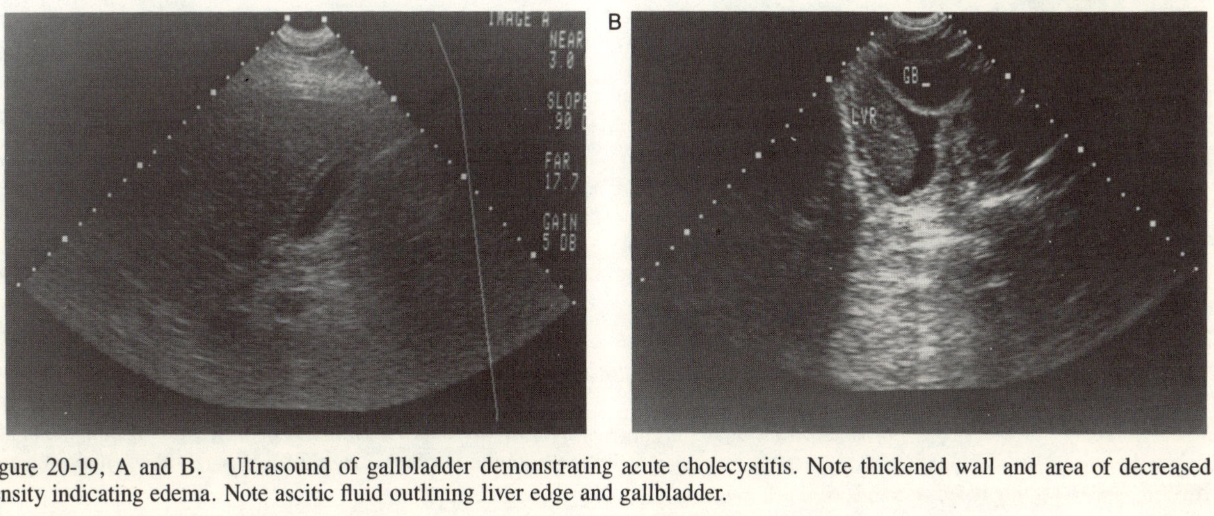

Figure 20-19, A and B. Ultrasound of gallbladder demonstrating acute cholecystitis. Note thickened wall and area of decreased density indicating edema. Note ascitic fluid outlining liver edge and gallbladder.

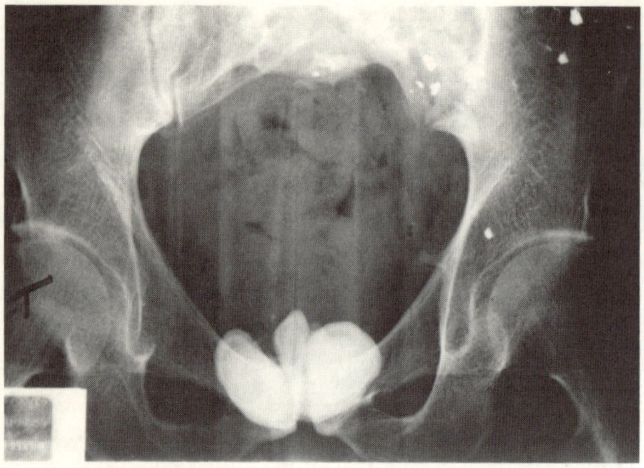

Figure 20-20. Enlarged and calcified prostate in a patient with sacral injury and post-traumatic neurogenic bladder.

The interventional radiologist plays a special role in these patients. By using techniques that are considerably less invasive and stressful to the patient, the interventionalist can often perform life-saving procedures at lesser risk to the patient. While all these procedures are not so dramatic in import, they may be therapeutic or temporizing.

Biliary tract drainage and decompression can be used prior to surgery for obstructing ductal malignancy. In the inoperable patient, the placement of a stent catheter (Fig. 20-22) can significantly improve the patient's status both physically and emotionally.

Dilatation of strictures may be therapeutic. Percutaneous cholecystotomy may make the difference between life and death in a cardiac patient with acute cholecystitis and abscess who is not amenable to surgery.

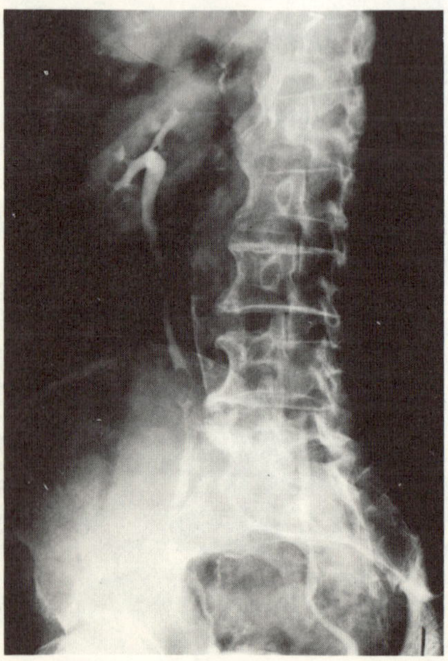

Figure 20-21. Oblique view from an intravenous pyelogram. Note the ureteral filling defect—transitional cell carcinoma.

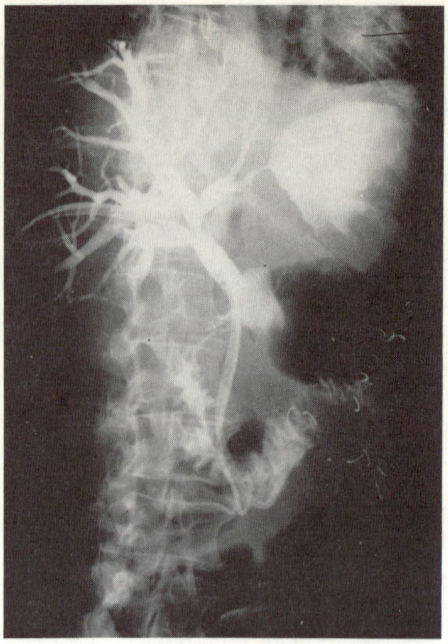

Figure 20-22. Percutaneous transhepatic internal drainage procedure for biliary obstruction resulting from pancreatic carcinoma.

Percutaneous drainage of abscesses, effusions, cysts, pseudocysts, and other collections may obviate the need for surgery. The improvement in these patients is often dramatic. Percutaneous gastrostomy can be performed by the radiologist.

Skinny needle percutaneous biopsy is another invasive diagnostic methodology that, in spite of possible complications, can significantly shorten the time to diagnosis without the inherent risks of open biopsy. Some useful areas are the workup of an isolated liver or lung nodule, pancreatic carcinoma, and breast biopsy. The major complication is bleeding, and, in the case of the lung, pneumothorax. The test can be performed in an outpatient setting.

Some other examples of interventional techniques are transrectal ultrasound-guided prostatic biopsy, percutaneous cystotomy, renal and biliary stone extraction, nephrostomy, and biliary and renal stent placement.

Vascular interventional studies range from the relatively low-risk peripheral venography to cardiac angioplasty. Arteriography as a diagnostic procedure is used less frequently today for many tumors since the advent of CT and MRI. This procedure still has a role, however, in peripheral and central circulatory evaluation prior to surgery. Additionally, balloon dilatation and small-vessel embolization are significant uses of arteriography. Carotid evaluation is often done through use of computer-enhanced digital arteriography.

21

Perioperative Risk and Preoperative Preparation of the Geriatric Surgical Patient

Charles H. McLeskey and Kenneth M. Janis

An absolute definition of a geriatric patient is impossible because arbitrary limits constantly change. For example, many studies of surgery in the elderly have been published since the early 1900's, but the definition of "elderly" has continually changed. In 1907, a report described 167 operations performed on patients older than age 50 and stated this advanced age was a contraindication to surgery (1). Twenty years later, Ochsner suggested that "an elective operation for inguinal hernia in a patient older than 50 years was not justified" (2). In 1937, Brooks reported a series of 293 operations in patients older than age 70, and subsequently most authors have considered patients older than 65 to 70 years as being elderly (3). In this chapter, geriatric patients will be considered those 65 years of age or older. However, with the not infrequent recent reports of anesthesia and surgery performed on patients older than the age of 80, there is no consensus today as to the definition of "geriatric" in medical practice. It is very likely that the arbitrary age that defines a geriatric patient will increase in the near future. For example, Djokovic and Hedley-Whyte have predicted the outcome after surgery in 500 patients older than age 80 (4). Miller et al. have described anesthesia and surgery in 147 patients ranging in age from 90 to 102 years (5). In 1985, Katlic reported on six patients older than the age of 100 who had anesthesia and surgery (6). Hosking, et al., recently reported on 795 patients over age 90 who underwent operative procedures at the Mayo Clinic. Of these, 13 patients were over the age of 100 (7). Katlic perhaps best reflected on the changed mood of medicine today when he stated that, "Elective surgery should not be deferred nor emergency surgery denied (even for) centenarians on the basis of chronologic age" (6).

Older patients are undergoing surgical procedures more frequently, in part due to medical advances, but also in part due to the aging of the American society. The 1980 census indicated that 11.3% of the American population was over age 65. By the early 21st century, it is predicted that the elderly will comprise 16% of the U.S. population (about 52 million). Inpatient operations performed on patients older than 65 increased by 43% from 1975 to 1980, while the overall increase for all age groups was only 11.5%. Patients in this age group accounted for 21% of all inpatient operative procedures and 38.4% of total hospital days. Surgical rates on patients 90 years of age or older have increased nearly five-fold over the past ten years (8). A specific example of the increasing age of the surgical population may be found in a series from the Cleveland Clinic, where over a 15-year period, greater than 5,000 patients over age 65 underwent coronary artery bypass surgery. Figure 21-1 illustrates the increasing percentage of the total bypass surgical population made up of patients greater than age 65 or greater than age 70 (9). Thus the trend is obvious: surgical procedures performed on older patients are becoming more widespread.

Linn and colleagues have suggested that our con-

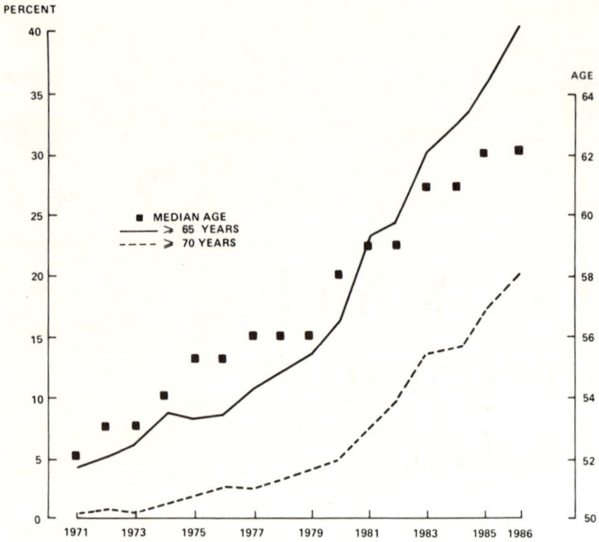

Figure 21-1. The median age of patients who underwent cardiac bypass surgery at the Cleveland Clinic in 1986 increased to age 62. The percentage of cardiac surgical candidates greater than age 65 exceeded 40% of the surgical volume, and there has also been an increase in the percentage of the surgical population above age 70, which in 1986 exceeded 20% of all surgical bypass patients. (Reprinted with permission from Loop, FD, et al. 1988. Coronary artery bypass graft surgery in the elderly. Indications and outcome. *Cleve Clin J Med* 55:23.)

cepts and understanding of risks in the perioperative period for geriatric patients are inconsistent (10). Dissimilar beliefs about these risks are commonly held by physicians. For example, some physicians believe extreme caution should be employed when operating on the elderly since they are at increased risk due to their age alone. An alternate view is that patients who have survived into old age are biologically preferred, and therefore surgical risk is not as great in them as in the general population. Finally, these authors suggest a third, more moderate opinion. They believe that elderly patients are at some increased risk due to their reduced physiologic reserve, but with proper perioperative monitoring and management, an acceptable outcome is possible.

Nevertheless, far more important than chronologic age is the patient's physiologic age. Because the aging process varies from person to person and from one organ system to another, elderly patients do not present to us as a homogeneous entity. There is little correlation between chronologic age and biologic age. People appear to reach their peak physiologic function in their late twenties or early thirties and from then on it is, in general, a "downhill course" (11). The amount of physiologic function that remains in people of advanced age varies greatly. For example, physiologically one patient may appear as a relatively young octogenarian when compared to another who appears physiologically as a relatively old septuagenarian. It is difficult to predict the physiologic function of an elderly patient simply from his or her chronologic age, which explains a primary reason why older citizens present a higher risk when undergoing anesthesia and surgery. Later, this chapter discusses some of the identifiable factors that increase their perioperative risk. The reliability of the American Society of Anesthesiologists physical status classification in predicting perioperative risk for geriatric patients will be emphasized. Also, risk factors, which may be identified preoperatively, that bear importance in predicting surgical risk will be described. In addition, suggestions will be made for preparing geriatric patients and thereby reducing their perioperative risk.

Because the average life expectancy has been extended, increasing numbers of elderly patients are having surgery. It is now estimated that 50% of Americans older than age 65 will have at least one operative procedure before death. This chapter summarizes the risks of anesthesia and surgery in this patient population and attempts to suggest techniques for their optimal preoperative preparation.

Age-Related Perioperative Risk

It is widely believed that, compared with younger patients, elderly patients (even those free from concomitant disease) having major surgery have a significantly higher incidence of complications or death. In an English survey, approximately 50% of intraoperative deaths occurred in geriatric patients, although this group of patients represented only 5% of the overall surgical population (12). As shown in Table 21-1, age, per se, appears to predict increased perioperative morbidity and mortality (13). A large study from Cardiff of 108,878 anesthetics between the years 1972 and 1977 also supported the concept of a

Table 21-1. Mortality within 7 days of anesthesia in consecutive surgical patients

Age		Deaths	
(yr)	Patients	No.	%
<1	3,396	56	1.6
1–10	3,650	30	0.8
11–20	5,608	25	0.45
21–30	5,192	41	0.8
31–40	3,962	55	1.4
41–50	4,129	97	2.3
51–60	4,063	126	3.1
61–70	2,941	130	4.4
71–80	1,162	79	6.8
>81	73	6	8.2
Total	34,140	645	1.9

Source: Marx et al. (13).

higher mortality for both men and women of older age groups (Table 21-2) (14). As shown in Table 21-3, Santos reviewed operative mortality within 10 days of surgery for patients aged 50 to 90+ years undergoing 2,186 operations (15). An apparently clear age-related mortality rate was observed. In addition, a large French survey conducted between 1978 and 1982 followed 190,389 anesthetic procedures in approximately 500 institutions (16). In this study, the overall frequency for anesthetic accidents was one death in 2,410 anesthetics or a 0.04% incidence. However, a sharp rise in incidence to approximately 2 to 3 deaths per 1,000 anesthetics occurs beyond age 65. As shown in Table 21-4, Gersh and colleagues have demonstrated a mortality rate in patients 75 years of age or older that is approximately twice that of patients 65 to 69 and far less than that of patients who are under age 65 (17). Similarly, Acinapura and colleagues compared 685 patients over age 70 with 3,142 patients under age 70 undergoing coronary artery bypass surgery (18). Hospital mortality was 8% for patients over age 75 compared to a mortality rate less than 2% for patients under age 70. Pottecher and colleagues surveyed 198,103 anesthetics in France and determined the overall frequency of cardiac arrest under anesthesia to be 1/1,665 anesthetics or 0.06% incidence (19). The greatest number of cardiac arrests occurred in patients between the ages of 55 and 74 years. These authors constructed a comparative risk coefficient (CRC), which was determined by dividing the incidence of occurrence of cardiac arrest by the number of anesthetics for patients of different ages. As shown in Figure 21-2, the CRC values were age-related and highest in patients over age 85. This age-related mortality also seems to be born out in the very oldest surgical patients. As Hosking and colleagues have observed (Table 21-5) the mortality rate of patients within 30 days of surgery was approximately 8% in patients in their early nineties, yet almost doubled in patients over age 100 (7).

However, not all studies concur with the notion that patients who are older will necessarily have a higher complication rate during the perioperative period. For instance, in a series of 500 patients having anesthesia and surgery, Djokovic and Hedley-Whyte found no consistent

Table 21-2. Mortality by age and sex

Age (yr)	Males Deaths	Males Total	Males Mortality (%)	Females Deaths	Females Total	Females Mortality (%)
0–14	105	8,041	1.3	59	4,601	1.3
15–24	46	5,695	0.8	27	9,683	0.3
25–44	121	9,488	1.3	94	22,411	0.4
45–64	428	14,174	3.0	331	15,925	2.1
>65	578	9,749	5.9	612	9,111	6.7

Source: Farrow et al. (14).

Table 21-3. Surgical mortality by age group

Age group (yrs)	No. of operations	Mortality: No. of deaths	Mortality: Percent
Under 50	212	2	0.9
50–59	220	7	3
60–69	467	15	3
70–79	603	21	3
80–89	568	33	5
90+	116	10	7
Total	2,186	88	3.9% (Avg)

Source: Santos and Gelperin (15).

increase in the incidence of death as patients' ages increased from 80 to 95 years (4). In 1983, Filzweiser and List reported a prospective study of 500 consecutive patients older than 70 and did not find a single intraoperative death (20). Similarly, Hatton et al., reported an actual reduction in deaths resulting from anesthesia in patients older than 80 (21). In view of the controversy, one wonders if there is a factor other than age alone that better predicts potential complications and deaths in geriatric patients undergoing the stress of anesthesia and surgery.

When the role that age plays as a risk factor for geriatric patients having anesthesia and surgery is examined, the distinction between physiologic age and chronologic age becomes important. Compared with younger patients, elderly patients may be at greater risk for perioperative complications and deaths because of two factors: first, a decline in basic organ function (independent of disease) resulting from aging per se, and second, an increased prevalence of age-related concomitant disease. Each of these factors will now be examined.

Physiologic Changes with Aging

Should aging, per se, influence perioperative morbidity and mortality in elderly patients? It likely does so, in part, as a result of the gradual decline in physiologic reserve in a variety of organ systems. For a review of these changes, the reader is referred to a more general text (22). Despite the progressive decline in physiologic function with age,

Table 21-4. Perioperative mortality in coronary artery bypass surgery patients

Age (yrs)	No. of patients	Deaths: No.	Deaths: %
<65	7,827	151	1.9
65–69	803	37	4.6
70–74	241	16	6.6
75–84	42	4	9.5

Source: Gersh et al. (17).

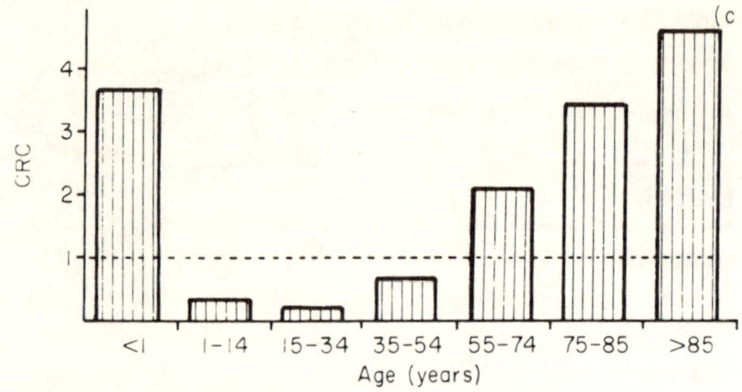

Figure 21-2. Comparative risk coefficient (CRC) related to age. *CRC* = cardiac arrests (percentage)/anesthetics (percentage) by age distribution. Older patients apparently have the highest risk for intraoperative cardiac arrest and perioperative complication. (Reprinted with permission from Pottecher T, et al. 1984. Cardiac arrest related to anesthesia: A prospective study in France (1978–1982). *Eur J Anaesth* 1:305.)

that which remains is nevertheless sufficient to allow the elderly person to carry out the normal requirements of living. However, the ability to respond to stress and to overcome complications is reduced. Response to cellular injury is impaired, and the ability to summon resources of increased organ function necessary to respond to complications after surgery is so dramatically limited that what would be a minor complication in a younger person may produce a domino-like cascade of progressive complications that frequently lead to death in the elderly surgical patient. These fatal complications often involve worsening of preexisting medical conditions which may or may not have been fully appreciated or stabilized preoperatively. Let us now discuss some of the more common age-related concomitant diseases and their impact upon morbidity and mortality during the perioperative period in elderly patients undergoing surgery.

Effects of Concomitant Disease

Multiple concomitant diseases are the rule, rather than the exception, in the elderly patient. A current surgical illness is likely to be present in patients in whom old injuries, prior illnesses, past operations, and a variety of chronic disorders, including cataracts, osteoarthritis, anemia, osteoporosis, and diabetes mellitus, may be observed. Malignancy, cerebral vascular accidents, Parkinsonism, dementia, and fractures of the femur are observed with increased frequency in this patient group. For instance, pathologic findings were observed on medical examination in 92% of patients 81 years of age or older (23). Of these, cardiovascular abnormalities, including arteriosclerosis and hypertension, were seen in 78% of patients, whereas mental dysfunction occurred in 30% and pulmonary, endocrine, and neurologic abnormalities were observed in 14%, 12%, and 10% of patients, respectively. Stephen has also reported on the frequency of abnormalities encountered in 1,000 patients older than age 70 as seen in Table 21-6 (24). Once again, hypertension, atherosclerosis, and renal disease led the list of concomitant disease states in geriatric patients interviewed before operation.

Which of the common preexisting conditions correlate most closely with an increased risk of perioperative complications and death in elderly patients? Rowe et al. found that ischemic heart disease, dementia, and diabetes seemed to correlate most closely with an increased risk (25). On the other hand, Farrow et al. found that cardiac failure, impaired renal function, and angina were the preoperative conditions most indicative of a high-risk perioperative death (Table 21-7) (14). These conditions were associated with mortality 10 to 30 times greater than the overall 0.5% mortality observed in patients without these preoperative medical conditions. Hosking et al. (7) observed that renal disease, central nervous system disease, or biliary tract disease contributed to poorer long-term survival in patients over age 90. They also noted that postoperative morbidity within 48 hours of surgery was more commonly observed in patients who had prior atrial arrhythmias. This is similar to another study demonstrating that patients with chronic atrial fibrillation have an increased mortality rate (26).

Thus, various preoperative medical conditions have been credited with producing increased risk in elderly pa-

Table 21-5. Surgical mortality in the very old

Age (yr)	Patients (n)	% Mortality (within 30 days)
90–94	671	8.1
95–99	111	9.4
100+	13	15.4

Source: Hosking et al. (7).

Table 21-6. Preanesthetic complications encountered in 1,000 elderly patients

Complications	Incidence (%)
Hypertension	46.6
Renal disease	31.4
Atherosclerosis	26.9
Myocardial infarction	18.5
Chronic obstructive pulmonary disease	14.0
Cardiomegaly	13.6
Diabetes	9.2
Liver disease	8.5
Congestive heart failure	7.5
Angina	6.4
Cerebrovascular accident	5.8

Source: Stephen (24).

Table 21-7. Mortality due to concomitant disease

Condition	Deaths	Operations	Mortality (%)
Cardiac failure	186	1,175	15.8
Impaired renal function	84	779	10.8
Angina, arteriosclerosis, or ischemic heart disease	544	7,776	7.0
Diabetes	82	1,452	5.7
Chronic lower respiratory tract infection	408	8,060	5.1
No preoperative condition	206	43,483	0.5

Source: Farrow et al. (14).

tients. Not only may the type of preoperative medical condition be important in determining the rate of perioperative complications, but so also may be the number of associated diseases. As mentioned above, Tiret and colleagues in a large study appeared to demonstrate that the rate of anesthesia-related complications correlated directly with the patient's age (16). On closer examination, however (as shown in Fig. 21-3), it is clear that the complication rate relates far more closely to the number of associated diseases with which the patient presented than to the patient's age per se.

The greater incidence of complications and death in older patients most likely reflects the fact that these patients more commonly present for surgery with a greater number of associated preexistent diseases. Stephen's analysis of a large number of elderly surgical patients showed that 36% developed a nonfatal complication and that 66% of these had three or more preoperative functional abnormalities (24). In addition, while he observed an overall mortality rate of 5.8% in elderly patients, of those who died, 84% had more than 3 preexistent medical conditions. Likewise, Denney and Denson reported a mortality rate of 29% among patients older than age 90 who had disease in multiple organ systems compared with a strikingly lower mortality of 4.9% in a group of healthy persons of similar age (27). The Goldman study of cardiac risk factors also suggests that preexistent medical condition may be more important than a patient's age when attempting to predict the risks associated with anesthesia and surgery (28). As shown in Table 21-8, "points" in the Goldman risk index are assigned to patients before operation, with greater point values given to those criteria more likely to result in perioperative complications and death. Age greater than 70 years is assigned a point value, indicating that age per se may be a risk. However, age is intermediate in value and carries a lesser value than that assigned to certain preoperative medical conditions such as a recent myocardial infarction or signs of congestive heart failure. Finally, Gersh (29) has also shown that long-term (5-year) survival in patients greater than 65 years was affected by the number of concurrent diseases. In patients with no concurrent diseases, there was an 89% 5-year survival in patients recovering from coronary artery bypass surgery compared to only 71% in patients presenting to surgery with two or more preexistent diseases (Fig. 21-4).

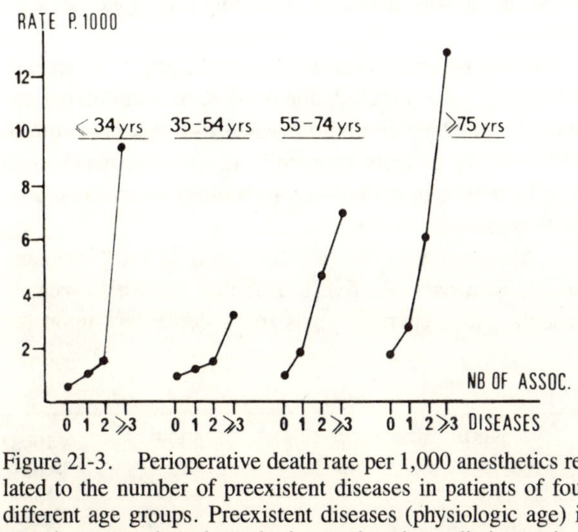

Figure 21-3. Perioperative death rate per 1,000 anesthetics related to the number of preexistent diseases in patients of four different age groups. Preexistent diseases (physiologic age) is more important than chronologic age alone in predicting perioperative morbidity and mortality. (Reprinted with permission from Tiret L, et al. 1986. Complications associated with anaesthesia—a prospective survey in France. *Can Anaesth Soc J* 33:336.)

What Factors Can Be Used to Predict Perioperative Complications in the Elderly Patient?

Perhaps the most productive question to ask is: what factors that increase risk can be identified preoperatively and what can be done with these findings to reduce risk? When reviewing various studies in elderly patients, it is evident that cardiovascular disease and infectious complications are the two most important factors in explaining perioperative deaths (Table 21-9). The two most frequent major cardiac complications postoperatively are myocar-

Table 21-8. Goldman risk index

Criteria	"Points"
Congestive heart failure	11
Myocardial infarction in previous 6 months	10
Rhythm other than sinus on ECG	7
Greater than 5 PVCs/min	7
Age greater than 70 yr	5
Emergency operation	4
General status	3
Intraperitoneal or intrathoracic operation	3
Valvular aortic stenosis	3

Source: Goldman et al. (28).

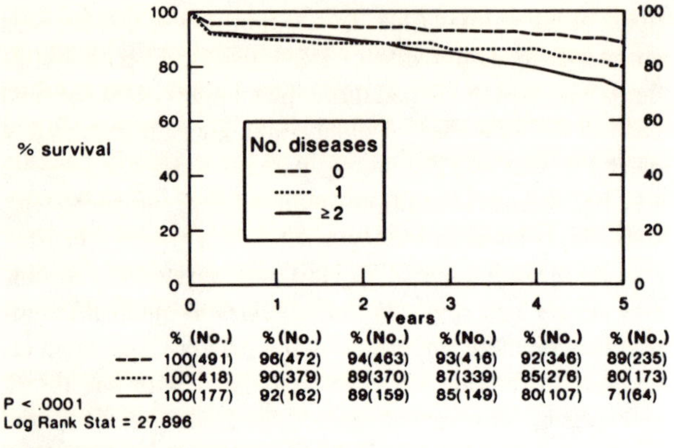

Figure 21-4. Cumulative 5-year survival of patients 65 years old or older. Three groups of patients with differing numbers of medical diseases are illustrated. Diseases included in this survey were diabetes mellitus, peripheral vascular disease, hypertension, cerebral vascular disease, and chronic obstructive pulmonary disease. An increasing number of preexistent diseases appears to predict reduced long-term survival following surgery. (Reprinted with permission from Gersh BJ, et al. 1983. Long-term (5 year) results of coronary bypass surgery in patients 65 years old or older: A report from the coronary artery surgery study. *Circulation* 68 (Supp II):II-190/II-199.)

dial infarction and congestive heart failure. In patients with previous *myocardial infarction,* the reinfarction rate associated with anesthesia and surgery results in a very high mortality rate (35). In a subsequent classic article by Rao and colleagues (36), reinfarction under anesthesia was compared in two groups of patients from two different time periods. The initial retrospective study found a reinfarction rate in patients greater than 65 years to be 11%. However, in a subsequent prospective study some years later where patients had more intensive monitoring and better postoperative care, the reinfarction rate was reduced significantly.

Congestive heart failure is also a major cause of perioperative morbidity and mortality. Preoperative enlargement of the heart seen on chest X-ray and reduced ejection fraction are two easily obtained, reliable, safe, and relatively inexpensive noninvasive predictors of the likelihood of postoperative heart failure (37). For example, ejection fraction relates directly to 5-year survival. Elderly patients with poor ejection fraction had a 47% survival rate when undergoing coronary artery bypass surgery compared to an 88% survival rate in those patients with normal ejection fractions preoperatively (17).

Interest has developed in methods to assess risk preoperatively, utilizing cardiovascular laboratory methods, such as exercise or stress evaluation of the ECG, echocardiography, and nuclide myocardial scanning. The exercise electrocardiogram allows some judgement to be made regarding the extent of coronary artery disease (38). However, many factors can confound the interpretation of exercise electrocardiography. Nuclide scanning of the myocardium has also been employed to determine patients at risk for perioperative complications. Boucher and colleagues (39) employed dipyridamole thallium scans for patients scheduled to undergo vascular surgery. By use of this technique, patients determined to have a normal response to "stress" thallium scanning or who showed a fixed abnormal area (suggestive of an old myocardial infarction) had no demonstrated episodes of perioperative ischemia. In contrast, of patients who showed a reversible defect on thallium scanning (suggestive of a myocardium at risk for ischemia) 50% demonstrated perioperative ischemic events.

A simpler testing scheme, the heart rate response or lack of response to supine bicycle riding, may be equally useful in stratifying high-risk elderly patients. Gerson and colleagues studying patients over age 65 who were scheduled to undergo major abdominal or thoracic surgical procedures found that patients over age 65 who were unable to raise their heart rate above 95 beats per minute during bicycle exercise had an 11-fold increased risk for postoperative complications, while abnormal nuclide myocardial scanning was associated with only a 1.3-fold increased risk (34).

Other preoperative cardiac conditions of interest in the elderly patient include the *arrhythmias* and hypertension. Ambulatory continuous EKG tracings in asymptomatic elderly patients frequently disclose a surprisingly high incidence of arrhythmia indicating an irritable conduction system.

Although *hypertension* has been labeled by many studies as a perioperative risk factor, anesthetic risk in patients with hypertension is more dependent upon the

Table 21-9. Causes of perioperative mortality of the elderly

No. of patients	500(30)	207(31)	443(32)	289(33)	77(33)	500(4)	100(34)
Age	>70	>80	>80	>70	>80	>80	>65
No. of operations	621	284	500	289	77	644	155
Mortality rate	12%	33%	22%	10%	16%	6%	5%
Cause of death							
MI/CHF	29%	12%	17%	13%		32%	100%
Sepsis	16%	14%	13%	9%		19%	—
Pneumonia	13%	29%	38%	26%		7%	—

end organ impairment produced by sustained increase in blood pressure rather than the actual level of blood pressure. However, in patients over 65 scheduled to undergo coronary artery bypass surgery, preoperative hypertension relates to 5-year survival. For example, patients without hypertension demonstrated an 85% 5-year survival rate compared to only 79% for those patients who demonstrated hypertension preoperatively (29). Hospital admission blood pressure is a reliable predictor of intraoperative and postoperative hypertension. In patients at risk for hypertension, attention can be focused upon preoperative control of blood pressure with the use of nitrates, beta blockers, and calcium channel blockers integrated with appropriate anesthetic selection specific for the hemodynamic profile of any given patient.

The other major perioperative complication is due to infection, primarily pulmonary infection (pneumonia) or sepsis. Sepsis is, of course, related to multiple factors and is frequently the final common pathway of pulmonary infection as well.

Postoperative *pneumonia* and ventilatory failure are most commonly observed in patients with chronic lower respiratory tract disease preoperatively. Other factors that increase the risk of perioperative pulmonary infections include factors that increase the risk of gastric aspiration during the perioperative period and impaired pulmonary function tests preoperatively. Pulmonary function tests, which demonstrate decreased maximal breathing capacity or decreased FEV_1, correlate with an increased incidence of postoperative pulmonary problems. The converse is true as well. Data suggest that optimization of pulmonary function decreases the incidence of pulmonary complications postoperatively in patients with chronic obstructive pulmonary disease (40).

Patients at increased risk for postoperative pulmonary infection, as a result of impaired pulmonary function preoperatively, may not reach normal levels of pulmonary function with therapy, but the goal should still be to improve their pulmonary function preoperatively as much as possible. Useful techniques for optimization of pulmonary function include cessation of smoking, administration of antibiotics if sputum is purulent, administration of bronchodilator drugs or inhalational therapy, and use of chest PT combined with postural drainage.

Sepsis in elderly patients may be explained in part by the reduced ability of elderly patients to combat infection. This underscores the concept that as an individual ages, organ function remains adequate for the needs of daily existence; however, the ability to increase function further in order to respond to stress may be impaired. Sepsis is an ever present part of perioperative care. It is often the final common pathway resulting in mortality following multisystem organ failure (41). Inciting events that eventually result in sepsis can range from respiratory and renal failure to hepatic dysfunction, coagulopathy, or GI bleeding. An assessment of risk in a geriatric patient who exhibits signs of multiple organ failure secondary to sepsis should focus on the concept that some of these elderly patients are "too sick" not to operate on rather than too sick to operate on. This suggestion was made by Hinsdale and Jaffe (42) who suggest that frequently the only hope for survival in patients with signs of intra-abdominal sepsis is abdominal re-exploration.

Other preoperative conditions that need attention include metabolic diseases such as diabetes. Attention also should be given to conditions of preoperative anemia or hypovolemia. Nutrition and dehydration of patients secondary to preoperative diagnostic procedures is easily overlooked.

Benefit of Exercise

Recent studies have touted the benefit of exercise in reducing the kinds of cardiac and pulmonary diseases related to surgical death rates. The theory of "hypokinetic disease" based upon "inactivity-induced somatic and mental derangements" is an increasingly attractive concept. This lifestyle in the elderly is associated with an increased prevalence of preoperative coronary artery disease, chronic obstructive pulmonary disease, metabolic disorders, and malnutrition, all of which render a patient more susceptible to postoperative complications such as myocardial infarction, heart failure, infection, and retarded rate of healing. Elderly men given vigorous exercise training have shown a reduced prevalence of asymptomatic coronary artery disease. Other studies have shown that maximal oxygen uptake, thallium scan scores, systolic volume, stroke volume, and cardiac output all were improved in men known to have coronary artery disease who were placed on a medically supervised exercise program. Radionuclide angiocardiography has shown improvement in left ventricular performance in elderly individuals undergoing a 12-week training program on a stationary bicycle (43). Very likely changes in lifestyle including exercise may delay the onset of chronic illness.

Preoperative control of medical illness by aggressive monitoring and medical consultation is important in minimizing the development of complications that limit survival during the perioperative period. Medical progress and changes in general lifestyle habits not only may delay the onset of chronic illness but also modify the influence of disease upon survival. In the future, we may expect that a larger proportion of elderly patients will approach an immunologically determined species-specific maximum life span, predicted to be approximately 85 years. Ideally, we may therefore expect that more elderly patients will come to surgery with fewer complicating multisystem diseases. There will be better control of the systemic disease processes that today contribute as primary causes of perioperative mortality in the elderly patient.

Predictive Value of American Society of Anesthesiologists Physical Status Classification System in Predicting Risk

The American Society of Anesthesiologists (ASA) Physical Status Classification is not affected by patient age but rather by the number and severity of preexistent medical conditions. A definition of these five classification types is illustrated in Table 21-10 (7). The ASA Classification system predicts with reasonable accuracy the risks of elderly patients undergoing anesthesia and surgery. For instance, in a study of 500 patients older than age 80, only 1 of 187 ASA Class II patients died in the perioperative period compared to 14 of 56 (25%) ASA Class IV patients (4). Similarly, a prospective study of almost 200,000 anesthetics demonstrated an incidence of complications that related directly to the patient's ASA physical status (16). Del Guercio and Cohn have shown a similar relationship in those of patients over age 65. Those that were ASA Class II had a mortality rate less than 10%, whereas ASA Class III patients had a mortality rate between 10% and 15%, and Class IV patients had a mortality rate greater than 20% (44). As shown in Table 21-11, in patients over 90 years of age, Hosking and colleagues found an increasing incidence of perioperative morbidity, and an increasing mortality rate (both at 48 hours and 30 days postoperatively) in patients of higher ASA classification (7). Similarly, in a large French study, ASA Physical Status Class I patients had an accident rate of approximately 1 per 1,000 anesthetics, which increased to a rate of 17 per 1,000 anesthetics for patients ASA Class IV and V. These authors found no deaths in ASA Class I patients but a death rate of 8.8 per 1,000 for physical status Class IV and V patients (21).

Table 21-10. American Society of Anesthesiologists Physical Status Classification

Class	Description
I	Healthy patient
II	Mild systemic disease—no functional limitation
III	Severe systemic disease—definite functional limitation
IV	Severe systemic disease that is a constant threat to life
V	Moribund patient unlikely to survive 24 hours with or without operation

Source: Hosking et al. (7).

Table 21-11. Patients > 90 years old

		Mortality (%)	
ASA Class	Morbidity (%)	<24 hr	30 days
II	3.2	1.3	5.6
III	8.5	0.8	5.6
IV	18.3	2.2	18.4
V	50.0	66.7	66.7

Source: Hosking et al. (7).

Marx, Mateo, and Orkin in 1973 found that increasing physical status classification indicated increased perioperative risk far more reliably than did increasing age (13). More recently, Cohen, Duncan, and Tate have shown the same phenomenon when observing more than 100,000 patients for the first 7 postoperative days. Although their data demonstrated that advanced age is an independent predictor of increased mortality, when viewed in comparison, the relative risk predicted by increased age was far less dramatic than the relative risk predicted by poor physical status (45). For example, as detailed in Table 21-12, advanced age increased the relative risk of perioperative deaths by approximately 13-fold; however, poor physical status as reflected by an ASA physical status score of III-V was an even more important determinant of relative risk.

From all of the information presented, it appears that the presence of age-related disease, especially as reflected in a higher ASA physical classification score, plays a greater role than does age itself in contributing to perioperative complications and death in elderly patients.

Importance of Type and Location of Surgery on Perioperative Mortality

As shown in Table 21-13, in a series of 500 patients over age 80 where an overall hospital mortality of 6.2% within 30 days of surgery was observed, a higher incidence of perioperative mortality was seen with specific and more complicated surgical procedures. The six procedures associated with the highest incidence of mortality were tabulated. Marx and colleagues have described similar data where patients undergoing cardiovascular or neurosurgical procedures demonstrated a 10% mortality rate compared to a 5% to 10% mortality rate in patients undergoing thoracic or intra-abdominal procedures. Surgical procedures of all other types were associated with a mortality rate less than 5% (13). Thus, similar to the observations in younger patients, older patients also have a far higher mortality rate when stressed with operations of greater magnitude.

Table 21-12. Relative risk

Variable	Rate of complications/1,000 pts	Relative risk
Age (yrs)		
< 1	3.5	8.7
1–14	0.4	1.0
15–44	0.6	1.5
45–54	1.3	3.2
55–64	1.9	4.7
65–74	3.2	8.0
> 75	5.2	13.0
ASA physical status		
I	0.5	1.0
II	2.9	5.8
III	7.2	14.4
IV & V	18.7	37.4

Source: Cohen et al. (45).

Effects of Emergency Procedures

The risk of perioperative complications and death is greatly increased in the elderly if surgery must be performed on an emergency basis (44, 46, 47). Gibson et al. suggested that death is four times more frequent in the elderly patient with coexistent disease compared to the healthy elderly patient and 20 times more frequent in those requiring emergency surgery (48). Farrow et al. showed that the crude mortality rate in a large series of patients increased 3.5-fold if the procedures were performed on an emergency rather than an elective basis (14). Hosking et al. found that emergency surgery resulted in a 12-fold increased incidence of mortality (7.8% versus 0.6%) during the 48-hour postoperative period in patients over age 90 when compared with the mortality rate in similar aged patients undergoing surgical procedures electively (7). They also found a marked increase in 30-day mortality as well (17.4% versus 6.8%). In addition, they observed a 10-fold increase in the frequency of prolonged postoperative mechanical ventilation following emergency procedures (13.8% versus 1.3%). Cogbill and colleagues (49) looked at survival for patients 80 years of age and older undergoing elective aortic reconstruction and found an 8%, 30-day mortality rate. However, when patients matched for age, sex, and race underwent a similar surgical procedure under emergency conditions (a ruptured abdominal aortic aneurysm), the 30-day mortality rate was 78% with no patients achieving 5-year survival.

Table 21-13. Mortality rate (within 30 days) in patients ≥ 80 years old determined by surgical procedure

Procedure	Incidence	%
AAA	1/4	25
Craniotomy	2/8	25
Thoracotomy	1/5	20
Wound abscess drainage	1/5	20
Exploratory laparotomy, bowel resection	7/37	19
Colectomy	5/40	13
Overall hospital mortality		6.2

Source: Djokovic and Hedley-Whyte (4).

Perhaps the best explanation of why elderly patients requiring emergency surgery have a higher incidence of perioperative complication and death is that they may have delayed seeking health care and may have more advanced pathologic conditions. Also, presentation for emergency surgery allows little time for control of preexisting disease. Although apparently healthy elderly patients may tolerate an elective operation, the initial stress of an emergency procedure, because of an acute exacerbation of preexistent disease or unexpected complication, can tax their limited physiologic reserve and lead to disastrous consequences. In general, it is wise to adequately prepare an elderly patient for elective surgery but unwise to defer surgery simply because of age. An unnecessary delay may result in complications that necessitate surgery under even more adverse emergency conditions, with a significantly increased risk of associated perioperative complications and death. This therefore strengthens the argument for performing elective surgical procedures, even major vascular surgical procedures, on patients who appear quite elderly, in order to avoid facing the dilemma of operating on these same elderly patients with reduced physiologic reserve under much less controlled emergency circumstances.

Role of Preoperative Monitoring in Reducing Perioperative Risk

Preoperative invasive monitoring can identify subgroups of elderly patients with severe multisystem dysfunction who require intensive physiologic preparation with monitoring continued intraoperatively and into the postoperative period. An example of the utilization of hemodynamic monitoring in the perioperative period (in an attempt to identify and reduce risk factors) has been published by Shoemaker and colleagues (50). These investigators demonstrated in patients over 70 years of age that by increasing cardiac index and oxygen delivery values to supranormal levels preoperatively, a decreased perioperative mortality was possible. They suggested that physiologic profiling of patients' responses to the infusions of vasoactive drugs coupled with measurement of oxygen supply and demand will allow more precise management of elderly patients.

Another example of the utilization of perioperative monitoring in defining and perhaps reducing operative risk in the elderly was published by Del Guercio and Cohn (44). In this study, 148 consecutive patients from 60 to 90 years of age underwent major monitoring prior to surgery. Parenthetically, all patients had been previously cleared for surgery by standard internal medical and surgical assessment techniques. Patients were then instrumented preoperatively with a pulmonary artery catheter and arterial line, and hemodynamic, respiratory, and oxygen transport functions were measured. Patients were classified into four stages. Stage I patients demonstrated no functional deficits. Stage II patients had mild physiologic impairment, whereas Stage III patients had moderate impairment that required a delay in order that blood volume replacement, treatment of infection, ventilatory support, or improvement in nutrition could be accomplished. Stage IV patients demonstrated advanced functional deficits that were uncorrectable. The overall findings were that 13% of the patient population had normal physiologic function when ventilatory, hemodynamic, and oxygen transfer measurements were made (Stage I). None of these patients died following surgery. Sixty-three percent of patients had mild to moderate aberrations in these measurements. These patients were managed either with a technique which produced no surgical delay (Stage II) or their surgery was delayed in order that medical management might improve their physiologic function preoperatively (Stage III). When these two groups were combined, a 5.4% postoperative mortality rate was observed. On the other hand, 23% of patients were assigned to Stage IV or were Stage III patients who became Stage IV patients when they did not improve with therapy. Of these very ill patients, the majority had their surgical procedures cancelled. A number underwent "lesser procedures" under local anesthesia and survived. However, in a small group in whom the defects determined by this pattern of invasive monitoring were uncorrectable and the original operation that was planned was undertaken anyway, *the mortality rate was 100%*. These data seem to justify the expense of intensive monitoring preoperatively to determine which elderly patients have uncorrectable physiologic defects, in whom a likely fatal outcome may be predicted.

Studies of patients who have a history of preoperative myocardial infarction also indicate that careful attention to preoperative hemodynamic preparation and intraoperative control with aggressive treatment of hypertension, tachycardia, myocardial failure, dysrhythmias, and oxygen availability influences the rate of perioperative reinfarction and associated mortality (51, 52). Similarly, Rao, Jacobs, and El-Etr have suggested that escalation of monitoring in a subgroup of primarily older patients in whom recent myocardial infarctions have occurred, has produced a decreased incidence of perioperative myocardial infarction (36). Thus, data are accumulating that suggest that elderly patients who are to undergo major surgical procedures may benefit from aggressive preoperative and intraoperative invasive monitoring.

Premedication of the Elderly

In general, premedicant drugs must be administered with caution to elderly patients, who will manifest a greater sensitivity and a longer duration of drug effect compared with their younger counterparts. Normal young adult premedication doses may produce an exaggerated effect in elderly patients and can create unwanted confusion and agitation. If there is doubt, premedication should be light or omitted. Most nonsedative type medications that are taken regularly should be continued during the perioperative period. For example, it is current practice to maintain therapy with beta blockers, antihypertensive drugs, vasodilating drugs, and calcium channel blocking agents. Recent speculation suggests that it even may be safe to continue monamine oxidase inhibitor medications up to the time of surgery. For the most part, preoperative drug therapy, originally considered to be a risk factor if continued perioperatively, has often been found to contribute to physiologic control and need not be discontinued. In fact, preoperative discontinuation of drug therapy has been found to be a greater source of risk than has maintenance of drug therapy up to and through the time of surgery. Thus, although there may be adverse interactions between various medications and anesthetic agents, nevertheless, it is current practice to continue almost all pharmacologic agents that a patient is taking preoperatively throughout the perioperative period.

Selection of Anesthesia

Although many articles suggest that no significant differences in short- or long-term survival were found between patients receiving regional versus general anesthesia (7), evidence is slowly accumulating that regional anesthesia may reduce anesthetic risk under certain surgical conditions. Although both general and regional anesthesia have been successfully employed, regional anesthesia appears to reduce the incidence of postoperative thromboembolic complications and mental confusion and enhance early ambulation and resumption of self care in elderly individuals undergoing repair of fractures of the femoral neck (53). In addition, short-term mortality and length of hospital stay are reduced by the use of regional anesthesia. In another study employing ^{125}I labeled fibrinogen in elderly patients undergoing open prostatic procedures, patients who received lumbar epidural anesthesia demonstrated a reduced incidence of deep vein thrombosis (54). Venous occlusion plethysmography studies in patients following total hip replacement indicate that arterial input, venous capacitance, and drainage rate are all increased after lumbar epidural anesthesia. These changes may explain the observation under certain surgical procedures that pulmonary embolus occurs three times more commonly postoperatively following general anesthesia than after epidural anesthesia. Probably the best morbidity and mortality statistics, however, are found in elderly patients who are able to undergo surgical procedures, such as a cataract operation, under local anesthesia with minimal or no sedation. Although elderly patients seem to benefit from regional anesthesia in certain specific surgical procedures, such as repair of fractured hips or total hip replacement, for most surgical procedures, there appears to be no difference in morbidity and mortality in the elderly population produced as a result of the type of anesthesia employed.

Importance of Postoperative Analgesia

The concept that postoperative analgesia may be an important factor in determining perioperative morbidity and mortality in elderly patients has been suggested by a number of recent studies. For example, Yeager and colleagues (55) observed "high-risk" elderly patients admitted to the ICU postoperatively. These patients with a mean age of 71 years were given an anesthetic protocol involving general anesthesia followed by routine parenteral narcotics postoperatively, and were then compared to a second group of patients who received epidural anesthesia and "light" general anesthesia intraoperatively and epidural analgesia postoperatively to reduce pain. These two regimens demonstrated a significant difference in morbidity and mortality, where 4 of 25 patients undergoing surgery with general anesthesia and routine postoperative pain management techniques died, compared to a mortality rate of 0 in 28 patients who received epidural anesthesia and postoperative epidural analgesia. In addition, patients treated with epidural anesthesia and epidural analgesia postoperatively had an overall 5-day shorter hospital stay with reduced physician and hospital costs. Although the data from Yeager and similar data from other centers are relatively preliminary, they offer the suggestion that perhaps the use of epidural analgesia or other techniques to reduce postoperative stress may contribute to an improved perioperative course in elderly patients.

Importance of Individual Physician Skill

In a recent article, Cohen et al. (45) ask, "Does anesthesia contribute to operative mortality?" Their retrospective study in Canada examined 100,000 anesthetics and concluded that management of patients by experienced anesthesiologists contributed to a lower patient mortality rate than that seen in patients cared for by less experienced physicians. Another study points to the troubling observation that variation in individual physician anesthetic management of intraoperative hemodynamic risk factors has been identified as an important variable in determining the infarction rate during coronary artery surgery (56). Individual anesthesiologist's control of intraoperative variables leading to myocardial ischemia was a more important factor in determining the incidence of postoperative infarction than were other factors in preoperative patient selection, such as the presence of left main coronary artery disease or reduced ejection fraction. Intraoperative tachycardia was a major determinant of myocardial ischemia and was felt to be a factor specifically controllable by the individual anesthesiologist. Although this study was performed in a series of patients undergoing cardiopulmonary bypass, some of whom were not elderly, the conclusions appear valid for elderly patients who have atherosclerotic heart disease undergoing noncardiac surgery as well. Many major surgical procedures are performed on elderly patients who have inoperable vascular disease. This study produces clear evidence that individual anesthesiologist's performance intraoperatively may directly influence outcome of patients with significant cardiac disease.

Postoperative management of patients is also critical. Postoperative hypertension is the main cause of neurologic sequelae after carotid endarterectomy. Individual physician differences in postoperative management techniques may also contribute to the incidence of perioperative morbidity and mortality.

Although physicians and patients have been hesitant to admit that there may be a difference in quality between physicians, data such as that from Slogoff and Keats (56) suggest that perioperative ischemia may vary by a factor of three depending upon the management by different anesthesiologists. There is little reason to believe that similar patterns would not be observed if surgical contribution to perioperative mortality were investigated.

Summary

In the year 2000, it is predicted that 16% of the United States population will be over age 65 and will account for greater than 33% of all health care costs (57). Further liberalization of surgical indications in the elderly may be expected due to further improvement in surgical outcomes.

Great advances in surgical outcome in the geriatric patient have already occurred. For example, perioperative mortality rate for patients 90 years of age or older have progressively decreased from 29% in the 1960s (27) to 9% by the late 1970s (4) to 1.6% in the 1980s (7). Although the operative mortality for the geriatric patient appears to have decreased over the last 20 years, it still remains at least one order of magnitude greater than the operative mortality in the overall surgical population.

A number of variables are important in contributing to mortality in the elderly. These include emergency surgery and certain types of procedures that have a greater operative mortality, including cardiothoracic and major vascular procedures. In addition, elderly patients have increased risk associated with surgery if they have preexistent medical conditions that are reflected in their ASA status. Although age, per se, influences perioperative morbidity and mortality in elderly patients as a result of the gradual decline in physiologic reserve of organ function that occurs during the aging process, the increased presence and severity of concomitant disease appears to have an even greater effect on perioperative morbidity and morality in the geriatric patient.

To limit anesthesia risk in the elderly patient, it is necessary to have a full recognition of the patient's preexisting medical condition and work to maximize organ function and correct abnormalities before surgery if possible. The use of preoperative major monitoring, to optimize cardiovascular and pulmonary function, intensive intraoperative and postoperative monitoring, and aggressive therapeutic intervention all contribute to improved outcome in elderly patients with preexistent severe disease processes. Efforts must be made to transform emergencies into planned procedures. Elective procedures should not be deferred except to improve function by direct intervention. There should be no reluctance to operate on patients simply because of their chronologic age, as a delay may allow the surgical disease to progress to become more profound, often requiring an emergency procedure of greater magnitude in a patient whose preexisting systemic abnormalities have worsened. Surgical treatment of disease thus appears to improve life for the elderly population if risk factors are controlled by meticulous attention to detail (58).

References

1. Smith, OC. 1907. Advanced age as a contraindication to operation. *Med Rec (NY)* 72:642.
2. Ochsner, A. 1927. Is risk of operation too great in the elderly? *Geriatrics* 22:121.
3. Brooks, B. 1937. Surgery in patients of advanced age. *Ann Surg* 105:481.
4. Djokovic, JL, and Hedley-Whyte, J. 1979. Prediction of outcome of surgery and anesthesia in patients over age 80. *JAMA* 242:2301.
5. Miller, R, Marlar, K, and Silvay, G. 1977. Anesthesia for patients aged over 90 years. *NY State J Med* 77:1421.
6. Katlic, MR. 1985. Surgery in centenarians. *JAMA* 253:3139.
7. Hosking, MP, et al. 1989. Outcomes of surgery in patients 90 years of age and older. *JAMA* 261:1909.
8. Warner, MA, Hosking, MP, and Lobdell, CM. 1988. Utilization of surgery among those ⩾ 90 years of age: A population-based study in Olmsted County, Minnesota, 1975–85. *Ann Surg* 207:26.
9. Loop, FD, et al. 1988. Coronary artery bypass graft surgery in the elderly. Indications and outcome. *Cleve Clin J Med* 55:23.
10. Linn, BS, Linn, MW, and Wallen, N. 1982. Evaluation of results of surgical procedures in the elderly. *Ann Surg* 195:90–96.
11. McLeskey, CH. 1985. Anesthesia for the geriatric patient. In *Advances in Anesthesia,* Eds., RK Stoelting, PG Barash, and TJ Gallagher, p. 31. Chicago: Year Book Medical Publishers.
12. Davenport, HT. 1983. Anesthesia for the geriatric patient. *Can Anaesth Soc J* 30:S51.
13. Marx, GF, Mateo, CV, and Orkin, LR. 1973. Computer analysis of post-anesthetic deaths. *Anesthesiology* 39:54.
14. Farrow, SC, et al. 1982. Epidemiology in anaesthesia. II: Factors affecting mortality in hospital. *Br J Anaesth* 54:811.
15. Santos, AL, and Gelperin, A. 1975. Surgical mortality in the elderly. *J Am Geriatr Soc,* XXIII(1):42–6, January.
16. Tiret, L, et al. 1986. Complications associated with anaesthesia—a prospective survey in France. *Can Anaesth Soc J* 33:336.
17. Gersh, BJ, et al. 1983a. Coronary arteriography and coronary artery bypass surgery: Morbidity and mortality in patients ages 65 years or older. *Circulation* 67(3):483; March.
18. Acinapura, AJ, et al. 1988. Coronary artery bypass in septuagenarians. *Circulation* 78(Suppl I):I-179/I-184, September.
19. Pottecher, T, et al. 1984. Cardiac arrest related to anesthesia: A prospective survey in France (1978–1982). *Eur J Anaesth* I:305.
20. Filzweiser, G, and List, WF. 1983. Morbidity and mortality in elective geriatric surgery. In *Mortality and Anesthesia,* Eds., MD Vickers and JN Lunn, p. 75, Berlin: Springer-Verlag.
21. Hatton, F, Tiret, L, and Vourc'h, G. 1983. Morbidity and mortality associated with anesthesia—French survey: Preliminary results. In *Mortality and Anesthesia,* Eds., MD Vickers and JN Lunn, p. 25. Berlin: Springer-Verlag.
22. McLeskey, CH. 1989. Anesthesia for the geriatric patient. In *Clinical Anesthesia,* Eds., PG Barash, BF Cullen, and RK Stoelting, p. 1301. Philadelphia: JB Lippincott.
23. Haljamae, T, Stefannsson, T, and Wickstrom, I. 1982. Preanesthetic evaluation of the female geriatric patient with hip fracture. *Acta Anaesthesiol Scand* 26:393.
24. Stephen, CR. 1984. The risk of anesthesia and surgery in the geriatric patient. In *Anesthesia and the Geriatric Patient,* Ed., SE Krechel, p. 231. New York: Grune and Stratton.
25. Rowe, JW, et al. 1976. The effect of age on creatinine

clearance in man: A cross-sectional and longitudinal study. *J Gerontol* 31:155.

26. Gajewski, J, and Singer, RB. 1981. Mortality in an insured population with atrial fibrillation. *JAMA* 245:1540.
27. Denney, JH, and Denson, JS. 1972. Risk of surgery in patients over 90. *Geriatrics* 27:115.
28. Goldman, L, et al. 1977. Multifactorial index of cardiac risks in non-cardiac surgical procedures. *N Engl J Med* 297:845.
29. Gersh, BJ, et al. 1983. Long-term (5 year) results of coronary bypass surgery in patients 65 years old or older: A report from the coronary artery surgery study. *Circulation* 68(Supp II):II-190/II-199.
30. Anglem, TJ, and Bradford, ML. 1953. Major surgery in the aged. *N Engl J Med* 249:1005.
31. Wilder, RJ, and Fishbein, RH. 1961. Operative experience with patients over 80 years of age. *Surg Gynecol Obstet* 113:205.
32. Marshall, WH, and Fahey, PJ. 1964. Operative complications and mortality in patients over 80 years of age. *Arch Surg* 88:896.
33. Palmberg, S, and Hirsjarvi, E. 1979. Mortality in geriatric surgery. *Gerontology* 25:13.
34. Gerson, MC, et al. 1985. Cardiac prognosis in noncardiac geriatric surgery. *Ann Int Med* 103:832.
35. Tarhan, S, et al. 1972. Myocardial infarction after general anesthesia. *JAMA* 220:1451.
36. Rao, TLK, Jacobs, KH, and El-Etr, AA. 1983. Reinfarction following anesthesia in patients with myocardial infarction. *Anesthesiology* 59:499.
37. Mangano, DT. 1985. Biventricular function after myocardial revascularization in humans. *Anesthesiology* 62:571.
38. Chaitman, BR. 1986. The changing role of the exercise electrocardiogram as a diagnostic and prognostic test for chronic ischemic heart disease. *J Am Coll Cardiol* 8:1195.
39. Boucher, CA, et al. 1985. Determination of cardiac risk by dipyridamole-thallium imaging before peripheral vascular surgery. *N Engl J Med* 312:389.
40. Stein, M, and Casssara, EL. 1970. Preoperative pulmonary evaluation and therapy for surgery patients. *JAMA* 211:787.
41. Fry, DE, et al. 1980. Multiple system organ failure: The role of uncontrolled infection. *Arch Surg* 115:136.
42. Hinsdale, JG, and Jaffe, BM. 1984. Re-operation for intra-abdominal sepsis: Indications and results in modern critical care setting. *Ann Surg* 199:31.
43. Schocken, DD, et al. 1983. Physical conditioning and left ventricular performance in the elderly. *Am J Cardiol* 52:359.
44. Del Guercio, LRN, and Cohn, JD. 1980. Monitoring operative risk in the elderly. *JAMA* 243:1350.
45. Cohen, MM, Duncan, PG, and Tate, RB. 1988. Does anesthesia contribute to operative mortality? *JAMA* 260:2859.
46. Johnson, JC. 1983. The medical evaluation and management of the elderly surgical patient. *J Am Geriatr Soc* 31:621.
47. Goldman, L, et al. 1978. Cardiac risk factors and complications in non-cardiac surgery. *Medicine* 57:357.
48. Gibson, JR, Mendelhall, MK, and Axel, NJ. 1985. Geriatric anesthesia: Minimizing the risk. In *Clinics in Geriatric Medicine,* Ed., GU Brindly, p. 313. Philadelphia: WB Saunders.
49. Cogbill, CL. 1967. Operation in the aged. Mortality related to concurrent disease, duration of anesthesia and elective and emergency operation. *Arch Surg* 94:202.
50. Shoemaker, WC, et al. 1988. Prospective trial of supranormal values of survivors as therapeutic goals in high-risk surgical patients. *Chest* 94:1176.
51. Schoeppel, SL, et al. 1983. Effects of myocardial infarction on perioperative cardiac complications. *Anesth Analg* 62:493.
52. Tinker, JH. 1982. Perioperative myocardial infarction. *Semin Anesth* 1:253.
53. McKenzie, PJ, Wishart, HY, and Smith, G. 1984. Long-term outcome after repair of fractured neck of femur. *Br J Anaesth* 56:581.
54. Modig, J. 1982. Thromboembolism and blood loss. *Reg Anesth* 7:S84.
55. Yeager, MP, et al. 1987. Epidural anesthesia and analgesia in high-risk surgical patients. *Anesthesiology* 66:729.
56. Slogoff, S, and Keats, AS. 1985. Does perioperative ischemia lead to postoperative myocardial infarction? *Anesthesiology* 62:107.
57. Craig, DB, et al. 1987. Panel summary: Geriatric anesthesia. *Can Anaesth Soc J* 34:156.
58. Anderson, B, and Ostberg, J. 1972. Long-term prognosis in geriatric surgery. *J Am Geriatr Soc* 20:225.

22

Geriatric Anesthesia

Norig Ellison

Definitions of Geriatrics and Aging

Despite the increased interest in aging, a universally accepted clinical definition of the terms "aging" and "geriatrics" has not evolved. While a tactful definition of the geriatric patient may be, simply, someone older than the patient to whom one is speaking, the vagaries of such a definition leave much to be desired. A medical dictionary definition of geriatrics is "that department of medicine which treats all problems peculiar to old age and the aging, including the clinical problems of senescence and senility" (1), but this definition merely substitutes the synonyms, old and senescence, for geriatrics. We choose to define aging in broad, conceptual terms as an inevitable phenomenon that represents the sum of the progressive changes in organ and cell structure and function, which occur in an individual with time, independent of recognizable disease or accident, and which eventually result in the increased probability of death (2). The utility of this definition for the clinician is, of course, questionable since it provides no markers that can be used to judge the extent of the aging process. Furthermore, this definition ignores the fact that function of various organ systems may decline at different rates. The difficulty in making a definition of aging more precise than this broad conceptual one explains why there remains a fixation on chronologic age. Nevertheless, clinicians must ever be alert to the fact that chronologic and physiologic age are not synonymous.

Definition of the age at which an individual enters the geriatric population is difficult. With the advent of Medicare in 1965, the federal government arbitrarily defined age 65 as the dividing line, but it is important to realize that such an arbitrary definition is not medically justified. Articles dealing with the subject of anesthesia and surgery in the aged have used age limits from 45 or 50 years to 80 or even 90 (3–6). While few would argue that those over 90 are aged, the selection of 50 as a limit may reflect the feeling prevalent 20 years ago, but no longer true today, that for cardiac surgery, 50 years is aged (7). Whatever definition is used for the age at which the geriatric population begins, it is certain that the size of this population is increasing.

The number of geriatric patients appearing on operating room lists increased sharply when Medicare coverage became available, with as many as 33% of beneficiaries undergoing surgical procedures annually. A further reason for the increase in geriatric surgery is the improved result attainable with modern surgical and anesthetic techniques. Advanced age is no longer an absolute or even a serious relative contraindication to surgery (8). The five most common procedures in this patient population are: 1) cataract extraction, 2) transurethral resection of the prostate, 3) herniorrhaphy, 4) cholecystectomy, and 5) reduction of fractured hip.

The steady increase in the number of older patients requiring surgery may continue. It is not necessarily true, however, that the need for medical care will increase as rapidly as the size of the older population. There may be factors that will ultimately increase the mean age of the population, without increasing their medical needs proportionally. Figure 22-1 shows how remaining life expectancy for different ages has changed since 1900. It can be seen that, for the newborn from 1900 to 1978, there was an increase in life expectancy of 27 years. However, in the 60-year-old group during the same period, the increase was only 7 years. In the 75-year-old group, the increase in life expectancy has been only 4 years between 1900 and 1978. Thus, people are not living a great deal longer. However, more people are living to their full life expectancy. Premature death, that which occurs before the natural life span is achieved, is being eliminated (Fig. 22-2).

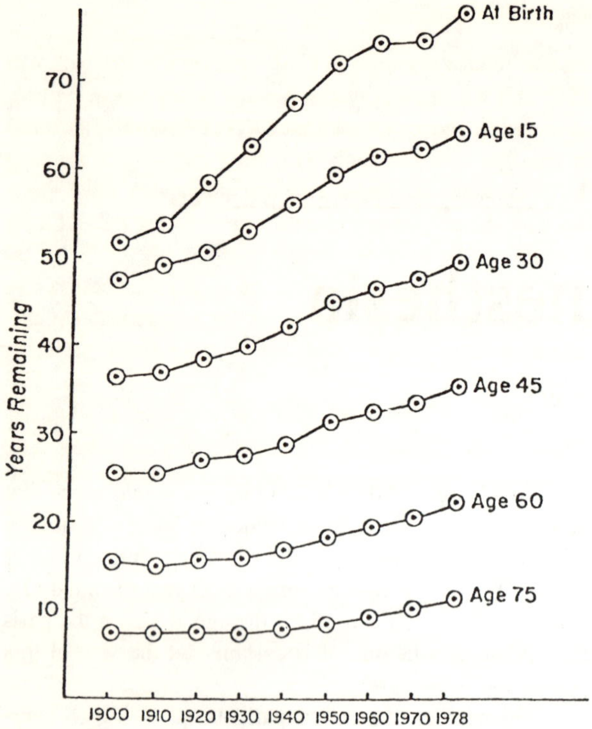

Figure 22-1. Life expectancy of white females by decade from 1900 to 1978. Life expectancy has continued to increase between 1900 and 1978, but the greatest increases have been in the young. Thus, the increase in life span has been small, but the percentage of individuals who will enjoy a normal life span is increasing dramatically. A graph showing the same tendencies could be plotted for males or for non-whites. (Data from: *U.S. Bureau of Census, Statistical Abstract of the United States*, 1981, 92nd edition. 1978 data from *Vital Statistics of the United States*, Lifetable 5-15, 1978. Washington, DC.)

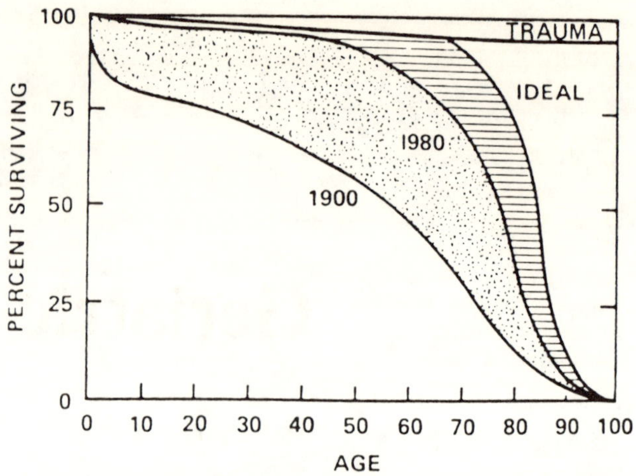

Figure 22-2. Comparison of survival curves. The curves illustrate the percentage of individuals still alive at each age from 0 to 100 years. Between 1900 and 1980, the elimination of most deaths due to disease has moved the survival curve far to the right, with the stippled area representing the difference due to elimination of deaths due to disease. Under ideal conditions most of the remaining instances of death before age 85 would also be eliminated, and the survival curve would be shifted even further to the right. The graph also illustrates the fact that deaths due to trauma occur at all ages at a relatively stable rate. (From Fries, JM. 1980. Aging, natural death and the compression of morbidity. *N Engl J Med* 303:130–135.)

Fries has pointed out that the elimination of much acute illness, which is usually quickly and relatively inexpensively treated, has left us with more chronic illness, which is more expensive to treat, requires a longer period of therapy, and may bring with it increased requirements for nursing homes and other public health costs (9). However, he goes on to suggest that chronic illness may be postponed by changes in life-style, resulting in the extension of adult vigor far into a fixed life span and compression of the period of senescence near the end of life. Fries' suggestion is based on the premise that premature organ dysfunction is due to disuse, not overuse. Thus, serum cholesterol, vital capacity, and systolic blood pressure—all of which can be viewed as markers of age—can be modified by exercise, weight control, or diet, resulting in the aged performing closer to peak performance. He suggests that under societal conditions more ideal than those that presently exist, mean age at death might be extended to 85 years. If the period of senescence can be compressed and chronic illness postponed, then most elderly would be able to live their natural life span in vigorous health.

While an exciting and attractive alternative to the promise of a nation of nursing homes caring for the aged, this proposal remains unproven and not universally accepted. Schneider and Brody caution that very large fractions of our aging population continue to suffer from chronic disease and remain a major health care burden as life expectancy moves into the ninth decade of life (10). Until such time as substantial inroads are made in the prevention, treatment, or management of the common chronic diseases associated with aging, the compression of senescence into a brief terminal period cannot be accepted as inevitable. Table 22-1 lists these chronic conditions.

Leaf has made extensive surveys in three isolated areas where long lives are characteristic (the Andean mountains of Ecuador, the Karakoram mountains in Pakistan, and the Caucasia region in Russia). Presumably genetic factors, specific dietary factors, and physical activity all play a part in explaining this longevity. Psychologic factors may also be important in that it is a characteristic of these isolated areas that the older people continue to be contributing, productive members of the society, in contrast to today's tendency in the United

Table 22-1. Chronic conditions contributing to limitation of activity in the population over 65 years of age

Condition	Incidence (%)
Heart disease	23.5
Arthritis	23.2
Impairment of vision	9.8
Diabetes mellitus	6.8
Cerebrovascular disease	4.9
Emphysema	4.4
Partial or complete paralysis	3.6
Psychiatric disease	3.4
Impairment of hearing	2.3
Malignant neoplasms	2.2

Source of data: U.S. Department of Health, Education and Welfare publication No. HRA 77-1537, *Limitation of Activity due to Chronic Conditions, United States, 1974.* National Center for Health Statistics, Hyattsville, MD, 1977.

States to "warehouse" the elderly in nursing homes (11). Leaf has concluded that rigorous, active life, involving physical and sexual activity, is possible for at least 100 years and in some instances for even longer.

In the last century, vigorous exercise was thought to damage the body and decrease longevity. Today, a wide variety of exercise regimens have been advocated to increase longevity. While there are no data that conclusively establish the effect of exercise on longevity, exercise clearly has beneficial effects on several aging processes and age-related disease, especially cardiovascular disease (12).

Organ System Function

The human body maintains homeostasis by varying cardiac, pulmonary, or renal function appropriately, as circumstances change. For example, cardiac output or minute ventilation may be increased as much as fivefold in a young male during exercise. Similarly, in a dehydrated patient, urine output may fall to less than 10 ml per kg per 24 hours, while a patient who has been volume overloaded may increase urine output tenfold. Unfortunately, the capacity to adapt by varying function over wide extremes is impaired with age. This decline in reserve capacity has been attributed to a decrease in the number of functioning parenchymal cells, particularly in tissues with poor capacity for division and replacement, such as those of the nervous system or kidney (13). The reduced reserve of various organs in the aged can be demonstrated usually only by stress testing. Nevertheless, even the healthy aged should never be viewed as younger than their chronologic age, since with the imposition of stress, they may be unable to maintain homeostasis.

Respiratory Function

An age-related decrease in vital capacity was first noted in 1846 and has been confirmed many times since. Subsequent studies have demonstrated a corresponding increase in residual volume, with total lung capacity remaining fairly constant. Comroe and his colleagues have summarized the pulmonary changes by defining the "elderly normal" as the man or woman over the age of 50 or 60 years whose lungs are normal upon physical and x-ray examination, who has no signs or symptoms of cardiopulmonary disease, and whose pulmonary function tests reveal the pattern outlined in Table 22-2 (14). The end result is a somewhat enlarged lung at rest, with decreased elasticity and reduced maximal movement. The decrease in vital capacity and maximal breathing capacity with age, due to diminished muscular power and physical training (15), are quantitated in males by the following equations:

$$\text{Vital Capacity (ml)} = 27.63 - (0.112 \times \text{age}) \times \text{heights (cm)}$$

$$\text{Maximum Breathing Capacity (L/min)} = 86.5 - (0.522 \times \text{age}) \times \text{Body Surface Area (m}^2\text{)}$$

A progressive loss of protective airway reflexes has been demonstrated with aging (16). This may explain the increase in silent aspiration seen in the elderly. The volume of the lung at which small airways begin to close, the closing volume, has been shown to increase with aging,

Table 22-2. Pulmonary function patterns in the elderly normal

Lung volumes
- Decreased vital capacity
- Increased residual volume and functional residual capacity
- Increased ratio of residual volume to total lung capacity

Ventilation
- Slight decrease in frequency, tidal volume, and minute volume
- Increase in anatomic dead space
- Decrease in oxygen consumption and carbon dioxide production
- Normal respiratory response to inhaled carbon dioxide

Distribution of inspired gas and blood
- Uneven with increased alveolar dead space

Pulmonary circulation
- Essentially normal

Diffusion
- Decreased maximal diffusion capacity for oxygen

Arterial blood gases
- Normal pH and carbon dioxide levels
- Decreased PaO_2

Adapted from Comroe, JH, et al. 1962. *The Lung: Clinical Physiology and Pulmonary Function Tests*, ed. 2, pp. 212–213. Chicago: Year Book Medical Publishers, Inc.

and this phenomenon is probably related to the decrease in arterial PO_2 observed with aging (17).

Respiratory changes in the elderly may also be due to alterations in other systems, such as arthritis in the spine, repeated pulmonary infections, or environmental factors, such as industrial pollutants in the air.

Cardiovascular Function

The cardiovascular changes seen with aging include progressive decrease in resting cardiac output (16), progressive increase in blood pressure, and prolongation of circulation time (13). The decrease in cardiac output is associated with longer duration of systole and reduced stroke volume. The increase in blood pressure results from an increase in peripheral vascular resistance greater than the decrease in cardiac output. Increased peripheral resistance is probably caused by atherosclerotic changes, especially in the larger arteries, producing a less compliant vasculature (18).

The prolonged circulation time has two pharmacologic implications for anesthesiologists. First, following bolus injection of an intravenous drug, interventions, such as laryngoscopy, might inadvertently be carried out before the patient is properly anesthetized and/or paralyzed. Second, a repeat bolus of the drug might be administered as a result of seemingly inadequate anesthesia or relaxation before the initial dose has had a complete effect, thus predisposing these patients to overdose of intravenous agents (19).

Baroreceptor reflexes, such as tachycardia and vasoconstriction, are blunted in the aged. As a result, warning signs of hypovolemia, which is poorly tolerated in the elderly, are less evident. However, when striving to maintain normovolemia with fluid administration, one must be careful to avoid hypervolemia, which is also poorly tolerated.

Renal Function

Decline in renal function with advanced age has long been recognized, manifested by decrease in glomerular filtration rate and concentrating ability (13). Such a reduction in renal function necessitates a larger urine volume to excrete a comparable nitrogen load in order to prevent nitrogen retention.

In response to salt deprivation, the renal response to sodium conservation occurs in 18 hours in the young and in 31 hours in the elderly. As a result, hyponatremia and impaired mental function are more likely to occur when the elderly are salt deprived (20). This fact necessitates special care in the administration of fluids and electrolytes to avoid abnormal saline levels.

Central Nervous System Function

Central nervous system changes include a decrease in brain weight and cell density. Bromage (21), in a study of the epidural lidocaine dose required per spinal segment anesthetized, and Gregory et al. (22) in their study of the relationship between halothane minimum alveolar concentration (MAC) and age, both demonstrated a decrease in anesthetic requirements with advancing age. These studies mention that decrease in requirement with aging is associated with decreased cell density in the central nervous system, decreased cerebral oxygen consumption, and decreased cerebral blood flow.

Gastrointestinal Function

Changes in gastrointestinal function reported to be associated with aging are controversial. An age-related increase in bromsulphalein (BSP) retention has been reported in one study but not confirmed in other animal and human studies (23, 24). Although age-related studies comparing rates of drug absorption and total recovery are lacking, numerous reports of reduction and/or delay in gastrointestinal absorption in the elderly can be used to infer alterations in drug absorption. Factors that help explain this decrease in absorption include decreased gastric acid output, reduced level of mesenteric blood flow, reduced absorptive surface, and impaired enzyme systems responsible for transport across the intestinal epithelial membrane (25).

Clinical Problems

Response to Drugs

Slower onset of drug action is characteristic in the elderly due to decreased rate of absorption from the gastrointestinal tract and slower uptake following injection, the latter being caused by decreased cardiac output and slower regional circulation. When renal or hepatic elimination is necessary for termination of effect, drugs may have longer actions in the elderly. In addition, a decreased number of receptors will result in greater effect for a given dose of drug. Thus, the probability of experiencing an adverse drug reaction increases with age, from 7.5% of hospitalized patients 40 to 49 years of age, to 21.3% in patients 70 to 79 years of age (26). Examples of adverse effects in the elderly include digitalis intoxication, potassium depletion with thiazide diuretics, extrapyramidal symptoms with phenothiazine therapy, and erratic responses to barbiturates. A peculiar coincidence is that drug responses in older persons are comparable to those in the very young. For example, serum antibiotic levels are elevated after intramuscular administration in the young because of undeveloped renal function and in the aged because of declining renal function.

One factor that might act to decrease the length of drug action in the elderly is that many of the aged are likely to be taking medications that can induce liver enzymes responsible for the metabolism of other drugs. Nevertheless, there is no evidence for increased drug requirements in the elderly. All the evidence, in fact, points the other way. Muravchick and Mandel have demonstrated that a thiopental sleep-inducing dose of 1.8 mg/kg was 100% effective in producing loss of consciousness in 31 patients over 65 years of age, and 0% effective in 17 control patients less than 40 years of age (27). This finding supports the admonition that reduced doses of anesthetic agents should be administered more slowly to the aged. Similarly, a recent pharmacokinetic analysis of lidocaine administered via caudal catheter demonstrated consistently higher serum levels in the group over 60 than in a group less than 40 (28). That analysis prompted the observation that, in the young, serum levels resemble those seen following a bolus injection, whereas in the aged, persistently higher levels resemble those seen during an infusion. The persistently high serum levels of lidocaine raise the possibility that with repeated injections toxicity may result.

Concomitant Disease

Figure 22-3 illustrates the average number of physician visits per year for males and females of all ages. With the exceptions of the first year of life and females during the childbearing years, there is a steady increase in the frequency with which patients seek medical attention as they age. Incidence of disease may reasonably be expected to parallel the number of physician visits per year. Thus, aged patients undergoing surgery can be presumed more likely to have pre-existing disease than their younger counterparts. The contribution of pre-existing disease to surgical mortality has been documented in numerous studies. Cogbill found a fourfold increase in surgical mortality in aged patients with acute pre-existing disease, mostly owing to pneumonia and acute urinary tract infection (29).

The chronic pre-existing diseases present in the aged are defined in part in Table 22-1, which lists the incidence of 10 chronic conditions contributing to limitation of activity in the aged. Table 22-3, which lists the 12 leading causes of death in the elderly, provides additional data on what the pre-existing disease is likely to be. Figure 22-4 depicts the prevalence of four illustrative diseases as a function of age. Each of these diseases can present problems for the anesthesiologist and the surgeon. The arthritic patient, for instance, brings a series of problems. He or she may be unable to assume the position required for the proposed surgery. Cervical arthritis may make intubation more difficult. Involvement of the temporomandibular joint in rheumatoid arthritis may result in airway management problems. In addition, patients with rheumatoid arthritis may be receiving steroids, and the need for supplementation must be considered during the pre- and postoperative periods.

Equivalent illustrations can be provided for the other diseases. The hypertensive patient may be in congestive heart failure on the basis of long-standing increased afterload. He or she may have atherosclerosis of vital circulatory beds, such as the cerebral and the coronary. The hypertensive patient is likely to manifest unusually wide swings in both pulse and blood pressure during anesthe-

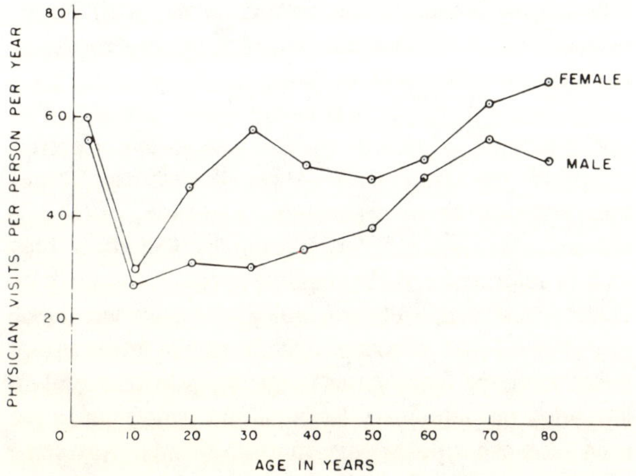

Figure 22-3. Number of physician visits annually by age for males and females. (From Ellison, N. 1975. Problems in geriatric anesthesia. *Surg Clin North Am* 55:936.)

Table 22-3. Twelve leading causes of death in persons over 65 years of age in 1977

Condition	Number of deaths
Heart disease	755,534
Malignant neoplasms	232,262
Cerebrovascular disease	154,379
Influenza and pneumonia	39,885
Accidents	24,181
Diabetes mellitus	23,604
Bronchitis, emphysema, and asthma	17,293
Hepatic cirrhosis	8,634
Nephritis and nephrosis	5,834
Hypertension	4,512
Hernia and intestinal obstruction	4,192
Septicemia	4,144

Source of data: Vital Statistics of the United States, 1977. Volume II: *Mortality*, Part B. Table 7-5. National Center for Health Statistics, Hyattsville, MD, 1980.

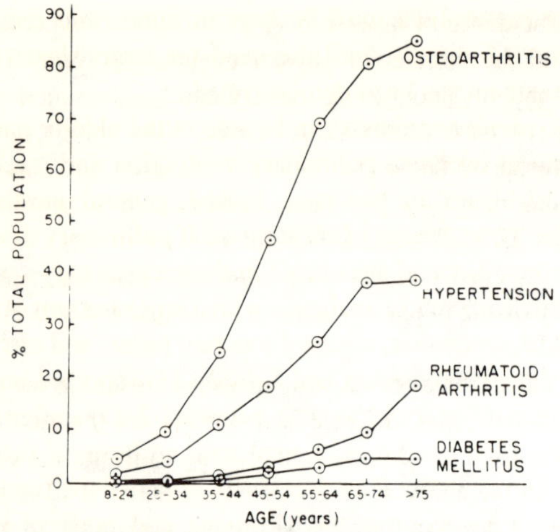

Figure 22-4. Prevalence of four illustrative diseases as a function of age. (From Ellison, N. 1975. Problems in geriatric anesthesia. *Surg Clin North Am* 55:937.)

sia, especially if time does not permit adequate preoperative control of the hypertension. In patients with diabetes mellitus, the need for insulin during the pre-, intra- and postoperative periods must be considered, even if the patient can usually control blood glucose with oral hypoglycemic agents. The atherosclerosis characteristic in these patients must be considered, as well as their tendency to become severely acidotic during starvation.

Emergency Procedures

The mortality rate in emergency surgery may be as great as five times that for elective procedures (30). Two main factors contribute to this increased mortality rate. First, the patient's tardiness in seeking medical attention results in a more advanced disease process than would be the case had elective repair been performed. Second, the lack of time permitted to control pre-existing disease may result in the patient being brought to the operating room in less than optimal condition. Furthermore, elderly patients have an especially poor tolerance for the complications that are more likely to occur during emergency procedures.

It is imperative, even in emergencies, that sufficient time be taken, albeit with a sense of urgency, to study and prepare these patients adequately. Examples would include preoperative digitalization of patients in congestive failure, correction of electrolyte imbalance, and cross matching and administration of blood to correct significant anemia. Lorhan found that in 60 patients with fractured hips operated upon within 12 hours of the fracture, the mortality rate was 42%; 491 patients operated upon more than 12 hours after the fracture had a 25% mortality rate. Intraoperative circulatory instability was recorded in most of the patients in the under 12-hour group. Treatment of volume deficits, electrolyte imbalance, and cardiac status could be expected to diminish the high mortality rate (31). To stress the need for urgency in adequately preparing the aged patient, Lorhan's study can be compared with that of Davie et al. (32), who found a twofold increase in mortality rate (18.5%) in patients hospitalized more than 48 hours after sustaining a hip fracture, as compared to those admitted within 48 hours following the fracture (8%).

Anesthetic Management

Preoperative Evaluation and Preparation

Careful preoperative evaluation and preparation are essential in managing the geriatric patient. The urgency of the contemplated surgery will of necessity influence the completeness of the preoperative evaluation. Nevertheless, thorough preoperative baseline evaluation of cardiac, pulmonary, renal, and neurologic status is desirable to detect underlying disease.

A complete history is the first requirement. If the patient is unable to provide sufficient coherent information, every effort must be made to obtain it from family, friends, neighbors, or nursing attendants. Especially important is any recent change in mental function. Symptoms of irritability, mental confusion, and severe depression should not be dismissed summarily as being due to organic brain syndrome or "senility." Symptoms of confusion can be caused by underlying systemic illness, especially cardiac or respiratory disease, resulting in inadequate oxygen transport to the brain. Vitamin deficiency and electrolyte imbalance are examples of other pathologic processes that may produce a similar picture. Labeling an ill elderly patient as senile may spell the end of diagnostic or therapeutic endeavor, thereby condemning the patient to a slow death.

As part of the physical examination, formal evaluation of the state of consciousness should always be carried out in the geriatric patient. A specific statement written preoperatively about orientation as to time, place, and person is often useful for postoperative comparison. Laboratory information that should be obtained routinely includes chest x-ray, electrocardiogram, complete blood count, blood urea nitrogen, and electrolyte levels. Additionally, arterial blood gases frequently provide useful information on pulmonary function and may point to the need for further pulmonary function testing. Any other laboratory tests appropriate for pre-existing disease should be obtained.

The importance of maintaining proper blood volume

in order to decrease overall mortality in the elderly has long been appreciated. In these patients, dehydration, anemia, and hypovolemia must be considered together. On admission, a patient may be dehydrated and have a hematocrit level within normal limits; however, rehydration would result in marked anemia and the requirement for preoperative blood transfusion. The patient's response to a tilt test is a useful sign in evaluating volume status. If more than a 10% increase in pulse rate or decrease in systolic blood pressure occurs when the patient sits upright for one minute, a volume deficit is most likely present. Dry mucosa, loss of tissue turgor, and oliguria are later signs of dehydration and hypovolemia. The importance of volume replacement prior to the induction of either a general or regional anesthetic must be emphasized, since both techniques may produce vasodilation. If time permits, correction of hypovolemia should be accomplished slowly to permit adequate adjustments in the patient's circulation. Central venous pressure and pulmonary artery pressure measurement may be useful guidelines in volume replacement. Whether volume deficits should be corrected preoperatively with red blood cells, balanced salt solution, or plasma protein fraction is a matter for debate; this is usually settled by personal preference. It has been our custom to tolerate a hemoglobin level of 10 mg per 100 ml before infusing whole blood or packed cells.

Preanesthetic medication should be used sparingly in the aged. The more ill, the more elderly, the less robust, and less active the patient, the smaller the appropriate doses of sedatives and analgesics. If the patient requires an analgesic for pain, this should be given. However, when a patient's grasp of reality is tenuous, one should not jeopardize that hold with a depressant or disassociative drug. Geriatric patients may be taking many other drugs, which do not fall within the definition of preanesthetic medication, and consideration must be given to whether they should be discontinued prior to induction of anesthesia and surgery.

Anesthetic Technique

General Anesthesia

Both data and clinical experience have documented an inverse relationship between the age and anesthetic requirement. Minimum alveolar concentration decreases from 1.08% halothane in the newborn to 0.64% for the octogenarian (22). In animals, the time for recovery from ether anesthesia has been shown to be markedly increased with advancing age, presumably reflecting a prolonged time for elimination of this inhalation agent by the lungs. The likelihood of prolonged retention times of other inhalation anesthetic agents or of intravenous adjuncts due to slower metabolism must be kept in mind, and reduced doses used initially until the need for larger doses in a given patient has been demonstrated.

General anesthesia can be safe in the elderly patient as long as adequate pulmonary ventilation and tracheobronchial toilet are provided. Indeed, general anesthesia may be the technique of choice even if pulmonary disease is present. General anesthesia in these cases may consist of a small amount of analgesia with a large amount of mechanical ventilation, tracheobronchial toilet, and circulatory support. Hamilton and Sokoll (33) reported on the case of a 75-year-old woman admitted 2 days after sustaining a hip fracture with near total collapse of the left lung. During general anesthesia for repair of the fracture, vigorous tracheobronchial cleansing and positive pressure inflation of the lungs produced dramatic improvement with almost complete clearing on repeat x-ray, demonstrating the efficacy of this technique.

General anesthesia usually involves the balanced use of several agents to produce analgesia, amnesia, sleep, muscle relaxation, and the alteration of reflexes. In many elderly debilitated patients, nitrous oxide inhalation may be sufficient to provide all of the elements of anesthesia with minimal cardiovascular depression. Supplemental barbiturates or narcotics given as premedicants or during anesthesia may provide the necessary balance if nitrous oxide alone is unsatisfactory. In some patients with respiratory disease, the cardiopulmonary effects of anesthesia—decreased functional residual capacity, increased closing volume, mismatching of ventilation and perfusion, and decreased cardiac output—may necessitate a high percentage of inspired oxygen. In these cases, a nitrous oxide/oxygen technique may not suffice. If halogenated agents are required, they will exert cardiovascular depressant actions through direct and reflex depression of myocardial activity and vascular tone.

Muscle relaxants are frequently required. *d*-Tubocurarine has been used effectively but may add the problem of vasodilation with hypotension. Pancuronium is less likely to exert this effect, and also less likely than gallamine to produce tachycardia. Succinylcholine is frequently used by intravenous drip since it is less likely to be associated with hypotension or tachycardia. Volume considerations sometime preclude use of this technique.

One of the most common complications of endotracheal intubation, chipping or dislodging of a tooth, is less prevalent in the aged due to the high incidence of edentulous patients. Whereas less than 20% of the population are edentulous at age 50, approximately 50% of patients above the age of 65 are edentulous. Unfortunately, the anesthetist merely trades one problem for another, since edentulous patients are notorious for their high incidence of upper respiratory obstruction if they are not intubated. We have found that leaving dentures in place is one way of overcoming this problem.

Regional Anesthesia

Gauthier and Hamelburg (34) reviewed the records of 200 patients with hip fractures, half of whom received spinal anesthesia and half general anesthesia; they were unable to find a significant difference in outcome between the two groups. However, regional anesthesia is often recommended in the elderly. The most significant problem in utilizing spinal or epidural anesthesia in the elderly is avoidance of hypotension due to sympathetic blockade. The solution to this problem may be approached in several ways. The lowest level of block consistent with good operating conditions should be used. A T-8 sensory level will provide adequate anesthesia for lower extremity or hip surgery. Since the level of sympathetic blockade is usually several dermatomes above the sensory level, a level higher than T-8 may prevent retention of sufficient sympathetic response to minimize cardiovascular depression. When unilateral sensory block is appropriate, it offers the advantage of a more unilateral sympathetic block, thus permitting more sympathetic reflex compensation. Epidural anesthesia may provide a lower onset of sympathectomy and allow more time for stabilization of blood pressure.

The muscle relaxation provided by spinal or epidural anesthesia may be beneficial in positioning the patient and applying traction for intraoperative maneuvers. Spinal headache is rare in the elderly. Some elderly patients prefer consciousness for fear of losing control of what they feel may be a slim grasp of life. The ability to monitor the sensorium and watch for agitation, restlessness, or confusion may be important in certain situations. Examples include monitoring for symptoms of hypoglycemia in a diabetic patient who is receiving insulin, or observing the need for nitroglycerin in a patient with angina pectoris. Unfortunately, the conscious state may be equally disadvantageous with a hostile, uncooperative patient attempting to get off the table or to move the upper half of his body uncontrollably. With regional anesthesia, this type of patient may require sedative-hypnotics to the point of general anesthesia, without the benefits of general anesthesia—that is, adequate ventilation and an opportunity to provide good tracheobronchial toilet. Furthermore, the sedative drugs may have a lingering effect after the operation, increasing the risk of complications. For such a patient, general anesthesia would be preferable.

Regional nerve block, field block, or local infiltration may be used for surgical procedures suitable for this technique, especially in patients considered too ill for other anesthetic techniques. Advantages include less fluctuation in blood pressure, more rapid ambulation, and a low rate of pulmonary complications. A regional anesthetic may be administered with the patient either in bed or on the operating table. The former procedure makes the move to the table easier if he or she is in pain as often occurs with a hip fracture. However, great care must be taken in monitoring the patient during the transfer.

Monitoring

In addition to routine monitoring of pulse rate, blood pressure, ventilation, and electrocardiogram, monitoring of central venous pressure and temperature should always be considered and is frequently done in the geriatric patient. Such additional monitoring may provide early warning of adverse trends. As adaptability to stress decreases because of limited reserve, it is especially important to avoid wide variations in vital functions. The presence of intraarterial or pulmonary artery catheters can permit direct monitoring of blood pressure, arterial blood gases, pulmonary capillary wedge pressure, and cardiac output, which may further help in early detection of adverse changes.

In every use of invasive monitoring, the benefits to be obtained must be weighed against the associated risks. Intelligent individualization in selection of patients and monitoring techniques is important. If a properly performed Allen's test reveals no abnormalities, the risk of radial artery cannulation is negligible. In our experience, the only two deaths in over 4,000 pulmonary artery catheterizations have been in octogenarians, who comprised a very small percent of that entire population. As a result, we have become extremely conservative in selecting elderly patients for pulmonary artery catheterization.

The often repeated admonition to avoid hypotension merits special comment. Target organs which might be expected to be especially sensitive to low perfusion pressure are the brain and heart. In an analysis of postoperative myocardial infarction in 365 patients with abnormal preoperative EKGs, Mauney et al. (35) found direct correlation between the incidence of infarction and both the length of operative procedure and the occurrence of intraoperative hypotension. While their definition of significant hypotension (30% reduction in the systolic pressure sustained for at least 10 minutes) seems reasonable, the multiple factors influencing blood pressure make any such analysis difficult. For example, the preoperative blood pressure may be elevated abnormally due to pain, and the decrease following induction of anesthesia may be from an elevated pressure rather than from a normal one. Dripps (36) cautioned against overtreatment of anesthesia-induced hypotension, since a moderate amount of hypotension may have some useful consequences. Vasodilation decreases cardiac work. Aggressive treatment with pressor drugs or fluid administration may produce hypertension, which can lead to increased cardiac work, arrhythmias, pulmonary edema, or cerebrovascular accidents. Anesthetists have thus come to fear hypertension as well as hypotension.

Even deliberate hypotension is possible in the elderly. Evaluation of the effects of hypotensive anesthesia on mental function in the elderly has demonstrated no appreciable difference from normotensive anesthesia when the two were compared using refined psychometric tests designed to detect brain damage (37). The issues were best summarized by Dripps (36) who stated that "the dictum should not be to treat a particular mm Hg blood pressure, but to respond appropriately when tissue perfusion is judged insufficient."

Summary

In 1948, Turville and Dripps wrote: "Until recently the aged were so few that little thought was given to them as a group. They were just old people, wise or foolish, feeble or well preserved. By the inescapable statistics of census takers, we are forced now to study the process of aging as well as care for the aged. . . . Anesthesia has much to offer the aged patient and this offer can be made with confidence." In fact, a more recent paper has suggested that nowhere are our geriatric patients safer than in the operating room in the hands of a competent anesthesiologist (6)!

References

1. *Dorland's Illustrated Medical Dictionary*, ed. 26. 1974. Philadelphia: WB Saunders.
2. Ellison, N, and Muravchick, A. 1986. An overview of geriatric anesthesia. *Semin Anesthesia* 5:1–7.
3. Spencer, FC, et al. 1964. Aortic valve replacement in elderly patients with cardiac failure. *JAMA* 189:103–107.
4. Vidne, B, and Levy, MJ. 1970. Heart valve replacement in the elderly patient. *Geriatrics* 25:136–139.
5. Mayo, CW, and Johnson, RA. 1962. Resection of the colon or rectum for malignant neoplasms in patients 80 years of age and older. *Surg Gynecol Obstet* 115:385–391.
6. Miller, R, Marler, K, and Silvay, G. 1977. Anesthesia for patients aged over ninety years. *NY State Med J* 77:1421–1425.
7. Edmunds, LH, Jr., Stephenson, LW, Edie, RN, Ratcliffe, MB. 1988. Open heart surgery in octogenarians. *N Engl J Med* 319:131–136.
8. Glenn, F. 1973. Pre- and postoperative management of elderly surgical patients. *J Am Geriatr Soc* 21:385–393.
9. Fries, JF. 1980. Aging, natural death, and the compression of morbidity. *N Engl J Med* 303:130–135.
10. Schneider, EL, and Brody, JA. 1983. Aging, natural death, and the compression of morbidity. Another view. *N Engl J Med* 309:854–856.
11. Leaf, A. 1973. Getting old. *Sci Am* 229:45–52.
12. Schneider, EL, and Reed, JD, Jr. 1985. Life extension. *N Engl J Med* 312:1159–1168.
13. Shock, NW. 1961. Physiologic aspects of aging. *Annu Rev Physiol* 23:97–122.
14. Comroe, JH, et al. 1962. *The Lung: Clinical Physiology and Pulmonary Function Tests*, ed. 2, pp. 212–213. Chicago: Year Book Medical Publishers.
15. Richards, DW. 1965. Pulmonary Changes Due to Aging. In *Handbook of Physiology: Respiration*, Eds., WO Fenn and H Rahn, pp. 1525–1529, vol 2. Washington, DC: American Physiological Society.
16. Ellison, N. 1975. Problems in geriatric anesthesia. *Surg Clin North Am* 55:929–945.
17. Smith, TC. 1986. Respiratory effects of aging. *Semin Anesthesia* 5:14–22.
18. Geer, RT. 1986. Cardiac effects of aging. *Semin Anesthesia* 5:23–30.
19. Evans, TI. 1983. The physiologic bases of geriatric general anesthesia. *Anaesth Intens Care* 1:319–322.
20. Epstein, M, and Hollenberg, M. 1976. Age as a determinant of renal sodium conservation in normal man. *J Lab Clin Med* 87:411–417.
21. Bromage, PR. 1969. Ageing and epidural dose requirements. *Br J Anaesth* 41:1016–1022.
22. Gregory, GA, Eger, EI, and Munson, ES. 1969. The relationship between age and halothane requirement in man. *Anesthesiology* 30:488–491.
23. Bender, AD. 1974. Pharmacodynamic principles of drug therapy in the aged. *J Am Geriatr Soc* 22:296–303.
24. Thompson, EN, and Williams, R. 1965. Effects of age on liver function with particular reference to bromsulphalein excretion. *Gut* 6:266–269.
25. Geokas, MC, and Javerback, BJ. 1969. The Aging Gastrointestinal Tract. *Am J Surg* 11:881–892.
26. Hurwitz, N. 1969. Predisposing factors and adverse reactions to drugs. *Br Med J* 1:536–539.
27. Muravchick, S, and Mandel, J. 1982. Thiopental sleep dosages in geriatric patients. *Anesthesiology* 57:A327.
28. Freund, PF, et al. 1982. Comparative lidocaine pharmacokinetics in caudal anesthesia in young and geriatric patients. *Anesthesiology* 57:A212.
29. Cogbill, CL. 1967. Operation in the aged: Mortality related to concurrent disease, duration of anesthesia and elective or emergency operation. *Arch Surg* 94:202–205.
30. Jegathesan, S, and Whitehill, JL. 1971. Surgery in the elderly. *Postgrad Med* 49:211–215.
31. Lorhan, PH, and Shelby, EA. 1964. Factors influencing mortality in hip fractures. *Anesth Analg (Cleve)* 43:539–543.
32. Davie, IT, McRae, WR, and Malcolm-Smith, NA. 1970. Anesthesia for the fractured hip–a survey of 200 cases. *Anesth Analg (Cleve)* 49:165–170.
33. Hamilton, WK, and Sokoll, MD. 1966. Choice of anesthetic technique in patients with acute pulmonary disease. *JAMA* 197:136.
34. Gauthier, JL, and Hamelburg, W. 1963. Hip fractures: Influence of anesthesia on the patient's hospital course. *Anesth Analg (Cleve)* 42:609–615.
35. Mauney, FJ, Ebert, PA, and Sabiston, DC. 1970. Postoperative myocardial infarction: A study of predisposing

factors, diagnosis, and mortality in a high risk group of surgical patients. *Ann Surg* 172:497–503.

36. Dripps, RD. 1970. Discussion following: Mauney FM, Albert, PA, and Sabiston, DC. Postoperative myocardial infarction. *Ann Surg* 172:497–503.

37. Rollason, N, et al. 1971. A comparison of mental function in relation to hypotensive and normotensive anaesthesia in the elderly. *Br J Anaesth* 43:561–566.

23

Perioperative Monitoring and Management of Normal, Stressed, and Elderly High-Risk Patients

William C. Shoemaker and Harry B. Kram

Shock

Traditional Approach to Shock

Traditional etiologic classifications of shock syndromes, which include hemorrhagic, cardiogenic, traumatic and septic shock, provide the basis for description, physiologic evaluation, and therapy. Clinical signs and symptoms, laboratory findings, and primary pathophysiologic derangements are listed for each of these etiologic types of shock (Table 23-1). From this analysis, therapeutic principles may be developed for each etiologic type. This approach assumes that each cause of shock has a characteristic clinical picture and diagnostic laboratory pattern; therapeutic principles are developed from this etiologic classification. This traditional approach is simple, clear, logical, straightforward, readily understandable, and wrong. The problem with this concept of shock is that real life is not this simple. Each primary etiologic event does not begin and end with a single pathophysiologic defect, which when corrected reverses the downhill lethal course.

The primary precipitating event of shock produces numerous physiologic compensatory reactions and decompensations that lead to lethal multiple organ failure. In hemorrhage, for instance, reduced blood volume reduces flow and oxygen (O_2) transport; in cardiogenic shock, diminished flow reduces blood pressure and oxygen transport. Traumatic and septic shock provoke increased flow, but these flow increases may not be adequate for the associated increased metabolism. Irrespective of the precipitating etiologic event, the interacting circulatory alterations of volume, flow, and oxygen transport lead to circulatory insufficiency, cardiac failure, shock, and death.

This traditional approach unfortunately leads to simplistic, one-dimensional therapy. Although each primary etiologic event affects the circulatory system in a unique way, there are a limited number of compensatory reactions, decompensations, and terminal pathways. A useful therapeutic plan must address the major problem produced by the primary event as well as the interaction of this primary event with compensatory and decompensatory responses. Maximally effective therapy must address all components of the disturbed circulation. A tire blowout that results in an automobile wreck is not corrected by replacement of the tire. The appropriate management of shock is to: (*a*) analyze the primary event in terms of circulatory dimensions, (*b*) describe the various clinical types of shock in terms of the temporal pattern of the primary event and its compensations, and (*c*) describe circulatory patterns of survivors and nonsurvivors in terms that will define criteria for therapy. An effective, coherent

Table 23-1. Approach to various etiologic types of shock

Hemorrhagic	Cardiogenic	Traumatic	Septic
Signs and symptoms			
Pallor, fainting	Pallor, fainting	History of injury	Fever, chills
Skin clammy, cold	Skin clammy, cold	Physical evidence of injury, fractures	Skin warm
Tachycardia	Arrhythmias	Oliguria	Tachycardia
Oliguria	Oliguria	Tachycardia	Oliguria
Collapse	Collapse	Collapse	Altered mental status
			Collapse
Laboratory			
↓ Hct, Hgb	↓ Cardiac enzymes	X-rays, CT scan	Positive smears and cultures
	ECG	Angiograms for organ and vascular injury	
Pathophysiology			
↓ Blood volume	↓ Cardiac output	Direct injury to organs and tissue	↓ Peripheral resistance
Therapy			
Fluids	Antiarrhythmics	Repair injuries	Antibiotics
Blood	Vasopressors	Fluids	Fluids
Control bleeding	Vasodilators	Blood	Drain abscesses

physiologic plan for therapy may be generated from analysis of the survivors' patterns (1–8).

In a large series of high-risk postoperative patients, the commonly monitored variables were restored to normal values in 75% of the survivors as compared with 76% of the nonsurvivors (Table 23-2) (4, 9). These variables are poor criteria for monitoring or predicting survival since they are not related to outcome. Unfortunately, mean arterial pressure (MAP), heart rate (HR), central venous pressure (CVP), urine output, hematocrit (Hct), arterial (PaO_2), and mixed venous oxygen tension ($P\bar{v}O_2$) are not well correlated with outcome (2–9).

Blood pressure, heart rate (HR), cardiac output, venous inflow pressures, stroke volume, stroke work, change in pressure over time (dP/dt), ejection fraction, and wall motion are used to measure cardiac hemodynamics. However, these extremely important measurements focus primarily on cardiac functions, which represent only one aspect of circulatory function. The basic function of the circulation is not cardiac hemodynamics, but transport of gases, nutrients, and other blood constituents; this is best tracked by the bulk movement and utilization of oxygen.

Table 23-2. Number and percent of patients with two or more values in the normal range

	Nonsurvivors		Survivors	
	Number	%	Number	%
Mean arterial pressure	29	78	68	89
Heart rate	30	81	66	87
Central venous pressure	35	95	72	95
Pulmonary wedge pressure	11	30	21	28
Cardiac index	35	95	64	84
Mean of these variables		76		75

Pathophysiology of Shock

The shock syndrome is a symptom complex whose recognition and diagnosis is based on signs and symptoms. As such, definitions and diagnoses are subjective and arbitrary. When definitions are imprecise, communications across disciplines and between institutions become difficult. Comparisons between clinical series of uncertain and heterogeneous composition become meaningless, and attempts to conceptualize shock pathophysiology are ambiguous and not generally accepted.

Hypotension is often the first clinically recognized manifestation of shock, but when hypotension is prevented or treated early by vasopressors, the pathophysiologic problem may be obscured until lethal complications occur.

The pathophysiology of clinical shock produced by hemorrhage, cardiac problems, accidental and surgical trauma, sepsis, and various combinations of these etiologies may be described by sequential changes in serial measurements of hemodynamic and oxygen transport variables obtained before therapy was begun or after the immediate direct effects of therapy were over.

Monitored physiologic variables can be readily and repeatedly obtained using a systemic arterial and a balloon-tipped pulmonary arterial (Swan-Ganz) catheter (1–10). Frequently repeated measurements of arterial and venous pressures in the systemic and pulmonary circulations, cardiac output, arterial and mixed venous gases, and hemoglobin or hematocrit (Hct) permit a number of directly measured and calculated hemodynamic variables, including cardiac index (CI), systemic and pulmonary vascular resistance index (SVRI and PVRI), left and right ventricular stroke work (LVSW, RVSW), and left and right cardiac work (LCW, RCW). When arterial and mixed venous gases are measured simultaneously with hemodynamic variables, it is possible to determine the bulk movement of oxygen: O_2 delivery ($\dot{D}O_2$), and O_2 consumption ($\dot{V}O_2$), as well as O_2 extraction, pulmonary venous admixture or shunting ($\dot{Q}sp/\dot{Q}t$), and the alveolar-arterial O_2 gradient ($P(A\text{-}a)O_2$). These variables can be readily calculated by a computer or a hand-held programmable calculator (Table 23-3).

Distinct cardiorespiratory patterns describe the natural history of the various clinical shock syndromes and characterize their pathophysiology. The confounding effects of various associated medical conditions and therapeutic interventions may be addressed by evaluating de-

Table 23-3. Cardiorespiratory variables: abbreviations, units, calculations, normal values, and preferred values; predictive capacity

Variables	Abbreviations	Units	Measurements or calculations	Normal values	Preferred values	Percent correct
Volume-related						
Mean arterial pressure	MAP	mm Hg	Direct measurement	82–102	> 84	76
Central venous pressure	CVP	cm H_2O	Direct measurement	1–9	< 5	62
Central blood volume	CBV	ml/m^2	CBV = MTT × CI × 16.7	660–1,000	> 925	61
Stroke index	SI	ml/m^2	SI = CI/HR	30–50	> 48	67
Hemoglobin	Hgb	g/dl	Direct measurement	12–16	> 12	66
Mean pulmonary artery pressure	MPAP	mm Hg	Direct measurement	11–15	< 19	68
Wedge pressure	WP	mm Hg	Direct measurement	0–12	> 9.5	70
Blood volume	BV	ml/m^2	BV = PV/(1 − Hct)^a × surface area	Men 2.74 Women 2.37	> 3.0 > 2.7	76
Red cell mass	RCM	ml/m^2	RCM = BV − PV	Men 1.1 Women 0.95	> 1.1	85
Flow-related						
Cardiac index	CI	liter/min•m^2	Direct measurement	2.8–3.6	> 4.5	70
Left vent stroke work	LVSW	g•M/m^2	LVSW = SI × MAP × 0.0144	44–68	> 55	74
Left cardiac work	LCW	kg•M/m^2	LCW = CI × MAP × 0.0144	3–4.6	> 5	76
Right vent stroke work	RVSW	g•M/m^2	RVSW = SI × MPAP × 0.0144	4–8	> 13	70
Right cardiac work	RCW	kg•M/m^2	RCW = CI × MPAP × 0.0144	0.4–0.6	> 1.1	69
Stress-related						
Systemic vasc resist	SVRI	dyne•s/cm^5•m^2	SVR = 79.92 (MAP − CVP)^b/CI	1,760–2,600	> 1,450	62
Pulmonary vasc resist	PVRI	dyne•s/cm^5•m^2	PVR = 79.92 (MPAP − WP)^b/CI	45–225	< 226	77
Heart rate	HR	beat/min	Direct measurement	72–88	< 100	60
Rectal temperature	temp	°F	Direct measurement	97.8–98.6	> 100.4	64
Oxygen-related						
Hemoglobin saturation	SaO_2	%	Direct measurement	95–99	> 95	67
Arterial CO_2 tension	$PaCO_2$	torr	Direct measurement	36–44	> 30	69
Arterial pH	pH	. . .	Direct measurement	7.36–7.44	> 7.47	74
Mixed venous O_2 tension	PvO_2	torr	Direct measurement	33–53	> 36	68
Arterial-mixed venous O_2 content difference	$C(a-v)O_2$	ml/dl	$C(a-v)O_2 = CaO_2 - CvO_2$	4–5.5	< 3.5	68
O_2 delivery	DO_2	ml/min•m^2	$DO_2 = CaO_2 \times CI \times 10$	520–720	> 550	76
O_2 consumption	VO_2	ml/min•m^2	$VO_2 = C(a-v)O_2 \times CI \times 10$	100–180	> 167	69
O_2 extraction rate	O_2 ext	%	$O_2\ ext = (CaO_2 - CvO_2)/\ CaO_2$	22–30	< 31	69

vasc resist = vascular resistance.

[a] Hematocrit: (Hct) value corrected for packing fraction and large vessel hematocrit to total body ratio.

[b] Venous pressures expressed in mm Hg.

veloping physiologic patterns of shock in patients with only one etiologic event as well as in patients with various combinations of etiologies and associated medical conditions (1–4).

Primary Pathophysiologic Mechanisms

Reduced oxygen consumption ($\dot{V}O_2$) was found to be the common denominator in each of these syndromes and the earliest pathogenic event, which occurred during or before the initial hypotensive crisis (1–9). From the physiologic viewpoint, reduced or inadequate $\dot{V}O_2$, which limits body metabolism and therefore may compromise survival, is the common pathophysiologic defect. It may be produced by: (*a*) low blood flow from cardiogenic shock and hemorrhage or other causes of hypovolemia; (*b*) maldistribution of flow particularly at the microcirculatory level from uneven vasoconstriction, neurohormonal mechanisms, and various mediator-induced responses; and (*c*) increased metabolic need (demand) exceeding the delivery (supply). In essence, the basic physiologic problem in acute circulatory crises is the imbalance between the supply ($\dot{D}O_2$) and demand of oxygen ($\dot{V}O_2$) as well as various nutrients transported by the circulation (1–9).

There is abundant evidence that: (*a*) oxygen transport is the major function of the circulation; (*b*) oxygen is the most flow-dependent blood constituent because it has the largest extraction ratio; (*c*) since oxygen cannot be stored, the net O_2 transported is the amount consumed by the tissues, and therefore it may be easily and repeatedly measured; and (*d*) oxygen transport is strongly related to survival or death (1–12). Thus, tissue perfusion, which reflects overall circulatory function, may be evaluated in terms of $\dot{V}O_2$ and oxygen delivery ($\dot{D}O_2$), which is calculated as the product of cardiac index (CI) and arterial O_2 content (Table 23-3).

Reduced or inadequate VO_2 is the common denominator of shock syndromes. More importantly, it is greater and more prolonged in patients who die than in those who survive. This was first suggested by Guyton and colleagues (10, 11), who found that when the cumulative deficit of $\dot{V}O_2$ in hemorrhaged dogs exceeded 140 ml/kg, all died; at 120 ml/kg, 50% died; and at < 100 ml/kg, all lived. This suggests that reduced or inadequate $\dot{V}O_2$ is not just associated with the development of shock, but the degree of $\dot{V}O_2$ deficit is associated with multiple organ failure and death. Recent evidence in clinical conditions indicates that inadequate $\dot{V}O_2$ also is a major determinant of outcome and, as such, it is the major pathogenic factor in the development of multiple organ failure and shock syndromes (3, 4, 8, 12).

The physiologic compensatory responses to the reduced $\dot{V}O_2$ include increased heart rate, increased myocardial contractility, increased cardiac output, hyperpnea, tachypnea, increased O_2 extraction rate, and altered vascular tone. These compensatory reactions to inadequate $\dot{V}O_2$ are usually the most apparent manifestations of shock syndromes and are often the first recognized clinical features. Unfortunately, these superficial manifestations, recognized for their association with the initial appearance of shock syndromes, may be misconstrued as being the essential problem of the shock syndrome, and therefore, therapy may be inappropriately and ineffectively directed against the compensations rather than the primary pathophysiology. The crucial missing information is the failure to define primary mechanisms of shock and to differentiate these from the compensatory responses that have survival value. When these important distinctions are ignored, therapy is directed against superficial manifestations of the shock syndromes.

Basic Concepts of Acute Circulatory Failure

Several concepts have been suggested by physiologic descriptions: the first is that reduced or inadequate $\dot{V}O_2$ leading to tissue hypoxia is the primary pathogenic mechanism for the shock syndromes. Second, $\dot{D}O_2$, the "supply-side" of the equation, may limit $\dot{V}O_2$ by either low flow, which occurs with hemorrhage and cardiogenic shock, unevenly distributed flow, which occurs with trauma and sepsis, or greater metabolic requirements that are present with severe trauma, sepsis, cirrhosis, and other hyperdynamic states. The third concept is that $\dot{V}O_2$ is the regulatory mechanism of circulatory failure in that decrements in $\dot{V}O_2$ stimulate compensations, including increases in heart rate, myocardial contractility, cardiac output, and increased respiratory functions. These two oxygen transport variables represent an exquisitely sensitive method for evaluating systemic perfusion: (*a*) $\dot{D}O_2$, the circulatory delivery system's ability to supply the required nutrients, and (*b*) $\dot{V}O_2$, the overall metabolic status (3, 4, 8, 12).

Circulatory Interactions

An appropriate and readily understandable conceptualization of the circulatory dynamics of shock syndromes will include the fundamental dimensions that physically characterize fluid systems: pressure, volume, flow, and function; the latter is best characterized by $\dot{V}O_2$. Figure 23-1 schematically represents each of these four dimensions as one side of a four-sided figure; the length of each dimension is represented as a percentage of the normal values. In the normal circulation, these dimensions may be represented as a square. This figure also illustrates average changes in these dimensions observed in a large series of patients with compensated septic shock. Figure 23-2

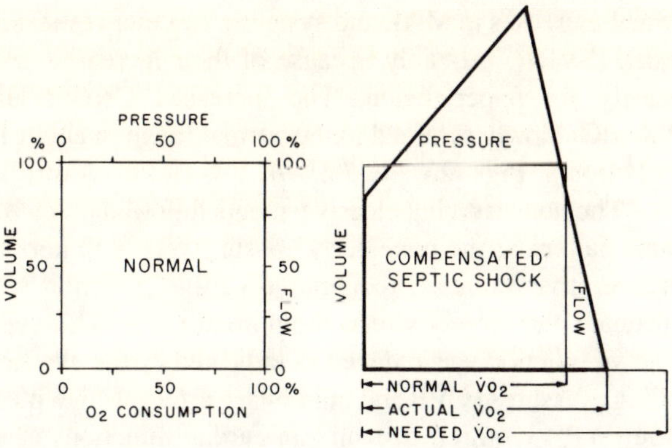

Figure 23-1. Left: Normal circulatory dimensions representing pressure, volume, flow, and function ($\dot{V}O_2$). Right: Average values of patients with compensated septic shock. The normal values shown by the fine lines of the square may be compared to the thicker lines representing changes of compensated septic shock, i.e., slightly decreased arterial pressure and blood volume due to dehydration and fever, as well as increased flow and $\dot{V}O_2$. The lower horizontal dimension representing $\dot{V}O_2$ shows the normal value, the actual observed mean value, and the $\dot{V}O_2$ values needed because of increased metabolism. (From Shoemaker (3) with permission.)

illustrates the interactions among circulatory dimensions produced by the primary event, the compensatory responses, the failure of compensatory responses (decompensation), and the terminal episode. These interactions may be illustrated in each of the common types of shock (3).

In hemorrhage, volume initially has the greatest reduction, but the other three dimensions are secondarily affected, although to a lesser extent (13). After volume therapy to restore normal or slightly greater than normal plasma volume, pressure is restored to the normal range, but compensatory flow responses and $\dot{V}O_2$ responses are considerably greater than normal, especially in the survivors. With decompensation of the nonsurvivors, the pressure, flow and $\dot{V}O_2$ fall; they continue to fall in the terminal state until death occurs.

The primary problem in cardiogenic shock is reduced flow, which secondarily affects pressure and $\dot{V}O_2$; some degree of hypovolemia may be present in acute myocardial infarction patients because of dehydration from nausea, vomiting, sweating, inadequate fluid intake, and diuretic therapy. Vasopressors together with compensations may restore pressure and flow. $\dot{V}O_2$ also may be increased because of the O_2 debt from earlier reductions in $\dot{V}O_2$ to levels below the actual metabolic need. In survivors, O_2 extraction and $\dot{V}O_2$ increased to meet the increased need; in nonsurvivors at the terminal state all dimensions progressively decreased.

With trauma, the blood volume, pressure and $\dot{V}O_2$ fall, while flow may be initially reduced. However, there is often an early compensatory flow increase. In the fully

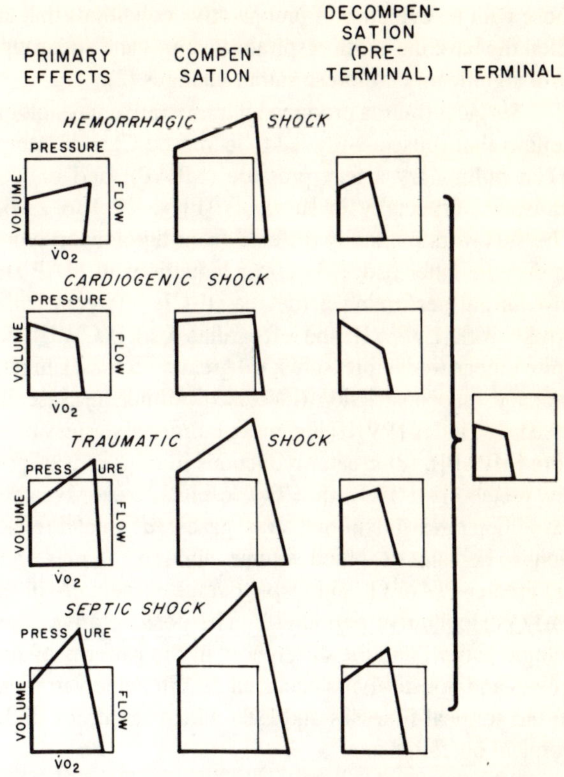

Figure 23-2. Circulatory dimensions of patients with various etiologic types of shock: The circulatory dimensions in various types of shock are schematically shown in Figure 23-2, hemorrhagic (upper tier), cardiogenic (second tier), traumatic (third tier), and septic shock (lowest tier). The initial primary changes of each etiologic type of shock are shown in the left column; the mean values of compensated shock are shown in the second column; the preterminal decompensations are shown in the third column; and the terminal state, which is often very similar in each etiologic type of shock, is shown on the extreme right.

compensated state, flow and $\dot{V}O_2$ are markedly increased. All four dimensions decrease with decompensation and even more in the terminal state.

In sepsis, pressure, volume, and $\dot{V}O_2$ decrease when there is dehydration, but with compensations, there are marked increases in flow and $\dot{V}O_2$; the latter is due to increased metabolic demands. With decompensation and also in the terminal state, all dimensions decrease (3).

Monitoring and Management of the Critically Ill Surgical Patient

Hemodynamic and Oxygen Transport Patterns in Patients with Normal Preoperative Values

To characterize the effects of surgical trauma without the problems of associated preoperative illnesses, 220 consecutively monitored high-risk patients were divided into those with no evidence of preoperative conditions that altered the baseline cardiorespiratory values and subgroups with significant cardiorespiratory changes (2).

Surgical trauma produced intraoperative physiologic deficits that subsequently led to increased CI, HR, temp, mean pulmonary artery pressure (MPAP), and oxygen transport, especially in survivors (Figs. 23-3 to 23-6). The survivors markedly differed from the nonsurvivors, in that the latter had: (*a*) greater reductions in MAP and myocardial performance (decreased CI, left ventricular stroke work [LVSWI], and left cardiac work [LCWI]), despite higher wedge pressures; (*b*) greater increases in pulmonary vasoconstriction (increased pulmonary vascular resistance index [PVRI] and mean pulmonary artery pressure [MPAP]); (*c*) greater reductions in oxygen transport and metabolism ($\dot{D}O_2$ and $\dot{V}O_2$) despite increased oxygen extraction rates and normal blood gases; (*d*) greater reductions in hematocrit, blood volume, and red cell mass; and (*e*) greater $P(A\text{-}a)O_2$ and $\dot{Q}sp/\dot{Q}t$ values especially in the early postoperative period (14). The postoperative physiologic pattern and the differences in the patterns of survivors and nonsurvivors occurred despite wide variations in the surgical illnesses and even wider variations in the surgical operations.

Specific Patient Categories

The Elderly Patient

Preoperatively, the hemodynamic and oxygen transport patterns of the elderly (> 65 years) patients for the most part were similar to the nonelderly (< 65 years) preoperative patient with normal values. The limitations in their cardiac and pulmonary function probably had been adequately compensated. Preoperatively and at their lowest point, the CI, $\dot{V}O_2$ and $\dot{D}O_2$ values of the elderly surviving patients were only slightly less than those of the nonelderly survivors with normal preoperative values; the elderly also had mild elevations in MPAP and right cardiac work (RCWI) (Figs. 23-7 and 23-8).

The elderly survivors' intraoperative and postoperative responses to surgical trauma were similar to those of the non-elderly survivors; however, these responses were somewhat blunted, probably reflecting some limitation of pulmonary and cardiac reserve functions and because their inherent metabolic needs may have been less. For example, the nonelderly patients had CI responses that averaged 40% greater than normal, while the elderly increased CI by 20%, and these values remained near the normal range. The elderly increased their $\dot{V}O_2$ an average of 55%; about half of this was supplied by the increased CI and $\dot{D}O_2$ and half by increased O_2 extraction. Unlike the nonelderly survivors, the elderly had early and sustained increases in MAP and systemic vascular resistance index (SVRI), probably because of their increased propensity for hypertension. The increased $\dot{Q}sp/\dot{Q}t$ and $P(A\text{-}a)O_2$ slowly returned to the normal range in about 12 to 24 hours (Figs. 23-7 and 23-8).

The nonsurviving elderly patients followed much the same pattern as the nonelderly nonsurvivors with normal preoperative values. Preoperative cardiac function was adequate and largely within the normal range. However, reserve function was reduced as indicated by the elevated filling pressures (CVP and pulmonary artery wedge pressure [WP]) required to maintain cardiac functions at or just slightly above normal. For example, LVSWI was substantially below normal values, while LCWI was within the normal range but only because of an elevated HR. Measurements of MPAP, $\dot{Q}sp/\dot{Q}t$, and $P(A\text{-}a)O_2$ were high preoperatively in the elderly probably as a result of prior illnesses, other stresses, or the aging process itself. Moreover, the elderly nonsurvivors tended to maintain these abnormally high values throughout their postoperative course (Figs. 23-7 and 23-8).

In essence, postoperative stress responses in the elderly were similar to the nonelderly patients in that there was increased cardiac function in response to surgical stress. They differ in that this augmented CI and LCWI did not exceed the normal range of values. This pattern of minimal cardiac function augmentation in elderly survivors and nonsurvivors was similar to that of the nonelderly nonsurvivors. The most striking cardiac function variable in the elderly patients was LVSWI, which remained low preoperatively and postoperatively, only transiently rising to within the normal range. A consistent pattern present in nonsurvivors was the fall in $\dot{D}O_2$, which despite compensatory increases in O_2 extraction, was not adequate to maintain $\dot{V}O_2$ at an optimal level.

Patterns in Patients with Preoperative Sepsis, Severe Trauma, and Advanced Cirrhosis

Patients who preoperatively had systemic manifestations of sepsis, severe stress from accidental injury, and advanced cirrhosis often had high cardiac output preoperatively. Postoperatively, pronounced increases in MAP, CI, $\dot{D}O_2$ and $\dot{V}O_2$ were observed in the survivors, with minimal changes in CVP, WP, MPAP, and PVRI. By contrast, the nonsurviving patients in these groups had little or no increases in CI, $\dot{D}O_2$, $\dot{V}O_2$ and flow-related variables despite higher CVP and WP. The PVRI and $\dot{Q}sp/\dot{Q}t$ were also higher in the nonsurvivors. In essence, they started from higher baseline cardiac output values preoperatively, but the patterns of changes of the survivors and nonsurvivors were similar to those with normal preoperative values (3, 5).

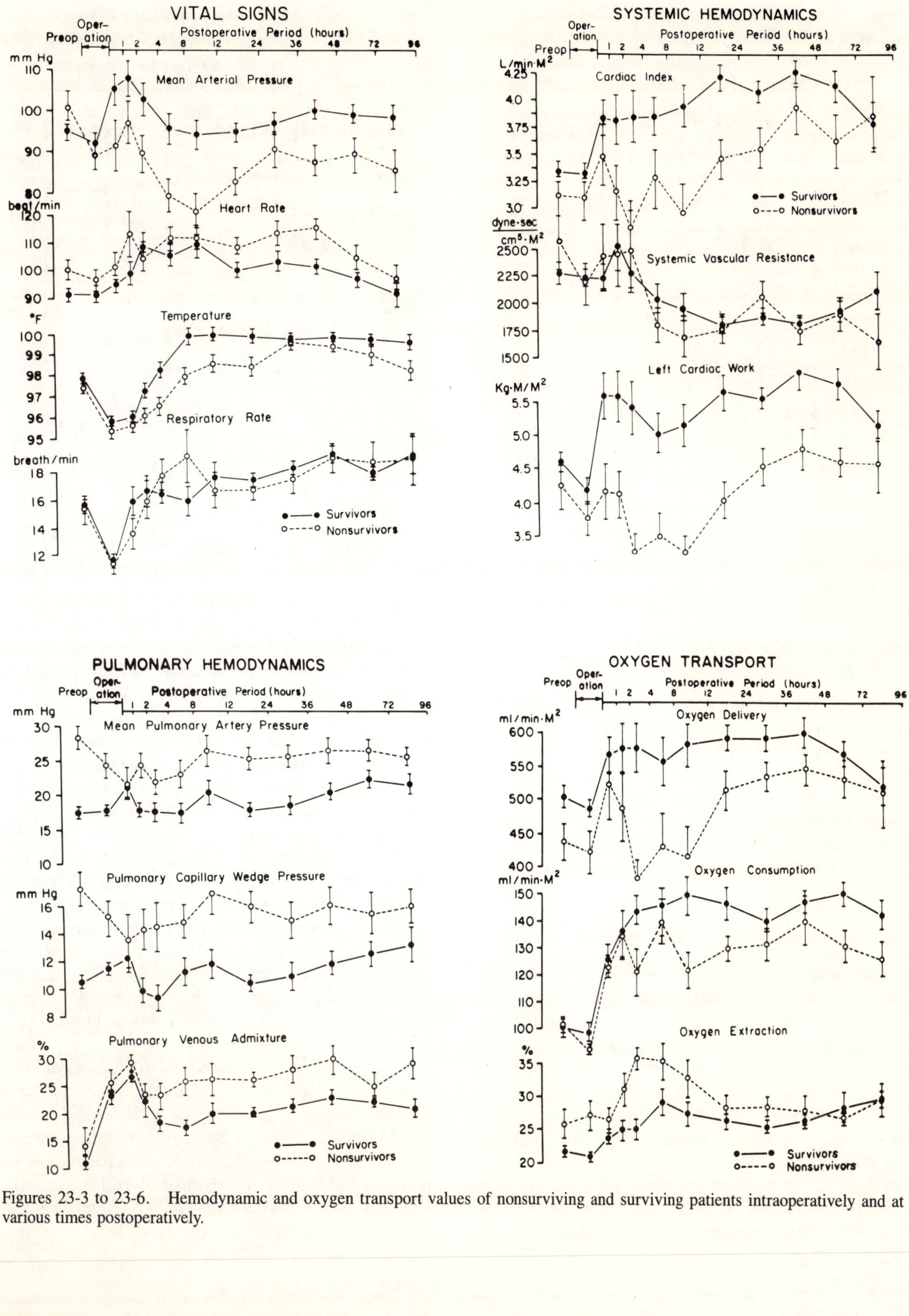

Figures 23-3 to 23-6. Hemodynamic and oxygen transport values of nonsurviving and surviving patients intraoperatively and at various times postoperatively.

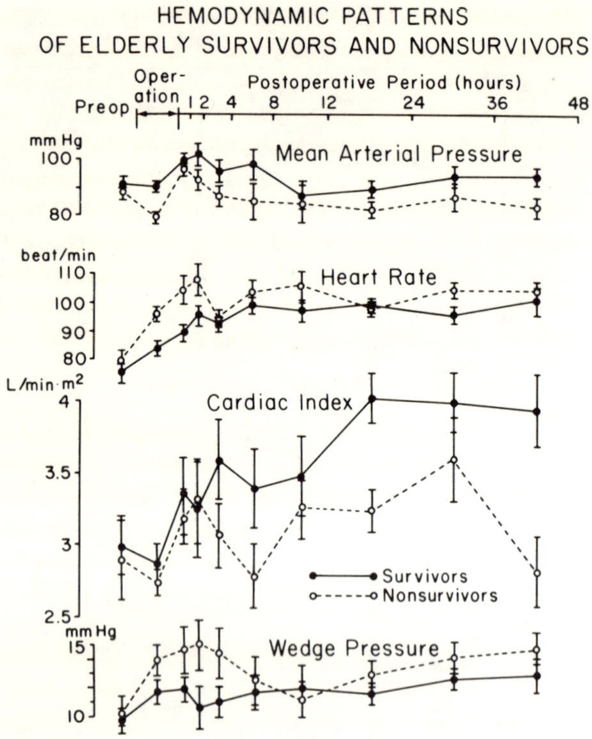

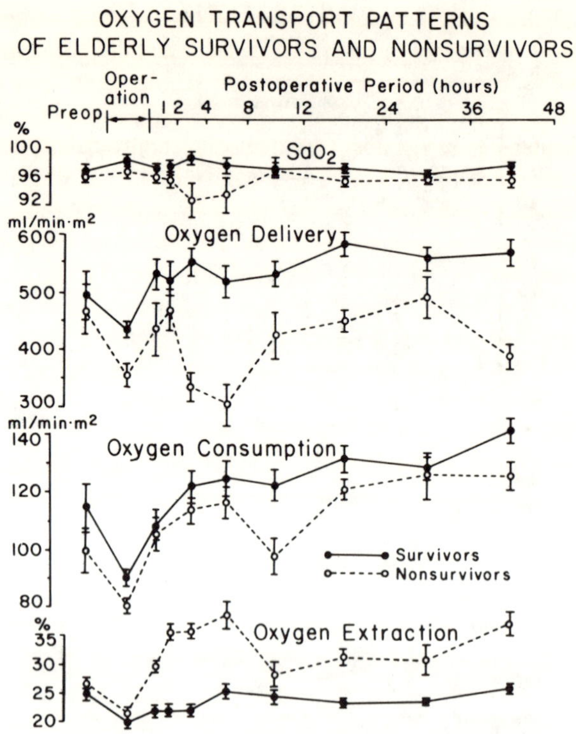

Figures 23-7 and 23-8. Hemodynamic and oxygen transport values in survivors and nonsurvivors who were elderly, had trauma, sepsis, shock, or cirrhosis.

Patterns in Patients with Preoperative Congestive Heart Failure or Shock

Preoperatively critically ill patients who had congestive failure or shock usually have the classic findings of low cardiac output, high WP, hypotension, reduced $\dot{D}O_2$ and low $\dot{V}O_2$. In the postoperative period, the average CI, $\dot{D}O_2$, and $\dot{V}O_2$ values of survivors predominantly increased with few exceptions. By contrast, the nonsurvivors had lower CI, $\dot{D}O_2$ and $\dot{V}O_2$ despite high WP; they also had significantly increased PVRI and $\dot{Q}sp/\dot{Q}t$ (3, 5).

Significance of Cardiorespiratory Patterns

Cardiovascular measurements have been increasingly used to monitor the surgical patient and to describe physiologic events during and after various surgical diseases and surgical operations. Presumably, patients have a finite number of physiologic compensatory responses to the various surgical diseases and to surgical trauma itself. These circulatory responses, developed in lower animals over time, have survival value. A comparison of physiologic patterns of the patients who have responded successfully to the stress of surgery with those who have died, provide insight into the nature and relevance of these cardiorespiratory compensations (3, 4, 8, 12).

Preoperatively, patients with advanced age or with underlying severe medical illnesses, such as cardiac failure, sepsis, hemorrhagic shock, trauma, nutritional debility, and cirrhosis, may have abnormal preoperative cardiorespiratory values and significantly greater risks of mortality and morbidity. Their postoperative cardiorespiratory patterns are similar, but they begin from different preoperative baselines. The survivors develop physiologic compensations for intraoperative tissue hypoxia including increased CI, $\dot{D}O_2$, and $\dot{V}O_2$, but the nonsurvivors are poorly compensated for oxygen deficits.

Induction of anesthesia is a stress on cardiovascular mechanics; inhaled anesthetics are known to depress myocardial function and to modify neural control of vascular tone. Besides having neural and vascular effects, anesthesia affects cellular function, which is reflected by diminished basal metabolic rate and $\dot{V}O_2$; this decline in $\dot{V}O_2$ is indicative of a tissue oxygen debt.

In the intraoperative period and to some extent in the immediate postoperative period, there may be minimal or variable compensatory responses because of the combined metabolic effects of anesthesia, including low cardiac output and low oxygen delivery with resultant tissue ischemia and hypoxia. Poorly maintained local vascular tone may lead to uneven distribution of flow in the systemic circulation further compromising local tissue metabolism. Tissue trauma causes leakage of fluid volume from the intravascular to the extracellular compartments, while hemorrhage produces hypovolemia; both lead to reduced intravascular loss, reduced cardiac output, and inadequate oxygen delivery that compromises tissue perfusion and limits $\dot{V}O_2$. These major life-threatening circulatory problems stimulate physiologic compensations that result in greater than normal cardiac and respiratory function. In short, surviving patients respond to surgical stress with compensatory reactions that restore tissue oxygenation and reduce mortality and morbidity (1–5).

In the clinical setting, a departure from the normal range may indicate a compensatory response, an unnoticed complication, a new physiologic process, or cardiorespiratory deterioration of the patient. For this reason, it is important to examine data obtained from patients with uncomplicated preoperative states and normal values in order to describe the basic response to surgical trauma not confounded by other medical problems. Characteristic patterns of survival and nonsurvival observed in a wide variety of surgical illnesses and surgical operations are responses to the stress of operative trauma plus the effects of anesthetics, blood and fluid losses, temperature, metabolic, and neurohormonal changes. Other patients with associated medical conditions may also be examined with regard to outcome patterns. Comparison of data from subsets of patients with different disease processes may also reveal important information on the pathophysiology of specific disease processes. Most nonsurvivors died of organ failure and other complications of their surgical trauma because of an inability to compensate for the added metabolic and cardiorespiratory demands of their postoperative state (12).

Relative Importance of Hemodynamic and Oxygen Transport Variables

The capacity to predict outcome is the most rigorous criterion for assessing the biologic importance of each cardiorespiratory variable. The monitored variables are most closely related to outcome in providing crucial information on the basic pathophysiology of shock syndromes and therefore must be considered for therapeutic management. In the aforementioned study, variables reflecting oxygen transport were found to have the greatest capacity to predict outcome and therefore were of utmost clinical importance (1–9). If a variable has little or no relation to outcome, then it should not have an important part in therapeutic decisions. The commonly monitored variables suggest where the patient has been, not where he is going.

$\dot{V}O_2$ increases about 30% in the uncomplicated general surgical postoperative patient. However, the postoperative increases in $\dot{V}O_2$ values with severe trauma, stress, sepsis, and hypercatabolic states may be considerably greater, indicating greater metabolic demands. The increased $\dot{V}O_2$ does not mean that all the patient's metabolic needs have been met. The adequacy of therapy cannot be measured directly, but tissue demand may be inferred indirectly by an empirical trial of therapy. Increased CI, $\dot{D}O_2$, and $\dot{V}O_2$ means that therapy opened up additional microcirculatory channels that perfused relatively hypoxic tissues, which then extracted more oxygen. Since tissues cannot take up more oxygen than they use, the increased $\dot{V}O_2$ after fluid challenge indicates a prior oxygen debt that was at least partially relieved.

Clinical Evaluation of Blood Volume Status

Restoration of blood volume is the most important goal in the treatment of shock and its sequelae, but criteria for achieving this goal have not been objectively defined. Experimental studies in anesthetized dogs subjected to sudden hemorrhage have been used to develop criteria for MAP, HR, CVP, WP, and Hct values to assess the blood volume status in patients. Unfortunately, the actual values on acute blood loss in anesthetized animals is not representative of most ICU patients, whose venous wall tension, over a period of time, accommodates to both excess blood volume and hypovolemia by CVP and WP that are usually in the range of 8–15 mm Hg (13). Most clinical reports have been inadequately controlled and have had poor documentation of blood volume status, although CVP and WP had fallen abruptly with acute hypovolemia. However, in critically ill postoperative patients, these commonly used clinical criteria were shown to be unreliable when compared with careful measurements of blood volume (13).

Therapeutic Goals

In acute catastrophes, fluid therapy is the first priority to restore blood volume. Therapeutic goals may be defined empirically from the median values for each cardiorespiratory variable of the survivors (2–8). Thus, therapy should restore physiologic defects not just to their normal values but to their optimal values, which are empirically defined by survivors of life-threatening critical illnesses. Criteria for optimal therapy include: (*a*) cardiac index (CI) 50% greater than normal (4.5 L/min·M^2); (*b*) oxygen delivery slightly greater than normal (600 ml/mn·M^2); (*c*) $\dot{V}O_2$ about 30% greater than normal (170 ml/min·M^2); and (*d*) blood volume 500 ml in excess of the norm, i.e., 3.2 L/M^2 for males, 2.8 L/M^2 for females. These increments are needed to supply the increased metabolism associated with the need for regeneration of ATP and tissue repair. Severely traumatized, cirrhotic, and septic patients may require even greater increments (1–4, 9).

Several multivariate nonparametric predictive indexes have been developed empirically from the frequency distributions of the survivors' and nonsurvivors' values. These analyses provide an objective outcome prediction based on the sequential physiologic patterns of the survivors and nonsurvivors early in the postoperative period (2–6, 8). The advantage of predictors is that they analyze the complex physiologic problems with no preconceptions and minimal assumptions. The criteria are heuristically determined, solely by observed values of critically ill surgical patients who survived as compared with the values of those who subsequently died. More recently, a simplified predictor was developed based on observed values of each cardiorespiratory variable at sequential time periods postoperatively (Figs. 23-9 and 23-10). This recent predictor based on the values of each variable was validated in a prospective series (Fig. 23-11) (2, 6).

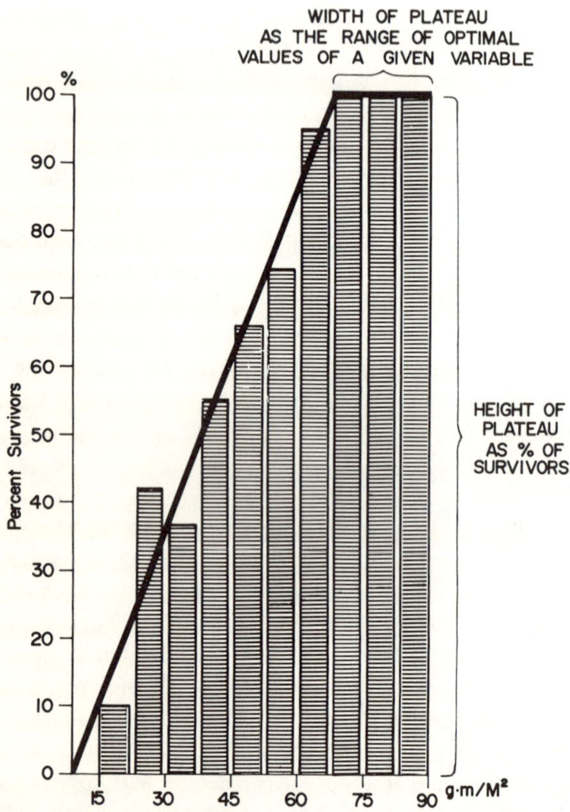

Figure 23-9. Distribution of observed values for left ventricular stroke work in the first 8 postoperative hours in our first series. The survival rates were calculated for the patients whose values fell into each of the ten divisions from the lowest to the highest value. Note the plateau at the top; the height of this plateau reflects how good the variable is as a predictor. The width reflects the values that are associated with good outcome. (From Shoemaker, WC, Bland, RD, and Appel, PL. 1985. Therapy of critically ill postoperative patients based on outcome prediction and prospective clinical trials. *Surg Clin North Am* 65:811.)

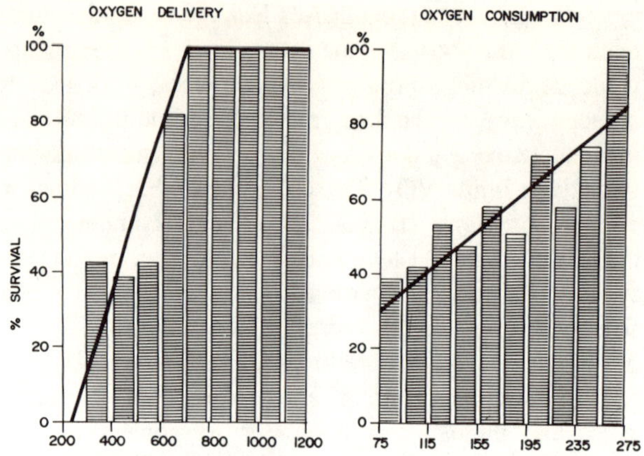

Figure 23-10. Distribution of values for oxygen delivery (left) and oxygen consumption (right) in the same series. (From Shoemaker, WC, Bland, RD, Appel, PL. 1985. Therapy of critically ill postoperative patients based on outcome prediction and prospective clinical trials. *Surg Clin North Am* 65:811.)

Branch Chain Decision Tree for Management of Surgical Patients

A branch chain decision tree (algorithm) for high-risk surgical patients was designed from decision rules based on predictor outcome data of several previous series and controlled clinical trials of various therapeutic agents (Fig. 23-12). Criteria for assignment of priorities were based solely on survival statistics (1–9). The strategy is, first, to give fluid volume rapidly and vigorously without exceeding a WP greater than 20 mm Hg. Plasma volume expansion with colloids is more effective than crystalloids, which unduly expand the interstitial water (3, 13–16). After the maximum effect of fluids has been obtained, dobutamine, an inotropic agent, is started at 2 μg/kg and increased with monitoring to obtain the optimal goals for CI, $\dot{D}O_2$ and $\dot{V}O_2$ defined above. If the patient has high MAP and systemic vascular resistance index (SVRI), vasodilation with labetalol, nitroglycerin, or nitroprusside is considered; the appropriate dose again is obtained by titration to improve CI, $\dot{D}O_2$ and $\dot{V}O_2$ without producing hypotension (i.e., MAP < 80, systolic pressure < 110 mm Hg). If fluids, inotropic agents, and vasodilators fail to achieve optimal goals, vasopressors such as dopamine or norepinephrine are then given in the smallest possible dose needed to maintain MAP at or slightly above 80 mm Hg and systolic pressure at or slightly above 110 mm Hg in patients who were normotensive in their pre-illness state. In hypertensive patients, 80% to 90% of pre-illness values are used as goals. Vasopressors are given last because they increase venous pressure, lactic acidosis, pulmonary vascular resistance, and pulmonary shunt in addition to increasing MAP, and thereby may limit optimal fluid administration.

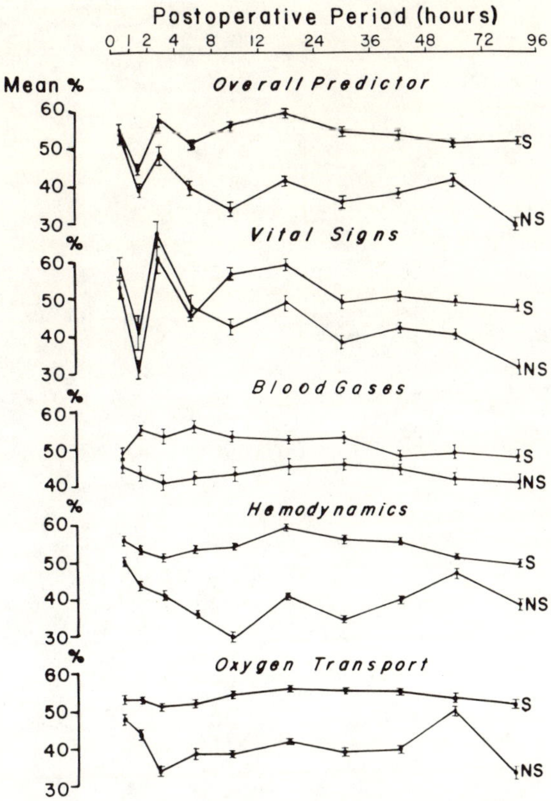

Figure 23-11. Upper section: overall predictor for survivors (S) and nonsurvivors (NS) at each time interval postoperatively. Second Section: Predictions calculated from the vital signs variables for S and NS. Third Section: Predictions calculated from the blood gas variables for S and NS. Fourth Section: Predictions calculated from the hemodynamic variables for S and NS. Lowest Section: Predictions calculated from the oxygen transport variables for S and NS. Dots represent mean values, vertical bars SEM. (From Bland, RD, et al. 1985. Probability of survival as a prognostic and severity of illness score in critically ill surgical patients. *Crit Care Med* 13:91; 10:390.)

This therapeutic plan was tested in prospective clinical trials against a control group that had normal values as the therapeutic goals (7, 8). Mortality was reduced from 35% in the control group to 12.5% in the protocol patients; there were also significant reductions in morbidity (7). Recently, we (8) completed a prospective trial of this concept which was preoperatively randomized to 3-legs: (*a*) CVP catheter, (*b*) pulmonary artery catheter with normal values as goals, and (*c*) pulmonary artery catheter with optimal values as goals of therapy. This trial showed no statistically significant difference between the mortality of patients managed with a CVP catheter (7/30, 23%) and those of the pulmonary artery catheter with normal values as therapeutic goals (10/30, 33%); however, use of the pulmonary artery catheter with supranormal "optimal goals" led to significantly reduced mortality (1/28, 4%) as well as morbidity (8).

Most surgical complications such as acute respiratory failure, acute renal failure, sepsis in the uncontaminated patient, and disseminated intravascular coagulation are the sequelae of shock; i.e., shock lung is a complication of shock, and without shock, there is no shock lung. Most postoperative deaths are attributable to physiologic changes that can be identified, described, predicted, and prevented. Therapy should be defined by physiologic criteria, given prophylactically, and monitored to obtain optimal physiologic goals rather than normal values.

Clinical Monitoring of the Elderly

From the practical clinical viewpoint, elderly surgical patients are preoperatively more likely to have associated medical conditions, such as hypertension, dysrhythmias, myocardial impairment, arteriosclerosis, congestive heart failure, diabetes, renal impairment, pulmonary disorders, infections, etc. Although many patients with advanced age have uneventful postoperative courses, there is, nevertheless, a greater mortality with age, not because of age per se, but because of associated medical illnesses. The elderly patient, therefore, may have less tolerance to hypovolemia, hypoxemia, and impaired tissue perfusion, all of which are commonly encountered perioperatively. For these reasons, invasive monitoring should be instituted preoperatively to optimize values prior to anesthetic induction and continued intraoperatively and postoperatively to prevent or promptly treat hypovolemia, hypoxemia, and suboptimal tissue perfusion.

Elderly patients share the same potentially life-threatening problems as the nonelderly, but are subject to a higher incidence, greater intensity, and higher morbidity. Moreover, their physiologic reserve capacity to compensate in terms of cardiodynamics is more likely to be limited. Therefore, they are treated similarly to the nonelderly in terms of specific therapeutic or pharmacologic interventions, but they are more carefully titrated to avoid under- or overtreatment. More importantly, they are more carefully monitored physiologically to prevent or to treat more vigorously hypovolemia and other correctable perioperative circulatory problems. The only difference is that the optimal postoperative goals of the elderly are somewhat less, i.e., 4 $L/min \cdot m^2$ rather than 4.5 $L/min \cdot m^2$ for the nonelderly.

Choice of Fluid Therapy in Shock

Efficacy comparisons of crystalloids with colloids were studied in prospectively randomized trials conducted in critically ill postoperative patients by Skillman, Restall, and Salzman (17) and Boutros et al. (18), in burn patients by Jelenko et al. (19), and in emergency hypotensive

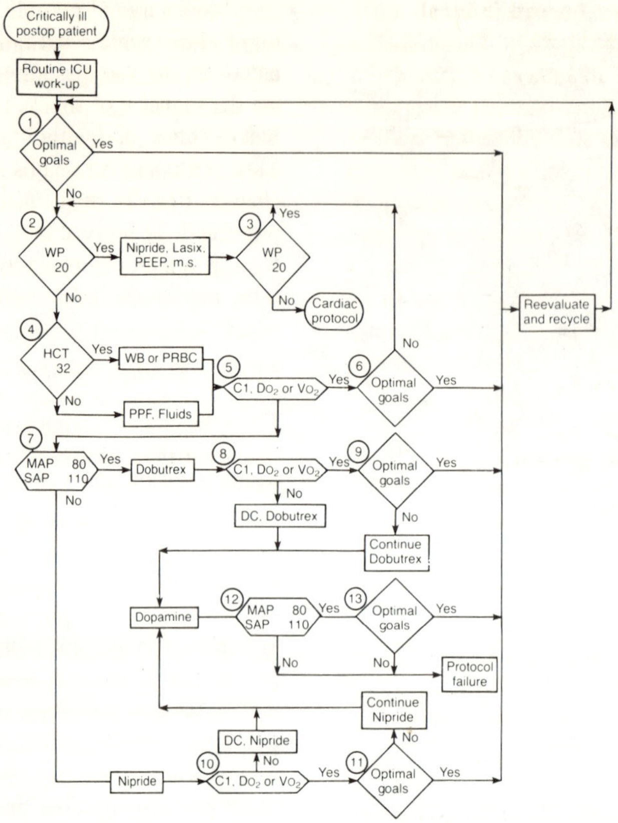

Figure 23-12. Branch chain decision tree for postoperative patients. Preliminary evaluation of high-risk critically ill patients by routine ICU work-up that includes arterial blood gases, chest x-ray, routine blood chemistries, ECG, and coagulation studies. These tests should be either performed or in process and the observed defects corrected; i.e., if $PaO_2 < 70$ torr, $7.3 > pH > 7.5$, $PaCO_2 > 55$ torr, or respiration rate (RR) > 30 breath/min, place on the respiratory protocol. If none of the above is present, proceed down the branch chain decision tree. *Step 1:* Determine if the patient has reached the optimal goals. Measure CI, $\dot{D}O_2$, $\dot{V}O_2$ and blood volume (BV). If CI < 4.5 L/min•m², < 600 ml/min•², $\dot{V}O_2$ < 160 ml/min•m², BV 3.2 L/m² for men or 2.7 L/m² for women, take Hct. If any of the preceding optimal values have not been reached, proceed to step 2. If the goals are reached, the objective of the algorithm has been achieved. Re-evaluate and recycle at intervals to maintain these goals. *Step 2:* Take the pulmonary wedge pressure (WP). If > 20 mm Hg, proceed to step 3; if < 20, proceed to step 4. *Step 3:* If WP > 20, give furosemide intravenously at increasing dose levels (20, 40, 80, 160 mg), particularly if there is clinical or x-ray evidence of salt and water overload or clinical findings of pulmonary congestion. If not, consider vasodilators, nitroprusside, or nitroglycerin if MAP > 80 and systolic pressure > 100 mm Hg. Recycle up to 5 times to titrate the dose needed to reduce WP < 10 mm Hg but maintain MAP > 80 mm Hg. If unsuccessful, place on cardiac protocol. *Step 4:* If hematocrit (Hct) < 32%, give 1 unit of whole blood (WB) or 2 units of packed red blood cells (Prbc). If Hct > 32%, give a fluid load (volume challenge), consisting of one of the following (depending on clinical indications of plasma volume deficit or hydration): 5% plasma protein fraction, 500 ml; 5% albumin, 500 ml; 25% albumin (25 g), 100 ml; 6% hydroxyethyl starch 500 ml; 6% dextran-60, 500 ml; D5RL, 1,000 ml. *Step 5:* If the blood or fluid load improved any of the optimal therapeutic goals defined in step 1, proceed to step 6; if none are improved, proceed to step 7. *Step 6:* If goals are not reached, recycle steps 2 through 6 until these goals are met or WP > 20 mm Hg. *Step 7:* If MAP > 70 or systolic arterial pressure (SAP) < 100 mm Hg, give dobutamine by constant intravenous infusion in increasing doses. *Step 8:* Titrate dobutamine beginning with 2 μg/min • kg and gradually increasing doses up to 20 μg/min • kg provided there is improvement in CI, $\dot{D}O_2$, or $\dot{V}O_2$ without further lowering of arterial pressure until goals are met. *Step 9:* If goals are reached, re-evaluate and recycle. If goals are not reached or if it becomes evident that higher doses of the drug are not more effective or that they produce hypotension and tachycardia, continue dobutamine at its most effective dose range. *Step 10:* If MAP > 80 mm Hg and SAP > 110 mm Hg, give sodium nitroprusside or nitroglycerin in gradually increasing doses. If the arterial pressures are lower than MAP > 80 mm Hg and SAP > 110 mm Hg, give vasopressors. *Step 11:* If there is no improvement in CI, $\dot{D}O_2$, $\dot{V}O_2$ with the vasodilator, or if hypotension (MAP < 80 mm Hg, SAP < 110 mm Hg) ensues, discontinue the vasodilator. If there is improvement in CI, $\dot{D}O_2$, or $\dot{V}O_2$, titrate vasodilator to its maximum effect consistent with satisfactory pressures. *Step 12:* If optimal goals are reached, re-evaluate and recycle at intervals. If these goals are not reached and MAP < 80 mm Hg, SAP < 110, give vasopressor. *Step 13:* Titrate doses of vasopressor (dopamine) in the lowest doses possible to maintain arterial pressures, MAP > 80, SAP > 110. If pressures cannot be maintained, the patient is considered to be a protocol failure. (Modified from Shoemaker, WC. 1989. Pathophysiology of shock syndromes. In *Textbook of Critical Care*, ed. 2. Eds., WC Shoemaker, WL Thompson, and PR Holbrook, pp. 977–993. Philadelphia: WB Saunders.)

shock and trauma patients by Shoemaker et al. (20), Rackow et al. (21, 22), and Modig (23). These studies showed statistically significant advantages of colloids.

The most important questions concern therapeutic criteria, on which there are few well controlled studies. The efficacy of alternative fluid therapies is best evaluated by the physiologic responses that are closely related to survival, rather than by the routinely monitored variables used because of convenience. The immediate, direct effects of sodium are increased blood pressure and urine output; if these two variables are used as the criteria of efficacy, then sodium-rich solutions will be judged as efficacious. If cardiac output, blood volume, $\dot{D}O_2$ and $\dot{V}O_2$ are the appropriate outcome measures, however, colloids and blood are the most effective agents (13–16).

The efficacy of alternative therapies was determined by hemodynamic and oxygen transport responses using the patient as his own control (13–16). Figure 23-13 illustrates data from a patient resuscitated from burn shock from a series of burn patients who were given various colloids and lactated Ringer's solution alternately (14). Colloids increased CI, $\dot{D}O_2$ and $\dot{V}O_2$ significantly more than crystalloids given in twice or four times the volume (13–16). Changes after one liter of lactated Ringer's solution were compared with those after 25 g of 25% albumin (100 ml) prospectively given in random order by a crossover design to a series of critically ill surgical patients with early shock lung (15); i.e., each patient reached each agent (Fig. 23-14). Albumin increased plasma volume 465 ± 47 (SE) ml by shifting over 350 ml of water from the interstitial compartment to the intravascular space. Albumin also increased CI, MAP, left ventricular stroke work, $\dot{D}O_2$ and $\dot{V}O_2$. Lung function variables were not worsened but in many instances actually improved. By contrast, one liter of Ringer's lactate expanded plasma volume only 194 ± 18 ml at their maxima which occurred at the end of infusion; over 80% of the infused crystalloid almost immediately equilibrated or "leaked" into the interstitial water, while only a small proportion of fluid remained in the plasma and then decreased exponentially. After Ringer's lactate administration, the pulmonary shunt and $\dot{V}O_2$ worsened despite the slightly increased $\dot{D}O_2$. The hemodynamic responses to the administered fluid were directly proportional to plasma volume expansion. Thus, colloids improve hemodynamics and oxygen transport by plasma expansion, while crystalloids principally expand interstitial volume; when tolerated, they may restore plasma volume if massive amounts are given (15).

Recently our series was expanded to include 400 fluid therapy interventions in 211 patients with early adult respiratory distress syndrome (ARDS), occurring postoperatively and with sepsis (16, 24). Figures 23-15 and 23-16 illustrate the flow and oxygen transport variables in: (*a*) patients during (ARDS), (*b*) these same patients

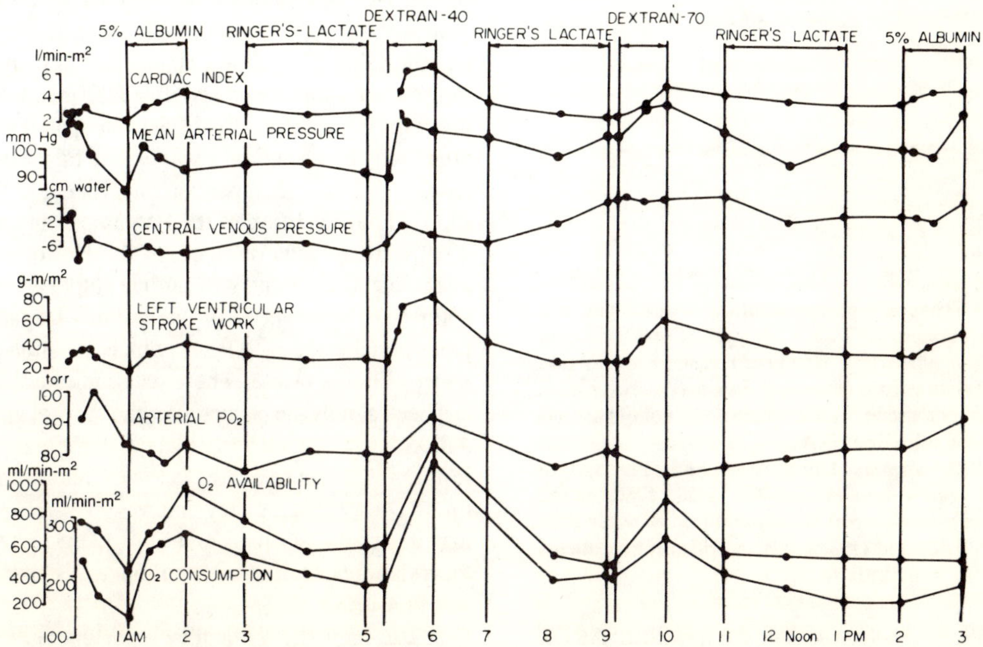

Figure 23-13. Cardiorespiratory values during resuscitation of a patient with severe burns. (From Shoemaker, WC, Matsuda, T, and State, D. 1977. Relative hemodynamic effectiveness of whole blood and plasma expanders in burned patients. *Surg Gynecol Obstet* 144:909.)

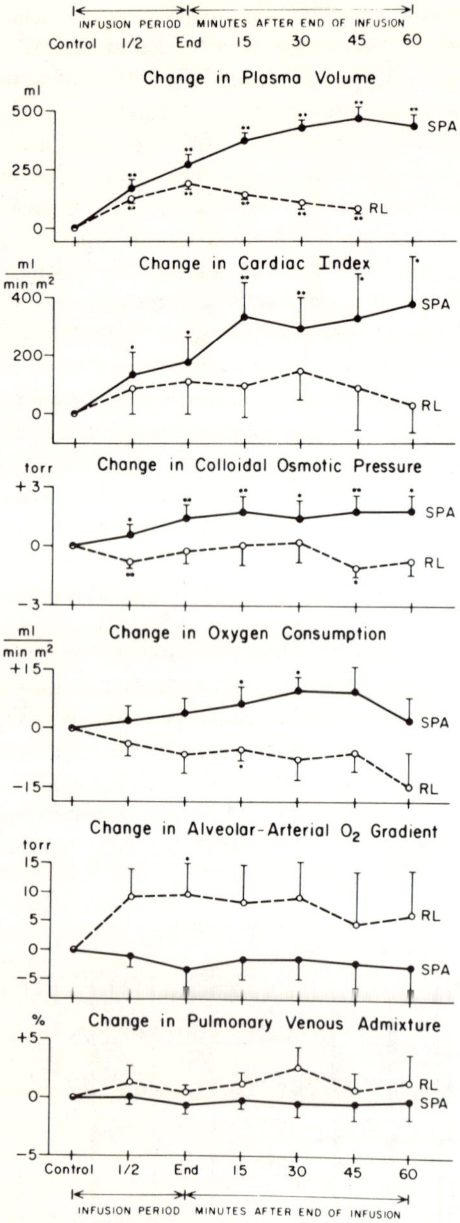

Figure 23-14. Changes in plasma volume, cardiac index (CI), colloid osmotic pressure, $\dot{V}O_2$, $P(A\text{-}a)O_2$, and $\dot{Q}sp/\dot{Q}t$ are compared after intervention with 1,000 ml of lactated Ringer's solution (RL) and 100 ml of 25% albumin (SPA) in a crossover study. Note the greater increase in plasma volume, CI, colloid osmotic pressure, and $\dot{V}O_2$ after SPA. $P(A\text{-}a)O_2$ as well as $\dot{Q}sp/\dot{Q}t$ were unaffected by SPA, whereas after infusion of RL, $P(A\text{-}a)O_2$ increased. $^*p < .05$. (From Hauser, CJ, et al. 1980. Hemodynamic and oxygen transport responses to body water shifts produced by colloids and crystalloids in critically ill patients. *Surg Gynecol Obstet* 150:811.)

without ARDS, i.e., before or after the episode of ARDS, and (*c*) a concurrent group of critically ill patients who did not develop ARDS. These data show significant increases in hemodynamic and oxygen transport after colloid infusion but insignificant changes after infusion of Ringer's lactate except in increased arterial pressure; there was a similar lack of changes when the data were stratified into groups with high, normal, and low initial cardiac index values. Table 23-4 shows changes in hemodynamic and oxygen transport variables after 500 ml of colloids was given during periods of ARDS as compared with changes after 500 ml of colloids was given to patients without ARDS. These therapeutic interventions were made shortly after insertion of the PA catheter in an average of 40 ± 48 hours after onset of ARDS. However, there were insignificant differences in cardiac output after infusion of colloids, whole blood, or crystalloids in patients in the preterminal stage of ARDS, which is defined as the last 24 to 48 hours of life. These data indicate that the capillary leak syndrome occurs after the clinical appearance of ARDS; evidence suggests that capillary leaks may be the result, not the cause of ARDS (24). Colloids may be given in ARDS as long as they improve physiologic variables that determine survival and until there is evidence that they significantly increase pulmonary shunting ($\dot{Q}sp/\dot{Q}t$ and $P(A\text{-}a)O_2$).

The high risk critically ill postoperative patient requiring fluid resuscitation should have a pulmonary artery catheter to define physiologic problems and to titrate fluid therapy to the optimal goals defined by the pattern of the

Table 23-4. Changes in cardiorespiratory variables after administration of colloids in acute respiratory distress syndrome patients during and not during their acute respiratory distress

Variables	During ARDS	Not during ARDS
Number	134	117
Mean arterial pressure	5.3 ±0.99**	2.9 ±1**
Mean pulmonary arterial pressure	2.6 ±0.4**	03.8 ±.6**
Cardiac index	0.66 ±0.98**	0.78 ±0.09**
Central venous pressure	02.5 ±0.4**	02.1 ±0.4**
Wedge pressure	2.6 ±0.4**	3.3 ±0.5**
Systemic vascular resistance	−247 ±39**	−378 ±50**
Pulmonary vascular resistance	−31 ±10**	−22 ±13*
Left ventricular stroke work	9.3 ±1.0**	9.6 ±1.2**
O_2 delivery	42 ±11**	45 ±12**
O_2 consumption	7.9 ±4.2*	7 ±4.8*
Pulmonary shunt (Qsp/Qt)	1.4 ±.6	1.4 ±1.0

* $p < .05$ compared with the corresponding control values.

** $p < .01$ compared with the corresponding control values.

Values represent mean ± 1 SEM changes from control measurements after all colloids, albumin, PPF, and Dextran-40. Positive numbers represent increases, and negative values represent decreases from the control values.

From Appel, PL, and Shoemaker, WC. 1981. Fluid therapy in adult respiratory failure. *Crit Care Med* 9:862.

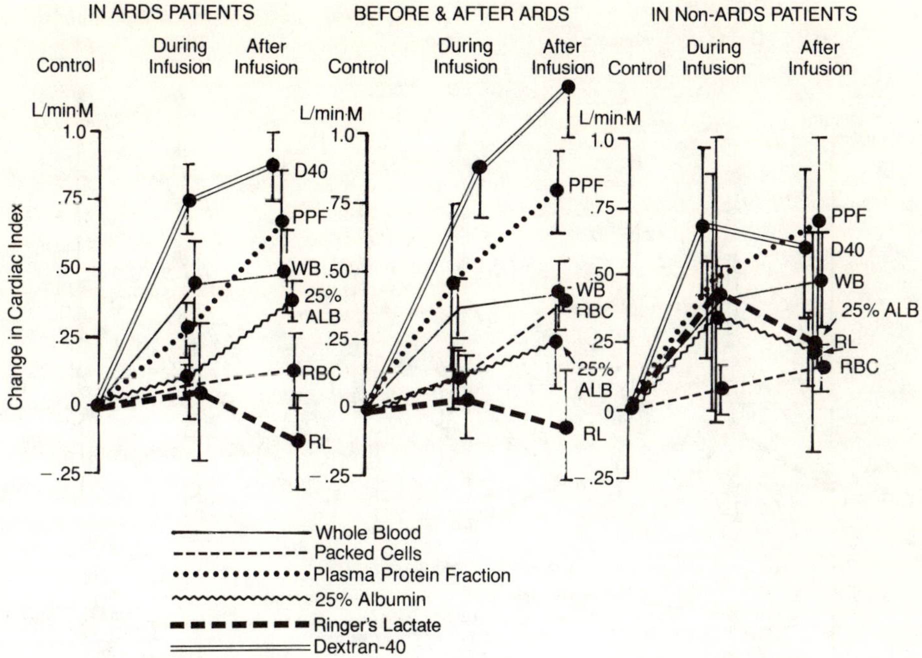

Figure 23-15. Cardiac index responses to various agents are shown in patients with ARDS during the episode of respiratory distress (left section), patients with ARDS not during the episode of respiratory distress (center section), and patients without ARDS (right section). The data represent changes in CI ± SEM during and after the administration of each agent. (From Appel, PL, and Shoemaker, WC. 1981. Fluid therapy in adult respiratory failure. *Crit Care Med* 9:862.)

survivors of life-threatening operations. The therapeutic agent used is less important than the achievement of these physiologic goals. Changes in the values of variables related to the bulk transport and utilization of oxygen provide more sensitive and specific criteria of circulatory performance.

Summary

The sequence of hemodynamic and oxygen transport events characterize various types of shock syndromes and demonstrate reduced $\dot{V}O_2$ as the earliest pathophysiologic event. Reduced or inadequate $\dot{V}O_2$, which may precede the initial hypotensive crisis, is produced by low flow or by maldistribution of flow, as well as by increased metabolic demand. Thus, low $\dot{V}O_2$ is the primary pathogenic event that produces the shock state. More importantly, $\dot{V}O_2$ is the regulatory mechanism that stimulates compensatory reactions including increases in heart rate, myocardial contractility, cardiac output, and minute ventilation. Sequential hemodynamic and oxygen transport patterns are related to the degree of the shock state and its outcome. Descriptions of survivors' and nonsurvivors' patterns were used to develop outcome predictors from these patterns by multivariate analyses. High-risk patients with normal preoperative values were primarily used to define the patterns before, during, and after surgical trauma. The patterns of patients who were elderly, stressed, and cirrhotic were similar but started at different baselines. A branch chain decision tree was developed for fluid resuscitation of critically ill postoperative patients from decision rules that were based on objective, physiologic, and heuristic data of survivors' hemodynamic and oxygen transport patterns. Criteria were defined for initiating and stopping fluids, inotropic agents, vasodilators and vasopressors. Empirically, colloids were found to be more effective than crystalloids in reaching the optimal hemodynamic and oxygen transport goals, especially in critically ill elderly patients.

Branch chain decision trees expeditiously help to achieve therapeutic goals by providing a coherent organized patient management plan. In prospective studies, therapy that supports compensatory increases in CI and $\dot{D}O_2$ produces the survivor pattern and was demonstrated to improve survival rates. This confirms the validity of an organized physiologic approach in contrast to the traditional approach whose objectives are to search for physiologic and biochemical abnormalities and then to restore them to normal, if and when they are discovered.

This approach emphasizes aggressive fluid management as unrecognized hypovolemia, delay in treatment of

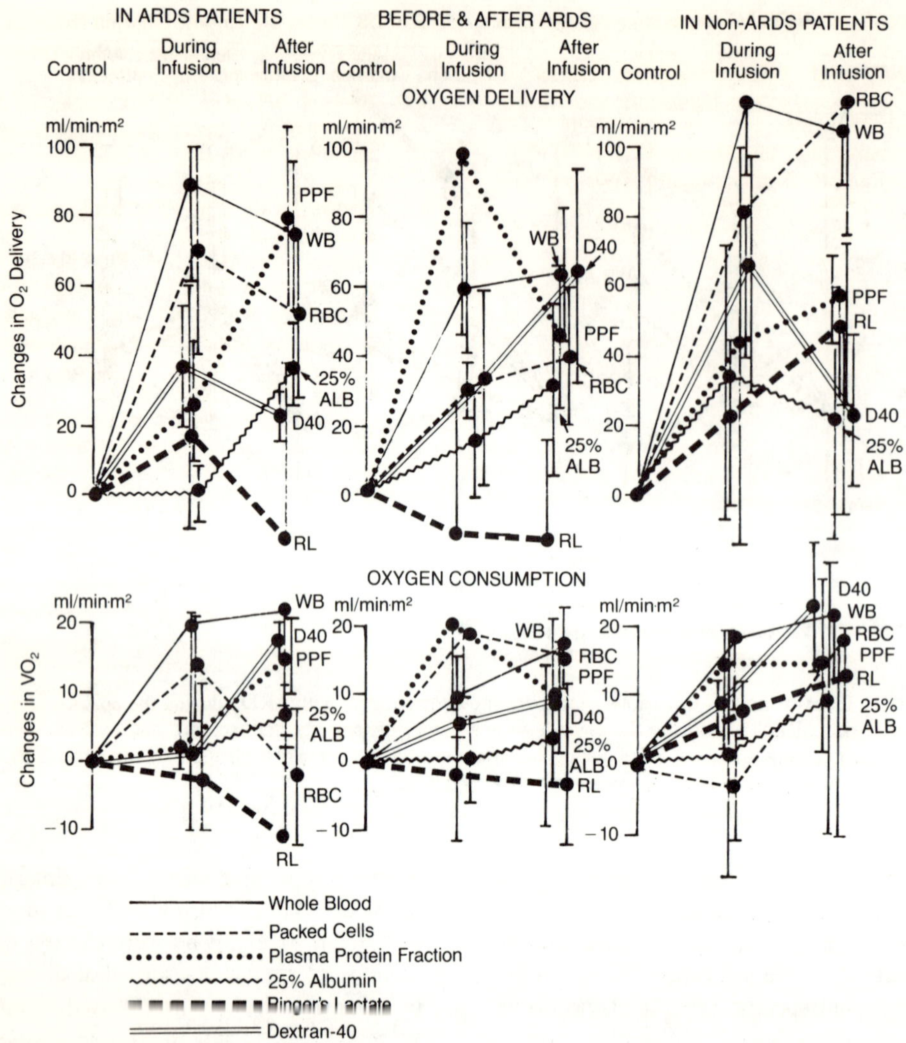

Figure 23-16. Changes in $\dot{D}O_2$ and $\dot{V}O_2$ during and after administration of various agents are shown, as described in Figure 23-15. (From Appel, PL, and Shoemaker, WC. 1981. Fluid therapy in adult respiratory failure. *Crit Care Med* 9:862.)

hypovolemia or inadequate volume therapy all lead to inadequate tissue perfusion reflected by low $\dot{D}O_2$ and $\dot{V}O_2$. Low $\dot{V}O_2$ is the primary pathophysiologic mechanism in postoperative, hemorrhagic, traumatic, and septic shock. This approach was found to be useful in elderly patients, but the therapeutic responses and cardiac reserve capacities were sometimes limited. The essence of this plan is to maintain the patient prophylactically in an optimal hemodynamic state that does not allow him to develop tissue hypoxia from blood volume, hemodynamic, and oxygen transport deficits.

References

1. Shoemaker, WC, et al. 1973. Physiologic patterns in surviving and nonsurviving shock patients. *Arch Surg* 106: 630–636.
2. Bland, RD, et al. 1985. Hemodynamic and oxygen transport patterns in surviving and nonsurviving postoperative patients. *Crit Care Med* 13:85–90.
3. Shoemaker, WC. 1989. Pathophysiology of shock syndromes. In *Textbook of Critical Care,* ed. 2. Eds., WC Shoemaker, WL Thompson and PR Holbrook, pp. 977–993. Philadelphia: WB Saunders.
4. Shoemaker, WC, Bland, RD, and Appel, PL. 1985. Therapy of critically ill postoperative patients based on outcome prediction and prospective clinical trials. *Surg Clin North Am* 65:811–833.
5. Bland, RD, and Shoemaker, WC. 1985. Common physiologic patterns in general surgical patients: *Surg Clin North Am* 65:793–810.
6. Bland, RD, et al. 1985. Probability of survival as a prognostic and severity of illness score in critically ill surgical patients. *Crit Care Med* 13:91; 10:390–394.
7. Shoemaker, WC, Appel, P, and Bland, R. 1983. Use of physiologic monitoring to predict outcome and to assist in

clinical decision in critically ill postoperative patients. *Am J Surg* 146:43–47.
8. Shoemaker, WC, et al. 1988. Prospective trial of supranormal values of survivors as therapeutic goals in patients. *Chest* 94:1176–1186.
9. Bland, R, Shoemaker, WC, and Shabot, MM. 1978. Physiologic monitoring goals for the critically ill patient. *Surg Gynecol Obstet* 147:833–838.
10. Guyton, AC, and Crowell, JW. 1961. Dynamics of the heart in shock. *Fed Proc* 10:51–58.
11. Crowell, JW, and Smith, EE. 1964. Oxygen deficit and irreversible hemorrhagic shock. *Am J Physiol* 216:313–317.
12. Shoemaker, WC, Appel, PL, and Kram, HB. 1988. Tissue oxygen debt as a determinant of lethal and nonlethal postoperative organ failure. *Crit Care Med* 16:1117–1123.
13. Shippy, CR, Appel, PL, and Shoemaker, WC. 1984. Reliability of clinical monitoring to assess blood volume in critically ill patients. *Crit Care Med* 12:107–112.
14. Shoemaker, WC, Matsuda, T, and State, D. 1977. Relative hemodynamic effectiveness of whole blood and plasma expanders in burned patients. *Surg Gynecol Obstet* 144:909–915.
15. Hauser, CJ, et al. 1980. Hemodynamic and oxygen transport responses to body water shifts produced by colloids and crystalloids in critically ill patients. *Surg Gynecol Obstet* 150:811–817.
16. Appel, PL, and Shoemaker, WC. 1981. Fluid therapy in adult respiratory failure. *Crit Care Med* 9:862–869.
17. Skillman, JJ, Restall, DS, and Salzman, EW. 1975. Randomized trail of albumin vs electrolyte solutions during aortic operations. *Surgery* 78:291–303.
18. Boutros, AR, et al. 1979. Comparison of hemodynamic, pulmonary and renal effects of use of three types of fluids following major surgical procedures on the abdominal aorta. *Crit Care Med* 7:9–13.
19. Jelenko, C, III, et al. 1979. Studies in shock and resuscitation. I: Use of a hypertonic, albumin-containing, fluid demand regimen (Halfd) in resuscitation: A physiologically appropriate method. *Crit Care Med* 7:157–167.
20. Shoemaker, WC, et al. 1981. Comparison of the relative effectiveness of colloids and crystalloids in emergency resuscitation. *Am J Surg* 142:73–84.
21. Haupt, MT, and Rackow, EC. 1982. Colloids osmotic pressure and fluid resuscitation with hetastarch, albumin, and saline solutions. *Crit Care Med* 10:159–162.
22. Rackow, EC, et al. 1983. Fluid resuscitation in circulatory shock. *Crit Care Med* 11:839–850.
23. Modig, J. 1983. Advantages of dextran-70 over Ringer's acetate solution in shock treatment and in prevention of adult respiratory distress syndrome: A randomized study in man after traumatic-hemorrhage shock. *Resuscitation* 10:219–225.
24. Shoemaker, WC, and Appel, PL. 1985. Pathophysiology of adult respiratory distress syndrome after sepsis and surgical operations. *Crit Care Med* 13:166–172.

24

Pain Management in the Geriatric Surgical Patient

Kim Shiu-Chin Yang and Russell K. Portenoy

Adequate postoperative pain management in the elderly surgical patient has benefits beyond the important goal of enhanced comfort. The rapid return of physical activity and normal pulmonary function demonstrated by the pain-free patient may prevent many of the postoperative complications to which this population is predisposed, including decubitus ulcers, atelectasis, pneumonia, and bone loss. Clinical experience suggests additionally that adequate analgesia may allow earlier discharge from the hospital. The expert application of analgesic techniques, therefore, is a fundamental aspect of the postoperative management of the elderly patient.

The goal of postoperative pain management in the elderly, as in all patients, is to provide analgesia without intolerable side effects. Pharmacologic approaches are the mainstay in this process, occasionally supplemented by other methods of pain control. Although successful analgesia is attainable in the vast majority of elderly patients, pain assessment and therapeutic intervention may be complicated in this population by age-related physiologic and psychologic changes. The management of these patients requires an understanding of the impact of aging on the neurophysiology of postoperative pain and the response to analgesic therapies.

Pathophysiology of Postoperative Pain

Pain has been defined by the International Association for the Study of Pain as "an unpleasant sensory and emotional experience associated with actual or potential tissue damage, or described in terms of such damage" (1). This definition emphasizes the fundamentally subjective nature of pain. Pain is a perception, loosely related to the sensation produced by activation of specific neurons sensitive to noxious stimuli, a process known as nociception. The experience and report of pain is profoundly influenced by psychologic state and traits, and may be out of proportion to the degree of nociception. For example, the equivalent degree of tissue damage has been shown to be associated with far less pain in soldiers who sustained injury in combat than civilians undergoing surgery (2).

Both nociceptive and non-nociceptive components to the pain experience vary enormously from patient to patient. This variability is the basis for the common observation that the same surgical procedure in different patients may be followed by markedly divergent pain complaints. An appreciation of this variability is a fundamental principal in the management of postoperative pain.

Ascending Pathways

Although non-nociceptive, specifically cognitive and emotional, factors can have a profound influence on the postoperative pain experience, nociception itself is the inciting cause and major contributor to pain in the vast majority of patients who sustain a surgical wound (3). This process involves the activation of primary afferent neurons sensitive to noxious stimuli, or nociceptors, that relay information into the central nervous system. This afferent barrage is associated with segmental and suprasegmental reflex responses, as well as cortical responses, which also influence the pain experience (4, 5). Nociceptors are present in skin, muscle, connective tissue, viscera, and possibly nerve trunks (6). They comprise a proportion of unmyelinated and lightly myelinated peripheral fibers and respond to one or more types of noxious mechanical, thermal, or chemical stimuli.

At its most basic level, therefore, the experience of postoperative pain begins with the activation of nociceptors by the tissue damage produced during the operation and the profuse inflammation following it. In the skin, lightly myelinated nociceptors subserve the sensation of sharp stinging pain, which is usually well localized to the incisional site, while unmyelinated nociceptors have been associated with more diffuse, dull burning or aching pain (5). Nociceptors in the connective tissue surrounding muscle fibers, tendons, or blood vessels typically produce a sensation interpreted as deep, poorly localized aching. A similar sensation probably arises from activation of nociceptors innervating the periosteum of bones and the pain-sensitive tissues surrounding joints. Finally, visceral nociceptors, which may be activated by irritation of the mucosal or serosal surfaces, torsion or traction of messentary, or distention or contraction of hollow viscus, produce a poorly localized, deep, cramping or achy pain (4, 5).

The importance of nociception in postoperative pain perception is suggested by the influence of the type of operation on the report of pain (4, 7). The severity and duration of pain is greater with intrathoracic and intra-abdominal procedures than with operations at other sites. Similarly, the same procedure performed through different incisions may result in different intensities of pain. For example, cholecystectomy through a midline incision is usually more painful than that using a subcostal approach. Finally, the degree of intraoperative trauma has been associated with variation in postoperative pain, with superficial operations often requiring minimal or no postoperative analgesic therapy. Thus, differences in nociception produce marked variation in postoperative pain and suggest again the importance of these basic processes in the overall pain experience.

From the therapeutic perspective, the important role played by nociceptor activation in postoperative pain suggests that interventions designed to attenuate this activity directly, either by reducing stimuli (for example, by diminishing inflammation) or by impeding the transmission of impulses into the central nervous system, may provide a highly effective means of analgesia. These interventions are discussed below.

The central connections of the primary afferent neurons subserving nociception are themselves multiplicative (5). Primary afferents originating from the body enter the spinal cord and synapse in the dorsal horn; those from the head, entering via cranial nerves V, VII, IX, and X, synapse with second order neurons in the trigeminal nucleus caudalis of the brainstem. Substantial evidence suggests that the peptide substance P is an important neurotransmitter at this first synapse (5, 8). The utility of substance P antagonists in the modulation of acute pain is currently under investigation.

Second order neurons originating in the dorsal horn or the nucleus caudalis send processes that ascend rostrally to the thalamus. Two distinct pathways have been identified. The neospinothalamic is a monosynaptic pathway that ascends in the contralateral anterolateral column of the spinal cord and terminates in the ventrobasal thalamus. This pathway appears to subserve the sensory-discriminative aspects of pain perception, such as localization and intensity. In contrast, the paleospinothalamic tracts are polysynaptic pathways that ascend bilaterally in the medial spinal cord and brainstem, and have extensive synaptic connections with nuclei in the brainstem, limbic system, and hypothalamus. These pathways ultimately synapse in nuclei of the medial thalamus and appear to subserve the arousal and affective concomitants of the pain experience. Multiple neurotransmitters have been identified in these ascending nociceptive pathways, but their precise functions remain obscure (5, 8).

In addition to these ascending nociceptive pathways, segmental reflex responses are important in the genesis of postoperative pain (6). Incoming nociceptive primary afferent neurons have collateral fibers that travel to the ventral horn of the same and adjacent segments of the spinal cord and stimulate motor neurons and sympathetic preganglionic neurons. This activity promotes segmental motor and autonomic reflex responses, respectively, that may in turn enhance nociception. Intense contraction of skeletal muscle may itself become nociceptive and may result in additional adverse effects, such as decreased chest wall compliance with impaired ventilation. Stimulation of sympathetic neurons can produce local vascular constriction, which may contribute to tissue ischemia and also result indirectly in the augmentation of nociception (9).

In addition to these segmental reflexes, a variety of suprasegmental reflex responses may also contribute to the aversive nature of the postoperative experience. Stimulation of neurons in the brainstem and limbic system results in the "fight or flight response," characterized in part by tachycardia and hypertension, effects that increase the cardiac work load and may be particularly serious in the elderly patient (10). These suprasegmental reflex responses also include the systemic secretion of hormones, such as catecholamines, cortisol, and others (10, 11), which may further add to the physiologic stress of the surgery (12) and delay the recovery of the elderly postoperative patient. The affect associated with these suprasegmental reflex responses is anxiety, which also increases postoperative pain and distress.

The ultimate perception of postoperative pain derives from a complex interaction between these processes and a large number of higher functions, such as cognition, memory, premorbid and current affective state, personality traits, ethnic background, social environment, and others. Recognition of these factors in the clinical setting can lead to improved understanding of the pain behaviors demonstrated by the individual patient and a more appropriate and sensitive targeting of pain-relieving interventions.

Endogenous Pain Modulation

Multiple segmental and descending pain modulating systems have been identified (8, 13). It is likely that future advances in postoperative pain control will be founded upon better understanding of these physiologic pathways.

The best characterized descending pain modulating system utilizes serotonin and enkephalin in a polysynaptic pathway that originates in the periaqueductal gray of the midbrain, synapses in the nucleus raphe magnus of the medulla, and descends to the dorsal horn of the spinal cord (13). The medullary pathway is serotonergic and activates inhibitory enkephalinergic interneurons in the dorsal horn, which in turn impede transmission of nociceptive inputs at the first synapse. Various other pathways have been identified, including one utilizing norepinephrine, and a large number of other neurotransmitters remain putative, such as dopamine, substance P, neurotensin, gamma aminobutyric acid, cholecystokinin, vasopressin, vasoactive intestinal peptide, oxytocin, and somatostatin (13). The sheer number of neurotransmitters involved in these systems suggest both their importance and complexity.

Enkephalin, which is involved in both segmental and descending pain modulating systems, is only one of many endogenous opioids or endorphins. These compounds are related to morphine and are widely distributed throughout the nervous system and extraneural sites (14–16). All bind specifically to endogenous opioid receptors, of which multiple subtypes have now been identified (15, 17–20). It is now known that three distinct subclasses of endorphins, representing a large number of individual compounds, interact with an opioid receptor network, which includes at least six separate receptor subtypes. Exogenous morphine-like drugs activate these endogenous systems, leading both to the desired effect of analgesia and many potential adverse consequences, as described below.

Recent advances in postoperative analgesia have been based upon better understanding of the physiology of this endorphinergic pain modulating system. The clinical use of spinal opioids developed from the identification of specific opioid receptors in the dorsal horn of the spinal cord, activation of which can provide segmental analgesia. The search for receptor-selective drugs, which may bind with high affinity to those receptors subserving analgesia and with low affinity to those receptors mediating adverse effects, is ongoing. Further elucidation of these endogenous pain modulating systems, both those mediated by endorphins and others, may provide the insights necessary to design analgesic interventions specifically directed to the activation of these antinociceptive pathways.

Determinants of Postoperative Pain

Surgical Determinants

Several clinically relevant influences on postoperative pain have been recognized, of which the type of surgical anesthesia and the occurrence of postoperative complications are most important. In addition to the age-related changes in pain perception described below, these may have a profound impact in the elderly population.

The influence of surgical anesthesia on nociceptive reflex responses depends first on whether modern balanced general anesthesia or regional anesthesia is used (4, 21). General anesthetics eliminate higher integrative functions, while the concomitant use of muscle relaxants prevents reflex muscle spasms. However, unless excessive concentrations of inhalation agents or anesthetic doses of opioids are used, the sympathetic, neuroendocrine, and biochemical responses provoked by the injury are reduced only slightly or not at all (11). The activity of reflex responses during general anesthesia may be reflected by an increase in cardiac output and blood pressure during surgery, or even by cardiac arrhythmias provoked by noxious stimulation. In addition, general anesthesia may be associated with subtle hypoxemia that may extend into the postoperative period for a variable time (22). As noted previously, these reflex responses may eventuate in greater postoperative pain intensity.

In regional anesthesia, the nociceptive input is blocked before it reaches the neuraxis (11). The various segmental and suprasegmental reflex responses are thereby prevented. Thus, while pain is reduced intraoperatively with both types of anesthesia, some of the physiologic accompaniments of nociception, which may later contribute to postoperative distress, are more likely to occur during general anesthesia. These phenomena suggest that attention to the reduction of nociceptive input may be worthwhile even in those settings where general anesthesia is employed, as discussed below.

Postoperative complications may also prolong and intensify the experience of pain. For example, atelectasis may produce reflex splinting of the thoracic or abdominal musculature, a process that may increase postoperative distress and perpetuate respiratory compromise; hypoxemia, if present, increases anxiety, which in turn further augments postoperative pain (23). The elderly are at particular risk for such pulmonary complications (24, 25). Other postoperative complications, such as incisional infection and ileus, may themselves be nociceptive (4). Clinical experience suggests that the elderly are also more predisposed to these complications and less likely to complain once they occur; additional attention to these factors in the aging population may provide another avenue for the amelioration of postoperative pain.

Individual Determinants

The endogenous pain transmission and modulation systems described above presumably play a major role in the ultimate experience of postoperative pain. Although there are yet no data to support such a hypothesis, it is likely that the process of aging alters these systems, and may thereby yield as yet poorly characterized changes in postoperative pain perception.

Investigations into the effect of aging on pain perception have produced conflicting results. Some studies of experimental pain have noted that pain sensitivity increases with age, while others have reported no change or a diminution (26). No age-related changes were found in the density or morphology of small subdermal nerve fibers in the human skin, many of which presumably subserve nociception (27). Overall, these experimental data do not strongly support the impression that aging is associated with a substantial reduction in pain perception.

A variety of clinical studies, however, suggest a different conclusion. A large epidemiologic survey noted that the prevalence of pain in all sites other than joints declines steadily with age (28). Other surveys have demonstrated that lesser analgesic medication is prescribed and consumed by elderly postoperative patients (29, 30) and that satisfaction with the pain relief provided by these analgesics is greater in the aged (31, 32). A study of pain responses after surgery reported lower pain scores among older patients (7). These clinical investigations suggest that elderly patients may experience less pain than their younger counterparts after a similar nociceptive insult, and that this physiologic change may combine with an enhanced therapeutic response to analgesic medications.

The impact of aging on psychologic and social status may also influence the experience of pain. Although nociception most likely underlies most postoperative pain behaviors (3), psychologic, social, and cultural factors also play a role (33). Of psychologic influences, perioperative anxiety provides the most important contribution to postoperative pain (34–37). The aged may be less prone to react with anxiety to stressful situations (38), which may in turn relate to the age-related reduction in postoperative pain described previously.

Current Status of Postoperative Pain Management

The inadequacy of current postoperative pain management has been stressed repeatedly (39–45). For example, Cohen (46) interviewed 109 patients during the postoperative period and discovered that 75% of those given opioid drugs continued to experience moderate to severe pain, and 70% indicated that pain interfered with sleep. This failure to respond to the analgesic needs of postoperative patients has been attributed to inadequate knowledge of clinical pharmacology, poor pain assessment during the postoperative period, and fear of opioid drugs (4, 47). Furthermore, the reluctance to administer analgesics may be exaggerated among elderly patients (48), further complicating the postoperative management of this group. Improved therapy of postoperative pain in the elderly will require a change in these attitudes and systematic instruction in pain assessment and analgesic pharmacology.

Pharmacokinetic and Pharmacodynamic Considerations

The process of aging greatly influences both the pharmacokinetic and pharmacodynamic responses to analgesic medications. Pharmacokinetics describe the movement of drugs through the body, comprising absorption, distribution, metabolism, and excretion. All phases can be affected by the aging process (40, 49, 50). Absorption may be influenced by an age-related decrease in gastric acid production, intestinal blood flow, mucosal cell mass, and gastrointestinal motility (51, 52). Perhaps more importantly, absorption may be diminished by various diseases associated with aging and by the concomitant use of other medications in elderly patients (53).

The distribution phase may be altered in the elderly by reduction in total body water, lean body mass, and serum protein, and by an increase in body fat (51). The effect of these changes on drug distribution depends on the lipid solubility of the specific drug and its degree of protein binding. In addition, the concurrent use of multiple drugs in many elderly patients may further alter distribution, with clinically significant effects (54).

Diminished hepatic mass and blood flow, as well as a reduction in enzymatic activity, may slow the metabolism of drugs in the elderly patient (55). These changes are most apparent with medications largely catabolized in the liver, including the opioids.

Finally, the excretion phase itself may be influenced by age-related impairment of renal function (53). This process, which is often subclinical, slows the clearance of drugs in the elderly patient and may also result in higher plasma drug concentrations.

Although these pharmacokinetic effects can be substantial, they may not account for all the changes in drug response observed in the aged (49). Pharmacodynamic factors, or the response to the drug after it reaches its site of action, must also be invoked to explain these observations. For example, a study of the psychotropic drug, nitrazepam, demonstrated a greater response at similar plasma concentrations and half-lives in elderly patients than in younger controls (56). The cellular mechanisms involved in this process have not been determined.

Of analgesic medications, an altered response in the elderly has been best demonstrated with opioid drugs. For example, Belleville et al (31) reported greater analgesia in elderly than in younger patients after 10 mg and 20 mg doses of morphine. This finding has been confirmed (57), and a similar effect has been described after epidural morphine administration (58).

Specific pharmacokinetic changes consonant with these observed effects have also been reported. After a single intramuscular injection of morphine, plasma levels were higher and the exponential rate of decline slower in elderly patients (59, 60). These data suggest that advanced age is associated with a decrease in morphine clearance. Similarly, plasma morphine concentrations were higher in the elderly 2 and 5 minutes after an intravenous injection (61), a finding indicative of a reduced volume of distribution in these patients. The latter study failed to demonstrate an age-related change in plasma half-life, further suggesting that age may affect the distribution of opioid drugs more prominently than their metabolism in some patients. More recently, Owen et al (62) demonstrated an age-related decrease in both the apparent volume of distribution and plasma clearance of morphine after a single intravenous injection. Similar changes in drug clearance and distribution have also been reported with other opioid drugs, including meperidine and alfentanil (63–65).

These pharmacokinetic and pharmacodynamic considerations are also relevant to the management of other postoperative analgesics, specifically local anesthetics and the nonsteroidal anti-inflammatory drugs (NSAIDs). For example, after caudal injection of 2% lidocaine, higher peak plasma levels were observed in older patients than in younger controls (66). In addition, an identical dose blocked a larger number of spinal nerves in elderly patients. Similarly, Bromage (67) demonstrated an inverse relationship between age and the epidural dose of lidocaine required to block a single spinal nerve. Although other local anesthetics have not been investigated, these studies suggest that aging is associated with higher plasma levels, slower elimination, and increased sensitivity to both therapeutic and adverse effects of the local anesthetics.

NSAIDs are highly protein bound, but are capable of saturating binding sites, resulting in rapidly increasing free drug concentrations after dosing has begun (68). Elderly patients may have both a diminished ability to bind these drugs (69–71) and relatively lower levels of plasma proteins. They are thus predisposed to develop a disproportionate increase in free drug concentration once dosing begins, potentially adding to the risk of adverse effects. Other studies (72, 73) have suggested that elimination of the NSAIDs may also be prolonged in the elderly. Although these kinetic changes have not been demonstrated uniformly (74), the extant data indicate that pharmacokinetic changes can also augment the aged patient's sensitivity to this class of drugs.

Management of Postoperative Pain

Increased understanding of pain physiology and analgesic pharmacology has direct impact on the clinical management of postoperative pain in the elderly. The development of rational, scientifically based guidelines for therapy is gradually becoming feasible, and the outlook for bettering postoperative analgesia in this population has improved commensurately. At the present time, the optimal therapeutic approach for most patients remains the repeated parenteral administration of opioid drugs. Selected patients are candidates for alternative methods of opioid delivery, supplemental NSAIDs, regional anesthetic techniques, or psychologic approaches to pain control.

Opioid Analgesics

The term *opioid* is used to designate any drug, either natural or synthetic, that binds specifically to any of the opioid receptors. The mainstay of postoperative pain management, these medications comprise a large group of compounds, varying in their receptor interactions and kinetics (Table 24-1). Expertise in the use of these agents for postoperative pain in the elderly requires familiarity with opioid pharmacology, appreciation for the variability of patient response and the impact of aging, and recognition of the various methods available for opioid delivery.

Influence of Opioid Pharmacology

Opioids can be broadly divided by their receptor interactions into the pure morphine-like agonists and the agonist-antagonists. The latter class can in turn be categorized into the mixed agonist-antagonist drugs pentazocine, nalbuphine, and butorphanol, and the partial agonists, of which buprenorphine is available clinically. While these two subclasses vary in their specific mechanisms, all

Table 24-1. Equianalgesic doses and half-lives of the opioid analgesics

Drug	Route	Equianalgesic dose	Half-life (hr)
Opioid agonists			
Morphine	IM	10	2–4
	PO	20–60 [a]	
Methadone	IM	10	15–57
	PO	20	
Levorphanol	IM	2	12–16
	PO	4	
Hydromorphone	IM	1.5	2–3
	PO	7.5	
Meperidine	IM	75	3–4
	PO	300	
Oxymorphone	IM	1	2–3
	PR	10	
Oxycodone	IM	15	–
	PO	30	
Codeine	IM	130	3–4
	PO	200	
Opioid agonist-antagonists			
Mixed agonist-antagonists			
Pentazocine	IM	60	2–3
	PO	180	
Nalbuphine	IM	10	5
Butorphanol	IM	2	2–4
Partial agonists			
Buprenorphine	IM	0.4	—
	SL	0.3	

Note: Equianalgesic doses were based on single-dose relative potency assays.

[a] An IM:PO relative potency of 1:6 is reported in single-dose studies of morphine, but uncontrolled data and clinical experience suggest that this changes to 1:2–3 with chronic dosing.

agonist-antagonist drugs share the ability to antagonize opioid effects at one or more receptor subtypes (75). This property explains the observation that the administration of an agonist-antagonist drug to a patient already physically dependent on an opioid medication may produce an abstinence syndrome identical to that caused by the pure antagonist, naloxone. This effect becomes a practical consideration only in the selection of a postoperative analgesic for those patients, usually with cancer pain, maintained on chronic opioid therapy.

In addition to the production of an abstinence syndrome in the physically dependent patient, the agonist-antagonists share other important properties (76–79). All have less abuse potential than the pure agonists, an observation with little clinical relevance in the aged population, and all possess a ceiling for respiratory depression. Drugs in the mixed agonist-antagonist subclass have significantly more psychotomimetic effects than the agonist drugs; of these agents, pentazocine is by far the worst offender. Finally, there is some evidence that agonist-antagonist drugs have a ceiling for analgesia at high doses, another effect without clinical relevance in the nontolerant, elderly postoperative patient.

The agonist-antagonist drugs also share the full gamut of opioid effects produced by the pure agonists. Although there is a clinical suspicion and some supportive data that the range of effects of individual drugs within each class can be distinguished from the others, these differences pale in comparison to the interindividual variability in patient response to the different agents. Thus, an individual patient may have a favorable response to morphine and intolerable side effects from meperidine, or vice versa. Clinical experience indicates that the most significant differences among drugs in the clinical setting are pharmacokinetic, with half-life the most salient. As explained below, these kinetic differences, in combination with relatively few caveats based on toxicity, form the basis for the few appropriate guidelines for opioid selection in the management of postoperative pain in the elderly.

Methods of Opioid Analgesia

Intramuscular. The intramuscular injection of an opioid is the most popular method of postoperative pain control, due to its convenience, efficacy, and relative low cost. Recent studies, however, have documented the difficulty inherent in providing continuous analgesia via intermittent injection. In pharmacokinetic studies of meperidine, for example, repetitive injection was associated with wide fluctuations in plasma concentration (80); individual patients demonstrated a twofold variation in peak plasma concentration and a threefold variation in time to peak concentration, while an interindividual variability in these parameters was fivefold and sevenfold, respectively. Overall, meperidine plasma levels were in excess of the minimal analgesic concentration for approximately 35% of each 4-hour-dosing interval (80). These data, in combination with the high prevalence of inadequate analgesia established through surveys of postoperative patients (39, 42, 46), have raised questions about the effectiveness of this traditional approach.

The variability observed with repeated intramuscular administration may be due to variability in drug absorption (81). Attempts to obviate this problem have included intramuscular infusions (82), intramuscular patient-controlled analgesia (83), and controlled-release intramuscular preparations of morphine (84). The efficacy and generalizability of these alternative approaches remain largely undetermined. Nonetheless, the availability of these, and the other alternative approaches described below, provides options for therapy in those patients with inadequate relief from the usual procedures.

Intravenous. Clinically, the intravenous route can be used in three distinct approaches to postoperative pain management: repeated intravenous injections, continuous intravenous infusion, and patient-controlled analgesia. Repetitive intravenous dosing has been used most often in the recovery room setting, where patients with severe pain can undergo rapid titration of the analgesic. In one approach (4, 85), small intravenous bolus injections are given every 15 to 20 minutes until effective analgesia ensues. After pain relief has occurred, the dosing interval is lengthened, usually to 1 hour or more. Although repeated intravenous injections are rarely possible after the patient is returned to the ward, the response to the initial titration can be used as a guide to determine the most suitable dose and dosing interval for subsequent intramuscular or oral administration of the same drug. This technique of repeated small intravenous doses has been reported to result in more stable analgesia, requiring a lesser quantity of opioid drug than that given in an intramuscular titration (86). Since any opioid drug that can be given intramuscularly can also be administered by intravenous bolus injection, this technique is possible with any of the opioid drugs. Its major disadvantage is the nursing time required for drug administration and patient monitoring. For this reason alone, the technique has relatively limited applicability in the management of postoperative pain.

Continuous intravenous infusion removes the peaks and troughs in plasma drug concentration and in theory permits maintenance of a continuous level somewhere between the minimum effective analgesic concentration and the toxic range. The approach also obviates the need for injections and may therefore add to patient comfort. Compared to repetitive intramuscular injections, several studies have claimed improved analgesia, reduced total consumption of opioid drug, and lower incidence of respiratory complications in patients treated with infusions (87–91). Although such favorable results have not been reported by all investigators (92), the technique is generally considered to be safe and effective.

The specific method of continuous opioid infusion may also influence outcome. An initial loading bolus provides a rapid rise of plasma concentration and thereby reduces the time necessary to approach steady state plasma levels. In the absence of pharmacokinetic studies, the size of the loading bolus is empirical, and is generally selected to be equal to the starting dose used in repetitive intramuscular administration. As an alternative to the loading dose, a loading infusion technique can be used. Rutter et al (91) infused morphine at 2 mg per minute until analgesia occurred, then 3 to 5 times this dose by continuous infusion over the ensuing 72 hours. In a similar approach, an initial morphine infusion rate of 6 mg per hour is gradually reduced to 1 to 3 mg per hour after several hours (4). These techniques require close observation initially and are perhaps best begun in the recovery room. After a stable intravenous infusion is in place, clinical experience suggests that adequate monitoring can be achieved in the ward, assuming that the infusion pump is reliable.

Additional analgesia may be required during maintenance infusions. A "rescue dose," a bolus injection usually selected to be equal to the loading dose, can be offered every 2 to 3 hours as needed to meet this requirement (93). Should frequent "rescue doses" be requested or analgesia become persistently inadequate, the infusion rate should be increased, using the sum of the "rescue doses" during the prior 12 to 24 hours as a guide. Each increment in the infusion rate should be preceded by a loading bolus. It is prudent to record vital signs hourly for at least 3 hours after every bolus dose given to patients receiving an infusion.

The final method of intravenous opioid administration is patient-controlled analgesia (PCA). This technique involves self-administration of analgesic medication by the use of a specialized infusion pump (85, 94, 95). These pumps are designed so that patients may activate an intravenous bolus injection, with the size of the dose, rate of delivery, and minimum time between doses preset by the physician. A variety of warning devices are installed to preclude accidental overdose, and both cumulative drug dose and number of attempts at drug delivery can be recorded, thereby providing a measure of postoperative analgesic use.

PCA using drugs such as morphine, meperidine, fentanyl, and buprenorphine has been studied extensively in recent years and has achieved some measure of clinical acceptance. Although most studies have demonstrated safety, efficacy and high level of patient and staff acceptance of the technique (94, 96), others have found no difference in analgesic effectiveness when compared to conventional methods (97). One study reported lesser satisfaction among those receiving PCA due to reduced nursing attention (98); in this investigation, the approach was least preferred by elderly patients, who as a group experienced the greatest difficulty in operating the pump. Thus, while PCA may have substantial advantages in selected patients by offering the opportunity for personal control and improved titration of analgesia, the older patient may be less comfortable with the technology and less able to achieve a maximal result. Should mild confusion occur after dosing begins, an effect to which the elderly patient is particularly predisposed, the use of the device will falter even more. Clinical experience therefore suggests that the role of PCA may be limited in the elderly population.

Oral. Oral administration of opioid analgesics, the preferred method in the management of cancer pain, can be used as premedication prior to surgery and, in selected settings, may be useful early in the postoperative period. Several factors must be considered, however, before oral administration is undertaken. First, the efficacy of oral analgesics will be compromised if absorption from the small intestine is impaired. This may be due to gastrointestinal dysmotility, either related directly to the surgery or to the use of anticholinergic drugs given prior to or during the operation. Second, equianalgesic doses (99) must be used in switching routes of administration (Table 25-1). Failure to consider this factor is a major cause of undertreatment in postoperative pain management.

Sublingual, buccal, and rectal. Alternative nonparenteral forms of opioid administration are occasionally useful in the elderly postoperative patient. For example, the safety and efficacy of sublingual administration has been established for the agonist-antagonist drug, buprenorphine (100), a formulation that will hopefully become available in this country soon. The efficacy of sublingual administration of other opioids has not been well established, although morphine was reported to be effective in one study (101). Buccal administration of morphine, in which a tablet is held against the buccal mucosa for up to 6 hours has also been determined to be efficacious in malignant pain (102), but has never been studied in the postoperative setting.

The efficacy of rectal administration is unquestioned, but its potency against the oral and intramuscular routes remains controversial (103). In this country, rectal formulations are available for morphine, hydromorphone, and oxymorphone. Administration by this route results in lower and more delayed peak analgesia with a longer duration of effect than intramuscular dosing. Clinical experience suggests that potency is similar to the oral route in most patients. The rectal route may provide an extremely useful alternative for elderly postoperative patients poorly tolerant of oral and parenteral administration of analgesic drugs.

Spinal opioids. The intraspinal administration of opioid analgesics in the clinical management of pain developed in response to the discovery of opioid receptors in the dorsal horn of the spinal cord. Advances in the technique have been extremely rapid, and both intrathecal and epidural approaches are now widely used (104).

Drugs injected into the cerebrospinal fluid (CSF) can reach adjacent neural tissues, ascend to higher cerebral structures by bulk flow of CSF, or enter the systemic circulation (105). Similarly, drugs administered into the epidural space also enter the CSF at high concentration, but are absorbed systemically to a much greater extent (106, 107). Segmental opioid effects include selective analgesia without motor, autonomic, or sensory effects (58, 104). Activation of receptors in the brainstem may both contribute to analgesia and result in side effects, as discussed below.

In the postoperative setting, the prototypical approach has utilized the instillation of morphine into the epidural space (104, 108, 109). Great clinical variability has been demonstrated in the effective dose, onset of action, duration of effect, and incidence of side effects (58, 104, 110, 111). Epidural doses of morphine as small as 0.5 mg may be effective, and the duration of effect may be 8 to 24 hours, rarely longer. Similar to parenteral dosing, equivalent doses appear to have greater effects in elderly than in youthful patients (58). A study of elderly patients reported that repeated epidural doses over a short period of time, specifically 4 mg followed by 2 mg every 30 minutes, provided effective analgesia, but was associated with an unacceptable incidence of side effects, especially sedation. These data and clinical experience suggest that a more useful approach in elderly patients who are candidates for epidural morphine begins with a relatively small initial dose (0.5–2 mg), followed by additional doses only after the effect of the first is fully assessed. The size of the injection is increased only if the peak effect is inadequate.

The epidural administration of opioid drugs other than morphine has theoretical benefits but is not widely used clinically. In particular, drugs with greater lipid solubility may be less likely to ascend in CSF or redistribute systemically, and may therefore produce fewer adverse effects. Although a comparative trial of epidural morphine, fentanyl, and meperidine reported no differences (112), additional studies are badly needed to clarify the efficacy and safety profile of the various opioids after spinal administration.

The intrathecal dose of morphine yielding analgesia is much less than that required epidurally; doses as low as 0.1 mg have been effective (113). The risk of adverse effects, including respiratory depression, may be somewhat higher than after epidural administration (114, 115), with the elderly again at particular risk. The additional liability renders this technique less favorable than epidural administration for postoperative pain management.

Less serious side effects following spinal opioid administration (both intrathecal and epidural) are common (104, 116). Urinary retention or pruritis may each occur in up to one-third of patients. Where analgesia is acceptable, these are typically managed symptomatically for the relatively brief period during which postoperative analgesia is required. If side effects are particularly severe or refractory to treatment, or if concomitant analgesia is inadequate, the technique usually needs to be abandoned and another approach pursued.

Prophylactic Use of Opioid Drugs

Several studies have assessed the potential value of premedication with opioid drugs in reducing postoperative pain. While shorter-acting opioids would likely have little impact in this respect, longer-acting drugs may be efficacious. While Ogg et al. (117) demonstrated no benefit and added side effects from the preoperative use of buprenorphine, others have noted improved pain relief in patients premedicated with a sustained-release morphine preparation (118, 119). Another prophylactic approach, intraoperative administration of an opioid, has also been evaluated as a method for reducing pain in the immediate postoperative period. A controlled comparison of 10 mg of intravenous morphine and 0.3 mg of intravenous buprenorphine at the end of surgery demonstrated a delay of more than 10 hours in the appearance of severe pain with the former and less than 5 hours with the latter (120). Thus, the concept of pain prophylaxis in the postoperative period may have validity. Studies are needed to compare the safety and efficacy of the approach against traditional therapies, and replication in the aged must be done before the technique can be recommended in this group.

Adverse Effects of Opioid Administration

The most serious adverse effect of opioid drugs is clearly respiratory depression. The risk of this effect is related to several factors, including age (116), size of the effective dose (121), and concurrent administration of other central nervous system depressants (113, 122). The earliest sign of opioid-induced respiratory depression is a slowed respiratory rate in a sedated patient. Sedation, therefore, should be viewed as a clinical signal, underscoring the potential for respiratory compromise. Patients who become markedly sedated after opioid administration should be closely monitored, and in most cases, subsequent doses should be decreased. Conversely, patients who develop respiratory compromise in the absence of sedation cannot be considered to have opioid toxicity and should be evaluated for the existence of a primary pulmonary process, such as pneumonia, atelectasis, or embolism.

While respiratory depression after oral or parenteral administration of opioid drugs occurs at peak plasma levels early in the dosing interval, this adverse effect can be delayed for many hours after spinal administration (122). The delayed onset is presumably due to the slow rostral spread of the opioid through the CSF to the respiratory centers of the brainstem. Although the incidence is extremely low (116), the potential for delayed respiratory compromise indicates the need for an extended period of monitoring in patients treated with spinal opioids.

Like other serious adverse effects of opioid drugs, respiratory depression can be promptly reversed by the specific opioid antagonist, naloxone. The only important exception to this rule occurs with buprenorphine, a drug with an extremely high affinity for the opioid receptor; repeated high doses of naloxone may still yield only partial reversal with this agent. Although administration of naloxone has been reported to treat respiratory depression without compromising analgesia (58, 110, 115), the typical effect is antagonism of all opioid effects. Thus, naloxone should only be considered in those patients with clinically significant respiratory depression; other adverse effects, such as sedation, are better managed by dose reduction. It must also be recognized that the duration of antagonism may be far shorter than the time required for the opioid effect to wane, particularly after spinal administration of the opioid, and that repeated doses of naloxone, or a naloxone infusion, may be required to maintain respiratory function until the opioid is metabolized.

Although respiratory depression is the most serious adverse effect, others are far more common. Sedation is a frequent occurrence and may be accompanied by confusion in the elderly patient, particularly if drugs with additive sedative or anticholinergic effects (e.g., hypnotics, tricyclic antidepressants, antiemetics, and antihistamines) are administered concurrently. Nausea and vomiting are also frequent and often require treatment with an antiemetic. Urinary retention occurs occasionally and is more common after spinal administration of opioid drugs. Although phenoxybenzamine has been reported to be useful in the management of this effect (123, 124), the drug may be poorly tolerated by the elderly patient. Inhibition of the cough reflex may be a problem in elderly patients who must clear secretions and reinflate atelectatic lung. Hypotension is an extremely uncommon complication, occasionally observed in the nontolerant, relatively dehydrated patient; intraspinal administration may predispose to this adverse effect (125, 126). Pruritus may complicate systemic opioids, but has been observed to be a frequent and troubling effect only after spinal administration (85, 104, 127). Clinical experience suggests that antihistamine therapy may not reliably reverse the effect, although these drugs are commonly utilized in this setting. Finally, the elderly are particularly prone to the constipating effect of opioid drugs. Although usually a minor problem in patients who have not undergone abdominal procedures, constipation can be significant in aged patients recovering from postoperative ileus, in whom the use of opioid drugs may prolong ileus and delay the recovery of normal bowel function.

Certain adverse effects occur more commonly with one drug than another. For example, chronic dosing with meperidine has been associated with the accumulation of a toxic metabolite, normeperidine, which may cause dysphoria, myoclonus, tremulousness, and seizures (128). Although these toxic effects are rare in postoperative patients, the elderly may be at particular risk due to subclinical renal insufficiency with impaired clearance of the toxic compound. This risk suggests that meperidine should be viewed as a second-line agent for the management of postoperative pain in the elderly patient.

Although psychotomimetic and dysphoric effects may occur with any of the opioids, the incidence is greater following administration of the agonist-antagonist drugs, with the exception of buprenorphine. Pentazocine is widely regarded as the most problematic and cannot be recommended for routine postoperative pain management.

Tolerance, Physical Dependence, and Psychologic Dependence

Concerns about tolerance, physical dependence, and psychologic dependence contribute heavily to the undertreatment of postoperative pain. Appropriate management of the elderly pain patient requires clear definition of these terms and an objective assessment of the risk involved.

Tolerance is a pharmacologic effect defined as the need for higher doses of opioid medication to maintain effects over time. Extensive clinical experience indicates that tolerance is not a significant problem in the postoperative period. The rapid need for higher doses of opioid medications in the absence of progressive disease is rare; in the postoperative period, during which the nociceptive lesion is gradually healing and opioid administration is typically short-lived, the need for escalation of opioid dosage due to declining effects is unlikely to occur. Should the patient become tolerant, the first sign of which is a reduction in the duration of effect after each dose of drug, the problem is easily managed by increasing the dosing frequency or the size of each dose. Thus, tolerance should not be considered to be a reason for limiting opioid doses to subtherapeutic levels during the postoperative period.

Physical dependence is also a pharmacologic effect, characterized by the occurrence of an abstinence syndrome upon abrupt cessation of opioid dosing or administration of an opioid antagonist drug. Like tolerance, this effect is not a significant problem during the postoperative period. Physical dependence is unlikely to develop during the brief period of analgesic dosing required by most patients with postoperative pain. Postoperative opioid doses, particularly in the elderly, are also relatively low, a second factor limiting the development of physical dependence. Finally, should the need for opioids continue long enough that some degree of physical dependence occurs, it can be simply managed by tapering the drug after the painful lesion has healed, rather than discontinuing it abruptly.

Tolerance and physical dependence are more likely to be a problem in patients with cancer pain who are chronically reliant on opioid drugs and who undergo surgery. These patients are often administered doses far too low to manage superimposed postoperative pain, given their degree of tolerance. Should respiratory depression develop postoperatively, the customary dose of naloxone may cause a severe abstinence syndrome, associated with recurrence of intolerable pain. The same outcome may occur if opioids are discontinued for surgery and reinstituted later at too low a dose. A similar error is made when patients physically dependent on opioid drugs are prescribed an agonist-antagonist drug, such as butorphanol, nalbuphine, or pentazocine, during the postoperative period. The antagonist effect of these drugs may also precipitate an abstinence syndrome. In these patients, naloxone should be used only in the setting of clinically significant respiratory depression, in which case repeated small doses of a dilute solution (e.g., 0.4 mg in 10 cc saline) is the safest approach.

A major impediment to improved postoperative management of pain is the fear, expressed by both practitioners and patients, of psychologic dependence. This term has been used synonymously with the frequently misapprehended "addiction" and denotes a psychologic and behavioral syndrome characterized by drug craving and intense involvement with securing its supply. Inappropriate use of prescribed medication, drug hoarding, or selling, and the acquisition of medication from multiple physicians are common elements. Clearly, a substantial risk of this syndrome among postoperative patients medicated with opioid drugs would warrant sharp curtailment of their use. Numerous surveys during the past two decades, however, have demonstrated an extremely low incidence of iatrogenic psychologic dependence in patients without a prior history of substance abuse (129–131). For example, one survey (130) identified only four cases of psychologic dependence among 11,882 patients without a prior history of substance abuse who received opioid drugs during a hospital admission. Psychologic dependence in the elderly after treatment with opioids is an extraordinary occurrence, and this consideration should not limit appropriate analgesic therapy in this population.

Guidelines for Opioid Use in the Elderly

Based on the above considerations and clinical experience, guidelines for the management of postoperative opioids in the elderly population can be provided, as follows.

Drug selection. Management is simplified with the use of an opioid analgesic with a short half-life (132). Steady state plasma drug concentrations are not approached for four to five half-lives after repetitive dosing has begun, and plasma levels of long half-life opioids, such as methadone or levorphanol, will continue to rise for several days after initiating or increasing the dose. Delayed toxicity may occur, which may be more significant in the older patient already sensitive to the adverse effects of these medications (133, 134).

Of the short half-life opioid drugs, meperidine and pentazocine should be considered second-line agents, due to their relatively high side effect liability. Clinical experience with fentanyl is very limited, and its kinetic profile suggests that it may be a difficult drug to manage in the postoperative period; it, too, is not recommended. Other short half-life agents include the agonist drugs, morphine and hydromorphone, and the agonist-antagonist drugs, butorphanol, nalbuphine and buprenorphine. There are neither controlled comparisons among these drugs, nor compelling individual characteristics that contraindicate the use of one or another in the postoperative period. Although butorphanol and nalbuphine are more likely to cause adverse psychotomimetic effects, these are unlikely to be a problem during the short duration of therapy at relatively low doses employed in treating the elderly surgical patient. Additionally, the risk of respiratory depression may be attenuated with these agents. Nonetheless, clinical experience is greatest with morphine and meperidine, and the choice among all these drugs remains in the realm of clinical judgement.

For mild to moderate pain, usually several days after surgery, codeine or oxycodone preparations (containing acetaminophen or aspirin) are customarily used. There are no controlled trials assessing the efficacy and side effect liability of these drugs against others, although extensive clinical experience suggest they are both safe and effective.

Dose. The initial opioid dose should be the lowest that provides analgesia. This is usually less than that required by younger patients. For example, morphine 5 mg or hydromorphonel 0.75 mg intramuscularly every 3 to 4 hours is a prudent and appropriate starting dose for the nontolerant elderly patient.

There is great interindividual variability in the response to opioid drugs, and it is often necessary to either increase or decrease the dose subsequently. After the response to the initial dose or two is observed, it should be adjusted, and the patient carefully monitored until the effect of this change can be ascertained. Again, it must be emphasized that plasma drug levels will not stabilize with repeated dosing until four to five half-lives have passed, usually 12 to 24 hours with these short half-life drugs.

Dosing should be initiated on an "as needed" basis in the elderly patient. This may be sufficient for the full period of administration if the patient can collaborate in the therapy and the nurses are responsive. After 24 hours, the analgesic requirement of the patient is indicated by the number of doses requested; should analgesia be inadequate at this time, consideration should be given to fixed dosing for the subsequent 24–48 hours.

If spinal opioids are selected, the initial dose for the elderly should also be lower than that used in the younger patient (e.g., morphine 2 mg epidurally or 0.5 mg intrathecally). As noted, additional doses should be withheld until the full effect of the first dose has be determined.

Route of administration. Repetitive intramuscular dosing can be adequate if attention is focused on the requirement of the patient (135). Continuous infusion of opioid drugs is an effective alternative approach, although the benefit of this technique over repetitive dosing has never been demonstrated (87, 91). Clinical experience suggests that patients who experience a significant "bolus effect" with repetitive dosing (adverse effects at the peak plasma level early in the dosing period and/or pain breakthrough toward the end) may obtain continuous analgesia from an infusion. As explained above, patient-controlled analgesia currently plays a limited role in the postoperative pain management of the elderly patient. Further evolution of this technique would be needed before it would be widely applicable to these patients.

Although epidural opioids are capable of providing prolonged analgesia with small doses of medication, the procedure requires an experienced clinician and skilled nursing staff. At the present time, it is most reasonable to consider this technique in patients undergoing surgery in the lower half of the body who develop significant central side effects from the systemic administration of opioid drugs. The additive risks involved in intrathecal administration limit the utility of this technique even more.

After the acute postoperative period has passed, it is advisable to switch to oral dosing if tolerated. Oral administration provides the simplist, least costly, and safest method of opioid administration. If necessary, oral administration of opioid drugs can be continued after discharge from the hospital.

Anticipate and treat side effects. Frequent monitoring of vital signs is necessary in elderly patients treated with opioids early in the postoperative period. Patients who become sedated should be closely followed for the potential development of respiratory depression. Nausea can be treated with small doses of hydroxyzine or prochlorperazine. Given the potential susceptibility of aged patients to additive side effects, prophylactic treatment with antiemetics is not recommended. This is true also of antihistamines for pruritus. In contrast, the extremely high prevalence of constipation and the relative safety of laxative drugs suggest that all patients administered opioids for more than 3 days should be provided laxatives, unless contraindicated.

Use drug combinations prudently. As noted, the administration of other drugs with opioids places the elderly patient at relatively high risk for adverse effects. Severe sedation or confusion may develop with the addition of tricyclic antidepressants, benzodiazepines, antihistamines, or neuroleptic drugs. Routine administration should be avoided, and if clinically indicated, one agent should be added at a time, beginning at low doses.

Several drugs produce additive postoperative analgesia when combined with the opioids. Should an indication for concurrent administration of another drug exist (e.g., nausea, anxiety, etc.) consideration should be given these agents first. Intramuscular injection of hydroxyzine 100 mg has been demonstrated to be analgesic and to potentiate the effects of morphine (136, 137). Co-analgesia from the doses used clinically (25–50 mg) has never been established, however. A similar effect has been observed with co-administration of 5 mg of diazepam (138), and a recent study of the benzodiazepine, midazolam, demonstrated a similar action (139). While these studies revealed no increased risk of respiratory depression, this complication has been observed with the combination of buprenorphine and lorazepam or diazepam (140, 141). Thus, the addition of an anxiolytic to morphine can have benefits, but the risks in elderly patients may be substantial, and the use of these compounds must be undertaken cautiously. Dextroamphetamine also potentiates morphine in the treatment of postoperative pain (142), but the risks of a potent sympathomimetic in the elderly limit the utility of this combination. In contrast to the above agents, neuroleptic drugs have never been demonstrated to be analgesic in the postoperative period (143). Finally, NSAIDs provide additive analgesia when combined with opioid analgesics (144, 145). These drugs should be considered to be important adjuvants in patients able to consume oral medications during the postoperative period. In addition, they may be used as primary analgesics in this setting for patients who complain of only mild to moderate pain, as discussed below.

Nonsteroidal Anti-inflammatory Drugs

NSAIDs (Table 24-2) inhibit the production of prostaglandins (146), important mediators of inflammatory pain. Although the precise mechanism of their analgesic effect is unknown (147), it is widely accepted that the primary site of action is in the periphery. This may explain the additive effects observed when these drugs are combined with the opioid analgesics, whose site of action is in the central nervous system.

The NSAIDS share several important properties. Except for acetaminophen, all of these compounds are both anti-inflammatory and antipyretic. The latter effect may be problematic for patients early in the postoperative period, when suppression of fever may obscure clinically important processes. While the anti-inflammatory effects could be of theoretical value in reducing local edema after surgery, the doses required for this effect are likely to be too high to consider this a primary indication for these drugs (148). Analgesia is the desired effect, and effective pain relief in the postoperative period has been demonstrated with indomethacin suppositories (149), oral ibuprofen (150–152) and naproxen (144), and an intravenous salicylate (153–155).

NSAIDs commonly produce side effects, although these are generally mild. The most frequent is gastric dysfunction, ranging from dyspepsia to frank ulceration. The incidence of this effect varies from drug to drug; the risk is minimal with acetaminophen, choline magnesium trisalicylate, and salsalate. With these three drugs again excepted, impairment of platelet aggregation is also an effect shared by all NSAIDs. Renal insufficiency, hepatotoxicity, and hypersensitivity reactions occur occasionally.

The use of NSAIDs in the treatment of postoperative pain in the elderly has not been specifically addressed. The metabolism of these drugs changes with age and the risk of adverse effects increases. While clinical experience suggests that safe and effective administration is possible in the elderly, further studies are needed to define their indications and clarify the side effect liability. At the present time, it is reasonable to use these agents in combination with an opioid when oral dosing is feasible following surgery. Mild to moderate residual pain may be manageable with an NSAID alone. In patients with a prior history of gastrointestinal intolerance to NSAIDs or in those with a potential or existent ulcer or bleeding diathesis, acetaminophen, choline magnesium trisalicylate, or salsalate should be considered first-line agents; with few exceptions, drug selection is otherwise empirical (Table 24-2).

Table 24-2. Nonsteroidal anti-inflammatory drugs

Class	Drugs	Comment
Salicylates	Aspirin Diflunisal Choline magnesium trisalicylate Salsalate	Choline magnesium trisalicylate and salsalate have no effect on GI tract or platelet aggregation
Propionic acids	Ibuprofen Fenoprofen Naproxen Naproxen sodium	Ibuprofen has short half-life
Pyrroles	Indomethacin Tolmetin Sulindac	Potent anti-inflammatory effects, but higher incidence of side effects
Fenamates	Mefenamic acid Meclofenamate	Use not recommended beyond 1 week
Oxicams	Piroxicam	Very long half-life
Pyrazoles	Phenylbutazone Oxyphenbutazone	Most toxic; use supplanted by newer agents
p-Aminophenol derivatives	Acetaminophen	Minimally anti-inflammatory; no effect on GI tract or platelet aggregation

Regional Anesthesia for Postoperative Pain

Local anesthetics bind to sodium channels, block nerve conduction, and at adequate concentration and dose, eradicate both the afferent and efferent function of the nerve. Regional anesthesia can thus provide complete or near complete relief of pain accompanied by inhibition of segmental and suprasegmental reflex responses. This is clearly advantageous in the elderly patient, for whom these responses may constitute a profound physiologic stress. In addition, regional anesthetics provide analgesia without impairing respirations or the cough reflex. This approach, therefore, may be especially indicated in elderly patients with localized wound pain in whom the use of a systemic opioid is contraindicated by advanced pulmonary, renal, or hepatic disease.

Regional anesthesia can be achieved in any part of the body. Local wound infiltration may occasionally be useful, but more often, individual nerves are blocked or a multisegmental epidural block, extending from 2 to 10 spinal segments, is produced. Although usually avoidable, high concentrations of local anesthetics, if required, can cause a complete sensory, motor, and autonomic blockade in addition to analgesia. Depending on the number and location of the nerves involved, paresis of one or more limbs or systemic hypotension may result (4, *156, 157*).

The most important toxicity from local anesthetic drugs occurs after systemic absorption. With the exception of hypersensitivity reactions, these adverse effects are all dose-rélated. Cardiac disturbances include bradycardia, conduction abnormalities, and reduced cardiac contractility; rarely, these effects can be life threatening (158). Central nervous system toxicity includes tremulousness, twitching, paresthesias, tinnitus, lethargy, and ultimately seizures (156). These adverse effects appear to occur with greater frequency in the elderly, although this has never been established unequivocally.

Regional blockade can be produced through one or more of a large and protean group of procedures. In the epidural space, for example, local anesthetics have been given as repeated injections or as a continuous infusion (157, 159). Supplemental injections during continuous epidural infusion are often required and can effectively manage transitory exacerbations of pain. Although a controlled comparison of the different anesthetics has not been performed, bupivacaine is usually preferred for this type of epidural anesthesia (Table 24-3).

Blockade of individual nerves, using local anesthetic or cryoanalgesia, is an extremely simple technique, potentially effective for localized wound pain. For example, intercostal nerve block may provide excellent analgesia after cholecystectomy, mastectomy, and other similar pro-

Table 24-3. Local anesthetic drugs

Shorter acting	Duration (min)
Chloroprocaine	30–60
Lidocaine	90–240
Mepivacaine	120–240
Pilocaine	120–240
Procaine	60–90
Longer acting	
Bupivacaine	180–600
Etiocaine	180–600
Tetracaine	180–600

cedures (160–164). Unilateral intercostal block after cholecystectomy has been demonstrated to provide equivalent analgesia with less respiratory depression than that of systemic opioids (161); bilateral intercostal blocks, however, can compromise respiration and are not recommended. The major potential complication from intercostal blockade is pleural puncture and pneumothorax (165). Similar to epidural injection, the risk of the procedure depends to a large extent on the skill and experience of the practitioner performing it. This is particularly true in the elderly population, where anatomical distortion, poor cooperation, and sensitivity to the systemic effects of local anesthetic drugs may combine to render the procedure more difficult and risky.

Blockade of other nerves can also be performed safely and may be useful in specific settings. For example, injection of the lateral cutaneous nerve of the thigh provided partial to complete analgesia in elderly patients undergoing repair of a fractured femur through a lateral incision (166). Inguinal procedures can be effectively managed by local blockade, and sciatic nerve block may be useful in the patient undergoing procedures of the leg, such as amputation (85).

Finally, local anesthetics can be used to infiltrate the wound at the time of surgery in an effort to reduce incisional pain and simplify postoperative analgesia. Single and repeated injections of long-acting local anesthetics into the wound (167, 168) and continuous wound perfusion (169) have been used effectively. Interestingly, several studies (170, 171) have demonstrated that intermittent injections of saline are almost as effective as local anesthetics, suggesting that dilution of noxious substances or the placebo effect may be operating in many of these cases. The most significant risks of local wound infiltration are infection and systemic absorption of the anesthetic, both of which can be minimized by careful technique. The procedure appears to be one with potentially much wider applicability in the elderly population.

The clinical experience described above suggests that regional anesthetic techniques may have utility in the aged postoperative patient at risk from the systemic administration of opioid analgesics. It must be recognized, however, that elderly patients commonly have concurrent cardiac, cerebral, or hepatic disease that increases the risk of the local anesthetics as well, particularly at the doses required to provide prolonged postoperative analgesia. Thus, the potential risks versus benefits of these techniques must be weighed on a case by case basis, and the decision to use one or another should be based on the type of operation, specific medical liabilities of the patient, and experience of the practitioner.

Other Methods of Analgesia

Transcutaneous Electrical Nerve Stimulation (TENS)

Electrical stimulation of the skin has been used as a method of pain control for almost two decades. The technique evolved from the Gate Control Theory of pain (172), in which stimulation of large diameter, heavily myelinated peripheral nerve fibers is postulated to inhibit the transmission of nociceptive information through activation of inhibitory interneurons in the dorsal horn of the spinal cord.

A number of studies have suggested that TENS may have salutary effects during the postoperative period. Most important, the need for opioid drugs is reduced in those using this approach (173–175). Although these data are highly suggestive of a potent analgesic effect, they derive from poorly controlled surveys, and the response of the elderly has never been assessed specifically. TENS has also been reported to improve respiratory function after cardiac surgery and cholecystectomy, and reduce postoperative ileus (173, 176). These benefits, however, have not been demonstrated in other series (174, 177). Thus, while TENS is widely considered to be potentially beneficial, additional studies are needed to establish its utility and define the scope of its effects.

There are no studies comparing the various methods of TENS; stimulation parameters and electrode placement remain empirical (178). Extensive experience with chronic pain patients suggests large interindividual variation in the response to different techniques. If this approach is selected, trials of multiple techniques are recommended should each fail to provide an analgesic effect.

Although studies of TENS in elderly patients are lacking, it is likely that the procedure would be useful in selected patients, providing analgesia adequate to allow a reduction or cessation of opioid consumption. Specialized equipment and well-trained staff are needed, but should not be a major obstacle to the wider use of this approach.

Cryoanalgesia

Application of a freezing probe to a peripheral nerve produces injury with minimal inflammatory reaction; a prolonged conduction block ensues, with consequent pain relief (179). Cryoanalgesia is only suitable for nerves in which the motor component is minimal or unimportant, such as the intercostal nerves. The technique can therefore provide excellent analgesia after thoracotomy (85, 180, 181). Although some investigators have observed less impressive results (182), it is now widely accepted that cryoanalgesia can be applied safely and may reduce opioid requirement after surgery. The prolonged analgesic effect, as well as the lack of significant pulmonary, cardiovascular, or central nervous system toxicity, suggests that the technique may have great potential in the elderly postoperative patient. Additional trials in the aged population are needed to confirm the safety of the technique and define its indications.

Psychologic Methods

Psychologic methods of pain control have been used to reduce anxiety, stress, and pain during the postoperative period. Mere encouragement and instruction about postoperative pain can reduce discomfort and the need for opioids (183–185). Specialized cognitive techniques, such as hypnosis (186), relaxation training (187), and distraction procedures (188, 189), have been used to reduce postoperative anxiety and pain. One investigator (187) trained elderly patients undergoing hip surgery in a relaxation technique and demonstrated a statistically significant reduction in pain and distress postoperatively. Although additional studies are needed to establish the applicability and effectiveness of these techniques in the elderly population, it appears likely that older, cognitively intact patients are candidates for psychologic interventions. At the least, these patients should receive the same explanations and instructions given their younger counterparts, since this alone may reduce the need for analgesic medications. Age itself should never be viewed as a limitation to the appropriate processing of information about surgery. The practice of withholding information from the elderly in the misapprehension that it would be misunderstood is countertherapeutic. Indeed, many elderly patients would benefit from longer preoperative sessions, during which the anticipated postoperative course is discussed in detail.

Conclusion

Clinician awareness of age-related changes in pharmacokinetics, pharmacodynamics, pain physiology, and psychologic reactions is increasing. In the management of postoperative pain, this has led to greater recognition of the potential value of local over systemic methods, improved use of systemic analgesics, and appreciation of nonpharmacologic techniques of analgesia. Additional research is needed in the elderly population to define the safety and efficacy of the various techniques available and determine the indications for each. These studies will complement the complex process of clinical judgment, by which the specific medical and psychologic needs of the aged patient are balanced against the anatomical and physiologic implications of the surgery to provide an approach for postoperative pain management appropriate to the individual.

References

1. Merskey, H. 1979. Pain terms: A list with definitions and notes on usage. *Pain* 6:249–252.
2. Beecher, HK, 1959. *Measurement of Subjective Responses*. New York: Oxford University Press.
3. Loeser, JD. 1983. Pain. In *The Clinical Neurosciences,* Ed., RN Rosenberg, vol 2. New York: Churchill Livingstone.
4. Benedetti, C, Bonica, JJ, and Bellucci, G. 1985. Pathophysiology and therapy of postoperative pain: A review. In *Advances in Pain Research and Therapy,* Eds., C. Benedetti, CR Chapman, and G Moricca, pp. 373–407, vol 7. New York: Raven Press.
5. Willis, WD. 1985. *The Pain System*. New York: S. Karger.
6. Zimmermann, M. 1979. Peripheral and central nervous mechanisms of nociception, pain and pain therapy: Facts and hypotheses. In *Advances in Pain Research and Therapy,* Eds., JJ Bonica, JC Liebeskind, and DG Albe-Fessard, pp. 3–32, vol 3. New York: Raven Press.
7. Famewo, CE. 1985. Study of incidence of post-operative pain among Nigerian patients. *Afr J Med Sci* 14:175–179.
8. Basbaum, AI. 1985. The generation and control of pain. In *The Clinical Neurosciences,* Ed., RN Rosenberg, pp. 301–324, vol 5. New York: Churchill Livingstone.
9. Nathan, PW. 1985. Pain in the sympathetic nervous system. *J Auton Nerv Syst* 7:363–370.
10. Wilmore, DW, Long, JM, and Mason, AD. 1976. Stress in surgical patients as a neurophysiologic reflex response. *Surg Gynecol Obstet* 142:257–269.
11. Kehlet, H. 1978. Influence of epidural analgesia on the endocrine metabolic response to surgery. *Acta Anaesthe Scand* (suppl) 70:39–42.
12. Bessman, FP, and Renner, VJ. 1982. The biphasic hormonal nature of stress. In *Pathophysiology of Shock, Anoxia and Ischemia,* Eds., RA Cowley and BF Trump. Baltimore: Williams & Wilkins.
13. Hammond, DL. 1985. Pharmacology of central pain—modulating networks (biologic amines and non-opioid analgesics). In *Advance in Pain Research and Therapy,* Eds., HL Fields, R Hubner, and F Cervero, pp. 499–512, vol 9. New York: Raven Press.

14. Akil, H, et al. 1984. Endogenous opioids: Biology and function *Annu Rev Neurosci* 7:223–255.
15. Millan, MJ. 1986. Multiple opioid systems and pain. *Pain* 27:303–348.
16. North, RA, and Egar, TM. 1983. Actions and distribution of opioid peptides in peripheral tissue. *Br Med Bull* 39:71.
17. Atweh, SF, and Kuhar, MJ. 1983. Distribution and physiological significance of opioid receptors in the brain. *Br Med Bull* 39:47.
18. Martin, WR, et al. 1976. The effects of morphine and nalorphine-like drugs in the non-dependent and morphine-dependent chronic spinal dog. *J Pharm Exp Ther* 197:517–532.
19. Patersen, SJ, Robson, LE, and Kosterlitz, HW. 1983. Classification of opioid receptors. *Br Med Bull* 39: 31–36.
20. Pert, CB, and Snyder, SH. 1973. "Opiate receptors": Demonstration in nervous tissue. *Science* 179:1011.
21. Pflug, AE, and Bonica, JJ. 1977. Physiopathology and control of postoperative pain. *Arch Surg* 112:773–781.
22. Marshall, BE, and Wyche, MQ. 1972. Hypoxemia during and after anaesthesia. *Anesthesiology* 37:178–209.
23. Parbrook, GD, Steel, DF, and Dalrymple, DG. 1973. Factors predisposing to postoperative pain and pulmonary complications. *Br J Anaesth* 45:21–32.
24. Craig, DB. 1981. Postoperative recovery of pulmonary function. *Anaesth Analg* 60:46.
25. Modig, F. 1976. Respiration and circulation after total hip replacement surgery. *Acta Anaesth Scand* 20:225–236.
26. Harkins, SW, Kwentus, J, and Price, DD. 1984. Pain and the elderly. In *Advances in Pain Research and Therapy,* Eds., C Benedetti, CR Chapman, and G Moricca, pp. 103–122, vol 7. New York: Raven Press.
27. Cauna, N. 1965. The effect of aging on the receptor organs of the human dermis. In *Advances in Biology of the Skin,* Ed., W Montagna, pp. 63–96. New York: Pergamon Press.
28. Sternbach, RA. 1986. Survey of pain in the limited states: The Nuprin pain report. *Clin J Pain* 2(1):49–53.
29. Portenoy, RK, and Kanner, RM. 1985. Patterns of analgesic prescription and consumption in a University-affiliated community hospital. *Arch Intern Med* 145: 439–441.
30. Faherty, BS, and Grier, MR. 1984. Analgesic medication for elderly people post-surgery. *Nurs Res* 33:369–372.
31. Belleville, JW, et al. 1971. Influence of age on pain relief from analgesics. *JAMA* 217:1835–1841.
32. Donovan, BD. 1983. Patient attitudes to postoperative pain relief. *Anesth Intens Care* 11:125–129.
33. Johnson, JE, Debbs, JM, and Leventhal, H. 1970. Psychosocial factors in the welfare of surgical patients. *Nurs Res* 19(1):18–29.
34. Chapman, CR. 1978. Psychological aspects of pain. *Hosp Prac* 13:15–19.
35. Graham, LE. 1971. Evaluation of anxiety and fear in adult surgical patients. *Nurs Res* 20(2):113–122.
36. Martinez-Urrutia, A. 1975. Anxiety and pain in surgical patients. *J Consul Clin Psychol* 43:4378–4442.
37. Spielberger, CD, et al. 1973. Emotional reactions to surgery. *Ann Consult Clin Psych* 40(1):33–38.
38. Scott, LE, Clum, GA, and Peoples, JB. 1983. Preoperative predictors of postoperative pain. *Pain* 15:283–293.
39. Angell, M. 1982. The quality of mercy. *N Engl J Med* 306:98–99.
40. Cohen, JL. 1986. Pharmacokinetic changes in aging. *Am J Med* 80 (Suppl. 5A):31–38.
41. Hug, CC. 1980. Improving analgesic therapy. *Anesthesiology* 53:441–443.
42. Tammisto, T, and Tigerstedt, I. 1982. Narcotic analgesics in postoperative pain relief in adults. *Acta Anaesth Scand* 74 (Suppl.):161–164.
43. Tracy, JB. 1976. Postoperative pain. *Br Med J* 2:1070.
44. Ulting, JE, and Smith, JM. 1979. Post-operative analgesia. *Anaesthesia* 134:320–332.
45. Weis, OF, et al. 1983. Attitudes of patients, housestaff, and nurses toward postoperative analgesic care. *Anaesth Analg* 62:70–74.
46. Cohen, FL. 1980. Postsurgical pain relief: Patients' status and nurses' medication choices. *Pain* 9:265–274.
47. Marks, RM, and Sachar, EJ. 1973. Treatment of medical inpatients with narcotic analgesics. *Ann Intern Med* 78(2):173–181.
48. Pilowsky, J, and Bond, MR. 1969. Pain and its management in malignant disease. *Psychosom Med* 31:400–404.
49. Morgan, J, and Furst, DE. 1986. Implications of drug therapy in the elderly. *Clin Rheum Dis* 12(1):227–244.
50. Reidenberg, MM. 1982. Drugs in the elderly. *Med Clin North Am* 66(5):1073–1078.
51. Bender, AD. 1965. The effect of increased age on the distribution of peripheral blood flow in man. *J Am Geriatr Soc* 13(3):192–196.
52. Geokas, MC, and Haverback, BJ. 1969. The aging gastrointestinal tract. *Am J Surg* 117:881–889.
53. Goldberg, PB, and Roberts, J. 1983. Pharmacologic basis for developing rational drug regimen for elderly patients. *Med Clin North Am* 67:315–331.
54. Wallace, S, Whiting, B, and Runcil, J. 1976. Factors affecting drug binding in plasma of elderly patients. *Br J Clin Pharmacol* 3:327–330.
55. Rafsky, HA, and Newman, B. 1965. Liver function tests in the aged. (The serum cholesterol partition, bromsulphalein, cephalin flocculation and oral and intravenous hippuric acid test). *Am J Digest Dis* 10(2):66–69.
56. Casteldan, CM, et al. 1977. Increased sensitivity to nitrazepam in old age. *Br Med J* 1:10–12.
57. Kaiko, RF. 1980. Age and morphine analgesia in cancer patients with postoperative pain. *Clin Pharmacol Ther* 28:823–826.
58. Modig, F, and Paalzow, L. 1981. A comparison of epidural morphine and epidural bupivacaine for postoperative pain relief. *Acta Anaesth Scand* 25:437–441.
59. Kaiko, RF, et al. 1982. Narcotics in the elderly. *Med Clin North Am* 66:1079–1089.
60. Kaiko, RF, et al. 1983. Sources of variation in analgesic responses in cancer patients with chronic pain receiving morphine. *Pain* 15:191–200.
61. Berkowitz, BA, et al. 1975. The disposition of morphine in surgical patients. *Clin Pharmacol Ther* 17:629–635.
62. Owen, JA, et al. 1983. Age-related morphine kinetics. *Clin Pharmacol Ther* 34:364–368.
63. Chan, K, et al. 1975. The effect of aging on plasma pethidine concentration. *Br J Pharmacol* 1:297–302.
64. Helmers, H, et al. 1984. Alfentanil kinetics in the elderly. *Clin Pharmacol Ther* 36:239–243.

65. Helmers, H, Noorduin, H, and Leeuwen, LV. 1985. Alfentanil used in the aged: A clinical comparison with its use in young patients. *Eur J Anaesth* 2:347–352.
66. Freund, PR, et al. 1982. Comparative lidocaine pharmacokinetics during caudal anesthesia in young and geriatric patients. *Anesthesiology* 57:212.
67. Bromage, PR. 1969. Aging and epidural dose requirements. *Br J Anesth* 41:1016–1022.
68. Schlegel, SI, and Paulus, HE. 1986. Non-steroidal analgesic therapy in the elderly. *Clin Rheum Dis* 12(1): 245–273.
69. Lesko, LJ, et al. 1983. Salicylate protein binding in young and elderly serum as measured by diafiltration. *Clin Pharmacol Ther* 33:257.
70. O'Malley, K, et al. 1971. Effect of age and sex on human drug metabolism. *Br Med J* 11:607–609.
71. Verbeeck, RK, and DeSchepper, PJ. 1980. Influence of chronic renal failure and hemodialysis on diflunisal plasma protein binding. *Clin Pharmacol Ther* 27(5): 628–634.
72. Cuny, G, et al. 1979. Pharmacokinetics of salicylates in the elderly. *Gerontology* 25:49–55.
73. Upton, RA, et al. 1984. Naproxen pharmacokinetics in the elderly. *Br J Clin Pharmacol* 18:207–214.
74. Albert, KS, et al. 1984. Effects of age on the clinical pharmacokinetics of ibuprofen. *Am J Med* 77(1A): 47–50.
75. Houde, RW. 1979. Analgesic effectiveness of the narcotic agonist-antagonists. *Br J Clin Pharmacol* 7:2975–3085.
76. Kantor, TG. 1986. Pentazocine: Clinical analgesic studies. In *Advances in Pain Research and Therapy,* Eds., KM Foley and CE Inturrisi, pp. 241–245, vol 8. New York: Raven Press.
77. Wallenstein, SL, et al. 1986. Nalbuphine: clinical analgesic studies. In *Advances in Pain Research and Therapy,* Eds., KM Foley and CE Inturrisi, pp. 247–252, vol 8. New York: Raven Press.
78. Caruso, FS. 1986. Butorphanol: Clinical analgesic studies. In *Advances in Pain Research and Therapy,* Eds., KM Foley and CE Inturrisi, pp. 253–257, vol 8. New York: Raven Press.
79. Heel, RC, et al. 1979. Buprenorphine: A review of its pharmacological properties and therapeutic efficacy. *Drugs* 17:81–110.
80. Austin, KL, Stapleton, JV, and Mather, LE. 1980. Multiple intramuscular injections: A major source of variability in analgesic response to meperidine. *Pain* 8: 47–52.
81. Rigg, JRA, et al. 1978. Variation in the disposition of morphine after intramuscular administration in surgical patients. *Br J Anaesth* 50:1125.
82. Davenport, HT, and Wright, BM. 1979. Relief of postoperative pain. *Br Med J* 1:1561.
83. Harmer, M, et al. 1983. Intramuscular on demand analgesia: Double blind, controlled trial of pethidine, buprenorphine, morphine and meptazinol. *Br Med J* 286: 680–682.
84. Johnson, CD. 1983. Methods for relief of postoperative pain. *Ann R Coll Surg Engl* 65:137.
85. Dodson, ME. 1985. *The Management of Postoperative Pain.* London: Edward Arnold.
86. Roe, BB. 1963. Are postoperative narcotics necessary? *Arch Surg* 87:912–916.
87. Briggs, GG, et al. 1985. Morphine: Continuous intravenous infusions versus intramuscular injections for postoperative pain relief. *Gynecol Oncol* 22:288–293.
88. Cundy, JM. 1981. Improved pain relief after thoracotomy. *Br Med J* 283:1185.
89. Fry, ENS. 1984. Postoperative analgesia: A technique using continuous intravenous infusion of buprenorphine. *Anaesthesia* 39:1134–1135.
90. Naymen, J. 1979. Measurement and control of postoperative pain. *Ann R Coll Surg Engl* 61:419.
91. Rutter, PC, Murphy, F, and Dubley, HAF. 1980. Morphine: Controlled trial of different methods of administration for postoperative pain relief. *Br Med J* 280: 12–13.
92. Marshall, H, et al. 1985. Relief of pain by infusion of morphine after operation: Does tolerance develop? *Br Med J* 291:19–21.
93. Portenoy, RK. 1987. Continuous intravenous infusion of opioid drugs. *Med Clin North Am* 71(2):233–242.
94. Bennett, RL, et al. 1982. Patient-controlled analgesia: A new concept of post-operative pain relief. *Ann Surg* 195:700–705.
95. Smith, G. 1984. Cardiff palliator. *Br J Anaesth* 56:311.
96. Tamsen, A, et al. 1982. Patient-controlled analgesic therapy: clinical experience. *Acta Anaethes Scand* 74 (Suppl.):157–160.
97. Welchew, EA. 1983. On-demand analgesia: A double-blind comparison of on-demand fentanyl with regular intramuscular morphine. *Anaesthesia* 38:19.
98. Gibbs, JM, Johnson, HD, and Davis, FM. 1982. Patient administration of I.V. buprenorphine for postoperative pain relief using the "Cardiff" demand analgesia apparatus. *Br J Anaesth* 54:279–284.
99. Houde, RW, Wallenstein, SL, and Beaver, WT. 1966. Evaluation of analgesics in patients with cancer pain. In *International Encyclopedia of Pharmacology and Therapeutics,* Ed., L. Lasagna, Section 6, pp. 59–99. New York: Pergamon Press.
100. Wallenstein, SL, et al. 1981. Clinical analgesic assay of sublingual buprenorphine and intramuscular morphine. *NIDA Mongr* 41:288–293.
101. Pannuti, F, et al. 1982. Control of chronic pain in very advanced cancer patients with morphine hydrochloride administered by oral, rectal and sublingual route. *Pharmacol Res Commun* 14:369–380.
102. Bell, MD, et al. 1985. Buccal morphine—a new route for analgesia? *Lancet* 1:71–72.
103. Beaver, WT, and Feise, GA. 1977. A comparison of the analgesic effect of oxymorphone by rectal suppository and intramuscular injection in patients with postoperative pain. *J Clin Pharmacol* 17:276–291.
104. Cousins, MJ, and Mather, LE. 1984. Intrathecal and epidural administration of opioids. *Anesthesiology* 61: 276–310.
105. Nordberg, G, et al. 1984. Pharmacokinetics aspects to intrathecal morphine analgesia. *Anesthesiology* 60:448.
106. Bromage, PR, et al. 1982. Rostral spread of epidural morphine. *Anesthesiology* 56:431–436.
107. Gustafsson, LL, et al. 1982. Disposition of morphine in cerebrospinal fluid after epidural administration. *Lancet* (1):796.
108. Klinck, JR, and Lindop, MJ. 1982. Epidural morphine in the elderly. *Anaesthesia* 37:907–912.

109. Reiz, S, et al. 1981. Epidural morphine for postoperative pain relief. *Acta Anaesth Scand* 25:111–114.
110. Crawford, RD, Batna, MS, and Fox, F. 1981. Epidural morphine dose response for postoperative analgesia. *Anesthesiology* 55:A150.
111. Pybus, DA, and Torda, TA. 1982. Dose-effect relationships of extradural morphine. *Br J Anaesth* 54: 1259–1262.
112. Rutter, DV, Skewes, DG, and Morgan, M. 1981. Extradural opioids for postoperative analgesia. A double blind comparison of pethidine, fentanyl and morphine. *Br J Anaesth* 53:915.
113. Kalso, E. 1983. Effects of intrathecal morphine, injected with bupivacaine, on pain after orthopedic surgery. *Br J Anaesth* 55:415–521.
114. Gjessing, J, and Tomlin, PJ. 1981. Postoperative pain control with intrathecal morphine. *Anaesthesia* 36: 268–276.
115. Glass, PSA. 1984. Respiratory depression following only 0.4 mg of intrathecal morphine. *Anaesthesiology* 60: 256–257.
116. Gustafsson, LL, Schildt, B, and Jacobsen, K. 1982. Adverse effects of extradural and intrathecal opiates: Report of a nationwide survey in Sweden. *Br J Anaesth* 54: 479–485.
117. Ogg, TW, et al. 1983. Day-case dental anesthesia: Evaluation of pre-operative sublingual buprenorphine. *Anaesthesia* 38:534–539.
118. Pinnock, CA, et al. 1985. Comparison of oral slow release morphine (MST) with intramuscular morphine for premedication. *Anaesthesia* 40:1082–1085.
119. Kay, B, and Healy, TEJ. 1984. Premedication by controlled-released morphine. *Anaesthesia* 39:587–589.
120. Kay, B. 1978. A double-blind comparison of morphine and buprenorphine in the prevention of pain after operation. *Br J Anaesth* 50:605–608.
121. Steppe, J, and Camu, F. 1982. Epidural morphine for postoperative analgesia following abdominal surgery in elderly patients. *Acta Anaesth Belg* 33:43–51.
122. Knill, RL, Clement, JL, and Thompson, WR. 1981. Epidural morphine causes delayed and prolonged respiratory depression. *Can Anaesth Soc J* 28:537.
123. Evron, S, Magora, F, and Sadovsky, E. 1984. Prevention of urinary retention with phenoxybenzamine during epidural morphine. *Br Med J* 288:190.
124. Murray, K. 1984. Prevention of urinary retention with phenoxybenzamine during epidural morphine. *Br Med J* 288:645–646.
125. Houlton, PG, and Reynolds, F. 1981. Epidural morphine and fentanyl for postoperative pain. *Anaesthesia* 36: 1144–1145.
126. Samii, K, Chauvin, M, and Viars, P. 1981. Postoperative spinal analgesia with morphine. *Br J Anaesth* 53: 817–820.
127. Scott, PV, and Fischer, HB. 1982. Intraspinal opiates and itching: A new reflex? *Br Med J* 284:1015–1016.
128. Kaiko, RF, et al. 1983. Central nervous system excitatory effects of meperidine in cancer patients. *Ann Neurol* 13:180–185.
129. Medina, JL, and Diamond, S. 1977. Drug dependency in patients with chronic headache. *Headache* 17:12–14.
130. Perry, S, and Heidrich, G. 1982. Management of pain during debridement: A survey of U.S. burn units. *Pain* 13:267–280.
131. Porter, J, and Jick, H. 1980. Addiction rare in patients treated with narcotics. *N Engl J Med* 302:123.
132. Portenoy, RK, and Foley, KM. 1985. Clinical and pharmacological considerations in the use of narcotic analgesics in the elderly. *Geriatr Med Tod* 4(5):32–37.
133. Braham, D. 1984. Death of patient participating in trial of oral morphine for relief of postoperative pain. *Lancet* 1:1083–1084.
134. Symonds, P. 1977. Methadone and the elderly. *Br Med J* 1:512.
135. Ellis, R, et al. 1982. Pain relief after abdominal surgery: A comparison of I.M. morphine, sublingual buprenorphine and self-administered I.V. pethidine. *Br J Anaesth* 54:421–428.
136. Hurpet, C. 1978. Treatment of postoperative pain—analgesic potentiation. *Hosp Prac* 13:27–31.
137. Stambaugh, JE and Lance, C. 1983. Analgesic efficacy and pharmacokinetic evaluation of meperidine and hydroxyzine, alone and in combination. *Cancer Invest* 1:111–117.
138. Singh, PN, et al. 1981. Clinical evaluation of diazepam for relief of postoperative pain. *Br J Anaesth* 53: 831–835.
139. Artru, AA. 1986. Midazolam potentiates the analgesic effect of morphine in patient with postoperative pain. *Clin J Pain* 2(2):93–100.
140. Forrest, AL. 1983. Buprenorphine and lorazepam. *Anesthesia* 38:598.
141. Faroqui, MH, Cole, M, and Curran, J. 1983. Buprenorphine, benzodiazepine and respiratory depression. *Anesthesia* 38:1002.
142. Forrest, WH, Jr., et al. 1977. Dextroamphetamine with morphine for the treatment of postoperative pain. *N Engl J Med* 296:712–715.
143. Judkins, KC, and Harmer, M. 1982. Haloperidol as an adjunct analgesic in the management of postoperative pain. *Anaesthesiology* 37:1118–1120.
144. Martans, M. 1982. A significant decrease of narcotic drug dose after orthopedic surgery. A double-blind study with naproxen. *Acta Orthopaedic Belgica* 48:900.
145. Raesbeck, PG, Rice, ML, and Raesbeck, JC. 1982. A double-blind trial of indomethacin as an adjuvant to narcotic analgesia after major abdominal surgery. *Lancet* 2:115.
146. Vane, JR. 1971. Inhibition of prostaglandin synthesis. A mechanism of action of aspirin-like drugs. *Nature New Biol* 231:232.
147. DiRosa, H, Papadimitriou, JM, and Willoughby, DA. 1971. A histopathological and pharmacological analysis of the mode of action of non-steroid anti-inflammatory drugs. *J Pathol Bacteriol* 105:239.
148. Skjelbred, P. 1984. The effects of acetylsalicylic acid on swelling, pain and other events after surgery. *Br J Clin Pharmacol* 17:379.
149. Keenan, DJM, et al. 1983. Comparative trial of rectal indomethacin and cryoanalgesia for control of early post thoracotomy pain. *Br Med J* 287:1335–1337.
150. Cooper, SA, Needle, SE, and Kruger, GO. 1977. Comparative analgesic potency of aspirin and ibuprofen. *J Oral Surg* 35:898.

151. Iles, JPH. 1980. Relief of postoperative pain by ibuprofen: A report of two studies. *Can J Surg* 23:288.

152. Squires, DJP, and Masson, EL. 1981. A double-blind comparison of ibuprofen, ASA-Codeine-Caffeine compound and placebo in the treatment of dental surgery pain. *J Int Med Res* 9:257.

153. Dundee, JW. 1981. Intravenous salicylates for postoperative pain. *Lancet* (1):154.

154. Kortilla, K, Penttig, OM, and Aurinen, J. 1980. Comparison of IM lysine acetylsalicylate and oxycodone in the treatment of pain after operation. *Br J Anaesth* 52: 613–617.

155. Kweekel, DE, et al. 1974. A new soluble acetylsalicylic acid derivative in the treatment of postoperative pain. *Br J Anaesth* 46:133–135.

156. Conacher, ID, et al. 1983. Epidural analgesia following thoracic surgery: A review of two years' experience. *Anaesthesia* 38:546–551.

157. Griffiths, DPG. 1981. Postoperative pain prevention by continuous epidural infusion. *Anaesthesia* 36:214.

158. Albright, GA. 1979. Cardiac arrest following regional anaesthesia with etidocaine or bupivacaine. *Anesthesiology* 51:285.

159. Tucker, GT, et al. 1977. Observed and predicted accumulation of local anesthetic agents during continuous extradural analgesia. *Br J Anaesth* 49:237–241.

160. Engberg, G. 1975. Single-dose intercostal nerve block with etidocaine for pain relief after upper abdominal surgery. *Acta Anaesth Scand* (suppl.) 60:43–49.

161. Engberg, G. 1978. Relief of postoperative pain with intercostal blockade compared with the use of narcotic drugs. *Acta Anaesth Scand* (suppl.) 70:36–38.

162. Murphy, DF. 1984. A new method of continuous intercostal nerve blockade: Clinical and anatomical studies. *Br J Anaesth* 56:425.

163. Nunn, JF, and Slavin, G. 1980. Posterior intercostal nerve block for pain relief after cholecystectomy: Anatomical basis and efficacy. *Br J Anaesth* 52:253–259.

164. O'Kelly, E, and Garry, B. 1981. Continuous pain relief for multiple fractured ribs. *Br J Anaesth* 53:989.

165. Moore, DC. 1975. Intercostal nerve block for postoperative somatic pain following surgery of thorax and upper abdomen. *Br J Anaesth* 47:284–286.

166. Jones, SF, and White, A. 1985. Analgesia following femoral neck surgery: Lateral cutaneous nerve block as an alternative to narcotics in the elderly. *Anaesthesia* 40:682–685.

167. Hashemi, K, and Middleton, MD. 1983. Subcutaneous bupivacaine for postoperative analgesia after herniorrhaphy. *Ann R Coll Surg Engl* 65:38–39.

168. Moss, G, Regal, ME, and Lichtig, L. 1986. Reducing postoperative pain, narcotics, and length of hospitalization. *Surgery* 99:206–210.

169. Levack, ID, Holmes, JD, and Robertson, GS. 1986. Abdominal wound perfusion for the relief of postoperative pain. *Br J Anaesth* 58:615–619.

170. Fry, ENS, 1984. The direct perfusion of surgical wounds with local anesthetics solution: An approach to postoperative pain. *Ann R Coll Surg Engl* 66:220.

171. Thomas, DFM, Lambert, WG, and Williams, GKL. 1983. The direct perfusion of surgical wounds with local anesthetic solution: An approach to postoperative pain. *Ann R Coll Surg Engl* 65:226.

172. Melzack, R, and Wall, PD. 1965. Pain mechanism: A new theory. *Science* 150:971–979.

173. Navarathnam, RG, et al. 1984. Evaluation of the transcutaneous electrical nerve stimulator for postoperative analgesia following cardiac surgery. *Anaesth Intens Care* 12:345–350.

174. Sodipo, JO, Adedeji, SA, and Olumide, O. 1980. Postoperative pain relief by transcutaneous electrical nerve stimulation (TENS). *Am J Clin Med* 8(2): 190–194.

175. Solomon, RA, Viernstein, MC, and Long, DM. 1980. Reduction of postoperative pain and narcotic use by transcutaneous electrical nerve stimulation. *Surgery* 87(2):142–145.

176. Ali, J, Yaffe, CS, and Serrette, C. 1981. The effect of transcutaneous nerve stimulation on postoperative pain and pulmonary function. *Surgery* 89:507–512.

177. Cuschieri, RJ, Morran, CG, and McArdle, CS. 1985. Transcutaneous electrical stimulation for postoperative pain. *Ann R Coll Surg Engl:* 67:127–129.

178. Tyler, E, Caldwell, C, and Ghia, JB. 1982. Transcutaneous electrical nerve stimulation: An alternative approach to the management of postoperative pain. *Anaesth Analg* 61(5):449–456.

179. Lloyd, JW, Bernard, JDW, and Glyn, CJ. 1976. Cryoanalgesia: A new approach to pain relief. *Lancet* 2:932.

180. Katz, J, et al. 1960. Cryoanalgesia for post-thoracotomy pain. *Lancet* 1:512.

181. Wood, GJ, et al. 1981. Postoperative analgesia for daycare herniorrhaphy patients: a comparison of cryoanalgesia, paravertebral blockade and oral analgesia. *Anaesthesia* 36:603.

182. Orr, IA, et al. 1983. Post-thoracotomy pain relief: Combined use of cryoprobe and morphine infusion. *Ann R Coll Surg Engl* 65:366–369.

183. Egbert, LD, et al. 1964. Reduction of postoperative pain by encouragement and instruction of patients: A study of doctor-patient rapport. *N Engl J Med* 270:825–827.

184. Langer, EJ, Janis, IL, and Wolfer, JA. 1975. Reduction of psychological stress in surgical patients. *J Exp Soc Psychol* 11:155–165.

185. Weis, OF, et al. 1983. Reduction of anxiety and postoperative analgesic requirements by audiovisual instruction. *Lancet* 1:43–44.

186. Bowen, DE. 1973. Transurethral resection under selfhypnosis. *Am J Clin Hypn* 16:132–134.

187. Ceccio, CM. 1984. Postoperative pain relief through relaxation in elderly patients with fractured hips. *Orthop Nur* 3(3):11–19.

188. Locsin, RG. 1981. The effect of music on the pain in selected postoperative patients. *J Adv Nurs* 6:19.

189. Ulrich, RS. 1984. View through a window may influence recovery from surgery. *Science* 224:420.

25

Rehabilitation of the Geriatric Surgical Patient

Chang-Zern Hong and Jerome S. Tobis

Terminology and Background

Rehabilitation medicine is the medical management of the disabled or the use of all methods of diagnosis and treatment that will restore the disabled individual to as nearly normal as possible (1).

Rehabilitation medicine is a new branch of modern medicine. The word *rehabilitation* was probably first mentioned in the mid-19th century (2). The term *Rehabilitation Medicine* did not exist before World War II. In 1947, the word *physiatrist* (physician who specializes in Physical Medicine and Rehabilitation; Physikos = physical, iatros = physician) was adopted by American specialists.

Even now, the term *Physical Medicine and Rehabilitation* (PM&R) is still used more frequently than Rehabilitation Medicine. This is because physical medicine modalities are still the most important tools for rehabilitation programs. In the 19th century, the three main physical agents used were exercise (with massage), water (with heat), and electricity. The three principal divisions of physical therapies were exercise/massage, hydrobalneology, and electrotherapy. At the turn of the century, these three groups became combined and called *physiotherapy,* then *physical therapy,* and in 1931, *physical medicine* (in England but not until 1946 in the USA) (1).

Geriatric Rehabilitation Programs

Rehabilitation medicine for the geriatric patient is usually concerned with the care of the severely disabled and chronically ill who often have multiple system disease with medical, psychologic, and social problems. Because of the multiplicity of problems, the evaluation of such patients often requires a multidisciplinary approach with the participation of several disciplines where feasible. This group forms a therapeutic team. The rehabilitation team usually includes a physiatrist, rehabilitation nurse, physical therapist, occupational therapist, speech pathologist, orthotist/prosthetist, psychologist, social worker, and vocational counselor. Other disciplines may be included as indicated, such as the primary care or family physician. Key participants should include the patient and patient's family. Initially, the patient will be evaluated by the physiatrist and other team members. The evaluation process emphasizes a functional assessment, which describes abilities and activities in order to measure an individual's skills in performing the tasks necessary for daily living, vocational pursuits, social interactions, leisure activities, and other required behaviors (3). Table 25-1 shows items of functional evaluation usually performed by a physiatrist.

Rehabilitation medicine is problem (functional limitation) oriented and requires specific goals as the guidance toward a successful outcome. The goals are usually established by the team members with the participation of the patient. The goals should be realistic and flexible. The patient's functional level should be assessed periodically to modify the goals as needed. Figure 25-1 shows the dynamic process of rehabilitation programs.

Advantages

The rehabilitation program should be initiated as early as possible. In the acute stage of illness, the program may facilitate functional improvement and/or prevent compli-

Table 25-1. Physiatrist evaluation

1. History
2. Physical examination
3. Functional assessment:
   a. Musculoskeletal function
      Strength
      Endurance
      Coordination
      Balance
      Skills
      Posture
      Gait
   b. Activities of daily living (ADL)
      Self-care activities
      Homemaking activities
   c. Speech and language function
   d. Bladder and bowel function
   e. Cardiopulmonary fitness
4. Electrodiagnosis
5. Evaluation for orthosis and prosthesis and other assistive devices/equipment
6. Psychologic assessment and psychosocial diagnosis
7. Vocational or recreational (for elderly) assessment

cations. For example, a stroke patient may be able to move his paralytic limbs in a few days through neuromuscular facilitation technique and thus shorten the period of being bedridden.

A rehabilitation program is usually cost effective. The cost of health care may be reduced through an appropriate rehabilitation program. An elderly patient may be

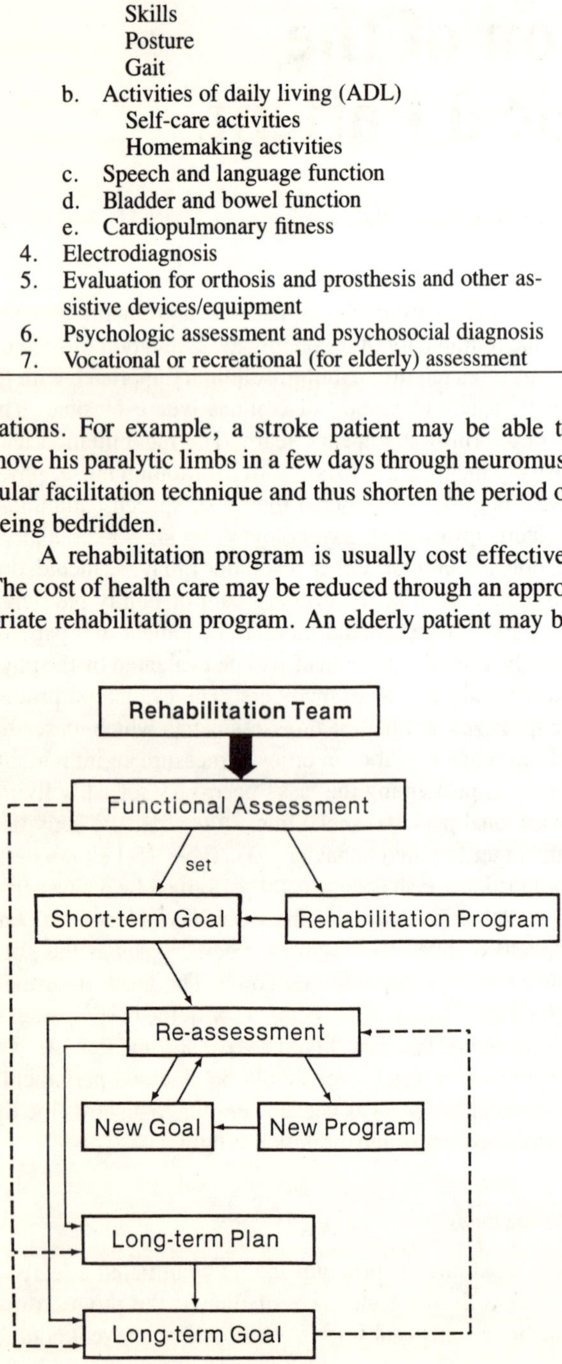

Figure 25-1. The dynamic process of a rehabilitation program—re-evaluation of patient's status and goals.

able to return home to live independently after a successful rehabilitation program rather than staying in a nursing home, which from a fiscal perspective alone is more expensive than being at home.

The rehabilitation program may also help to improve the quality of life for a geriatric patient. This is certainly important from an ethical point of view. Through an effective rehabilitation program, an elderly hemiplegic can avoid many complications—pressure sores, joint contractures, recurrent pneumonia, recurrent urinary tract infection—which would interfere with his or her well being.

Risks

On the other hand, one should not disregard the risk of possible accident during the rehabilitation process for the geriatric patient. Physical activities as part of the rehabilitation program may subject a geriatric patient to the risk of trauma or significant stress (4). For example, an active ambulatory patient may fall, with resultant injury, whereas the bedridden patient is not exposed to such danger. However, it may be worth it to take such risk since immobilization has its own complications including osteoporosis, venous thrombosis, hypostatic pneumonia, and depression.

What Is Aging?

Recent geriatric research suggests that "aging" itself is not a disease. Much of what has been termed the "changes of aging" may represent the unrecognized disease processes that are so often more widespread in the elderly. For example, osteoporosis may in part represent a disease phenomenon in old age rather than the intrinsic phenomenon of aging. The physician may tell an elderly patient that his right knee pain is due to his age. However, this patient may ask the doctor, "How about my left knee? It is just the same as my right one, but it never bothers me."

In summary, geriatric rehabilitation has to consider the following factors: (*a*) team approach; (*b*) functional assessment; (*c*) specific and realistic goals; (*d*) a dynamic process; (*e*) early rehabilitation management; (*f*) cost effectiveness; (*g*) medical ethics; (*h*) risk factors.

Levels of Rehabilitative Care

The different levels of rehabilitation care are summarized in Table 25-2. Rehabilitation programs may be conducted in the acute care hospital immediately after the stage of acute illness or once the acute illness has been stabilized. Depending upon the diagnosis, the patient may begin an

Table 25-2. Levels of rehabilitation care

Stage	Acute I	II	Subacute III	Chronic IV	V
Programs	Bedside care	Comprehensive rehab	Comprehensive rehab	Long-term rehab	Maintenance rehab
Site	Acute general hospital—acute ward	Acute general hospital—rehab ward	Acute general hospital—rehab ward or rehab center	Rehab center or ambulatory care or extended care facilities	Nursing home or ambulatory care
Emergency services	Available	Available	Not immediately available	Not immediately available	Not immediately available
Rehab staff involved	Limited	All	All	All	Very limited
Therapy time	Limited	As needed	As needed	Limited	Very limited
Criteria:					
1. Rehab potential	Uncertain	Good	Good	Fair	Poor
2. Function improved	Uncertain	Significant	Significant	Some	No
Cost	Moderate	High	High	Moderate	Low
Outcome	Uncertain	Good	Good	Fair	Poor

intensive rehabilitation program. This should only be carried out in a general hospital where all acute care resources are available.

At a later stage, a comprehensive rehabilitation program can be done in either the rehabilitation unit of the acute care hospital or in the rehabilitation center. A patient selected for this program should have a good potential to improve his or her functional level. The program is not only intensive (many hours of therapy in a day) but also extensive (with several therapists or staff involved). This is the most critical part of rehabilitation; through such a program the severely impaired patient may be able to become independent in daily living. There are patients in whom a trial of rehabilitation is warranted, even if the outcome is uncertain. Thus, an elderly debilitated patient with cancer of the breast and metastasis who has had a mastectomy may be started on an activity program, even though the risk of fracture may be high.

Sometimes we see patients who may have potential to improve their functional level, but the improvement is so slow that they are unable to stay in the program since it is not cost effective. Unfortunately, decisions regarding such care may be determined by health insurance coverage rather than by medical judgment. For such a patient, we are opposed to forfeiting the opportunity for further rehabilitation. There are two options: either the patient may be placed in a skilled nursing home to continue a long-term rehabilitation program (with limited time of therapies), or the patient may stay at home (if feasible) and receive home care or outpatient services.

For those patients placed in a custodial care setting, a maintenance rehabilitation program should be provided to prevent medical complications and reduce dependency as much as possible. Without this minimum rehabilitation care, patients may deteriorate rapidly. This program can also be carried out at home if the patient's family is supportive.

It is important that the patient be placed in the appropriate setting at the right time. Figure 25-2 shows the relationship of different environments for rehabilitation care at different times for different individuals.

Rehabilitation Modalities

Therapeutic Modalities in Physical Medicine

Therapeutic Exercise

Physiology of exercise. Knowledge of exercise physiology has advanced rapidly in the past two decades. With a sound physiologic basis, organized exercise programs have been well developed in medical settings. The important physiologic effects of exercise training that have clinical implications are listed in Table 25-3. The most basic clinical application of therapeutic exercise is to improve muscle function (strength, endurance, speed, and motor skills) (5–9). With the advancement of research technology, many metabolic, cardiopulmonary, and endocrine effects have been studied extensively.

Types of exercise. Passive exercise is prescribed for the maintenance of range of motion or the stretching of tight muscles or soft tissue contractures. Active nonresistive exercise is employed for severely weakened muscles, poor cardiopulmonary fitness, or difficulty in mobility due to pain (such as postoperative). Active resistive exercise can be static (isometric) or dynamic (isotonic or isokinetic). Static exercise is usually not recommended

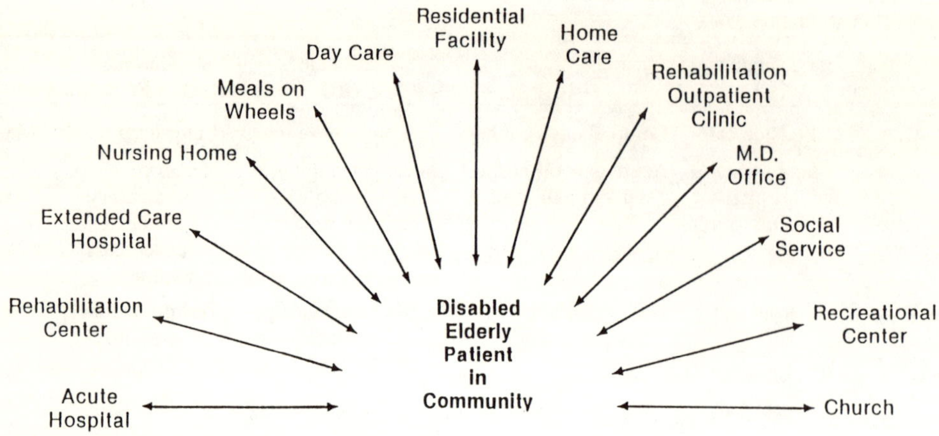

Figure 25-2. Spectrum of services to provide comprehensive care of the elderly-disabled.

for the hypertensive or cardiac patient because of its high pressure load on the cardiovascular system. Static exercise may cause significant elevation of mean arterial blood pressure (10). Dynamic exercise usually causes an increase of cardiac output but little change in blood pressure. Isokinetic (constant velocity) exercise (Fig. 25-3) is a newly developed rehabilitative technique for muscle training and testing. Some of the alleged advantages of isokinetic exercise include safety, accommodating resistance, and the facility for muscle force analysis (11).

Therapeutic exercise to increase strength and endurance. High resistance and high repetition activities are required for increasing strength. On the other hand, low resistance, low rate, and long duration of activities are required for improving muscle endurance. In geriatric reha-

Table 25-3. Physiologic effects of exercise training

Organ system	Structural changes	Biochemical changes	Functional changes
Skeletal muscle	Number of myofibrils ↑	Contractile protein ATP and CP ↑	Strength ↑
	Connective tissue thickening	Glycolytic enzyme ↑	
	Capillarization ↑	Myoglobin ↑	Endurance ↑
		Glycogen store ↑	
		Oxidative enzyme ↑	
	Number of mitochondria ↑		
		Myosin ATPase ↑	Speed ↑
Central nervous system			Coordination ↑
			Motor skills ↑
			Neurologic recovery ↑
		Serum endorphines ↑	Pain tolerance ↑
Skeletal system	Bone density ↑	Mineral content ↑	Strength to stress ↑
Heart	Hypertrophy (Athletic heart)		At Rest:
		Myocardial enzyme ↑	Bradycardia,
	Vascularity ↑		stroke volume ↑
	Size of coronary artery ↑		
			During Exercise:
			Less tachycardia
			Higher stroke volume
Vascular System			At Rest:
			Diastolic BP ↓
			During exercise:
			Less BP ↑
			Cardiac output ↑
			Peripheral resistance ↓
			Coronary blood flow ↑
Pulmonary			Pulmonary ventilation ↑
			Diffusion capacity ↑

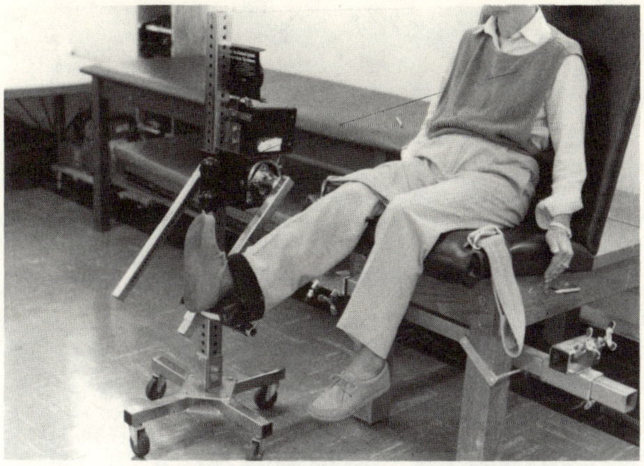

Figure 25-3. "Othotron" for isokinetic exercise.

bilitation programs, both types of activities should be emphasized to improve muscle function to its optimal state. Usually, the intensity and the duration of the exercise are increased gradually as required. This change should be based on the physician's judgment of the individual case and observations by a well-trained physical or occupational therapist. Figure 25-4 shows some equipment used for improving strength and endurance.

Therapeutic exercise to increase or maintain range of motion. The maintenance of joint and muscle flexibility is also very important in geriatric rehabilitation programs. A contractured joint cannot work efficiently even with normal strength, speed, and endurance. This is particularly important in the geriatric patient recovery from trauma or surgery. If motion is maintained during healing of a traumatic or surgical wound, connective tissue of the areolar type develops, which is essential for wound healing. If the wound is immobilized, a dense contracted scar forms that leads to contracture (12). However, vigorous range of motion is not recommended, especially during the first few postoperative weeks, to avoid delay of wound healing. If there is associated fracture, immobilization is required and motion should be avoided. An intensive therapeutic exercise should be started as soon as motion is permitted to stretch the contracture resulting from immobilization (i.e., the cast is removed).

Therapeutic exercise for central nervous system recovery. Neuromuscular facilitation techniques (13) have been well developed to facilitate motor recovery in upper motor neuron damage cases, such as head injury, cerebral infarction, or other brain lesions. These techniques are based on neurophysiologic principles, including spinal reflex patterns, brain stem reflex phenomena, or higher center reflex circuits, sensory feedback, and cortical integration. Classical training methods including Bobath technique (neurodevelopmental approach), Brunnstrom technique (central facilitation with initiating and shaping abnormal synergic pattern), Knott and Voss technique (proprioceptive neuromuscular facilitation or PNF), and Rood's approach (application of cutaneous stimuli) are still valuable if they are combined, coordinated, and modified depending on the individual problem. The modern biofeedback training technique based on "central EMG" has been proven to be effective (6). The plasticity of the central nervous system has been well studied and has clinical implications for recovery after CNS injury (14–16).

Therapeutic exercise for coordination. Motor skill and coordination may be improved by practice, such as repetitive patterns of motor activity. Sensory feedback is also important for both conscious and subconscious levels. Frenkel exercise is a classical method for training of coordination impairment. It is still useful in some cases of cerebellar ataxia. Each movement is done slowly and with repetition. The physiologic basis of this exercise is to improve coordination by sensory compensation, by voluntary relearning of functions lost, and by retraining of functional patterns (17).

Therapeutic exercise for gait training. The gait deviations usually seen in the aged include reduced free walking speed, short stride, wide base, slow cadence, low swing-to-stance time ratio, poor floor-to-foot clearance, diminished ability to use the determinants of gait, which results in greater energy cost, difficulty in using gravity, inertia in ambulation, and difficulty in regaining their balance once they start to fall (18). Considering the safety factor, one should allow the geriatric patient to walk slowly and stably in ambulation training.

Generally, older individuals adopt a gait that is most economical for them. If patients have a neurologic or orthopedic problem, which makes them unable to walk independently, the gait training should be initiated with parallel bars. Patients should experience the feeling of weight bearing before they are allowed to take steps in the bars. When they are able to balance themselves well, they can try to walk outside the bars. A cane, a walker, or a pair of crutches may be given to improve stability. Sometimes a splint or brace may be required for a better gait pattern and for energy-saving purposes. Therapeutic exercises may be emphasized for certain groups of muscles as an adjunct program to improve the gait pattern.

Therapeutic exercise for soft tissue lesions and arthritis. Chronic soft tissue lesions, such as myalgia, fibrositis, or myofascial pain syndrome, as well as degenerative joint diseases, are common problems in the geriatric population. Surgical procedures for other organ systems generally aggravate symptoms of soft tissue lesions or arthralgias. Pain, stiffness, spasmodic tightness, or reduced

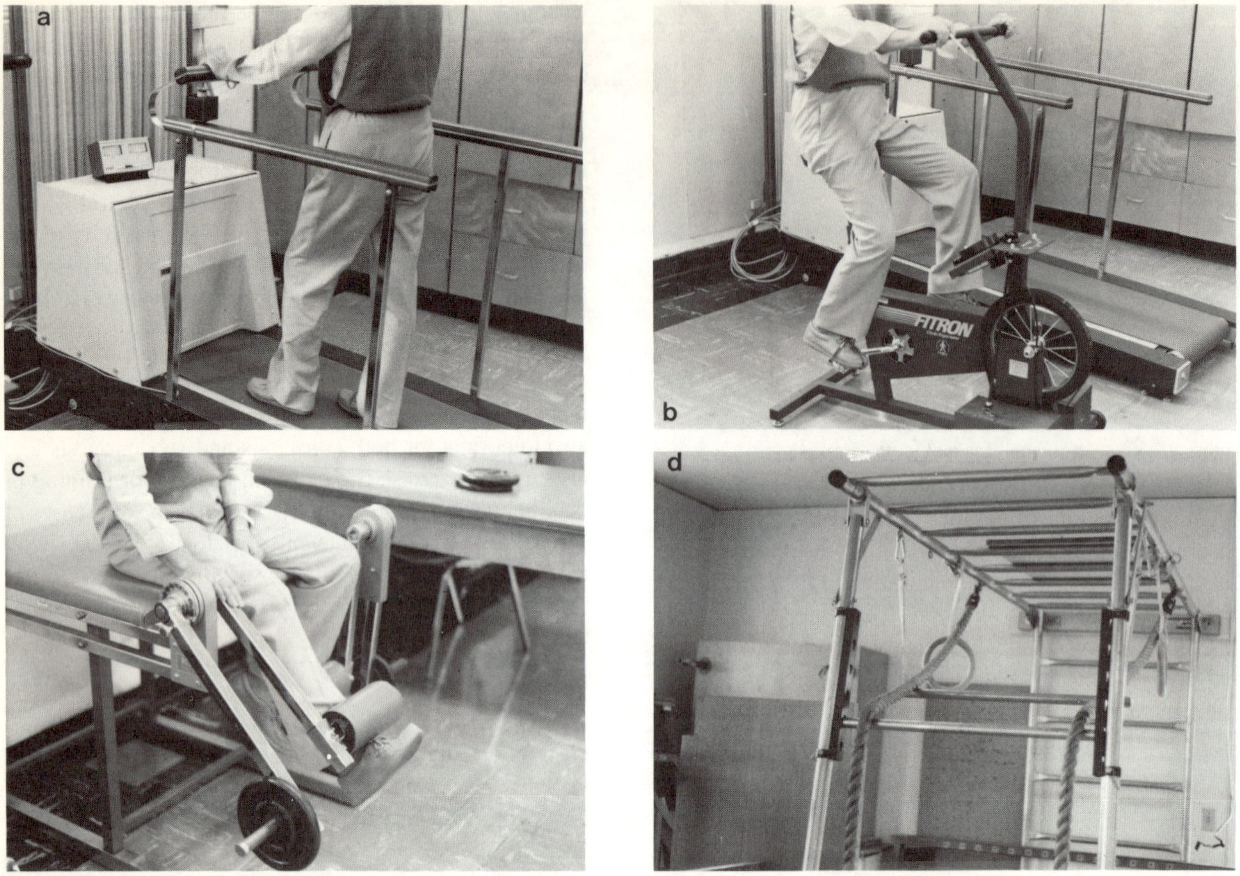

Figure 25-4. a, Treadmill; b, exercise bicycle; c, N–K table for quadriceps strengthening exercise; d, overhead bar for suspension exercise, climbing, reaching, or other functional activities;

range of motion are the usual complaints. Therapeutic exercise, if performed appropriately, not only can help reduce stiffness and increase range of motion, but also can prevent the occurrence of stiffness postoperatively. A specific exercise program should be based on the diagnosis.

In general, gentle and progressive stretching to improve mobility, and gradual strengthening exercise to the involved muscles or periarticular muscles are the common principal exercises. For arthritis, isometric exercise is usually recommended rather than dynamic strengthening in order to avoid excessive articular motion, which may aggravate an inflammatory reaction of the synovial or periarticular tissue. Isometric exercise is also easier to do when arthritic pain is too severe to allow joint movement. The recent discovery of increase in serum concentrations of endorphins during exercise may create a new field of pain management (19). Exercise is highly encouraged for the patient with chronic pain.

Therapeutic exercise to increase cardiopulmonary fitness. Many physiologic effects on cardiovascular function have been studied (5, 20–23). In animal studies, following repeated strenuous dynamic exercise for an extended period of time, there is an increase in the size of the major coronary arteries and a corresponding change in the number of capillaries (24). It thus appears that exercise may play both a preventive and rehabilitative role with respect to coronary heart disease. With prolonged exercise, the activities of some myocardial enzymes, including glycogen synthetase, some oxidative and glycolytic enzymes, and myosin ATPase, were increased in animal studies (23, 25). These changes may partly explain the improvement in myocardial function from exercise training.

It is well known that well-trained human subjects have a lower heart rate and higher stroke volume at rest and during submaximal exercise than normal sedentary people due to improvement of myocardial contractility (5, 20, 21). Decrease of total peripheral resistance with increase of muscle blood flow during exercise results in a lowering of blood pressure. There is evidence that long-term exercise training might reduce blood pressure in hy-

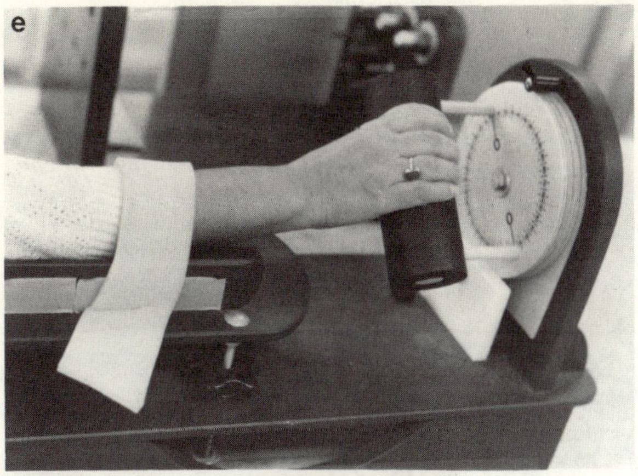

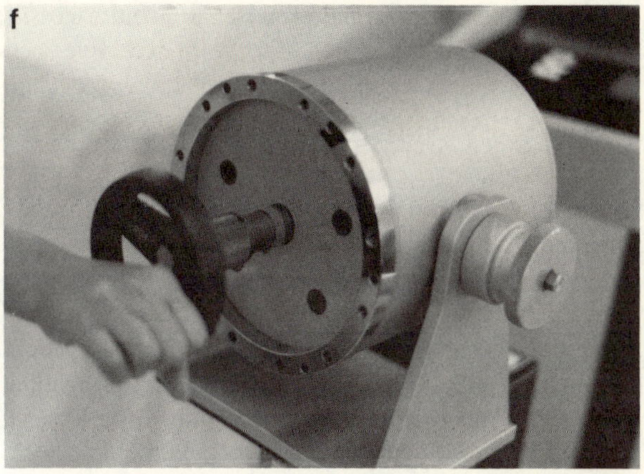

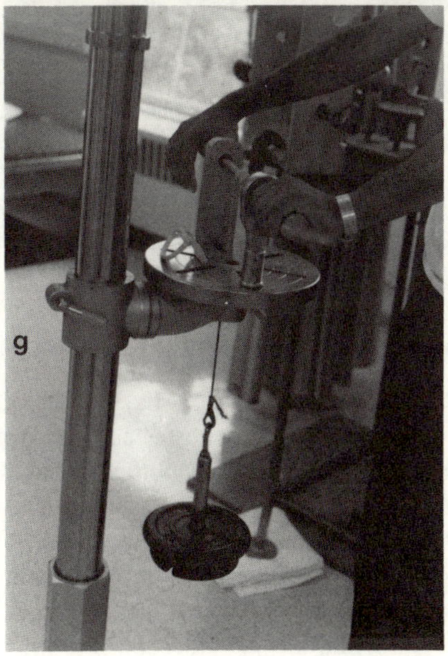

Figure 25-4. e, supination-pronation machine for forearm; f, Baltimore Therapeutic Equipment (BTE) for strength, endurance, skill and dexterity training of the hand; g, weight well for training of various aspects of hand function.

pertensive subjects, but not in normotensive individuals (26).

Exercise training produces an increase in maximal oxygen uptake (aerobic capacity) and oxygen debt (anaerobic capacity) (5, 21). The improvement of aerobic capacity is due to many factors, including pulmonary function, oxygen transport, and tissue oxygen utilization. Changes of pulmonary function due to exercise training are usually not as remarkable as that of cardiovascular function. The maximal pulmonary ventilation and pulmonary diffusion capacity may be increased by training. Biochemical changes in skeletal muscle fibers cause improvement in tissue oxygen utilization. On the other hand, there is no significant change in hemoglobin concentration from exercise training (27). The mechanism of increase in anaerobic capacity is probably due to an increased physiologic tolerance for lactic acid with its side effects, such as tachypnea, dyspnea, and tachycardia, or a greater psychic ability to exert onself (5).

Physical training may increase the ability to utilize fat as an energy source for exercise. Long-term heavy exercise can produce a decrease of serum levels of triglyceride, low density lipoprotein, and total cholesterol (5, 28, 29). This is another benefit of exercise for patients with a high risk of coronary artery disease or cerebral vascular disease.

Principles of exercise prescription. The general principles of the exercise prescription for the geriatric patient to improve cardiopulmonary fitness are: (*a*) generalized exercise involving all limbs and trunk rather than local exercise to one part of the body; (*b*) dynamic exercise rather than static exercise to avoid undesired excessive elevation of blood pressure; (*c*) aerobic rather than anerobic, i.e., submaximal exercise, to avoid excessive stress on an impaired myocardium from excessive accumulation of serum lactic acid and lack of oxygen; (*d*) intermittent rather than continuous exercise to allow longer duration of activities with a heavy load (30).

Exercise training for the elderly. Shephard (31) has pointed out the importance of physical fitness in the elderly. This includes: (*a*) extended physical independence in activities of daily living due to increase of muscular and cardiopulmonary fitness; (*b*) improved general life-style; (*c*) opportunities for social interaction, with an elevation of mood; and, most importantly, (*d*) a lessened risk of certain medical disorders, including obesity (32–34), adult-onset diabetes (35), hypertension (26), bone demineralization (36–38), coronary heart disease (20, 39–41), and chronic obstructive lung disease (42).

The optimal frequency, intensity, duration and mode of exercise for older adults depends to a large degree on the specific individual for whom it is prescribed (43). Many older persons with cardiovascular disorders are limited to low-intensity exercise and need to increase the frequency and duration of exercise to achieve the desired training benefits. However, many frail elderly may improve their physical performance without achieving a training effect. Other older persons with musculoskeletal problems may be limited to modes of exercise, such as swimming or stationary bicycling.

The risk of exercise itself for the elderly is another concern. It is usually related to cardiac dysfunction. The cardiac risk can be reduced by careful evaluation and monitoring. Musculoskeletal complications are non-life-threatening risks in the geriatric patient. The type of exercise and the exercise load should be carefully selected.

Therapeutic Heat and Cold

Physiology of thermotherapy. The physiologic basis of thermal therapy is summarized in Table 27-4. Lehmann and De Lateur (44) described the physiologic effects of therapeutic heat as follows: (*a*) increase of extensibility of the collagen tissues (for treatment of joint contracture); (*b*) decrease of visco-elastic properties of tissues (for treatment of joint stiffness); (*c*) increase of Ia primary afferent discharges but decrease of most of II secondary afferent discharges from muscle spindles, and increases of Ib afferent discharges from Golgi tendon organs (for treatment of muscle spasm); (*d*) increase of local blood flow probably due to reflex phenomena via the autonomic nervous system or a local mechanism, such as one or more of the following: a direct effect on vascular smooth musculature, stimulation of histamine-like substances and bradykinin, increase of metabolic rate, or an axonal reflex; (*e*) analgesic and sedative effects probably due to local effects upon free nerve endings or other indirect effects; (*f*) facilitation of the resolution of inflammatory reactions (subacute or chronic); (*g*) increase of enzymatic activity and chemical reaction rate.

Table 25-4. Physiologic basis of therapeutic heat

Organ system	Physiologic effects	Clinical application
Connective tissue	Extensibility of collagen tissue ↑	Relief of joint contracture
	Visco-elastic property ↑	Relief of joint stiffness
Nervous system	Ia afferent discharges ↑ II afferent discharges ↓ Ib afferent discharges ↑	Relief of muscle spasm
	Analgesic effect ↑	Relief of pain
	Sedative effects ↑	General relaxation
Vascular system	Local blood flow ↑	Relief of active inflammation

Several types of thermal therapy may be given.

Superficial heat. Superficial heat may be applied through the use of conductive heat transfer devices. Hot packs, electric heating pads, hot water bottles, Aqua-K pads, and hot paraffin wax belong in this category. They are easy to apply, but the effects are limited to superficial or to reflex phenomena. Clinically, this type of heat therapy is useful and convenient for the bedridden geriatric patient who has a pain syndrome of soft tissue or arthritic origin that is exacerbated postoperatively.

Convecting heat may be delivered through hot water hydrotherapy with either whirlpool or Hubbard tank. This type of heat therapy is helpful in many musculoskeletal disorders, particularly when it is applied in conjunction with therapeutic exercise. It is useful for the geriatric patient who has stiffness of a joint or soft tissue postoperatively (especially after orthopedic surgery), when the operative wound is completely healed and the patient is allowed to have some degree of mobility of the affected limb(s).

Radiation heat modalities, such as infrared or radiant heat, provide only superficial heating effects. Since this is a type of dry heat, it may be useful in treating the open wound or pressure sore to facilitate the healing process. It is currently not used as often as it once was.

Deep heat. Shortwave diathermy and microwave diathermy are the only two modalities of electromagnetic energy used frequently in physical medicine. Ultrasound heat therapy is the application of mechanical energy to generate heating effects to the deep tissue. Both forms of deep heat therapy are used frequently to treat arthritis or soft tissue lesions, such as bursitis, capsulitis, tendonitis, sprain, and strain. However, the application of electromagnetic energy on an area with metallic implantation is contraindicated as tissue burns may occur easily.

Heat therapy for the elderly patient. Heat therapy is prescribed to the geriatric patient frequently due to the increased incidence of degenerative arthritis and soft tissue lesions. This should be applied carefully due to the following special considerations:

Some aged patients may have reduced thermal sensation and may get burns easily, especially of the lower extremities in the presence of peripheral vascular disease or neuropathy.

Some patients with heart failure or other cardiac disease may not be able to tolerate increased metabolism from generalized heat therapy, such as hot water hydrotherapy.

Patients with generalized edema may have an exacerbation from vigorous heat therapy.

Patients with a bleeding disorder may risk a massive bleed if the heat therapy is applied over the hemorrhagic site.

Patients with malignancy may risk spread of the malignant cells if heat is applied directly over the area with malignant growth.

Patients with local infection may risk bacteremia or septicemia if the heat is applied directly over the site of infection.

Heat applied to an ischemic area, such as in peripheral vascular disease, may precipitate gangrene due to a rise in local metabolism without concomitant increase in local blood flow and oxygenation of the local tissues.

Physiology of cryotherapy. a) *Effects on blood vessels:* Vasoconstriction produced by cold application can be due to direct effect of cooling on the blood vessels or via the sympathetic fibers (45). This is the physiologic basis for cryotherapy in trauma and inflammation.

b) *Effects on peripheral nerves and receptors:* The sensitivity of the muscle spindle and nerve fibers (especially the small myelinated fibers, such as the gamma fibers) is reduced at low temperature. Some spastic hemiplegic patients complain of increased spasticity in the winter, which is probably due to a systemic effect rather than the local effect to the nerve. Therefore, cold therapy may be effective in relief of spasticity. There is also a local anesthetic effect of cryotherapy if the sensitivity of the small C fiber or A-delta fiber is reduced at low temperature.

Clinical application of cryotherapy. A cold pack is used very frequently for postoperative wound pain, tissue swelling, or edema. For any acute soft tissue lesion, cold therapy is the first choice of a physical therapy modality to reduce the inflammatory reaction, pain, and reflex spasmodic reaction of muscles.

Therapeutic Electromagnetic Energy

Therapeutic electricity—Electrical stimulation. The clinical application of electricity for therapeutic purposes can be based on muscle, nerve, or bone stimulation. Modern electrical stimulators can generate direct or alternating currents of various intensities, durations, and frequencies. The minimal duration of an effective stimulus for muscle is about 1 msec and that for nerve is only about 0.03 msec (46, 47). Therefore, in most cases of electrical stimulation, the nerve or the nerve endings near the motor point are stimulated before the muscle itself is excited from electrical stimulation if the innervation of the muscle is intact. However, if the muscle is denervated, the duration of the current should be long enough to stimulate the denervated muscles.

The physiologic basis of therapeutic electricity is summarized in Table 25-5. Stimulation of the denervated muscle is applied for preparation of re-innervation, prevention of complications, such as muscle fibrosis, muscle contracture, or deep vein thrombosis, and neuromuscular re-education (46). It may be useful after nerve grafting. Whether it has beneficial or adverse effects is still controversial. An animal study demonstrated that chronic electrical stimulation of a denervated muscle accelerated the recovery of normal function in re-innervated muscle fibers (48).

Stimulation of the sensory nerve is widely used for pain relief, such as transcutaneous electrical nerve stimulation (TENS) or acupuncture (47, 49). Our experience is that acupuncture is not very effective unless electrical stimulation is used concomitantly.

Motor or sensory nerve stimulation is applied in treating spasticity from spinal cord injury by using strong tetanizing current (50, 51), the treatment of scoliosis with implanted electrodes in the paraspinal muscles (52), and for phrenic nerve stimulation. Phrenic nerve stimulation may be used to enhance respiratory function when paralysis of the diaphragm has resulted from bulbar palsy. Liberson was the first one to apply functional electrical stimulation on the peroneal nerve of the hemiplegic patient to prevent foot drop during ambulation (electrophysiologic orthosis). Later, he and other authors developed various techniques, including an upper extremity functional splint

Table 25-5. Physiologic basis of therapeutic electricity

Site of stimulation	Physiologic effects	Clinical application
Skeletal muscle stimulation	Maintain normal function	Retard atrophy in denervated muscles
	Full range of muscle fiber contraction	Prevent muscle contracture in denervated muscle
	Maintain muscle pumping	Prevent deep vein thrombosis in flaccid paralytic limb
Sensory nerve stimulation	Large fiber impulses ↑ Small fiber impulses ↓ (Gate control)	Relief of pain
Motor nerve stimulation	Contraction of partially paralyzed muscles, or upper-motor-neuron-induced paralyzed muscles	Diaphragm pacing, correction of scoliosis, electrophysiologic splint, treatment of neurogenic bladder

and multichannel stimulation, to produce the desired motor pattern (47, 53).

As to electrical stimulation of bone, recent research has shown that electrical currents can facilitate healing in non-union fractures (54, 55). Most of the studies have used DC current or a time-varying, magnetic-field-induced current.

Ultraviolet. Physiological effects of ultraviolet therapy include erythema, pigmentation, exfoliation, sterilization, antirachitic effect, and counterirritation (56, 57). Traditionally, ultraviolet was used in various conditions, including many dermatological lesions. However, it is now used less frequently than it once was. This is partly because it can be replaced by other more convenient or more effective methods of therapy. It is still used clinically for treatment of chronic ulcer, psoriasis, and sterilization.

Magnetotherapy. In the late 19th and early 20th century, magnetotherapy with a static magnetic field was very popular in Europe for the treatment of chronic pain. Today, it is not used in this country, as heat therapy is simple and effective in managing pain. The mechanism of magnetotherapy is still unknown, although Hong et al. (58, 59) found increased nerve excitability from exposure to a high density static magnetic field.

Diathermy. See therapeutic heat.

Massage

The physiologic effects of massage may be classified as either reflex or mechanical (60). The reflex effects of massage are induced from skin stimulation and are transmitted through the spinal cord or higher centers of the central nervous system. The final effects are sedation, relaxation of muscles, and vasomotor changes (either vasoconstriction or vasodilation). The direct mechanical effects consist of: (*a*) an increase of flow of blood and lymph in the deep tissues, and (*b*) intramuscular motion to stretch adhesions between muscle fibers and to mobilize accumulations of fluid (60, 61).

Massage may be applied to treat the geriatric patient who has pain, muscle spasm, or tissue swelling postoperatively. The contraindications for massage are infection, skin lesions, burns, thrombophlebitis and malignancy, many of which may be seen more frequently in the geriatric patient.

Manipulation

Manipulation is the mechanical restoration of the joint or soft tissue by a second party, either gently and slowly (so-called mobilization) or forcefully and quickly with dynamic thrust (62, 63). The physiologic basis of manipulation is considered to be the stretching of spasmodic muscles (62, 64).

Geriatric patients have a high incidence of degenerative and demineralized changes in the spine. Therefore, spinal manipulation to these subjects should be performed cautiously.

Diagnostic Tools in Physical Medicine

Electromyography

The electromyographic (EMG) technique examines the electrical activity of the muscle fibers to detect the disorder involved at any site of the motor unit (the lower motor neuron, its axon and the neuromuscular junction, and its innervated muscle fibers). This is accomplished by inserting a needle electrode into the muscle. The muscle action potential is recorded extracellularly from the needle tip and transmitted through a preamplifier, a small box outside the EMG machine. The function of the preamplifier is to intensify the desired muscle action potential, which occurs near the needle tip, and to reject the interfering electrical activity from other sources. The recorded signal is further magnified by the amplifier inside the EMG machine. The wave form of the electric activity is displayed on the oscilloscope. The sound of the waves of the electrical activity can also be recorded and magnified through the loudspeaker. Figure 25-5 shows the basic components of a typical EMG machine.

During the EMG test, the needle electrode is inserted into the muscle in various directions. For each sampling, the following parameters should be observed during the EMG test (Table 25-6):

Insertional activity—Some electrical activities are elicited during the movement of the EMG needle. A train of muscle action potential up to 300 msec duration is usually observed in the normal insertional activity. A reduced insertional activity can be seen if the amount of viable muscle fibers is reduced, such as might occur with muscle necrosis or fibrosis. A prolonged insertional activity can be seen in some forms of myopathy, especially in myotonic disease due to hyperirritability of the muscle membrane.

Resting state—If the needle is placed in a certain area with no relative movement between the needle and the muscle, normally there is electrical silence as long as the patient is completely relaxed. Spontaneous activities, such as fibrillation potentials and positive sharp waves, may be observed if the muscle is denervated for longer than 2 weeks. These potentials also can be seen in polymyositis. Fasciculation is the spontaneous activity from a group of muscle fibers usually seen in chronic long-standing neurogenic lesions, such as motor neuron disease, chronic radiculopathy, or neuropathy.

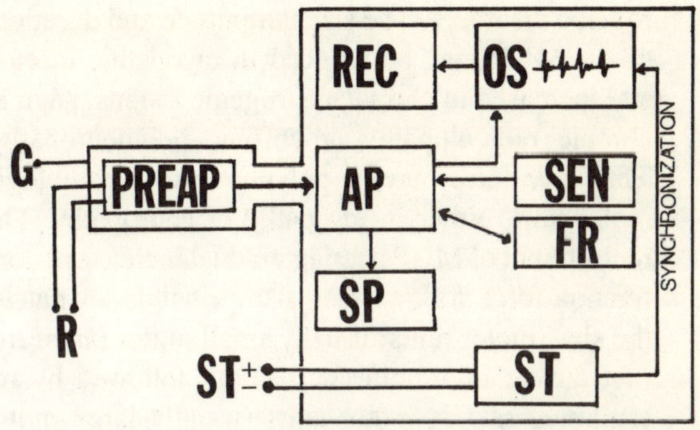

Figure 25-5. Basic components of an electromyographic (EMG) machine. G, ground electrode; R, recording electrodes; ST, stimulating device and electrodes; PREAP, preamplifier; AP, amplifier; SP, loudspeaker; SEN, sensitivity control; FR, frequency response; OS, oscilloscope; REC, recording.

Motor unit potential (MUP)—When the subject is doing minimum contraction of the muscle, the individual motor unit potential (summation of action potentials from all muscle fibers innervated by the same motor neuron) can be identified easily. The morphologic patterns, including amplitude, duration, and wave form, and the recruitment patterns should be analyzed carefully to distinguish various types of neu-

Table 25-6. Electromyographic (EMG) test

Procedures	Items examined	Normal EMG	Neurogenic lesion: Acute	Neurogenic lesion: Chronic	Myogenic lesion: Dystrophy	Myogenic lesion: Myotonia	Myogenic lesion: Polymyositis
Needle insertion	Insertional activity	Few hundred msecs	Increased	Decreased	Increased	Increased	Increased
Rest	Resting potential	Silent	Fibrillation, positive sharp waves	Fibrillation, positive sharp waves (less), fasciculation	Silent	Myotonic discharges	Fibrillation, positive sharp waves
Minimum contraction	Motor unit potentials (MUPs):						
	Size	0.1–3.0 mV	Normal	Large	Small	Small	Small
	Form	2–4 phases	Normal	Polyphasic	Polyphasic or normal	Polyphasic or normal	Polyphasic or normal
	Motor unit recruitment	Early-slow MUPs, later-fast MUPs, gradual increase of number of MUPs	Early-fast MUPs	Early-fast MUPs	Early full	Early full	Early full
			Early decrease of number of MUPs	Early decrease of number of MUPs	Early increase of number of MUPs	Early increase of number of MUPs	Early increase of number of MUPs
Maximum contraction	Interference pattern	100% (full)	Reduced	Reduced	Full	Full	Full

rogenic disorders. The size (amplitude and duration) of the MUP may be reduced in myopathic disease and increased in chronic neurogenic lesions, such as chronic radiculopathy or chronic polyneuropathy. The wave form may be polyphasic in a pathologic motor unit, either in myopathy or neuropathy. The recruitment of MUPs during gradual increase of contraction force follows the "size principle." That is, the slow motor units, usually small motor units, fire first during minimum contraction, followed by recruitment of fast motor units (usually large motor units). In neurogenic disease, the fast motor units fire earlier than normal (increase of temporal recruitment), and the number of motor units are reduced (decrease of spatial recruitment), with further increased force of contraction. In myogenic disorders, however, the recruitment is full even with a weak force of contraction.

Interference pattern (maximal recruitment of MUPs)—When a normal person is asked to perform a maximal contraction, the MUPs completely fill the screen of the oscilloscope without an observed baseline. This is a full interference pattern (or 100% interference). The pattern may be reduced in any disease involving the motor unit or even in the presence of an upper motor neuron lesion.

Nerve Conduction Study

The nerve conduction study can be done with an EMG machine, when a stimulator is connected to the machine and triggers the sweep in the oscilloscope synchronously with the delivery of the stimulating current. For the motor nerve conduction study, the nerve is stimulated at two or more points along the course of the nerve, and a compound muscle action potential is recorded from the muscles innervated by this nerve (Fig. 25-6). The latency from the time of stimulation to the onset of the compound action potential can be measured for each point of stimulation. The nerve conduction velocity (NCV) can be calculated easily by dividing the distance between any two points of stimulation by the difference in latencies between these two points. The sensory nerve conduction study follows the same principle, but the nerve action potential is recorded rather than the muscle action potential as in a motor nerve conduction study (Fig. 25-7).

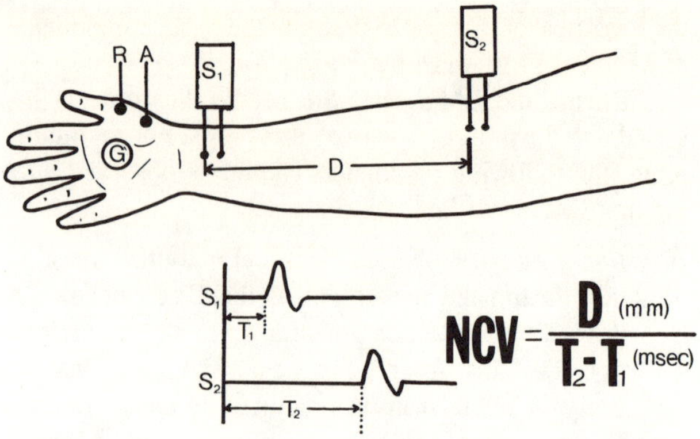

Figure 25-6. Motor nerve conduction study on the median nerve. R, reference electrode; A, active electrode; G, ground electrode; S_1, distal stimulation; S_2, proximal stimulation; NCV, nerve conduction velocity; D, distance; T_1, distal latency; T_2, proximal latency.

Clinical Application of EMG and Nerve Conduction Studies

Many neurologic lesions can be identified or confirmed by doing EMG and nerve conduction studies (65). This is summarized in Table 25-7. For a geriatric patient with neurogenic disease, EMG and nerve conduction studies may be helpful to confirm the diagnosis, determine the prognosis, and, more importantly, help in the determination and location of the surgical intervention. There is a high incidence of peripheral neuropathy in the geriatric patient due to many factors, including poor nutrition, accident, alcohol abuse, diabetes, uremia, etc. EMG and NCV study may be helpful in distinguishing different types of neuropathy and then in determining the treatment plan. Cervical or lumbosacral radiculopathy is another common problem in the geriatric patient. EMG examination is an important procedure for determining the degree of nerve root lesion (65).

Other Electrophysiologic Studies

The classical nerve conduction studies measure the conduction of the distal segment of nerve. In the last 10 to 20 years, many techniques have been developed to measure the proximal segments.

The H-reflex study measures the conduction time

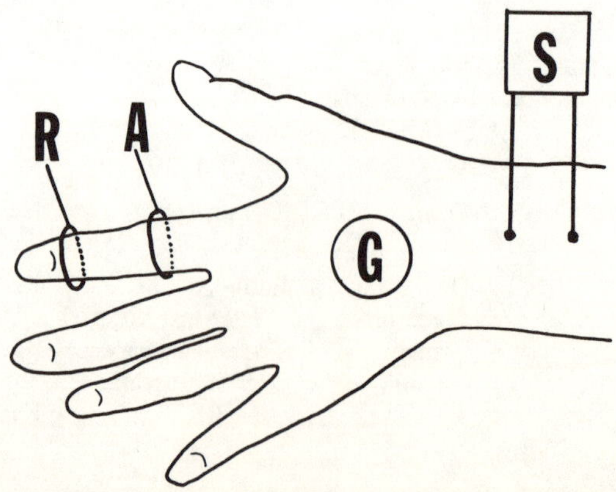

Figure 25-7. Sensory nerve conduction study on the median nerve. R, reference electrode; A, active electrode; G, ground electrode; S, stimulation.

Table 25-7. Electromyographic (EMG) and nerve conduction tests for differential diagnosis

Diagnosis	EMG findings, pattern and distribution	Nerve conduction study: NCV	Amplitude of evoked potential	Wave form of evoked potential	Distribution of abnormality
Upper motor neuron lesion	Normal except for reduced recruitment and interference	Normal	Normal	Normal	—
Motor neuron disease	Neurogenic pattern, diffuse	Normal	Reduced	Normal	Diffuse
Radiculopathy	Neurogenic pattern in muscles innervated by specific root	Normal	Reduced	Normal	In nerves derived from involved root
Polyneuropathy, axonopathy	Neurogenic pattern in distal muscles of all limbs	Normal	Reduced	Normal	In distal nerve segment of all limbs
Polyneuropathy, demyelinative	Normal	Slow	Reduced	Temporal dispersion	In all nerves
Polyneuropathy, combined	Neurogenic pattern in distal muscles of all limbs	Slow	Reduced	Temporal dispersion	In all involved nerves
Mononeuropathy, entrapment	Neurogenic pattern in muscles innervated by certain nerve	Slow	Reduced	Temporal dispersion	In the nerve segment with lesion
Myopathy	Myopathic pattern	Normal	Normal or reduced	Normal	—

from the site of stimulation on the sensory fibers to the motor neuron through the monosynaptic reflex, and then on to the motor fibers and muscles (Fig. 25-8). Unfortunately, this technique can only be applied in a study on the tibial nerve by picking up from the soleus muscle, and on the median nerve by picking up from the flexor carpi radialis muscle. The H-wave is difficult to record from the other muscles.

Measurement of F-wave is also a useful technique for evaluating proximal segment conduction (65–67). The F-wave study measures the time from the site of stimulation proximally to the motor neuron, and then back to the motor fibers and muscle fibers (Fig. 25-9). Unlike the H-wave, the F-wave can easily be recorded from any of the muscles, especially from the distal muscles. However, it measures only the motor fibers but not the sensory ones.

The somatosensory evoked potential (SSEP) can measure the conduction of the sensory fibers in the proximal segment (65). Since the potential recorded from the scalp is so small, an "averager" is required to pick up these very small potentials. The function of the "averager" is to intensify the recorded potentials from nerve stimulation and to cancel the random noise.

Blink reflex has also been used to measure the time from the forehead to brain stem and then back to the facial

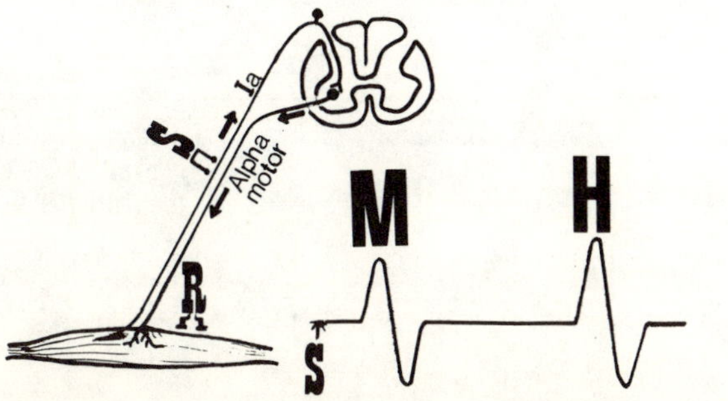

Figure 25-8. Neural pathway for H-reflex. S, stimulation; R, recording; M, main wave of compound muscle action potential recorded as the direct response via the motor fiber; H, H-wave of the compound muscle action potential recorded as the indirect response from Ia sensory afferent via the monosynaptic reflex to the motor neuron and then return to the alpha motor fiber.

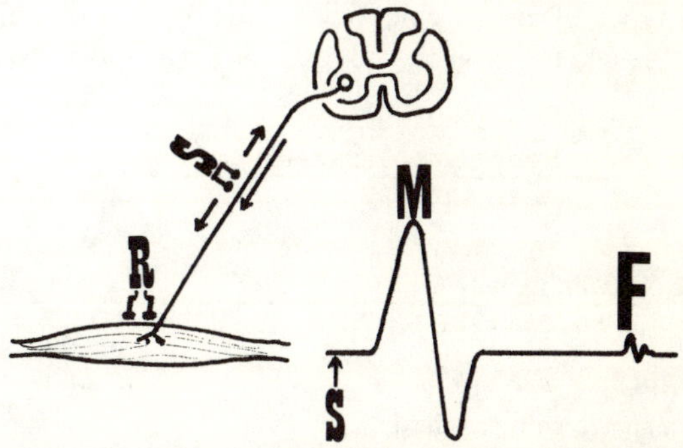

Figure 25-9. Neural pathway for F-response. S, stimulation; R, recording; M, main wave of compound muscle action potential recorded as the direct response via the motor fiber; F, F-wave of the compound muscle action potential recorded as the indirect response from proximal propagation of impulse to the motor neuron and then return to the motor nerve fiber of the same neuron (only about 5% of motor fibers can leave such responses).

muscles (65). It is a useful technique to distinguish facial palsy of various sites of lesions.

Devices, Equipment, Orthosis, and Prosthesis

After surgery, particularly after orthopedic surgery, the elderly patient often requires a device, equipment, orthosis, or prosthesis to become independent in activities of daily living (ADL). The following items are prescribed frequently in rehabilitation medicine: wheelchair, walker, crutches, cane, ADL devices (such as reacher, feeding devices, etc.), splints, hemisling, braces, spinal support, shoe support, and prostheses. The purposes of using these are either for energy conservation or for substitution of lost function. The energy cost (kcal/min) of ambulation using various devices or equipment (68) is listed in Table 25-8. One can see how important the wheelchair is in saving the energy of patients with cardiopulmonary disease.

Postoperatively, a geriatric patient may need a wheelchair temporarily for transportation. It is important to evaluate the patient's ability for transfer to and from a wheelchair, ability to control the wheelchair, sitting balance, sitting tolerance, and visual, perceptual, and cognitive function. Physical therapy may be required to help the patient to become "wheelchair independent." If ambulation is encouraged after surgery, a walker is much safer than any other ambulatory device for a geriatric patient because of its stability. However, the patient should have fair strength of trunk muscles for stability and good strength of the upper extremities to lift and move the walker. A hemiwalker may be used if the patient is hemiplegic.

Other ambulatory devices are available when the stability has improved to a certain level. Crutches are convenient and inexpensive, and are usually prescribed for the geriatric patient after orthopedic surgery. There are several types of crutch gaits for various degrees of weight bearing and for various types of mobility due to unilateral or bilateral limitations of the lower extremities. "Swing-to" or "swing-through" gait can be used if the patient has weakness or limitation of mobility of both lower extremities, with good strength in the upper extremities. In the swing-to gait pattern, the patient slides both feet forward, but does not reach the two supporting points of the crutches. The patient moves the crutches forward and then repeats the same movement. In the swing-through pattern the patient lifts and swings the legs through to a heel strike ahead of the crutches, and then moves the crutches forward and repeats the same cycle.

Three-point gait (Fig. 25-10a) allows different degrees of weight bearing (0% to 100%) of the affected lower extremity. The patient moves both crutches and the affected leg forward to new positions and then moves the unaffected leg when the weight bearing is placed on both crutches and the unaffected leg (3-point support). Four-point gait (Fig. 25-10b) allows weight bearing of $1/3$ of body weight for either leg. The patient moves one crutch forward and the contralateral leg forward, then the other crutch followed by the other leg. For each movement, there are always three points of support. So the weight bearing on each leg is $1/3$ of the body weight. Two-point (Fig. 25-10c) gait allows weight bearing of $1/2$ of the body weight for either leg. The patient moves one crutch and the contralateral leg at the same time, and then moves another crutch and another leg simultaneously. Therefore, the number of supporting points is always two, and the weight bearing for each leg is $1/2$ of the body weight. With these principles, the patient can be taught the appropriate pattern of crutch walking.

When the patient has better stability during the postoperative recovery period, a cane can be used instead of a walker or crutches. There are several different types of canes. The most common types are the standard or J cane with only one supporting point, the small based quad-cane with four supporting points but a small supporting base, and the large based quad-cane with four supporting

Table 25-8. Energy cost of ambulation

Type of disability	Speed (M/min)	Energy expenditure per unit time (kcal/min/kg B.W.)	Energy expenditure per unit distance (cal/M/kg B.W.)
Normal	80	0.04–0.06	0.6–0.8
BK Amputee with prosthesis	50–60	0.04–0.07	1.0–1.2
AK amputee with prosthesis	40–60	0.05–0.08	1.0–1.7
Hemiplegics—no brace	40	0.04–0.06	1.0–1.5
Hemiplegics with brace	50	0.07	1.4
Paraplegics with brace and crutches	20–30	0.05–0.09	2.3–2.4
Wheelchair (disabled)	67	0.04	0.5

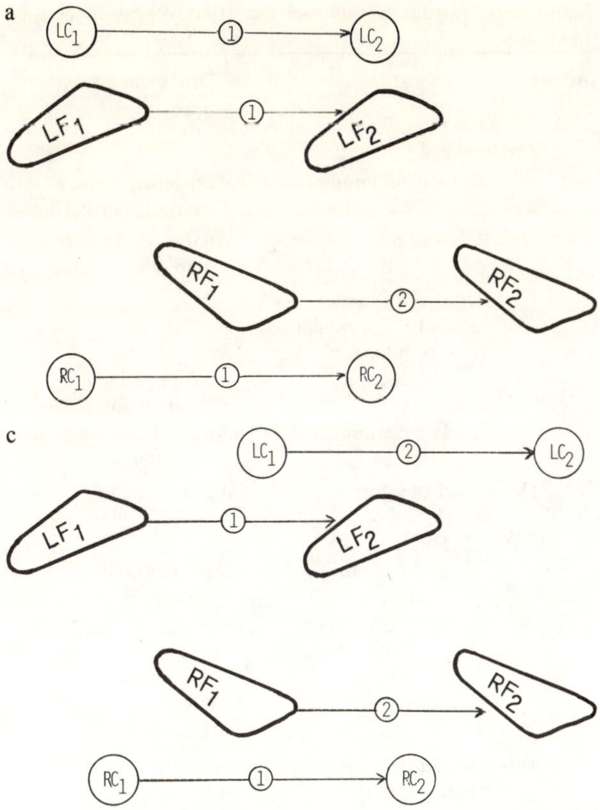

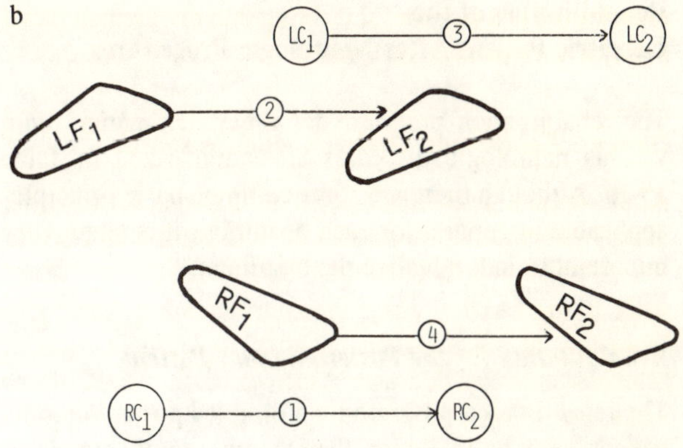

Figure 25-10. a, The sequence of 3-point gait; b, the sequence of 4-point gait; c, the sequence of 2-point gait. LC, left crutch; LF, left foot; RC, right crutch; RF, right foot.

points and a large supporting base. The cane should be held by the hand contralateral to the involved leg. If both legs are similarly affected, the cane should be held by the stronger hand for safety.

Some ADL devices may be helpful for postoperative care. Due to pain over the surgical site, the patient may be unable to move certain parts of the body for daily living activities. A reacher is useful for the patient to pick up something or to perform an activity without movement of the operated region (Fig. 25-11). Other devices may be made by an experienced occupational therapist, depending on the patient's need. ADL devices are also useful for patients with limited range of motion of any joints, motor weakness, or incoordination.

Prescription of a splint, brace, or prosthesis should be individualized. An effective orthosis or prosthesis may prevent complications, may improve motor function, and may be helpful for independent ADL. However, an inappropriate or poorly fitting device may create complications or reduce function. For example, if a tight splint is applied continuously on a patient with poor sensory function postoperatively, a pressure sore may develop. The same may occur with an ill-fitting artificial limb on an amputee. This is particularly important for elderly patients since they have a higher risk of many complications postoperatively.

Pharmacologic Tools

Some medications commonly used in conjunction with a rehabilitation program to enhance the effectiveness of physical medicine modalities are listed in Table 25-9.

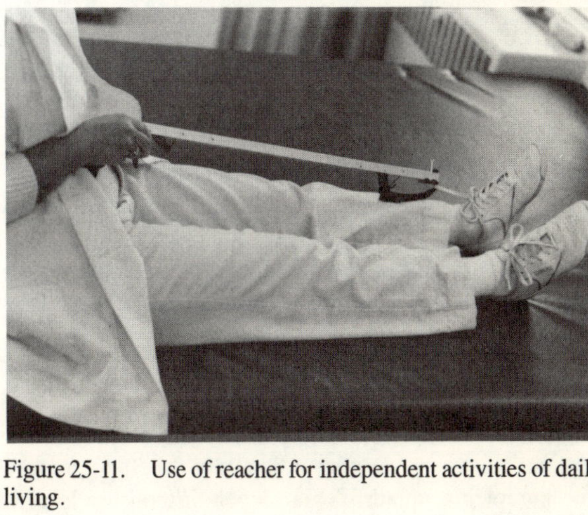

Figure 25-11. Use of reacher for independent activities of daily living.

Rehabilitation of the Geriatric Patient After Neurologic Procedures

The rehabilitation programs for a geriatric patient with various neurologic disorders are summarized in Table 25-10. Although there are some common basic principles applicable in general for each condition, it is again very important to individualize the treatment.

Rehabilitation for the Postcraniotomy Patient

The rehabilitation program for a disabled postcraniotomy patient with brain injury (hematoma), brain tumor, or other space-occupying lesions varies with the phase of recovery. In the acute stage the functional disability is either due to extensive postoperative brain edema or due to brain tissue damage or defect. The rehabilitation program is directed toward facilitating functional recovery and preventing complications of bed rest, such as contracture, pressure sores, or circulatory complications due to immobilization. The initial neurologic recovery may be related to the relief of brain edema or diaschisis (69).

In the later stage, the anatomical lesion causing functional impairment becomes more clear cut. The regeneration of the dead neurons is very limited or unlikely (70). However, axonal sprouting may play an important role in neurologic recovery (69). Further neurologic recovery may depend on the unmasking of previously unused pathways (15, 16). In this stage, both neurologic facilitation and compensatory mechanisms are important for the rehabilitation therapies. The residual functions should be reinforced through training to compensate for the lost function. Substitution of a paralyzed dominant hand to the contralateral side through occupational therapy is important in improving function. In addition, some adaptive devices or equipment may be required in order to achieve independent living.

The rehabilitation program should also include the management of the patient's and family's psychosocial stress.

The rehabilitation goal should be organized based on the anatomic lesion (CT scan or MRI), the residual neurologic function, the cognitive deficit, the general medical status, and other related factors, such as educational level, vocational training and experience, and the family support systems (71).

Rehabilitation for the Patient with Spinal Cord Injury

A geriatric patient receiving spinal surgery for trauma, infection, tumor, or vascular lesion may develop paraparesis, paraplegia, quadriplegia (depending on the level of the lesion), or an exacerbation of previously existing neurologic deficits. In the early postoperative stage the rehabilitation program should begin with passive range of motion, strengthening of residual muscles, bed positioning, and care for the neurogenic bladder and bowel dysfunction.

A patient with an established complete spinal cord lesion (e.g., a transected cord) will not have significant neurologic recovery. Therefore, the rehabilitation program for such a patient emphasizes training of compensatory or substitutive mechanisms rather than techniques of neurologic facilitation. A complete paraplegic patient can

Table 25-9. Drugs to enhance the effectiveness of physical medicine

Action	Drugs categories
I. Drugs to improve physical performance through:	
A. Relief of inflammation	Anti-inflammatory—steroid, nonsteroid
B. Relief of pain	Analgesic—non-narcotic, narcotic
C. Removal of casual factors of 2nd weakness	
1. For infection	Antibiotics
2. For anemia	Iron supplement, vitamin supplement
3. For neuromuscular diseases	Anticholinesterase (for myasthenia)
D. Relief of abnormal muscle tone:	
1. For spasticity	
a. Systemic	Diazepam, baclofen, dantrium
b. Motor point block or nerve block	Phenol
2. For rigidity	Anticholinergics, L-DOPA
II. Drugs to improve mental performance through:	
A. Relief of depression	Antidepressants
B. Relief of anxiety	Tranquilizers
C. Decrease of agitation	Haloperidol
III. Drugs to improve social performance through:	
A. Improvement of bladder function	
1. For hypotonic bladder	Cholinergics—urecholine
2. For hypertonic bladder	Anticholinergics
3. For tight sphincter	Sympatholytics—alpha blockers
B. Improvement of bowel function	
1. For constipation	Stool softeners
2. For diarrhea	Anticholinergics

Table 25-10. Rehabilitation for neurologic disorders

Possible disabilities	Rehabilitation programs
Impairment of motor function	
Weakness, paralysis	Therapeutic exercise, orthosis
Ataxia, poor balance	Exercise
Spasticity	Medicine, cold, heat, exercise, intramuscular neurolysis (motor point block)
Impairment of perceptual function	Perceptual training (OT)
Impairment of cognitive function	Cognitive training (OT, psychology, speech therapy, rehab nurse)
Impairment of speech and language function	Speech therapy
Impairment of sphincter function	Bladder and bowel training (rehab nurse)
Impairment of activities of daily living (ADL)	ADL training (OT, rehab nurse)
Poor adjustment to disability	Psychologic assessment and management
Others	

Diseases: CVA, head injury, parkinsonism, spinal cord injury, multiple sclerosis, ALS, peripheral neuropathy, polymyositis, muscular dystrophy, etc.

be trained to become totally independent in daily living at the wheelchair level. Ambulation with crutches is not a priority, considering the mechanical efficiency and the energy cost. In the young with great physical prowess, ambulation with crutches or participation in wheelchair sports are occasionally achieved. In the elderly, such goals are unrealistic if not dangerous. Table 25-11 shows the functional significance of the spinal cord lesion level.

Some complications from neurologic deprivation, such as pressure sores, problems from neurogenic bladder and bowel, orthostatic hypotension, autonomic hyperreflexia, heterotropic ossification, spasticity, and loss of normal thermoregulatory mechanism, can be prevented through judicious care. If they occur, they should be treated early. With normal cognitive function but loss of motor function, a spinal cord injured patient characteristically has severe depression during the early stages of the disability. Psychologic counseling by the physician, the psychologist, or psychiatrist is important in dealing with such problems. The social worker also plays an important role in helping the patient to overcome environmental, social, and family problems.

The rehabilitation team has a role in helping patients

Table 25-11. Maximal functional achievement in relation to the level of spinal cord lesion

	C-4	C-5	C-6	C-7	T-1	T-6	T-12	L-4
Feeding	−	+	+	+	+	+	+	+
Grooming	−	−	±	+	+	+	+	+
Dressing								
Upper	−	−	+	+	+	+	+	+
Lower	−	−	−	+	+	+	+	+
Bed mobility	−	−	±	+	+	+	+	+
Wheelchair management	−	−	+	+	+	+	+	+
Regular	−	−	+	+	+	+	+	+
Power	±	+	+	+	+	+	+	+
Transfer	−	−	±	+	+	+	+	+
Toilet	−	±	±	+	+	+	+	+
Ambulation	−	−	−	−	−	±	±	+

set realistic goals based on their medical, psychological, and social status.

Rehabilitation in Cardiac Surgery

General Principles in Cardiac Rehabilitation

Disability from heart disease in the geriatric patient is usually related to reduced cardiac fitness due to the hemodynamic impairment of the cardiovascular system or general deconditioning from prolonged bedrest. In the patient who has recently undergone open heart surgery, the same principles apply, although the additional duties of the healing wound may delay or extend the rehabilitation program. Well-programmed therapeutic exercise is one of the most important aspects of cardiac rehabilitation. Physiological effects of exercise for the myocardium have been discussed in the previous section. The quality and quantity of the exercise should be adjusted carefully to obtain optimal effects and to avoid undue risks (72). The general principles of exercise prescription for the cardiac patient are as follows: (*a*) readily accessible programs with practical and simple protocols, with little or no exercise equipment required; (*b*) avoidance of excessive stress to the myocardium; and (*c*) measurable data to document improvement and to adjust the exercise program. An outline of cardiac rehabilitation programs is shown in Table 25-12.

Preoperative Programs

Evaluation

In elective cardiac surgery, it is desirable that the patient be evaluated not only in regard to his cardiopulmonary function and medical status, but also his psychologic and social function. This will be very helpful in preparing for the postoperative period.

Education

The patient should be informed about the anticipated postoperative deterioration in fitness and the need for a rehabilitation program.

Exercise

If feasible, the practice of therapeutic exercises before surgery is desirable. Patients can learn these exercises more easily before surgery than after surgery when postoperative pain may limit their mobility.

Postoperative Program

Re-evaluation

Soon after surgery, patients can be evaluated in the intensive care unit so that their general functional impairment can be assessed and an early exercise program can be started.

Early Exercise Program

In order to prevent complications and to facilitate postoperative recovery, early exercise programs are important. Patients can start abdominal breathing exercises, which have been taught before surgery, as soon as they wake up from general anesthesia. Passive range of motion or active assistive exercise can be done cautiously when there is no cardiac contraindication. Early ambulation is encouraged as soon as patients are discharged from the intensive care unit if it is not contraindicated for any reason.

Functional Assessment and Training in Activities of Daily Living

Functional impairment after cardiac surgery may be a serious problem, especially for the geriatric patient. An occupational therapy program may help the patient become independent in daily living activities with minimum energy consumption. Some devices or equipment may be required for such purposes. For example, use of a stool in the shower may be helpful.

Rehabilitation in Chest Surgery

General Principles in Pulmonary Rehabilitation

Pulmonary disorders in the geriatric patient may cause significant functional limitation in daily living activities. Rehabilitation programs may be of help in improving cardiopulmonary fitness, efficiency, and the functional level in activities of daily living. Breathing exercises improve the efficiency of the respiratory excursion by utilizing improved diaphragmatic abdominal control. Research has shown that the pulmonary patient can improve work capacity in an exercise training program (42). Training also alleviates the emotional problems and social isolation frequently present in the geriatric patient with pulmonary disease.

Table 25-12. Rehabilitation for cardiopulmonary disorders

Possible disabilities	Rehabilitation programs
Impairment of cardiopulmonary fitness	Assessment of fitness level and general conditioning exercise with the following principles: Submaximal rather than maximal; Aerobic rather than anaerobic; Dynamic (isotonic) rather than static (isometric) Intermittent rather than continuous; and, Large group muscle activities
Impairment of ADL	ADL training, energy-saving techniques
Others	

Diseases: Coronary artery diseases, chronic obstructive lung diseases, congestive heart failure, etc.

Geriatric patients who have had chest surgery may develop functional limitations even if their premorbid pulmonary function has been normal. The limitation is even more remarkable if lobectomy or pneumonectomy is performed. For such patients, rehabilitation may have an important role in the recovery phase.

Preoperative Program

Before the operation the evaluation for cardiopulmonary fitness, pulmonary function testing, and arterial blood gas analysis may be used as a guide for the postoperative rehabilitation program. Other important data will include other medical problems that affect the cardiopulmonary fitness and functional capability, the patient's mental function, and psychologic and social status. As in the case of cardiac surgery, the patient's education and preoperative practice of therapeutic exercise are also important for the preparation of the postoperative rehabilitation program.

Postoperative Program

When the patient is still on the ventilator, passive range of motion of all extremities should be done daily. Bed positioning is also important in preventing complications, such as pressure sores or retention of pulmonary secretions. Respiratory therapy is the most important pulmonary rehabilitation program during this stage.

As soon as the patient can be weaned off the ventilator, breathing exercises, postural drainage, and active exercise of the limbs should begin. Gradually, the patient should be helped to sit up. Early ambulation is important when feasible with vital signs stable, chest tube removed, and pulmonary function permitting. Pulmonary function should be monitored periodically to assess and design the program.

Occupational therapy should be involved if activities of daily living are impaired. Devices or equipment may be prescribed as required. For example, a "reacher" may be useful for a patient with pneumonectomy when the mobility of the ipsilateral arm is limited due to pain (Fig. 25-11).

Rehabilitation in the Geriatric Patient After Orthopedic Surgery

Rehabilitation for the Geriatric Patient with a Fracture or Dislocation

Fracture or dislocation may be associated with falling in the geriatric patient. In the case of a fracture the emergent care is provided by the orthopedic surgeon for either open reduction or external fixation. Rehabilitation should start as early as the day after surgery (73). After surgery, physical medicine modalities are helpful to facilitate recovery, to relieve pain, to maintain range of motion and strength, and to prevent complications. As mentioned in the previous section, electrical stimulation may facilitate the healing in a non-union fracture (54, 55). Heat therapy, transcutaneous nerve stimulation, and hydrotherapy may be helpful for the relief of postoperative pain. Therapeutic exercise, either passive or active, should start as soon as possible. The muscles originating from or inserting on the fractured bone should be exercised isometrically. The nearby joints without immobilization should have full range of motion (either actively or passively) within the patient's tolerance. Other groups of muscles should be strengthened by general conditioning exercises to maintain normal fitness. As soon as the period of immobilization is over, the contractured joint should be stretched gradually to increase its range of motion, accompanied by heat therapy or hydrotherapy. If the lower extremity is involved, ambulation should begin as soon as weight bearing is allowed. Crutches or cane should be prescribed at an early stage of ambulation training to help the stability and to reduce weight bearing on the affected leg.

Occupational therapy may help the patient to become independent or to reduce the dependency in self-care activities if the patient is disabled during the healing phase.

Hip fractures are a major source of morbidity among the elderly (73). The rehabilitation programs for the geriatric patient with hip fracture are listed in Table 25-13.

Rehabilitation for the Geriatric Patient with Total Joint Replacement

General Considerations

Due to the higher incidence of degenerative joint disease and aseptic necrosis of the hip in the geriatric patient, total joint replacement has become a common procedure in the elderly. About 60% of the total hip replacements are performed in patients older than 65 years of age (74). The purposes of such a procedure are to reduce pain and to improve motor function of the involved joint. However, these goals may not be able to be reached without an appropriate postoperative rehabilitation program.

The common postoperative problems are pain, weakness, and limited range of motion. The postoperative pain is not only from the operation wound but also may be related to misuse of the surrounding muscles (75). As pointed out by Opitz, the patient usually has had years of progressive pain about the joint in question, with resultant long-term expectation and experience of joint pain. These induce changes in the coordination and motor behaviors of the periarticular muscles, with disuse in some muscles and overuse in others. Therefore, decreased range of motion and strength may occur. In addition, an overuse syndrome related to certain muscle groups may result, leading to a myofascial pain syndrome (76), tenosynovitis, or tendinitis. All these problems may persist, even though the original joint pain has been relieved after total joint replacement. The rehabilitation program should also be emphasized because of the retraining of the misused muscle groups (75). Table 25-14 summarizes the general rehabilitation program for total joint replacement.

Total Hip Arthroplasty

Due to the high incidence of deep vein thromboembolic disease after total hip replacement, the immediate postoperative care should emphasize prevention of this complication (77). Isometric exercise of all muscle groups in the lower extremity, especially gluteal muscles, hamstrings, and calf muscles, should begin as early as possible after the surgery. The involved lower extremity should be elevated. To avoid dislocation, the hip joint should not be moved excessively in the direction of adduction, flexion, and internal rotation. Passive exercises or active assistive exercise should be done carefully to avoid dislocation. Upper extremity and contralateral lower ex-

Table 25-13. Rehabilitation programs for the geriatric patient with hip fractures

Postoperative days	Physical medicine modalities	Physiologic basis
1st–4th day	Exercise: Sitting up Quadriceps, hamstring and upper extremity strengthening Passive or active assistive exercise for hip and knee, both flexion and extension, but avoid rotations	To avoid complications such as contractures, thromboembolic disorders, disuse weakness, edema, osteoporosis, etc. To facilitate soft tissue recovery after surgery, and to prepare for ambulation
	Cold therapy	To reduce pain and swelling
	Transcutaneous nerve stimulation	To reduce pain
5th–9th day	Exercise (As in day 1–4, and add:) Straight-leg raising (active or active assist) Standing and ambulation training with walker, with weight-bearing up to 50% of total body weight Isometric exercise of hip muscles	As above under "Exercise"
	Cold or heat therapy or electrical stimulation	To reduce pain
	ADL training	For independent daily living activities

Modified from Kumar, VN, and Redford, JB. 1984. Rehabilitation of hip fractures in the elderly. *Am Fam Physician* 29:173–180.

tremity strengthening exercises should also be performed early after surgery. Sitting and transfer training usually begin on the 3rd or 4th postoperative day, and more aggressive physical therapy programs including standing and ambulation training on the 5th postoperative day (77). ADL training is often needed for those patients with other complicated medical problems, such as arthritis or cardiac disease. A home program should be provided before discharge from the hospital.

Total Knee Arthroplasty

As in the case of total hip replacement, there is also a relatively high risk of deep vein thromboembolic disease after the total knee replacement, and therefore the immediate postoperative rehabilitation program focuses on prevention (78). The principles are the same as those for total hip replacement. Early isometric exercise, elevation of the leg, range of motion exercise, and dynamic strengthening exercises of the contralateral lower extremity and of both upper extremities should be carried out. Ambulation training can begin during the 3rd to 4th postoperative days (78). ADL training should be carried out when indicated and should begin as soon as the patient starts to walk. A home program is also required after discharge.

Other Joints

Patients requiring replacement of a joint other than the hip or knee will have less problems in daily living activities. However, appropriate application of physical medicine modalities and certain types of occupational therapy are still indicated to facilitate recovery for optimal functional status.

Rehabilitation for the Geriatric Patient with Amputation

Lower Extremity Amputation

Preoperative care. Before surgery, the patient should ideally have an orientation to postoperative realistic expectations and plans, education on stump care, strengthening exercise for the trunk and upper extremities, and breathing exercises. The phenomenon of phantom sensation should also be discussed.

Table 25-14. Rehabilitation programs for total joint replacement

Problems	Rehabilitation programs
Pain	Cold (early), heat (later), massage, TENS, motor re-education
Edema	Cold, massage, elastic bandage, limb elevation, active exercise (such as calf pumping), electrical muscle stimulation
Limited range of motion	Exercise (passive stretching, active, motor re-education), mobilization, dynamic orthosis
Weakness	Exercise (isometric, dynamic), motor re-education, orthosis
Focal muscle spasm	Cold, heat, massage, manipulation, exercise (passive stretching, isometric), medicine
Gait deviation	Ambulation training, orthosis
Dependence in ADL	ADL training, devices, equipment
Environmental difficulty	Home evaluation, equipment, home reconstruction
Depression, emotional disturbance, etc.	Psychologic counseling
Placement (discharge difficulty)	Social service

Early postoperative care. In the first few days after surgery, the patient usually experiences severe stump pain. The rehabilitation program emphasizes stump care and general conditioning. Bedside exercise, for strengthening of the upper extremities and the contralateral lower extremity, and breathing exercises can be started as early as feasible. Gentle range of motion of the hip and knee (if a below-knee amputation) and appropriate positioning of the stump may prevent complications, such as a contracture or excessive edema. An above-knee (AK) amputee is encouraged to sleep in the prone position to avoid flexion contracture of the hip joint, and a below-knee (BK) amputee is advised to straighten the knee by not permitting a pillow under the stump and thereby avoiding flexion contracture. Transcutaneous electric nerve stimulation (TENS) may help by applying it above the site of amputation for pain relief.

As soon as the bandage can be removed to check the stump wound, the stump should be wrapped with an elastic bandage or with a rigid dressing to maintain good shaping and to avoid excessive swelling (which may also reduce pain). Therapeutic exercises for upper and contralateral lower extremity strengthening, trunk balancing, and stump mobility and strengthening should be done gradually and progressively. The patient should continue to maintain the appropriate position of the stump. For example, prolonged sitting in a wheelchair is not encouraged (79). Standing and ambulation training can be started within 1 week if no stump complications (such as wound maceration, infection, or excessive edema) occur. When the sutures are removed, the patient should be taught stump wrapping.

Occupational therapy is important for ADL training. In our experience, all geriatric patients with lower extremity amputation have the potential to become independent in dressing, transfer, personal hygiene and bathroom activities, at least at the wheelchair level, unless complicated with other disability.

Immediate postoperative pylon fitting (80) has become popular for certain uncomplicated amputations, such as an amputation for a bone tumor or a clean traumatic amputation. The stump is dressed in a rigid case to which the pylon is attached, and the patient can stand on the pylon for early (often the 1st postoperative day) ambulation training. The advantage is to reduce postoperative edema and pain and to offer early ambulation training, thereby shortening the period of hospitalization (80). Unfortunately, it is infrequently done in geriatric amputations, probably due to debilitation and the high incidence of vascular insufficiency of the contralateral limb. However, it is believed to be valuable in the elderly where complications due to prolonged bedrest are more prone to occur.

Preprosthetic training. The majority of amputations in geriatric patients are due to peripheral vascular disease in the lower extremity (81). They frequently have other medical problems, such as diabetes, heart disease, hypertension, or renal insufficiency. Therefore, the time required for rehabilitation is usually longer than that for the young amputee. However, age itself is not a factor in determining the indication for prosthesis fitting. The authors have fitted many prostheses, both above and below the knee, to geriatric patients 80 years of age and older with excellent results. The factors that may affect the success of prosthesis fitting are cognitive function, vision, motivation, cardiopulmonary fitness, medical problems, and the condition of the stump and the contralateral extremity.

Once patients are considered to be candidates for prosthetic fitting, they should begin preprosthetic training. Therapeutic exercise and stump care are the primary programs. Besides the general conditioning exercise, crutch walking should be begun as soon as feasible. Endurance for crutch walking is the determinant of the capability for ambulation with a prosthesis. A patient wearing a BK prosthesis requires 20% to 40% higher energy cost for ambulation than for normal ambulation; for an AK amputation, the energy cost is 60% to 100% higher (Table

25-8). The patient should be able to do daily stump care independently, including wrapping, hygiene, and exercise. A pylon or temporary prosthesis may be prescribed early as soon as the wound is healed. The patient may need several temporary prostheses before a permanent one can be prescribed.

Prosthetic fitting. As soon as the stump shrinkage is mature and the patient is able to use a temporary prosthesis, a permanent prosthesis can be prescribed. This may take an average of 6 weeks. The type of prosthesis should be selected carefully, based on both clinical judgment and the patient's desire.

For the AK amputation, a pelvic suspension belt is usually required for a geriatric patient (81). The quadrilateral socket is the standard one for most patients. A Bock knee joint is the choice for most geriatric patients for safety reasons. A new type of molded SACH (solid ankle-cushion heel) light-weight foot is recommended for the geriatric patient (79). For the BK amputation, a patellar-tendon weight-bearing (PTB) socket with cuff suspension is usually the choice for the elderly (81). And again, the light SACH foot is usually given to the elderly amputee.

Upper Extremity Amputation

The major cause of upper extremity amputation is due to trauma (82). This occurs less often in the elderly than in young adults who are physically active.

A rehabilitation program should start immediately after surgery. Therapeutic exercises, including range of motion and strengthening exercises for the shoulder, the elbow (for below-elbow amputation), and the contralateral upper extremity, should be instituted (82). For the above-elbow (AE) amputee, strengthening exercises for the shoulder girdle muscles is essential, as these muscles are needed for operating the prosthesis. For the below-elbow (BE) amputee, both shoulder girdle and elbow muscles are important for effective control of the prosthesis, and these muscles should be trained intensively. Stump care is also important as in the lower extremity amputation; stump wrapping and stump hygiene should be taught to the patient. Occupational therapists should become involved on the first day after surgery, since they are key persons in giving prosthetic training.

The successful rate of prosthesis fitting is lower in the upper extremity amputation than in the lower one. The upper extremity prosthesis is usually used only as an assistive device. Many patients discard the prosthesis as they obtain better sensory feedback from the bare stump. Cosmesis is usually the greatest benefit (83). In terms of the decision on prosthetic fitting, the age of the patient should not be a determinant as long as the mental status is satisfactory, since the energy cost of prosthetic use is of little or no consequence (83).

Rehabilitation for the Geriatric Patient with Burns

Burns are not uncommon and usually cause significant disability in the geriatric population. Once the patient has survived moderate or severe burns, the rehabilitation program becomes very important in the medical care. The main goal is to restore optimal function as quickly as possible through a well-organized and coordinated program (84).

The rehabilitation programs are summarized in Table 25-15, based on the description from Helm et al. (85). In order to prevent serious complications, rehabilitation should start during the acute phase. Splinting is an important tool for supporting the involved limb in a desirable position to avoid complications. Splints are usually made by an occupational therapist. Exercise may be very difficult to perform due to severe pain, and is usually combined with hydrotherapy when the patient is medically stable. Exercises are performed emphasizing isolated joint motion, followed by patterned movement involving groups of joints (85). When feasible, some basic self-care activities should be started even in the acute phase. In the chronic stage, scar control and training activities of daily living become the most important aspects of care. Many kinds of functional splints or special orthoses are very helpful in controlling the scar and improving motor func-

Table 25-15. Rehabilitation programs for the geriatric patient with burns

Programs		Purpose
Acute phase		
Positioning Range of motion Splinting Active exercise	→	To reduce edema and pain To avoid contracture, abnormal scarring, and deformity
Convalescent phase		
Skin care Splinting/orthosis Massage Therapeutic exercise Stretching Active exercise General conditioning Hydrotherapy	→	Scar control To avoid contracture To improve motor function Cosmetic To avoid other medical complications
Psychotherapy	→	Emotional support
Occupational therapy	→	Independent daily living activities

tion. Figure 25-12 shows some samples of splints for the care of the patient with burns.

The importance of psychologic support for such a traumatized elderly person should not be ignored. After all, successful rehabilitation is based on the motivation and cooperation of the patient.

Once the wounds are healed, more vigorous programs should be given to reduce the scar contracture and to improve motor function. Patients should be encouraged to increase their physical activities progressively. Some patients can be treated on an outpatient basis. Regular use of a pressure garment or face mask is very helpful in controlling the scar.

Rehabilitation for the Geriatric Patient Receiving General Surgery

In general, a patient undergoing abdominal surgery will not become disabled except under special circumstances or if complications occur. However, due to reduced reserve or compromised organ systems, a geriatric patient more often may develop a functional disability postoperatively. The most common problem is general deconditioning.

During the acute stage, intercostal breathing exercise is helpful in avoiding postanesthetic complications, such as atelectasis or pneumonia. Active exercise of all limbs for mobility, strength, and endurance should be done early at the bedside with the help of a physical therapist. As soon as the stitches of the abdominal wound are removed, abdominal exercises can be started gradually. At the beginning, the patient can do isometric exercise gently, just by raising the head or the legs slightly. Sitting up in bed or in a chair is encouraged, but should be done carefully as the abdominal pressure is significantly higher for the sitting position. Standing and ambulation training should be allowed as long as the patient can tolerate the activity.

For patients with severe deconditioning, occupational therapy for ADL training is desirable to help them to become independent.

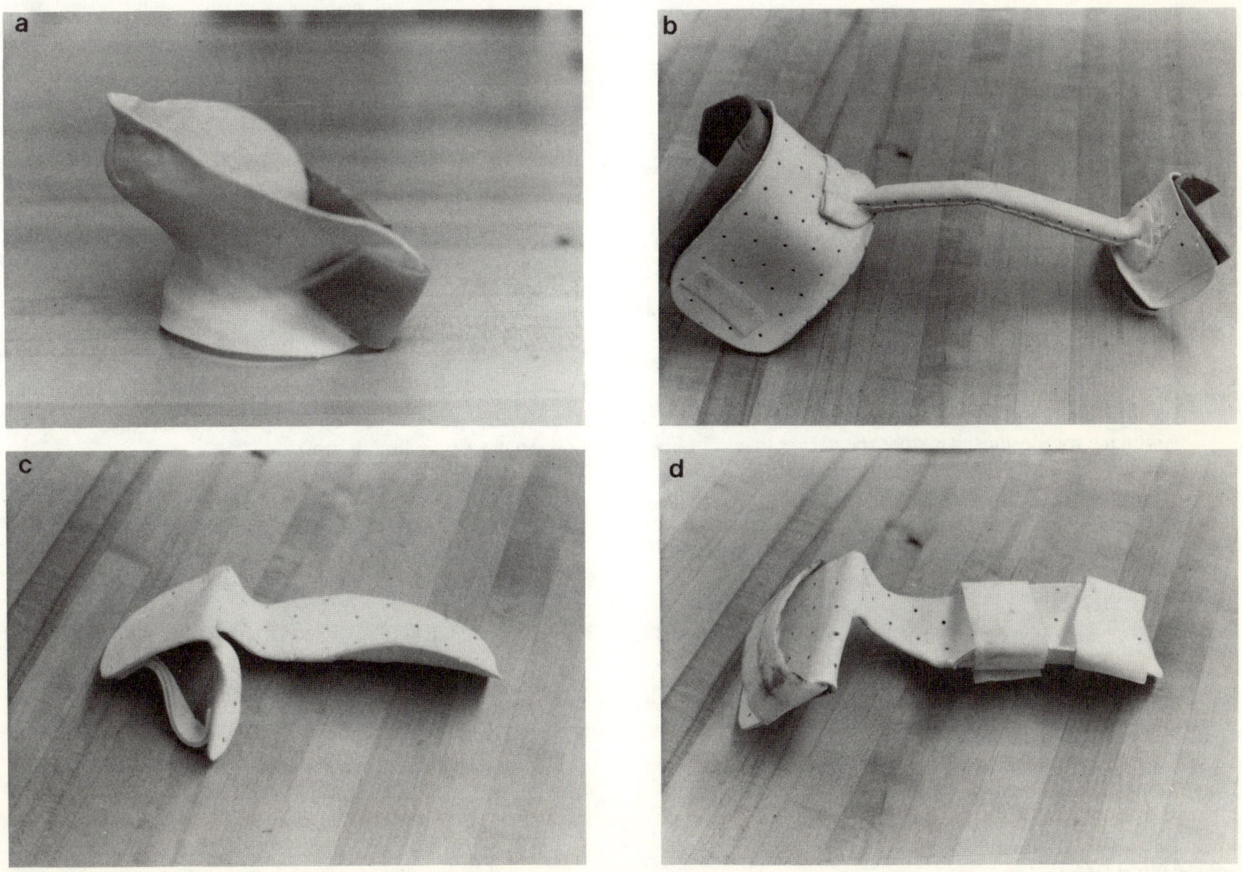

Figure 25-12. a, Neck splint to maintain hyperextension of cervical spine to avoid scar contracture in the anterior skin of neck; b, modified airplane splint to keep shoulder abduction to avoid scar contracture in the axillary area; c and d, wrist resting splint to keep the hand in functional position.

References

1. Gullickson, G, and Licht, S. 1968. Definition and philosophy of rehabilitation medicine. In *Rehabilitation and Medicine*, Ed., S. Licht. Baltimore: Waverly Press.
2. Licht, S. 1984. In *Therapeutic Exercise*, ed. 4, Ed., JV Basmajian. Baltimore: Williams & Wilkins.
3. Granger, CV. 1984. A conceptual model for functional assessment. In *Functional Assessment in Rehabilitation Medicine*. Eds., CV Granger, and GE Gresham. Baltimore: Williams & Wilkins.
4. Tobis, JS. 1979. Rehabilitation of the Geriatric Patient. In *Clinical Geriatrics*, ed. 2, Ed., I Rossman. Philadelphia: J.B. Lippincott Co.
5. Astrand, P-O, and Rodahl, K. 1977. Physical Training. In *Textbook of Work Physiology*, ed. 2. Eds., P-O Astrand and K Rodahl. New York: McGraw-Hill Book Company.
6. Basmajian, JV. 1984. Biofeedback in therapeutic exercise. In *Therapeutic Exercise*, ed. 4, Ed., JV Basmajian. Baltimore: Williams & Wilkins.
7. de Lateur, BJ. 1984. Exercise for strength and endurance. In *Therapeutic Exercise*, ed. 4, Ed., JV Basmajian. Baltimore: Williams & Wilkins.
8. Holloszy, JO, et al. 1977. Physiological consequences of the biochemical adaptations to endurance exercise. *Ann NY Acad Sci* 301:440–450.
9. Matoba, H, and Gollnick, PD. 1984. Response of skeletal muscle to training. *Sports Med* 1:240–251.
10. Petrofsky, JS, and Phillips, CA. 1986. The physiology of static exercise. *Exercise Sport Sci Rev* 14:1–44.
11. Osternig, LR. 1986. Isokinetic dynamometry: Implications for muscle testing and rehabilitation. *Exercise Sport Sci Rev* 14:45–80.
12. Kottke, FJ. 1982. Therapeutic exercise to maintain mobility. In *Krusen's Handbook of Physical Medicine and Rehabilitation*, ed. 3, Eds., FJ Kottke, GK Stillwell, and JF Lehmann. Philadelphia: W.B. Saunders.
13. Harris, FA. 1984. Facilitation techniques and technological adjuncts in therapeutic exercise. In *Therapeutic Exercise*, ed. 4, Ed., JV Basmajian. Baltimore: Williams & Wilkins.
14. Yu, J. 1980. Neuromuscular recovery with training after central nervous lesions: An experimental approach. In *Behavioral Psychology in Rehabilitation Medicine: Clinical Applications*. Ed., IP Ince. Baltimore: Williams & Wilkins.
15. Yu, J. 1982. Instrumental conditioning and plasticity of motor function. In *Changing Concepts of the Nervous System*, Eds., AR Morrison and PL Strick. New York: Academic Press, Inc.
16. Yu, J. 1982. Animal models of recovery with training after central nervous system lesions. *Int Rehab Med* 4:190–194.
17. Cailliet, R. 1984. Exercise in multiple sclerosis. In *Therapeutic Exercise*, ed. 4, Ed., JV Basmajian. Baltimore: Williams & Wilkins.
18. Corcoran, PJ, and Peszczynski, M. 1984. Gait and gait retraining. In *Therapeutic Exercise*, ed. 4, Ed., JV Basmajian. Baltimore: Williams & Wilkins.
19. Sutton, JR. 1985. Endorphins in exercise. *Med Sci Sports Exerc* 17:73.
20. Clausen, JP. 1977. Circulatory adjustments to dynamic exercise and effect of physical training in normal subjects and in patients with coronary artery disease. In *Exercise and Heart Disease*, Eds. EH Sonnenblick and M Lesch. New York: Grune & Stratton.
21. Hammond, HK, and Froelicher, VF. 1985. The physiologic sequelae of chronic dynamic exercise. *Med Clin North Am* 69(1):21–39.
22. Leon, AS. 1985. Physical activity levels and coronary heart disease—analysis of epidemiologic and supporting studies. *Med Clin North Am* 69(1):3–20.
23. Scheuer, J, and Tipton, CM. 1977. Cardiovascular adaptations to physical trainings. *Annu Rev Physiol* 39:221–251.
24. Thomas, DP. 1985. Effects of acute and chronic exercise on myocardial ultrastructure. *Med Sci Sports Exerc* 17:546–553.
25. Baldwin, KM. 1985. Effects of chronic exercise on biochemical and functional properties of the heart. *Med Sci Sports Exerc* 17:522–528.
26. Tipton, CM. 1984. Exercise, training and hypertension. *Exercise Sport Sci Rev* 12:245–306.
27. Martin, RP, Haskell, WL, and Wood, PD. 1977. Blood chemistry and lipid profiles of elite distance runners. *Annu Rev Physiol* 39:345–360.
28. Haskell, WL. 1984. The influence of exercise on the concentrations of triglyceride and cholesterol in human plasma. *Exercise Sport Sci Rev* 12:205–244.
29. Hong, C-Z, and Lien, I-N. 1984. Metabolic effects of exhaustive training of athletes. *Arch Phys Med Rehabil* 65:362–365.
30. Zohman, LR, and Tobis, JS. 1970. *Cardiac Rehabilitation*. New York: Grune & Stratton.
31. Shephard, RJ. 1986. Physical training for the elderly. *Clin Sports Med* 5:515–533.
32. Buskirk, ER. 1986. Introduction to the symposium: Exercise in the treatment of obesity. *Med Sci Sports Exerc* 18:1–2.
33. Lampman, RM, Schteingart, DE, and Foss, ML. 1986. Exercise as a partial therapy for the extremely obese. *Med Sci Sports Exerc* 18:19–24.
34. Pacy, PJ, Webster, J, and Garrow, JS. 1986. Exercise and obesity. *Sports Med* 3:89–113.
35. Richter, EA, and Galbo, H. 1986. Diabetes, insulin and exercise. *Sports Med* 3:275–288.
36. Stillman, RJ, et al. 1986. Physiological activity and bone mineral content in women aged 30 to 85 years. *Med Sci Sports Exerc* 18:576–580.
37. Smith, EL. 1981. Bone changes in the exercising older adult. In *Exercise and Aging: The Scientific Basis*, Eds., EL Smith and RC Serfass. New Jersey: Enslow Publishers.
38. Aloia, JF. 1981. Exercise and skeletal health. *J Am Geriatr Soc* 29:104–107.
39. Shephard, RJ. 1986. Exercise in coronary heart disease. *Sports Med* 3:26–49.
40. Sidney, KH. 1981. Cardiovascular benefits of physical activity in the exercising aged. In *Exercise and Aging: The Scientific Basis*, Eds., EL Smith and RC Serfass. Hillside, New Jersey: Enslow Publishers.
41. Long, C. 1980. Exercise in the prevention and rehabilitation of ischemic heart disease. In *Prevention and Rehabilitation in Ischemic Heart Disease*, Ed., C Long. Baltimore: Williams & Wilkins.
42. Shayevitz, MB, and Shayevitz, BR. 1986. Athletic training in chronic obstructive pulmonary disease. *Clin Sports Med* 5:471–491.

43. Morse, CE, and Smith, EL. 1981. Physical activity programming for the aged. In *Exercise and Aging: The Scientific Basis*, Eds., EL Smith and RC Serfass. Hillside, New Jersey: Enslow Publishers.
44. Lehmann, JF, and De Lateur, BJ. 1982. Therapeutic heat. In *Therapeutic Heat and Cold*, ed. 3, Ed., JF Lehmann. Baltimore: Williams & Wilkins.
45. Lehmann, JF, and De Lateur, BJ. 1982. Cryotherapy. In *Therapeutic Heat and Cold*, ed. 3, Ed., JF Lehmann. Baltimore: Williams & Wilkins.
46. Jacobs, SR, et al. 1983. Electrical stimulation of muscles. In *Therapeutic Electricity and Ultraviolet Radiation*, ed. 3, Ed., GK Stillwell. Baltimore: Williams & Wilkins.
47. Liberson, WT. 1984. Electrotherapy. In *Current Therapy in Physiatry*, Ed., AP Ruskin. Philadelphia: W.B. Saunders.
48. Eberstein, A, and Pachter, BR. 1986. The effect of electrical stimulation on reinnervation of rat muscle: Contractile properties and endplate morphology. *Brain Res* 384:304–310.
49. Thorsteinsson, G. 1983. Electrical stimulation for analgesia. In *Therapeutic Electricity and Ultraviolet Radiation*, ed. 3, Ed., GK Stillwell. Baltimore: Williams & Wilkins.
50. Mooney, V, Wileman, W, and McNeal, DR. 1969. Stimulation reduces spastic activity. *JAMA* 207:2199–2200.
51. Petajan, JH. 1987. Sural nerve stimulation and motor control of tibialis anterior muscle in spastic paresis. *Neurology* 37:47–52.
52. Bobechko, WP, Herbert, MA, and Friedman, HG, 1979. Electrospinal instrumentation for scoliosis: Current status. *Orthop Clin North Am* 10:927–941.
53. Gracanin, F. 1982. Functional electric stimulation. In *Krusen's Handbook of Physical Medicine and Rehabilitation*, ed. 3, Eds., FJ Kottke, GK Stillwell, and JF Lehmann. Philadelphia: W.B. Saunders.
54. Brighton, CT, et al. 1981. A multicenter study of the treatment of non-union with constant direct current. *J Bone Joint Surg* 63(A):2–13.
55. De Haas, WG, Watson, J, and Morrison, DM. 1980. Noninvasive treatment of ununited fractures of the tibia using electrical stimulation. *J Bone Joint Surg* 62(B):465–470.
56. Stillwell, GK. 1982. Ultraviolet Therapy. In *Krusen's Handbook of Physical Medicine and Rehabilitation*, ed. 3, Eds., FJ Kottke, GK Stillwell, and JF Lehmann. Philadelphia: W.B. Saunders.
57. Scott, BO. 1983. Clinical uses of ultraviolet radiation. In *Therapeutic Electricity and Ultraviolet Radiation*, ed. 3, Ed., GK Stillwell. Baltimore: Williams & Wilkins.
58. Hong, C-Z, Harmon, D, and Yu, J. 1986. Static magnetic field influence on rat tail nerve function. *Arch Phys Med Rehabil* 67:746–749.
59. Hong, C-Z. 1987. Static magnetic field influence on human motor nerve function. *Arch Phys Med Rehabil* 68:162–164.
60. Knapp, ME. 1982. Massage. In *Krusen's Handbook of Physical Medicine and Rehabilitation*, ed. 3, Eds., FJ Kottke, GK Stillwell, and JK Lehmann. Philadelphia: W.B. Saunders.
61. Wakim, KG. 1980. Physiologic effects of massage. In *Manipulation, Traction and Massage*, ed. 2, Ed., JB Rogoff. Baltimore: Williams & Wilkins.
62. Maigne, R. 1980. Manipulation of the spine. In *Manipulation, Traction and Massage*, ed. 2, Ed., JB Rogoff. Baltimore: Williams & Wilkins.
63. Mennell, JM. 1975. History of the development of medical manipulative concepts; Medical terminology. In NINDS Monograph No. 15: *The Research Status of Spinal Manipulative Therapy*, Ed., M Goldstein. Bethesda: U.S. Department of Health Education and Welfare, NIH.
64. Tobis, JS, and Hoehler, F. 1986. *Musculoskeletal Manipulation, Evaluation of the Scientific Evidence*. Springfield, Illinois: Charles C Thomas.
65. Kimura, J. 1983. Nerve conduction studies and electromyography. In *Peripheral Neuropathy*, vol. I, Eds., P Dyck et al. Philadelphia: W.B. Saunders.
66. Hong, C-Z, Lee, S, and Lum, P. 1986. Clinical, radiological and electromyographic findings in cervical radiculopathy. *Orthop Rev* 15:433–539.
67. Hong, C-Z, et al. 1981. Axillary F-loop latency of ulnar nerve in normal young adults. *Arch Phys Med Rehabil* 62:565–569.
68. Fisher, S, and Gullikson, G. 1978. Energy cost of ambulation in health and disability: Literature Review. *Arch Phys Med Rehabil* 59:124–133.
69. Lynch, GS, Smith, RL, and Cotman, CW. 1976. Recovery of function following brain damage: A consideration of some neural mechanisms. In *Neurophysiologic Aspects of Rehabilitation Medicine,* Eds., AA Buerger and JS Tobis. Springfield: Charles C Thomas.
70. Kelly, JP. 1985. Reactions of neurons to injury. In *Principles of Neural Science*, ed. 2, Eds., ER Kandel and JH Schwartz. Amsterdam: Elsevier.
71. Tobis, JS, and Lowenthal, M. 1960. *Evaluation and Management of the Brain-damaged Patient*. Springfield, IL: Charles C Thomas.
72. Foster, C. 1986. Exercise training following cardiovascular surgery. *Exercise Sport Sci Rev* 14:303–323.
73. Kumar, VN, and Redford, JB. 1984. Rehabilitation of hip fractures in the elderly. *Am Fam Physician* 29:173–180.
74. NIH Consensus Conference. 1982. Total hip-joint replacement in the United States. *JAMA* 248:1817–1821.
75. Optiz, JL. 1982. Reconstructive surgery of the extremities. In *Krusen's Handbook of Physical Medicine and Rehabilitation*, ed. 3, Eds., FJ Kottke, GK Stillwell, and JF Lehmann. Philadelphia: W.B. Saunders.
76. Travell, J, and Simons, D. 1983. *Myofascial Pain and Dysfunction: The Trigger Point Manual*. Baltimore: Williams & Wilkins.
77. Duncan, BF. 1982. The postoperative total hip—a patient-oriented rehabilitation program. *Contemp Orthop* 5:41–47.
78. Duncan, BF. 1982. Rehabilitation for total knee arthroplasty patients. *Contemp Orthop* 5:41–47.
79. Stoner, EK. 1985. Management of the lower extremity amputee. In *Krusen's Handbook of Physical Medicine and Rehabilitation*, ed. 3, Eds., FJ Kottke, GK Stillwell, and JF Lehmann. Philadelphia: W.B. Saunders.
80. Burgess, EM. 1969. The management of lower extremity amputation: Surgery. Immediate postsurgical prosthetic fitting: Patient care. VA publication TR-10-6. Washington, DC: Government Printing Office.
81. Oh, SH. 1982. Rehabilitating the geriatric amputee: What the primary MD should know. *Geriatrics* 37:91–94.
82. Bender, LF. 1982. Upper extremity prosthetics. In *Krusen's Handbook of Physical Medicine and Rehabilita-*

tion, ed. 3. Eds., FJ Kottke, GK Stillwell, and JF Lehmann. Philadelphia: W.B. Saunders.

83. Cummings, V, Alexander, J, and Gans, SO. 1984. Management of the amputee. In *Current Therapies in Physiatry*, Ed., AP Ruskin. Philadelphia: W.B. Saunders.

84. Koepke, GH. 1970. The role of physical medicine in the treatment of burns. *Surg Clin North Am* 50:1385–1399.

85. Helm, PA, et al. 1982. Burn injury: Rehabilitation management in 1982. *Arch Phys Med Rehabil* 63:6–16.

SECTION IV
Operative Management and Results in Geriatric Surgery

26

Burns in the Elderly

Anne E. Missavage, William F. McManus, and Basil A. Pruitt, Jr.

Causes of Burns

About two million people are burned each year. Although most burns are of limited extent, a major burn is a relatively common traumatic event that, during a lifetime, will affect 1 of every 50 people and be responsible for the death of 10% of the victims. Elderly individuals are excessively represented in these statistics, since they suffer more burn injuries than younger persons due to decreased mobility and decreased awareness of danger. In addition, the ability to survive burn injury is influenced by age, so that the risk of death from a given burn injury is greater for the aged than for young adults. Linn reviewed hospitalized patients in Florida for 1980 and found that patients age 65 or greater presented with larger, more severe burns, suffered more complications, and had decreased survival (1). In 1981, Slater and Gaisford found that the number of elderly burn patients was increasing. Twenty percent of their patients were age 65 or older and the mortality rate of these patients was 63%. Preexisting pulmonary and cardiac disease contributed to the excess mortality (2).

A mortality predictor model based on age and burn size has been developed at the US Army Institute of Surgical Research (USAISR) from patient outcome data. In adults, as age increases, mortality for a given sized burn increases. Figure 26-1 displays the LA50 (the body surface area burned associated with a 50% mortality), which has continued to increase as improvements in intensive care and burn care occur. The increased mortality of burn injury in the elderly is a consequence of both age-related deterioration of organ function and the presence of chronic disease. Because of the increased risk of death from burn injury, most elderly individuals suffering burns should be considered for in-hospital care, and burn center care is advised for all those with burns associated with predicted mortality of 20% or more (Table 26-1). The increased risks of complications and mortality in the elderly require that they have rapid initiation of treatment when first seen even when transfer to a burn unit or center is anticipated.

The hospital course and outcome of 432 burn patients 50 or more years of age who were admitted to the US AISR between January 1976 and December 1985 have been reviewed (Table 26-2). The average burn covered 34% of the total body surface with an average estimated full thickness injury of 19% of the total body surface. Two hundred twenty patients survived, 209 patients expired, and three patients were transferred early in their care. Autopsy examination was carried out on 129 patients, 62% of deaths. The most common cause of burn injury in these patients was mishandling of gasoline and other flammable fuels; many of these accidents were contributed to by dementia or mobility problems. Other causes of burns in this group appeared to be related to decreased awareness of hazards and decreased mobility; these involved cooking accidents, explosions of natural gas stoves, accidental ignition of clothes, and smoking in bed. Housefires were responsible for 65 burns; automobile and recreational vehicle accidents with fires were responsible for 32 burns. Twenty-six patients were burned by explosions while working on oil rigs, gas lines, transformers, electrical units, and welding jobs.

General Considerations

Physiologic Changes with Burns and Age

The elderly individual has greater risks of burn injury and severe burn injury because of the physiologic changes associated with aging. The older person may be more likely

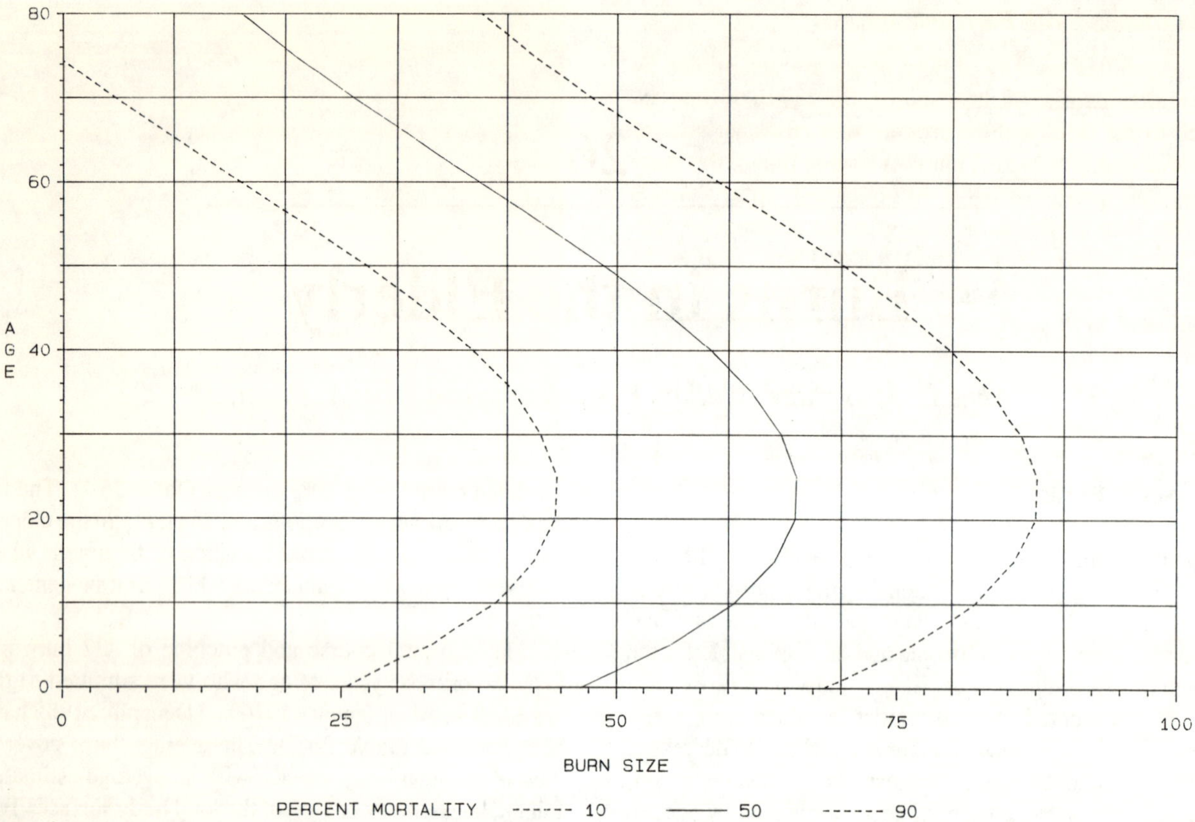

Figure 26-1. Burn mortality is displayed from a probit analysis of patients treated at the U.S. Army Institute of Surgical Research during a recent period. The highest rate of survival is observed in the young adult. For any size burn, increased age is associated with a decrease in survival.

to be burned due to loss of sensation, loss of mobility, or loss of judgement. The burn injury may be more severe due to slow reflexes and inability to escape the heat source. The stress of any such burn will be confounded by the loss of physiologic reserve due to aging as well as any preexisting disease. The early phase of fluid resuscitation is complicated by cardiac and renal disease; pulmonary disease will impair the ability to tolerate inhalation injury. Diabetes and prior malnutrition will complicate the metabolic changes associated with burn injury. Cancer and immunologic problems may increase the burn-induced impairment of immune function and the risk of infection. Neurologic problems or musculoskeletal conditions, such as arthritis, may make early positioning and physical therapy difficult and will hinder rehabilitation after healing.

Table 26-1. Triage criteria for burn patients

Minor Burn Injury—can be treated as outpatient
- Second-degree burn of less than 15% of body surface in adult; of less than 10% of body surface in child
- Third-degree burns less than 2% of body surface

Moderate Burn Injury—requires hospitalization
- Second-degree burn of 15–25% of body surface in adult; 10–20% of body surface in child
- Third-degree burns more than 10% of body surface

Major Burn Injury—requires treatment in a specialized burn center
- Second-degree burn of more than 25% of body surface in adult; of more than 20% of body surface in child
- Third-degree burn of more than 10% of body surface
- Any complicating conditions
  - Age less than 5 years or more than 60 years
  - Burns of hands, feet, face, or perineum
  - Inhalation injury
  - Significant preexisting disease
  - Associated trauma

From American Burn Association recommendations.

Table 26-2. Elderly burn patients at the U.S. Army Institute of Surgical Research, January 1976–December 1985

	Age	Total burn (% of total body surface)	Full-thickness burn (% of total body surface)
432 Patients	62 years (50–97)	34% (1–100%)	19% (0–97%)
220 Survivors	59 years (50–97)	20% (1–64%)	8% (0–49%)
209 Nonsurvivors	65 years (50–93)	49% (1–100%)	31% (0–97%)

Skin Changes with Burn and Age

The depth and severity of burn injury are determined by the temperature of the heat source, the length of time applied to the skin, and the specific skin characteristics of the area that is burned. Thin skin such as that of the inner arms can easily suffer a full-thickness injury, while thicker skin of palms or soles is more resistant to full-thickness injury. Areas with high blood flow, such as the face, can dissipate heat and suffer less damage from equivalent heat sources. Aged skin is thinner and less elastic, which renders it susceptible to greater injury by an equivalent amount of heat than the skin of young adults. Histologic changes seen in aging skin include dermal atrophy; fewer fibroblasts, blood vessels, capillary loops, and sweat and oil glands; loss of hair; and flattening of the dermoepidermal junction. The deterioration of skin structure leads to irregular thinning of the skin, decreased resistance to shearing, and decreased nutrient transfer to the epidermis (3). These changes increase the depth of injury in response to a given heat load, and with age-associated decreases in epidermal turnover and repair, slow the rate of healing of burns in the elderly, and decrease the resistance of the epidermis to infection. Preexisting atherosclerotic changes in the blood vessels of elderly individuals limit skin blood flow and can increase burn depth by diminishing heat removal from injured tissues and permitting prolongation of the heat exposure. Hypotension during resuscitation may combine with the flow deficits produced by atherosclerotic lesions and further impair skin blood flow, converting partial-thickness to full-thickness injuries (Fig. 26-2). Infection that occurs later in the post-burn course may also impair local wound blood flow and cause the conversion of a partial-thickness injury to full-thickness necrosis.

The diminution of healing that occurs in the elderly patient is manifested by a delay in the separation of eschar and formation of granulation tissue. Delayed healing of partial-thickness injuries may necessitate skin grafting for closure in the elderly patient. Once grafted, the graft may be slow to vascularize from the recipient bed, and the donor site may be slow to re-epithelialize. Decreased perfusion, decreased metabolic reserve, and alteration of neuroendocrine control of tissue synthesis probably all contribute to this impairment of healing and response to injury.

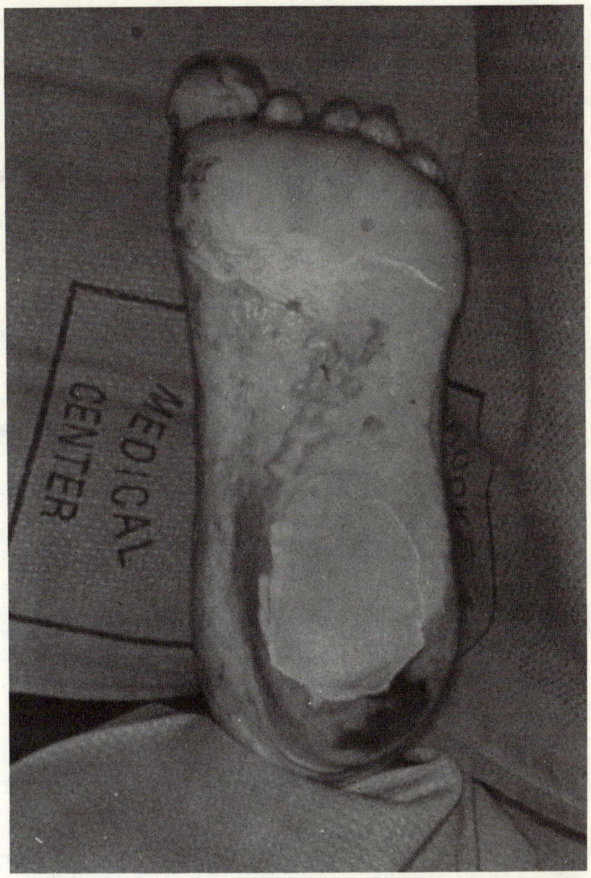

Figure 26-2. A 65-year-old woman suffered a 69.5% burn in a housefire. She had preexisting diabetes and vascular disease and had femoral-popliteal bypass of the right leg performed 5 months prior to the burn injury. The left leg, which had not had arterial reconstruction, showed evidence of decreased circulation and gangrene of the skin of the heel developed, shown here. The decreased blood flow in the left leg delayed healing of this extremity.

Resuscitation—Early Phase

Fluids

The early phase of burn care is focused on the maintenance of circulation and oxygenation. An initial phase of fluid sequestration starts immediately after the burn, continues for the first 24 hours, and is manifested by a trans-capillary fluid loss into the interstitium proportional to the extent of the burn. The plasma volume deficit that occurs is replaced by the administration of electrolyte containing fluids for the first 24 hours. Various replacement formulas have been used and found to be effective, which suggests that imprecision in volume, electrolyte, and protein composition of the fluid administered for resuscitation is tolerated by most burn patients. Elderly patients do not have the same physiologic reserve and the same tolerance of imprecision and will be more difficult to manage. In view of the sensitivity of the elderly patient to volume overload, the authors use the Modified Brooke formula for resuscitation, which recommends 2 ml of lactated Ringer's solution/kg/percent burn for the first 24 hours post-burn, and 25% albumin diluted to physiologic concentration in normal saline at 0.3 to 0.5 cc/kg/percent burn to replace the plasma volume deficit, plus 5% dextrose in water to maintain urinary output in the second 24 hours (Table 26-3). Urinary output is measured hourly with adjustment of the infusion rate to obtain a urine output of 30 to 50 ml per hour. As is true when using any formula, the rate of fluid administration during resuscitation must be monitored closely and adjusted according to the response of the patient.

During the first 24 hours when the increase in capillary permeability causes loss of blood and plasma volume, vasoconstriction and a decrease in cardiac output occur. Vasoconstriction is a hemodynamic response that attempts to maintain perfusion pressure during the period of loss of fluid through leaky capillaries and abates as fluids are replaced. The decreased plasma volume is responsible for an initial fall in the cardiac output. Increases in heart rate and contractility, however, return the cardiac output to near normal levels in adequately resuscitated patients during the latter half of the first 24 hours, despite the fact that blood and plasma volumes are incompletely replaced at this time. Since the maximum heart rate that can be sustained decreases with age and further decreases with underlying cardiac disease, the elderly patient may not be able to augment the cardiac output as easily as the young adult.

Underlying cardiac disease, such as prior myocardial infarctions, ischemia, or arrhythmias, may prevent the elderly heart from responding appropriately to the demand created by the thermal injury. In the series of 432 patients, a history of cardiac-related disease (hypertension, congestive heart failure, or myocardial infarction) was obtained in more than 25% of the patients. Arrhythmias, acute myocardial infarctions, and cardiac failure were observed in 20 patients who died during the first 7 days after injury. Vasoconstriction, another hemodynamic response to improve perfusion while hypovolemic, may further depress cardiac function, decrease cerebral perfusion, increase pre-renal azotemia, or produce thrombotic occlusion particularly when a preexisting fixed atherosclerotic lesion exists. Renal failure, manifested by elevated blood urea nitrogen and creatinine and low urine output, was a common finding in elderly patients dying shortly after their burn injury despite appropriate fluid resuscitation. Impairment of peripheral circulation and extremity ischemia occurred in three patients who expired within 48 hours post-burn, with emergency amputation attempted in one patient. Nine other patients who survived the early resuscitation went on to require amputations of extremities for ischemia. Ten additional elderly patients required amputation of digits when ischemia due to impaired perfusion produced gangrene of fingers or toes.

Table 26-3. Modified Brooke resuscitation formula

First 24 hours
Adult: Lactated Ringer's solution 2 ml/kg/percent burn
Urine output 30–50 ml/hour[a]
Second 24 hours
5% albumin containing plasma substitute
0.3 ml/kg/percent burn for 25–50% burn
0.4 ml/kg/percent burn for 50–70% burn
0.5 ml/kg/percent burn for > 70% burn
5% dextrose in water to maintain urinary output
0.5–1.0 ml/kg/hour

[a]75–100 ml/hour in patients with significant urinary hemochromogen concentrations.

Airway

The first priority in the care of the thermally injured elderly patient should be the evaluation of the patency of the airway and the adequacy of ventilation. The flow of air in the upper airway and the depth of respirations are immediately assessed. Patients who demonstrate apnea or stridor should be intubated as soon as this is identified. The nasotracheal route of intubation is preferred for most burn patients because the endotracheal tube is more easily and securely immobilized, and is more comfortable if prolonged intubation is necessary. Most other patients should have oxygen supplied by mask starting during the transport from the scene of burn injury.

An arterial blood sample for blood gases and carboxyhemoglobin determination is obtained as soon as possible in patients who have had significant facial burns, were burned in a closed space, or have had burns due to plastics or chemical fires, with the results used to determine the need for continued oxygen therapy. Carbon monoxide inhalation can occur in any patient who is injured in a fire. Inhaled carbon monoxide is avidly bound to hemoglobin and reversibly inhibits the normal binding and release of oxygen by hemoglobin. Levels of carboxyhemoglobin greater than 40% may be associated with collapse or coma due to tissue hypoxia; elderly persons with preexisting pulmonary or cardiac disease may be threatened by any such reduction of oxygen-carrying capacity. Since the binding and dissociation of carbon monoxide from hemoglobin is proportional to the partial pressures of carbon monoxide and oxygen in the blood, administration of 100% oxygen by a nonrebreathing mask hastens the removal of carbon monoxide. Administration of higher partial pressures of oxygen in a hyperbaric chamber is potentially useful for continued therapy of those patients with coma and carboxyhemoglobin levels greater than 40%.

Another cause of respiratory compromise that can occur in the early phase of resuscitation is an encircling full thickness burn of the torso. Tight, unyielding eschar overlying the thorax progressively limits respiratory excursion, and mechanical ventilation with high inspiratory pressures is necessary to produce adequate air flow and tidal volumes and reduce respiratory acidosis and hypercarbia. To relieve the limitation of chest wall motion, the eschar is incised along the anterior axillary lines. If diaphragmatic excursion is limited by eschar of the anterior abdominal wall as well as the chest, the escharotomies are continued down the anterior axillary line to the iliac crest, and then connected by a third incision along the costal margin. When the escharotomy has been sufficient, peak inspiratory pressure will fall.

Pulmonary edema is another cause of respiratory insufficiency for which mechanical ventilatory support may be necessary. Pulmonary edema will most commonly occur during the 3rd or 4th post-burn day following resuscitation, at the time of resorption of edema fluid, which expands the intravascular volume. Pulmonary edema may rarely occur during the first 24 to 48 hours of resuscitation in the elderly burn patient with limited cardiac reserve, if large volumes of resuscitation fluid are required to treat extensive burn injury. Pulmonary edema that occurs after the 1st week post-burn is likely to be iatrogenically produced. This can occur when the evaporative losses from the burn wound and donor sites decrease due to grafting and healing, and the fluid replacement is not proportionally reduced. Pulmonary edema may also occur when a large volume of fluid is infused subcutaneously to facilitate harvesting of split thickness skin graft donor areas; such fluid is resorbed within approximately 24 hours. For this reason, the total volume of fluid used for such purposes should be limited to the minimum volume necessary to accomplish the autograft removal, and in no case should more than one blood volume be administered.

The need for mechanical ventilation in the thermally injured patient may be caused by excessive production of carbon dioxide. Increased oxygen consumption and carbon dioxide production occur due to the hypermetabolism caused by the thermal injury and produce hyperventilation beginning on the 2nd post-burn day. The hyperventilation characteristically peaks late in the 1st post-burn week at levels that are 2 to $2^1/_2$ times normal (4). The use of a topical agent containing mafenide acetate, a carbonic anhydrase inhibitor, may impair carbon dioxide elimination and accentuate hyperventilation. Increased carbon dioxide production as a result of feeding diets with high carbohydrate content may further increase ventilatory requirements, but such was not identified in this group of 432 elderly burn patients. However, elderly patients with limited pulmonary reserve may not be able to increase their spontaneous ventilation to the level necessary and may require mechanical ventilatory support more frequently than younger patients.

Inhalation injury, another cause of respiratory embarrassment, should be suspected in patients with a history of being burned in a closed space, with or without a history of having breathed fire or smoke, or being burned by ignition of petroleum products. Physical findings in patients with inhalation injury include facial burns, singed nasal vibrissae, pharyngeal burns, carbonaceous sputum, and stridor. Any such patient should be evaluated by fiberoptic bronchoscopy and/or ^{133}Xenon ventilation perfusion scintiphotographic scan. Bronchoscopy will demonstrate laryngeal edema; tracheal mucosal edema, erythema, or ulcerations; and carbonaceous particulate matter in the bronchial tree—all indicative of inhalation injury of the larger airways. The ^{133}Xenon scintiphotographic lung scan is complementary to bronchoscopy and will demonstrate trapping of inhaled gas in the distal airway, but may be falsely positive in patients with chronic obstructive pulmonary disease. If evidence of inhalation injury is obtained, the patient must be closely watched during the first 24 hours of resuscitation for the development of respiratory compromise due to laryngeal edema and bronchial mucous plugging. In patients with significant laryngeal edema, early intubation should be carried out to prevent laryngeal obstruction and respiratory arrest.

Inhalation injury may also produce respiratory compromise later in the course of the patient, since it appears to predispose the patient to the development of pneumonia. One hundred fifty-six of these elderly patients (44 survivors, 112 nonsurvivors) were diagnosed as having inhalation injury by bronchoscopic examination or by ^{133}Xenon lung scan, and pneumonia developed in 97 (62%). Early intubation and clearing of tracheal secretions, mucosal epithelial casts, and mucous plugs may help to prevent the development of such pneumonia. After the patient has been intubated, continuous positive airway pressure will assist in maintaining expansion of alveoli and clearance of secretions. The therapy for a patient with inhalation injury should include administration of humidified oxygen and aerosolized saline to help mobilize secretions and frequent coughing and deep breathing. Prophylactic antibiotics and steroids have been shown to be of no benefit in the treatment of inhalation injury, and their use may predispose to the development of resistant pneumonias (5).

Endotracheal intubation is readily used for airway access in the elderly burn patient with respiratory compromise, and early tracheostomy is not usually required, unless secretions and necrotic debris cannot be cleared from the airway through the endotracheal tube. Tracheostomy is reserved for those patients requiring prolonged ventilation who are unable to be weaned from mechanical ventilation due to copious secretions or inadequate pulmonary reserve. In patients with severe facial or pharyngeal burns, tracheostomy will facilitate cleansing of the burns and oral care by eliminating the endotracheal tube and its securing mechanism. Autografting of facial burns may be easier with a tracheostomy in place, allowing airway access for anesthesia. At the USAISR during the 10-year period reviewed, 57 elderly patients required tracheostomy, with 13 survivors and 44 nonsurvivors. Only one patient who underwent tracheostomy in the 1st week for inability to clear secretions survived. Four of 27 patients who had tracheostomies performed during the 2nd week after burn injury lived, and 8 of 25 patients who had tracheostomies after the 2nd week survived. The authors do not recommend an early tracheostomy unless the patient will not tolerate the transtracheal route of intubation or cannot clear copious secretions. When respiratory failure is present and prolonged mechanical ventilation appears necessary, there is little benefit of conversion of intubation by the translaryngeal route to tracheostomy before the 2nd to 3rd week after burn injury (6). Tracheal stenosis, tracheal malacia, and tracheo-esophageal fistula have been reported to occur with both tracheal and transtracheal tubes, but were not identified in the 432 patients in this study, perhaps due to universal use of soft, low-pressure cuffed tubes.

Circulation

The increase in capillary permeability in the thermally injured patient and administration of fluid to maintain perfusion of the carcass and viscera leads to edema of the burn wound. In limbs with circumferential full thickness burns and tight, unyielding eschar, the edema fluid may accumulate to the point that the circulation is diminished to distal and underlying viable tissues. Therefore, the circulation in all burned extremities is evaluated using the ultrasound flow meter upon admission and rechecked hourly for the first 48 to 72 hours post-burn. The upper extremity pulses are monitored in the palmar arch and digital vessels, and the lower extremity pulses are monitored at the ankle in the dorsalis pedis and posterior tibial arteries. The burned extremity is elevated and actively exercised hourly to improve the lymphatic and venous return. Escharotomy is necessary when the pulses are absent or progressively diminish on serial examinations. Escharotomy is performed by placing medial and lateral incisions through anesthetic burned skin into the subcutaneous fat. The return of pulses demonstrates the sufficiency of the escharotomy in restoring circulation to the limb. Some thermally injured elderly patients who have preexisting fixed atherosclerotic lesions may have significant impairment of blood flow with only minor amounts of edema and may require escharotomy even when the burns are less than full thickness in depth.

Fasciotomy is rarely required for the burn patient. Monitoring muscle compartment pressures has not been routinely performed for fear of contamination of the deep tissue planes, since the usual escharotomy is adequate to restore flow to the burned extremity. Only patients with electrical injury, deep burns involving muscle, or burns with associated fractures and soft tissue trauma will have a significant chance of requiring fasciotomy due to the development of edema in the injured muscle. When these conditions are present, the clinical impression of increased pressure on palpation of the injured extremity confirms the need for prompt fasciotomy.

Monitoring

The goal of monitoring in the elderly burn patient is to anticipate, prevent, or modify complications, while producing no increased risk from the monitoring devices. Cardiac monitoring to detect arrhythmias during resuscitation is used for most burn patients, particularly the elderly patient who may have underlying cardiac disease. Hourly urine output is used to monitor the adequacy of visceral perfusion during resuscitation, but may not correlate in the elderly patient because of preexisting renal or cardiac disease. In these cases, additional measurement of hemodynamic indices will be necessary to optimize fluid administration. Central venous catheters are used to administer fluids and to record trends in the central venous pressure. Low or decreasing central venous pressure indicates that cardiac filling may be impaired and that more fluid may be required; conversely, elevated central venous pressure may indicate excessive rates of fluid administration or development of cardiac failure. Pulmonary artery pressure, pulmonary artery wedge pressure, and cardiac output are measured with a flow-directed intracardiac thermodilution catheter that will permit the indirect measurement of cardiac function, the optimization of fluid administration, and the administration of cardioactive drugs. When decreased filling pressure is identified, additional fluids should be administered to improve cardiac output. If an elderly burn patient continues to show low filling pressures while requiring high rates of fluid administration, colloid may be added to the resuscitation regimen to limit the total amount of salt and water required for resuscitation.

Elderly patients with diminished cardiac reserve can rapidly develop heart failure during resuscitation for moderate or major thermal injuries. Profound hypotension and cardiac arrest occurred in six elderly burn patients who died in less than 24 hours after the burn, and preexisting heart disease or acute myocardial infarction was blamed. High filling pressures with low cardiac output indicates the development of cardiac failure and the need for vasoactive drug therapy. Dopamine is used for inotropic support and is begun at 5 μg/kg/min with the dosage adjusted according to the response of the cardiac output. In some patients with preexisting hypertension, the usual vasoconstriction seen in the first 24 hours post-burn may be excessive, and depressed cardiac output and blood pressure will be produced as a result of the increased afterload and elevated systemic vascular resistance. When the blood pressure and cardiac output fail to respond despite additional fluids, small doses of vasodilators, such as hydralazine (0.5 mg/kg) or nitroprusside (0.01 mg/min), can be cautiously used with continuous arterial blood pressure monitoring to improve tissue blood flow. If such treatment is associated with further decrease in cardiac output, additional crystalloid- and colloid-containing fluids should be administered to increase cardiac filling. While intravenous and intracardiac catheters are in place, sterile techniques must be used to abate the increased risk of infection from such devices.

After the initial resuscitation, complicated monitoring is required in the elderly burn patient only if complications develop or sepsis supervenes. Hypotension and plasma volume deficits may occur with the development of sepsis, and the rapid infusion of large volumes of electrolyte containing solutions may be necessary to maintain blood pressure, cardiac output, and urine output. The elderly septic patient who fails to respond adequately to such treatment with fluids should have a flow-directed intracardiac thermodilution catheter placed for careful titration of the fluids required, and assessment of the need for inotropic support.

Complications from the use of monitoring devices should always be considered prior to their use. Urinary catheters are extremely useful for the monitoring of fluid administration, but can lead to bacteriuria and infection, or trauma to the urethra, particularly when placed in an elderly man with prostatic hypertrophy. The insertion of intravenous cannulae into central veins for monitoring of central venous pressure, pulmonary artery pressure, and cardiac output is associated with the risk of pneumothorax, malplacement of the catheter, arrhythmias, and infection. Technical errors in placement decrease with increased experience of the operator, but infection associated with the use of central venous lines continues to threaten burn patients. The incidence of suppurative thrombophlebitis is proportional to the duration of residence of intravenous catheters, and can be nearly eliminated when all intravenous catheters are changed every three days. Infection with intra-arterial cannulae has not been identified despite longer duration of cannulation, probably due to the increased blood flow in these vessels. Because of the risk of complications, particularly in the elderly patient, all invasive monitoring devices should be removed as soon as warranted by the condition of the patient.

Later Care

Nutrition

The metabolic demand in a thermally injured patient is proportional to the extent of the injury and reaches higher levels than occur in other surgical patients. The initial ebb phase characterized by the hypometabolism seen in the first few hours after injury is replaced by hypermetabolism, which develops by the 2nd or 3rd post-burn day. In patients with extensive burns (>45% of the total body surface), the metabolic rate peaks at 2 to 2½ times normal requirements at the end of the 1st post-burn week and gradually decreases towards normal levels as the burns heal or are grafted. Hypermetabolism in burn patients is temperature sensitive but not temperature dependent. Additional cold stress should be avoided by nursing the burn patient in an environment with the temperature maintained at 30°C and with 50% to 60% humidity. The normal, unburned elderly person has been shown to have impaired thermoregulatory responses and accelerated heat loss in a cool environment and is more prone to hypothermia than a normal young adult (7). The elderly burn patient with significant burns may require external heating in addition to a warm environment if the core body temperature cannot be maintained.

Without nutritional support, the metabolic demands of the burn patient preferentially drive catabolism of lean body protein stores, causing nitrogen loss and weight loss. The amount of protein and calories required to decrease tissue wasting and weight loss are calculated by nomograms, which estimate the increased requirements from the initial basal metabolic rate, modified by age (Table 26-4). The ability to feed burn patients will be limited in the early post-burn period by the development of ileus in most patients with burns of more than 20% of the total body surface. When the post-burn ileus abates, oral alimentation is the preferred route for providing the required nutritional support if the patient is able to consume the quantity of food required. The elderly burn patient's ability to consume the needed nutrients is often compromised by poor appetite, preexisting nutritional problems, and the need to cease oral intake for surgery. Special oral supplements that are formulated to provide high concen-

Table 26-4. Nutritional needs in an elderly patient

Age: 65 years	Sex: Female	Total burn: 69.5%
Height: 166 cm	Preburn weight: 69.7 kg	
Body surface area: 1.78 square meters		
Basal metabolic rate: 33.93 kcal/m²/hour (unburned)[a]		
Estimated metabolic rate: 73.09 kcal/m²/hour (burned)[a]		
Estimated caloric needs: 3893 kcal/day		
Estimated protein needs: 162 g/day		

Note patient in Figure 26-2.

[a]Due to age correction, calories required decreased 16% from Curreri formula.

trations of calories and protein in a palatable form should be offered around the clock to increase the spontaneous oral intake of nutrients when the tolerance of an increased quantity of food is poor.

Many patients will require additional supplementation with tube feedings administered through a nasogastric or nasoenteric tube. A nasogastric tube is more easily placed than a nasoenteric tube, but small bowel feeding is better tolerated without emesis than gastric feeding when gastric emptying is impaired by anesthetic administration or the development of sepsis. To avoid emesis and the potential for aspiration into the respiratory tree, gastric residuals are aspirated prior to each bolus gastric feeding. They may be aspirated continuously with enteric feedings, and the quantity of tube feeding may be decreased or discontinued if the majority of the previous feeding is returned from the stomach. Relative contraindications to the use of enteric feeding include incompetence of the gastroesophageal sphincter or prone positioning, which increase the risks of aspiration. In general, the authors have avoided operative placement of jejunal tubes for enteric feeding because of the poor wound healing and increased incidence of anastomotic disruption that are seen in burn patients following laparotomy.

When the patient is unable to consume adequate calories and protein by the oral or enteral route, additional nutrition can be provided by parenteral feeding. Intravenous alimentation using solutions containing hypertonic glucose and amino acids as well as emulsified fat solutions (to provide up to 30% of calories) is administered by central vein. Glucose is more effective than fat in decreasing the nitrogen loss in the burn patient; however, post-injury insulin resistance may make the patient intolerant of the large glucose loads necessary to provide the calories required in the patient with a large burn. The increased incidence of diabetes in elderly patients will increase the chance that insulin will be needed to treat hyperglycemia. The sudden appearance of hyperglycemia in a patient previously normoglycemic is a harbinger of the development of infection or sepsis and mandates a search for the site of infection and prompt treatment thereof. When hyperglycemia fails to respond to the continuous or bolus administration of insulin, the rate of glucose administration is decreased to prevent osmotic diuresis and hyperglycemic coma.

Burn Wound Care

Because stress and hypermetabolism persist until the patient is resurfaced with epithelium, control of bacterial density, prevention of invasive infection, debridement of nonviable tissue, maintenance of mobility and function, and timely operative closure are the goals of wound care in the elderly burn patient. After the admission assessment of adequate respiration and the initiation of fluid resuscitation, attention may be turned to the burn wound. The wounds are gently cleansed with a surgical detergent, and nonviable tissue and bullae are gently debrided. An initial estimate of the extent of injury is made to guide the administration of resuscitation fluids, and assessment of the depth of injury is performed to anticipate the need for operative excision. A topical antibiotic agent is then selected and applied to control microbial proliferation.

Daily wound therapy begins with gentle cleansing with a surgical detergent disinfectant, such as chlorhexidine glucuronate solution. Iodine-containing disinfectant solutions are avoided in the burn patient because significant absorption of iodine through the open burn wound has been reported to produce suppression of lymphocyte activity (8) and cytotoxicity to fibroblasts (9). To prevent exposure of the entire burn wound to the patient's enteric flora, the patient is cleansed with a shower device, and immersion is avoided. Patients who are physically able ambulate to the shower where they can cleanse themselves with assistance as needed. Nonambulatory patients are cleansed in bed or while lying on a plinth suspended over a Hubbard tank. Since evaporation from the entire body surface can cause significant cooling, the patient should be quickly dried and warmed after the cleansing procedure. Analgesics are sufficient for such cleansing and debridement of nonviable tissue, and anesthetics are not generally required.

There are three available topical agents of documented effectiveness, 11.1% mafenide acetate burn cream, 1% silver sulfadiazine burn cream, and 0.5% silver nitrate soaks. All appear to be capable of limiting microbial proliferation in burn wounds when application is begun in the immediate post-burn period, but significant penetration of the wound and diffusion into nonviable eschar, which is necessary to control infection in a heavily colonized wound, is only observed with mafenide acetate. An understanding of the advantages and limitations (Table 26-5) of these topical agents permits one to employ the

Table 26-5. Topical antimicrobial burn wound agents

	Advantages	Limitations
Mafenide acetate sulfamylon cream), 11.1% Cream	Penetrates eschar Wound visible Associated injuries visible No gram-negative resistance Motion of joints maintained	Painful for 20–30 min after application to second degree burns Inhibition of carbonic anhydrase activity may predispose to metabolic acidosis Hypersensitivity (7%) Delays eschar separation
Silver nitrate, 0.5% occlusive dressings	No hypersensitivity Painless except for dressing change No gram-negative resistance Decreases heat loss	No eschar penetration Loss of NA^+, K^+, $C1^-$, Ca^{2+} Dressings limit motion Discolors unburned skin of patient, skin of personnel, and environment
Silver sulfadiazine (silvadene cream), 1% Cream	Painless Wound visible when used without dressings Associated injuries visible Motion of joints maintained	Poor eschar penetration Bone marrow suppression Hypersensitivity (rare) Resistance of many *Enterobacter cloacae* and *Pseudomonas* sp. Plasmid-mediated resistance to multiple antibiotics

best choice for the wound care needs of a given patient. To minimize agent-related limitations and complications and to discourage the development of resistant organisms, the authors presently alternate application of mafenide acetate and silver sulfadiazine burn creams on a 12-hour basis. Mafenide acetate burn cream is applied after the morning wound cleansing, and silver sulfadiazine is applied 12 hours later in the evening. Hypersensitivity to either or both of those agents mandates the use of 0.5% silver nitrate soaks that are changed twice or thrice daily and periodically moistened with additional 0.5% silver nitrate solution to prevent evaporation from increasing the concentration of silver nitrate to cytotoxic levels.

Topical antimicrobial agents do not sterilize the burn wound. Topical chemotherapy limits microbial proliferation and maintains the bacterial density at levels below 10^5 organisms per gram of tissue that are seldom associated with invasive infection. In patients in whom the topical therapy is ineffective in controlling microbial proliferation or those with severe immunologic compromise, the dreaded complication of invasive burn wound infection can occur. Early detection of burn wound infection is accomplished by daily complete examination of the entire burn surface for signs of burn wound invasion (Table 26-6). If any of the clinical signs of burn wound infection are present, a burn wound biopsy of that area showing the most prominent changes must be performed to assess the microbial status of the wound (Fig. 26-3). The biopsy is obtained from that area of the wound showing the most pronounced changes and must include underlying viable subcutaneous tissue as well as the eschar (Fig. 26-4). The specimen is divided for histologic examination and quantitative culture. Neither surface culture monitoring nor quantitative burn wound culturing are reliable in making a diagnosis of invasive bacterial infection of the burn wound (10). The results of the culture merely identify the inhabitants of the burn wound and the predominant organism for which antibiotic sensitivities should be determined. The specimen for histologic examination can be processed by either the frozen section technique in one-half hour or by the rapid technique in 4 hours. The pathologist examines the prepared section to identify the microscopic criteria of burn wound invasion (Table 26-7) and make the critical differentiation between burn wound colonization and invasive burn wound infection (Fig. 26-5).

Table 26-6. Clinical signs of burn wound infection

Focal black, dark brown, or violaceous areas of discoloration
Conversion of second-degree burn to full-thickness necrosis
Hemorrhagic discoloration of subeschar fat
Unexpectedly rapid eschar separation and/or marked subeschar suppuration
Edema, violaceous discoloration, or superficial ulceration of unburned skin at wound margins
Erythematous nodular lesions in unburned skin (may ulcerate or escharify in time)
Vesicular lesions in healing or healed second-degree burn[a]

[a]Characteristic of herpes simplex virus infection.

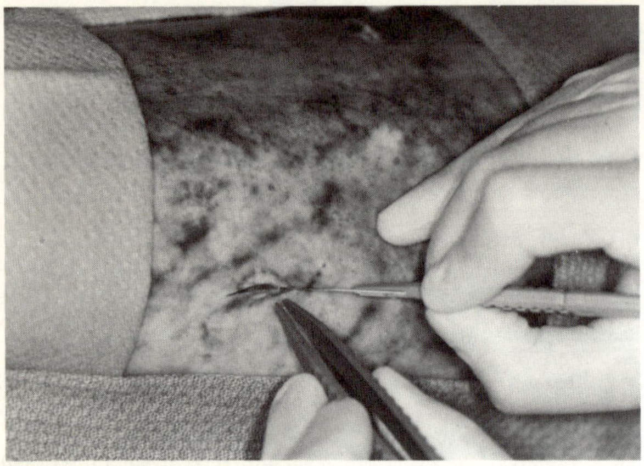

Figure 26-3. A 65-year-old woman with a 69.5% burn and inhalation injury (note Fig. 26-2) developed signs of sepsis. Careful examination of the full-thickness burn wound of the left leg demonstrated focal areas, which had become darkly discolored, and one such area on the anterolateral aspect of the leg was biopsied. The histologic specimens showed invasion of the wound by fungal elements.

A diagnosis of burn wound infection mandates a change in wound care. Subeschar antibiotic clysis and administration of systemic antibiotics followed by excision of the burn wound and definitive autografting is the optimum management. If autograft donor sites are not available or one is uncertain about the removal of all infected

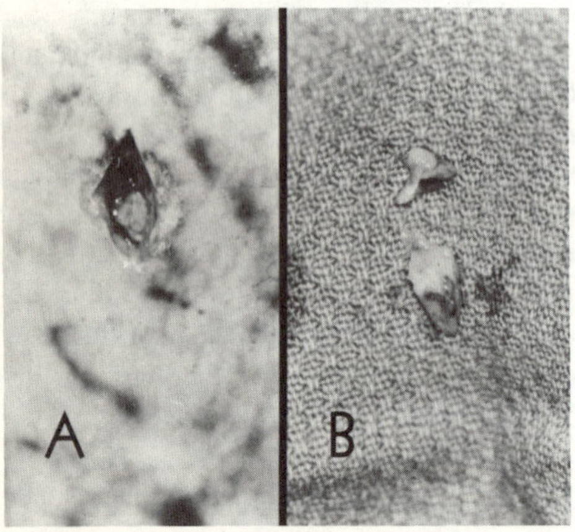

Figure 26-4. A, Biopsy site in full-thickness burn of anterior thigh of a 65-year-old female. Dark linear discolorations represent thrombosed superficial veins. The biopsy was taken from an expanding circular area of wound discoloration. Note area of light discoloration surrounded by a semicircular rim of hemorrhagic change just to the right of the biopsy wound and a similar but smaller area just to the left of wound. B, The biopsy specimen has been divided following harvest. The smaller fragment will be sent for culture identification of microorganisms. The larger fragment, showing hemorrhagic discoloration indicative of invasive infection, will be sent to pathology for processing and histologic examination. The thickness of this specimen verifies inclusion of underlying unburned tissue.

Table 26-7. Histologic classification of burn wound infection

Stage I: Colonization in nonviable tissue	
(I,a)	Superficial colonization
(I,b)	Penetration of nonviable tissue
(I,c)	Proliferation at the viable-nonviable tissue interface
Stage II: Invasion into viable tissue	
(II,a)	Micro-invasion
(II,b)	Generalized invasion
(II,c)	Microvascular involvement

tissue, temporary coverage of the excised wound bed can be obtained by applying cutaneous allografts or another biologic membrane. Spread of infection to the local blood vessels is a harbinger of systemic blood-borne infection. If microvascular involvement in the septic process has permitted blood-borne dissemination of the causative organism, hematogenous pneumonia or acute bacterial endocarditis may eventuate. If the primary and secondary septic foci cannot be controlled, systemic sepsis may evoke multiple organ failure leading to death.

Surgical Excision

Early operative excision and skin grafting to effect closure of burn wounds is becoming the preferred method for care of the burn wound, particularly for the elderly patient, where separation of eschar and epithelialization of wounds are delayed by the age-associated decrease in blood flow. The elderly patient was previously managed with daily debridement and prolonged application of topical antibiotics until a sufficiently vascularized bed of granulation tissue was produced over the wound and skin grafts could be applied. The major disadvantages of this method remain the continued loss of fluid and protein from the wound and the continued risk of invasive infection if microbes escape from control by topical antibiotics. However, this method may offer some advantages for selected elderly burn patients with moderate size burns of up to 40% of the total body surface and significant underlying illness and disability. Housinger et al. used this conservative treatment with emphasis on meticulous burn wound care, adequate nutrition, early return to normal activities, and close outpatient supervision in a selected group of elderly patients (burns of 4% to 40% of the total body surface with mean burn size of 11.2%) and demonstrated fewer complications, shorter hospital stays, and equivalent functional results when compared to a similar group that underwent excision and grafting (11).

Advocates of excision and grafting suggest that the early removal of eschar and skin grafting can reduce the duration and magnitude of physiologic stress in the burn patient. The work of Deitch shows that elderly patients can tolerate early excision and grafting of burn wounds,

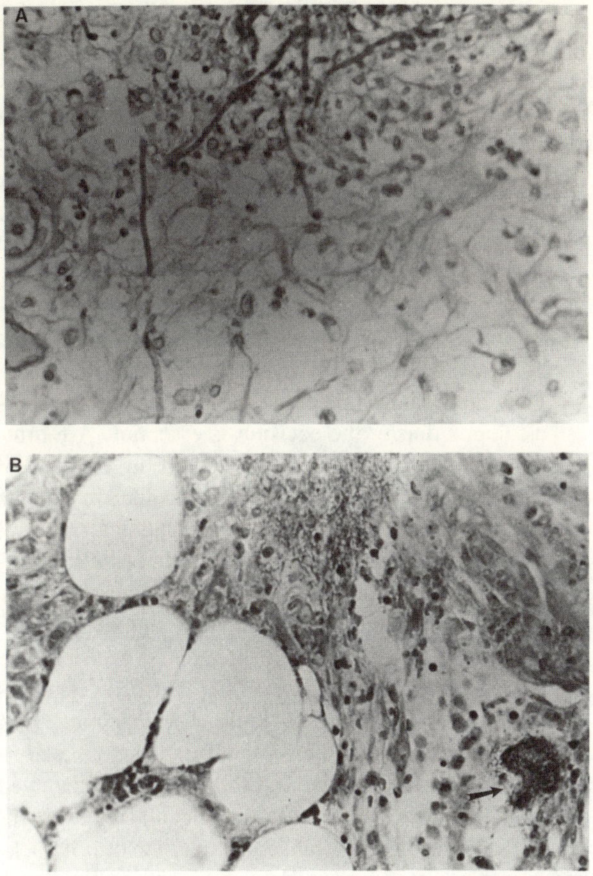

Figure 26-5. A, This histologic specimen from a burn wound biopsy demonstrates *Aspergillus* filaments invading into viable subcutaneous tissue (Stage II,c). B, Perivascular "cuffing" (arrow) typical of *Pseudomonas* burn wound invasion (Stage II,c) is seen in another burn wound biopsy specimen. Both specimens were prepared by the rapid technique.

and that early definitive closure of burns decreases the risk of infection in the wound, decreases hospital stay, and promotes survival when compared to historical controls (12, 13). Elderly patients with extensive burns may continue to manifest hemodynamic or respiratory instability after the first 48 hours and may not tolerate early excision and skin grafting. One hundred fifty-seven patients (36.6%) of the 432 elderly patients reviewed could not be stabilized sufficiently for surgery and succumbed to their injury without excision having been performed. Fifty-one (11.9%) of the elderly patients healed their burns (in less than 21 days in most cases) and were able to be discharged. The remaining 221 (51.5%) patients, 169 survivors with average burns of 22% (10% full thickness), and 52 nonsurvivors with average burns of 34% (20% full thickness), underwent debridement and skin grafting. More than half of these elderly patients were first operated on within 3 weeks of injury. The post-burn day of the first excision decreased during the period reviewed, and fewer patients were allowed to undergo spontaneous eschar separation. Despite earlier and more frequent excision and skin grafting of the burn wound, no decrease in hospital stay was seen in the survivors and no improvement in survival was observed in the elderly patients whose wounds were excised.

To prepare an elderly patient for successful surgical closure of the burn wound, adequate ventilation must be established and an adequate blood volume maintained. Persistence of hypoxia despite maximum mechanical ventilation suggests the patient will not tolerate transport to the operating room and will not withstand the increased oxygen demand and hemodynamic changes associated with surgical excision. The patient should be able to maintain an arterial partial pressure of oxygen of at least 70 torr with supplementation and hemoglobin saturation of at least 90%. The minute ventilation required to maintain a normal pCO2 (35–45 torr) and pH (7.35–7.45) is determined and will have to be continued during the operative procedure. If the usual ventilator used for anesthesia cannot provide that level of support, the ventilator from the burn unit should be moved with the patient to the operating room for surgery.

When an elderly patient has adequate cardiac and renal function, these serve as clinical indices of adequate blood volume. Stable values in the normal range for serum sodium (130–140 meq/L), urea nitrogen (10–20 mg/dl), and creatinine (0.5–1.5 mg/dl), as well as weight loss appropriate for the post-burn time, are markers suggesting adequate hydration. Dehydration, manifested in the burn patient by hypernatremia, hyperosmolality, elevated urea nitrogen and creatinine, as well as excessive weight loss, necessitates administration of supplemental fluids prior to surgery. Some elderly patients who have had renal or cardiac disease and have been previously treated with antihypertensives and cardiac drugs may not excrete the resuscitation fluid as rapidly as usual, and may require treatment with diuretics to aid in the off-loading of excess water. In the elderly patient with more severe preexisting cardiac disease or those with hemodynamic instability, monitoring by means of central venous, arterial, or pulmonary arterial catheters may be required. Vasoactive drugs and diuretics can be safely administered when such catheters are placed preoperatively, and fluid infusions, both preoperatively and during surgery, can be optimized.

Consultation by the anesthesiologist is mandatory prior to any operation on an elderly patient, in order to plan the procedure, choose the least toxic anesthetics, and anticipate problems in monitoring and positioning. Impaired pulmonary function will necessitate modification of ventilatory support during anesthesia and may require continuation of support postoperatively. When airway problems are present, control of the airway should be obtained while the patient continues spontaneous respirations, prior to the administration of muscle relaxants. Succinylcholine is best avoided since it has been reported to cause life-threatening arrhythmias due to the release of intracellular potassium when used between the 18th and 66th post-burn days. Other preexisting disease may influence the choice of anesthetic agents, e.g., the preferential use of narcotic agents in the elderly patient with cardiac disease. Altered metabolism may increase the dosages necessary to maintain anesthesia in patients who have developed increased tolerance to narcotic analgesics.

Because of the large expected blood losses during excision, adequate amounts of cross-matched blood products should be ordered and must be available prior to operation. Blood losses are concomitantly replaced by packed red cells and crystalloid solutions. Fresh frozen plasma is not used unless deficiencies of coagulation factors and clinical bleeding develop. Thrombocytopenia, defined as a platelet count less than 50,000/mm^3, may occur in burn patients with sepsis and should be corrected by platelet transfusions prior to excision; additional platelets are transfused during surgery if excessive bleeding occurs.

Since manipulation of the burn wound may cause bacteremia and thereby produce hematogenous infections in remote organs and tissues (commonly the lungs or heart), perioperative antibiotics are used for all patients. The antibiotic used is chosen on the basis of the extent of the burn and the predominant members of the institution's flora as determined by the microbial surveillance program. During the period reviewed for this report, elderly patients undergoing excision of extensive burns were treated with vancomycin and amikacin to provide coverage against *Staphylococcus aureus* and gram-negative bacilli, the organisms commonly isolated from the burn wounds. Patients with smaller, less heavily colonized burns were treated with perioperative penicillin to prevent streptococcal graft infection. Unless antibiotics are necessary for treatment of a coexisting infection, the administration of antibiotics is continued for only 24 hours. This limits the risk of antibiotic toxicity and reduces the chance of producing antibiotic-resistant flora or superinfections with fungi or yeasts.

Planning for operation on an elderly patient should also consider the extent of surgery. The length of the procedure should be limited so that heat loss and blood loss are not excessive. Elderly patients appear to tolerate excision of up to 20% of the total body surface area, 2 hours of surgery, or replacement of one blood volume. More extensive surgery may produce too much physiologic instability necessitating termination of the procedure to apply resuscitative efforts. The rapidity of surgical excision is limited only by the ability of the anesthesiologist to replace blood loss and prevent hypotension. Any hemorrhage from visible blood vessels is controlled as it is identified to minimize blood loss and maintain cardiovascular stability. Hemorrhage from the excised wound is controlled sequentially with topical thrombin, warm dressings, and pressure followed by electrocautery of the larger bleeding points. Two surgical teams can accomplish the excision and autograft harvesting rapidly, but the ongoing blood loss from the combined sites of excision may overwhelm the capacity of the anesthesiologist to replace the loss. To avoid significant hypovolemia and its consequences, good communication between surgeon and anesthesiologist during the excision is essential. A tourniquet may be used to limit blood loss during excision of burns on the extremities, but is usually avoided in patients more than 60 years old due to the potential for arterial damage and thrombosis of atherosclerotic vessels.

The technique of excision, typically chosen on the basis of depth of the burn, influences significantly the functional and cosmetic result. Tangential excision, the sequential removal of thin layers of escharified dermis, is performed with a guarded skin knife. The appearance and function are good when the wound does not extend completely through the dermis, and the function of involved joints is enhanced by the residual subcutaneous tissue, which facilitates motion. Tangential excision of full thickness burns results in a wound bed within the subcutaneous fat. Tangential excision can be associated with significant blood loss from the deep dermal plexus of capillaries and the small subcutaneous vessels. Skillful judgment as to the viability of the subcutaneous fat is required, since the color of some of the burned and ischemic fat may mimic that of viable adipose tissue. Newly placed autografts will not survive on such necrotic tissue. Blood loss may be limited by excision at the level of the investing fascia using a scalpel or electrocautery; however, the loss of the dermis and subcutaneous tissues typically results in greater limitation of motion and a less satisfactory cosmetic result. Perforating vessels are controlled prior to arborization as they penetrate the investing fascia by this technique of excision, and the blood loss is much less than that associated with tangential excision. Since all the subcutaneous fat is removed by this technique the difficulty of judging the viability of adipose tissue is avoided. This form of excision can be accomplished very rapidly.

The consistency of the skin of the elderly patient with thermal injury must be considered in order to select appropriate autograft donor sites. Since the skin thins with age, care must be taken to insure that thick dermal or full thickness skin grafts are not harvested, which would necessitate further split-thickness skin grafting to close the donor sites. The dermatome setting is adjusted and visually inspected to ensure removal of appropriately thin skin grafts.

The postoperative positioning of the elderly patient must be planned to allow air-drying of skin graft donor sites; dependent or posteriorly placed donor sites may be elevated or the patient placed in an air-fluidized bed to promote drying and healing and prevent maceration and excessive pressure, which can convert a split-thickness donor site to a full-thickness skin loss. The plan for postoperative positioning of the elderly patient must also ensure the immobilization necessary for autograft "take." With immobilization of the grafted areas by splints and appropriate positioning, shear of the newly applied grafts is avoided and prompt vascularization occurs. However, prolonged immobilization will progressively limit joint motion, foster the development of decubitus ulcers, and accentuate the development of dependent edema. Supine bedrest limits the capacity of the lungs, and atelectasis or pneumonia may develop. For these reasons, the grafted areas are immobilized for only about 7 days, at which time vascularization of the grafts is usually adequate. Thereafter, mobility is encouraged by daily exercise and other physical therapy modalities to regain as much lost motion as possible. Splinting and protective dressings after this time are used only to prevent damage to fragile grafts and maintain position during sleep.

Prior to the introduction of topical antimicrobials in the early 1960s, invasive burn wound sepsis occurred commonly in the thermally injured patient. The incidence of burn wound sepsis, which decreased initially in response to topical therapy, has remained low during the past 10 years with only 24 of the 432 elderly patients identified as having burn wound sepsis. Twenty of those cases occurred in the first 5 years of this review, and only one of those patients with invasive burn wound sepsis survived. The specific reason for the decrease in invasive burn wound sepsis is not apparent, but improved wound care and earlier excision of the burn wounds may have contributed.

Complications

Pneumonia

As burn wound infection has decreased, pneumonia has emerged as the most common form of infection in the burn patient. The majority of pneumonias in the burn patient occur as a complication of inhalation injury and are frequently the cause of death of patients who suffer burns and inhalation injury. Inhalation injury causes impairment of ciliary function and a decrease in surfactant production, as well as increased exudation from damaged respiratory mucosa. The inability to clear the secretions leads to atelectasis, which may progress to pneumonia in the involved pulmonary segments. Bronchoscopy is diagnostic in cases of pharyngeal, tracheal, or bronchial injury and reveals tenacious endobronchial exudates, necrotic ulcerations, and sloughing bronchial mucosa. When mechanical obstruction of larger bronchi is present and the patient is unable to clear secretions and cellular debris, repeated bronchoscopy may be used to clear the airways and permit adquate ventilation. When pneumonia occurs, the diagnosis is confirmed when a gram stain of a specimen of endobronchial secretions shows significant number of organisms and white blood cells. Initial antibiotic therapy is based on the gram stain, with confirmatory antibiotic susceptibilities obtained from culture results.

Inhalation injury and pneumonia are responsible for increases in mortality that are age and burn size related. Inhalation injury will increase burn-related mortality up to a maximum of 20%, and pneumonia will increase the mortality in burn patients by up to a maximum of 40%. Since pneumonia occurs frequently following inhalation injury, and these increases are cumulative, the mortality with both conditions is enhanced by up to a maximum of 60% (14). Because of the additive effects, the combination of inhalation injury and pneumonia has a significant effect on mortality even in the elderly patient with smaller burns.

Immobilization for associated trauma, following skin grafting or that necessitated by monitoring devices, may produce pneumonia in the susceptible elderly patient, particularly those who require prone positioning for posteriorly placed skin grafts. Atelectasis and impaired clearance of secretions are produced by bedrest due to impaired chest wall motion, and aspiration may also occur in patients who are kept supine. Both of these sequelae of immobility may progress to pneumonia. Avoidance of immobilization is the best course, but when immobilization is required for postoperative positioning, the duration must be minimized, pulmonary function must be carefully monitored, and the patient must be repositioned if significant compromise of pulmonary function develops.

Hematogenous pneumonia that presents as a single rounded peripheral infiltrate on chest roentgenogram may also occur in the elderly burn patient. This type of pneumonia commonly results from bacteremia astray from infection elsewhere such as a site of suppurative thrombophlebitis, an infected burn wound, an intra-abdominal or other soft tissue abscess, or the urinary tract. With the decreased tolerance to infection of the elderly burn patient, the lungs may filter out the blood-borne organisms and not clear them as effectively as in a younger patient. Whenever this type of pneumonia is identified, appropriate blood cultures are obtained, the origin of the bacteria is identified and controlled, and antibiotic therapy effective against the causative organism is initiated.

During the 10-year period of this review, 153 patients were diagnosed as having pneumonia during their hospitalization, and only 29 (19%) survived. Pneumonia was a consequence of inhalation injury in 97 patients (21 survivors, 76 nonsurvivors). The other 56 elderly patients who developed pneumonia did not have inhalation injury but had other causes of pneumonia identified including aspiration or other sites of infection (the burn wound, suppurative thrombophlebitis, and the urinary tract), and only 8 of these patients survived. Because the mortality of the elderly burn patient with pneumonia is increased significantly, prompt identification and supportive treatment of inhalation injury, prevention of aspiration, and treatment of other infections prior to hematogenous dissemination should improve survival.

Gastrointestinal

Gastrointestinal complications have become less frequent in the elderly burn patient as prevention of gastric hyperacidity has become possible. Before 1976, the most frequent complication requiring surgery was bleeding Curling's ulcer that occurred in 11% of elderly burn patients (15). Since the previous review, routine pH monitoring of aspirated gastric secretions, prophylactic treatment with histamine H2 receptor antagonists, and intragastric instillation of antacid when the pH of gastric aspirate is less than 5.0 has prevented the development of significant stress ulcers. Only one of the current series of 432 elderly patients required surgery for a bleeding ulcer.

Gastrointestinal ileus is a more frequent complication in the elderly burn patient. Most patients with a burn of more than 20% of their total body surface will develop ileus in the early phase of resuscitation, making nasogastric decompression necessary to remove gastric secretions and prevent aspiration. Gastrointestinal function is expected to return by the 3rd or 4th post-burn day. When patients develop ileus of the small or large intestine later in their post-burn course, sepsis is the most likely cause, and a search for unsuspected invasive infection should be carried out in any such patient. Ileus can impair gastric emptying and may decrease tolerance of enteral feeding. If significant impairment of gastrointestinal motility develops, nasogastric suction should be reinstated to prevent gastric distention or aspiration. Seven of this group of 432 elderly patients were found to have aspiration and succumbed to the resulting pneumonia. Conversely, 8 of the elderly burn patients who had concurrent pneumonia had recurrent problems with gastrointestinal motility and distention. Of these 8 patients, unsuspected perforation of the small bowel in one and the sigmoid colon in another was found at autopsy. The remaining 6 patients underwent celiotomy with bowel perforation identified in 2, and cecal distention identified in the other 4. Neither patient with perforation survived after bowel resection or attempted closure, but 2 of the patients with cecal distention survived, 1 of whom underwent cecostomy.

The high mortality associated with intra-abdominal infection in the elderly burn patient is in large part due to the difficulty in diagnosis. Burns of the anterior abdominal wall make evaluation of peritonitis difficult, and impairment of immune function in elderly burn patients may limit their ability to localize intra-abdominal infection. Sepsis in the elderly burn patient frequently produces confusion or obtundation, which limits cooperation with the examiner. Because the diagnosis of intra-abdominal pathology in the elderly burn patient is so difficult and the consequences are so severe, the likelihood of intra-abdominal infection should be considered in any elderly burn patient with abdominal distention or ileus accompanied by signs of sepsis.

Another manifestation of intra-abdominal pathology seen in the elderly burn patient is jaundice. In 1975, Czaja prospectively reviewed nonpediatric burn patients without prior history of liver failure and found clinical and laboratory evidence of abnormal liver function in many of the patients with extensive burns. Abnormal transaminase values were documented early in the post-burn course and were correlated to autopsy findings of hepatocellular injury. In contrast, hyperbilirubinemia occurred later and was consistent with intrahepatic cholestasis (16). The evaluation of abnormal liver function tests and liver disease in this group of 432 elderly patients was further confused by the admission history of heavy ethanol consumption or delirium tremens in 75 patients. Severe preexisting liver disease was identified on admission in 5 patients with cirrhosis and 3 with prior porto-caval shunts; these 8 patients all expired. Six of these patients who had small burns died as a result of their liver disease, 4 with ascites and jaundice and 2 of bleeding varices. Another cause of jaundice, acalculous cholecystitis, has been identified in critically ill patients with sepsis, shock, ileus, hemolysis, and dehydration. The diagnosis is made by ultrasonic imaging or computerized tomography of the gallbladder, with demonstration of thickening of the gallbladder wall. It can be confirmed with radiolabelled white blood cell scintiphotographic scanning in patients without burns of the abdominal wall overlying the gallbladder. Two of the 432 elderly patients had this condition diagnosed, underwent cholecystectomy, and survived. Because the abdominal exam can be unreliable in the elderly burn patient with laboratory evidence of abnormal liver function, treatable causes of sepsis such as cholecystitis must be excluded in such patients.

Thrombophlebitis

Suppurative thombophlebitis is an intravenous infection that, in burn patients, commonly occurs at the site of intravenous cannulation. Trauma to the intima of the vein by the indwelling catheter produces thrombus on the wall of the vein and on the catheter, which is seeded by microbes that circulate during cleansing or manipulation of the burn wound. Suppurative thrombophlebitis may be manifested by purulence or erythema at the site of intravenous cannulation. Fewer than one-half of the patients will have local signs of infection and the signs of systemic sepsis, toxicity, or even hematogenous pneumonia or acute bacterial endocarditis may be the first manifestations of the disease. The diagnosis is confirmed by biopsy of the involved vein, which will demonstrate intraluminal purulence, inflammatory infiltrate and bacteria, or culture of bacteria from the intraluminal thrombus. When the process is diagnosed, the treatment for involved peripheral veins involves excision of the entire extent of the process, even to the junction with central veins. When central veins are involved with suppurative thrombophlebitis, excision can rarely be accomplished, and the treatment consists of prolonged antibiotic therapy until the process is sterilized. Because suppurative thrombophlebitis is associated with a high mortality rate, the best therapy is prevention, which is accomplished by aseptic handling of intravenous lines and infusates and by changing the site of intravenous catheter residence every 3 days.

Suppurative thrombophlebitis was identified in 16 of 432 elderly burn patients (3.7%) in this review. The average burn size of these patients was 35.8% with 22.4% full-thickness burns, which corresponds to the average size burns in the entire group. Seven of the 16 patients had suppurative thrombophlebitis diagnosed only at autopsy, with other types of infection usually suspected premortem. Nine of the 16 patients underwent biopsy, excision of involved veins, and treatment with antibiotics, and 5 survived. Associated complications were frequent with pneumonia present in 13 of the patients, heart failure in 5, and renal failure, respiratory failure, and gastrointestinal complications in others. Most of these patients had prolonged intravenous cannulation, with 9 patients requiring cannulae for more than 1 month, or had complications that required intravenous monitoring devices, and these predisposed the patients to the development of infection in the central veins. Since the complications of suppurative thrombophlebitis associated with intravenous catheterization can be so devastating, and the mortality is so significant, any benefits expected from the use of intravenous catheters or monitoring devices should be weighed against the risks.

Prevention of Burns

Improvements in burn care continue to decrease the risk of death from burns, but the most effective mechanism to decrease burn-related death in the elderly is prevention of thermal injury. Many burn injuries can be avoided if the elderly person recognizes his development of infirmity and increases his awareness of danger. In the series of 432 elderly patients, 48 were found to have been burned by careless handling of cigarettes, matches, and cigarette lighters (11%). In addition to their pre-injury history of smoking, many had preexisting pulmonary disease that predisposed them to the development of pulmonary complications following burn injury. Cessation of smoking earlier in life would have prevented these injuries. Heavy alcohol intake was identified on admission in 79 patients (18%). Associated chronic liver failure was responsible for decreased survival of this subgroup. Sobriety would have prevented the acute impairment in judgement that was the cause of many of these accidents. Cooking accidents produced 39 scalds and flame burns (9%) and frequently occurred when clothing ignited from contact with a hot stove or caught on protruding objects on a hot stove. Because of the decrease in agility associated with age, elderly persons should not wear voluminous sleeves or flammable fabrics when cooking and should exercise care around the hot stove. Hot tap water scalds occurred in eight elderly patients (2%), all avoidable by maintaining water heater settings below 120°F (49°C), which extends the time needed to cause full-thickness burns to approximately 10 minutes (17). Elderly persons with sensory deficits should test the temperature of hot water with a thermometer prior to immersing themselves, or equip faucets with anti-scald devices. Other warning devices, such as smoke detectors, may help alert the elderly person to the presence of unanticipated fires and help expedite escape.

To optimize the survival of the elderly burn patient, care is best provided in a burn center where a broadly experienced multidisciplinary burn care team is available to manage the special problems of the elderly burn patient. Many of the concerns of the elderly burn patient occur in younger patients, but the complications are more devastating in the elderly due to the effects of aging and chronic disease. Cardiovascular instability during resuscitation, pulmonary compromise from inhalation injury and pneumonia, fragility of skin and poor healing, nutritional needs for healing, and impaired resistance to infection require early, skilled intervention by the experienced members of a burn center team. Burn center care of the elderly patient allows anticipation of the impaired physiologic responses, prompt institution of the treatment modifications necessary to protect and restore organ function, and early control of the microorganisms in the burn wound with timely wound closure which will prevent the development of complications, ensure optimum functional results, and maximize survival.

References

1. Linn, BS. 1980. Age difference in the severity and outcome of burns. *J Am Geriatr Soc* 28(3):118–123.
2. Slater, H, and Gaisford, JC. 1982. Burns in older patients. *J Am Geriatr Soc* 29(2):74–76.
3. Gilchrist, BA. 1982. Age-associated changes in the skin. *J Am Geriatr Soc* 30(2):139–143.
4. Petroff, PA, Hander, EW, and Mason, AD. 1975. Ventilatory patterns following burn injury and effect of sulfamylon. *J Trauma* 15(8):650–656.
5. Levine, BA, et al. 1978. Prospective trials of dexamethasone and aerosolized gentamicin in the treatment of inhalation injury in the burned patient. *J Trauma* 18(3):188–192.
6. Lund, T, et al. 1985. Upper airway sequelae in burn patients requiring endotracheal intubation or tracheostomy. *Ann Surg* 201(3):374–382.
7. Wagner, JA, and Horvath, SM. 1985. Influences of age and gender on human thermoregulatory responses to cold exposures. *J Appl Physiol* 58(1):180–186.
8. Ninnemann, JL, and Stein, MD. 1981. Suppressor cell induction by povidone-iodine: In vitro demonstration of a consequence of clinical burn treatment with betadine. *J Immunol* 125(5):1905–1908.
9. Lineaweaver, W, et al. 1985. Topical antimicrobial toxicity. *Arch Surg* 120(3):267–270.
10. McManus, AT, et al. 1987. Comparison of quantitative microbiology and histopathology in divided burn-wound biopsy specimens. *Arch Surg* 122:74–76.
11. Housinger, T, et al. 1984. Conservative approach to the elderly patient with burns. *Am J Surg* 148:817–820.
12. Deitch, EA, and Clothier, J. 1983. Burns in the elderly: An early surgical approach. *J Trauma* 23(10):891–894.
13. Deitch, EA. 1985. A policy of early excision and grafting in elderly burn patients shortens the hospital stay and improves survival. *Burns* 12:109–114.
14. Shirani, KZ, Pruitt, BA, and Mason, AD. 1987. The influence of inhalation injury and pneumonia on burn mortality. *Ann Surg* 205(1):82–87.
15. Pruitt, BA, Mason, AD, and Hunt, JL. 1976. Burn injury in the aged or high-risk patient, In *The Aged and High-Risk Surgical Patient,* Eds., J Siegel and P Chodoff, p. 523–546. Orlando, FL: Grune & Stratton, Inc.
16. Czaja, AJ, et al. 1975. Acute liver disease after cutaneous thermal injury, *J Trauma* 15(10):887–893.
17. Katcher, ML. 1981. Scald burns from hot tap water, *JAMA* 246(22):1219–1222.

27

Endocrine Surgery in the Elderly

Randall D. Gaz

In general, the clinical presentation, diagnosis, and management of surgical diseases of the parathyroids, thyroid, and adrenal glands for the elderly are similar to that of other ages (1–3). The surgical anatomy of the glands, diagnostic approaches, and operative procedures do not differ for the aged. Chronologic age alone is not a contraindication for surgical treatment of endocrine disorders (4). Clinical wisdom is necessary, nevertheless, to optimize quality of life, maximize prolongation of survival, and minimize costs of care (5–7).

The risks presented by the individual disease process may, however, have variable age-dependent consequences. Coexisting chronic obstructive pulmonary disease or asthma may make it difficult to assess the severity of upper airway compromise by obstructive goiters. The differentiated thyroid carcinomas appear to behave more aggressively with regards to recurrence and survival in the high-risk category of older patients. Some of the subtle changes in mentation or personality caused by primary hyperparathyroidism and hypothyroidism may be masked because of similar changes commonly occurring with senescence (8, 9). Previous or concurrent nonparathyroid malignancies may obscure or complicate the evaluation and management of hypercalcemia in the aged. The concomitant postmenopausal acceleration of osteoporosis in females is accentuated by coexisting hyperparathyroidism. Preexisting cardiovascular or cerebrovascular disease, which is more frequently encountered in the geriatric population, increases the dangers of pheochromocytoma in the aged.

This chapter focuses on the management of parathyroid, thyroid, and adrenal surgical diseases of the elderly. Special attention is made to those factors encountered with the aged patient.

Parathyroid

Anatomy and Physiology

In comparison to other ages, the parathyroid glands have similar locations in the elderly. However, chronically enlarged parathyroid glands may become ptotic with time and migrate down into the anterior or posterior superior mediastinum, attached to a vascular pedicle in the neck region. Some senior citizens with obesity have increased amounts of adipose tissue in the deep cervical compartment that may camouflage or mask the parathyroid glands when the surgeon performs a neck exploration. With aging, the histology of the parathyroids may reveal a progressive increase in the fat content of the normal glands (10, 11, 24). The plasma parathyroid hormone (PTH) level increases in advanced age with an associated fall in the calcitonin, 25(OH) vitamin D, and $1,25(OH)_2$ vitamin D levels. With a diminution in renal 1 alpha hydroxylase activity, the activation of vitamin D is decreased. This results in less gastrointestinal absorption of calcium. In the elderly, this may contribute to or accelerate the physiologic progressive osteoporosis (12, 13).

Hypoparathyroidism

Hypofunction of the parathyroid glands in the elderly is uncommon. The causes of hypoparathyroidism include neck surgery, radioiodine therapy for hyperthyroidism, hemosiderosis, Wilson's disease, secondary neoplasia, amyloidosis, tuberculosis, trauma, sarcoidosis, hypomagnesemia, and autoimmune polyglandular syndrome. Surgical hypoparathyroidism is the most common cause, especially in those patients undergoing total thyroidectomy, subtotal parathyroidectomy (excision of $3^1/_2$ glands) for parathyroid hyperplasia with damage to the blood supply of the parathyroid remnant, and total parathyroidectomy with parathyroid autotransplantation with potential parathyroid graft failure. The diagnosis is made by the clinical findings (paresthesias, tetany, Chvostek and Trousseau reflexes) and biochemical determinations (low calcium, high phosphorus, and low or absent parathyroid hormone). The treatment is outlined below in the section on surgical complications.

Pseudohypoparathyroidism (peripheral target-organ resistance to PTH) is manifest by symptoms of tetany (carpopedal spasm, tetanic convulsions, paresthesias, muscle cramps, laryngospasm, and stridor), hypocalcemia, hyperphosphatemia, and elevated levels of PTH. Some patients have Albright's hereditary osteodystrophy, a genetic disorder manifest by round faces, short stature, obesity, brachydactyly, and heterotopic subcutaneous ossification. Rare patients with these physical features but with normal calcium and normal PTH levels and responsiveness have what is termed pseudo-pseudohypoparathyroidism.

Hyperparathyroidism

Etiology

There are numerous etiologies of hyperparathyroidism (HPTH). The majority (85%) of cases are due to benign neoplasms (adenomas). The cause of primary hyperplasia remains obscure, while secondary hyperplasia appears to be a compensatory growth in the glands due to renal calcium wasting. Hyperplasia accounts for about 14% of the cases of HPTH. The remainder (1%) are due to rare malignant neoplasms (parathyroid carcinomas) (14). Rarely, patients who have received prior neck irradiation develop neoplasms of the parathyroids similar to the tumor induction of the thyroid gland. There are kindreds of familial HPTH without other associated endocrine tumors. Multiple endocrine neoplasia Type 1 (MEN I) with associated pituitary and pancreatic tumors seems to involve a genetic predisposition for parathyroid disease (hyperplasia) (15). Vitamin D resistant rickets may have associated HPTH.

Epidemiology

Parathyroid hyperfunction is rare in the young, more common in the middle-aged population, and not uncommon in the aged. The general prevalence is about 1 in 1,000 patients (16–18). Because of the bone densitometry and other diagnostic evaluations for the high-risk osteoporotic population of postmenopausal women, this may be a frequent source of referrals to the surgeon. Simultaneous multichannel analyzer (SMA) blood determinations of calcium frequently detect individuals with asymptomatic hypercalcemia found to be due to HPTH. The aged are at greater risk for developing life-threatening hypercalcemic crisis due to HPTH when other illnesses or injuries cause dehydration and prolonged immobilization, both of which contribute to hypercalcemia.

Clinical Presentation

Aged patients with HPTH may present in many ways. As mentioned above, asymptomatic hypercalcemia is detected during the evaluation of other illnesses or routine SMA blood screening. Patients with hypertension treated with thiazide diuretics may have unmasking (augmentation of the serum calcium) of latent HPTH by the renal calcium retention loop effects of the medication. Longstanding mild HPTH may progress in the face of worsening renal function, immobilization, or dehydration. Thus other acute illnesses, requiring bed rest or causing fluid losses, may accentuate the hypercalcemia. This occasionally results in life-threatening hypercalcemic crisis (19, 20). This may be an argument for early surgical intervention in the elderly prior to potential future problems. Some patients with previous malignancy develop coexisting HPTH. This may pose a diagnostic challenge to differentiate the hypercalcemia of malignancy from coexisting parathyroid disease. Patients who have undergone previous parathyroid surgery may develop recurrent or persistent HPTH. Growth of a remaining hyperplastic gland fragment or missed parathyroid tumor may present a challenging management situation for the surgeon.

Differential Diagnosis

The differential diagnosis of hypercalcemia in the elderly includes malignancy (21) (the most common cause in hospitalized patients), HPTH (the most common cause for otherwise healthy ambulatory patients), sarcoidosis, multiple myeloma, milk alkali syndrome, hyperthyroidism, thiazide therapy, Addison's disease, vitamin D intoxication, renal failure, and familial hypocalciuric hypercalcemia (FHH) (22).

Clinical Evaluation

The evaluation for hypercalcemia begins with a careful history. A long history of elevation in serum calcium argues for the diagnosis of HPTH. A recent acute development of hypercalcemia suggests possible malignancy. Direct questioning for evidence of cancer may help differentiate the two diagnoses. Have there been any weight loss, unexplained fever, cough, hemoptysis, chronic tobacco use, blood in the stool, breast mass, hematuria, or other symptoms or signs of malignancy? Classic symptoms of HPTH include stones (nephrolithiasis), bones (osteoporosis, arthralgias, or pathologic fractures), groans (pancreatitis, ulcer disease, or dyspepsia), and moans (depression, fatigue, muscle weakness, psychiatric problems). Other frequent symptoms include polyuria, polydipsia, constipation, and nonspecific malaise.

Physical Examination

The physical exam may reveal a palpable neck mass, suggestive of parathyroid carcinoma or another head and neck tumor. However, less than 5% of parathyroid tumors are palpable. Some manifestations of hypercalcemia are not specific for HPTH. These include medial and lateral arcus (senile arcus is totally circumferential), hypotonia and muscle weakness, and calcified soft tissues.

Laboratory Findings

The laboratory evaluation should include calcium metabolism (calcium, phosphorus, albumin, alkaline phosphatase, magnesium, and parathyroid hormone [23]), renal function (urinalysis, blood urea nitrogen, creatinine, 24-hour urine calcium and creatinine), and thyroid function tests (T_4, T_3 resin uptake, free T_4 index, and TSH, $+/-TT_3$). If the clinical situation suggests possible multiple myeloma, the serum immunoelectrophoresis (IEP) may reveal an M (myeloma) spike, and urine IEP may disclose Bence Jones proteins. Measurement of the serum angiotensin converting enzyme (ACE) and chest X-ray are helpful in making the diagnosis of sarcoidosis. The Dent test (daily administration of corticosteroids with serial measurements of calcium) may distinguish the hypercalcemia of malignancy from HPTH. Hypermagnesemia and a low urinary calcium in association with hypercalcemia suggest the diagnosis of FHH. Evidence of osteoporosis, by Panorex dental films revealing loss of the lamina dura or hand films showing subperiosteal resorption of the distal phalanges, may help confirm the presence of HPTH. Excretory urography (IVP) is useful in documenting the presence of renal or ureteral calculi in patients with urinary tract symptomatology, and in identifying renal cell carcinoma (hypernephroma).

Operative Indications

Selection of those patients who require surgical intervention may sometimes be difficult (24–31), especially in the case of normocalcemic (calcium <10.5 mg% with an elevated PTH) or asymptomatic mild hypercalcemia (calcium 10.5 to 11 mg%). For those patients who are symptomatic with nephrolithiasis, renal insufficiency, ulcer disease, pancreatitis, joint and bone pain, fatigue, or depression, the decision to operate is usually straightforward. Asymptomatic patients require clinical wisdom and careful individual case examination (32). Those patients with serum calcium levels consistently over 11 mg% or progressively increasing calcium and PTH levels may be at greater risk for future problems. These patients may benefit from correction of the disease before complications ensue. Younger patients who face a lifetime of observation and risk also may be better off undergoing early intervention. Those patients who are noncompliant or unable to continue close observation for any reason should consider parathyroidectomy. Accelerated progressive bone loss documented by serial densitometry is a relative indication to proceed with an operation.

Preoperative Localization

Parathyroid localization tests are beneficial in several situations. High resolution (10 MHz) cervical ultrasound and thallium technetium scanning have proven helpful for identifying hyperfunctioning parathyroid tumors. Ultrasound can confirm the diagnosis of HPTH if a large hypoechoic nodule is identified behind the thyroid, suggesting a parathyroid adenoma. The distinction of thyroid nodules and parathyroid tumors can sometimes be made. However, the presence of thyroid nodules may make the ultrasound exam more difficult. Multiple enlarged parathyroid-like sonolucent nodules by sonogram may point to the diagnosis of parathyroid hyperplasia (multiple gland disease). Reoperative cases involving recurrent or persistent HPTH may require thyrocervical and internal mammary arteriography with digital subtraction for localization of mediastinal parathyroid tumors. Computerized tomography (CT) scanning or magnetic resonance imaging (MRI) have been less rewarding in locating missing parathyroids. In rare instances, selective venography with PTH sampling has been employed to localize hyperfunctioning parathyroids by pinpointing a step-up in PTH levels. These sophisticated tests should only be performed in centers with established expertise with these procedures.

Preoperative Management

The management preoperatively for HPTH may require treatment of severe hypercalcemia. These measures are listed in Table 27-1. A neck ultrasound or thallium-technitium scan may help confirm the diagnosis, localize the enlarged gland(s), and guide the surgeon during the neck exploration. Confirmation of the diagnosis by clinical (history, physical, and X-ray exams) as well as biochemical (elevated serum calcium, depressed phosphorus, elevated urinary calcium, and inappropriately high PTH) should be made. A discussion of the risks, benefits, and alternatives (medical management, close

Table 27-1. Management of life-threatening hypercalcemia

1. Hydration
   IV saline (as much as 200–500 cc/hr or 4–10 liters per 24 hours may be necessary)
   Foley catheter to facilitate accurate fluid balance input and output measurements
   Caution: In the presence of underlying heart disease (congestive failure, myocardial ischemia, pulmonary edema) hemodynamic monitoring with a pulmonary arterial catheter in an intensive care setting may be required.
2. Calciuresis
   Furosemide 20–40 mg IV; 40–80 mg PO q4–6h as necessary
   Caution: Monitor potassium and magnesium to avoid dangerous hypokalemia or hypomagnesemia with replacement as necessary.
   Caution: Avoid thiazides because they increase serum calcium!
3. Chemotherapy
   Mithramycin (Plicamycin) doses of 25 μg/kg IV in 100 ml NS or D5W are administered over 1 hour with results in 24–36 hours.
   Caution: Monitor hematologic status (Hct, WBC and platelet count), renal and liver function, as administration may result in hypocalcemia, renal or liver toxicity.
4. Hormonal therapy
   Calcitonin 4 MRC units/kg q12h to 8 MRC units/kg q6h given subcutaneously or intramuscularly with rapid response, short duration (2–3 days)
   Caution: Side effects in 10% of patients include nausea, vomiting, and local injection site irritation.
   Corticosteroids: Prednisone 40–60 mg PO per day; Prednisolone 40 mg IM q8h
   Caution: These drugs are not helpful with HPTH, but are helpful in other forms of hypercalcemia such as myelomas, lymphomas, lymphocytic leukemias, and possibly breast cancer. It may take 5–10 days to see a response.
5. Phosphate therapy
   Orthophosphate (Neutraphos) 250–500 mg PO TID
   Caution: Monitor for renal insufficiency. This drug is contraindicated if serum phosphorus is greater than 3.0 mg% because of risk of renal precipitation of calcium.
   Diphosphonates: Dichloromethylene diphosphonate 300–500 mg/day or 5 mg/kg/day IV or aminohydroxypropylidine diphosphonate 30 mg/day. These agents will usually bring about a fall in calcium within 6–7 days.
6. Hemodialysis
   Patients with refractory life-threatening hypercalcemic crisis, impaired renal function, or failure with other measures to reduce serum calcium may require hemodialysis.
7. Questionable treatments
   Prostaglandin synthesis inhibitors: Indomethacin

(*continued*)

Table 27-1 (*continued*)

   25–50 mg PO TID or aspirin 650 mg PO q4-6h are rarely effective.
   Chelating agents (EDTA) are transient in benefit, nephrotoxic, may induce renal failure, and should be avoided in the treatment of hypercalcemia.
8. Diagnostic measures
   PTH (Intact 1–84 hormone radioimmunoassay can be performed in 24 hours or less.)
   Cervical ultrasound (Documentation of enlarged parathyroid gland or glands confirms the diagnosis of HPTH.)
   Serial calcium determinations with simultaneous albumin (correct for hypoalbuminemia). Adjusted calcium = measured calcium − measured serum albumin + normal mean lab serum albumin.
9. Surgical intervention
   If the diagnosis of HPTH is confirmed, then the patient should be prepared for exploration and parathyroidectomy within 48 hours. If some other tumor is the cause (ectopic hyperparathyroidism or humoral hypercalcemia or malignancy) then excision may be beneficial. Surgical correction of the underlying cause is the goal.
10. Mobilization
   If possible, avoid bedrest and immobility, which accelerate bone resorption and may augment hypercalcemia.
11. Calcium restriction
   Maintain a low calcium diet, avoiding dairy products and other calcium-containing foods and medications.
   Discontinue vitamin D or any other tachysterol or calciferol containing medications.
   Avoid using Ringer's lactate (1 liter contains about 60 mg of calcium) or other calcium-containing fluid.

observation with serial blood tests) should occur between the surgeon and the patient (and the family). The possibility of an unsuccessful exploration, postoperative hypocalcemia, or a laryngeal nerve palsy should be entertained. If necessary the need for mediastinotomy may arise and should be explained to the patient. The operative management of coexisting thyroid nodules or masses may be necessary at the time of surgery for parathyroid disease. The nutritional status of the patient should be assessed with attention to possible hypomagnesemia, which may complicate the management of postoperative calcium homeostasis. Extensive osteoporosis with elevation of alkaline phosphatase may predict hungry bone syndrome and the need for prolonged calcium and vitamin D replacement postoperatively. Medications that are affected by or that alter calcium and phosphate metabolism should be reviewed: diuretics (thiazides lower and furosemide raises calcium), digoxin (hypercalcemia lowers the threshold for toxicity), antacids (Amphojel and Basaljel bind phosphate, and increase urinary calcium loss, thus lowering phosphate), and vitamins (vitamin D may augment hypercalcemia). Associated thyroid disease should be evaluated by the appropriate thyroid scan, blood tests, or needle biopsy.

Anesthesia

The operations for parathyroid disease usually require general anesthesia. However, the use of local cervical block anesthesia has been described. The preoperative evaluation for anesthesia is similar to that for other surgical procedures. The stresses for the operation are minimal as far as blood loss and fluid shifts are concerned. Meticulous dissection on or around the trachea, which is very sensitive, may require special efforts to maintain an adequate depth of anesthesia by increasing the level of inhalation agent or by the use of narcotics or depolarizing agents.

Surgical Treatment

The operative strategy has several goals: (*a*) removal of hyperfunctioning parathyroid tissue, (*b*) preservation of adequate normally functioning parathyroid tissue, (*c*) avoidance of injury to the nerves, and (*d*) treatment of any coexisting incidental thyroid abnormalities. These goals are usually achieved by a systematic, meticulous approach. Adequate exposure of the thyroid and tracheoesophageal regions can be performed via a low collar transverse cervical incision with development of subplatysmal flaps and division of the strap muscles (sternohyoid and sternothyroid). Careful, bloodless dissection with preservation of the normal tissue planes facilitates identification of the oftentimes elusive parathyroid glands. All four glands should be identified. Then all abnormally enlarged glands should be removed or biopsied. Care should be taken to avoid injury to the often closely associated recurrent laryngeal nerves. Capsular rupture and failure to remove a small fragment or lobule of the tumor should be avoided. This is accomplished by gentle technique and thorough skeletonization of the parathyroid vascular pedicle prior to excision. A single enlarged gland with three small associated glands suggests the diagnosis of parathyroid adenoma. Removal of the enlarged neoplastic gland should be curative. Multiple enlarged glands suggest the diagnosis of parathyroid hyperplasia. In the case of four gland disease, three glands are totally excised. The fourth gland is partially resected, carefully leaving about 50 mg of viable tissue on the intact vascular pedicle. An attempt should be made to leave a gland fragment which is well away from the recurrent nerve should future reoperation be necessary. Additional parathyroid tissue may be cryopreserved. In the event of prolonged (greater than 6 months) postoperative hypocalcemia from hypoparathyroidism, autotransplantation may be necessary. Remaining parathyroid tissue may be marked with a surgical clip or permanent suture flag. Examination of the thyroid gland may disclose a mass or nodule. This may be biopsied or excised simultaneously, thereby foregoing the need for reoperation. Closure of the wound anatomically without a drain is then performed. The management of those cases in which only three normal glands are identified or in which there is recurrent/persistent hyperparathyroidism, is discussed in references 5 to 7.

Surgical Complications

The major life-threatening complication involves airway or respiratory problems. The immediate postoperative period is the time to watch closely for airway or breathing problems. Respiratory distress may represent laryngeal obstruction from vocal cord palsy (from recurrent laryngeal nerve injury or hypocalcemic laryngospasm), laryngeal edema from intubation, or difficulty clearing secretions due to postoperative odynophagia, tracheal compression from hematoma, or some other pulmonary or medical problem such as COPD, asthma, or congestive failure. Air hunger, agitation, or respiratory distress in the immediate postoperative period require urgent evaluation. If inspection of the wound suggests a hematoma, then the incision should immediately be opened and the clot evacuated. This usually immediately relieves the airway obstruction. Bilateral cord palsy suggested by stridor or strained respiratory muscle movements without satisfactory ventilation necessitate reintubation or emergency tracheostomy. Hypocalcemia may occur rapidly (within 4 hours) postoperatively if all the parathyroids are removed or injured. This is usually accompanied by tetany, positive Chvöstek's and Trousseau's signs, and the patient's sensation of impending doom and dyspnea. Prompt administration of intravenous calcium chloride (½ to 2 amps of 10% solution over 5 to 10 minutes) usually relieves the crisis. This should be followed by a constant infusion of intravenous calcium (40 to 50 ml of 10% calcium solution in 500 to 1000 ml of fluid given at 50 to 100 ml per hour). Monitoring of the pre- and post-treatment serum calcium will help in making the diagnosis and adjusting the calcium administration rate.

Postoperative hypocalcemia due to "hungry bone syndrome" (rapid calcium deposition in bones) or transient temporary hypoparathyroidism (bruised hypofunctioning parathyroid remnants) usually becomes manifest within 24 to 72 hours postoperatively. A daily early morning fasting (nadir) determination of the calcium, phosphorus, and albumin is helpful. Paresthesias of the digits and circumoral region, positive Chvöstek's and Trousseau's signs, muscle weakness, and general malaise are the most frequent diagnostic clues. This is treated successfully by the measures listed in Table 27-2. Occasional refractory hypocalcemia is due to coexisting profound hypomagnesemia requiring replacement therapy. Other less common postoperative complications include gout, pancreatitis (rare), temporary odynophagia (common), neck and occipital myalgias (not infrequent), phenothiazine-induced tardive dyskinesias and oculogyric crisis (rarely caused by antiemetic drug administration in the presence of hypocalcemia), wound seroma or infection, and hoarseness.

Postoperative Management

In general, a successful parathyroidectomy results in permanent cure of the hypercalcemia without morbidity. Attention to details in the preoperative, intraoperative, and postoperative management of elderly patients is rewarded by a smooth and uncomplicated hospitalization and recuperation. Patients are typically discharged on the morning of the third day after operation if the calcium is stable. Examination of the neck incision is performed about 2 or 3 weeks following discharge. Those patients requiring temporary oral calcium replacement can usually be tapered off therapy after 4 to 6 weeks, guided by periodic serum calcium determinations as the calcium replacement dosage is reduced.

Summary

Hyperfunctioning parathyroid disease of the aged is not uncommon. The diagnosis of hyperparathyroidism should be considered in those patients with unexplained mental status deterioration, nephrolithiasis, hypercalcemia on screening test, or severe osteoporosis (osteitis fibrosa cystica). The diagnosis is confirmed by serial blood tests showing hypercalcemia, hypophosphatemia, and elevated PTH levels. Surgical intervention by an experienced surgeon can be expected to cure the disease in over 95% of cases.

Table 27-2. Treatment of postoperative hypocalcemia

1. Evaluation by history and physical examination. Are there paresthesias, positive Chvöstek's or Trousseau's signs, tetany, carpopedal spasm, or laryngospasm?
2. Biochemical investigation with blood tests: ionized calcium and/or total serum calcium with phosphorus, albumin, and magnesium.

Asymptomatic or mild hypocalcemia (Ca<8.5)

3. Dietary calcium replacement with dairy products: milk, ice cream, yogurt, cheese, cottage cheese, etc. for mild hypocalcemia without severe symptoms or other problems.

Mildly symptomatic or moderate hypocalcemia (Ca<8.0)

4. Oral pharmacologic calcium replacement: 250–500 mg QID

OsCal:	250–500 mg/tablet
Tums:	200 mg/tablet
Titralac:	115 mg/5 mls
Neocalglucon:	400 mg/5 mls

Markedly symptomatic or severe hypocalcemia (Ca<7.0)

5. Intravenous calcium replacement: 25–80 mg/hr IV*
   10% calcium chloride: 273 mg/10 ml
   10% calcium gluconate: 93 mg/10 ml

   *Typical intravenous mix consists of four 10 ml amps of 10% calcium gluconate in 500 cc of D_5W at a rate of 50–100 cc/hr as necessary to correct the hypocalcemia and alleviate symptoms. In life-threatening emergencies, rapid (over 5–10 minutes) intravenous administration of 10% calcium chloride may be necessary.
6. Vitamin D administration for refractory hypocalcemia.
   Calcitriol (Rocaltrol): 25–100 μg per day (onset of action in 1 day)
   Dihydrotachysterol (DHT): 0.25 mg QID for 2 days (loading dose), then 0.25–0.5 mg daily (onset of action in 1 week)
7. Magnesium replacement as necessary for refractory hypocalcemia with associated hypomagnesemia.
   magnesium sulfate: 8 mEq/2 ml IM
   magnesium chloride: 5 mEq/5 ml PO

Thyroid

Anatomy and Physiology

With aging the thyroid gland diminishes in size and undergoes atrophic changes, including the increase in connective tissue (fibrosis) and decrease in follicular tissue. Histologically, the follicular cells change from columnar to more cuboidal in shape. There is an increased incidence of thyroid nodules and inflammatory cellular infiltration (thyroiditis) (33, 34).

The changes in the function of the thyroid reflect an overall diminution in the synthesis of levothyroxine (T_4). There is a fall in the basal metabolic rate (BMR) of 15% to 20% from the fourth to the ninth decade (35). Those individuals over age 70 have a decrease in T_4 production to 50 to 70 μg/day in comparison to 80 to 100 μg/day in young adults (36). When one adjusts for total body water changes, however, there appears to be no significant change (37). Iodine accumulation falls 40% when comparing young adults with those over 90 (38). Laboratory thyroid function tests show the following changes with advanced age: decrease in triiodothyronine (T_3) levels, decrease in T_4 to T_3 conversion, and decrease in T_4 clearance. TSH appears to be unchanged as is pituitary feedback response to thyroid hormones (35–46).

Epidemiology

Many thyroid disorders are more frequently encountered in the elderly. These include thyroid nodules, thyroiditis, large goiters with obstructive airway complications, primary thyroid lymphoma, anaplastic (undifferentiated) and medullary thyroid cancer. Hypothyroidism is more common in the aged, occurring in from 2.1% to 3.8% (47, 48). Other problems become less common, such as differentiated thyroid cancers and thyroglossal duct tract remnants and cysts. Thyroid cancer, which is the second most common malignancy in 20- to-30-year-olds, is relatively rare in the elderly with respect to other malignancies. There will be only an estimated 11,300 (8300 females and 3000 males) new thyroid cancers during the year 1989 in the United States (49–51). This is in comparison to a total of about 1,010,000 new cancers (142,900 breast, 151,000 colorectal, 155,000 lung, and 47,000 uterine). It is estimated that there will be only 1025 thyroid cancer related deaths (375 men, 650 women) for 1989. The prognosis for thyroid cancer is generally good as manifested by the 82% observed (88% relative when actuarial adjustments are made) 5-year survival and 75% (88%) 10-year survival of patients from 1973 to 1975 when one takes all age groups together. The 5-year survival has improved from 83% for patients from 1960 to 1963 to 93% for patients from 1979 to 1984. Differentiated thyroid carcinoma behaves much more aggressively in the aged (52). Consequently, the prognosis is much worse for elderly patients with thyroid malignancies. More advanced disease often necessitates multimodality treatment for cancers.

Clinical Considerations

The symptoms of hypothyroidism are more subtle or masked by senescence. In addition, coexisting diseases may obscure the diagnosis.

Thyroid suppression or replacement therapy is often employed in the management of both benign and malignant thyroid diseases in the elderly. The aged are much more sensitive to levothyroxine (T_4) and triiodothyronine (T_3) therapy. Overdosage may result in exacerbation of hypertension, cerebrovascular accidents, tachyarrhythmias, congestive heart failure, angina pectoris, or myocardial infarction. T_4 has a serum half life of about 7 days. Gastrointestinal absorption is variable from 50% to 75%. Therefore it must be used cautiously, starting with lowered doses, which are increased gradually with monitoring of the thyroid function and cardiovascular response. Certain drugs alter the bioavailability of levothyroxine: cholestyramine inhibits absorption, while phenytoin enhances biliary excretion. In the presence of preexisting congestive heart failure, digoxin and diuretics should be administered first. As T_4 is instituted, the requirement for digoxin may increase. With coronary artery disease and angina, consideration of the use of beta blockers and T_3 with its shorter half life (36 hours) should be made.

Indications for Surgical Intervention

The diseases requiring surgical treatment fall into several categories, including abnormalities of function, inflammatory processes, problematic benign and malignant neoplasms, obstructive and substernal goiters, and cosmetic neck disfigurement (53, 54). Hyperthyroidism may be due to a diffuse exophthalmic goiter (Graves' disease), the thyrotoxicosis associated with thyroiditis (Hashitoxicosis), or a "hot" (hyperfunctioning) nodular goiter (Plummer's disease). Hypothyroidism associated with a myxedematous goiter rarely requires surgical intervention other than for the diagnosis of associated suspicious nodules. Thyroiditis may manifest itself in various forms: acute, subacute, and chronic with associated goiter, nodules, inflammatory or compressive symptoms, or associated malignancy requiring operative intervention. Those benign neoplasms of the thyroid that may become problematic due to suspicion of malignancy or compressive symptoms include follicular adenoma, fetal adenoma, embryonal adenoma, oxyphilic (Hürthle) cell adenoma, and colloid goiter. Thyroid cysts may be benign or malignant and can present as chronic (usually asymptomatic) or acute (often tender) nodules. Among the primary thyroid malignancies we find papillary, mixed papillary-follicular, follicular, medullary (sporadic and familial/MEN forms), and anaplastic (undifferentiated) carcinoma. Primary thyroid lymphoma, sarcoma, squamous cell carcinoma, and metastatic tumors to the thyroid gland are less common. Enlargement of thyroid nodules or a diffuse goiter may result in obstructive symptoms, especially when the goiter has a substernal component or bilateral (vise-like book-ends) compression of the airway or esophagus (55).

Hypothyroidism

A knowledge and awareness of hypothyroidism is important in the care of elderly patients for several reasons (47). Operations on patients with undiagnosed hypothyroidism may result in serious consequences due to the hypersensitivity to anesthetic medications and slowed metabolism. Any patients undergoing operations who have symptoms or signs of hypothyroidism and all thyroid surgery patients should undergo preoperative thyroid function testing. Numerous thyroid surgical diseases have associated hypothyroidism including Hashimoto's thyroiditis, extensive malignancy such as lymphoma or anaplastic carcinoma with replacement of the majority of normal thyroid tissue with tumor, and thc occasional nodular goiter with associated hypothyroidism.

The classic symptoms of hypofunction include cold intolerance, lethargy, a low-pitched, crackly voice, alopecia, dry skin, loss of auditory acuity, constipation, and generalized mental deterioration. Autoimmune phenomena are sometimes seen with hypothyroidism, including conditions such as pernicious anemia, achlorhydria and vitamin B_{12} deficiency. Other associated conditions include hypercholesterolemia, fecal impaction, ileus, megacolon, congestive heart failure, cardiomegaly, convulsions, syncope, dementia, and myxedema coma.

The laboratory diagnosis is made by the detection of a low T_4 and FT_4I with a high thyroid stimulating hormone (TSH). The treatment is by the administration of T_4 or T_3 with monitoring of the thyroid function and cardiovascular response.

Hyperthyroidism

The recognition of hyperthyroidism is usually made preoperatively with subsequent medical control prior to operations. Thus the incidence of intraoperative or postoperative thyroid storm has become nearly nonexistent. Nevertheless, thyroid function testing in all thyroid surgical patients should be performed to obviate this life-threatening complication. Thyrotoxicosis due to Graves', Plummer's, or Hashimoto's disease may be clinically apparent preoperatively, or latent and detected only by blood testing with new supersensitive TSH measurements. The preoperative medical management of hyperthyroidism is described in Table 27-3. About 20% to 30% of all hyperthyroid patients are elderly, with about a third being over 60 (56, 57).

Graves' disease (exophthalmic goiter) occurs more often in women than men and in as many as 1% of the elderly. The symptoms of associated hyperthyroidism may include palpitations, tremor, diarrhea, sweating, nervousness, irritability, insomnia, and weight loss despite a normal appetite. The classic signs are those of exophthalmos, thyroid bruit, and diffuse firm gland with prominence of the isthmus, tachycardia, and hyperdynamic heart sounds. The laboratory diagnosis is made by confirmation of an elevated T_3, T_4, T_3RU, and a low TSH. The treatment in the United States consists usually of antithyroid drugs such as propylthiouracil (PTU) or methimazole (Tapazole) and ^{131}I-radioiodine therapy (RAI), which is effective in over 95% of patients. Subtotal thyroidectomy is reserved for pediatric or adolescent patients, young women of childbearing age, cases with huge goiters, medical treatment failures, and those who prefer not to receive radioiodine (58). The operative treatment involves subtotal thyroidectomy, preserving about 3 to 5 g of thyroid parenchyma, with either bilateral subtotal lobectomy, preserving the thyroid tissue near the entry of the recurrent laryngeal nerve into the larynx and the blood supply to the parathyroid glands, or unilateral total lobectomy with contralateral subtotal lobectomy. The surgeon must ensure that the nerves are not injured and that normal functioning parathyroid glands are preserved. If performed by an experienced, skilled thyroid surgeon, there should be minimal risk (less than 1%) of permanent vocal cord palsy or hypoparathyroidism in this operation for benign disease.

Plummer's disease (toxic adenomatous goiter) is manifest by hyperthyroidism with an associated nodular

Table 27-3. Preoperative management of hyperthyroidism

1. Thionamide antithyroid medications

	initial dose	maintenance dose
Carbimazole:	30–60 mg/day	5–20 mg/day
Methimazole (Tapazole):	30–60	5–20
Propylthiouracil (PTU):	300–600	50–200

It usually requires 1–3 months to achieve the euthyroid state using these medications.

Caution: Some patients are allergic to these agents and develop skin rashes, rarely agranulocytosis.

2. Beta blockers

Propranolol (Inderal): 40 mg Q6H

For thyroid storm: 1–2 mg IV test dose with cardiac monitoring followed by an IV drip with 50–100 μg/min.

Atenolol (Tenormin): 50–200 mg QD
Metoprolol (Lopressor): 50–200 mg BID

Caution: Avoid using these agents in patients with congestive heart failure, asthma, bradyarrhythmias, Raynaud's syndrome, or malignant hypertension.

3. Iodine

Lugol's solution: 3–5 gtts TID for 10–14 days
SSKI: 1 gtt TID

Caution: Some patients may develop angioedema, hemorrhagic skin lesions, or serum sickness.

4. Antipyretics

Tylenol: 650–1200 mg q4–6h

Chlorpromazine: 25–50 mg q6h

Caution: Avoid aspirin, which displaces thyroid hormone from the blood-binding protein and worsens thyrotoxicosis.

(solitary or multiple) goiter. The presenting symptoms are those of hyperthyroidism (similar to Graves' disease) and may include cardiac arrhythmias, tachycardia, or congestive heart failure. The diagnosis is confirmed by a "hot" nodular goiter on thyroid scan and low TSH with elevated thyroid hormone levels. The treatment of choice is subtotal thyroidectomy, removing the hyperfunctioning tissue or RAI for small toxic nodules (59).

Thyroiditis

Fibrous thyroiditis (Riedel's struma) usually occurs in the elderly. It is a rare surgical finding (1 in 2000 thyroidectomies). The clinical signs include a firm to hard, fixed thyroid gland that may mimic malignancy and can cause obstructive symptoms. The treatment involves biopsy to confirm the diagnosis and exclude malignancy, and on rare occasions, alleviation of obstructive compression of the trachea or esophagus by debulking the goiter with subtotal lobectomy and/or isthmectomy. Aspirin and occasionally steroids are necessary for inflammatory symptoms (60–62).

Subacute granulomatous thyroiditis (de Quervain's thyroiditis) may present with symptoms of pain and a tender mass with spontaneous resolution. The treatment is conservative observation with needle or open biopsy for suspicious lesions and steroids for severe cases.

Lymphocytic thyroiditis (Hashimoto's thyroiditis) is found more commonly in the aged. It may present with symptoms of hyperthyroidism or hypothyroidism in association with occasional neck tenderness and pain. The thyroid size may be normal to enormous, with a rubbery texture and diffuse nodular surface including the isthmus, which is usually prominent. The diagnosis may be supported by elevations in circulating thyroid colloid and microsomal antibodies, although these may be normal with this disease. The treatment includes observation with needle or open biopsy of any suspicious dominant nodules and aspirin for inflammatory symptoms. Associated hypothyroidism or hyperthyroidism may require the appropriate medical therapy. Thyroid suppression therapy with T_4 is often beneficial for those patients who have hypothyroidism or inflammatory symptoms without associated hyperthyroidism. Close follow-up is mandatory because of the risk of associated thyroid lymphoma and carcinoma. A coexisting cold nodule by scan has a 25% risk of malignancy. Therefore, needle biopsy and thyroidectomy often become necessary for suspicious dominant nodules in the setting of Hashimoto's disease (63). Otherwise, surgery is rarely necessary unless the patient develops crippling localized pain or obstructive symptoms from a constricting firm goiter.

Solitary Thyroid Nodules

The incidence of thyroid nodules increases with age: 70% of women over 60 have nodules, 90% of women over 70. Similarly, 80% of men over 80 have nodules. At necropsy, as many as 50% of cases have thyroid nodules, of which 2.8% were thyroid carcinoma and 2% were metastatic carcinoma from non-thyroid primary malignancies. Of those patients screened by thyroid scanning, about 10% of cold nodules are malignant. Although more elderly than younger patients have thyroid nodules, they are more commonly benign in the aged.

The management of the solitary thyroid nodule is outlined in Table 27-4. This begins with a careful history

Table 27-4. Management of thyroid nodules

1. History
   - What factors have associated higher risk of malignancy?
     (Neck irradiation, family history of MTC, MEN)
   - Are there symptoms of thyrotoxicosis, obstruction, inflammation?
2. Physical examination
   - Are there signs of malignancy? (Rapidly enlarging, hard, fixed, irregular goiter with adenopathy or vocal cord palsy)
   - Are there signs of tracheal deviation or narrowing, or a substernal component to the goiter?
3. Thyroid function testing
   - What is the hormone synthetic function of the gland? (Euthyroid, hyperthyroidism, or hypothyroidism)
   - Is there evidence of autoimmune disease by circulating thyroid antibodies? (Graves' or Hashimoto's disease)
4. Thyroid scanning
   - What is the characteristic uptake pattern of the nodule? (Functioning [warm], toxic or autonomous [hot], or nonfunctioning [cold])
5. Needle biopsy
   - What is the cytologic and/or histologic appearance of the nodule? (Benign, suspicious, malignant, equivocal or nondiagnostic)
6. Levothyroxine suppression
   - 0.1 mg to 0.15 mg PO daily is usually adequate.
   - Check thyroid function tests in 6 weeks (goal is subnormal TSH with normal T_3 and T_4).
   - Periodic physical examination of the nodule.
   - Is the nodule diminishing or increasing in size?
7. Observation
   - If appropriate, re-examine the nodule in 2–3 months, documenting the size by physical exam or ultrasound.
8. Surgical excision
   - Those lesions that are suspicious for malignancy by clinical evaluation or biopsy, enlarging in size during periodic observation, unresponsive to suppression therapy, or causing obstructive symptoms should be removed surgically.

and physical examination. Are there obstructive (dysphagia, dyspnea, stridor, or odynophagia) or inflammatory (discomfort, pain, or tenderness) symptoms which warrant surgical treatment? Is the appearance of the nodule disfiguring, such that removal for cosmesis is justified? Relative risk factors for malignancy and/or indications for surgery include a family history of medullary carcinoma or MEN, coexisting hyperparathyroidism or pheochromocytoma, or prior head or neck region irradiation therapy. Other worrisome signs include hoarseness (suggestive of recurrent laryngeal nerve invasion) and a recent onset, rapidly enlarging, stony hard, fixed lesion with an irregular shape and surface and associated cervical lymphadenopathy. The risk of a thyroid nodule being cancer is greater in males and younger patients.

The assessment also includes thyroid function testing and radioiodine (^{123}I) or technetium (Tc^{99m}) thyroid scanning. If the nodule is warm or functioning, then the likelihood of malignancy is negligible and, if clinically appropriate, the nodule may be followed with observation. If the functioning nodule subsequently enlarges, then further evaluation is pursued. If the nodule is "cold" (hypofunctioning) by scan, then excision if the clinical situation warrants (see above) or needle biopsy to obtain a tissue diagnosis is indicated. The diagnostic gold standard is the cytologic or histologic information obtained by needle biopsy. Fine needle aspiration with experienced cytologic examination can be accurate in 70% to 90% of cases. Large needle cutting or core biopsy requires more expertise on the part of the surgeon but provides a more accurate histologic diagnosis with greater than 95% accuracy. If a hypercellular neoplasm (microfollicular, fetal, embryonal, oxyphilic) pattern is identified, then surgical excision of the nodule is indicated to exclude the possibility of malignancy. These hypercellular lesions may be malignant in as many as 15% of cases. Those biopsies suggesting obvious carcinoma mandate thyroidectomy. The patients with benign diagnoses such as macrofollicular adenoma or colloid goiter may be followed on levothyroxine suppression. However, there is controversy regarding the relative benefit of T_4 treatment (64). Patients with autonomous hyperfunctioning nodules should not be treated with T_4 because of the risk of hyperthyroidism. Reassessment of the nodule should be made in two or three months. If the nodule has failed to diminish in size, then surgical removal should be considered.

Other tests are rarely beneficial in the evaluation of cold thyroid nodules. Ultrasound is usually unnecessary because it provides little additional information not ascertained with the needle biopsy. (Occasionally, it may detect additional nodules not palpable by physical exam.) Those patients with a family history of thyroid cancer or multiple endocrine neoplasia should undergo calcitonin testing to look for evidence of medullary thyroid carcinoma. Conventional neck films are usually unrewarding except in those patients with thyroid calcifications (psammomma bodies) due to papillary carcinoma. Inflammatory symptoms, associated autoimmune phenomena (dyslexia, premature graying of the hair, diabetes, vitiligo, anemia, arthritis, exophthalmos), or hypothyroidism indicate the need for testing for thyroid antibodies often seen with Graves' disease or Hashimoto's thyroiditis.

Benign Thyroid Neoplasms and Cysts

Nontoxic multinodular goiter (NTMNG) is common in the elderly (65). When evaluating these patients, the clinician tries to answer several questions. Is the patient euthyroid, hypothyroid, or hyperthyroid? Is the patient symptomatic with obstructive or inflammatory signs? Is there a suspicious dominant nodule that warrants biopsy or intervention? Would the patient benefit from levothyroxine suppression therapy? Does the patient have any signs suggestive of thyroid malignancy? Evaluation by careful interview, physical exam, thyroid function tests, thyroid scanning, and periodic reexamination usually answers these questions. Observation with goiter dimension measurements and occasional blood tests are usually sufficient.

Cystic thyroid nodules are encountered in the evaluation of solitary lumps in the thyroid region of the neck. They appear cold on thyroid scan and are almost always in euthyroid patients. They commonly arise from degeneration of benign thyroid neoplasms. The patient may describe the sudden onset of a painful, tender neck lump. This is usually a hemorrhagic degenerative cyst. With time, the blood may resorb and the cyst spontaneously disappear. If it does not, then needle aspiration is indicated. Insertion of a needle documents that the nodule is cystic. Aspiration of fluid is also ideally accompanied with curettage and multiple needle punctures of the cyst wall or adjacent thyroid tissue to obtain a tissue diagnosis. Cytologic examination of the cyst fluid may also provide a diagnosis. The cyst usually collapses and disappears following aspiration. If it returns, reaspiration may be necessary. The tissue diagnosis obtained by needle biopsy will guide in the decision about whether or not to operate.

Obstructive goiters are more common in the elderly. The aged patient often has neglected a slowly growing goiter that ultimately begins to produce symptoms of compression manifested by dysphagia, dyspnea, stridor, or pressure-like discomfort in the neck. Occasionally, the goiter has a substernal extension. Chest X-ray often reveals tracheal deviation and a widened superior mediastinum. For those patients with underlying pulmonary disease, it is sometimes difficult to determine to what extent their symptoms are due to the goiter. Pulmonary function testing with flow-volume loops may show an upper airway obstructive defect due to tracheal narrowing. CT scanning of the neck and mediastinum also provide more precise information about the degree of tracheal narrowing and deviation. Barium swallow elucidates the diagnosis of those patients with impaired deglutition.

Substernal goiters present as a chest X-ray abnormality or as obstructive symptoms as described above (66). Since the chest is a closed compartment, the enlargement of a mediastinal goiter may ultimately result in compressive complications. It is unsafe to attempt needle biopsy of large obstructive substernal goiters because of the risk of hemorrhage and swelling of the mass which is already encroaching the airway.

Thyroid Malignancies

The incidence of all thyroid cancers combined is about 6 in 100,00 per year. Thyroid malignant neoplasms are more common in women than in men (67–69). However, a male with a thyroid nodule has a greater risk of associated malignancy. The frequency of the various types of malignant tumors is as follows: papillary (including mixed papillary-follicular) 70%, follicular 15%, medullary 5%, anaplastic 5%, and other 5%.

Papillary carcinoma is the most common thyroid cancer. It occurs more frequently in the young. It has a generally indolent course often remaining intrathyroidal. The tumor spreads by the lymphatics with the local cervical lymph nodes being the most common site of metastasis. Patients less than 40 years of age have an excellent prognosis. The extent of treatment has little bearing on the outcome. Therefore, a conservative approach with total lobectomy on the side of the lesion with isthmectomy and optional contralateral subtotal or subtotal lobectomy is usually adequate for intrathyroidal disease, less than 3 cm in size, without distant spread (70, 71). Rare pulmonary, liver, brain, or bone metastases have been described. In those patients older than 40 or with extraglandular spread, the disease has a more virulent, aggressive behavior with increased risk of recurrence and mortality. Therefore, the treatment should be more thorough in the aged or in those patients with large tumors (> 3 cm), local invasion of structures outside the thyroid capsule, or distant metastases. Near total thyroidectomy (preserving a small amount of posterior capsule on the side opposite the bulk of the tumor) or total thyroidectomy with postoperative thyroid scanning and RAI treatment for residual disease may be indicated. All patients should subsequently receive postoperative levothyroxine suppression therapy.

Follicular carcinoma is the second most common thyroid cancer. It disseminates by hematogenous spread with pulmonary, osseous, hepatic, and cerebral metastases. Intrathyroidal disease, less than 3 cm in size, that has not crossed the thyroid capsule into extraglandular structures such as the strap muscles, thyroid cartilage, and trachea has a good prognosis. Thyroidectomy (similar to that for papillary carcinoma) with preservation of the recurrent laryngeal nerves and parathyroid glands can be expected to have excellent results (55, 72). Those patients with bulky tumors with extrathyroidal disease (local extraglandular invasion or distant metastases) have a much worse prognosis. Total thyroidectomy with postoperative RAI treatment for any residual disease is indicated.

Medullary thyroid carcinoma (MTC) has several forms including sporadic cases (73) with no associated endocrinopathy or family history of thyroid cancer, familial cases with a family history of MTC but without other endocrine tumors, and the multiple endocrine neoplasia syndrome (MEN IIa) with associated hyperparathyroidism and pheochromocytoma and the MEN IIb syndrome with a marfanoid habitus, mucosal neuromas, and pheochromocytoma (74, 75). The MEN syndromes are transmitted genetically as autosomal dominant traits. MTC has an associated tumor marker of calcitonin that facilitates screening of the kindred and postoperative surveillance of the patient. The treatment for this form of thyroid cancer is total thyroidectomy and middle compartment neck dissection, removing all apparent lymphatic tissue from carotid sheath to the opposite carotid sheath from the level of the hyoid bone to the sternum and clavicles. If lateral neck lymph nodes are clinically suspicious, they should be biopsied and if positive a modified radical (function preserving) neck dissection should be performed on the involved side, sparing the spinal accessory nerve, internal jugular vein, and sternocleidomastoid muscle. If both sides of the neck are involved with lymph node metastases then it may be prudent to stage the neck dissections at different times. Coexisting pheochromocytoma should be treated first (prior to thyroid surgery) to prevent hypertensive catastrophe.

Anaplastic or undifferentiated carcinoma occurs primarily in women over 60. It presents as a rapidly enlarging goiter, often arising in patients with a long history of previously stable goiter. It has an exceedingly poor prognosis, with the majority of patients dying within 6 months of diagnosis. The disease is often extensive at the time of presentation, with bulky tumors that are locally invasive and therefore usually unresectable. Smaller tumors may be resected, but the disease invariably recurs locally, so radical en bloc resections are not indicated in principle. The treatment often involves open biopsy to confirm the diagnosis, limited resection to palliate obstructive symptoms, and consideration of tracheostomy to protect the airway if necessary. Postoperative external beam radiation therapy provides limited transient palliation for some patients. Chemotherapy, RAI, and T_4 suppression are generally ineffective.

Primary thyroid lymphoma occurs usually in women over the age of 60 (76). It often presents as an enlarging neck mass in a patient with previously diagnosed thyroiditis. Commonly the goiter is very large and firm or stony hard. Other associated symptoms may include dysphagia, hoarseness with vocal cord paralysis, and dyspnea. About half the patients exhibit hypothyroidism and three-fourths have elevated thyroid antibodies. The most frequently encountered histology is diffuse histiocytic lymphoma. Associated chronic lymphocytic thyroiditis is apparent in about three-fourths of the cases. Capsular invasion with extrathyroidal extension is generally found at the time of diagnosis. Occasionally the diagnosis can be made by large needle biopsy. Alternatively, an open biopsy with limited debulking of the tumor to alleviate any obstructive symptoms and tracheostomy if necessary is usually performed. Lymphoma cell surface marker analysis may help classify the tumor and guide in the choice of treatment. Staging is carried out by thoracic and abdominal CT scan and bone marrow biopsy. Depending on the stage and tumor type, the definitive treatment usually involves external beam radiation therapy and/or chemotherapy. The overall 5-year survival is about 40%.

Summary

The most common endocrine surgical problems encountered in the elderly are diseases of the thyroid gland. These include large obstructive or substernal goiters, suspicious cold thyroid nodules, and obvious thyroid malignancies. Although papillary carcinoma is less frequent in the elderly, other cancers including anaplastic, medullary, and lymphoma are more frequent. Differentiated carcinomas (papillary and follicular) tend to be larger and more extensive with consequent worse prognosis in the elderly. Early diagnosis is paramount in the successful management of thyroid neoplasms. Therefore screening by scan and needle biopsy are advocated for all clinically suspicious goiters. There is no chronologic age limit for the surgical treatment of thyroid diseases. With careful preoperative preparation, meticulous thorough operative treatment, and appropriate postoperative management, thyroid surgery for the elderly can be safe and efficacious (77).

Adrenal

Anatomy and Physiology

The adrenal cortex decreases in weight in the elderly, while the frequency of nodules increases (78). The adrenocortical cells decrease in number and accumulate lipofuscin granules. There is also a thickening of the capsular connective support tissue and the perivascular fibrous infiltrations.

With aging there is reduced production, utilization, and clearance of cortisol and its metabolites. However, the circulating level of cortisol remains unchanged. There is also a tendency toward blunting of the nocturnal drop in serum cortisol. Circulating adrenocorticotropic hormone (ACTH) levels remain unchanged, and the pituitary-adrenal axis feedback and response is intact. The sex hormone dehydroepiandrostenedione (DHEA) declines with age. Aldosterone levels remain normal unless there is associated potassium deficiency in the diet or underlying renal disease. Aldosterone secretion, urinary excretion, and hepatic metabolism all decrease in the aged. Plasma epinephrine appears to be unchanged; however, there is an age-associated increase in norepinephrine. This may be related to decreased responsiveness to catecholamines in the aged (79–88).

Adrenal Insufficiency

Many elderly patients have illnesses or conditions requiring corticosteroid therapy. These include asthma, chronic bronchitis, arthritis, inflammatory bowel disease, transplant immunosuppression, and some neoplasms such as lymphoma or leukemia. Long-term therapy often predisposes to secondary adrenocortical insufficiency. These patients are at risk for developing adrenal (Addisonian) crisis when stressed by surgery (82), sepsis, trauma, myocardial infarction, or other illnesses requiring increased amounts of glucocorticoids. Other causes of adrenal insufficiency include Addison's disease (primary adrenal insufficiency), pituitary tumors that have altered

Table 27-5. Glucocorticoid medications

Medication	Relative activity	Duration (hrs)
Cortisol	1	4–8
Cortisone	8	4–8
Prednisone	4	6–12
Prednisolone	4	6–12
Triamcinolone	5	6–12
Methylprednisolone	6	6–12
Dexamethasone	3–4	12–20
Fludrocortisone	10	12–20

the normal ACTH (adrenocorticotropin) release, hypothalamic disease with altered corticotropin releasing hormone (CRH) secretion, and infection or metastatic disease that has destroyed or replaced the adrenal glands. During times of hospitalization for severe illness or surgery, these patients require increased steriod therapy (89, 90). See Tables 27-5 and 27-6 for information regarding glucocorticoid stress treatment.

Incidentaloma

With the increased use of computerized tomography (CT) scanning of the abdomen, there are numerous instances of the detection of previously occult asymptomatic nonfunctioning adrenal masses known as "incidentalomas" (91–93). This has raised a management dilemma. When such a tumor is detected, a survey for evidence of any primary malignancies is made. Metastasis to the adrenal glands is common in disseminated malignancy of all types, particularly with lung, breast, melanoma, stomach, and kidney tumors. A search for evidence (by history or physical examination) of Cushing's syndrome, virilization, feminization, menstrual changes, weight change, mineralocorticoid excess (hypokalemia), and catecholamine excess (hypertension) is made. When appropriate, biochemical screening is then performed to exclude the possibility of a functioning adrenal tumor. The screening tests may include a fasting cortisol and/or dexamethasone suppression test, serum estrogen or testosterone, renin and aldosterone, 24-hour urine collection for 17-hydroxycorticosteroids, 17-ketosteroids, metanephrine, and vanillylmandelic acid (VMA). Cystic lesions can be needle aspirated with cytologic examination if there is no suspicion of pheochromocytoma. If the tumor is greater than 6 cm in size, then surgical exploration is advisable. If the tumor is less than 6 cm, then observation with a repeat CT scan is performed in 6 months. If the tumor size remains stable, then continued observation is recommended. Enlarging lesions should be removed. These growing tumors often represent nonfunctioning adrenocortical carcinomas (more frequent in the elderly), adrenal adenomas, or lipomas. Adrenal adenomas occur in about 1.5% of autopsied patients. Adenomas larger than 6 cm are rare. About 30% of adrenal masses in patients with known carcinoma at other sites are adenomas. Adrenocortical carcinoma is rare, and most are biochemically active and larger than 6 cm.

Hypercortisolism (Cushing's Syndrome and Disease)

Except for ectopic ACTH secretion, hyperadrenocorticism (Cushing's syndrome) is very uncommon in the elderly. Spontaneous hyperfunction of the adrenal cortex from unilateral adenoma or carcinoma or bilateral adrenocortical hyperplasia and hyperfunction due to pituitary overproduction of ACTH (Cushing's disease) are uncommon in the aged. Severe hypokalemia in the older population is most often due to diuretic therapy or gastrointestinal losses from laxative abuse. High anti-inflammatory

Table 27-6. Glucocorticoid administration for major illness or surgery

Addisonian crisis (acute life-threatening adrenal insufficiency)

1. Establish large bore intravenous access.
2. Obtain stat electrolytes, glucose, and cortisol values.
3. Give dexamethasone 4 mg IV or hydrocortisone 100 mg IV followed by hydrocortisone 100 mg IV q8h.
4. Rapidly infuse 1–3 liters of normal saline or 5% dextrose in normal saline. Observe filling pressures (CVP or PCWP) and watch for signs of congestive failure. Continue fluid administration at a slower rate.
5. Provide supportive measures as necessary.
6. Identify and treat underlying cause.

Emergency surgery

(For those patients with known or suspected adrenal insufficiency who require urgent operations, steroid administration is mandatory to prevent potentially lethal complications.)

1. Institute resuscitative and supportive measures as outlined above for Addisonian crisis.
2. Give hydrocortisone 100 mg IV preoperatively.
3. Give another dose of 100 mg IV intraoperatively.
4. Monitor electrolytes and fluid balance closely.
5. Continue steroid administration postoperatively (100 mg IV q8h) as necessary, tapering the dosage as the patient recovers.

Elective surgery

Preoperatively

1. Assess the need for steroid therapy by interview, review of previous medical history, and physical examination.
2. Consider Cortrosyn stimulation testing to evaluate the adrenal gland responsiveness to ACTH.

Day of surgery (total of 300 mg of cortisol hemisuccinate)

1. On the morning of surgery give 100 mg IV hydrocortisone or its equivalent.
2. At the time of anesthetic induction, give an additional 100 mg IV.
3. Eight hours later, give a third dose of 100 mg.

1st postoperative day (total of 150 mg)

1. If there are no problems, give 50 mg every 8 hours.
2. If there is ongoing stress, maintain higher dosage.

2nd postoperative day (total of 75 mg)

1. If there are no complications give 25 mg in three divided doses.
2. Individualize the dose for those patients with ongoing needs.

3rd postoperative day

1. Resume maintenance dose of steroids.
2. Discontinue the steroids for those healthy uncomplicated patients not requiring continued use.

doses of corticosteroids may cause iatrogenic cushingoid features. The classic clinical presentation includes centripetal obesity, moon facies, buffalo hump, striae, purpura, diabetes mellitus, osteoporosis, hypertension, acne, hirsutism, renal stones, emotional lability, and oligomenorrhea. The etiology is a pituitary adenoma in 65% of cases, ectopic ACTH in 15%, adrenal carcinoma in 10%, and adrenal adenoma in 10%. The biochemical confirmation of Cushing's syndrome is obtained by documenting the presence of marked elevation of 24-hour urinary free cortisol and failure to suppress the morning plasma cortisol below 5 μg/dl with dexamethasone (1 mcg at midnight). Cushing's disease is diagnosed using the high-dose dexamethasone suppression test (2.0 mg q6h for 2 days) with a fall (less than 50% of baseline) in the urinary 17-hydroxysteroids (17-OHS) (94, 95). Treatment is by transphenoidal hypophysectomy or proton beam irradiation. Ectopic production of ACTH is documented by high levels of ACTH that are not suppressed with high-dose dexamethasone. Treatment is directed toward the primary tumor, often an oat cell carcinoma of the lung with very poor prognosis. Patients who have an adrenal tumor (adenoma or carcinoma) usually have undetectable levels of ACTH. CT scanning will localize 95% of the neoplasms. If the lesion is less than 5 cm is size, the posterior approach adrenalectomy may be possible. If a large (> 5 cm) or malignant lesion is anticipated, then the anterior abdominal or thoracoabdominal approach is required. Total excision of an adenoma is curative (96). En bloc resection of adrenal carcinomas and the invaded adjacent tissues is the only curative treatment (97). Unresectable or recurrent disease is treated with mitotane. Chemotherapy with 5-fluorouracil, adriamycin, and cisplatin has been reported. The mean overall duration of survival for carcinoma is about 3 years, with a 25% 5-year survival.

Primary Hyperaldosteronism (Conn's Syndrome)

Primary aldosteronism is caused by a benign adenoma in approximately 60% of patients and by hyperplasia of the zona glomerulosa in 40%. Of those with adenomas, about 10% are bilateral. The clinical manifestations include hypertension, hypokalemia, muscle weakness, paresthesias, or cardiac irritability. The diagnosis is confirmed by elevated plasma aldosterone level and low plasma renin activity. The evaluation is carried out with the patient off diuretics and antihypertensives and on a normal salt intake diet. Preoperative medical management can often be obtained with spironolactone. CT scan will localize about 90% of tumors. Surgical excision of an adenoma by the posterior approach is curative (98). Hyperplasia may respond to unilateral adrenalectomy. Bilateral adrenalectomy is not advised because of the unpredictable response and morbidity.

Pheochromocytoma

Pheochromocytoma is rare in older persons (99, 100). The signs and symptoms are similar to those in the young. Because of underlying cardiovascular or neurologic disease, however, the elderly may be much less tolerant of catecholamine excess. Tachycardia (palpitations), hypertension (paroxysmal or sustained), headache, diaphoresis, tremor, sleep disorders, and changes in psyche may be of greater significance in the elderly. The diagnosis is confirmed by finding elevations of the plasma or urine catecholamines (epinephrine and norepinephrine) or their metabolites (metanephrine and VMA). Localization can be obtained by CT scan (101), magnetic resonance imaging (MRI) (92, 102, 103), or ^{131}I-metaiodobenzylguanadine (MIBG) scanning (104). In the familial form the disease is usually bilateral, especially with MEN II (105). Therefore, it is standard practice to examine both adrenal glands at the time of surgery. About 10% of all pheochromocytoma cases are multiple, malignant, or extra-adrenal (paragangliomas). The most common sites of paragangliomas are near the renal veins, the bifurcation of the aorta (organ of Zuckerlandl), and along the paravertebral sympathetic chains. Cervical, thoracic, bladder wall, spermatic cord, vaginal, and sacrococcygeal sites have also been described. Preoperative medical treatment is instituted with phenoxybenzamine alpha blockade starting with a dose of 10 mg a day and increasing until nasal stuffiness and orthostatic hypotension are obtained over the course of 1 or 2 weeks. This may require doses as high as 200 mg per day. In addition, hydration may be necessary to compensate for preexisting volume contraction. Beta blockade may be helpful for tachycardia or arrhythmias. Intraoperative pulmonary arterial (Swan-Ganz) catheter monitoring is generally valuable for elderly patients with pheochromocytoma. Expert intraoperative anesthetic management of hypertension with nitroprusside and/or nitroglycerin, and administration of lidocaine and propranolol or atenolol for arrhythmias or tachycardia is frequently necessary. Surgical excision of the tumor is the treatment of choice. The transabdominal (if bilateral or extra-adrenal disease is anticipated) or the thoracoabdominal (if bulky malignant disease is expected) approach is advised for optimal exposure. Early ligation of the adrenal veins with minimal manipulation of the tumor during the mobilization is important. A thorough exploration for other paragangliomas and examination of the contralateral adrenal is performed. In patients with MEN II, the pheochromocytomas are usually bilateral, and bilateral total adrenalectomy with adrenal replacement therapy may be necessary. Postoperative urine output observation and adequate volume replacement are crucial. Inoperable patients or those with recurrent malignant disease may be treated with alpha and beta blockade, ^{131}I-MIBG, or methylparatyrosine. Rarely, chemotherapy with streptozotocin, cyclophosphamide, vincristine, and adriamycin has been employed. The operative risk for pheochromocytoma is significantly greater for the aged because of not infrequently associated pulmonary, renal, cardiac and/or cerebrovascular disease, and therefore warrants precision in the surgical technique, anesthetic management, and perioperative care.

Adrenocortical Carcinoma

Carcinoma of the adrenal cortex is quite rare to begin with, representing only about 0.2% of all cancers. It is most unusual in patients over 65 years of age. The presentation may be that of hormonal excess (roughly half the tumors are functional, mostly Cushing's but often multiple hormone abnormalities), abdominal pain, an abdominal mass, and rapid onset of the disease. Anatomic evaluation of both adrenal glands is obtained by CT scan. The treatment is surgical excision with care not to violate the tumor capsule, thus avoiding seeding of the malignancy in the operative wound and inevitable recurrence (97). Adjuvant or palliative treatment with o,p'DDD (mitotane), metyrapone, or aminoglutethemide has been described (106). Because most adrenocortical carcinomas are advanced when discovered, only about 50% are amenable to resection. The overall 5-year survival has been reported to be 10% to 20%.

Summary

Surgical disease of the adrenal glands in the elderly is very unusual. It may be difficult to diagnose because of the normal senescent body changes and often coexisting medical disease, which may mimic or obfuscate the signs and symptoms of hormone excess. The treatment should be carefully individualized to the patient.

References

1. Davis, PJ, and Davis, FB. 1986. Endocrine diseases. In *The Practice of Geriatrics*, Eds., E Calkins, PJ Davis, and AB Ford, pp. 451–465. Philadelphia: WB Saunders.
2. Green, MF. 1985. The endocrine system. In *Principles and Practice of Geriatric Medicine* Ed., MSI Pathy, pp. 909–913. New York: John Wiley & Sons.
3. Cryer, PE. 1983. *Endocrinology*. In *Care of the Geriatric Patient*, ed. 6, Ed., FU Steinberg, pp. 275–290. St. Louis: CV Mosby.
4. Adkins, RB, and Scott HW (Eds.) 1988. *Surgical Care for the Elderly*. Baltimore: Williams & Wilkins.
5. van Heerden, JA (Ed.). 1989. *Common Problems in Endocrine Surgery*. Chicago: Year Book Medical Publishers.
6. Edis, AJ, Grant, CS, and Egdahl, RH. 1984. *Manual of Endocrine Surgery*, ed. 2. New York: Springer-Verlag.
7. Bardin, CW (Ed.). 1988. *Current Therapy in Endocrinology and Metabolism*, ed. 3. Philadelphia: B.C. Decker Inc.
8. Gambert, SR, and Escher, JE. 1988. Atypical presentation of endocrine disorders in the elderly. *Geriatrics* 43(7):69–78.
9. Davis, PJ. 1977. Endocrines and aging. *Hosp Pract* September: 113–128.
10. Castleman, B, and Roth, SI. 1978. Tumors of the parathyroid glands. *Atlas of Tumor Pathology*, Fascicle 14. Bethesda, MD: Armed Forces Institutes of Pathology.
11. Oertel JE, and Anderson, WAD. 1971. Parathyroid glands. In *Pathology*, ed. 6. Ed., WAD Anderson. St. Louis: CV Mosby.
12. Orwoll, E, and McClung, MR. 1984. Disorders of calcium and mineral metabolism. In *Geriatric Medicine*, Eds., CK Cassel and JR Walsh. New York: Springer-Verlag.
13. Eastell, R, and Riggs, BL. 1987. Calcium homeostasis and osteoporosis. In *Endocrinology and Aging, Endocrinology and Metabolism Clinics*, Vol. 16, No. 4, pp. 829–842. Philadelphia: WB Saunders.
14. Wang, CA, and Gaz, RD. 1984. Natural history of parathyroid carcinoma. *Am J Surg* 149:522–527.
15. van Heerden, JA, et al. 1983. Primary hyperparathyroidism in patients with multiple endocrine neoplasia syndromes. *Arch Surg* 118:533–536.
16. Heath, H, Hodgson, SF, and Kennedy, MA. 1980. Primary hyperparathyroidism: Incidence, morbidity, and potential economic impact in a community. *N Engl J Med* 302:189.
17. Mundy, GR, Cove, DH, and Fisken, R. 1980. Primary hyperparathyroidism: Changes in the pattern of clinical presentation. *Lancet*. i:1317.
18. Bounstra, CE, and Jackson, CE. 1965. Hyperparathyroidism detected by routine serum calcium analysis. *Ann Intern Med* 63:468–474.
19. Wang, CA, and Guyton, SW. 1979. Hyperparathyroid crisis. *Ann Surg* 190:782–790.
20. 1986. Case Reports of the MGH, Case 44-1986. *N Engl J Med* 315:1209–1219.
21. Mundy, GR, Wilkinson, R, and Heath, DA. 1983. Comparative study of available medical therapy for hypercalcemia of malignancy. *Am J Med* 74:421–432.
22. Marx, SJ, et al. 1981. The hypocalciuric or benign variant of familial hypercalcemia: Clinical and biochemical features in fifteen kindreds. *Medicine* 60:397–412.
23. Nussbaum, SR, et al. 1987. Highly sensitive two-site immunoradiometric assay of parathyrin, and its clinical utility in evaluating patients with hypercalcemia. *Clin Chem* 33:1364–1367.
24. Alveryd, A, et al. 1976. Indications for surgery in the elderly patient with primary hyperparathyroidism. *Acta Chir Scand* 142:491–494.

25. Purnell, DC, et al. 1971. Primary hyperparathyroidism: A prospective clinical study. *Am J Med* 50:670–678.
26. Peskin, GW, Greenburg, AG, and Salk, RP. 1978. Expanding indications for early parathyroidectomy in the elderly female. *Am J Surg* 136:45–48.
27. Lifschitz, BM, and Barzel, US. 1981. Parathyroid surgery in the aged. *J Gerontol* 36(5):573–575.
28. Block, MA, Xavier, A, and Brush, BE. 1975. Management of primary hyperparathyroidism in the elderly. *J Am Geriatr Soc* 23:385–389.
29. Tibblin, S, Palsson, N, and Rydberg, J. 1983. Hyperparathyroidism in old age. *Ann Chir Gynaecol* 72: 135–138.
30. Riddick, FA. 1967. Primary hyperparathyroidism in the aged. *Geriatrics* 22:94–98.
31. Scholz, DA, and Purnell, DC. 1981. Asymptomatic primary hyperparathyroidism: 10 year prospective study. *Mayo Clinic Proc* 56:473.
32. Gaz, RD, and Wang, CA: Management of asymptomatic hyperparathyroidism. *Am J Surg* 147:498–502.
33. Meissner, WA, and Warren, S. 1969. Tumors of the thyroid gland. *Atlas of Tumor Pathology*, Fascicle 4. Bethesda, MD: Armed Forces Institutes of Pathology.
34. Meissner, WA. 1984. Tumors of the thyroid gland. Supplement. *Atlas of Tumor Pathology*, Fascicle 4, Bethesda, MD: Armed Forces Institutes of Pathology.
35. Keys, A, Taylor, HL, and Grande, F. 1973. Basal metabolism and age of adult man. *Metabolism* 22:579–587.
36. Gregerman, RI, Gaffney, GW, and Shock, NW. 1962. Thyroxine turnover in euthyroid man with special reference to changes with age. *J Clin Invest* 41:2065–274.
37. Shock, NW, et al. 1963. Age differences in the water content of the body as related to basal oxygen consumption in males. *J Gerontol* 18:1.
38. Hansen, JM, Skovsted, L, and Siersboek-Neilsen, K. 1975. Age dependent changes in iodine metabolism and thyroid function. *Acta Endocrinol* 79:60–65.
39. McClung, MR. 1984. Thyroid disorders. In *Geriatric Medicine*, Eds., CK Cassel and JR Walsh, pp. 354–385. New York: Springer-Verlag.
40. Spaulding, SW. 1987. Age and the thyroid. In *Endocrinology and Aging, Endocrinology and Metabolism Clinics*. Vol. 16, No. 4,, Philadelphia: WB Saunders.
41. Sawin, CT, et al. 1979. The aging thyroid. *JAMA* 242(3):247–250.
42. Melmed, S, and Hershman, JM. 1982. *The thyroid and aging*. In *Endocrine Aspects of Aging*. Ed., SG Korenman. New York: Elsevier Biomedical.
43. Pittman, JA. 1962. The thyroid and aging. *J Am Geriatr Soc* 10:10–21.
44. Havard, CWH. 1981. The thyroid and aging. *Clin Endocrinol Metab* 10:163–178.
45. Felicetta, JV. 1987. Thyroid changes with aging: Significance and management. *Geriatrics* 42:86–92.
46. Solomon, DH. 1987. The elderly patient with thyroid disease. *Geriatric Consultant* March/April, 20–23.
47. Bahemuka, M, and Hodkinson, HM. 1975. Screening for hypothyroidism in elderly patients. *Br Med J* 2: 601–360.
48. Jefferys, PM, et al. 1972. Thyroid function tests in the elderly. *Lancet* 1:924–927.
49. Silverberg, E, and Lubera, JA. 1989. Cancer Statistics 1989. *CA: Canc J Clin* 39:3–20.
50. Myers, MH, and Ries, LAG. 1989. Cancer patient survival rates: SEER program results for 10 years of follow-up. *CA: Canc J Clin* 39:21–32.
51. Baranovsky, A, and Myers, MH. 1986. Cancer incidence and survival in patients 65 years of age and older. *CA: Canc J Clin* 36:26–41.
52. Rossi, RL, et al. 1986. Current results of conservative surgery for differentiated thyroid carcinoma. *World J Surg* 10:612–622.
53. Kaplan, EL (ed.). 1983. *Surgery of the Thyroid and Parathyroid Glands*. New York: Churchill Livingstone.
54. Clark, OH. 1985. *Endocrine Surgery of the Thyroid and Parathyroid Glands*. Toronto: CV Mosby.
55. 1987. Case Records of the Massachusetts General Hospital, Case 15-1987. *N Engl J Med* 316:931–937.
56. Gambert, SR. 1985. Atypical presentation of thyroid disease in the elderly. *Geriatrics* 40:63–69.
57. Davis, PJ, and Davis, FB. 1974. Hyperthyroidism in patients over the age of 60 years. *Medicine* 53:161–181.
58. Simms, JM, and Talbot, CH. 1983. Surgery for thyrotoxicosis. *Br J Surg* 70:581–583.
59. Jensen, MD, et al. 1986. Treatment of toxic multinodular goiter (Plummer's disease): Surgery or radioiodine? *World J Surg* 10:673–680.
60. Hurley, JR. 1977. Thyroiditis. *Disease a Month* 24:3.
61. Woolf, P. 1985. Thyroiditis. *Med Clin North Am* 69: 1035–1049.
62. LiVolsi, VA, and LoGerfo, P. 1981. *Thyroiditis*. Boca Raton, Fla: CRC Press.
63. Clark, OH, Greenspan, FS, Dunphy, JE. 1980. Hashimoto's thyroiditis and thyroid carcinoma: Indications for operation. *Am J Surg* 140:65–71.
64. Gharib, J, James, EM, and Charbonneau, JW. 1987. Suppressive therapy with levothyroxine for solitary thyroid nodules: A double blind controlled clinical study. *N Engl J Med* 317:70–75.
65. Clark, OH, and Demling, R. 1976. Management of thyroid nodules in the elderly. *Am J Surg* 132:615–619.
66. Katlic, MR, Grillo, HC, and Wang, CA. 1985. Substernal goiter. *Am J Surg* 149:283–287.
67. Hamburger, JI. 1980. The presentation of thyroid malignancy in the geriatric patient. *Henry Ford Hosp Med J* 28:158–160.
68. Woolner, LB, et al. 1961. Classification and prognosis of thyroid carcinoma. *Am J Surg* 102:354–387.
69. Simpson, WJ. 1982. Thyroid malignancy in the elderly. *Geriatrics* 37:119–125.
70. Vickery, AL, Wang, CA, and Walker, AM. 1987. Treatment of intrathyroidal papillary carcinoma of the thyroid. *Cancer* 60:2587–2595.
71. Hay, ID, et al. 1987. Ipsilateral lobectomy versus bilateral lobar resection in papillary thyroid carcinoma: A retrospective analysis of surgical outcome using a novel prognostic scoring system. *Surgery* 102:1088–1095.
72. Schmidt R, and Wang, CA. 1986. Encapsulated follicular carcinoma of the thyroid: Diagnosis, treatment, and results. *Surgery* 100:1068–1076.
73. Rossi, RL, et al. 1979. Nonfamilial medullary thyroid carcinoma. *Am J Surg* 139:554–560.
74. Brunt, LM, and Wells, SA. 1987. Advances in the diagnosis and treatment of medullary thyroid carcinoma. *Surg Clin North Am* 67:623–679.

75. Russell, CF, et al. 1983. The surgical management of medullary thyroid carcinoma. *Ann Surg* 197:42–48.
76. Rasbach, DA, et al. 1985. Malignant lymphoma of the thyroid gland: A clinical and pathologic study of twenty cases. *Surgery* 98:1166–1170.
77. Falk, SA, Birken, EA, and Baran, DT. 1988. Temporary postthyroidectomy hypocalcemia. *Arch Otolaryngol Head Neck Surg* 114:168–174.
78. Page, DL, DeLellis, RA, and Hough, AJ. 1986. Tumors of the adrenal. *Atlas of Tumor Pathology*, Fascicle 23.Bethesda, MD: Armed Forces Institutes of Pathology.
79. Abrass, IB. 1984. Adrenal disorders. In *Geriatric Medicine*, Eds., CK Cassel and JR Walsh, Jr. New York: Springer-Verlag.
80. Sapolsky, R, et al. 1987. Stress and glucocorticoids in aging. In *Endocrinology and Aging, Endocrinology and Metabolism Clinics*, vol. 16, no. 4, pp. 965–980. Philadelphia: WB Saunders.
81. Lakatta, EG. 1987. Catecholamines and cardiovascular function in aging. In *Endocrinology and Aging, Endocrinology and Metabolism Clinics*, vol. 16, no. 4, pp. 877–891. Philadelphia: WB Saunders.
82. Wolfsen, AR. 1982. Aging and the adrenals. In *Endocrine Aspects of Aging*, Ed., SG Korenman. New York: Elsevier Biomedical.
83. Kelly, J, and O'Malley, K. 1984. Adrenoceptor function and ageing. *Clin Sci* 66:509–515.
84. Hegstad, R, et al. 1983. Aging and aldosterone. *Am J Med* 74:442–448.
85. Wallace, EZ, et al. 1980. Pituitary-adrenocortical function in chronic renal failure: Studies of episodic secretion of cortisol and dexamethasone suppressibility. *J Clin Endocrinol Metab* 50:46–51.
86. Touitou, Y, et al. 1982. Adrenal circadian system in young and elderly human subjects: A comparative study. *J Endocrinol* 93:201–210.
87. Sapolsky, R, et al. 1987. Stress and glucocorticoids in aging. *Endocrinol Metab Clin* 16:965–981.
88. Lakatta, EG. 1987. Catecholamines and cardiovascular function in aging. *Endocrinol Metab Clin* 16:877–891.
89. Byyny, RL: 1980. Preventing adrenal insufficiency during surgery. *Postgrad Med* 67:219–226.
90. Tzagournis, M. 1978. Acute adrenal insufficiency. *Heart Lung*, 7:603–609.
91. Mitnick, JS, et al. 1983. Non-functioning adrenal adenomas discovered incidentally on computed tomography. *Radiology* 148:495–499.
92. Copeland, PM. 1983. The incidentally discovered adrenal mass. *Ann Intern Med* 98:940–945.
93. Seddon, JM, Baranetsky, N, and van Boxel, PJ. 1985. Adrenal incidentalomas. *Urology* 25:1–7.
94. Sharp, NA, Devlin, JT, and Rinmer, JM. 1986. Renal failure obfuscates the diagnosis of Cushing's disease. *JAMA* 256(18):2564–2565.
95. Carpenter, PC. 1986. Cushing's syndrome: Update of diagnosis and management. *Mayo Clin Proc* 61:49–58.
96. Watson, RGK, et al. 1986. Results of adrenal surgery for Cushing's syndrome: 10 years' experience. *World J Surg* 10:531–538.
97. Henley, DJ, et al. 1983. Adrenal cortical carcinoma—A continuing challenge. *Surgery* 94:926–931.
98. Granberg, PO, et al. 1982. The management of patients with primary aldosteronism. *World J Surg* 6:757–764.
99. van Heerden, JA, et al. 1982. Pheochromocytoma: Current status and changing trends. *Surgery* 91:367–373.
100. Wheeler, MH, et al. 1982. The Management of the patient with catecholamine excess. *World J Surg* 6: 735–747.
101. Welch, TJ, et al. 1983. Pheochromocytoma: Value of computed tomography. *Radiology* 148:501–503.
102. Reinig, JW, et al. 1986. Adrenal masses differentiated by *MR. Radiology* 158:81–84.
103. Glazer, GM, et al. 1986. Adrenal tissue characterization using MR imaging. *Radiology* 158:73–79.
104. Thompson, NW, et al. 1984. Extra-adrenal and metastatic pheochromocytoma: The role of ^{131}I MIBG in localization and management. *World J Surg* 8:605–611.
105. van Heerden, JA, et al. 1984. Surgical management of the adrenal glands in the multiple endocrine neoplasia type II syndrome. *World J Surg* 8:612–621.
106. Kvols, LK, and Buck, M. 1987. Chemotherapy of endocrine malignancies: A review. *Semin Oncol* 14(3): 343–353.

28

Breast Disorders in the Elderly

James E. Devitt

Symptoms

The symptoms of breast disorders in the elderly are the same as those in younger women: lumps, pain, discharge, and deformity. Because of the involutional changes in the breast that follow the menopause, a lump discovered by a woman over age 60 is much more likely to be a cancer than is a breast lump found by a premenopausal woman (1). However, approximately half of the women over age 60 who report a breast complaint in fact will have a benign disorder and not carcinoma (2). The less common complaint of a deformity of the breast or nipple must be assumed to be due to a breast cancer until it has been proven to be otherwise. While it is not uncommon for a transient pain or distress to draw a patient's attention to a malignant breast lump, when pain is a dominant symptom, it is unusual for a carcinoma to be present (3). Nipple discharge is usually the result of nonmalignant disease even in the elderly (4).

Physical Examination of the Breast

The physical examination differs in no way from the examination of the breast in younger patients, except that the clinical diagnosis of carcinoma is easier because of the lessened physiologic nodularity.

The examination should be commenced with the patient in a comfortable sitting position on the side of the examining table or the side of the bed (5). The breasts, nipples, and areolae are inspected for any deformity or asymmetry. While various movements of the arms will occasionally reveal dimpling that cannot be observed in any other way, this is uncommon and is usually a waste of both the patient's and the clinician's time. Approximately 75% of patients over age 60 with breast cancer will have a visible sign, though this may only become evident when the breast is palpated (6). Thus, palpation should commence with the patient in the sitting position. Although the breast is more easily palpated when spread out over the chest wall when the patient is recumbent, there are occasional lumps that are best felt in the sitting position. More important, dimpling may sometimes be observed more easily when the breast and the mass are palpated with the patient upright (7).

The axilla and supraclavicular gland areas are palpated while the patient is sitting. Though palpation is an inexact way to assess the presence of axillary lymph node metastases, it is least inaccurate when done with the patient sitting.

The breast is then palpated with the patient reclining. It does not matter whether it is palpated in a radial or a circumferential fashion or with the arms at the side or above the head, so long as all parts of both breasts are examined thoroughly. Particular attention is paid to any transitory, visible change in the skin surface in the area of the breast mass while it is palpated. Any unilateral dimpling or flattening of contour during this procedure almost always indicates that the lesion being examined is a carcinoma.

Investigation of Breast Disorders

In the office, aspiration biopsy with cytologic examination of the specimen is easily performed. A 10-cc syringe and a number 20 needle and the appropriate fixative solution and container are all that are necessary. No local anesthetic is needed. While a Tru-cut needle biopsy technique which obtains a histological specimen is somewhat more accurate (8), the improved accuracy is almost certainly limited to larger tumors where the diagnosis is obvious clinically. In any event, the decision to recommend biopsy must be made on clinical grounds. This decision will only be changed by the aspiration biopsy report when either suspicious or positive cells are found in a patient whose lesion was clinically thought to be benign and formal biopsy believed to be unnecessary.

Mammography when it is done in a dedicated unit and interpreted by a skilled and experienced radiologist can be of help. Because of the involutional breast changes after the menopause, false negative reports become less common and small carcinomas as well as in situ lesions may be discovered. On the other hand, all too often the mammography available does not meet the aforementioned standards, with a resulting increase in unnecessary surgery or less commonly, in delayed diagnosis. A surgeon must determine the quality of the mammography available to him if it is to be used as a helpful adjunct. Negative mammography does not rule out cancer as the cause of a dominant mass.

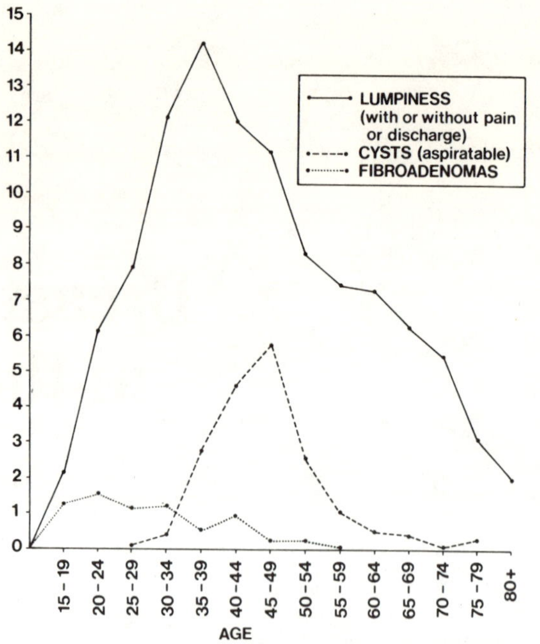

Figure 28-1. Relative age-specific incidence of benign breast findings: lumpiness, cysts, and fibroadenomas. (From Devitt, JE. 1983. Lumpy breasts: Normal. *Can J Surg* 26:6–7.)

Benign Breast Disorders

The benign breast disorders are usually diagnosed, not because they require treatment, but rather to exclude the existence of cancer. Clinicians must avoid applying inaccurate labels to patients who only have lumpy, sore, or discharging breasts (9).

Breast Nodularity

This is by far the most common benign clinical finding in older patients (2). It characteristically is vague, multiple, diffuse, and sometimes roughly symmetrical. Pain and sensitivity may or may not be associated. It is most easily found at the areolar edge or at the edge of the mammary disc, particularly in the lower inner quadrant along the inferior margin of the breast. It is rarely as prominent as it is in premenopausal women, nor is the firmness as evident. Approximately 25% of patients will have associated pain, which is characteristically intermittent and episodic. The distress may be likened to the distress that can occur premenstrually.

While the relative age-specific incidence of clinical benign disorders diminishes dramatically after the menopause (Figs. 28-1 and 28-2), they do continue to occur in older women (10) and indeed, up to the age of 75, they are more likely than cancer to be responsible for an individual seeking consultation with a breast surgeon. On the other hand, autopsies of patients not dying of breast cancer reveal *histologic* benign breast disorders to continue at the same frequency, if not to increase in older women (11, 12). This only demonstrates the poor correlation between the histologic observations seen by pathologists and the clinical lumps and sensitive areas for which patients seek advice.

No treatment is required for breast nodularity and sensitivity. The natural history of these findings is for them to spontaneously disappear, although they can wax and wane. Their only significance relates to the confusion that they may cause clinically in diagnosing breast cancer. Surgery is only indicated if there is genuine concern about the possible presence of breast cancer. Usually, clinical examination with or without aspiration biopsy or mammography will suffice to make a diagnosis. There is no association between these changes and the taking of hormonal supplements, even though the changes are almost certainly the result of continuing endogenous hormonal activity. There is no contraindication to the use of hormonal supplements if these conditions are present. Nor is the patient at greater risk of developing breast cancer (9).

Specific Benign Lumps (Cysts and Fibroadenomas)

Cysts do occur in older women, usually to the surprise of the clinician. They are diagnosed by aspiration. The withdrawal of some green, brown, or yellow, watery fluid with

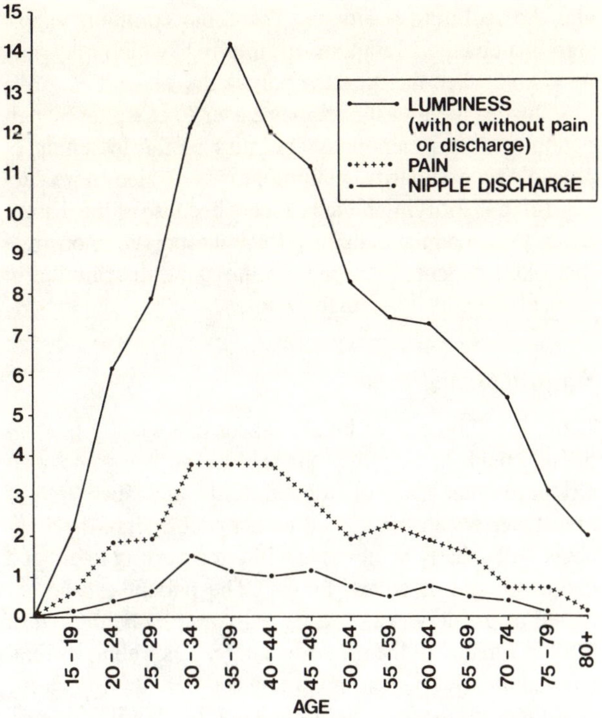

Figure 28-2. Relative age-specific incidence of benign breast findings: lumpiness, pain, and nipple discharge. (From Devitt, JE. 1983. Lumpy breasts: Normal. *Can J Surg* 26:6–7.)

the disappearance of the lesion and its failure to recur allows a confident diagnosis of benign cyst. Cystic carcinomas (which are quite uncommon) will usually have an aspirate that is blood-tinged, and either will not disappear completely on aspiration or will promptly recur (13). There is an association between the taking of supplemental hormones and benign cyst formation. Such a patient may have to choose between occasional breast cyst aspirations or the "benefit" of her supplemental hormones. There is no particular breast cancer risk. Again there is no need for surgery.

Fibroadenomas also occasionally occur in elderly women. These cannot be confidently diagnosed clinically and will be encountered as a pleasant surprise when excisional biopsy is carried out for what is thought to be a breast cancer. Though calcified fibroadenomas may be suspected by their hardness on palpation, excision is usually recommended for confident diagnosis (6).

Nipple Discharge

The symptom of nipple discharge (which the patient will frequently describe as bleeding from the nipple) is usually a sign of a benign breast phenomenon. The most common cause in older women is duct ectasia. Duct ectasia is an involutional change in the breast which, with the cessation of ovarian cycles, results in a dilation of one or more of the duct systems which are filled with a black or dark green fluid. The fluid resembles the fluid that is seen in some breast cysts. The condition presents with nipple discharge. Usually, the inflammatory features that are associated with duct ectasia in premenopausal women are absent (14). Careful inspection will reveal that more than one duct is involved, and often both nipples will have several ducts from which a few drops of dark greenish-black discharge can be extruded. There is absolutely nothing convincing to feel in the breast or the subareolar area. Occasionally, the discharge can be produced from only a single duct.

Nothing useful is achieved by forwarding a specimen of nipple discharge for either bacteriologic or cytologic examination. The management is one of reassuring the patient of the nonthreatening nature of the disorder. Eventually, it will stop spontaneously, although possibly not for many months. No intervention is required.

Approximately one-third of elderly patients with nipple discharge will be suffering from a duct papilloma (2). These present with discharge which is either serous, serosanguineous, black, or bloody. Its most characteristic feature, however, is that it comes from a single duct and is relatively profuse in amount. Once again there is usually absolutely nothing to feel since the papilloma is often only a few millimeters in size and is a friable soft lesion. Such discharge will continue unless there is surgical intervention. Thus, biopsy is indicated to rid the patient of the inconvenience of the discharge. The patient should be reassured that there is no threat of malignancy.

The lesion is most easily identified by inserting a fine blunt probe into the duct from which the discharge exudes (4). A straight skin needle serves admirably for the purpose, and if rotated over the duct, will usually enter the duct system easily. An incision is made down through the nipple and the areola to the needle, so that the dilated duct can be laid open. Hemostasis has to be precise and gentle. The papilloma can usually then be seen as a small friable, reddish-purple lesion of only a few millimeters in size. Rough sponging can inadvertently remove it. If the papilloma is recognized, it is excised conservatively. If no papilloma is seen, the duct system is excised, again relatively conservatively.

On those rare occasions when a carcinoma is associated with nipple discharge, there will almost invariably be a palpable mass. The mass is dealt with by the appropriate surgical procedure.

Carcinoma of the Breast

The risk of developing breast cancer increases with age. Indeed over 50% of all breast cancers will occur in women over the age of 60 (6). This is predominantly a phenomenon of women living in the affluent world (15). Prior to the menopause, age-specific death rates are similar in all parts of the world. Those countries with a low incidence of breast cancer after menopause tend to have either stationary or even falling age-specific breast cancer mortality rates. But in the affluent countries, the rate steadily increases with age.

There is still an incorrect belief that breast cancer in older women is an indolent and relatively unthreatening disorder. Unfortunately, the calculation of survival rates has been distorted by an attempt to correct for the greater death rates from other causes that are naturally seen in a population of older women. If, however, the breast cancer mortality rate is studied, it can be seen that the rates are at least as bad as those experienced by younger women. Indeed, there are many studies that suggest that the breast cancer mortality rates are actually worse in older patients (16). It appears that the older woman does not survive metastatic disease as well as the younger person (17).

Pathology

There are some pathologic differences in the breast cancers of older women. They are more likely to have a mucinous or tubular carcinoma. Medullary and lobular carcinomas are relatively less common. The differences, however, are not substantial and are of comparatively little clinical significance (18). Multicentricity has no association with age. The distribution of tumors of histologically low- and high-grade malignancy is similar at all ages. On the other hand, with increasing age breast cancers are more likely to have steroid receptors found, and the levels are likely to be higher (19).

Symptoms and Signs

As with younger women, in ordinary clinical practice the carcinoma is most likely to be found by the patient herself. Her attention is usually attracted by the finding of a lump 90% of the time (6). The remainder will be found by the patient recognizing a deformity of some sort or occasionally pain or nipple discharge. In most practices tumors recognized by screening examination will usually be found by identifying a lump, or less commonly, deformity or a suspicious mammographic shadow.

A physical examination of the older patient is always easier because the nodularity associated with the menstrual cycles tends to disappear after the menopause so that the breast is softer and neoplasms are more easily identified on palpation. Also, 75% of patients over the age of 60 will have a visible breast sign if inspection and palpation are careful and are carried out both in the sitting and the reclining positions. The most common visible sign is a change in contour or dimpling, which may only be visible when the breast is palpated.

Just as the breast becomes easier to examine by palpation after the menopause because of the lessening of physiologic nodularity, mammography is also more successful in identifying breast cancers because of the lessening of these nodular densities. Recent reports demonstrate that older patients present with the same distribution of clinical stage as do younger women.

Surgical Management

Thus, the diagnosis of breast cancer can usually be confidently made in the office. Since older women do not usually have other kinds of isolated lumps and since 75% of breast cancers are associated with a visible sign, the diagnosis will usually be obvious without resorting to either a diagnostic aid or formal biopsy. The patient can be apprised of the diagnosis and be reassured by being told of the exact nature of the proposed surgery as well as its relative simplicity. By recommending segmental mastectomy when it is appropriate, the patient and her family will perceive the operation to be much less demanding and will therefore be able to accept surgery with much less anxiety.

If the clinical diagnosis is not confident, then the biopsy can be done as a segmental mastectomy as it is awkward to do this procedure after a biopsy. The surgical purpose and the operation is no different from that which is appropriate for younger patients. There are two objectives. First, there is the adequate staging of the tumor to determine the extent of the threat (and hence the treatment) that it poses to the patient. Second, there is the attempt to achieve local control. Thus, segmental mastectomy is indicated if the tumor can be grossly excised and yet a breast of reasonable size and shape be preserved. If, because of the large size of the tumor or its location, or the small size of the breast, gross excision with a reasonable breast remaining cannot be achieved, then total mastectomy is done.

Although it is common to subject breast cancer patients to extensive imaging and laboratory staging procedures, these have a disappointingly low yield (20, 21). In any event, they will not change the need for or the nature of the surgery or the subsequent management (22). In addition, they can be a significant source of unnecessary morbidity.

Breast surgery is easily tolerated by the elderly, as the anesthesia required is relatively simple and no body cavity is entered. There is no physical upset such as that associated with intra-abdominal or intrathoracic surgery. As the raising of the flaps of skin denervates the incisions, postoperative pain is minimal. If reasonable attention is paid to hemostasis, breast surgery should be quite possible to perform, except under the most unusual circumstances, without the need for blood transfusion. Most patients will be ready for discharge on the third postoperative day, the suction catheters being removed in the outpatient clinic at a later date. Usually in addition to the breast surgery, the ipsilateral axillary lymph nodes should be excised. Although this will not change the survival rates, (23), it will identify or confirm those patients who have axillary lymph node metastases and who are therefore at risk of suffering further from their breast cancer. And while delayed regional lymph node dissection does not seem to worsen the prognosis, the relatively minor addition of the axillary dissection at the time of the initial surgery will save the patient a subsequent anesthetic and operation, a point of significance in these elderly patients.

Segmental Mastectomy

Most authors recommend that segmental mastectomy be done through a circumferential incision if the lesion is in the upper half of the breast. A radial incision is recommended for lower half lesions without excising skin and without repairing the breast disc defect. Failure to rigidly follow these rules can still produce acceptable cosmetic results. The difficult part is being sure that one has grossly excised the tumor. This can be achieved by raising skin flaps for a centimeter or two around the lesion. The lesion is constantly held by the fingers to maintain orientation. Incision through the breast is carried down to and through the pectoral fascia. This is best commenced peripherally (there is less tissue to go through). Dissection is then carried along at the level of the pectoralis major, completing the surrounding lateral incisions until the desired segment has been excised. Orientation is maintained by holding the tumor by the fingers throughout. The specimen should be examined grossly by the pathologist and the surgeon in the operating room. The lines of resection should only be considered to be involved when the cancer has been transected (24).

Axillary Dissection

This is most conveniently done through a vertical 7- to 8-cm incision behind the pectoral fold, starting at the apex of the axilla. Flaps are raised to demonstrate the pectoral muscles in front and the latissimus dorsi behind. The clavipectoral fascia is divided along the edge of the pectoralis minor and below and parallel to the axillary vein. Division of a lateral pectoral vein will allow the axillary contents to be separated from the axillary vein, revealing the subscapular vein coming off the inferior aspect of the axillary vein. This is the landmark that identifies the nerve to the latissimus dorsi, a nerve which runs downward to join the medial side of the neurovascular bundle. The axillary contents can be separated by gentle finger dissection from this bundle, taking care to coagulate the occasional tiny branches that course forward into the axillary pad from the subscapular vessels. The nerve to the serratus anterior can be recognized in the fascia against that muscle by gentle finger dissection high in the axilla against the chest wall (the nerve is actually more likely to be injured lower down). The axillary contents contained between the above muscles can thus be removed preserving the identified nerves. Some large veins require securing in the area of the axillary tail of the breast. The skin alone is closed over a suction catheter, using a subcuticular stitch. Semipressure dressings are used to encourage adherence of the skin to the underlying muscle.

Total Mastectomy and Axillary Dissection

This is best done through a transverse, elliptical incision, calculating carefully, to leave enough skin to achieve easy closure. Skin flaps are raised between the subcutaneous fat and breast fat. They should not exceed 5 mm thickness. They are raised to the first interspace above and the abdominal wall (anterior rectus sheath and external oblique) below. Dissection is from the midline medially to the latissimus dorsi laterally. The mastectomy is commenced medially at the level of the pectoralis major muscle, removing the pectoral fascia, but not the anterior rectus sheath. Coagulation with the Shaw Scalpel and/or diathermy minimizes blood loss. The breast is mobilized to the edge of the pectoralis minor when the axillary dissection begins as described above. Because of the size of the mastectomy incision, the axilla is much more comfortably excised than what it is done through a small axillary incision. The skin flaps are approximated with non-absorbable loosely tied simple sutures. Semipressure dressings over suction catheters are desirable.

Postoperative Management

The suction catheters should be left in place for 1 week. Patients can be discharged with the suction apparatus in place, to be removed as an outpatient. It is usual for serum to gather in the axilla for a few weeks afterward. This can easily be aspirated as necessary.

After segmental mastectomy, most local "recurrences" will reappear in the operative site (25), so that it is here that they must be most diligently sought. Recognition of reactivation will usually result from physical examination (26). At first, the local postoperative reaction will be confusing, but this should fade within 3 months. If the defect in the breast was not repaired, its edges may be palpable and feel like a lump. There is often edema of the breast early on, particularly after axillary dissection. There may be peau d'orange and even an inflammatory appearance. The edema may persist. Careful physical examination and judicious use of aspiration biopsy will be required as experience is gained.

Adjuvant Therapy

Postoperative radiation is not indicated after mastectomy and axillary dissection or after segmental mastectomy unless there is serious doubt about the total excision of the primary tumor. Radiation should probably be reserved for those patients who have local recurrent disease or who have local disease sufficiently advanced that primary surgery is inappropriate. The clinical trials and retrospective reviews available do not suggest that survival rates will be threatened by this approach (25, 27).

While automatic adjuvant chemotherapy is probably not indicated in any older patient because of the lack of benefit and the questionable tolerance of it, efforts must still be made to diagnose the relative threat that the breast cancer poses to the patient. At this time, the axillary lymph node status is perhaps the most useful indication of this, but the record should include the tumor size, presence of grave signs, steroid receptor status, and histological type, in anticipation of an era when adjuvant chemotherapy will be available that will be effective. Tamoxifen (10 mg twice daily) is probably indicated in patients with axillary lymph node metastases, since it does appear that survival rates are improved with it (28). Therefore, patients who appear to be at risk from the nature of their breast cancer should be provided with it. If the lymph node status is negative, the outlook is sufficiently favorable to probably not justify the economic cost of adding tamoxifen.

For elderly patients who are unfit for surgery or primary radiotherapy, tamoxifen will induce a regression in two-thirds (including those whose steroid receptor status is unknown). There may be a slow response time (median 16 weeks), however (29).

Screening Detection

Because half of breast cancers occur in women over age 60 and because the breast is relatively easy to examine in elderly women, greater attention should be paid to this age group by providing screening examinations. Although at this time there is no good scientific study that shows that screening detection is effective in older women, it would seem appropriate to recommend it at least for those who are fit and otherwise well (6). Aside from the comparatively easier diagnosis, anxiety will not be created from the discovery of nonmalignant physiologic symptoms or signs, as is the case in premenopausal patients. Such efforts, of course, must be shown to be of benefit by prospective randomized clinical trials before they are too vigorously enforced. There would seem to be more justification for performing a screening breast examination on a healthy elderly patient, where there is a substantial risk of breast cancer occurrence, than there is in patients in their thirties, where cancer is uncommon and nonmalignant lumpiness almost the rule.

References

1. Devitt, JE. 1977. Value of the history in the office diagnosis of breast cancer. *Can Med Assoc J* 116:1127–1128.
2. Devitt, JE. 1986. Benign disorders of the breast in older women. *Surg Gynecol Obstet* 162:340–342.
3. Haagensen, CD, Bodian, C, and Haagensen, DE. 1981. Breast carcinoma: Risk and detection. Philadelphia: WB Saunders.
4. Devitt, JE. 1985. The management of nipple discharge by clinical findings. *Am J Surg* 145:789–792.
5. Rush, BF. 1984. Breast. In *Principles of Surgery, ed. 4*, Ed., SI Schwartz. New York: McGraw-Hill.
6. Devitt, JE. 1987. Unpublished data.
7. Bassett, AA. 1982. Technique of clinical screening for breast cancer. *N Engl J Med* 307:826–827.
8. Owen, AWMC, Anderson, TJ, and Forrest, APM. 1980. "Closed" biopsy for breast cancer. *J R Coll Surg Edinb* 25:237–241.
9. Hutter, RVP. 1985. Goodbye to "Fibrocystic Disease." *N Engl J Med* 321:179–181.
10. Devitt, JE. 1983. Lumpy breasts: normal. *Can J Surg* 26:6–7.
11. Frantz, VK. et al. 1951. Incidence of chronic cystic disease in so-called "normal breast." *Cancer* 4:765–783.
12. Sandison, AT. 1962. *Autopsy Study of the Human Breast.* Natl Cancer Inst. Monograph, No. 8, U.S. Dept. of Health, Education and Welfare. Washington: U.S. Dept. of Health, Education and Welfare, Public Health Service.
13. Devitt, JE, and Barr, JR. 1984. The clinical recognition of cystic carcinoma of the breast. *Surg Gynecol Obstet* 159:130–132.
14. Dixon, JM. 1983. Forrest, APM: Mammary duct ectasia. *Br J Surg* 70:601–603.
15. de Waard, F. 1979. Premenopausal and postmenopausal breast cancer: One disease or two? *JNCI* 63:549–552.
16. Mueller, CB, Ames, F, and Anderson, GD. 1978. Breast cancer in 3558 women: Age as a significant determinant in the rate of dying and causes of death. *Surgery* 83: 123–132.
17. Rutquist, LE, Wallgren, A, and Nilsson, B. 1984. Is breast cancer a curable disease? *Cancer* 53:1793–1800.
18. Fisher, ER, et al. 1975. The pathology of invasive breast cancer. *Cancer* 36:1–85.
19. Wittliff, JL. 1984. Steroid-hormone receptors in breast cancer. *Cancer* 534:630–643.
20. Monypenny, IJ, et al. 1984. The value of serial bone scanning in operable breast cancer. *Br J Surg* 71: 466–468.

21. Pandya, KJ, et al. 1985. A retrospective study of earliest indicators of recurrence in patients on Eastern Cooperative Oncology Group adjuvant chemotherapy trials for breast cancer. *Cancer* 55:202–205.
22. Mueller, CB. 1983. Asymptomatic metastases—to treat or not to treat? *Surgery* 93:328–329.
23. Fisher, B, et al. 1985. Ten-year results of a randomized clinical trial comparing radical mastectomy and total mastectomy with or without radiation. *N Engl J Med* 312: 674–681.
24. Fisher, ER, et al. 1986. Pathologic findings from the National Surgical Adjuvant Breast Project (protocol 6). II. Relation of local recurrence to multicentricity. *Cancer* 57:1717–1724.
25. Clark, RM, et al. 1982. Breast cancer: A 21 year experience with conservative surgery and radiation. *Int J Radiat Oncol Biol Phys* 8:967–975.
26. Mahoney, LJ. 1986. Methods for detecting locally recurrent and contralateral second primary breast cancer. *Can J Surg* 29:372–373.
27. Fisher, B, et al. 1985. Five-year results of a randomized clinical trial comparing total mastectomy and segmental mastectomy with or without radiation in the treatment of breast cancer. *N Engl J Med* 321:665–672.
28. Baum, M, et al. 1985. Controlled trial of Tamoxifen as single adjuvant agent in management of breast cancer. *Lancet* 1:836–840.
29. Allan, SG, et al. 1985. Tamoxifen as a primary treatment of breast cancer in elderly or frail patients: A practical management. *Br Med J* 290:358.

29

Thoracic Surgery in the Elderly

Mark R. Katlic

Present-day thoracic surgery is, *au fond,* geriatric surgery. The predominant disorders that occupy a modern chest surgeon's time and interest—lung and esophageal cancer, pleural disease and effusion, esophageal diverticulum, and others—tend to afflict the elderly. In addition, the thoracic surgeon must routinely probe the limits of his or her patient's cardiopulmonary reserve and general nutritional state. This specialty confronts the many faces of age in daily practice.

It was not always so. The earliest recorded chest surgical treatments, from the Smith papyrus (about 1700 to 2000 B.C.) to the writings of Hippocrates (about 400 B.C.), concerned traumatic wounds, thoracic empyema necessitatis, and even induced pneumothorax for pleurisy (Fig. 29-1); however, these were all in young men and women (1). The older patients, including a woman with bronchiectasis and clubbed fingers, were treated medically or not at all. For the next 2000 years, conditions amenable to chest surgery remained principally confined to the categories of trauma, empyema, and foreign body. As late as 1864, Gross devoted only 30 pages of his 2136-page *System of Surgery* (2) to injuries and diseases of the lungs, heart, and esophagus, and surgery played little role in these. Agnew, in his lengthy and detailed textbook, listed 36 cases of esophagotomy for foreign body, with the oldest patient being 49 years (3).

The introduction of endotracheal anesthesia by Meltzer and Auer (4) supplanted the ponderous pressure chambers of Sauerbruch (5) and allowed safer intrathoracic surgery. By 1926, Lilienthal could write his two-volume *Thoracic Surgery* (6). Surgeons were still operating chiefly to combat the sequelae of infections, e.g., tuberculosis and bronchiectasis, but their patients were older, at least by the standards of the day. This was a period during which surgeons were taught that "an elective operation for inguinal hernia in a patient older than 50 years was not justified" (7).

Lung cancer was a clinical rarity then (8), but automated rolling machines already had increased cigarette availability to a larger public, and by the 1930s and 1940s, the explosion in bronchogenic carcinoma had begun. Now, lung cancer has become the leading cause of cancer death in both men and women (9). Its incidence and prevalence generally increase with increasing age (10, 11), and surgery provides the principal means toward a cure. Accordingly, 20th century thoracic surgeons have become geriatric surgeons.

This chapter begins by presenting aspects of physiology and perioperative care that affect all chest surgery patients. Then it discusses specific disease entities and operations, which are arbitrarily organized by regional anatomy.

Anatomy and Physiology

The fact that age has an effect on pulmonary function was recognized by the earliest respiratory physiologists. When the inventor of the spirometer, John Hutchinson, presented his "On the Capacity of the Lungs and On the Respiratory Functions" before the Royal Medical And Chirurgical Society of London in 1846, he noted "The vital capacity of man may be considered as a constant quantity, but this quantity is disturbed or modified by four circumstances—1st. By Height, 2ndly. By Weight, 3rdly. By Age, and 4thly. By Disease" (12). Whether lung function in the elderly is more the result of the aging process itself

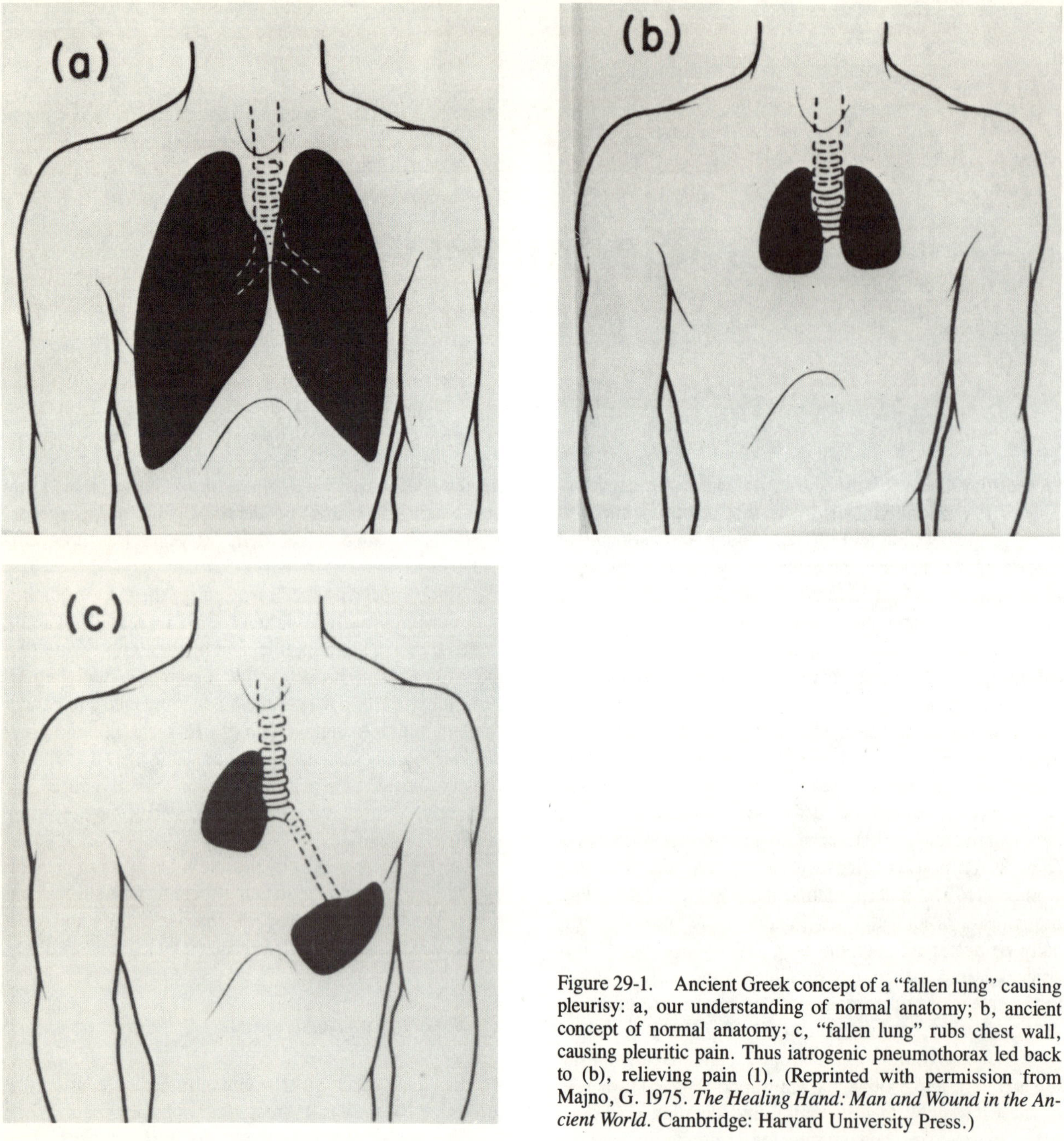

Figure 29-1. Ancient Greek concept of a "fallen lung" causing pleurisy: a, our understanding of normal anatomy; b, ancient concept of normal anatomy; c, "fallen lung" rubs chest wall, causing pleuritic pain. Thus iatrogenic pneumothorax led back to (b), relieving pain (1). (Reprinted with permission from Majno, G. 1975. *The Healing Hand: Man and Wound in the Ancient World*. Cambridge: Harvard University Press.)

or of the cumulative effects of the environment (pollutants/smoking, daily mechanical stress, subclinical infection) is unclear, but a picture of the end result can be drawn. These changes have been discussed in previous chapters and by others (13, 14) and will simply be summarized here.

Recognized structural changes in lung parenchyma in the elderly resemble emphysema, with enlargement of respiratory bronchioles and alveolar ducts; there may be true loss of septae. Similar but less marked than in emphysema is a decrease in lung elastic recoil (Fig. 29-2). Decreased elastic recoil allows airway closure at higher lung volumes, thus increasing residual volume. The reduction in vital capacity that Hutchinson observed over a century ago is felt to result primarily from this increase in residual volume, with total lung capacity remaining unchanged. The forced expiratory volume in 1 second (FEV_1) decreases by about 30 ml/yr in nonsmoking patients, again due chiefly to elastic recoil decrements (13). The phenomenon of airway closure at higher lung volumes is particu-

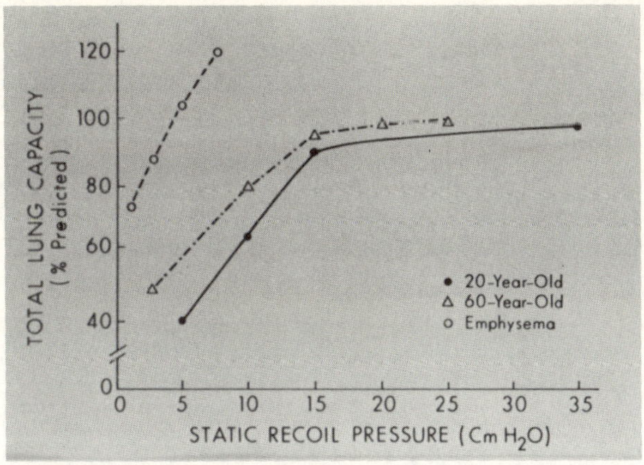

Figure 29-2. Relation of static recoil pressure to lung volume. Elderly lung resembles emphysematous lung in this regard (less recoil pressure at a given lung volume) but to a lesser degree (13). (Reprinted with permission from Lefrak, SS and Campbell, EJ. 1981. Structure and function of the aging respiratory system. In *Pulmonary Disease In The Adult,* Ed., DR Gracey. Chicago: Yearbook Medical Publishers.)

larly evident at the lung bases in elderly patients, leading to decreased basilar ventilation, ventilation/perfusion mismatch, increased physiologic dead space, and decreased arterial oxygenation; this is accentuated in the recumbent position.

Other changes in the elderly include a diminished central response to both hypoxemia and hypercapnia, predominantly in the form of decreased tidal volume rather than lowered respiratory rate (15). The chest wall stiffens and respiratory muscle strength decreases with age.

The cardiovascular system in the elderly individual manages well at rest. In the healthy, conditioned subject, it also responds well to exercise, with increases in stroke volume (16) compensating for a blunted heart rate response to hypoxemia or hypercapnia (17). Most elderly individuals have some cardiovascular disease and are not conditioned to exercise, however, and their maximum exercise capacity is clearly reduced (18).

The chief message regarding chest physiology is that the elderly are fine at rest but, with diminished reserve, respond suboptimally to stress.

Diagnostic Procedures

Although most diagnoses are evident to the thoracic surgeon following careful history, physical examination, and radiologic studies, the need for histologic proof and for staging generally leads to endoscopy, needle biopsy, or open biopsy. These procedures are well tolerated even by nonagenarians, and only the exceptionally ill patient should be denied the definitive diagnosis that will allow his or her best chance for cure or palliation.

Introduced by Killian (19) and popularized by Jackson (20, 21), rigid bronchoscopy allows a large biopsy to be taken and, when coupled with a straight telescope system, provides the best view of the airways down to segmental bronchus size; it is usually carried out under general anesthesia now. Since its development by the Japanese in 1967 (22), the flexible fiberoptic bronchoscope has surpassed the rigid in popularity; this type of bronchoscopy is performed with local anesthesia and allows visualization of subsegmental airways. Both rigid and flexible procedures can be done on an outpatient basis and are quite safe: 0.08% major complications, 0.01% deaths (23). The author believes that thoracic surgeons should be facile with both instruments and use each where most appropriate. The elderly patient should be gently positioned due to possible cervical arthritis and should be given judicious doses of intravenous sedation. They should also be carefully monitored by electrocardiogram and pulse oximeter.

Peripheral lung lesions are unlikely to be reached by the bronchoscope but can be biopsied percutaneously under fluoroscopic or computed tomographic (CT) guidance. Improvements in radiologic equipment, needles, and cytopathology have greatly advanced this technique since its first use a century ago (24). Presently, diagnostic accuracy is good, with 2% false positive and 14% false negative (25), although specificity as to cell type—particularly small cell undifferentiated carcinoma—is less reliable. Pneumothorax occurs in 20% to 30%, with one-third to one-half of these requiring tube thoracostomy; minor hemoptysis occurs in 2% to 5% (25, 26).

Esophagoscopy is of great value in esophageal disease, providing a histologic diagnosis in 96% of patients with esophageal carcinoma (27) and allowing inspection and dilatation in benign disorders. This procedure's chief complication, perforation, occurs in about 0.1% of patients (28) and is most common at the narrowest area, the introitus (29). This cricopharyngeal region is particularly dangerous in the elderly patient, who may have little esophageal muscle at and above the cricopharyngeus posteriorly and who may have osteoarthritic spurs of the cervical spine (Fig. 29-3). Care and correct positioning are mandatory (Fig. 29-4).

Other diagnostic procedures—thoracentesis, needle biopsy of pleura, thoracoscopy, open pleural biopsy, mediastinoscopy, Chamberlain mediastinotomy, open lung biopsy—will be discussed where appropriate below.

Thoracic Incisions

Incisions commonly employed by thoracic surgeons include cervical, upper sternotomy, full median sternotomy,

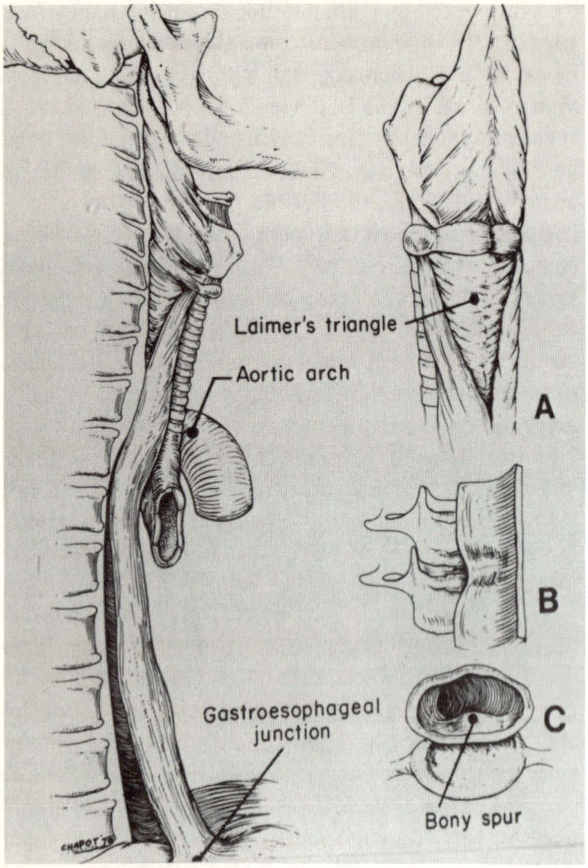

Figure 29-3. Areas of anatomical esophageal narrowing: introitus, aortic arch, gastroesophageal junction. A, Laimer's triangle in posterior cervical esophagus; B, and C, bony spurs indenting cervical esophagus (147). (Reprinted with permission from Rubin, JW. 1979. Complications of esophageal diagnostic procedures. In *Complications of Intrathoracic Surgery,* Eds., AR Cordell and RG Ellison. Boston: Little, Brown.)

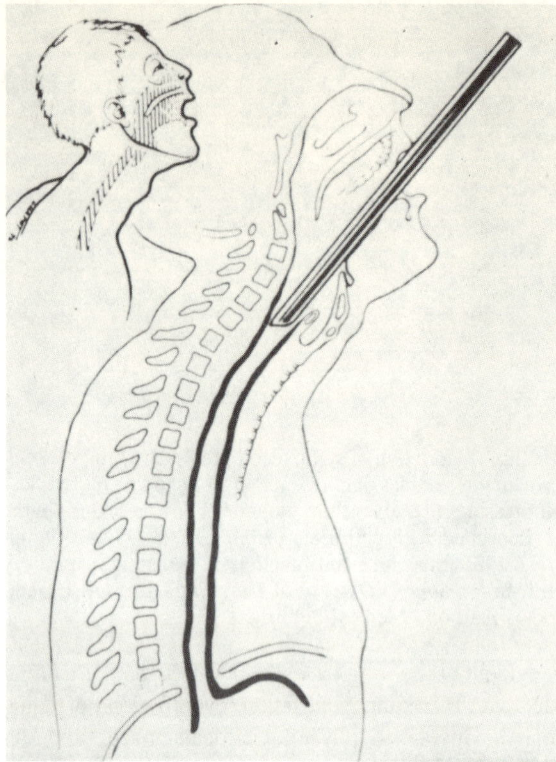

Figure 29-4. Proper esophagoscopy positioning: head extension and neck flexion relax the strap muscles and open the retrolaryngeal hypopharynx (147). (Reprinted with permission from Rubin JW. 1979. Complications of esophageal diagnostic procedures. In *Complications of Intrathoracic Surgery,* Eds., AR Cordell and RG Ellison. Boston: Little, Brown.)

anterolateral thoracotomy, posterolateral thoracotomy, thoracoabdominal, and laparotomy.

Cervical incisions cause relatively little discomfort and minimal effect on pulmonary function, and they should be used in the geriatric patient when possible. Most tracheal resections (30), for example, and virtually all resections of substernal goiter (31, 32) can be performed through collar incisions; an upper sternotomy can be added if additional mediastinal exposure is needed (Fig. 29-5). Although cervical incisions are advocated by some for thymectomy in myasthenia gravis as well (33), the author prefers a short vertical upper sternotomy to ensure complete resection.

Full median sternotomy, used routinely in cardiac surgery, can also provide access to the mediastinum and both pleural cavities. Its added benefit for the elderly is the somewhat decreased adverse effect on pulmonary function compared to thoracotomy (34), particularly in the latter half of the first postoperative week (Fig. 29-6); this is generally attributed to differences in postoperative pain. Frequently used in resection of bilateral lung metastases or blebs (35), sternotomy will allow virtually any type of resection (36) although some, e.g., left upper sleeve lobectomy and left lower lobectomy, may be difficult. One complication of sternotomy, brachial plexus injury, may be due to occult fracture of the first rib. Although one study found no correlation of these fractures with patient age (37), it is still prudent to place the sternal retractor low and to use the minimum needed spread of the sternum.

Anterolateral thoracotomy is often used for open lung biopsy and pericardial window procedures, but can be employed readily for larger pulmonary resections. Perhaps due to lessened traction on intercostal nerves or less muscle division, it, too, seems to be better tolerated than posterolateral thoracotomy (38) (Fig. 29-7). Posterolateral thoracotomy, however, must be considered the standard approach for most chest surgeons, for it allows excellent exposure of the entire pleural cavity and facilitates the addition of sleeve resection of the bronchus or *en bloc* chest wall resection. This type of thoracotomy can be per-

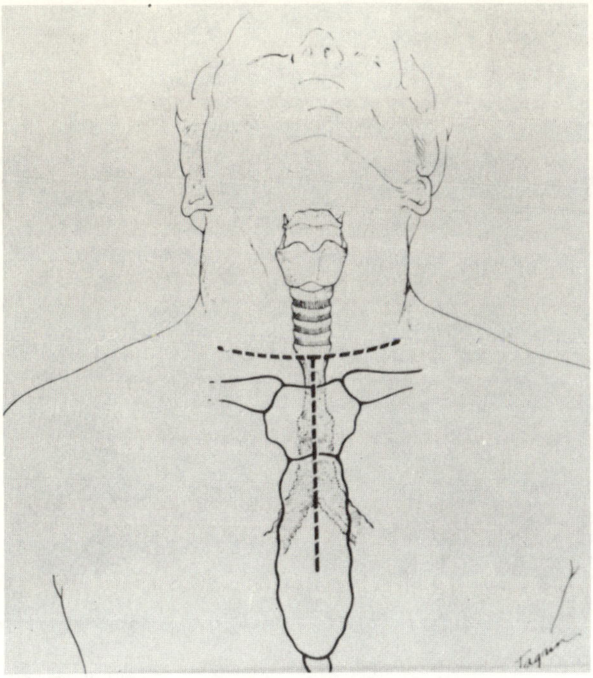

Figure 29-5. Collar incision and extension for upper sternotomy (148). (Reprinted with permission from Grillo, HC. 1970. Surgery of the Trachea. In *Current Problems In Surgery,* Ed. MM Ravitch. Chicago: Yearbook Medical Publishers.)

formed with division only of the latissimus dorsi and with sparing of the serratus anterior, trapezius, and rhomboid muscles; even the latissimus can be retracted undivided in many patients (39). The ribs should be slowly spread for access, although resection of a brittle rib in the elderly patient may be best, for this enhances exposure and adds no morbidity.

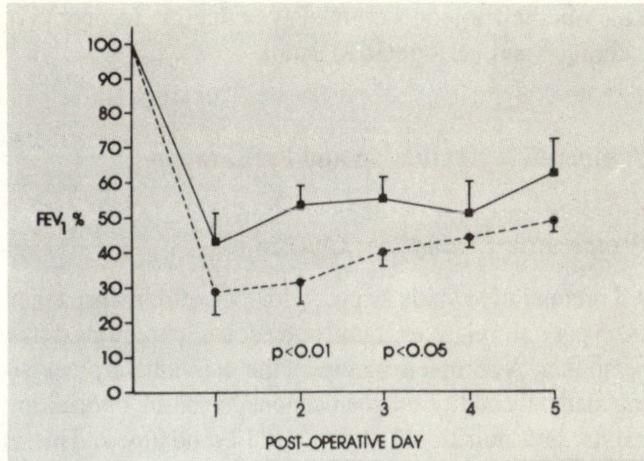

Figure 29-7. Comparison of FEV_1 values between posterolateral thoracotomy (●---●) and anterolateral thoracotomy (■—■). Results differed significantly during the 2nd and 3rd postoperative days (38). (Reprinted with permission from de la Rocha, AG and Chambers, K. 1984. Pain amelioration after thoracotomy. *Ann Thorac Surg* 37:239–242.)

Some surgeons abhor the thoracoabdominal incision—generally used for resection of gastroesophageal junction carcinoma—for it adds division of the diaphragm and costal arch to the combined debility of thoracotomy and laparotomy. It does offer unequaled access, however, to this particular area of the body and in the author's experience is well tolerated by patients in their seventies and eighties.

The author believes that an incision least disruptive to chest wall function should be planned for the elderly patient, as long as it is *consistent with good exposure*. The aged tolerate complications poorly, and the best determinant of a smooth postoperative course is still a well-conducted operation. More important than the specific in-

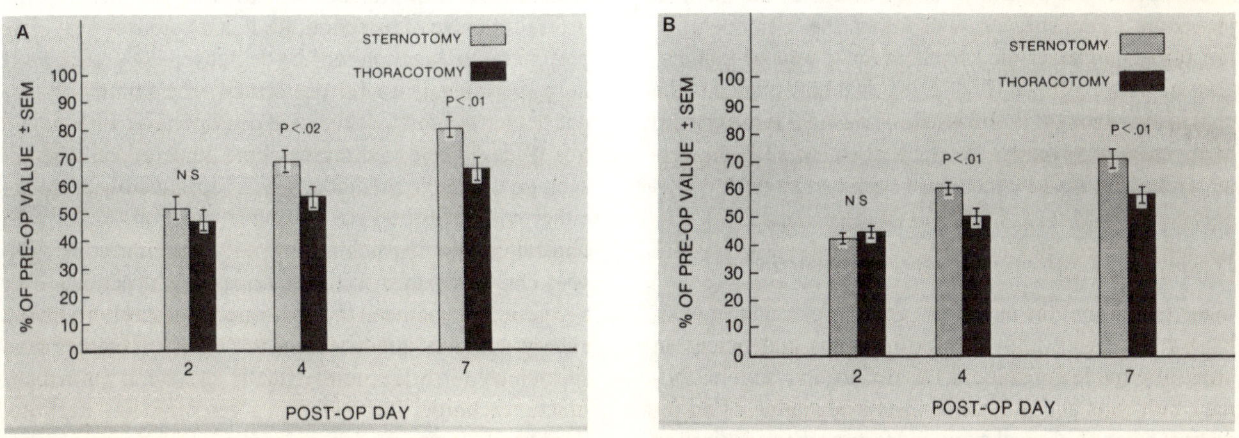

Figure 29-6. Pulmonary function studies as a percent of the preoperative value in 14 patients undergoing sternotomy and 14 lateral thoracotomy. A, Peak flow measurements; B, vital capacity (34). (Reprinted with permission from Cooper, JD, et al. 1978. Extended indications for median sternotomy in patients requiring pulmonary resection. *Ann Thorac Surg* 26:413–420.)

cision is the surgeon's compulsive attention to operative technique and perioperative detail.

Preoperative Evaluation and Preparation

Preoperative Evaluation: General

All preoperative study begins with a careful history taken from patient, relatives, family physician, or nursing home personnel. A complete picture of the individual's preexisting medical conditions, medications, smoking or drinking habits, and nutritional state should be obtained. This is done not as much to discover contraindications to surgery as to adequately prepare the patient for the needed operation, since there is surprisingly little documentation that clinical factors per se influence mortality in the elderly chest surgery patient. Yellin et al. (40), for example, found no correlation between operative risks and preexisting conditions such as coronary disease, hypertension, and diabetes mellitus in 58 patients over age 70 undergoing thoracotomy. In Breyer's 150 resections for lung cancer in the elderly, the only historical factors statistically related to death or major complication were prior resection and congestive heart failure (41). Nevertheless, cardiopulmonary complications predominate in all series of surgery in the elderly, and it is best to be forewarned by knowledge of the patient's baseline state.

Physical examination, conversely, may uncover a contraindication to operation, e.g., nodal metastasis, hepatomegaly, Horner's syndrome. Blood sampling for anemia, coagulation abnormality, dehydration, or renal dysfunction is mandatory. It also cannot be overemphasized that the thoracic surgeon must personally review all radiographs, for the radiologist will not have the same knowledge of the patient or of the details of the planned procedure. The surgeon will know the intraoperative functional and anatomic correlates and potential implications of what is shown (Fig. 29-8). Just how dilated is the proximal esophagus in the achalasia patient? Is the cricoid likely to be involved by the tracheal stenosis? Is the vertebral body eroded by the apical lung carcinoma?

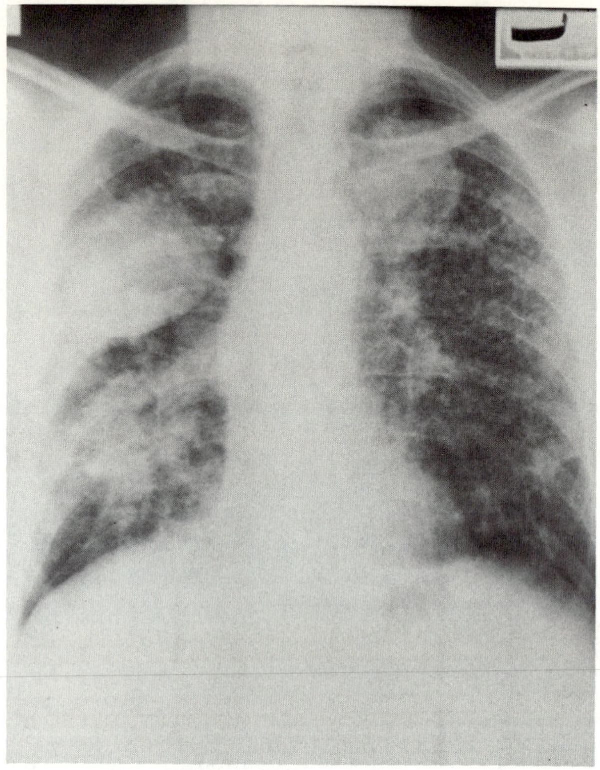

Figure 29-8. Chest radiograph of elderly patient with anthracosilicosis and early carcinoma. Carcinoma itself not visible on this radiograph. This degree of anthracosilicosis is a strong relative contraindication to resection; the thoracic surgeon can weigh the risks only after seeing the radiograph itself, not just the radiologist's report.

Preoperative Evaluation: Pulmonary Function

In ancient Rome, the augur was a public official responsible for observing and interpreting signs and omens in order to provide guidance. Like modern-day augurs, thoracic surgeons and pulmonologists evaluate an often indistinct array of clinical signs and test results to determine whether their patient will tolerate lung resection or even thoracotomy. The most commonly used of these indicators are also the most readily available: spirometry, arterial blood gas sampling, quantitative ventilation/perfusion scanning, and subjective judgment.

Most patients with a forced expiratory volume in 1 second (FEV_1) of 1.0 liter will tolerate the thoracotomy itself, exclusive of resection, for it is recognized that early postoperative function will be decreased 20% to 30%. If lung resection is to be performed, the commonly espoused lower limit for predicted postoperative FEV_1 is 0.8 to 1.0 liter. There is disagreement, however, on whether such preoperative predictions will reproducibly correlate either with measured postoperative function (42) or with clinical end points such as mortality and morbidity (43–45). One study examining this question in patients over age seventy concluded that postoperative mortality in the elderly could be predicted on the basis of preoperative spirometry (46). If spirometrically measured pulmonary function is borderline to allow a given resection, quantitative ventilation/perfusion scanning is worthwhile, since the portion of lung to be removed may be found to contribute little to overall function.

Preoperative arterial blood gas sampling should be done in all elderly thoracic surgery patients since they may have worse degrees of hypoxemia or hypercapnia than is clinically evident. Resting pCO_2 is particularly valuable, with a value greater than 45 mm Hg worrisome, since it will likely only be worsened by operation. Hypoxemia is a less reliable predictor and could actually be improved by surgery if obstructed but perfused lung segments are removed.

Subjective clinical evaluation still has a role in assessment of suitability for thoracic surgery. Spirometry is an effort-related test, and some patients appear better than the objective tests indicate; other patients test well but have ominous signs such as prominent wheezes on auscultation or copious secretions. Each patient must be evaluated individually.

Finally, cardiac function cannot be separated entirely from lung function, and tests that consider this may prove to be more valuable yet. Pulmonary artery catheterization is straightforward, as is echocardiography and dynamic cardiac scanning. Although the author can still occasionally be seen climbing hospital stairs with a patient—and there is recent corroboration of the method in the literature, with three flights allowing lobectomy and five flights pneumonectomy (47)—this form of exercise evaluation may be supplanted by the more standardized determination of maximal oxygen consumption or MVO_2 (48).

Preoperative Preparation

Emergency operations in the elderly carry threefold greater risk for mortality compared to elective surgery (49–51), and they also embody increased chance of complications (52, 53); this relates in great part to the lack of preoperative preparation in the emergency cases. Fortunately, most thoracic surgery in the aged is elective, and few patients should be brought to the operating room in suboptimal shape.

Cessation of smoking is paramount, even for a period of days. Experienced bronchoscopists are familiar with the smoker's rubber cement-like mucus, which clings tenaciously to the bronchial mucosa and stretches before snapping into the bronchoscope suction apparatus. It is exceedingly difficult for the elderly postoperative patient to clear this type of secretion. Bronchitis should be aggressively treated and bronchodilators instituted if auscultation or spirometry point to their need. These measures will occasionally improve lung function to the point that an initially inoperable patient can undergo resection.

The elderly patient, particularly one with carcinoma and weight loss, may be dehydrated, and such dehydration itself can mask anemia. Fluid and sometimes blood must be given, if necessary with Swan-Ganz catheter monitoring, to prevent intraoperative hemodynamic instability and its postoperative consequences. For the healthy elderly individual in whom operative blood loss is anticipated, revisions in blood bank arbitrary age limits should soon allow preoperative donation of autologous blood (54).

The question as to whether the elderly lung surgery patient should receive prophylactic preoperative digoxin cannot be scientifically answered at the present time. About 5% of lobectomies and 10% to 30% of pneumonectomies will experience postoperative atrial dysrhythmias and, although most can be readily treated, there is increased mortality in those in whom the rhythm disturbance occurs—25% versus 7% in a recent Mayo Clinic series (55). However, it is not established that preoperative digitalization would change this. Some researchers have found the elderly to be at increased risk for this complication (56) and others have not (57); some routinely digitalize all elderly chest surgery patients (58). Future studies into possible risk factors such as intrapericardial dissection or subclinical fluid overload may help the surgeon select specific groups that would benefit from digitalization. At present, the author does not use prophylactic digitalization but does rapidly treat postoperative dysrhythmias, for the elderly will likely tolerate the new rhythm poorly.

Intraoperative Management

With the exception of cervical procedures and endoscopy, chest surgery in the aged should be carried out with a full complement of monitoring devices: EKG, Foley catheter, arterial line, temperature probe, pulse oximeter, and possible end tidal CO_2 monitor. Swan-Ganz catheterization is useful in selected patients and is best done preoperatively; if lung resection is planned, catheter position must be radiographically or fluoroscopically checked to be certain the line is directed into the contralateral lung. Time should be taken to gently position the patient due to potential arthritis, decreased muscle mass, and easy bruisability.

Intrathoracic surgery is greatly facilitated by the use of double-lumen endotracheal tubes, which allow selective collapse of the ipsilateral lung (59, 60); this minimizes retraction trauma to the lung and enhances exposure. Continuous communication with the anesthesiologist will allow the earliest detection of any problem. Although some investigators have found increased mortality related to longer time spent in the operating room (50, 61), speed is less important than gentle handling of tissues, meticulous technique, and secure anastomosis. The elderly patient will handle a longer operation better than he will postoperative bleeding, bronchopleural fistula, or anastomotic leak. The surgeon should have a low threshhold for performing therapeutic bronchoscopy at the end of the case, particularly if secretions or endobronchial blood are suspected.

Methods for reducing postoperative pain can begin in the operating room. Each of the many techniques—intercostal block, cryoanalgesia of intercostal nerves, transcutaneous electrical nerve stimulation (TENS), epidural narcotics—has its advocates and critics; this subject is reviewed by Coleman (62). The author has experience with all of the above and presently prefers long-acting or continuous epidural morphine for the first 24 hours or so in the intensive care unit, followed by patient-controlled analgesia or intermittent oral or parenteral narcotics.

Postoperative Care

Attentive nursing care, with an eye sensitive to subtle changes, must be added to the routine monitoring of the intensive care unit (continuous EKG, arterial line, hourly urine output, oximetry). Postoperative respiratory failure from cardiac or pulmonary causes is poorly predictable (63), and the elderly may not develop the usual clinical signs such as tachypnea and tachycardia until late.

Peters has drawn attention to the phenomenon of postpneumonectomy pulmonary edema (64, 65): following pneumonectomy, all of the cardiac output must traverse the remaining lung and the lymphatic pump cannot keep up with the high filtered volume (Fig. 29-9). Warning signs are high perioperative fluid infusions, high urine output, and high pulmonary artery pressure combined with high cardiac output; the pulmonary artery wedge pressure may be falsely low since inflation of the Swan-Ganz catheter balloon can result in occlusion of a sizable part of the remaining cross-sectional area of the pulmonary vasculature (66). Cautious fluid administration can prevent this. Diuretics and mechanical ventilation may or may not successfully treat it.

The physiologic changes in the aged respiratory system noted earlier in the chapter—decreased elastic recoil, decreased expiratory flow rate, decreased chest wall compliance—coupled with postoperative pain, significantly lower the elderly patient's ability to clear secretions and prevent atelectasis. The surgeon and nurses must first walk the line between adequate analgesia, allowing deep breathing and coughing, and oversedation; epidural analgesia may prove optimal here. Encouragement, nasotracheal suction (Fig. 29-10), and liberal use of therapeutic flexible bronchoscopy at the bedside are in order. Other metabolic demands such as fever should be treated. Despite the fact that mechanical ventilation increases airway pressure against a bronchial closure, the surgeon should not hesitate to institute it as early as the necessity becomes clear (63).

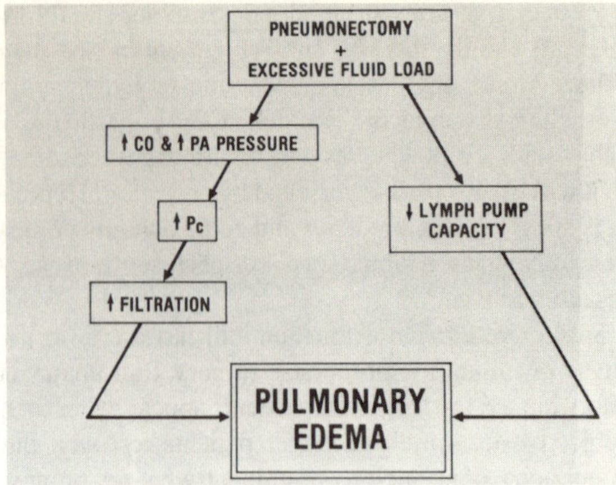

Figure 29-9. Mechanism of pulmonary edema formation. Increased pulmonary capillary pressure (P_c) and decreased lymph pump capacity in remaining lung after pneumonectomy predispose to pulmonary edema. CO, cardiac output; PA, pulmonary artery (64). (Reprinted with permission from Peters, RM. 1984. Pulmonary resection and gas exchange. *J Thorac Cardiovasc Surg* 88:872–879.)

The elderly patient must be mobilized early, not just to sitting in a chair but to walking with assistance. A longer postoperative stay than that of a younger counterpart is not mandatory but is likely (67).

Chest Wall

Primary tumors of the chest wall, such as fibrosarcoma, chondrosarcoma, chondroma, etc., are uncommon overall and are exceptionally rare in the elderly. Much more likely is rib cage involvement by bronchogenic carcinoma, breast cancer recurrence, or metastatic disease.

The chest wall is involved by extension of lung cancer in 2% to 8% of patients who come to operation (68) (Fig. 29-11). The best treatment for this is *en bloc* resection at the time of lobectomy or pneumonectomy, despite the fact that the elderly have increased operative mortality and decreased survival compared to their younger equivalents. The one death and two of the three cases of severe respiratory failure in Keagy's series of lung resections in patients older than 70 had had concomitant chest wall resection (57). In Piehler's study of 66 patients undergoing *en bloc* chest wall and pulmonary resection, operative mortality was 19.6% (age over 60 years) versus 5.0% (age under 60 years); in patients without nodal metastasis, $T_3 N_0 M_0$, only age had a significant correlation with long-term survival (69) (Fig. 29-12). Age is not a contraindica-

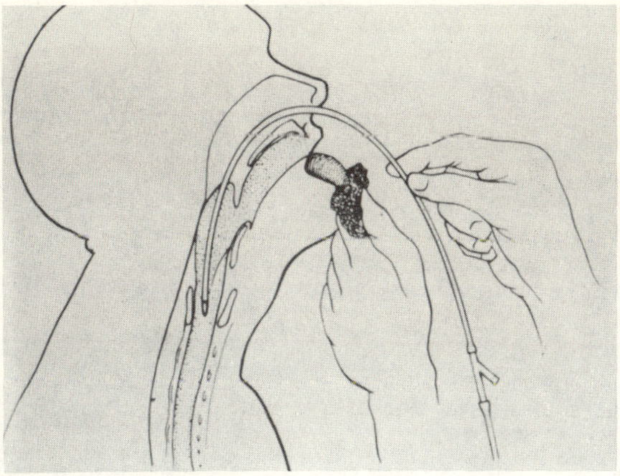

Figure 29-10. Method of nasotracheal aspiration (149). (Reprinted with permission from Pairolero, PC, and Payne, WS. 1983. Postoperative care and complications in the thoracic surgical patient. In *Thoracic and Cardiovascular Surgery,* 4th ed., Ed., WWL Glenn. Appleton-Century-Crofts.)

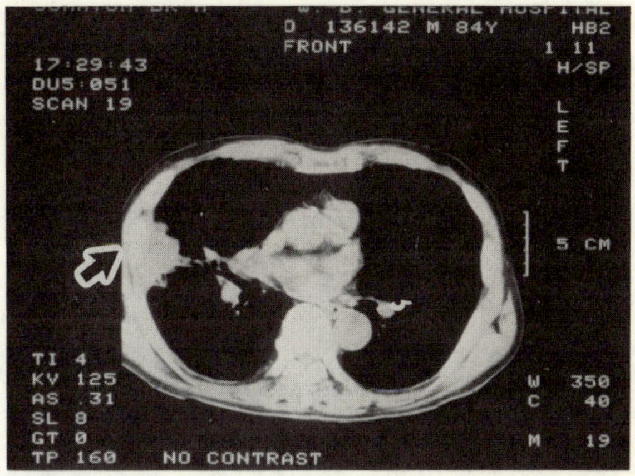

Figure 29-11. Squamous cell carcinoma (arrow) invading right chest wall in 84-year-old man.

tion to this operation, however, since the 5-year survival in the older age group with T_3 N_o M_o lesions, 27.7% is still superior to that offered by any other treatment. Most patients do not require replacement of this portion of chest wall, but if the defect is large or is not covered by the scapula, it can be stabilized by Marlex® mesh, Gore-tex® patch, or a sandwich of Marlex® and methylmethacrylate (Fig. 29-13).

Although chest wall resection for locally recurrent breast cancer or osteoradionecrosis rarely cures the patient, it can prolong survival and increase quality of life (70, 71). Reconstruction is facilitated by myocutaneous flaps (pectoralis, rectus, latissimus), pedicled omentum with skin graft (Fig. 29-14), or rotation flaps of skin or contralateral breast (72). Patients with breast or other carcinoma may require biopsy of a "hot" rib on radionuclide scan or radiograph; this can be done under local or general anesthesia after preoperative localization (73).

Infectious problems can also involve the chest wall and are often recalcitrant to nonoperative management. Sternotomy wound infections occur in less than 1% of open heart operations, but their incidence does increase significantly with age (74); costal chondritis can also occur after systemic infection, trauma, burns, or surgery (75). These, too, require complete debridement with advancement of well-vascularized tissue, such as muscle flap or omentum, into the area.

Pleura

Means of diagnosing pleural disease include thoracentesis, Cope needle biopsy, thoracoscopy, and open biopsy. These techniques differ little with the age of the patient. Both thoracoscopy (76) and open biopsy are usually done under general anesthesia but can be done under local,

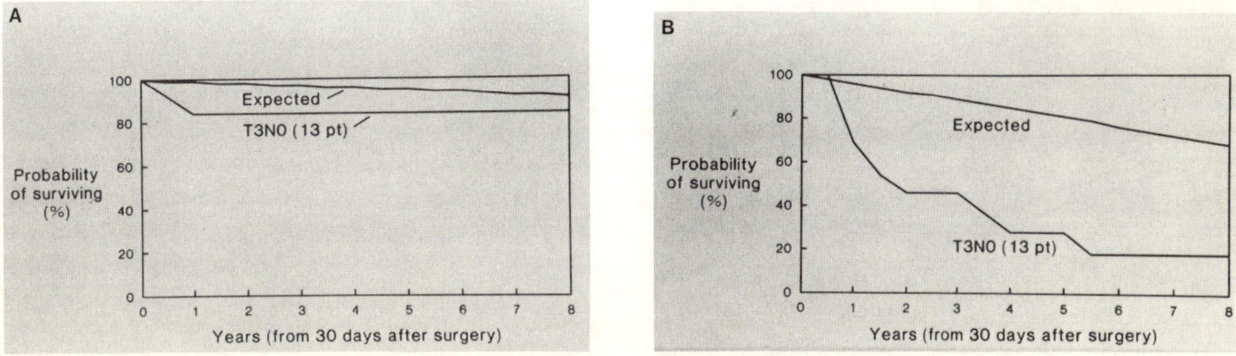

Figure 29-12. Survival in patients with postsurgical T_3 N_o M_o bronchogenic carcinoma invading the chest wall. A, 13 patients 60 years of age or less; B, 13 patients greater than 60 years of age (69). (Reprinted with permission from Piehler, JM, et al. 1982. Bronchogenic carcinoma with chest wall invasion. *Ann Thorac Surg* 34:684–691.)

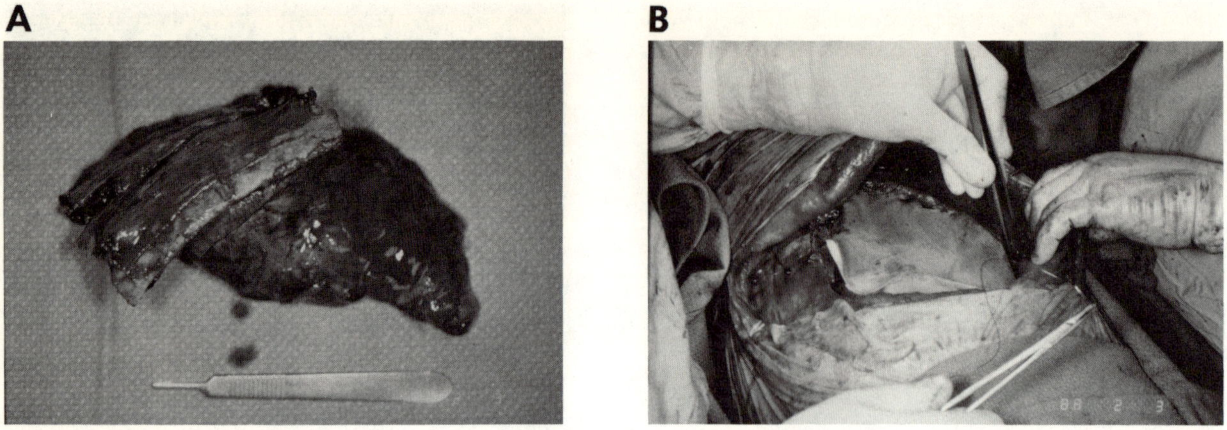

Figure 29-13. 84-year-old man with squamous cell carcinoma invading right chest wall (see Fig. 29-11). A, resected right middle lobe with attached ribs 5, 6, and 7; B, reconstruction using Marlex® mesh.

with assisted ventilation by mask or by endotracheal tube placed via awake intubation.

The chief causes of pleural effusion in the elderly are malignancy, congestive heart failure, and infection (including tuberculosis). Chest surgeons are often called to provide palliation for the dyspneic patient with recurrent effusion secondary to lung carcinoma, breast carcinoma, lymphoma, or other malignancy. Repeated thoracentesis is acceptable if life expectancy is short or the interval between reaccumulation long, otherwise chest tube placement and chemical pleurodesis (1–2 g tetracycline in 250 cc saline given once each day for 3 days) can be per-

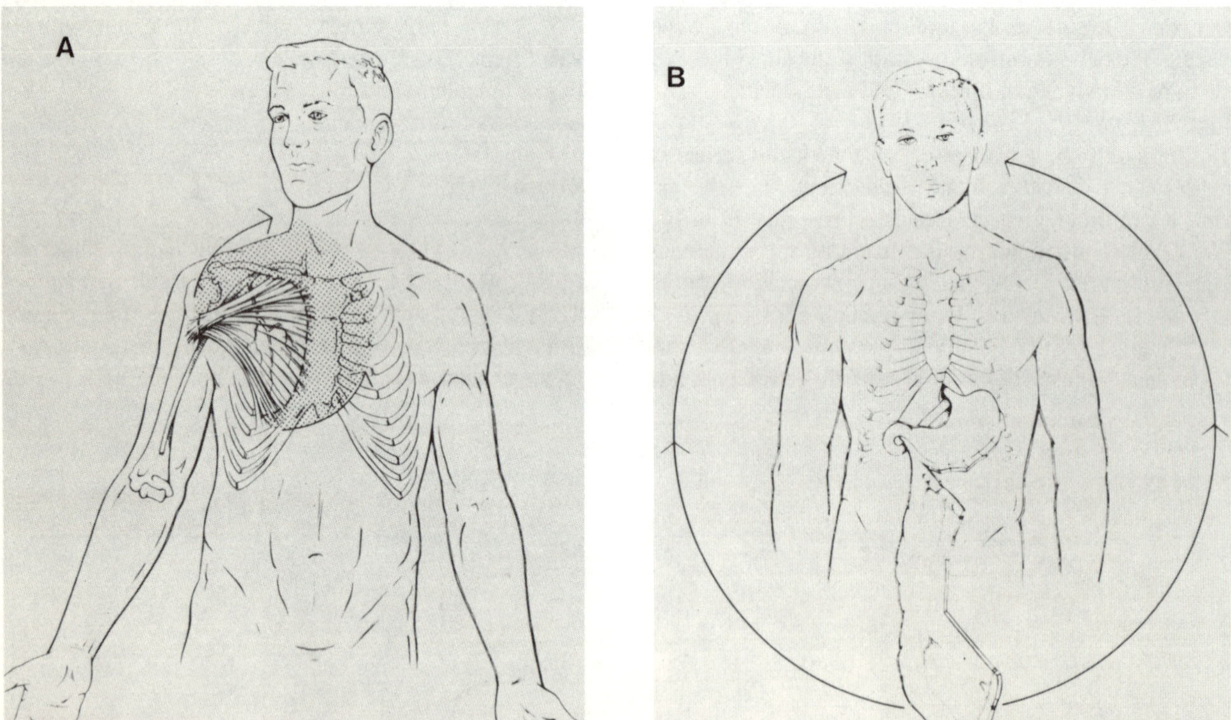

Figure 29-14. Chest wall reconstruction facilitated by the use of pectoralis major myocutaneous flap (A) or omental flap (B) (72). (Reprinted with permission from Dingman, RO, and Argenta, LC. 1981. Reconstruction of the chest wall. *Ann Thorac Surg* 32:202–208.)

formed (77). Options for dealing with the 20% to 25% that still recur are operative pleurodesis/partial pleurectomy in the good-risk patient—99% effective but with 6% to 10% mortality (78, 79)—or pleuroperitoneal shunt under local anesthesia (Fig. 29-15)—100% effective with no mortality in small series (80) and author's experience.

Recent reports show that pleural tuberculosis has become a disease of older patients and must be considered in the elderly patient with effusion, even if the patient has other potential causes for the fluid. Skin tests, pleural fluid culture, and pleural biopsy should be performed for any undiagnosed effusion (81). Both thoracic empyema (82, 83) and chylothorax (84, 85) occur in all age groups and will not be discussed here. Evidence in the literature shows, however, that early operative treatment results in decreased mortality and morbidity in both conditions.

In most series, the mean age of patients with primary pleural neoplasm is about 55 years, but Martini et al. (86) in a recent review relate an increased incidence with age up to ages 70 to 79 years. Pleural mesothelioma can be localized benign (pleural fibroma, fibrous mesothelioma)

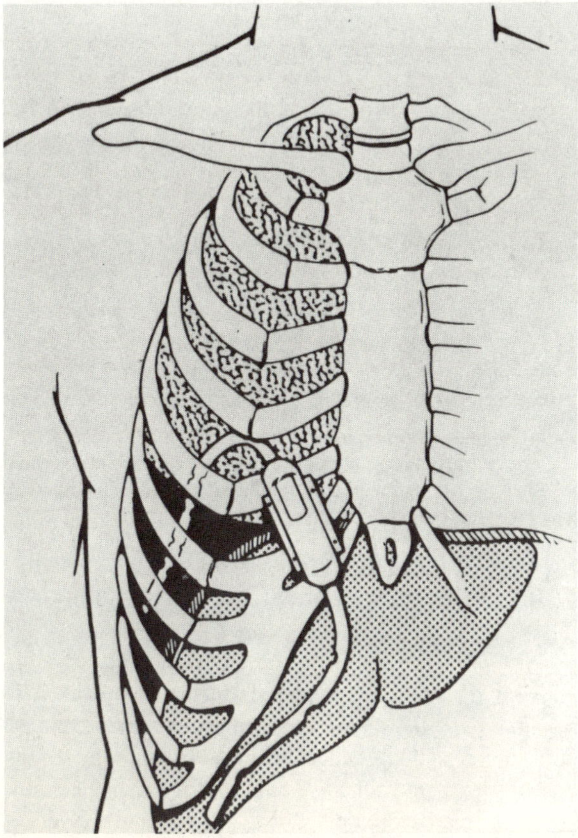

Figure 29-15. Pleuroperitoneal shunt for refractory pleural effusion (80). (Reprinted with permission from Cimochowski, GE, et al. 1986. Pleuroperitoneal shunting for recalcitrant pleural effusions. *J Thorac Cardiovasc Surg* 92:866–870.)

localized malignant, and diffuse malignant. Treatment of the benign type is straightforward resection. The localized malignant form should be widely resected, with *en bloc* resection of lung or chest wall if necessary, to prevent the recurrence that usually follows incomplete removal. Diffuse malignant mesothelioma is more often associated with asbestos exposure and almost always requires open biopsy for definitive diagnosis; even multi-modality treatment is invariably unsatisfactory, although some surgeons have reported somewhat increased survival in the good-risk patients who can tolerate pleuropneumonectomy (87) or pleurectomy (88).

Trachea and Bronchi

From the time of Chevalier Jackson's classic *Diseases Of The Air And Food Passages Of Foreign Body Origin* (89)—which tabulates 3266 foreign bodies with 2000 illustrations—to the present (90), it has been recognized that less than 20% occur in adults. These will often be chicken or fish bones or loose dental fillings (Fig. 29-16) and, if discovered early, can be removed via rigid bronchoscopy. Delay in diagnosis can lead to impaction, inflammation, and the rare need for bronchotomy or even pulmonary resection.

Grillo, emphasizing a straightforward approach to eliminating anastomotic tension and preserving blood supply, has shown that extensive tracheal resections for neoplasm (91), or stenosis (30) can be carried out in all age groups. Whereas half the trachea may be resectable in the young, long-necked patient, increased kyphosis and decreased tissue resiliency will allow far less in the elderly (Fig. 29-17). This kyphotic posture also has implications for tracheostomy in the elderly: if the surgeon routinely uses the sternal notch rather than the cricoid cartilage as his reference point in selecting a tracheotomy site, the tube may be placed too high in the trachea. A more widely used outgrowth of this tracheal reconstruction experience, bronchial sleeve resection, is particularly valuable in the aged, for it will preserve functioning lung tissue (92) (Fig. 29-18).

An unusual condition of the trachea, tracheopathia osteoplastica, may or may not be a lesion of "old age" (93).

Lung

Bronchogenic Carcinoma

Lung cancer incidence (10) and prevalence (11) increase with increasing age, and this malignancy is now the lead-

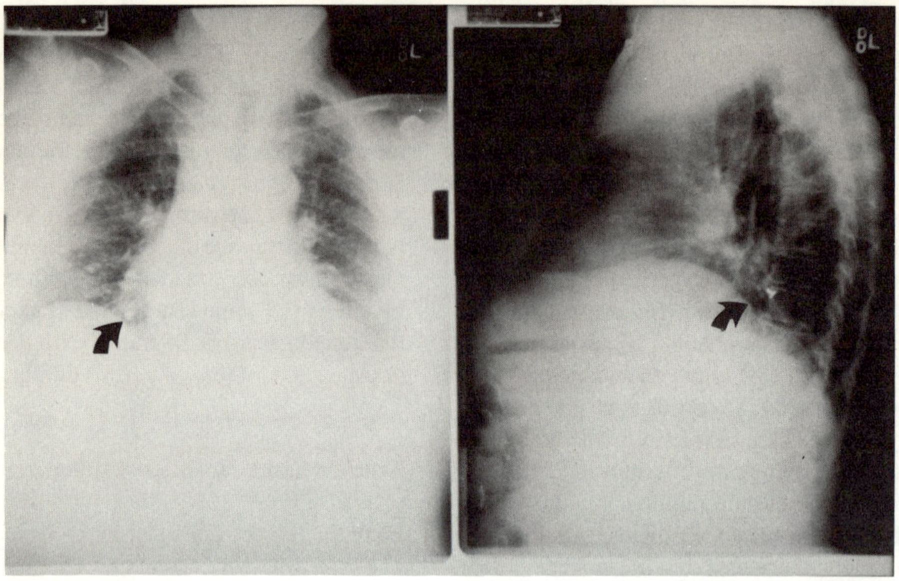

Figure 29-16. Aspirated loose dental filling (arrow) in right lower lobe segmental bronchus.

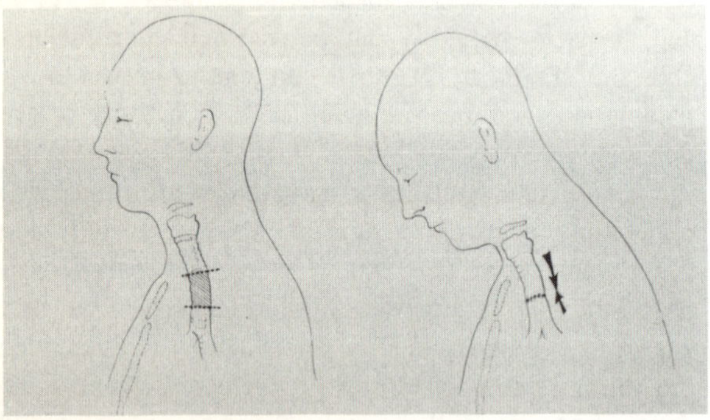

Figure 29-17. Cervical flexion rather than upward traction on carina allows tension-free tracheal anastomosis following tracheal resection. The kyphotic elderly neck begins somewhat flexed, thereby diminishing the value of this maneuver and promoting smaller resection (150). (Reprinted with permission from Grillo, HC. 1983. Congenital lesions, neoplasms, and injuries of the trachea. In *Gibbon's Surgery of the Chest,* 4th ed., Eds., DC Sabiston Jr and FC Spencer. Philadelphia: WB Saunders.)

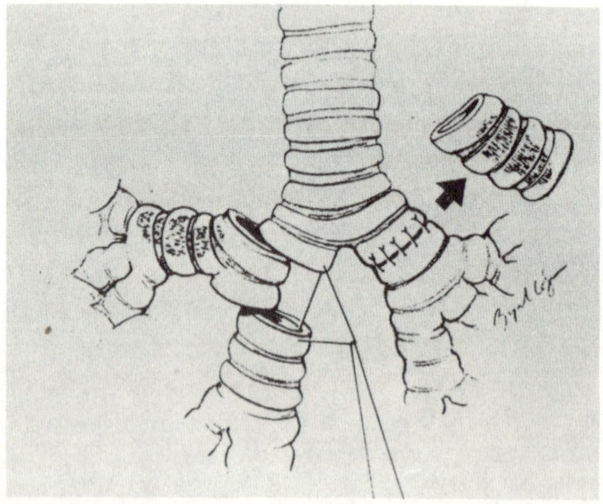

Figure 29-18. Two common types of bronchial sleeve resection, one with right upper lobectomy (e.g., for carcinoma) and the other of left main bronchus without pulmonary resection (e.g., for carcinoid) (92). (Reprinted with permission from Frist, WH, et al. 1987. Bronchial sleeve resection with and without pulmonary resection. *J Thorac Cardiovasc Surg* 93:350–357.)

ing cause of cancer death in both men and women (9). Thirty-five percent of cancer deaths in men, 93,000 cases, and 20% in women, 46,000 cases, are due to bronchogenic cancer; 30,000 of these deaths in 1985 were in patients older than 75 years (9). Interestingly, while the elderly are at greater risk for lung cancer, they are also more likely to have it detected at a localized stage (94, 95). O'Rourke and colleagues (96) found this to pertain regardless of sex, race, histologic subtype, and whether clinically or surgically staged. Selective screening for lung cancer may, therefore, be worthwhile in the elderly.

Similarly, age should not be a barrier to accurate diagnosis and staging, although the data of Teeter et al. (97) show that in reality there is marked decrease in histologic confirmation of lung cancer with increasing age. Bronchoscopy or percutaneous needle biopsy will generally provide a microscopic diagnosis and staging may commence. With small cell undifferentiated carcinoma, a search for distant metastases (bone, liver, and brain scans; bone marrow aspirate) is worthwhile, but with non-small cell carcinoma—in the absence of symptoms, signs, or abnormal blood studies—this evaluation is less productive. One should have a low threshhold, however, for assessing the mediastinum in the elderly patient, for this will allow selection for surgery, and its attendant risks, those who will most benefit. Both mediastinoscopy (98) and anterior mediastinotomy (99) are safe in all age groups and can be complemented by CT and other scans (100).

Untreated lung cancer in the elderly leads to a 7% survival at 1 year (101)—a time period far exceeded by the life expectancy of even octogenarians and nonagenarians (102). Hence, treatment in the form of resection, radiotherapy, chemotherapy, or a combination should be offered. Few would disagree that resection presents the best chance for cure in lung cancer, as well as the highest risk of morbidity and mortality. Is this risk higher in the elderly? Is the chance of cure less?

Most, but not all, studies have found an increased risk of perioperative complications, particularly cardiorespiratory ones in the elderly. Keagy et al. (44), in their review of elective pulmonary lobectomy, reported that 50% of patients over 60 years had complications compared to 35% of those under 60; this did not, however, lead to increased mortality, as the problems resolved with good postoperative care. In Nagasaki's (103) series, patients over the age of 70 had a significantly higher major complication rate, 18%, compared to those under 70, 9%. The majority of complications occurring in the 33% of patients aged 70 to 93 in Breyer's (41) report were minor (atrial fibrillation, retained secretions, air leak for over 1 week) and responded well to treatment. A more recent study (104) found no statistical difference in complications or length of hospital stay between a group over age 70 and one under age 70.

Operative mortality for lung cancer resections performed in the 1940 to 1980 decades range from 5% to 9% for lobectomy to 11% to 16% for pneumonectomy (105, 106); more recent data from the Lung Cancer Study Group (LCSG) (107) showed a 2.9% mortality for lobectomy, 6.2% for pneumonectomy, 3.7% overall. Although comparable rates for the elderly vary a great deal by series (Table 29-1), it is clear that the risk of operative death does increase with age, to the 7% to 10% range. The LCSG study directly compared three different age groups and found the following mortality rates: age less than 60 years, 1.3%; 60 to 69 years, 4.1%; 70 years or greater, 7.1% (107). Virtually all deaths are from cardiopulmonary causes such as pneumonia, respiratory insufficiency, myocardial infarction, and congestive heart failure.

Extent of resection appears to be a strong determinant of operative mortality in the older patient, with decreasing risk from pneumonectomy to lobectomy to segmentectomy and wedge resection (the last two often termed "limited resections"). Breyer et al. (41), for example, performed segmentectomy on 52 patients over age 70 with 2% operative mortality. There is also accumulating evidence that, for the selected small, early-stage lesion in which it is appropriately employed, limited resection does not sacrifice the chance of cure (41, 108–110) (Fig. 29-19). In keeping with this principle of sparing functioning lung tissue, sleeve lobectomy should be performed where possible instead of pneumonectomy. Finally, it is again noted that concomitant *en bloc* chest wall resection, while often appropriate, does add more to the operative

Table 29-1. Pulmonary resection for bronchogenic carcinoma, age ≥ 70 years

Author (reference)	Number of cases	Operative mortality (%)	5-Year survival (%)
Sensenig (1966) (157)	33	12	30
Golebiowski (1971) (158)	50	8	—
Didolkar (1974) (159)	50	36	—
Kirsh (1976) (160)	58	14	30
Harviel (1978) (161)	22	18	—
Breyer (1981) (41)	150	4	27
Ginsberg (1983)[a] (107)	453	7	—
Raychaudhury (1983) (162)	16	19	—
Berggren (1984) (46)	82	16	35
Keagy (1984) (57)	43	2.3	—
Yellin (1985) (40)	58	10	40
Sherman (1987) (104)	63	10	36
	1078	10	—

[a]Combined Lung Cancer Study Group (LCSG) data.

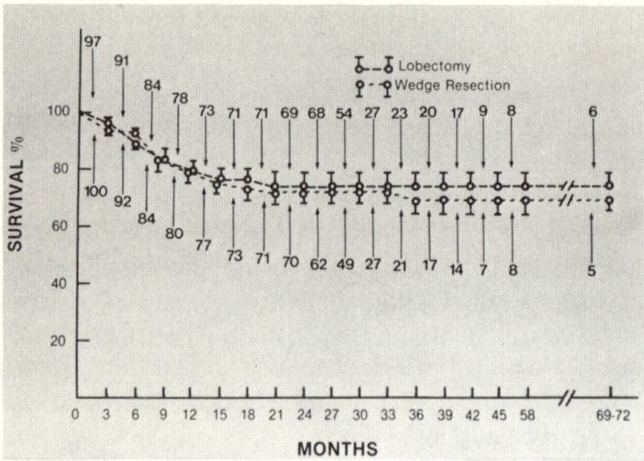

Figure 29-19. Cumulative survival rates (life table analysis) in patients undergoing either lobectomy or wedge resection for Stage I non-small cell bronchogenic carcinoma. Numbers indicate patients at risk at the start of each interval (108). (Reprinted with permission from Errett, LE, et al. 1985. Wedge resection as an alternative procedure for peripheral bronchogenic carcinoma in poor-risk patients. *J Thorac Cardiovasc Surg* 90:656–661.)

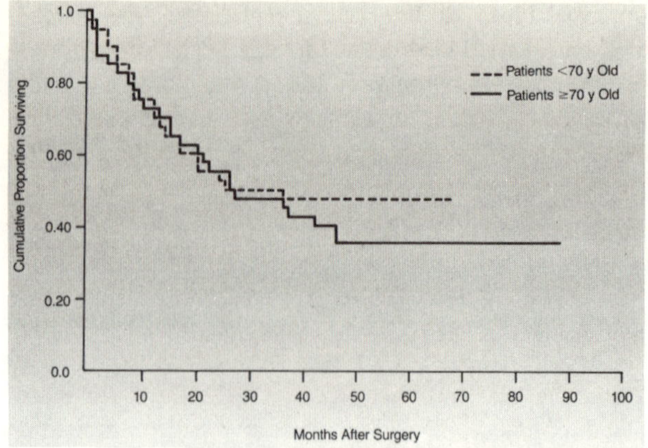

Figure 29-20. Actuarial survival curves following lung cancer resection for 75 patients under age 70 and 64 patients age 70 or older. No significant difference was demonstrated, $p = .55$ (104). (Reprinted with permission from Sherman, S and Guidot, CE. 1987. The feasibility of thoracotomy for lung cancer in the elderly. *JAMA* 258:927–930. Copyright 1987, American Medical Association.)

risk in the elderly than in their younger counterparts (see earlier section on "Chest Wall").

Technical aspects of lung resection in the elderly that merit emphasis are one-lung anesthesia; proper exposure with resection of a rib if necessary; delicate handling of tissues, especially pulmonary artery branches; use of the linear stapling device without blade to divide incomplete fissures or in wedge resections where the lung is emphysematous (this leaves four rows of fine staples on the remaining lung instead of two); and postoperative therapeutic flexible bronchoscopy if needed. Prevention of poorly tolerated complications is foremost in this age group.

The good news is that the chance of long-term survival following resection in the elderly is equivalent to that in the younger patient (Table 29-1 and Fig. 29-20): 30% to 35% 5-year survival. This lack of difference pertains regardless of the stage of the cancer (104).

The use of radiotherapy—either as adjunct to resection in the patient with nodal involvement or as primary treatment—differs little from its use in a younger patient. Great care must be taken, however, to limit the dose to surrounding lung tissue (111). Brachytherapy (i.e., endobronchial radiotherapy) shows promise in its ability to deliver reasonable doses to the tumor while limiting that given to normal tissues (Fig. 29-21). Combination chemotherapy for metastatic non-small cell carcinoma (112) or as primary treatment for small cell carcinoma (113) can benefit even the elderly patient with multiple medical problems. For the patient with recurrence of endobronchial carcinoma, laser bronchoscopic resection with or without subsequent brachytherapy may be indicated (114). To date, the author has performed over 80 such re-

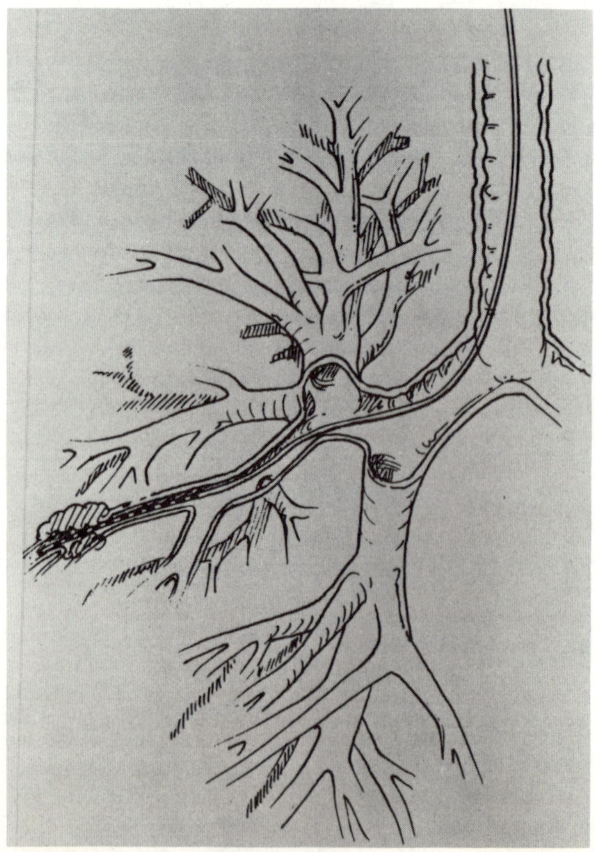

Figure 29-21. Endobronchial radiotherapy (brachytherapy) through a bronchoscopically placed catheter delivers high doses to the lung cancer while limiting radiation to normal tissues (151). (Reprinted with permission from Speiser, BH. 1987. Remote afterloading at Humana Hospital, Phoenix. *Activity Newsletter* (Nucletron Corporation 1:3–4.)

sections with two deaths (intraoperative bleeding; respiratory failure at 2 weeks) and fair to excellent palliation in the remainder (Fig. 29-22).

Surgery, therefore, has much to offer the geriatric patient with bronchogenic carcinoma. Although the risks of morbidity and mortality are somewhat higher than in younger patients, they are still acceptable and are equal to the risks surgeons were relating to all patients in the recent past. Moreover, the chance of cure is equivalent to that in the young and remains superior to any other treatment. Resection should be offered to the appropriately staged, well-informed elderly patient with lung cancer.

Tuberculosis

Tuberculosis can affect the elderly in atypical ways and may be underdiagnosed in this age group generally. Stead and To (115) found that in Arkansas the age-specific rate for persons over 65 living at home was three times greater than that for individuals aged 40 to 60 years; for the elderly in nursing homes, the age-specific rate increased another four times. This has implications for differential diagnosis in the elderly patient with hemoptysis or upper lobe infiltrates, but also may result in a larger group of patients with less typical presentations. Pleural tuberculosis, for example, is more common in older adults, often causing exudative pleural effusions (81). Lower lung field tuberculosis also occurs more often in older patients and frequently has endobronchial involvement (116). One cannot depend on skin testing to suggest the diagnosis, since there is significant, progressive loss of tuberculin sensitivity with advancing age (117). Pleural fluid culture and pleural biopsy should therefore be performed in the older adult with undiagnosed effusion, and tuberculosis should be remembered in the elderly individual with mucosal ulceration, stenosis, or submucosal infiltration at bronchoscopy.

Other Lung Disease

Spontaneous pneumothorax occurs in the young and is associated with subpleural blebs. In an older group, it is associated with bullous emphysema. Treatment of the pneumothorax itself does not differ greatly between the two, but physicians need to be aware of the possible association of carcinoma with the bleb in the older patient. Scannell (118), after finding four such cases in his practice, treats with suspicion any parenchymal lesion associated with large bullae in the elderly. Steinhäuslin and Cuttat (119) discovered 6 carcinomas in 338 patients with spontaneous pneumothorax and analyzed 46 others from the literature; they recommend cancer evaluation for the adult smoker with bullous emphysema and incomplete lung expansion after tube thoracostomy.

A group of patients can be selected who will benefit from resection of pulmonary metastases of carcinomas or sarcomas. The elderly tolerate such resections well (120).

Esophagus

Esophageal Carcinoma

Cancer of the esophagus represents only 1% to 2% of all cancers in the United States. It is a particularly morbid disease, and if left untreated, leads to a wasting death from dysphagia, malnutrition, and then pneumonia. It accounts for 9800 new cases and 9100 deaths annually (9). This has long been considered a disease of the elderly. The first patient to undergo successful transthoracic resection

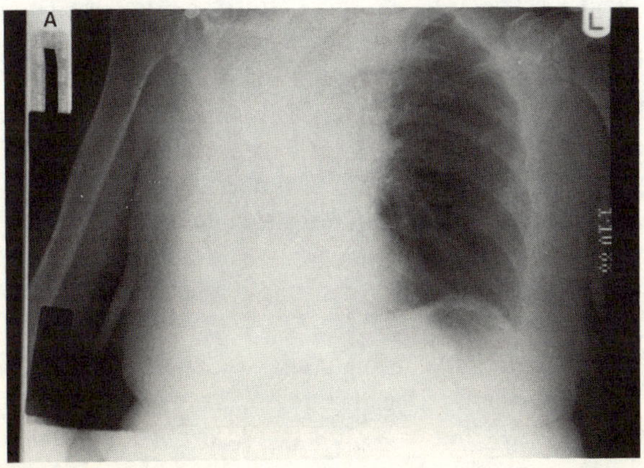

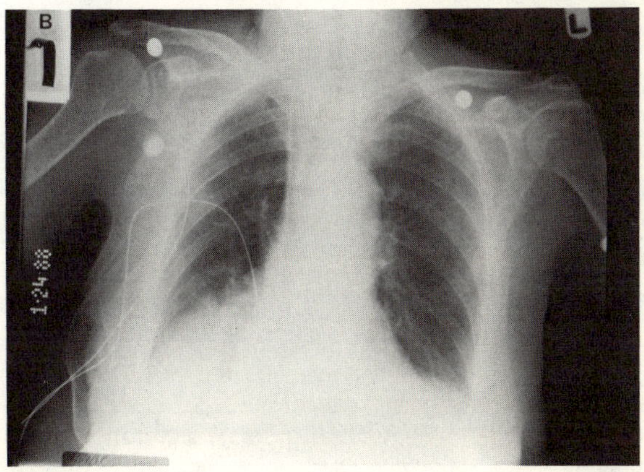

Figure 29-22. 72-year-old woman with inoperable obstructing carcinoma in right main stem bronchus and severe dyspnea. A, Chest radiograph before laser bronchoscopy showing complete right lung collapse; B, after laser bronchoscopy showing re-expansion of right lung.

(121) was a 67-year-old woman (Fig. 29-23); in Sweet's (122) pioneering series of esophageal resections with high intrathoracic esophagogastric anastomosis, half of the patients were older than 65 years. Although the mean age of these patients presently remains 63 to 65 years, it is common to see patients in their 80s and 90s (27, 123).

True esophageal cancer is squamous cell carcinoma (124), but adenocarcinoma arising at the gastroesophageal junction is often included since its surgical treatment is similar. Most patients are smokers and/or drinkers and suffer from dysphagia and weight loss. Barium swallow (Fig. 29-24) and esophagoscopy are nearly always diagnostic, for the cancer is rarely in an early stage. For an overview of esophageal cancer, the reader is referred to general review articles (27, 125). As in bronchogenic carcinoma, surgery remains the mainstay of treatment, although the goal of treatment here is as much palliation of dysphagia as it is cure. Can the elderly patient, however, tolerate such extensive surgery?

Referring to Sweet's work in his 1948 Shattuck Lecture, "Surgery in the Aged," C. Stuart Welch stated that "The results obtained in the surgical treatment of cancer of the esophagus not only are remarkable in themselves but also offer the most convincing evidence supporting a contention that advanced age is not at all an insurmountable obstacle to radical extirpative surgery for cancer" (126). More recently Sugimachi et al. (127) studied 231 resected patients and compared three different age groups (under age 59; 60 to 69; over 70). Resectability did not differ, averaging 59%. Pulmonary complications were significantly higher in the over-70 group (55% versus 34% and 37%) but other complications, including anastomotic leakage, did not differ. Mortality was higher in the over-70 group (14% versus 4% and 6%), chiefly from pneumonia in patients with poor preoperative lung function, and survival rate did not differ, averaging 26% at 5 years after curative resection. Other authors have confirmed the increased risk of pulmonary complications after esophagectomy in the elderly (128, 129), although in the studies of Mohansingh (130), and Williamson (129), advanced age did not increase the risks of either anastomotic leak or death. Nishi et al. (131) found that preoperative degree of organ impairment, rather than age per se, was most predictive of postoperative problems.

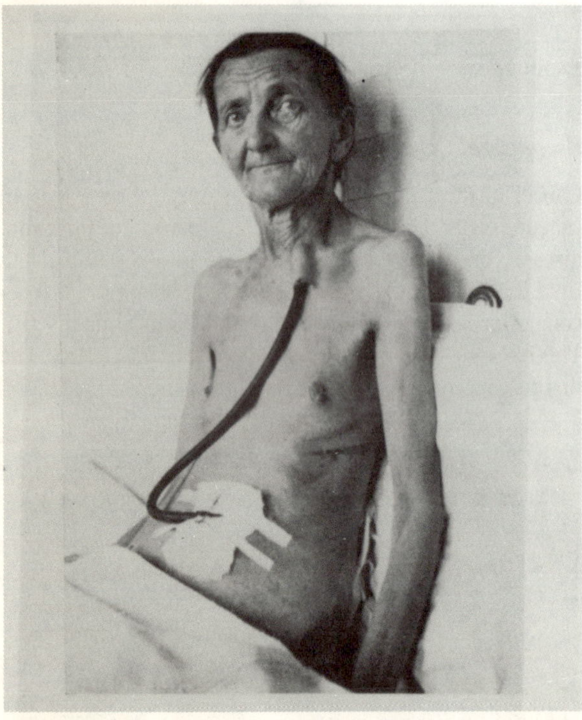

Figure 29-23. Torek's first transthoracic esophagectomy patient. This 67-year-old woman was able to eat bread, cereal, potatoes, and eggs through the removable external tube connecting cervical esophagostomy and gastrostomy; she died of pneumonia 13 years following resection of her Stage III midesophageal carcinoma (121). (Reprinted with permission from Torek, F. 1913. The first successful case of resection of the thoracic portion of the esophagus for carcinoma. *Surg Gynecol Obstet* 16:614–617.)

There are advocates of stapled anastomoses and of transhiatal resections to spare the patient a thoracotomy, but the author prefers transthoracic resection under direct vision and a careful hand-sewn, two-layer anastomosis of fine silk. Mathisen et al. (132) recently presented their results using this approach in 104 consecutive resections: there were 3 deaths (2.9%) and no anastomotic leaks.

Alternatives to resection in the poor-risk patient include radiotherapy, chemotherapy, endoesophageal prosthetic tube placement, endoscopic laser resection, brachytherapy, or combinations of these; these treatments are similar regardless of patient age.

It appears, then, that the elderly patient undergoing esophagectomy is at increased risk for pulmonary complications, particularly if he or she already has impaired lung function, but this may or may not lead to increased mortality. The chances of long-term cure and relief of dysphagia do not differ from those of a younger patient and are better with resection than with the alternatives. Adjunctive radiotherapy and chemotherapy regimens may further improve survival in the near future.

Hiatus Hernia and Gastroesophageal Reflux

Hiatus hernia, protrusion of the stomach through the esophageal hiatus of the diaphragm, is often classified according to whether or not the gastroesophageal junction remains intra-abdominal: Type I (sliding), Type II (paraesophageal), Type III (combined sliding and paraesophageal) (Fig. 29-25). The prevalence of *Type I or sliding hernias* increases with age, and patients with this disorder

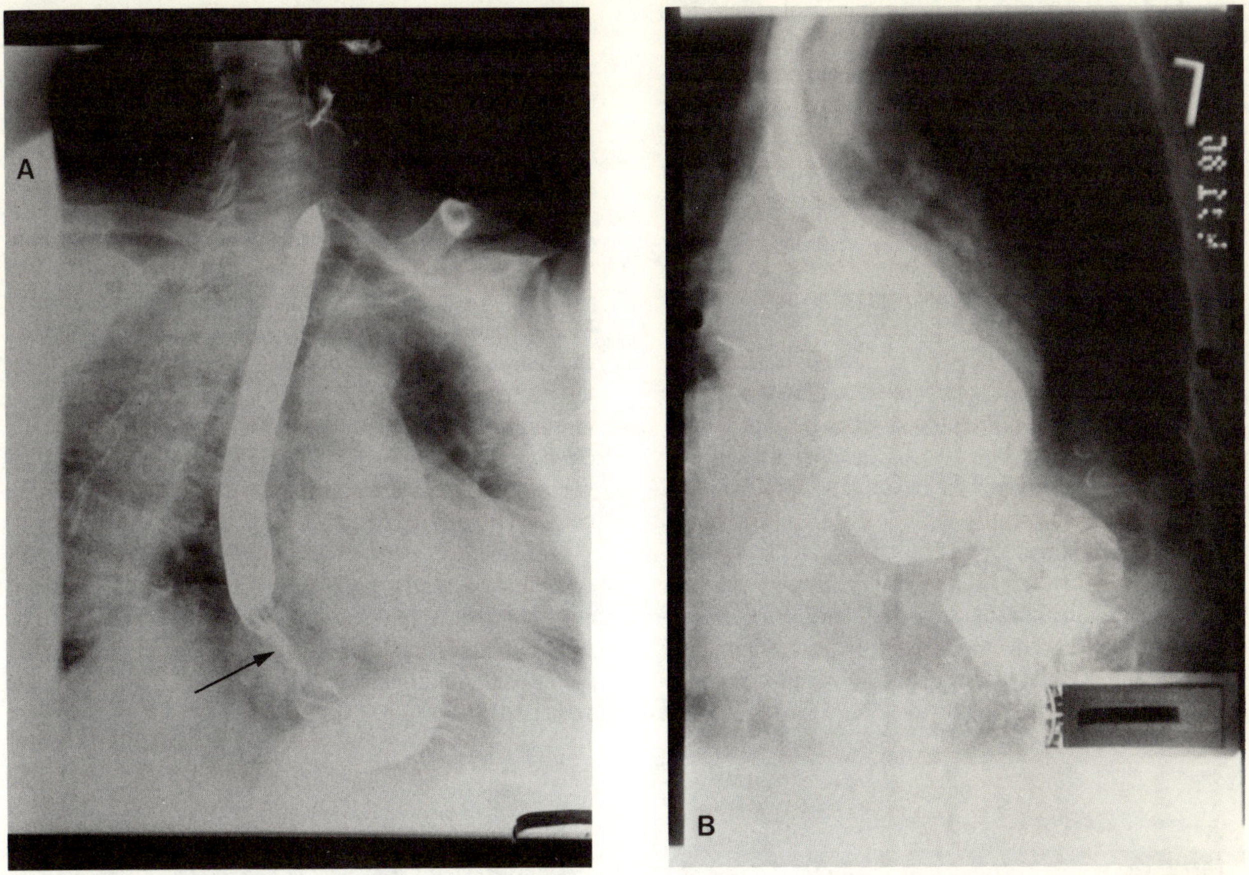

Figure 29-24. Barium swallows of esophageal carcinoma (arrow) in an 82-year-old woman. A, Preoperative radiograph; B, following left thoracoabdominal esophagogastrectomy and esophagogastrostomy in chest.

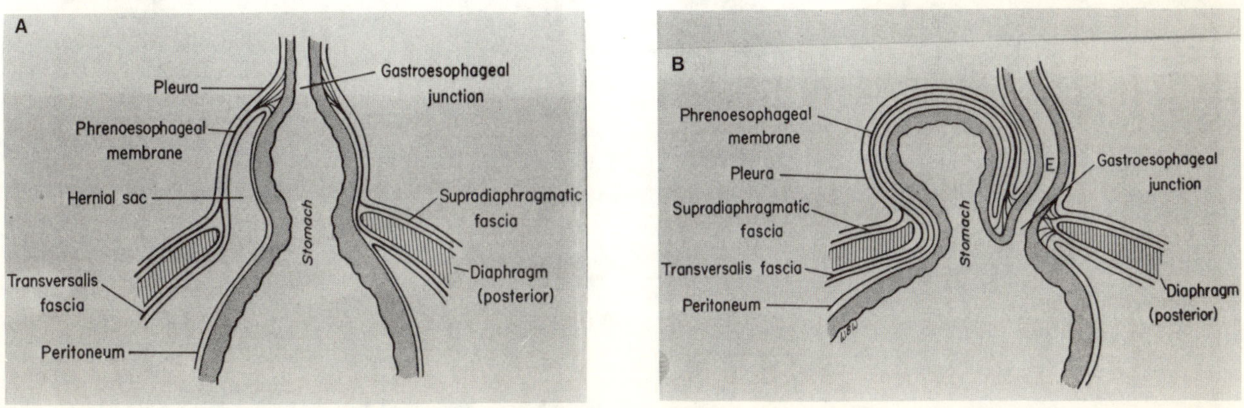

Figure 29-25. Types of hiatus hernia. A, Sliding (Type I) hiatus hernia; B, paraesophageal (Type II) hiatus hernia. Note normal position of gastroesophageal junction in B (152). (Reprinted with permission from Andersen, HA, and Payne, WS. 1974. Esophageal hiatal hernia, gastroesophageal reflux, and their complications. In *The Esophagus,* Eds., WS Payne and AM Olsen. Philadelphia: Lea & Febiger.)

may or may not experience gastroesophageal reflux. It is beyond the scope of this chapter to fully discuss the pathophysiology of reflux or its medical and surgical management (133, 134). Advanced age does not, however, appear to significantly increase the risk of hiatus herniorrhaphy. Mohansingh (130) had no mortality in 35 patients over age 70 who underwent hiatus herniorrhaphy, and had one death from pulmonary embolus in 10 patients who required esophageal resection for benign peptic stricture.

Whereas non-operative management may offer an alternative for the poor-risk patient with sliding hernia and reflux, the individual with a large *Type II (paraesophageal) or Type III (combined) hernia* should have operative repair. Often the entire stomach becomes incarcerated in the chest (Fig. 29-26), leading not only to symptoms of dysphagia, nausea, or substernal pain but also to potential catastrophe in the form of acute bleeding, aspiration pneumonia, or gastric strangulation and gangrene. Hill (135) had no mortality with elective repairs or in acute cases where nasogastric decompression was successful, allowing adequate preoperative correction of dehydration and anemia; when emergency repair was necessary, mortality was 50%. Pearson et al. (136) found that postoperative complications in their 53 cases (52 elective, one emergency) were few despite the advanced age of the patients; there was one death, from massive aspiration.

Other Esophageal Disorders

Esophageal perforation can be caused by iatrogenic instrumentation, forceful or prolonged emesis (Boerhaave's syndrome), foreign body, or external trauma. In separate Mayo Clinic studies of instrumental perforations and Boerhaave's syndrome, the mean patient age was an identical 62 years (137, 138). The strongest determinant of morbidity and mortality is delay in operative repair and drainage (29), although Postlethwait (139) found that advanced age also increased risk of death in 191 collective cases of Boerhaave's rupture (Fig. 29-27).

Motor disorders of the esophagus and *esophageal diverticula* occur in the elderly but are treated no differently from those in the young. *Cervical spondylotic dysphagia* is a rare condition caused by the osteophytes common to older individuals; spur excision may occasionally be needed (140).

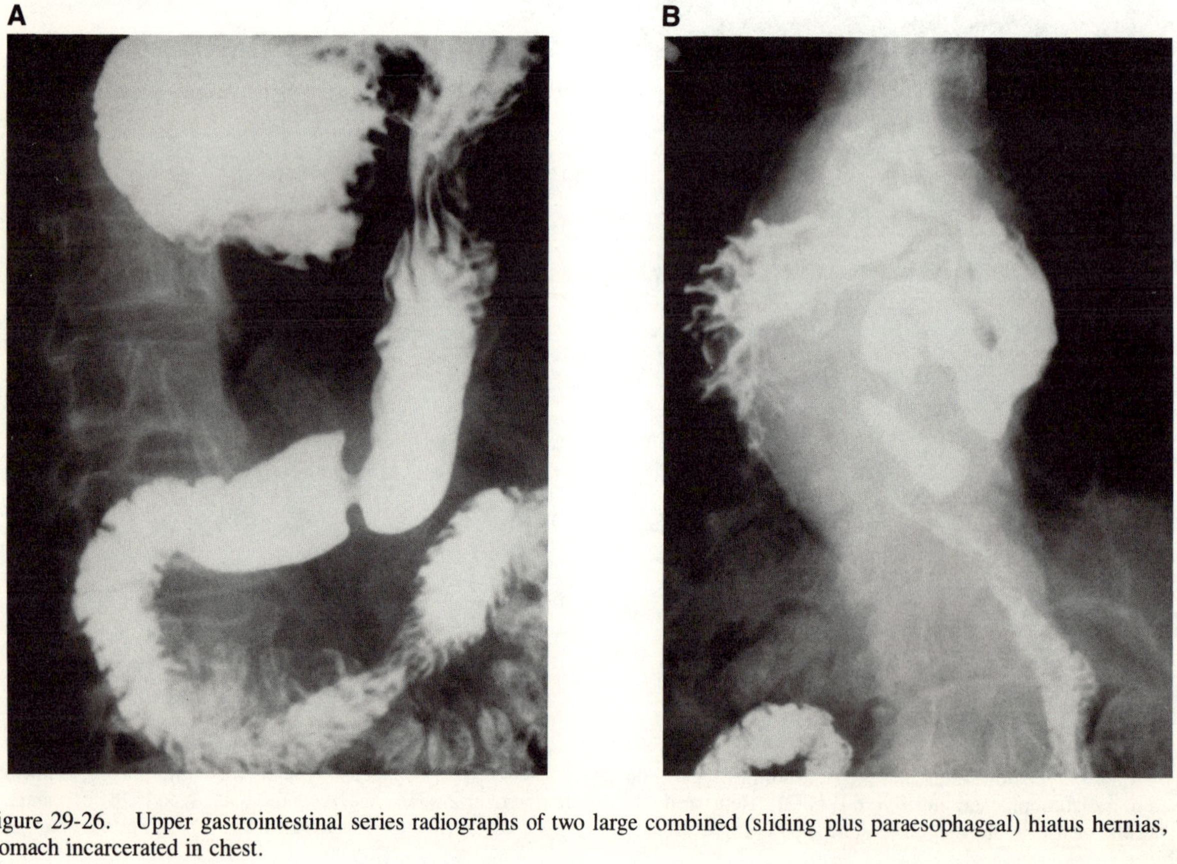

Figure 29-26. Upper gastrointestinal series radiographs of two large combined (sliding plus paraesophageal) hiatus hernias, with stomach incarcerated in chest.

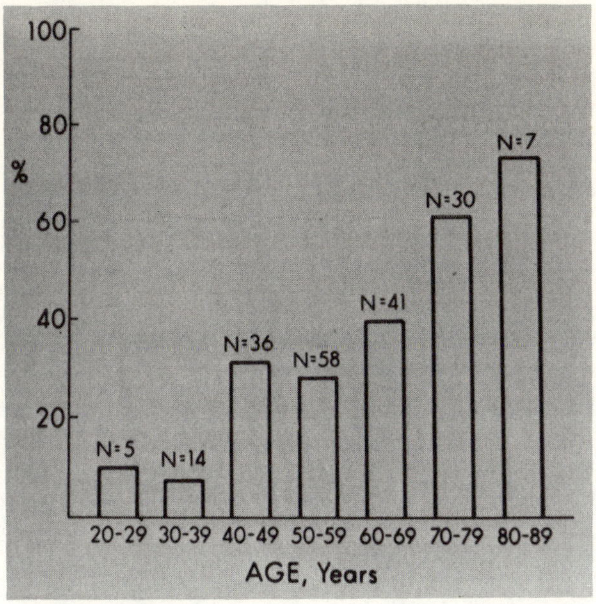

Figure 29-27. Mortality as a function of age in 191 collected cases of spontaneous (post-emetic) esophageal rupture (139). (Reprinted with permission from Postlethwait, RW. 1979. Perforation and rupture. In *Surgery of the Esophagus*, Ed., RW Postlethwait. New York: Appleton-Century-Crofts.)

Mediastinum

Thymus

The two chief indications for thymectomy are thymoma and myasthenia gravis, and occasionally the two coexist. The incidence of myasthenia gravis in patients with thymoma is about 30% to 35%; the incidence of thymoma in patients with myasthenia is about 15% (141).

Located in the anterior and superior mediastinum—thus often detected on chest radiograph or CT scan (Fig. 29-28)—*thymoma* is among the most common mediastinal masses. Its bland cytologic appearance and slow growth belie an unpredictable behavior. Consequently "malignancy" in a thymoma is based more on its extent (e.g., invasion of surrounding structures, lack of a capsule, rare metastasis) than on its histology (142). Thymomas generally affect middle-aged and elderly individuals (although the presence of myasthenia gravis seems to lead to earlier detection) (Fig. 29-29). Thymomas should be widely resected with total thymectomy via sternotomy or thoracotomy, and operative risk is unrelated to age alone. Fifty-two resections over 10 years at the Toronto General Hospital resulted in no operative deaths (143). Radiotherapy is worthwhile perioperatively for the exten-

A

B

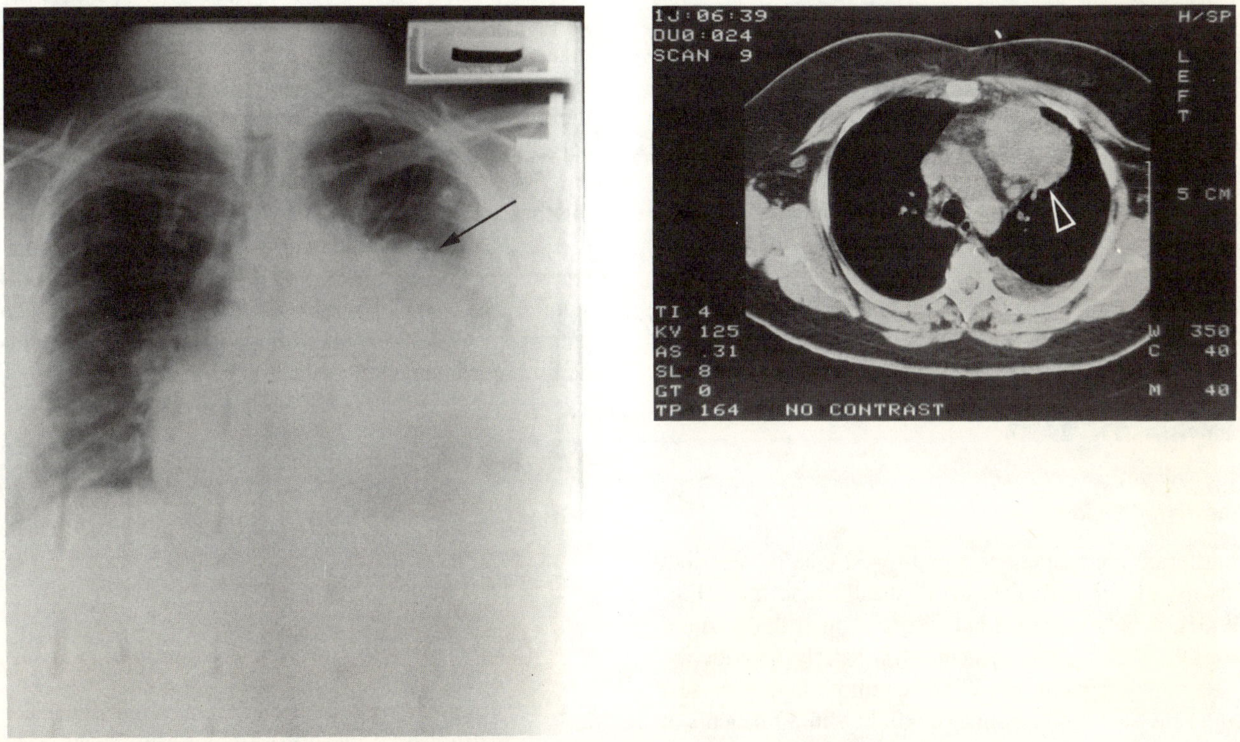

Figure 29-28. Spindle cell thymoma (arrows) of left anterior mediastinum. A, Chest radiograph; B, computed tomographic scan.

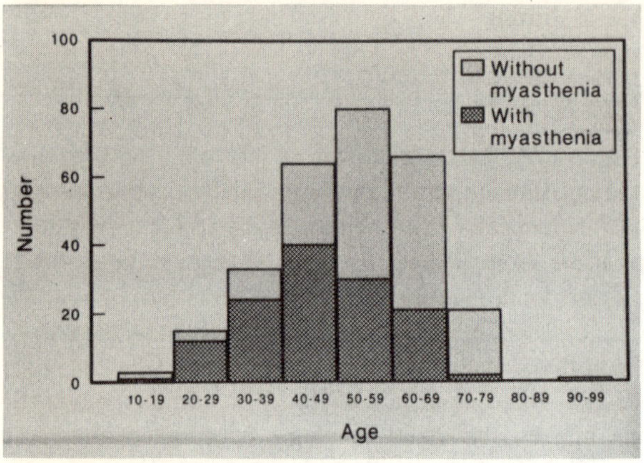

Figure 29-29. Age at time of diagnosis of thymoma. The presence of myasthenia gravis may lead to earlier detection (142). (Reprinted with permission from Lewis, JE, et al. 1987. Thymoma: A clinicopathologic review. *Cancer* 60:2727–2743.)

sive tumor and as primary treatment in the inoperable patient. Although it was once thought that the presence of myasthenia gravis adversely affected prognosis in these patients, recent reports have disputed this (143, 156). Improved medical management of myasthenia and better postoperative care may be responsible.

In 1941, Blalock presented six patients in whom thymectomy had been performed, not for evidence of any mediastinal mass, but simply to affect the course of *myasthenia gravis* (144). This procedure is now an accepted treatment for myasthenia gravis and, although precise patient selection criteria may be debated, it appears that the patient population that will potentially benefit is broadening (145). Monden et al. (146), in a clinical study and literature review, found that the clinical effects of thymectomy in elderly subjects did not differ statistically from those in young patients and concluded that "Thymectomy should be performed in all elderly patients with myasthenia gravis." Both transcervical and transsternal approaches are safe for all ages; the author prefers a short upper sternotomy to ensure complete resection under direct vision (Fig. 29-30).

Substernal Goiter

Substernal goiter, defined as a thyroid enlargement that has its greater mass inferior to the thoracic inlet (Fig. 29-31), is most common in patients in the fifth decade of life but is frequently seen in more elderly individuals. With rare exceptions, these can be removed via a cervical collar incision with minimal morbidity. In 80 patients at the Massachusetts General Hospital, for example, there were no deaths or major complications and patients were discharged in 3 to 4 days (31). Given the small but present risks of acute stridor and occult malignancy and a negligible operative risk, resection can be recommended for patients of any age. A collective review of this subject has been published (32).

Other Mediastinal Masses

Other types of mediastinal masses include neurogenic tumors, cysts, lymphoma, germ cell tumors, and metastatic carcinoma. The incidences of these masses in general and of malignant ones in particular appear to peak in middle age, but they are still commonly seen in the elderly. Open biopsy or resection are usually indicated and can be considered safe regardless of age per se. Of 400 cases in a recent report from Duke University, mortality was 0.8% overall, and there were no deaths in the last 26 years (155).

Summary

Aging cardiopulmonary physiology is such that the elderly are often well at rest but, with diminished reserve, respond suboptimally to stress. It can be anticipated that the procedures most likely to apply such stress (e.g., pneumonectomy with *en bloc* chest wall resection, thoracoabdominal esophagogastrectomy, etc.) will embody concomitant increased risk of complications, particularly pulmonary complications. For most chest surgical conditions, however, surgery still offers survival and palliation significantly superior to the alternatives. Thus, modern thoracic surgeons must become, of necessity, geriatric surgeons.

Most chest surgery in the elderly is elective, allowing time for optimal preoperative preparation. This, combined with compulsive attention to operative technique and to every detail of postoperative care, will lead to results in the aged comparable to those in the young. The patient's age should neither be ignored nor feared by today's thoracic surgeon.

References

1. Majno, G. 1975. *The Healing Hand: Man and Wound in the Ancient World.* Cambridge: Harvard University Press.
2. Gross, SD. 1864. *System of Surgery,* ed. 3. Philadelphia: Blanchard and Lea.
3. Agnew, DH. 1881. *The Principles and Practice of Surgery.* Philadelphia-London: JB Lippincott.
4. Meltzer, SJ, and Auer, J. 1909. Eine Vergleichung der "Volhardschen Methode der Kunstilichen Atmung." Mit der von Meltzer und Auer in der Kontinuelichen Bewegungen Verwendeten Methode. *Zentrable Physiol* 22:442.

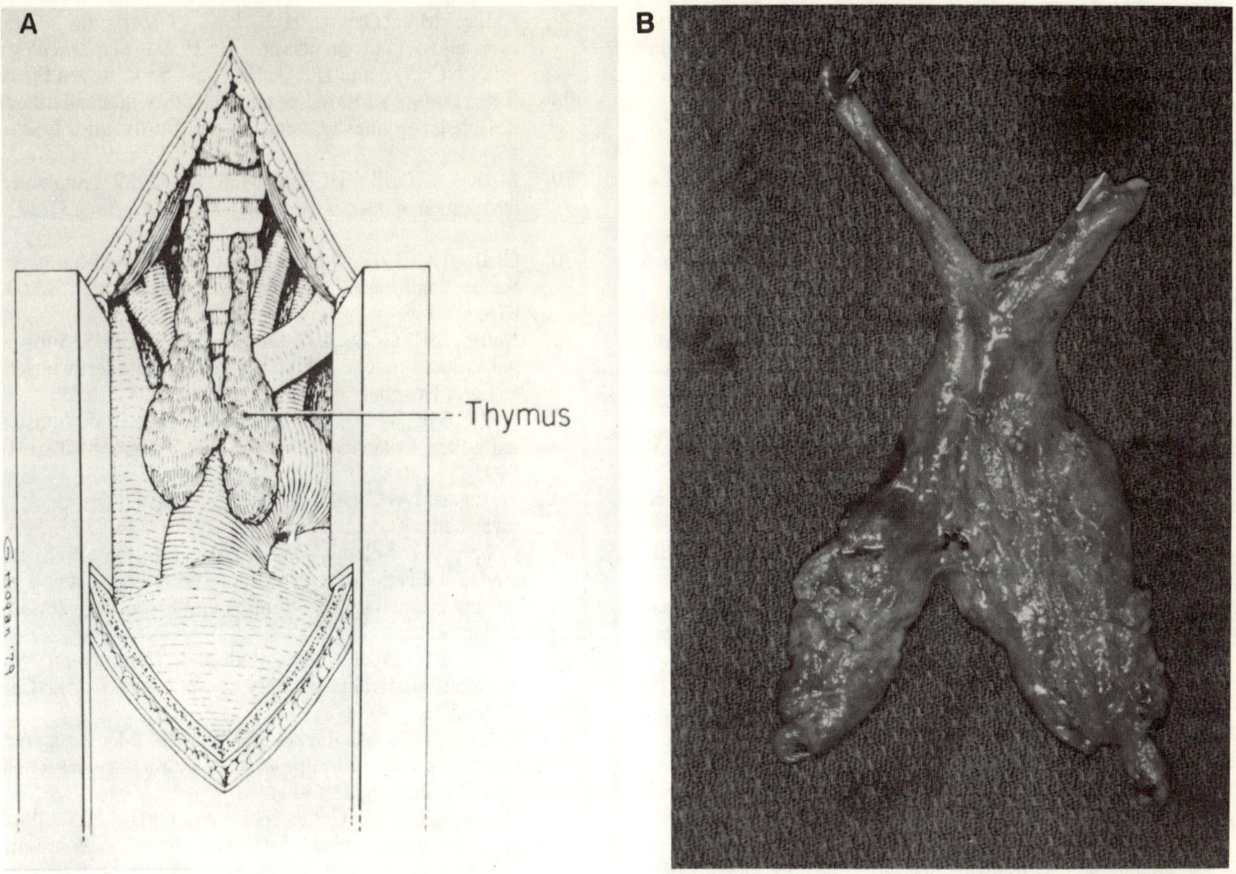

Figure 29-30. Thymectomy via upper sternotomy. A, Operative exposure with small retractor in place (153). (Reprinted with permission from Miller JI, et al. 1982. Median sternotomy T incision for thymectomy in myasthenia gravis. *Ann Thorac Surg* 34:473–474.) B, resected thymus gland.

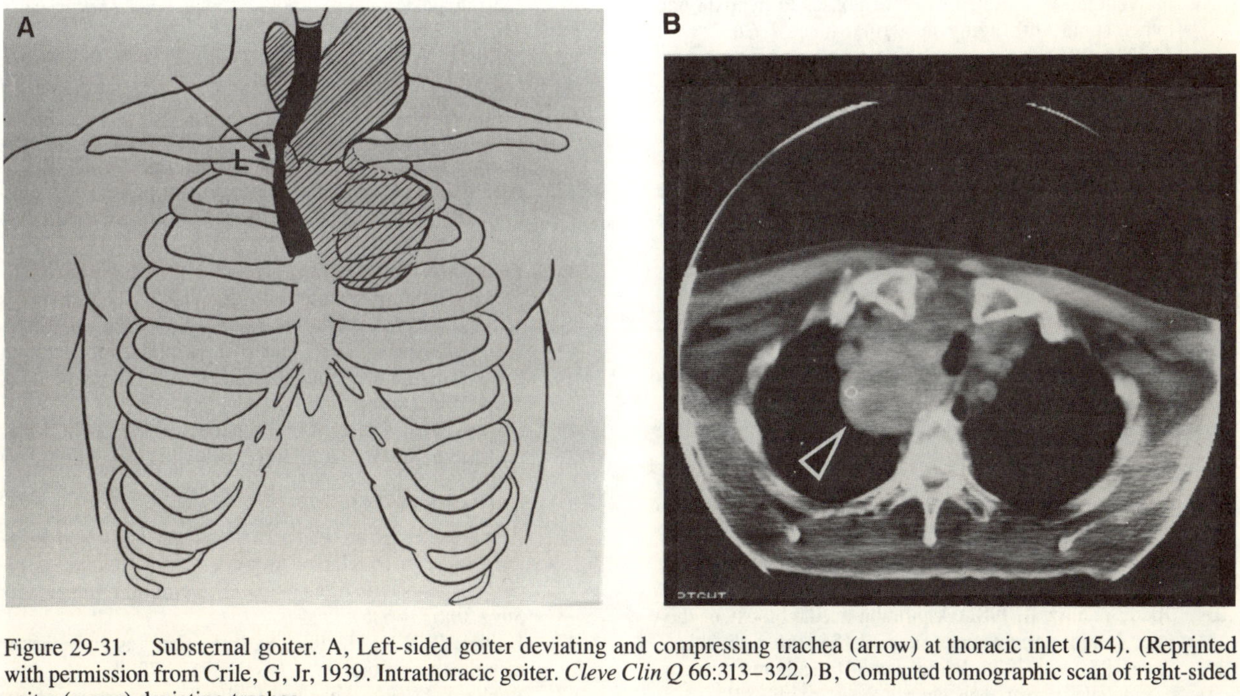

Figure 29-31. Substernal goiter. A, Left-sided goiter deviating and compressing trachea (arrow) at thoracic inlet (154). (Reprinted with permission from Crile, G, Jr, 1939. Intrathoracic goiter. *Cleve Clin Q* 66:313–322.) B, Computed tomographic scan of right-sided goiter (arrow) deviating trachea.

5. Sauerbruch, F. 1904. Über die physiologischen und physikalischen Grundlagen bei intrathorakalen Eingriffen in meiner pneumatischen Operationskammer. *Arch Klin Chir* 77:977–987.
6. Lilienthal, H. 1926. *Thoracic Surgery.* Philadelphia: WB Saunders.
7. Ochsner, A. 1967. Is risk of operation too great in the elderly? *Geriatrics* 22:121–130.
8. Ochsner, A. 1978. The development of pulmonary surgery, with special emphasis on carcinoma and bronchiectasis. *Am J Surg* 135:732–746.
9. Silverberg, E, and Lubera, J. 1988. Cancer Statistics, 1988. *CA* 38:5–22.
10. Baranovsky, A, and Myers, MH. 1986. Cancer incidence and survival in patients 65 years of age and older. *CA* 36:27–41.
11. Feldman, AR, et al. 1986. The prevalence of cancer. *N Engl J Med* 315:1394–1397.
12. Hutchinson, J. 1846. On the capacity of the lung, and on the respiratory functions, with a view of establishing a precise and easy method of detecting disease by the spirometer. *Med Chir Trans Lond* 29:137–232.
13. Lefrak, SS, and Campbell, EJ. 1981. Structure and function of the aging respiratory system. In *Pulmonary Disease in the Adult.* Ed., DR Gracey. Chicago: Yearbook Medical Publishers.
14. Murray, JF. 1976. Aging. In *The Normal Lung*. Philadelphia: WB Saunders.
15. Peterson, DD, et al. 1981. Effects of aging on ventilatory and occlusion pressure responses to hypoxia and hypercapnia. *Am Rev Respir Dis* 124:387–391.
16. Rodeheffer, RJ, et al. 1984. Exercise cardiac output is maintained with advancing age in healthy human subjects: Cardiac dilation and increased stroke volume compensate for diminished heart rate. *Circulation* 69:203–213.
17. Kronenberg, RS, and Drage, CW. 1973. Attenuation of the ventilatory and heart rate responses to hypoxia and hypercapnia with aging in normal men. *J Clin Invest* 52:1812–1819.
18. Gerstenblith, G, Lakatta, EG, and Weisfeldt, ML. 1976. Age changes in myocardial function and exercise response. *Progr Cardiovasc Dis* 19:1–21.
19. Killian, G. 1902. Direct endoscopy of the upper air passages and oesophagus: Its diagnostic and therapeutic value in the search for and removal of foreign bodies. *J Laryngol Rhinol Otol* 18:461.
20. Jackson, C. 1905. Foreign bodies in the trachea, bronchi, and oesophagus: The aid of oesophagoscopy, bronchoscopy and magnetism in their extraction. *Laryngoscope* 15:247.
21. Jackson, C. 1928. Bronchoscopy: Past, present and future. *N Engl J Med* 199:759.
22. Ikeda, S, Yawai, N, and Ishikawa, S. 1968. Flexible bronchofiberscope. *Keio J Med* 17:1.
23. Credle, WF Jr, Smiddy, JF, and Elliott, RC. 1974. Complications of fiberoptic bronchoscopy. *Am Rev Respir Dis* 109:67–72.
24. Leyden, H. 1883. Über infektios Pneumonie. *Dtsche Med Wochenschr* 9:52–54.
25. Todd, TRJ, et al. 1981. Aspiration needle biopsy of thoracic lesions. *Ann Thorac Surg* 32:154–161.
26. Sagel, SS, et al. 1978. Percutaneous transthoracic aspiration needle biopsy. *Ann Thorac Surg* 26:399–405.
27. Katlic, MR, Grillo, HC. 1983. Carcinoma of the esophagus: A current perspective. In *Thoracic Oncology,* Eds., NC Choi and HC Grillo. New York: Raven Press.
28. Katz, D. 1969. Morbidity and mortality in standard and flexible gastrointestinal endoscopy. *Gastrointest Endosc* 15:134.
29. Michel, L, Grillo, HC, and Malt, RA. 1982. Esophageal perforation: Collective review. *Ann Thorac Surg* 33:203–210.
30. Grillo, HC, 1979. Surgical treatment of post-intubation tracheal injuries. *J Thorac Cardiovasc Surg* 78:860–875.
31. Katlic, MR, Grillo, HC, and Wang, CA. 1985. Substernal goiter: Analysis of 80 patients from Massachusetts General Hospital. *Am J Surg* 149:283–287.
32. Katlic, MR, Wang, CA, and Grillo, HC. 1985. Substernal goiter: Collective review. *Ann Thorac Surg* 39:391–399.
33. Papatestas, AE, et al. 1975. Transcervical thymectomy in myasthenia gravis. *Surg Gynecol Obstet* 140:535–540.
34. Cooper, JD, Nelems, JM, and Pearson, FG. 1978. Extended indications for median sternotomy in patients requiring pulmonary resection. *Ann Thorac Surg* 26:413–420.
35. Meng, RL, et al. 1980. Median sternotomy for synchronous bilateral pulmonary operations. *J Thorac Cardiovasc Surg* 80:1–7.
36. Urschel, HC, and Razzuk, MA. 1986. Median sternotomy as a standard approach for pulmonary resection. *Ann Thorac Surg* 41:130–134.
37. VanderSalm, TJ, Cutler, BS, and Okike, ON. 1982. Brachial plexus injury following median sternotomy: Part II. *J Thorac Cardiovasc Surg* 83:914–917.
38. de la Rocha, AG, and Chambers, K. 1984. Pain amelioration after thoracotomy: A prospective randomized study. *Ann Thorac Surg* 37:239–242.
39. Bethencourt, DM, and Holmes, EC. 1988. Muscle-sparing posterolateral thoracotomy. *Ann Thorac Surg* 45:337–339.
40. Yellin, A, Hill, RL, and Lieberman, Y. 1985. Pulmonary resections in patients over 70 years of age. *Isr J Med Sci* 21:833–840.
41. Breyer, RH, et al. 1981. Thoracotomy in patients over age seventy years. *J Thorac Cardiovasc Surg* 81:187–193.
42. Ali, MK, et al. 1980. Predicting loss of pulmonary function after pulmonary resection for bronchogenic carcinoma. *Chest* 77:337–342.
43. Keagy, BA, et al. 1983. Correlation of preoperative pulmonary function testing with clinical course in patients after pneumonectomy. *Ann Thorac Surg* 36:253–257.
44. Keagy, BA, et al. 1985. Elective pulmonary lobectomy: Factors associated with morbidity and operative mortality. *Ann Thorac Surg* 40:349–352.
45. Boysen, PG, Block, AJ, and Moulder, PV. 1981. Relationship between preoperative pulmonary function tests and complications after thoracotomy. *Surg Gynecol Obstet* 152:813–815.
46. Berggren, H, et al. 1984. Hospital mortality and long-term survival in relation to preoperative function in elderly patients with bronchogenic carcinoma. *Ann Thorac Surg* 38:633–636.
47. Bolton, JWR, et al. 1987. Stair climbing as an indicator of pulmonary function. *Chest* 92:783–788.
48. Bechard, D, and Wetstein, L. 1987. Assessment of ex-

ercise oxygen consumption as preoperative criteria for lung resection. *Ann Thorac Surg* 44:344–349.

49. Linn, BS, Linn, MW, and Wallen, N. 1982. Evaluation of results of surgical procedures in the elderly. *Ann Surg* 195:90–96.
50. Palmberg, S, and Hirsjärvi, E. 1979. Mortality in geriatric surgery. *Gerontology* 25:103–112.
51. Keller, SM, et al. 1987. Emergency and elective surgery in patients over age 70. *Am Surg* 53:636–640.
52. Katlic, MR. 1985. Surgery in centenarians. *JAMA* 253: 3139–3141.
53. Greenburg, AG, et al. 1981. Mortality and gastrointestinal surgery in the aged. *Arch Surg* 116:788–791.
54. Pindyck, J, et al. 1987. Blood donation by the elderly: Clinical and policy considerations. *JAMA* 257:1186–1188.
55. Krowka, MJ, et al. 1987. Cardiac dysrhythmia following pneumonectomy: Clinical correlates and prognostic significance. *Chest* 91:490–495.
56. Mowry, FM, and Reynolds, EW. 1964. Cardiac rhythm disturbances complicating resectional surgery of the lung. *Ann Intern Med* 61:688–695.
57. Keagy, BA, et al. 1984. A review of morbidity and mortality in elderly patients undergoing pulmonary resection. *Am Surg* 50:213–216.
58. Wellington, JL, and Lynn, RB. 1966. Thoracic surgery in the elderly. *Can Med Assoc J* 95:252–256.
59. Carlens, E. 1949. A new flexible double-lumen catheter for bronchospirometry. *J Thorac Surg* 18:742.
60. Robertshaw, FL. 1962. Low resistance double-lumen endobronchial tubes. *Br J Anaesth* 34:576.
61. Lewin, I, et al. 1971. Physical class and physiologic status in the prediction of operative mortality in the aged sick. *Ann Surg* 174:217–231.
62. Coleman, DL. 1987. Control of postoperative pain: Nonnarcotic and narcotic alternatives and their effect on pulmonary function. *Chest* 92:520–528.
63. Hirschler-Schulte, CJW, Hylkemn, BS, and Meyer, RW. 1985. Mechanical ventilation for acute postoperative respiratory failure after surgery for bronchial carcinoma. *Thorax* 40:387–390.
64. Peters, RM. 1984. Pulmonary resection and gas exchange. *J Thorac Cardiovasc Surg* 88:872–879.
65. Zeldin, RA, et al. 1984. Postpneumonectomy pulmonary edema. *J Thorac Cardiovasc Surg* 87:359–365.
66. Wittnich, C, et al. 1986. Misleading "pulmonary wedge pressure" after pneumonectomy: Its importance in postoperative fluid therapy. *Ann Thorac Surg* 42:192–196.
67. Kohman, LJ, et al. 1986. Random versus predictable risks of mortality after thoracotomy for lung cancer. *J Thorac Cardiovasc Surg* 91:551–554.
68. Grillo, HC, Greenberg, JJ, and Wilkins, EW. 1966. Resection of bronchogenic carcinoma involving thoracic wall. *J Thorac Cardiovasc Surg* 51:417–421.
69. Piehler, JM, et al. 1982. Bronchogenic carcinoma with chest wall invasion: Factor affecting survival following *en bloc* resection. *Ann Thorac Surg* 34:684–691.
70. Snyder, A. et al. 1968. Chest wall resection for locally recurrent breast cancer. *Arch Surg* 97:246–253.
71. McKenna, RJ, et al. 1984. A perspective on chest wall resection in patients with breast cancer. *Ann Thorac Surg* 38:482–487.
72. Dingman, RO, and Argenta, LC. 1981. Reconstruction of the chest wall. *Ann Thorac Surg* 32:202–208.
73. Shih, WJ, et al. 1984. Open rib biopsy guided by radionuclide technique. *Ann Thorac Surg* 38:59–62.
74. Breyer, RH, et al. 1984. A prospective study of sternal wound complications. *Ann Thorac Surg* 37:412–416.
75. Talucci, RC, and Webb, WR. 1983. Costal chondritis: The costal arch. *Ann Thorac Surg* 35:318–321.
76. Bloomberg, AE. 1978. Thoracoscopy in perspective (collective review). *Surg Gynecol Obstet* 147:433–442.
77. Austin, EH, and Flye, MW. 1979. The treatment of recurrent malignant pleural effusion (collective review). *Ann Thorac Surg* 28:190–203.
78. Jensik, R, et al. 1963. Pleurectomy in the treatment of pleural effusion due to metastatic malignancy. *J Thorac Cardiovasc Surg* 46:322–330.
79. Martini, N, Bains, MS, and Beattie, EJ Jr. 1975. Indications for pleurectomy in malignant effusion. *Cancer* 35:734–738.
80. Cimochowski, GE, et al. 1986. Pleuroperitoneal shunting for recalcitrant pleural effusions. *J Thorac Cardiovasc Surg* 92:866–870.
81. Epstein, DM, et al. 1987. Tuberculous pleural effusions. *Chest* 91:106–109.
82. Lemmer, JH, Botham, MJ, and Orringer, MB. 1985. Modern management of adult thoracic empyema. *J Thorac Cardiovasc Surg* 90:849–855.
83. Mavroudis, C, et al. 1981. Improved survival in management of empyema thoracis. *J Thorac Cardiovasc Surg* 82:49–57.
84. Strausser, JL, and Flye, MW. 1981. Management of nontraumatic chylothorax. *Ann Thorac Surg* 31:520–526.
85. Milsom, JW, et al. 1985. Chylothorax: An assessment of current surgical management. *J Thorac Cardiovasc Surg* 89:221–227.
86. Martini, N, et al. 1987. Pleural mesothelioma (current review). *Ann Thorac Surg* 43:113–120.
87. De Laria, GA, et al. 1978. Surgical management of malignant mesothelioma. *Ann Thorac Surg* 26:375–382.
88. Hilaris, BS, et al. 1984. Pleurectomy and intraoperative brachytherapy and postoperative radiation in the treatment of malignant pleural mesothelioma. *Int J Radiat Oncol Biol Phys* 10:325–331.
89. Jackson, C, and Jackson, CL. 1937. In *Diseases of the Air and Food Passages of Foreign Body Origin*. Philadelphia: WB Saunders.
90. Weissberg, D, and Schwartz, I. 1987. Foreign bodies in the tracheobronchial tree. *Chest* 91:730–733.
91. Grillo, HC. 1978. Tracheal tumors: Surgical management. *Ann Thorac Surg* 26:112–125.
92. Frist, WH, et al. 1987. Bronchial sleeve resection with and without pulmonary resection. *J Thorac Cardiovasc Surg* 93:350–357.
93. Young, RH, Sandstrom, RE, and Mark, GJ. 1980. Tracheopathia osteoplastica. *J Thorac Cardiovasc Surg* 79:537–541.
94. Holmes, FF, and Hearne, E. 1981. Cancer stage-to-age relationship: Implications for cancer screening in the elderly. *J Am Geriatr Soc* 29:55–57.
95. Ershler, EB, Socinski, MA, and Greene, CJ. 1983. Bronchogenic cancer, metastases, and aging. *J Am Geriatr Soc* 31:673–676.
96. O'Rourke, MA, et al. 1987. Age trends of lung cancer stage at diagnosis. *JAMA* 258:921–926.
97. Teeter, SM, Holmes, FF, and McFarlane, MJ. 1987. Lung carcinoma in the elderly population: Influence of

histology on the inverse relationship of stage to age. *Cancer* 60:1331–1336.
98. Carlens, E. 1959. Mediastinoscopy: A method for inspection and tissue biopsy in the superior mediastinum. *Dis Chest* 36:343–352.
99. McNeill, TM, and Chamberlain, JM. 1966. Diagnostic anterior mediastinotomy. *Ann Thorac Surg* 2:532–539.
100. Unruh, H, and Chiu, RC. 1986. Mediastinal assessment for staging and treatment of carcinoma of the lung: Collective review. *Ann Thorac Surg* 41:224–229.
101. Evans, EWT. 1973. Resection for bronchial carcinoma in the elderly. *Thorax* 28:86–88.
102. Bureau of the Census, United States Department of Commerce. 1984. Current population reports (series P-25, no 952). Washington, D.C.: GPO.
103. Nagasaki, F, Flehinger, BJ, and Martini, N. 1982. Complications of surgery in the treatment of carcinoma of the lung. *Chest* 82:25–29.
104. Sherman, S, and Guidot, CE. 1987. The feasibility of thoracotomy for lung cancer in the elderly. *JAMA* 258: 927–930.
105. Wilkins, EW, Jr, Scannell, JG, and Craver, JG. 1978. Four decades of experience with resections for bronchogenic carcinoma at the Massachusetts General Hospital. *J Thorac Cardiovasc Surg* 76:364–368.
106. Belcher, JR. 1983. Thirty years of surgery for carcinoma of the bronchus. *Thorax* 38:428–432.
107. Ginsberg, RJ, et al. 1983. Modern thirty-day operative mortality for surgical resections in lung cancer. *J Thorac Cardiovasc Surg* 86:654–658.
108. Errett, LE, et al. 1985. Wedge resection as an alternative procedure for a peripheral bronchogenic carcinoma in poor-risk patients. *J Thorac Cardiovasc Surg* 90:656–661.
109. Hoffmann, TH, and Ransdell, HT. 1980. Comparison of lobectomy and wedge resection for carcinoma of the lung. *J Thorac Cardiovasc Surg* 79:211–217.
110. Jensik, RJ, Faber, LP, and Kittle, CF. 1979. Segmental resection for bronchogenic carcinoma. *Ann Thorac Surg* 28:475–483.
111. Green, N, and Weinstein, H. 1983. Reassessment of radiation therapy for the management of lung cancer in patients with chronic pulmonary disease. *Int J Radiat Oncol Biol Phys* 9:1891–1898.
112. Begg, CB, Cohen, JL, and Ellerten, I. 1980. Are the elderly predisposed to toxicity from cancer chemotherapy? *Cancer Clin Trials* 3:369–374.
113. Clamon, GH, Audeh, MW, and Pinnich, S. 1982. Small cell lung carcinoma in the elderly. *J Am Geriatr Soc* 30:299–302.
114. Schray, MF, et al. 1988. Management of malignant airway compromise with laser and low dose rate brachytherapy. *Chest* 93:264–269.
115. Stead, WW, and To, T. 1986. Tuberculosis, a special problem for the elderly. *Chest* 89 (Supplement): 5295.
116. Chang, SC, Lee, PY, and Perng, RP. 1987. Lower lung field tuberculosis. *Chest* 91:230–232.
117. Dorken, E, Grzybowski, S, and Allen, EA. 1987. Significance of the tuberculin test in the elderly. *Chest* 92: 237–240.
118. Scannell, JG. 1980. "Bleb" carcinoma of the lung. *J Thorac Cardiovasc Surg* 80:904–908.
119. Steinhäuslin, CA, and Cuttat, JF. 1985. Spontaneous pneumothorax: A complication of lung cancer? *Chest* 88:709–713.
120. Wilkins, EW, Jr, Head, JM, and Burke, JF. 1978. Pulmonary resection for metastatic neoplasms in the lung. *Am J Surg* 135:480–483.
121. Torek, F. 1913. The first successful case of resection of the thoracic portion of the esophagus for carcinoma. *Surg Gynecol Obstet* 16:614–617.
122. Sweet, RH. 1946. Carcinoma of midthoracic esophagus: Its treatment by radical resection and high intrathoracic esophagogastric anastomosis. *Ann Surg* 124:653–666.
123. Katlic, MR, Wilkins, EW, Jr, and Grillo, HC. Three decades of esophageal carcinoma at the Massachusetts General Hospital. *J Thorac Cardiovasc Surg* (in press).
124. Raphael, HA, Ellis, FH Jr, and Dockerty, MB. 1966. Primary adenocarcinoma of the esophagus: 18-year review and review of the literature. *Ann Surg* 164:785–796.
125. Postlethwait, RW. 1979. Squamous cell carcinoma of the esophagus. In *Surgery of the Esophagus,* Ed., RW Postlethwait. New York: Appleton-Century-Crofts.
126. Welch, CS. 1948. Surgery in the aged. *N Engl J Med* 238:821–832.
127. Sugimachi, K, et al. 1985. Evaluation of surgical treatment of carcinoma of the oesophagus in the elderly: 20 years' experience. *Br J Surg* 72:28–30.
128. Fan, ST, et al. 1987. Prediction of postoperative pulmonary complications in oesophagogastric cancer surgery. *Br J Surg* 74:408–410.
129. Williamson, RCN. 1985. Abdominocervical oesophagectomy in the elderly. *Ann R Coll Surg Engl* 67:344–348.
130. Mohansingh, MP. 1976. Mortality of oesophageal surgery in the elderly. *Br J Surg* 63:579–580.
131. Nishi, M, et al. 1988. Risk factors in relation to postoperative complications in patients undergoing esophagectomy or gastrectomy for cancer. *Ann Surg* 207:148–154.
132. Mathisen, DJ, et al. 1988. Transthoracic esophagectomy: A safe approach to carcinoma of the esophagus. *Ann Thorac Surg* 45:137–143.
133. Cooper, JD, and Jeejeebhoy, KN. 1981. Gastroesophageal reflux: Medical and surgical management (collective review). *Ann Thorac Surg* 31:577–593.
134. Skinner, DB. 1985. Pathophysiology of gastroesophageal reflux. *Ann Surg* 202:546–556.
135. Hill, LD. 1973. Incarcerated paraesophageal hernia: A surgical emergency. *Am J Surg* 126:286–291.
136. Pearson, FG, et al. 1983. Massive hiatal hernia with incarceration: A report of 53 cases. *Ann Thorac Surg* 35:45–51.
137. Bradley, SL, et al. 1981. Spontaneous rupture of the esophagus. *Arch Surg* 116:755–758.
138. Sarr, MG, Pemberton, JH, and Payne, WS. 1982. Management of instrumental perforations of the esophagus. *J Thorac Cardiovasc Surg* 84:211–218.
139. Postlethwait, RW. 1979. Perforation and rupture. In *Surgery of the Esophagus,* Ed., RW Postlethwait. New York: Appleton-Century-Crofts.
140. Gohel, VK, Karasick, S, and Canino, C. 1976. Cervical spondylotic dysphagia. *JAMA* 235:935–936.
141. Rosenow, EC III, and Hurley, BT. 1984. Disorders of the thymus: A review. *Arch Intern Med* 144:763–770.
142. Lewis, JE, et al. 1987. Thymoma: A clinicopathologic review. *Cancer* 60:2727–2743.
143. Shamji, F, et al. 1984. Results of surgical treatment for thymoma. *J Thorac Cardiovasc Surg* 87:43–47.
144. Blalock, A, et al. 1941. The treatment of myasthenia

gravis by removal of the thymus gland: Preliminary report. *JAMA* 117:1529.
145. Papatestas, AE, et al. 1987. Effects of thymectomy in myasthenia gravis. *Ann Surg* 206:79–88.
146. Monden, Y, et al. 1985. Myasthenia gravis in elderly patients. *Ann Thorac Surg* 39:433–436.
147. Rubin, JW. 1979. Complications of esophageal diagnostic procedures. In *Complications of Intrathoracic Surgery,* Eds., AR Cordell and RG Ellison. Boston: Little, Brown.
148. Grillo, HC. 1970. Surgery of the trachea. In *Current Problems in Surgery,* Ed., MM Ravitch. Chicago: Yearbook Medical Publishers.
149. Pairolero, PC, and Payne, WS. 1983. Postoperative care and complications in the thoracic surgical patient. In *Thoracic and Cardiovascular Surgery,* ed 4, Ed., WWL Glenn. CT: Appleton-Century-Crofts.
150. Grillo, HC. 1983. Congenital lesions, neoplasms, and injuries of the trachea. In *Gibbon's Surgery of the Chest,* ed. 4, Eds., DC Sabiston Jr and FC Spencer. Philadelphia: WB Saunders.
151. Speiser, BH. 1987. Remote afterloading at Humana Hospital, Phoenix: Bronchial treatment. *Activity Newsletter* (Nucletron Corporation) 1:3–4.
152. Andersen, HA, and Payne, WS. 1974. Esophageal hiatal hernia, gastroesophageal reflux, and their complications. In *The Esophagus,* Eds., WS Payne and AM Olsen. Philadelphia: Lea & Febiger.
153. Miller, JI, Mansour, KA, and Hatcher, CR Jr. 1982. Median sternotomy T-incision for thymectomy in myasthenia gravis. *Ann Thorac Surg* 34:473–474.
154. Crile, G Jr. 1939. Intrathoracic goiter. *Cleve Clin Q* 6:313–322.
155. Davis, RD, Jr, Oldham, HN, Jr, and Sabiston, DC, Jr. 1987. Primary cysts and neoplasms of the mediastinum: Recent changes in clinical presentation, methods of diagnosis, management, and results. *Ann Thorac Surg* 44:229–237.
156. Wilkins, EW, Jr, and Castleman, B. 1979. Thymoma—A continuing survey at the Massachusetts General Hospital. *Ann Thorac Surg* 28:252–256.
157. Sensenig, DM, Rossi, NP, and Ehrenhaft, JL. 1966. Pulmonary resection for bronchogenic carcinoma in geriatric patients. *Ann Thorac Surg* 2:508–513.
158. Golebiowski, A. 1971. Pulmonary resection in patients over 70 years of age. *J Thorac Cardiovasc Surg* 61:265–270.
159. Didolkar, MS, Moore, RH, and Takita, H. 1974. Evaluation of the risk in pulmonary resection for bronchogenic carcinoma. *Am J Surg* 127:700–703.
160. Kirsh, MM, et al. 1976. Major pulmonary resection for bronchogenic carcinoma in the elderly. *Ann Thorac Surg* 22:369–373.
161. Harviel, JD, McNamara, JJ, and Straehley, CJ. 1978. Surgical treatment of lung cancer in patients over the age of 70 years. *J Thorac Cardiovasc Surg* 75:802–805.
162. Raychaudhury, T. 1983. Mortality in pulmonary resection for bronchogenic carcinoma. *J R Coll Surg Edinb* 28:182–187.

30

Cardiac Surgery in the Elderly

Mark S. Hochberg

In 1968, the *British Medical Journal* flatly stated that "surgical treatment for valvular disease is not at present feasible in elderly patients, and any treatment must therefore be medical" (1). Since that time, cardiac surgery in general and cardiac surgery for the elderly in particular has reached the age of maturity.

The 1950s witnessed the development of blood oxygenators for cardiopulmonary bypass. At that time, the first cardiac operations using cardiopulmonary bypass were undertaken. The initial operations were simple congenital cardiac defects or repair of end-stage valvular lesions. Soon prosthetic valves were developed, and the disc oxygenator was rapidly replaced by a second generation oxygenator—the bubble oxygenator. Cardiac surgery became more widespread, and by the early 1960s, over a score of centers were performing cardiac operations with cardiopulmonary bypass techniques. The late 1960s witnessed the first tentative steps of coronary artery bypass grafting. As the 1960s turned into the 1970s, explosive growth of cardiac surgery in three major areas occurred: (*a*) coronary bypass, (*b*) valvular replacements, and (*c*) congenital heart surgery. Further refinements of technique included the introduction of membrane oxygenators, vastly improved methods of myocardial preservation, and more durable cardiac valve designs. Equally important, the newer cardiac surgeons were being formally trained in residency programs. The technical advances and improved surgical training combined to bring about the rapid growth of cardiac surgery. By 1980, over 200,000 open heart operations were being performed yearly in the United States, and cardiac surgery was a routine tool in the care of the heart patient.

General practitioners, cardiologists, and surgeons alike now feel quite comfortable in extending the potential benefits of cardiac surgery to the extremes of cardiac disease. Specifically, patients in the elderly population with more hemodynamic impairment, more extensive coronary artery disease, and even end-stage cardiac disease are now being routinely offered cardiac operation. Despite the anticipated increased risks of elderly individuals undergoing cardiac surgery, the results have been impressive. For the well-selected elderly patient with cardiac disease in the 1980s, cardiac surgery can offer improved quality and quantity of life in sharp contrast to the *British Medical Journal's* pronouncement of 1968.

Physiologic Consequences of the Aging Heart

Cardiac performance in the aging heart has come under increased scrutiny in the recent past. Nixon and colleagues (2) studied the effects of increasing and decreasing cardiac preload by 15% in patients aged 61 to 73 years when compared to a similar hemodynamic challenge in patients aged 21 to 28 years. The report found that alterations in preload produced changes in left ventricular (LV) end-diastolic pressure and stroke volume of those older patients that conform to normal LV function curves, but the responses were diminished compared with changes in younger patients. This suggests an age-related change in diastolic ventricular stiffness.

A basic tenet of normal cardiac function is that increasing ventricular volume (preload) leads to improved cardiac contractility (usually measured by cardiac output). This mechanism, known as the Frank-Starling relationship, is preserved in the elderly patient (3–6). However, the Frank-Starling mechanism is preserved at a lower level of left ventricular ejection fraction in older individuals. Using radionuclide measurements, Port et al. (4) showed that, at rest, left ventricular end-diastolic volume and regional wall motion did not significantly vary in 77 healthy volunteers aged 20 to 95 years of age. However, during exercise the ejection fraction was less than 60% in 45% of the subjects over age 60. This compares to an ejection fraction of less than 60% in only 2% of the subjects aged 60 or below. Apparently, wall motion abnormalities occur with increasing frequency in patients who are 60 years and older. A substantially reduced cardiac output in older subjects with exercise was a consistent finding in older subjects as far back as Brandfonbrenner's report in 1955 (3).

The cause of the reported decrease in cardiac response to exercise in the elderly heart has not been defined. However, some interesting clues have been provided by a chemical evaluation of senescent animal hearts. Lakatta and Yin (7), in an invited review in the *American Journal of Physiology,* studied the level of excitation-contraction, the properties of myofilaments and energy metabolism in senescent rat hearts. They concluded that maximum myocardial oxygen consumption and substrate oxidation rates declined approximately 20% from adulthood to senescence and may result from the effect of age on workload, coronary blood flow, and mitochondrial respiration. This would suggest that the effect of age on the myocardium is not simply generalized decline in myocardial function but rather certain specific changes in cardiac biochemistry and in particular excitation-contraction coupling in the aging heart.

In evaluating cardiac function in the aging heart, it must be remembered that the observed decreased cardiac output in the older heart cannot be viewed in isolation without also evaluating preload and afterload characteristics. These latter are determined by vascular volume and peripheral resistance. Ebert et al. (8) feel that the decreased hemodynamic response to exercise in the elderly patient is a function of higher baseline peripheral resistance levels on both the arterial and venous sides of the peripheral circulation. They conclude that the preload (peripheral venous volume) is higher in older individuals. The peripheral arterial and arteriolar resistance (afterload) is also increased in the elderly. This presumably is due to stiffening of the arterial vasculature accompanying the aging process.

Thus, when evaluating cardiac performance in the elderly, one must look at all four components of cardiac output: preload, afterload, myocardial contractility, and heart rate—not simply myocardial contractility alone. This was clearly demonstrated by a comprehensive report by Rodeheffer et al. (5). They found that there are no age-related changes in cardiac output. However, there were significant changes in the constituents that comprised the cardiac output in elderly versus younger patients. Specifically, there was an age-related *increase* in end-diastolic volume and stroke volume and an age-related *decrease* in heart rate in older individuals.

In summary, these authors confirmed earlier findings that older individuals have a decreased ejection fraction. To maintain a similar cardiac output with younger cohorts, however, older individuals have a slower heart rate, a higher end-systolic volume (preload), and consequently an increased stroke volume. Thus, although aging does not limit cardiac output per se, the hemodynamic profile accompanying this cardiac output is significantly altered by age.

Valve Replacement

Life expectancy for healthy 70-year-old men and women is 10 and 12 years, respectively (9). Ross and Braunwald (10) collected data on the natural life history of patients with aortic stenosis in 1968. Their analysis revealed that the average age of death in patients with isolated aortic stenosis is 63 years. Eighty percent of those dying have symptoms existing for less than 4 years. On average, death occurred 3 years after the onset of angina, 3 years after the onset of syncope, and only 2 years after the onset of congestive heart failure. Their conclusion was that with the onset of symptoms of angina, syncope, or left ventricular dysfunction in adults with valvular aortic stenosis, the outlook for survival is extremely limited. The confirmation of these data is provided by Harken et al. (11) who reported 61 patients in whom operation was not performed. Fifty-five of the 61 (90%) died within 6 months of diagnosis. Rotman et al. (12) similarly estimated the average life span of patients with aortic stenosis alone or combined with aortic regurgitation to be approximately 4 years after the development of the major symptoms of angina, syncope, or left ventricular dysfunction. Frank and Ross (13) noted an 83% mortality within 5 years in patients shown to have an aortic valve gradient of at least 50 mm Hg.

Thus, symptomatic aortic valve disease may severely curtail life expectancy in otherwise healthy patients 70 years of age or older. It is against this curtailed life expectancy that one must balance the normal life expectancy of a 70-year-old when making the surgical decision.

Mitral valve disease in the elderly has received much less attention than aortic valve disease. Presumably, this is due to the fact that symptoms of mitral stenosis or regurgitation tend to occur at an earlier decade than isolated disease of the aortic valve. As will be discussed next, the predominant pathologic lesion of the mitral valve is due to rheumatic fever; this is in contradistinction to the predominant pathology of the aortic valve, which tends to be the aging process of valve sclerosis with or without an underlying bicuspid valve. The symptoms of mitral disease tend to be more insidious in onset compared to the symptoms of aortic valvular disease. Mitral stenosis has a less predictable natural history (14). In a report of the natural history of 271 patients with mitral stenosis under medical treatment, Olesen (15) found that for patients in the New York Heart Association functional Class IV, the complications and deaths climbed noticeably unless the process was interrupted by operation. When lesions of the aortic and mitral valve occur simultaneously (especially regurgitant lesions), they are especially dangerous because they are tolerated only at the severe expense of myocardial damage (16).

Pathologic Anatomy

Considerable differences in the pathologic anatomy of the stenotic aortic valve in the elderly, as compared to that of younger patients, were found by Roberts and his colleagues (17, 18). Stenotic aortic valves in the older population were tricuspid (90%) rather than bicuspid (10%) and had large amounts of calcium superimposed. They believed these findings suggest that the aortic stenosis in the elderly was caused largely by fibrotic and sclerotic changes of valve wear and tear, rather than any specific disease entity. A rheumatic etiology (signified by associated mitral valve disease) was rare in the elderly population. Subacute bacterial endocarditis rarely, if ever, caused pure stenosis. In contrast, for younger patients undergoing aortic valve replacement only 45% of the valves were tricuspid, 45% were bicuspid, and 10% were unicuspid. The higher percentage of younger patients than older patients coming to aortic valve replacement with bicuspid valves suggests that bicuspid valves develop degenerative changes earlier than tricuspid valves.

In contrast, Roberts and co-workers (18) also found that the cause of aortic regurgitation in the older patients was rarely "wear and tear." They observed that aortic regurgitation was more commonly due to rheumatic disease, subacute bacterial endocarditis, or a dilated annulus. The latter was usually due to cystic medial necrosis, with or without Marfan's syndrome and syphilis.

The predominant pathologic change in mitral valve disease in the elderly is myxomatous degeneration of the leaflets. Rheumatic mitral valve disease usually becomes symptomatic in the younger age groups, making its repair rare in patients over 70. In addition to myxomatous degeneration of the mitral valve, ischemic and/or infarcted papillary muscles frequently cause mitral regurgitation. Infarction in the distribution of the right coronary artery particularly is associated with papilllary muscle dysfunction leading to mitral regurgitation.

Operative Results of Valve Replacement

Twenty-four reports of valve operations in the elderly are listed in Table 30-1 (19–38). Because cardiac operations in the elderly are reported in vastly different ways, it is sometimes difficult in reviewing the literature to determine which elderly patients in a series underwent aortic or mitral valve replacement. Table 30-1 attempts to be as inclusive as possible in reporting the significant series and the key data. Most of the reports deal with aortic valve replacement. Only 7 of the 24 reports deal with mitral valve replacement in the elderly. Presumably this is due to the fact that disease of the mitral valve requiring operative intervention usually presents itself before age 60.

The results of operations reported in the last decade are amazingly similar. In general, hospital mortality ranged from 5% to 10% in patients 70 years of age or older, and the late mortality was sporadically reported but appears to be approximately 20%.

There is no clear reason why mortality from the mid-1970s until now is significantly better than the reports prior to 1975, however, changes in intraoperative techniques must be considered. Specifically, the mid-1970s saw the development of routine instillation of cold cardioplegia as the preferred method of myocardial preservation. The widespread use of intra-aortic balloon pumping has been invaluable in removing critical patients from cardiopulmonary bypass. This is especially true in elderly individuals who undergo mitral valve replacement. In addition to improved myocardial preservation and the intra-aortic balloon pump, newer techniques of cardiac anesthesia, intraoperative monitoring, and postoperative care have all contributed to halving valve replacement mortality from the decade prior to 1975 to the decade since 1975, when it has reached its low 5% to 10% operative rate.

In attempting to justify valve replacement in individuals over age 70, virtually all the reports in Table 30-1 compare the older patients to a similar cohort of younger patients undergoing valve replacement. This technique is useful because it provides an adequate control group in the same hospital setting operated upon by the same team. In virtually every circumstance, the hospital mortality for the older patient exceeds the hospital mortality for the younger cohort of patients undergoing valve surgery. However, these differences are not significant and in most cases are attributed to the ability of the younger patients to

Table 30-1. Survey of literature of valve operations in elderly patients

Author	Year	Number of patients	Age		Operation	Mortality		Follow-up months
			Range	Mean		Hosp	Late	
Hildner	1969	35	≥60	64.3	ALL VALVE	26%	NR	NR
Finegan	1969	70	60–80	64	AVR	11.5%	20%	25
Ahmad	1969	91	≥60	64.6	ALL VALVE	17.5%	10%	NR
Austen	1970	40	70–85	74.6	AVR	20%	7.5%	28
Grondin	1971	38	≥60	NR	AVR	24%	NR	NR
Gurhrie	1972	16	≥65	NR	MVR	37%	NR	NR
Shanahan	1972	31	≥60	NR	MVR	23%	16%	NR
Bensaid	1973	43	≥60	NR	AVR	7%	10%	NR
Oh	1973	22	≥60	NR	MVR	18%	14%	NR
Barnhorst	1974	60	≥65	NR	MVR	20%	NR	NR
Barnhorst	1974	158	≥65	NR	AVR	11%	NR	NR
Bessone	1977	21	≥70	73	MVR	4.7%	5%	12.6
Bessone	1977	14	≥70	73	AVR	0	0	12.6
Copeland	1977	196	65–84	70.2	AVR	12%	29%	36
Hochberg	1977	73	60–77	64.6	AVR	2.7%	21%	56
Stephenson	1978	27	≥70	NR	AVR	11%	NR	NR
Stephenson	1978	14	≥70	NR	AVR	57%	NR	NR
Canepa-Anson	1979	29	70–75	71	ALL VALVE	10%	4%	38.6
Hochberg	1979	43	60–75	65.0	MVR	14%	14%	54
Jones	1979	38	65–86	70	AVR	10%	16%	NR
Nicoloff	1984	213	70–87	NR	ALL VALVE	8%	7.7%	NR
Craver	1984	98	70–83	73.4	AVR	5.1%	22%	24
Arom	1984	41	≥70	NR	AVR	9.8%	NR	NR
Arom	1984	24	≥70	NR	MVR	8.3%	NR	NR

NR, not reported.

withstand postoperative complications in a more satisfactory way.

Complications and Causes of Death

The causes of hospital death following valve replacement in the elderly are at times difficult to isolate. For patients who die in the operating room, the death is usually attributed to ventricular failure. Whether the cause of this ventricular dysfunction is inability to adequately preserve the myocardium during crossclamp, preexisting left ventricular failure that worsened under the stress of cardiopulmonary bypass, or a technical failure of valve implantation, it is impossible to know. Similarly, patients who die in the hospital days or weeks following their valve replacement usually die of generalized sepsis following multi-organ failure. Indeed, Craver et al. (27), in their report of aortic valve replacement in 152 patients over age 70, list "multiple organ failure/sepsis" as the single largest cause of death in their 21 patients (33% of the deaths). Their second most frequent cause of death (28%) is left ventricular pump failure. The other causes of death are neurologic, pulmonary, arrhythmia, hemorrhage, gastrointestinal bleed, renal failure, and hepatic encephalopathy. All of these causes of death occur as very small percentages of the total deaths in the large series. Thus, it is hard to extrapolate from one series to another. Clearly, decreased cardiac output is usually the source of most of the organ failures just listed.

Following valve replacement in the elderly, morbidity is usually more frequent than in younger patients undergoing the same procedure. Difficulty in pulmonary toilet is the single most frequent cause of morbidity in the elderly patient. Generalized weakened condition coupled with many more years of cigarette smoking tend to make clearing secretions and pulmonary exercise more difficult in the older individual. These individuals require more attentive nursing care than their younger cohorts.

Because the elderly patient requires more pulmonary, emotional, and exercise support in the postoperative period, it is not surprising that in most of the series the length of stay following valve replacement for older patients is usually 4 to 6 days longer than younger patients undergoing the same procedure (25, 27, 33).

Special Postoperative Problems of Individuals Undergoing Mitral Valve Replacement

Stephenson et al. (38) found a 57% hospital mortality in 14 patients aged 70 or over undergoing mitral valve replacement. Two of the patients died of left ventricular rupture. They reported that in both patients the papillary muscles were not cut and at autopsy there was no evidence of fresh myocardial infarct. In both patients, the site of rupture was distant from the valve annulus in an area that Stephenson felt was unlikely to have been injured at the time of operation. He concluded that a weakened, thin ventricular wall led to the rupture in the setting of increased afterload. He felt that it is crucial to reduce afterload in these elderly patients in the immediate postoperative period following mitral valve replacement. This was further confirmed by Bjork et al. (39) who reported on left ventricular rupture in 26 patients following mitral valve replacement. Bjork found this complication more common in older patients.

Although left ventricular rupture is dramatic and memorable, a more frequent cause of death in elderly patients following mitral valve replacement is low cardiac output. This is due to reduced left ventricular contractile reserve in older patients, especially in the circumstance where mitral valvular incompetence is predominant. Kirklin (40) and Kouchoukos et al. (41) have shown that valve replacement for mitral insufficiency is associated with an acute increase in left ventricular afterload leading to decreased cardiac output. Reduction of afterload may be particularly important in elderly patients to reduce the incidence of left ventricular rupture and low cardiac output.

Choice of Valve Prosthesis in Elderly Patients Undergoing Valve Replacement

For many years, the choice of prosthetic valve model usually focused on whether the patient was a candidate for Coumadin therapy and whether the life expectancy of the patient was greater than the life expectancy of the specific valve model. The rule of thumb in the 1970s was that younger patients should have a more durable prosthesis, which was usually a mechanical valve requiring Coumadin. The thinking was that the younger patient was less accident prone, less likely to need an emergency operation (hip repair, etc.), and should have the benefit of a valve with the longest durability. Conversely, the bioprosthetic valve was recommended for the older individual who perhaps could not be as reliable in the taking of Coumadin, and who might suffer more seriously from a hemorrhagic situation than a younger patient. Indeed, Craver et al. (27) in their report of 152 patients undergoing valve replacement over age 70, state that greater than 93% of all the elderly patients underwent insertion of a bioprosthesis.

However, the impressive durability characteristics of the latest generation of mechanical prostheses have made more surgeons consider their implantation for the older individual (20, 35). Nicoloff (35) reported a series of 213 patients aged 60 years or greater who underwent implantation of the St. Jude mechanical prosthesis. Of these 213 patients, 86 were 70 years of age or older. The St. Jude short-term and long-term results are impressive. The operative mortality of patients aged 60 to 69 was 5% and of patients 70 years of age or greater was 11.5%. Late mortality from 6 months to 6 years (mean not provided) was 7% in individuals aged 60 to 69 and 12.5% in individuals aged 70 or greater. These numbers are certainly impressive for a mechanical prosthesis implanted in an elderly individual. The incidence of thromboembolism in patients aged 70 or greater was 1.1% per year. Similarly, the incidence of hemorrhagic complications in the older individuals following valve replacement was low and not dissimilar from a matched cohort of younger patients.

If a bioprosthetic valve is indicated, the choice is usually between the Carpentier-Edwards prosthesis, the Hancock prosthesis, the Ionescu-Shiley pericardial prosthesis, or the homograft valve. While the homograft valve is very appealing for a host of theoretical reasons, its availability is obviously limited. Of the other valves, the Carpentier-Edwards low-pressure, fixed-gluteraldehyde-preserved valve is the most widely used by American cardiac surgeons (42, 43). Thus, the indications for mechanical versus bioprosthetic implantation in elderly patients requiring valve replacement are still as unclear as ever. There are champions with good supporting data emphasizing the benefits of either bioprosthetic or mechanical valves in the older age group. The decision must be made by the surgeon and patient based on a variety of considerations. However, the big difference now versus 20 years ago is that either prosthesis can be expected to serve the elderly patient very well for a long period of time.

Coronary Artery Bypass Grafting

The timing of operative intervention for coronary artery disease in elderly patients is more difficult than determining when operation is indicated for valvular lesions. This is true for younger as well as older patients. The natural history of aortic and mitral valve disease unoperated upon is predictable and has been reviewed in the previous section. In contrast, the onset and progression of coronary artery disease is more insidious than valvular disease, and consequently there has been more reluctance to recommend coronary artery bypass grafting in the elderly population.

It was not until the early 1970s that coronary angiography to evaluate coronary artery disease was available to large segments of the American population. Not until coronary angiography defined the precise extent of coronary artery disease could decisions on surgical intervention be made. It was not until the mid-1970s that both cardiologists and cardiac surgeons felt it feasible to extend the new coronary artery bypass grafting technique to the elderly population.

Most cardiologists would agree that the symptom of angina pectoris is at best a poor marker of the anatomic extent of coronary disease. In contradistinction to valvular disease, where symptoms closely correlate with the extent of anatomic disease, the anatomic extent of atherosclerotic disease is insidious and poorly correlates with the patient's complaint. Consequently, many general practitioners and internists, when confronted with the elderly patient with angina, have tended to delay catheterization and possible coronary bypass surgery in the hope that the natural aging process will antecede coronary disease as the cause of death.

Life Expectancy of Elderly Population

The 1980 United States census (44) revealed interesting and surprising information on the length of life of older individuals. It found that the life expectancy of patients 70 years of age and older is substantial. For individuals aged 70 to 74 years, life expectancy was 12.4 years (women 13.9 years, men 10.7 years). For those aged 75 to 79 years, the average life expectancy was 9.8 years (women 10.8 years, men 8.4 years).

As if these absolute life expectancy numbers are not convincing enough, Fries (45) attempted to evaluate the quality of life in this older age group. He studied physical, emotional, and intellectual vigor of patients from 70 to 84 years of age. The average remaining years of "active" life expectancy were defined as the duration of well-being, with the endpoint being the loss of independence in the activities of daily living. The number of years of "active life" remaining was 8.1 years for individuals aged 70 to 74, 6.8 years for patients 75 to 79, and 4.7 years for individuals aged 80 to 84.

Results of CABG

The early results of coronary artery bypass grafting in elderly patients were not impressive. Table 30-2 details the reports of isolated coronary artery bypass grafting in the elderly population from 1973 through 1985 (46–69). Although the numbers of patients in the reports varies greatly, several trends become apparent.

In the early years of coronary bypass, only the severely ill elderly patients underwent coronary artery bypass grafting. Not surprisingly, the mortality rates were quite high in these patients. These unacceptably high mortality rates led Kirklin et al. (60) to conclude that hospital mortality increases exponentially in patients aged 70 years or older. They found mortality was 20% in patients aged 70 to 79. Kirklin questioned the advisability of coronary bypass graft operations in this age group. However, as the newer intraoperative techniques including myocardial preservation, optical magnification, finer sutures, membrane oxygenation, etc., became widely applied in the mid- and late 1970s, the results of the operation improved markedly.

Three reports of over 1000 patients each of isolated coronary artery bypass grafting in elderly patients were reported by Gersh in 1983 (the CASS data) (70), Cosgrove in 1984 (48), and Elayda in 1984 (49). Hospital mortality of coronary bypass grafting was 5.2%, 3.3%, and 5.8%, respectively. Although these large groups of 1000 patients each showed a slightly higher operative mortality than younger matched cohorts undergoing the same procedure at the same institution, the differences were barely significant.

In reviewing all the reports in Table 30-2, it becomes apparent that the number of bypass grafts per patient increased significantly from 1973 and 1985. Despite this more extensive revascularization, the mortality steadily declined over the past 10 years. The low mortality for coronary artery bypass grafting in the elderly certainly compares favorably to the life expectancy data described at the beginning of this section. There certainly is now no longer any excuse for hesitating in recommending coronary artery bypass grafting in the elderly population since the data suggest that the elderly patient has many remaining years of independent active life.

Results of the CASS (Coronary Artery Surgical Study)

Once it is determined that the therapy of coronary artery disease in the elderly can improve life expectancy beyond what these individuals could otherwise expect, medical versus surgical therapy must be evaluated. From 1974 to 1979, 15 medical centers in the United States collaborated in the Coronary Artery Surgery Study (CASS) registry. It is of interest to note that when the CASS study was designed in the early 1970s, perioperative mortality in the elderly was felt to be unacceptably high (Table 30-2). Therefore, the randomization process on which the great mass of the CASS study was based specifically excluded

Table 30-2. Survey of literature of coronary artery bypass operations in elderly patients

Author	Year	Number of patients	Age Range	Age Mean	Avg.# grafts	Mortality Hosp	Mortality Late	Follow-up months
Hamby	1973	17	65–79	68	NR	6%	NR	NR
Ashor	1973	78	≥65	NR	2.0	3%	4%	3.5
Garcia	1975	265	≥65	NR	NR	3%	2%	NR
Meyer	1975	95	70–79	71.9	2.0	22%	NR	NR
McCallister	1975	48	70–78	73	1.7	6%	5%	20.4
Stringer	1975	207	≥65	NR	NR	14%	6%	NR
Smith	1976	47	≥65	NR	NR	19%	NR	NR
Gann	1977	30	70–76	71.5	2.3	7%	0	15
Kirklin	1979	19	70–79	NR	NR	21%	NR	NR
Berry	1981	65	70–78	72.4	3.4	3%	6%	16
Knapp	1981	121	≥70	NR	2.9	1.6%	4.1%	6
Kennedy	1981	227	≥70	NR	NR	8%	NR	NR
Hochberg	1982	75	70–79	74.2	2.8	12%	3%	23.7
Gersh	1983	1036	≥65	NR	2.6	5.2%	11.8%	57
Gooch	1983	86	70–80	NR	NR	5.8%	6.2%	27
Hibler	1983	115	65–81	67.5	NR	5%	4%	12
Faro	1983	105	70–81	72.5	2.4	10.5%	3%	NR
Cosgrove	1984	1114	≥70	NR	NR	3.3%	NR	NR
Elayda	1984	1275	70–90	NR	3.1	5.8%	15%	60
Jeffrey	1985	71	70–85	74	3.4	7%	4.5%	26
Montague	1985	597	70–87	73.1	3.4	2.7%	NR	NR
Rose	1985	201	70–83	73.8	2.5	5.9%	NR	NR
Roberts	1985	66	≥65	70	2.7	7.6%	NR	NR
Tsai	1986	33	≥80	NR	3.7	6.0%	6.4%	28

NR, not reported.

patients past the age of 65 (53, 70). Thus, the results of the CASS randomization in patients under 65 cannot and should not be applied to patients over age 65 who were not randomized.

However, many patients over age 65 were entered into the CASS registry for further evaluation despite their exclusion from the younger randomized CASS group. Gersh (71) compared the results of coronary artery bypass surgery with those of medical therapy alone in 1,491 of these *nonrandomized* patients 65 years of age or older at the 15 CASS centers. Surgical treatment was given to 861 of these patients and 630 were given medical therapy. It is important to point out that there was a crucial exclusion of patients from this study. Gersh states that "because the superiority of surgery over medical therapy for left main coronary disease is well established, we also excluded patients with stenosis of the left main coronary artery of 70% or more." This point is crucial since in evaluating an older individual with angina, the presence of left main stenosis is a definite indication for coronary surgery. For this reason alone, older patients with angina should undergo catheterization to define the extent of their disease.

Despite excluding the left main patients from the medical or surgical group, the 6-year survival was 79% in the surgical group and 64% in the medical group ($p <$ .0001) (Fig. 30-1). At 5 years, chest pain was absent in 62% of the surgical group and only 29% of the medical group ($p < .0001$). All 1491 patients entered the study with angina as their primary symptom. The superiority of surgical therapy in both long-term survival as well as freedom from chest pain is clearly significant by the p values.

Flaws in the design of the CASS study have been widely discussed (72). Of interest, it is felt that if anything, the flaws have biased the results against surgical therapy in favor of medical therapy. However, despite this prejudice, the CASS data impressively comes down on the side of surgical therapy for both improving the *quality* and *quantity* of life in individuals aged 65 or older who have angina as their primary symptom. In another study of a nonrandomized but high-risk patient population from

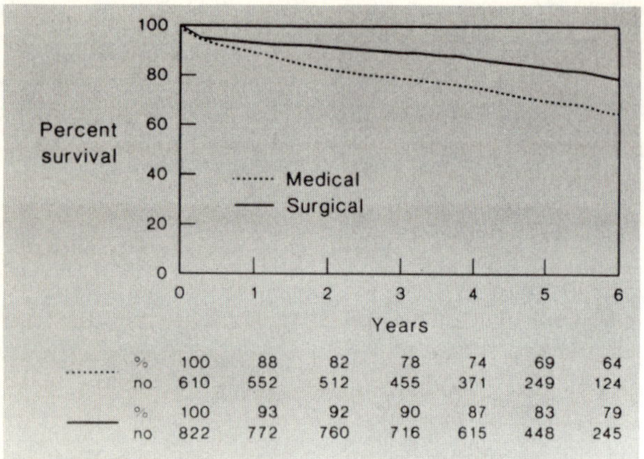

Figure 30-1. Cumulative 6-year survival in surgical and medical groups for the Coronary Artery Surgical Study (CASS). (Reproduced with permission from Gersh, BJ, et al. 1985. Comparison of coronary artery bypass surgery in medical therapy in patients 65 years of age or older. A non-randomized study from the Coronary Artery Surgery Study Group (CASS) registry. *N Engl J Med* 313:217–224.)

the CASS registry, Alderman et al. (73) showed a substantial benefit for coronary artery bypass in patients with severe ventricular dysfunction.

The major exclusion group from the CASS registry were patients with left main disease. This topic was specifically addressed by Jeffery et al. (58) in 71 consecutive patients 70 to 85 years of age (mean 74 years of age) with left mainstem disease. These patients underwent an average of 3.4 coronary bypasses per patient. The hospital mortality was 7% and the late mortality (mean 26 months) was 4.5%. Given the advanced age of these individuals and significant expected curtailment of life due to the left mainstem lesion, these results are certainly impressive.

Complications Following Coronary Bypass Operations

All of the reports of coronary artery bypass grafting in elderly patients noted in Table 30-2 deal with postoperative complications. It is fair to say that older individuals in general have a larger measure of infirmity than younger individuals. Morbidity as well as mortality must be taken into account in projecting the results of an older individual undergoing bypass surgery. Severe pulmonary dysfunction is generally reported in the 5% to 10% range for elderly patients undergoing bypass surgery. This usually means prolonged postoperative ventilation. The causes are the cumulative effect of many years of smoking as well as the inability to adequately perform independent pulmonary toilet. Other factors such as diabetes, obesity, hypertension, etc. tend to be more widespread and have a higher morbid effect in the older versus the younger population. Mental confusion resulting in disorientation affects 3% to 6% of the elderly population. Cerebral vascular accidents (strokes) tend to afflict 2% to 4% of the elderly patients following operation. The increased prevalence of carotid artery disease in older versus younger patients as well as the increased prevalence of intracranial atherosclerosis presumably account for this level of stroke in older patients. In contrast, reoperation for bleeding or tamponade (2% to 5%), bradyarrhythmia requiring permanent pacemaker (1% to 2%), perioperative myocardial infarction (2% to 6%), and chest wound infection (1% to 2%) do not significantly differ from comparative cohorts of younger individuals undergoing coronary bypass surgery by the same team at the same institution.

Ventricular Failure as an Indication for CABG

Although angina pectoris is the symptom that guides an elderly patient to evaluation and therapy for coronary artery disease, an interesting report by Kunis et al. (74) detailed four patients aged 76 to 84 who presented with acute pulmonary edema as their symptom of ischemia (angina equivalent). Ischemic pulmonary edema without concurrent infarction is associated with an extremely poor prognosis, and according to the authors, the 2-year mortality is 70% in patients over 70 years of age. Often, solely because of their age, elderly patients with ischemic heart disease presenting with pulmonary edema do not undergo angiography and are thus treated nonoperatively after their pulmonary congestion resolves. The four patients described in the report all underwent coronary bypass surgery with good result.

Conclusions of CABG

Consideration of the "physiologic" as opposed to the "chronologic" age is an intrinsic part of clinical evaluation. The reports detailed in Table 30-2 demonstrate that over the last decade there has been a significant improvement in mortality for elderly patients undergoing coronary bypass surgery. The CASS study and others noted above have documented substantial relief of angina in the majority of elderly patients undergoing CABG, results that do not differ substantially from comparable younger groups of cohorts. Equally important is the finding of the CASS study that improvement in survival and freedom from angina can be definitely shown to be superior in elderly patients treated surgically as opposed to medically. There should now be no question that the elderly patient presenting with angina (or a clear angina equivalent) should undergo appropriate evaluation including angiography, and if indicated should undergo coronary bypass surgery for improved quantity and *quality* of the remaining years of active life.

Complex Cardiac Surgical Procedures

The extensive literature on isolated valvular or isolated coronary cardiac surgical procedures in the elderly has been reviewed in the previous two sections. More complex cardiac surgical procedures have not been reported in large numbers in any specific series. Combined coronary and valvular procedures, repair of left ventricular aneurysms, procedures on the ascending, transverse, and descending thoracic aorta, and repair of congenital cardiac defects in the elderly population has not been extensively reviewed. In general, most of the reports cited previously include occasional patients with these complex cardiac surgical procedures. However, because the numbers of these patients undergoing complex procedures in each of these reports is relatively small, it is difficult to draw significant comparisons.

Combined Coronary and Valvular Procedures

Tsai et al. (69) reported 23 patients aged 80 or older undergoing various combinations of coronary bypass and valvular procedures. These 23 patients had a 30% hospital mortality and a 21% late mortality. This is in stark contrast to another group of patients over 80 undergoing isolated coronary bypass surgery or isolated valve replacement at the same hospital with mortalities of 6% and 6.5% respectively.

In contrast, Arom et al. (20) reported on 59 patients who underwent combined valve and coronary procedures with a 4.8% hospital mortality. The fairest conclusion in looking at these and other reports of patients undergoing combined coronary plus valve procedures is that there is no conclusion (Table 30-3). In most of the papers the numbers of patients are small. The early and late mortalities vary significantly. The results clearly depend on the specific lesions for which correction is undertaken and must include associated illnesses, especially pulmonary, renal, and neurologic. Surgical judgment on the part of the referring cardiologist and surgeon must be on an individual case basis, because one cannot find support in the literature that will confirm the correct approach for a specific elderly patient requiring valve plus bypass. However, it is fair to say that if the operation includes a mitral valve for an individual with the diagnosis of mitral regurgitation, this is the most serious valvular lesion when taken in comparison to the other valvular lesions and bypass.

Procedures on the Aorta

Operations on the aorta itself are usually considered for acute dissections and sacular or fusiform aneurysms. It is important to differentiate between an acute dissection and a slow-growing aortic aneurysm in surgical decision making.

An acute dissection of the ascending aorta (Stanford Type A) is a clear surgical emergency. The most common presenting symptom is sharp, searing substernal chest pain. This is usually confused with an acute myocardial infarction. Accordingly, patients are usually admitted to coronary care units and treated conservatively with nitroglycerin, sedation, oxygen, etc. while the severest part of the infarction is presumably occurring. The tipoff for these patients is that the pain does not improve with intravenous nitroglycerin, and there are no significant ECG changes.

These individuals should in general undergo rapid arteriography of the ascending aorta. It is important that a pigtail catheter be passed into the ventricle before any injection is performed. This would obviate a power injection of contrast into a false lumen, which can lead to the immediate demise of the patient. Once one is sure that the catheter is in the true lumen, an attempt should be made to identify the tear. Usually it is located 1 to 3 cm above the aortic annulus. This patient should be rapidly transferred to the operating room and put on cardiopulmonary bypass via the groin. Various techniques have been employed. Najafi et al. (76) recommend rapid cross-clamping of the ascending aorta. Rarely, if ever, must the aortic valve be replaced. Resuspension of the leaflets from the annulus is all that is required. The ascending aorta is then replaced with a graft. The results of this operation are frequently gratifying. Since only about 10% of patients with an acute ascending aortic dissection survive to make it to the hospital, it is important that the evaluation and operation proceed with the utmost dispatch. Although the diagnosis can be strongly suggested by CT scanning, aortography is still the "gold standard" and should be performed before the operation.

Dissections of the descending thoracic aorta (Stanford Type B) usually originate beyond the left subclavian artery and extend distally. The diagnosis is more subtle. Usually pain or simply a chronically enlarging aortic silhouette can suggest this diagnosis. Again, aortography must be performed. If the patient is stable and the blood pressure is brought under control, medical therapy may be preferable in an older patient. Indeed, there is active debate in the surgical literature about whether *any patient,* regardless of age, with a stable descending thoracic dissection should undergo operation since the results with medical and surgical therapy are not all that dissimilar. It is important to point out that in choosing medical therapy it is important that the patient be stable with no evidence of ischemia to any major organ system. Medical therapy should include both afterload reduction with nitroprusside and decreasing the strength of ventricular contraction

Table 30-3. Survey of literature of CABG and valve operations in elderly patients

Author	Year	Number of patients	Age Range	Age Mean	Mortality Hosp	Mortality Late	Follow-up months
Bessone	1977	19	⩾70	73.3	5.2%	5.5%	12.6
Craver	1984	54	70–92	74.8	5.6%	6%	24
Arom	1984	59	⩾70	NR	4.8%	NR	NR
Akins	1985	33	50–79	66.7	12%	28%	40.7
Tsai	1986	23	⩾80	NR	30%	21%	28

NR, not reported.

(dp/dt) with inderal. Certainly if the treatment for descending dissections points towards medical therapy in the younger age groups, then in the older age group this would be an even more persuasive argument to proceed with nonsurgical therapy.

Saccular or fusiform aneurysms of the ascending or descending thoracic aorta do not present a surgical emergency of the magnitude of acute dissections but again must be evaluated to determine the benefits versus the risks of surgical or medical therapy. The important issue is that these aneurysms tend to grow. The rate of growth is variable. In the younger patient who may well expect many years of life, an aneurysm in the ascending aorta that measures 6 or more centimeters is a suitable candidate for repair. Many of these are associated with cystic medial necrosis or Marfan's syndrome. The usual therapy for these individuals is a conduit that incorporates a valve attached to a Dacron graft (77). In these circumstances, the ascending aorta and valve are removed and the coronary ostia are implanted back into the conduit. In the younger patient, the aneurysm will certainly grow, so the question of surgical therapy is not really an issue but is clearly the best route given an expected normal life span. However, in the elderly age group, each patient must be evaluated separately vis-à-vis the expected course of aneurysmal growth. An otherwise healthy patient in the 70-year age range should undergo ascending aortic replacement with a risk below 10%. Similarly, an aneurysm of the descending thoracic aorta should be considered for surgical replacement if it exceeds 5 cm in greatest diameter. While the surgical decision should be tempered by the overall condition of the patient, an aneurysm of the descending thoracic aorta can usually be done with a Gott bypass shunt and need not subject the patient to cardiopulmonary bypass. The operation can usually be performed without heparinization, further mitigating the risks. Prior to repair of ascending or descending thoracic aneurysms in elderly patients, it would be advisable to study the coronary arteries in the angiography suite as part of the full evaluation.

Other Cardiac Disease

Occasionally, a patient aged 70 or older is referred with a history of congestive heart failure and found to have an atrial septal defect (ASD). For an individual to survive to advanced age without any ill effects from an ASD is certainly rare and probably suggests that the shunting is not great. However, if the failure is not well controlled and the left to right shunt is greater than 2:1, then operation should be considered. Before proceeding with repair, it is advisable to study the coronary arteries for associated disease.

Left ventricular aneurysms occur following infarction of that region of the heart. Usually these aneurysms are repaired at the time of coronary artery bypass grafting as an adjunct to the bypass procedure. Repair of these aneurysms usually adds little morbidity or mortality to the coronary bypass procedure. In fact, they can confer a great deal of benefit on the procedure in that aneurysmal repair will markedly improve ventricular function immediately. Occasionally, patients are operated upon solely for ventricular aneurysms presenting with recurrent failure. One must be very selective about which patients are appropriate candidates for aneurysm repair. Too aggressive an approach can lead to fatal compromise of left ventricular chamber size. However, in the selected patient, significant improvement of ejection fraction can be achieved with gratifying results.

Myocardial infarction leading to ventricular septal defect is a rare but catastrophic complication. It usually occurs several days after a myocardial infarction, usually when the patient seems to be well on the way to recovery. Sudden symptoms of congestive heart failure associated with a new murmur are usually the first indication. The diagnosis can be easily made by passing a Swan-Ganz catheter and measuring the saturation of blood in the right atrium versus the right ventricle and pulmonary artery. At this point, it is crucial to stabilize the patient by reducing afterload with nitroprusside. If this is unsuccessful, an intra-aortic balloon pump may be required. The patient should be rapidly transferred to the catheterization laboratory to both document the VSD and evaluate the coronary arteries because they may have to be treated surgically along with the VSD. Daggett and Buckley (78) have described repair of ventricular septal defects both in the anterior and posterior septum. Their double patch technique permitted markedly improved survival in place of the previously dismal surgical outcome.

Special Postoperative Problems

The psychiatric morbidity of older individuals undergoing coronary artery bypass grafting was assessed in a report by Folks et al. (79). The authors attempted to assess whether age causes greater risk for postoperative psychiatric symptoms in 58 patients over age 60 compared to a matched group under age 60. The authors specifically evaluated preoperative and postoperative anxiety, depression, and cognitive function in the elderly and the younger groups. They found no difference in anxiety or depression levels in the older versus the younger patients. However, they found a significant difference in cognitive function in the older patients.

A report by Gallagher et al. (80) attempted to evaluate extravascular water in older patients compared to a younger cohort during cardiopulmonary bypass for coronary bypass grafting. During extracorporeal bypass, pulmonary extravascular volume increased in both age groups. The older group accumulated 6.38 ml/kg during bypass and the younger cohort accumulated 5.15 ml/kg of extracellular lung water. The difference was significant. However, by the next morning, extravascular water had returned to preoperative levels in both cohorts with little clinical significance being observed in either group. Consequently, it appears that the aging process does not adversely effect pulmonary function or vasculature at the time of cardiopulmonary bypass.

Early exercise training was evaluated in 76 patients aged 65 or older following myocardial infarction or coronary artery bypass grafting. Williams et al. (81) found that following a 12-week exercise program (within 6 weeks of infarction or bypass grafting) the benefits of early exercise seen in young cardiac patients could also be found in elderly cardiac patients.

Future Trends

The techniques of cardiac surgery have been refined to such a degree that there have been no major changes in the conduct of cardiac operations in the past 5 years. The use of a single continuous period of aortic cross-clamping protected by blood cardioplegia has gained widespread acceptance at the major cardiac surgical centers. Perfusion technology has similarly advanced to the stage that virtually all centers are using a clear prime solution and a majority are using membrane oxygenators. Patient selection for cardiac surgery has been refined to such a degree that the indications for coronary or valve surgery at most major centers are virtually superimposable. The use of 7-0 suture material and magnification loops for the performance of coronary surgery is now standard. There is even little debate among the type of valvular prostheses that surgeons implant for valvular lesions.

Probably the most exciting new developments in the field of cardiac surgery have not been developed by the surgeons but rather the cardiologists. Percutaneous transluminal coronary angioplasty (PTCA) has proven to be effective in selected circumstances. Individuals with discrete single- or double-vessel coronary artery disease with good distal vessels can expect a 70% chance of 1-year improvement in symptoms and presumably freedom from myocardial infarction. This is in contrast to single- or double-vessel coronary artery bypass graft surgery, which can expect a 90% to 95% 1-year patency rate. The difference, of course, is that to achieve the higher patency rate one must undergo the operation. However, once one gets beyond the discomfort of the operation, surgery clearly gives a superior long-term result. However, for the older individual who can expect a higher degree of morbidity with surgery, the short-term success rate of balloon angioplasty without surgery may be more advantageous. Individuals with three or more vessel disease are not candidates for percutaneous transluminal coronary angioplasty at most large centers. The results in these individuals for coronary bypass are excellent as described earlier in this chapter. Many surgical centers are seeing younger individuals with one- or two-vessel disease undergoing successful angioplasty. The hope is that PTCA will buy time for disease to develop in other distributions so a single multiple coronary bypass operation could be performed at a later date. There seems to be a great deal of merit in PTCA being a "temporizing bridge" to coronary bypass surgery for complete revascularization at a later time when it becomes necessary. However, if anatomic and symptomatic relief of coronary artery disease can be achieved for a number of years in an elderly patient, the morbidity and mortality of surgery may be obviated for the selected individual.

Balloon dilatation is also being expanded to individuals with valvular stenoses. An early report by Lock et al. (82) reported on balloon dilatation of children with pulmonary valvular stenoses. In the 5 children in whom this procedure was attempted, the RV pressure fell from a mean of 104 to 80, and the gradient cross obstruction fell from 61 to 32 mm Hg. The authors felt that 3 of the 5 patients had anatomic improvement at the time of the followup study, 2 to 12 months later.

Balloon dilatation of the aortic valve was attempted in 2 patients, aged 93 and 85, with long-standing calcific aortic stenosis (83). The balloon was passed retrograde across the aortic valve. In a 93-year-old woman, the aortic valve area was increased from 0.4 cm^2 to 0.6 cm^2 with the cardiac index improving from 2.1 liters/min/m^2 to 2.4 liters/min/m^2. In the 86-year-old patient, the aortic valve area was increased from 0.5 cm^2 to 0.7 cm^2 with a cardiac index increasing from 2.2 to 2.7 liters/min/m^2. In both patients aortic regurgitation increased from trace to 1+. Palacios et al. (84) passed a balloon across the atrial septum and across a stenotic mitral valve in a 57-year-old man, who was not a surgical candidate for medical reasons. Using this trans-septal technique, the procedure resulted in a decrease of the diastolic transvalvular gradient from 20 to 4 mm Hg. The mitral valve area increased from 0.7 to 2.5 cm^2. These two reports certainly herald a new approach to individuals who may not otherwise be candidates for cardiac surgery. It is disappointing to see that the balloon valvuloplasty technique cannot open valves more than slightly. However, relieving valvular gradients even slightly may be enough to increase longevity and improve older patients symptomatically. Further developments in both balloon dilatation of coronary arteries and heart valves may impact significantly on the treatment of heart disease in the older individual.

Conclusions

Although most organs undergo functional decline with aging, none is compromised sufficiently even in extreme age for death to result in the absence of disease (85). Consequently, even the compromised physiology of the elderly still requires a specific pathologic insult such as pulmonary edema, myocardial infarction, or aspiration for death to occur. The body does not simply "wear out" but rather succumbs to a specific disease process. Demographic data clearly show that the number of very old people is increasing rapidly, that the average period of diminished vigor will probably increase, and that chronic diseases will probably occupy a larger proportion of one's life span (86). The conclusion is obvious—the need for medical care in later life is likely to increase substantially.

The surgical treatment of cardiac disease in the elderly in the United States is well beyond the stage of clinical investigation. Report after report cited in this chapter suggest that the current techniques of preoperative, operative, and postoperative care can be successfully applied to the elderly patient in the same manner as younger individuals. More importantly, the expected result in patients aged 70 or older is not all that dissimilar from younger cohorts. This holds true for the treatment of the more straightforward disease processes, of coronary artery disease or valvular heart disease as well as the more complex procedures involving both of these disease processes, as well as operations on the aorta itself. This statement could not be made with certainty 15 or even 10 years ago. To deny a patient a cardiac operation solely on the basis of age can simply no longer be justified.

References

1. Editorial. 1968. Systolic murmurs in the elderly. *Br Med J* 4:530–531.
2. Nixon, JV, et al. 1985. Ventricular performance in human hearts aged 61 to 73 years. *Am J Cardiol* 56:932–937.
3. Brandfonbrenner, M, Landowne, M, and Shock, NW. 1955. Changes in cardiac output with age. *Circulation* 12:557–566.
4. Port, S, et al. 1980. Effect of age on the response of the left ventricular ejection fraction to exercise. *N Engl J Med* 303:1133–1137.
5. Rodeheffer, RJ, et al. 1984. Exercise cardiac output is maintained with advancing age in healthy human subjects: Cardiac dilatation and increased stroke volume compensate for a diminished heart rate. *Circulation* 69:203–213.
6. Weisfeldt, ML. 1980. Left ventricular function. In *The Aging Heart,* Ed., ML Weisfeldt. New York: Raven Press.
7. Lakatta, EG, and Yin, FCP. 1982. Myocardial aging: Functional alterations and related cellular mechanisms. *Am J Physiol* 242:H927–H941.
8. Ebert, TJ, et al. 1982. Effect of age and coronary heart disease on the circulatory responses to graded lower body negative pressure. *Cardiovasc Res* 16:663–669.
9. Feinleib, M. 1975. Changes in life expectancy since 1900. *Circulation* 51 (Supp. III): 16–17.
10. Ross, J Jr., and Braunwald, E. 1968. Aortic stenosis. *Circulation* 38 (Supp. V) V61–V67.
11. Harken, DE, et al. 1962. Aortic valve replacement with a caged ball valve. *Am J Cardiol* 9:292–297.
12. Rotman, M, et al. 1971. Aortic valvular disease. Comparison of types and their medical and surgical management. *Am J Med* 51:241–257.
13. Frank, S, and Ross, J Jr. 1967. The natural history of severe, acquired valvular aortic stenosis. *Am J Cardiol* 19:128.
14. Selzer, A, and Cohn, KE. 1972. Natural history of mitral stenosis. *Circulation* 45:878–890.
15. Olesen, KH. 1962. The natural history of 271 patients with mitral stenosis under medical treatment. *Br Heart J* 24: 349–357.
16. Hildner, FJ, and Kouchoukos, NT. 1973. Problems in mitral valve replacement. In *Advances in Cardiovascular Surgery,* Ed., JW Kirklin. New York: Grune & Stratton.
17. Roberts, WC. 1970. The structure of the aortic valve in clinically isolated aortic stenosis. An autopsy study of 162 patients over 15 years of age. *Circulation* 42:91–97.

18. Roberts, WC, Perloff, JK, and Costantino, T. 1971. Severe valvular aortic stenosis in patients over 65 years of age. A clinicopathologic study. *Am J Cardiol* 27:497–506.
19. Ahmad, A, and Starr, A. 1969. Valve replacement in geriatric patients. *Br Heart J* 31:322–326.
20. Arom, KV, et al. 1984. Should valve replacement and related procedures be performed in elderly patients? *Ann Thorac Surg* 38:466–472.
21. Austen, WG, et al. 1970. Surgical management of aortic valve disease in the elderly. *JAMA* 211:624–626.
22. Barnhorst, DA, et al. 1974. Open heart surgery in patients more than 65 years old. *Ann Thorac Surg* 18:81–90.
23. Bensaid, J, Lasry, JM, and Maurice, P. 1973. Results of aortic valve replacement by a ball-valve prosthesis in 43 subjects aged more than 60 years. *Arch Mal Coeur* 66: 971–973.
24. Bessone, LN, et al. 1977. Valve replacement in patients over 70 years. *Ann Thorac Surg* 24:417–421.
25. Canepa-Anson, R, and Emanuel, RW. 1979. Elective aortic and mitral valve surgery in patients over 70 years of age. *Br Heart J* 41:493.
26. Copeland, JG, et al. 1977. Isolated aortic valve replacement in patients older than 65 years. *JAMA* 237:1578–1581.
27. Craver, JM, et al. 1984. Clinical, hemodynamic and operative descriptors affecting outcome of aortic valve replacement in elderly versus young patients. *Ann Surg* 199:733–741.
28. Finegan, RE, Gianelly, RE, and Harrison, DC. 1969. Aortic stenosis in the elderly. Relevance of age to diagnosis and treatment. *N Engl J Med* 281:1261–1263.
29. Grondin, CM, Meere, C, and Castonguay, Y. 1971. Cardiac surgery in the aged: A review of 120 cases. *Int Cardiol* 2:234–245.
30. Guthrie, RB, et al. 1972. Open heart valve surgery in patients 65 and older. *Arch Surg* 105:42–43.
31. Hildner, FJ, et al. 1969. Clinical and hemodynamic comparisons of valve replacement in patients over and under age 60. *Ann Thorac Surg* 7:438–445.
32. Hochberg, MS, et al. 1979. Mitral valve replacement in elderly patients: Encouraging postoperative clinical and hemodynamic results. *J Thorac Cardiovasc Surg* 77:422–426.
33. Hochberg, MS, et al. 1977. Aortic valve replacement in the elderly. Encouraging postoperative clinical and hemodynamic results. *Arch Surg* 112:1475–1480.
34. Jones, TW, et al. 1979. Aortic valve replacement and the senior citizen. *Am Surg* 45:684–699.
35. Nicoloff, DM, et al. 1984. Valve replacement in the geriatric patient using the St. Jude Medical prosthesis. In *Cardiac Valve Replacement: Current status,* Ed., JM Matloff. Boston: Martinus Nijhoff Publishing.
36. Oh, W, et al. 1973. Heart valve surgery in 114 patients over the age of 60. *Br Heart J* 35:174–180.
37. Shanahan, MY, Windsor, HM, and Golding, L. 1972. Open heart surgery in the elderly. *Aust NZ J Surg* 42:107–112.
38. Stephenson, LW, MacVaugh, H, III, and Edmunds, LH. 1978. Surgery using cardiopulmonary bypass in the elderly. *Circulation* 58:250–254.
39. Bjork, VO, Henze, A, and Rodriguez, L. 1977. Left ventricular rupture as a complication of mitral valve replacement. Surgical experience with eight cases and a review of the literature. *J Thorac Cardiovasc Surg* 73:14–22.
40. Kirklin, JW. 1972. Replacement of the mitral valve for mitral incompetence. *Surgery* 72:827–836.
41. Kouchoukos, NT, Sheppard, LC, and Kirklin, JW. 1972. Effect of alterations in arterial pressure on cardiac performance early after open intra-cardiac operations. *J Thorac Cardiovasc Surg* 64:563–572.
42. Carpentier, A, et al. 1982. Continuing improvements in bioprostheses. *J Thorac Cardiovasc Surg* 83:27–42.
43. Jamieson, WRE, et al. 1984. Five year evaluation of the Carpentier-Edwards porcine bioprosthesis. *J Thorac Cardiovasc Surg* 88:324–333.
44. Katz, S, et al. 1983. Active life expectancy. *N Engl J Med* 309:1218–1224.
45. Fries, JF. 1980. Aging, natural death and the compression of morbidity. *N Engl J Med* 303:130–135.
46. Ashor, GW, et al. 1973. Coronary artery disease—Surgery in 100 patients 65 years of age and older. *Arch Surg* 107:30–33.
47. Berry, BE, et al. 1981. Coronary artery bypass operation in septuagenarians. *Ann Thorac Surg* 31:310–313.
48. Cosgrove, DM, et al. 1984. Primary myocardial revascularization. Trends in surgical mortality. *J Thorac Cardiovasc Surg* 88:673–684.
49. Elayda, MA, et al. 1984. Coronary revascularization in the elderly patient. *J Am Coll Cardiol* 3:1398–1402.
50. Faro, RS, et al. 1983. Coronary revascularization in septuagenarians. *J Thorac Cardiovasc Surg* 86:616–620.
51. Gann, D, et al. 1977. Coronary artery bypass surgery in patients seventy years of age and older. *J Thorac Cardiovasc Surg* 73:237–241.
52. Garcia, JM, Cheanvechai, C, and Effler, DB. 1985. Myocardial revascularization in patients aged 65 and older. *Cardiovasc Clin* 7:83–91.
53. Gersh, BJ, et al. 1983. Coronary arteriography and coronary artery bypass surgery: Morbidity and mortality in patients ages 65 years or older. *Circulation* 67:483–490.
54. Gooch, JB, et al. 1983. Coronary artery bypass surgery in the septuagenarian. *Texas Heart Inst J* 10:137–141.
55. Hamby, RI, et al. 1973. Intractable angina pectoris in the 65 to 79 year age group: A surgical approach. *Chest* 64:46–50.
56. Hibler, BA, et al. 1983. Coronary artery bypass surgery in the elderly. *Arch Surg* 118:402–404.
57. Hochberg, MS, et al. 1982. Isolated coronary artery bypass grafting in patients 70 years of age and older. *J Thorac Cardiovasc Surg* 84:219–223.
58. Jeffery, DL, et al. 1985. Coronary bypass for left main disease in patients over 70 years of age. *J Cardiovasc Surg* 26: 212–216.
59. Kennedy, JW, et al. 1981. Clinical and angiographic predictors of operative mortality from the collaborative study in coronary artery surgery (CASS). *Circulation* 63:793–801.
60. Kirklin, JW, et al. 1979. Research related to surgical treatment of coronary artery disease. *Circulation* 60:1613–1618.
61. Knapp, WS, et al. 1981. Efficacy of coronary artery bypass grafting in elderly patients with coronary artery disease. *Am J Cardiol* 47:923–930.
62. McCallister, BD, et al. 1975. Coronary artery bypass in patients over the age of 70: Initial and late results. *Circulation* 52 (Supp II):II 91.
63. Meyer, J, et al. 1975. Coronary artery bypass in patients over 70 years of age: Indications and results. *Am J Cardiol*

36:343.
64. Montague, NT, et al. 1985. Morbidity and mortality of coronary bypass grafting in patients 70 years of age and older. *Ann Thorac Surg* 39:552–557.
65. Roberts, AJ, et al. 1985. Mortality, morbidity, and cost-accounting related to coronary artery bypass graft surgery in the elderly. *Ann Thorac Surg* 39:426–432.
66. Rose, DM, et al. 1985. Analysis of morbidity and mortality in patients 70 years of age and over undergoing isolated coronary artery bypass surgery. *Am Heart J* 110:341–346.
67. Smith, JM, et al. 1976. Cardiac surgery in geriatric patients. *Surgery* 80:443–448.
68. Stringer, RJ, et al. 1975. Coronary bypass grafting in the older age group. *Circulation* 52 (Supp II):245.
69. Tsai, TP, et al. 1986. Cardiac surgery in the octogenarian. *J Thorac Cardiovasc Surg* 91:924–928.
70. Gersh, BJ, et al. 1983. Long term (5 year) results of coronary bypass surgery in patients 65 years old or older: A report from the coronary artery surgery study. *Circulation* 68 (Supp II):II 190–II 199.
71. Gersh, BJ, et al. 1985. Comparison of coronary artery bypass surgery and medical therapy in patients 65 years of age or older. *N Engl J Med* 313:217–224.
72. Kaiser, GC. 1986. CABG: Lessons from the randomized trials. *Ann Thorac Surg* 42:3–8.
73. Alderman, EL, et al. 1983. Results of coronary artery surgery in patients with poor left ventricular function (CASS). *Circulation* 68:785–795.
74. Kunis, R, et al. 1985. Coronary revascularization for recurrent pulmonary edema in elderly patients with ischemic heart disease and preserved ventricular function. *N Engl J Med* 313:1207–1210.
75. Akins, CW, et al. 1985. Myocardial revascularization with combined aortic and mitral valve replacements. *J Thorac Cardiovasc Surg* 90:272–277.
76. Najafi, H, et al. 1972. Acute aortic regurgitation secondary to aortic dissection. Surgical management without valve replacement. *Ann Thorac Surg* 14:474–482.
77. Crawford, ES, and Crawford, JL. 1984. Aneurysms of degenerative origin. In *Diseases of the Aorta,* Eds., ES Crawford and JL Crawford. Baltimore: Williams & Wilkins.
78. Daggett, WM, and Buckley, MJ. 1980. The surgical treatment of post infarction ventricular septal defect. In *Surgery for the Complications of Myocardial Infarction,* Eds., JM Moran and LL Michaelis. New York: Grune & Stratton.
79. Folks, DG, et al. 1986. Coronary artery bypass surgery in older patients: Psychiatric morbidity. *South Med J* 79:303–306.
80. Gallagher, JD, et al. 1985. Effects of advanced age on extravascular lung water accumulation during coronary artery bypass surgery. *Crit Care Med* 13:68–71.
81. Williams, MA, et al. 1985. Early exercise training in patients older than age 65 years compared with that in younger patients after acute myocardial infarction or coronary artery bypass grafting. *Am J Cardiol* 55:263–266.
82. Lock, JE, et al. 1983. Balloon dilatation angioplasty of hypoplastic and stenotic pulmonary arteries. *Circulation* 67:962–967.
83. McKay, RG, et al. 1986. Balloon dilatation of calcific aortic stenosis in elderly patients: Postmortem, intraoperative and percutaneous valvuloplasty studies. *Circulation* 74:119–125.
84. Palacios, IF, et al. 1986. Percutaneous transvenous balloon valvotomy in a patient with severe calcific mitral stenosis. *J Am Coll Cardiol* 7:1416–1419.
85. Shock, NW. 1977. Systems integration. In *Handbook of the Biology of Aging,* Eds., CE Finch and L. Hayflick. New York: Van Nostrand Reinhold Co.
86. Schneider, EL, and Brody, JA. 1983. Aging, natural death and the compression of morbidity: Another view. *N Engl J Med* 309:854–856.

31

Abdominal Surgery in the Elderly

Ronnie Ann Rosenthal, Nonyelu Chukwuogo, and Thomas M. Scalea

General Considerations

Abdominal surgery in the elderly presents special problems and challenges to the surgeon. "Acute" and "atypical" are the terms that best describe the abdominal surgical disorders in these patients. "Acute" presentation leads to urgent or emergent surgery, which is associated with an operative mortality rate of approximately three times that for comparable elective procedures. "Atypical" presentation leads to delay in treatment and error in diagnosis, which further compound the underlying illness and favor the development of complications. Postoperative complications are poorly tolerated in these patients; operative mortality rates have been reported to increase from 10% in certain uncomplicated procedures to over 60% in similar cases where complications have occurred (1).

Also important is the presence of coexisting pathologic conditions of other major organ systems found in 65% to 75% of elderly patients who undergo abdominal operation. In a study of colon surgery in patients over age 50 years, Boyd et al. (2) documented the incidence of coexisting pathology and its effect on the outcome of surgery. The preoperative incidence of coexisting diseases rose steadily with age so that by age 80 only 5% of patients had no pathologic condition other than the primary surgical illness (Table 31-1). Cardiovascular disease was the most common and was present in 85% of octogenarians. Mortality rates rose from 0% in patients under 70 years of age with less than two coexisting disorders, to over 16% in patients over 70 with two or more additional conditions.

It should not be surprising that emergency abdominal operations, which place great demands on cardiovascular and pulmonary reserves, are associated with a high incidence of postoperative complications and death in the elderly. To improve the outcome, emergency circumstances must be avoided as much as possible by the appropriate early selection of patients for elective surgery. Delays in treatment must also be minimized by an awareness of the atypical presentation of surgical illness and by an aggressive approach to diagnosis. Limitations imposed by coexisting pathology, particulary of the cardiovascular and pulmonary systems, must be ameliorated by expeditious preoperative assessment and treatment through the use of invasive monitoring and pharmacological intervention when indicated.

Distribution of Abdominal Disorders

The distribution of specific abdominal surgical disorders in the elderly is difficult to determine with certainty from the literature. Reports that do provide some useful data include a study from Sweden which quantified the causes of nearly 10,000 visits to a surgical emergency room for acute abdominal complaints (3). Gallbladder disease, intestinal obstruction, acute diverticulitis, gastrointestinal bleeding, and hernia all demonstrated an increased incidence in elderly patients (Table 31-2). Surprisingly, appendicitis, which occurs typically in the first three decades of life, demonstrated a second peak in the elderly with an incidence of 3/1,000 population per year in men over 80.

In another recent report from Israel (4), 1,000 consecutive major abdominal procedures in patients over 70 were reviewed. Table 31-3 shows the distribution of be-

Table 31-1. Percent of patients with additional preoperative pathologic conditions

Number of additional pathologic conditions	Age (years) 50–59	60–69	70–79	Over 80	Total
0	46	33	21	5	30
1	37	34	28	37	33
2	13	27	23	41	24
3 or more	3	8	22	15	11

Reprinted with permission from Boyd BJ, Bradford B, and Watne AL. 1980. Operative risk factors of colon resection in the elderly. *Ann Surg* 192:743–746.

nign and malignant disorders found at operation. Biliary tract disease was responsible for 46% of the procedures performed for benign disease and nearly one third of all procedures. Obstruction of both small and large bowel, due to postoperative adhesion, incarcerated hernia, or malignancy, in that order, accounted for nearly 25% of all procedures. Peptic ulcer disease was the operative indication for nearly 20% of all procedures performed for benign disease. Over half of these ulcer operations were undertaken emergently for complications such as bleeding or perforation.

Malignant disease was present in 45% of all operations. Tumors of the colon and rectum accounted for 56% of malignancies, while tumors of the stomach and esophagus were next most common, occurring in 23% of cancer cases.

While the pattern of diagnosis and operative procedure performed differ somewhat with geographic location, most series concur that biliary tract disease is the most common cause of acute abdominal complaints and accounts for approximately one-third of abdominal surgical procedures in the elderly (3–8).

Colonic disorders appear to be second most common; cancer and diverticular disease account for the majority of colonic procedures. Colonic volvulus, pseudo-obstruction, stercoral perforation, and rectal prolapse are less common but are peculiar to this age group and are therefore of special interest. Gastric disorders, including ulcer and malignancy, and small bowel disorders, including obstruction, are next most common, and each accounts for approximately 10% of abdominal operations. While hernia operations are generally not true abdominal procedures, the frequent presentation of incarceration and small bowel obstruction, which may require laparotomy and bowel resection, is a special concern. Finally, while acute appendicitis is responsible for only 5% of all abdominal procedures in the elderly, it, too, deserves special attention because of the pecularities in presentation in this age group.

Table 31-2. Etiology of abdominal complaints in the elderly

Disorder	Incidence per 1000 population per year	
Biliary	16	(women >80)
Intestinal obstruction	6.8	(women >80)
Acute diverticulitis	3.5	(all patients >70)
GI hemorrhage	5.7	(men 70–79)
Hernia	4–6	(men >70)
Appendicitis	3	(men >80)

Adapted from Janzon L, Ryden CL, and Zederfeldt B. 1982. Acute Abdomen in the surgical emergency room. Who is taken care of when for what? *Acta Chir Scand* 148:141–148.

Table 31-3. Operative procedures performed

Procedures	Cases	(%)
Benign cases—547		
Simple cholecystectomy	162	(30)
Cholecystectomy + choledochotomy	92	(17)
Stomach and duodenum (vagotomy included)	98	(18)
Appendectomy	34	(6)
Lysis of adhesions	43	(8)
Miscellaneous procedures	118	(21)
Malignant cases—453		
Resections		
Colon and rectum	216	(47)
Stomach and esophagus	66	(14)
Miscellaneous	31	(8)
Palliative procedures	68	(15)
Laparotomy only, with or without biopsy	72	(16)

Reprinted with permission from Reiss, R, Deutsch AA, and Nudelman L. 1987. Abdominal surgery in elderly patients: Statistical analysis of clinical factors prognostic of mortality in 1000 cases. *Mt Sinai J Med* 54:135–140.

Operative Management of Biliary Tract Disease

Biliary tract disease is the most common cause of acute abdominal complaints in the elderly and accounts for 26% to 40% of all acute abdominal disorders (3, 5, 6). It is also the most common indication for abdominal surgery in patients over age 60 (7, 8).

It is well known that there is a rise in the incidence of gallstones with aging. In a frequently quoted autopsy study, Crump (9) demonstrated the presence of gallstones in more than 50% of all patients over age 70 years. Another more recent autopsy study by Newman (10) confirmed the steady age-related increase in cholelithiasis in white females (Table 31-4).

It is less well known, however, that there is also a clear rise in the incidence of acute and complicated biliary tract disease with aging. Forty to sixty percent of patients over age 70 present with an acute complication of biliary tract disease and require emergency surgery (4, 11–16). These complications include acute cholecystitis, em-

Table 31-4. Incidence of gallstones in white females proven at autopsy

Age in years	Number of autopsies	Number with calculi	Percentage
Under 20	399	0	
20–29	49	5	10.2
30–39	92	17	18.4
40–49	171	44	25.7
50–59	237	78	32.9
60–69	290	112	38.6
70–79	134	55	41.0
80–89	30	16	53.3
All ages	1402	327	23.3

Reprinted with permission from Glenn F. 1981. Surgical management of acute cholecystostomy in patients 65 years of age and older. *Ann Surg* 193:56–59.

pyema, perforation, and abscess. The overall incidence of these complications in the general population is only 7% to 20% (14, 17, 18). The mortality for emergency surgery in the older age group is 5% to 19% compared to an elective mortality rate of 0% to 3% (11, 13–20). It is therefore important to carefully evaluate every elderly patient with gallstones and to consider elective treatment before complicated disease occurs.

Cholelithiasis and Chronic Cholecystitis

Efforts are now underway to identify a form of treatment that will obliterate or dissolve gallstones and thus make surgery for cholelithiasis unnecessary. Unfortunately, to date no such treatment has been proven safe and effective for all types of stones. The efficacy of the bile acids chenodeoxycholic and ursodeoxycholic acid on cholesterol stones has been studied extensively (21, 22), and this form of dissolution therapy is presently being used. Small, radiolucent stones in a functional gallbladder must be demonstrated before therapy is initiated (Fig. 31-1). With proper patient selection and adequate dose and length of therapy, these agents have proven somewhat efficacious and safe. The need for prolonged treatment and reports of high failure and recurrence rates, however, have prevented widespread acceptance of these agents. Furthermore, specific data regarding the use and results of these potentially toxic agents in patients over 65 years old is not yet available. Other approaches such as percutaneous instillation of methyl tert-butyl ether (23) or lithotripsy (24) in combination with dissolution therapy are under investigation but are not yet routinely available.

At present, cholecystectomy is still the best accepted treatment for chronic cholelithiasis. Controversy exists, however, about when and in whom cholecystectomy should be advised. A distinction has been made between

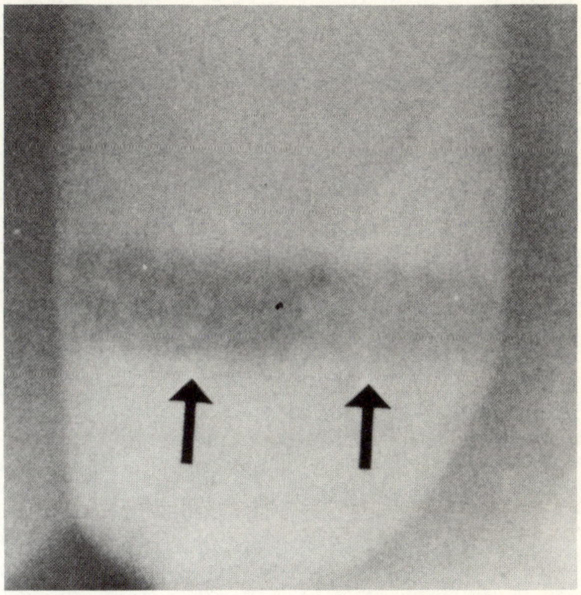

Figure 31-1. Multiple small, floating, radiolucent gallstones in a functioning gallbladder. (Reprinted, with permission, from: Hatfield PM, and Wise RE., 1976. *Radiology of the Gallbladder and Bile Ducts*. Baltimore, Md: Williams & Wilkins.) (277).

"symptomatic" and "asymptomatic" stones, and several studies have been undertaken to determine the natural history of each (25–28).

Extreme caution must be used when drawing conclusions relevant to the elderly from the seemingly benign results of conservative or expectant therapy of "asymptomatic" gallstones in younger patients. In the aged, this distinction between "symptomatic" and "asymptomatic" disease is often quite difficult. Although no study has specifically examined the experience in elderly patients, some age-related data is available. Wenckhert and Robertson (25) followed 781 patients with documented gallstones for 1 to 11 years. Of these, 223 were over age 60 years at the time of diagnosis. During the follow-up period, a significantly higher percent of the older patients developed complications of their stone disease (29% versus 14%). The authors attribute this high incidence of complications in part to the smaller number of elderly patients undergoing elective cholecystectomy (Fig. 31-2). However, even when the influence of elective operation was excluded, the complication rate in these patients was still significantly higher.

In another frequently quoted study, Lund (26) followed 526 patients with unoperated gallstones for 5 to 20 years and determined that 50% of "asymptomatic" females and 30% of "asymptomatic" males developed more severe symptoms or a complication of their stone disease. In approximately 25% of these patients, an acute complication occurred without preceding symptoms. In this

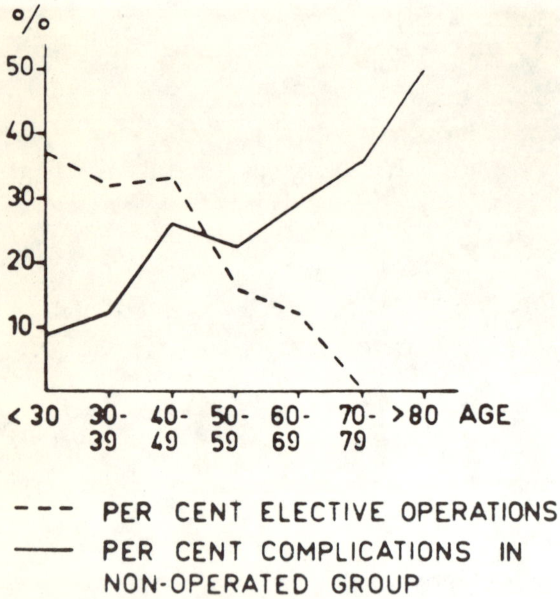

Figure 31-2. Percent of complications and elective operations in various age groups. (Reprinted, with permission, from Wenckhert A, and Robertson B. 1966. The natural course of gallstone disease. *Gastroenterology* 50: 376–381.) (25).

study, there appeared to be no significant difference in outcome between the "symptomatic" and "asymptomatic" patients. Unfortunately, there were too few patients over age 65 in the "asymptomic" category to allow analysis of the outcome in this group. While not conclusive, both of these studies support the view that "asymptomatic" or "mild" biliary tract disease is not a benign condition, particularly in elderly patients.

More recent studies dispute this contention. In 1982, Gracie and Ransohoff (27) studied the natural history of silent gallstones in a group of predominately male faculty members, mean age 54. These silent stones were detected on routine screening oral cholecystograms. The results showed that one-third of patients remained "asymptomatic," one-quarter had "prophylactic" cholecystectomy, one-quarter died of nonrelated causes, and one-sixth developed biliary symptoms. Although a substantial number of these patients did remain "asymptomatic," it is difficult to apply the conclusions drawn from the data on this select group of relatively young patients to the much more diverse elderly population in general.

In 1985 McSherry et al. (28) published a retrospective review of the natural history of gallstones, in which the mean age of the study group was 65 years. While this study was not confined to elderly patients, some interesting and relevant observations are presented. The patient population consisted of 556 (80%) "symptomatic" and 135 "asymptomatic" patients. The "symptomatic" patients were younger than the "asymptomatic" patients, with a mean age of 63 compared to 73 years. Of the "symptomatic" patients, 44% underwent operation within a median of 2½ years, and 21% of those operations were performed for acute cholecystitis. The fact that a large number of these "symptomatic" patients required emergency surgery suggests a failure to predict which patients would develop acute complications of gallstone disease based on the history of their symptomatology. Of the "asymptomatic" patients, only 10% required biliary surgery in nearly 4 years of follow-up. However, the incidence of complicating diseases, such as significant coronary artery disease, hypertension, and malignancy was also higher in this group. The overall mortality rate during the follow-up period for "asymptomatic" patients was 18.5% compared to only 4.5% for the "symptomatic" patients. In addition, only 11% of the "symptomatic" patients in this study demonstrated radiopaque gallstones compared to 64% of the "asymptomatic" patients. It would appear that the terms "symptomatic" and "asymptomatic" in this study may describe two somewhat different patient populations. The "symptomatic" group was found to be younger, "healthier," and had a higher incidence of radiolucent stones, while the "asymptomatic" group was older, had more coexisting diseases, and more frequently documented calcified stones. Whether or not the presence of calcium in the gallstones portends a more benign progression of disease in this group of patients remains to be elucidated.

It was concluded from this study that "symptomatic" patients should be advised to undergo cholecystectomy. There is now general agreement that early operative intervention is warranted even in the very oldest "symptomatic" patients. The significant incidence of acute complications despite careful surveillance strongly supports this decision. It was also concluded that all "asymptomatic" patients can be treated nonoperatively and followed with reasonable safety. Should a safe and efficacious treatment for stone dissolution become available, these patients would be ideal candidates. Whether or not these recommendations can be applied to elderly patients, however, remains questionable. Although enthusiasts of dissolution therapy suggest it as the treatment for "asymptomatic" stones in high-risk elderly patients, the predominance of calcified stones in this age group disqualifies the majority of these patients from presently available forms of medical therapy. Furthermore, the safety of nonoperative management in this age group is not well documented.

A strong argument against the benign nature of "asymptomatic" gallstones in the elderly can be made from studies of the pathophysiology of gallbladder perforation. This entity, which is principally a disease of elderly males, is associated with a mortality rate of 15% to

23%. In a study by Roslyn and Busuttil (29), only one quarter of the patients with perforation had a prior history of biliary symptoms, in spite of the pathological finding of chronic cholecystitis underlying the acute inflammation in 70% of cases. Therefore chronic cholecystitis may be present but undetected in the elderly and may have devastating consequences.

A final consideration favoring a more liberal use of surgery in the elderly with "asymptomatic" stones is the association of chronic stone disease with gallbladder carcinoma. While cancer develops in only about 1% of patients with stones (11, 26), we agree with Lund (26) who states, "the risk of cancer, per se, does not indicate prophylactic cholestectomy, but it intensifies the operative indication."

Whether or not "asymptomatic" stones are benign, no study of the natural history of gallstones explains why elderly patients have such a high incidence of complicated biliary tract disease. The distinction between "symptomatic" and "asymptomatic" stones must be made with extreme care in these patients, whose abdominal complaints are often vague, poorly localized, and ill described. Until a reliable method exists for predicting which elderly patient with gallstones will develop complicated disease, every elderly patient should be evaluated for therapeutic intervention. If the patient is a reliable historian capable of distinguishing symptoms and is aware enough to respond to new symptoms quickly, noninterventional follow-up may be prudent. If this is not so, but the patient is otherwise in good health, then operative therapy should be considered. Clearly each such patient must be evaluated on an individual basis.

Diagnosis

Diagnostic techniques to determine the presence of gallstones in the elderly do not differ from those used in younger patients. Ultrasound of the abdomen will establish the presence of gallbladder stones in over 90% of cases (30). The function of the gallbladder can be assessed by oral cholecystography. Due to the high incidence of radiopaque stones in the elderly, a plain roentgenogram of the abdomen alone may be diagnostic (Fig. 31-3).

Operative Treatment

In elderly patients, the technique of cholecystectomy does not differ from that in younger patients. However, because of the finding of common bile duct stones in well over 20% of elderly patients (18, 31), intraoperative cholangiography should be performed routinely regardless of the presence of absence of other indicators of stones on preoperative chemical studies. Prophylactic antibiotics are also indicated because of the high incidence of infected bile and the increased complications associated with positive bile cultures (32). The operative management of common bile duct stones will be discussed separately.

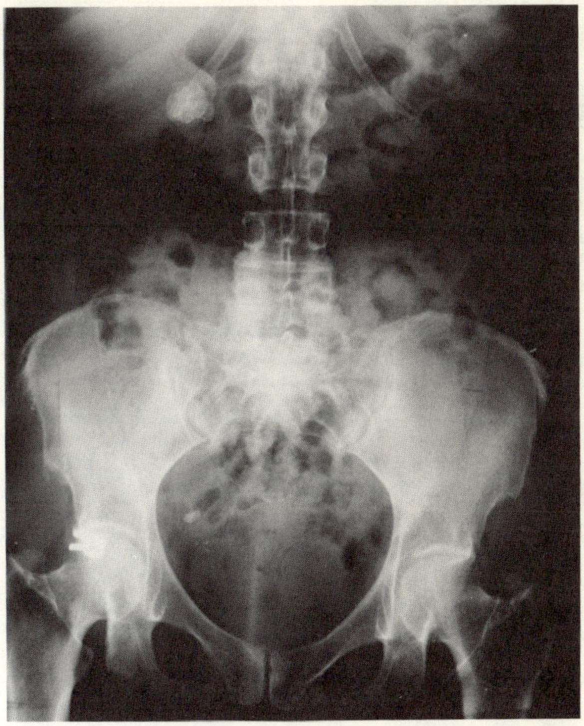

Figure 31-3. Calcifications in the right upper quadrant on this flat plate of the abdomen representing radiopaque gallstones.

Results

Cholecystectomy for the treatment of uncomplicated gallstones is well accepted as a safe surgical procedure. Mortality for all ages ranges from 0.5% to 1.8% and is reported as low as 0.1% for those under age 50 (17, 18). Although it appears that the mortality for elective cholecystectomy in the elderly is higher (up to 3%), age itself is not thought to be the cause. In a prospective analysis of elderly patients undergoing biliary surgery, Houghton (19) divided patients into two groups: the "old" (65–74) and the "aged" (over 74). The overall elective mortality was 0.8% and was not significantly different between the two age groups.

As with all intra-abdominal procedures in the elderly, the incidence of other unrelated disorders increases with age in patients undergoing operations for cholelithiasis (32) (Table 31-5). It is the presence of these conditions and not age alone that is thought to be responsible for the small apparent increase in mortality. It has also been stated that the presence of infected bile at the time of cholecystectomy is associated with a higher mortality in elderly patients, even in the elective clinical setting (32).

The principal cause of death after elective cho-

Table 31-5. Incidence of preoperatively associated diseases in percent

	Age (years)			
Condition	65–75	76–85	86–98	Total
Cardiovascular	38	64	85	53.2
Pulmonary	12	34	36	26
Renal	10	19	28	21
Hepatic	13	21	27	20
Nutritional	4	17	23	15
Others	14	21	22	19

Reprinted from Lydigakis NJ. 1983. Operative risk factors of cholecystectomy—choledochotomy in the elderly. *Surg Gynecol Obstet* 157:15–19 (By permission of Surgery, Gynecology & Obstetrics.).

lecystectomy is cardiovascular, usually due to myocardial infarction (11, 14). Complications occur in approximately 20% of elderly patients. Half of these are minor (12, 14, 33). Cardiovascular problems are most common and usually the most serious. Pulmonary, urinary, and wound infections also occur.

It appears that elective cholecystectomy in the elderly can be accomplished with acceptable risk of mortality and morbidity. The decision to operate must include assessment and correction, if possible, of factors which predispose to increased surgical mortality in this age group in general.

Acute Cholecystitis

Acute cholecystitis in patients over age 65 is viewed by most surgeons as a surgical emergency. In a study by McSherry and Glenn (18), of 2347 patients treated for acute cholecystitis, the percent of patients over age 65 at the time of operation increased from 5.3% in the 1930s to 39.8% in the 1970s. During this same interval, the percent of the population over age 65 just slightly more than doubled. This increase in elderly patients undergoing operation not only reflects less reluctuance to operate on the elderly in general, but more importantly, also indicates the realization that nonoperative management of acute cholecystitis carries an extraordinarily high failure rate in this age group.

A detailed discussion of the etiology and pathogenesis of acute cholecystitis can be found elsewhere (34, 35). However, it is generally accepted that the initiating factor is cystic duct obstruction. In 95% of cases, this obstruction is caused by stones. The remaining 5% of cases occur in the absence of stones and are usually associated with sepsis, trauma, and prolonged fasting. Although the cause for the increased incidence of acute cholecystitis in the elderly is not completely understood, several possible explanations have been suggested. Changes in bile composition that promote lithogenesis may also cause chemical irritation of the gallbladder mucosa (34) and alter mucosal function. Bacteria have been implicated, and positive bile cultures are found in over 75% of elderly patients with this disease (33). Altered host defenses that occur with aging may also promote or facilitate development of acute inflammation (36). Changes in the gallbladder wall itself, due to aging or to repeated episodes of inflammation from the long-standing presence of stones, may render it more susceptible to chemical, bacterial, or ischemic injury.

Diagnosis

As with many other sources of intra-abdominal pathology in the elderly, acute biliary tract disease can often present in a misleading manner. Delays in diagnosis and treatment further promote the development of acute disease. Initial symptoms are usually vague and poorly localized and are often ignored by patients. In a frequently quoted study of elderly patients with acute cholecystitis, Morrow et al. (33) documented that nearly 33% of acutely ill patients had a delay in diagnosis of more than 24 hours because of inconsistencies in presentation. Over one-third of patients were afebrile, one-quarter had no abdominal tenderness, and more than one-half had no signs of peritoneal inflammation despite advanced intra-abdominal sepsis. As a result of this benign presentation, only 25% of patients reached the operating room within the first 24 hours of admission.

Laboratory findings can also be misleading. In over one-third of patients in this study, the white blood cell (WBC) count was less than 10,000 cell/mm^3. Jaundice, usually found in 10% to 15% of patients with acute cholecystitis (34), was more common than expected and occurred in 28% of patients.

Methods used to confirm the diagnosis of acute cholecystitis in the aged do not differ from those used in younger patients. However, the absence of physical findings in the elderly should not delay the use of studies to image the biliary tract. The presence of stones or an enlarged gallbladder with thickened walls on sonogram is often diagnostic (37). If there is a question, radionuclide imaging with one of the technetium-99 labeled iminodiacetic acid (IDA) compounds can be used. Failure to visualize the gallbladder in the presence of a visualized common bile duct has an accuracy of 95% for the diagnosis of acute cholecystitis (38).

Although the diagnosis of acute cholecystitis can usually be made accurately once it is suspected, the status of the gallbladder wall itself and the extent of intra-abdominal sepsis is often difficult to assess preoperatively. Only 44% of elderly patients in the series by Morrow et al. (33) had simple acute cholecystitis at operation; 21% had empyema, 10% had perforation, 8% had gangrenous cholecystitis, and 15% had intra-abdominal or liver abscess. A total of 54% of these elderly patients had findings which could not have been easily assessed nonoperatively. In other studies, gangrene of the gallbladder wall at the time of operation was found in over 50% of cases of acute cholecystitis in elderly patients (12, 19) (Fig. 31-4).

Operative Treatment

Operative intervention should be expeditious. Time is allowed preoperatively to correct fluid and electrolyte abnormalities and to optimize cardiac performance. With the liberal use of invasive monitoring and pharmacologic intervention, these deficits can be rapidly identified and corrected. Throughout the perioperative period, the patient should receive broad-spectrum antibiotics because of the high incidence of positive bile cultures and concomitant perioperative bacteremia (11, 33).

The options for surgical treatment depend on the ability to improve the patient's general condition and on the findings at operation. In general, the procedure of choice for acute cholecystitis is cholecystectomy. In the vast majority of cases, this can be accomplished quickly and safely with acceptable blood loss. At operation the gallbladder is usually found to be large, tense, and edematous. It is often necessary to decompress the gallbladder before attempting to remove it to facilitate exposure of the cystic duct area. Most often, however, the area of the cystic duct is surrounded by inflamed, edematous tissue, and early control of the cystic artery and duct is hazardous. Dissection is therefore begun at the fundus and carried down toward the duct. While some bleeding may be encountered, the dissection usually proceeds rapidly because edema in the tissue planes facilitates the separation of gallbladder from the enveloping peritoneum. Since the incidence of common bile duct stones in association with acute cholecystitis is high in the elderly (39), intraoperative cholangiography should be performed if technically feasible. If stones are found and the duct is accessible, exploration with removal of stones and drainage with a large bore t-tube should be performed. Gallbladder bile should be cultured routinely as well.

Recent developments in endoscopic approaches to the common bile duct have made it possible to avoid exploring the duct operatively in technically difficult circumstances (40, 41). When acute cholecystitis is present, the use of additional duct drainage procedures, such as choledochoenterostomy, is controversial and should be reserved for special circumstances. (See Choledocholithiasis.)

Cholecystostomy under local anesthesia may be the procedure of choice in those patients for whom the risk of general anesthesia is prohibitive. These include patients with recent myocardial infarct, severe uncorrectable congestive heart failure, or severe pulmonary compromise. Cholecystostomy may also be necessary for those patients in whom cholecystectomy is technically hazardous (i.e., patients with cirrhosis and portal hypertension). Cholecystostomy is performed through a small subcostal incision placed over the fundus of the gallbladder. Once the gallbladder is decompressed, the stones are removed, and

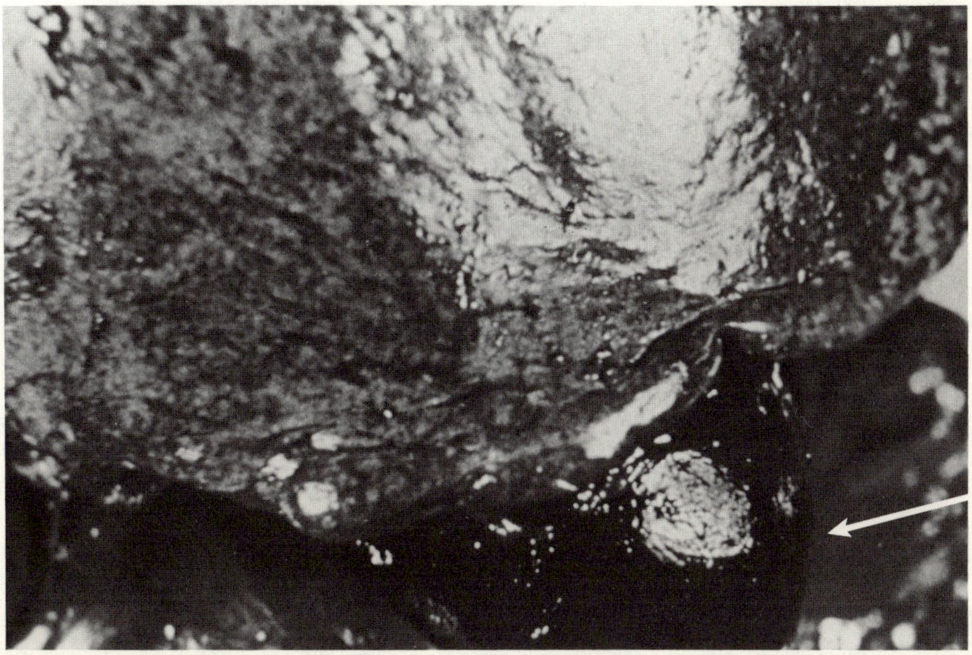

Figure 31-4. Intraoperative photograph of acute gangrenous cholecystitis. The arrow points to the fundus of the necrotic gallbladder.

drainage is established through a large bore balloon or mushroom catheter. Occasionally, cholecystostomy is performed under general anesthesia, usually when a planned cholecystectomy has to be abandoned for technical reasons. Recently, reports of percutaneous transhepatic cholecystostomy have appeared in the literature (42). While the advantage of this technique over conventional cholecystostomy is not well established, it may prove to be a valuable alternative in the high-risk elderly.

Results

Recent results of operative therapy support the use of cholecystectomy as the procedure of choice in acute cholecystitis in the elderly. In the past many older patients were treated with cholecystostomy. In a large series by Glenn (43) (1932–1979), 82% of patients under 50 years of age had cholecystectomy alone compared to only 48% of patients over 65 (Table 31-6). Cholecystostomy alone was performed in 30% of elderly patients in this study. As expected, there was an increased need for choledochotomy in patients over 65. In the more recent study by Morrow (33) (1971–1975), 100% of elderly patients underwent cholecystectomy, and 36% required choledochotomy as well. No patients in this series had a cholecystostomy. Several other recent reports confirm the infrequent need for cholecystostomy (13, 14). The declining use of this procedure in recent years reflects improvement in the ability to safely anesthetize and operate on elderly patients. Nearly 50% of the operative deaths in Glenn's series occurred in patients undergoing cholecystostomy alone. Mortality rates for this procedure are still high and range from 10% to 30% in the recent literature (13). While the use of cholecystostomy has declined significantly, it still has a place in therapy and can be a useful and lifesaving procedure.

The overall operative mortality rate for acute cholecystitis in elderly patients ranges from 5% to 16.7% (14, 16, 18, 30, 33). Mortality by age group from Glenn's study was 9.8% for patients older than age 65 compared to 1.6% for those younger than age 65. Sepsis and resultant multi-organ system failure is the most common cause of death. Cardiovascular causes, including myocardial infarction, congestive heart failure, and cerebrovascular accident are second most common, while pulmonary causes, including pulmonary embolism, also frequently occur.

The morbidity rate for acute cholecystitis in the elderly is high and ranges from 18% to 45% (6, 14, 18, 33). Complications typically include wound infections, pulmonary infections, and nonfatal cardiac events.

Although the mortality and morbidity rates for the operative treatment of acute cholecystitis in the elderly appear to be high, surgery is still the treatment of choice. The mortality for non-operative management of acute cholecystitis in this age group approaches 100% (33).

Choledocholithiasis

In an American College of Surgeons study of over 28,000 cholecystectomies in Ohio, the overall incidence of choledocholelithiasis was reported as 7.3% (17). More recent estimates approach 10% to 15% (44). In the elderly, the incidence of common bile duct (CBD) stones rises steadily, reaching 15% to 22% in patients over age 60 (18, 33), 31% to 33% over age 80 (15, 45), and 60% over age 90 (46). Herman et al. (31) reported an even higher incidence, documenting CBD stones at the time of cholecystectomy in over 50% of patifs-3ents over 70 years old, and in 96% of patients over age 80.

In young patients, cholesterol stones found in the CBD appeared to be identical to the typical cholesterol stones found in the gallbladders of these patients. This finding supports the theory that the majority of this type of ductal stone arise by migration into the CBD from the gallbladder (44). In contrast, stones found in the CBD of elderly patients frequently contain pigment. While the incidence of pigment stones in the gallbladder also increases with age, the percentage of pigmented CBD stones is higher than would be expected from migration alone. Bernhoft et al. (47) studied the morphology and chemical composition of gallbladder stones and CBD stones from the same patient. They found that the stones in the pigment-containing pairs differed from each other in composition and appearance more than did the stones

Table 31-6. Operative procedure performed for acute cholecystitis (in percent)

Age	Cholecystectomy	Cholecystostomy	Cholecystectomy + dochotomy	Cholecystostomy + dochotomy
Greater than 65 years	48	30	21	0.9
64–50	73	13	14	0.9
less than 50 years	82	7	11	0.2

Adapted from Glenn F. 1981. Surgical management of acute cholecystostomy in patients 65 years of age and older. *Ann Surg* 193:56–59.

in cholesterol-containing pairs (Fig. 31-5). Pigment CBD stones are also frequently found in association with infected bile, possibly implicating bacteria in their etiology. It has been postulated that B-glucuronidase from *E. coli* increases the concentration of unconjugated bilirubin, which in turn joins with calcium to form insoluble calcium bilirubinate (48). The high incidence of infected bile in the elderly may partially explain the increased incidence of pigment CBD stones in this age group.

Diagnosis

The diagnosis of CBD stones in the absence of jaundice is usually made at operation. Unfortunately, preoperative chemical indicators of CBD stones, such as elevated alkaline phosphatase or bilirubin, are very unreliable predictors in the aged (33). Preoperative sonographic demonstration of mild enlargement of the common hepatic duct or common bile duct is also an unreliable indication of bile duct stones in the elderly, due to the normal age-related increase in ductal diameter (49). The sonographic demonstration of actual stones in the CBD is possible in only about 20% of cases in most hands (50). For these reasons, operative cholangiography is recommended routinely in elderly patients. With careful technique, false positive and false negative results can be minimized. Recent reports suggest that intra-operative sonography may prove superior to contrast cholangiography for the detection of small CBD stones (51).

In the presence of obstructive jaundice, accurate methods of imaging the biliary tree preoperatively become necessary. Although sonography is an excellent method for determining the presence of markedly dilated ducts and establishing biliary obstruction as the cause of jaundice (52), it is far less successful in delineating the nature and location of the obstructing lesion. Computerized tomography (CT) is now thought to be superior to sonography in determining the level and etiology of biliary obstruction (53). It is not, however, a definitive study for the identification of CBD stones. Endoscopic retrograde cholangiopancreotography (ERCP) (Fig. 31-6) or percutaneous transhepatic cholangiography (PCT) (Fig. 31-7), using the skinny needle technique, are both excellent methods of demonstrating the presence of CBD stones (see Acute Cholangitis).

Treatment

The management of common duct stones at the time of cholecystectomy changes with advancing age. There is a liberalization of the indications for choledochoenterostomy and a trend away from simple t-tube drainage. The reasons for this shift toward permanent bile duct drainage include the increased incidence of multiple stones in a dilated ductal system, the increased possibility of retained or recurrent primary CBD stones, and the desire to avoid additional invasive procedures in elderly patients. Data by Lygidakis (32) showing lower morbidity and mortality af-

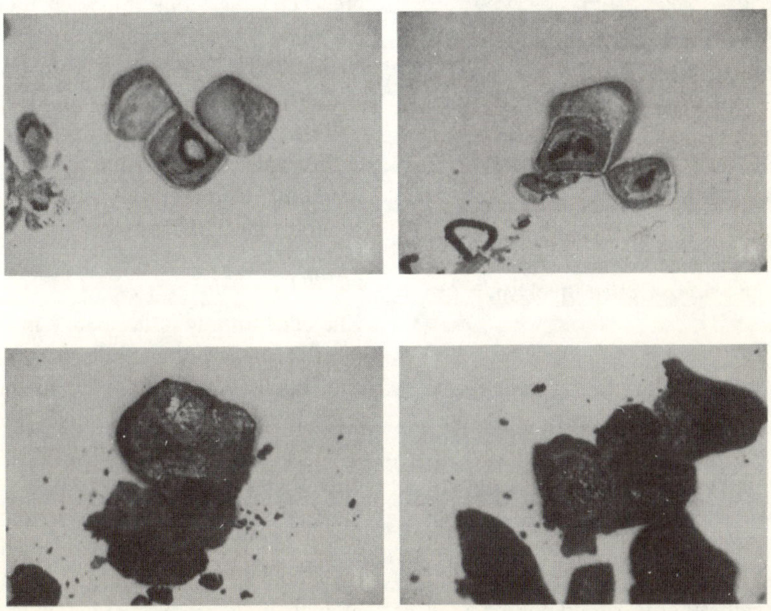

Figure 31-5. *Top,* Cholesterol stones from the gallbladder (left) and the common duct (right) from one patient. Visually and chemically the stones were identical. *Bottom,* Pigment stones from the gallbladder (left) and the common duct (right) from another patient. These stones are less similar in appearance and chemical composition than the above cholesterol pair. (Reprinted, with permission, from Bernhoft RA, et al. 1984. Composition and morphologic and clinical features of common duct stones. *Am J Surg* 148: 77–85.) (47).

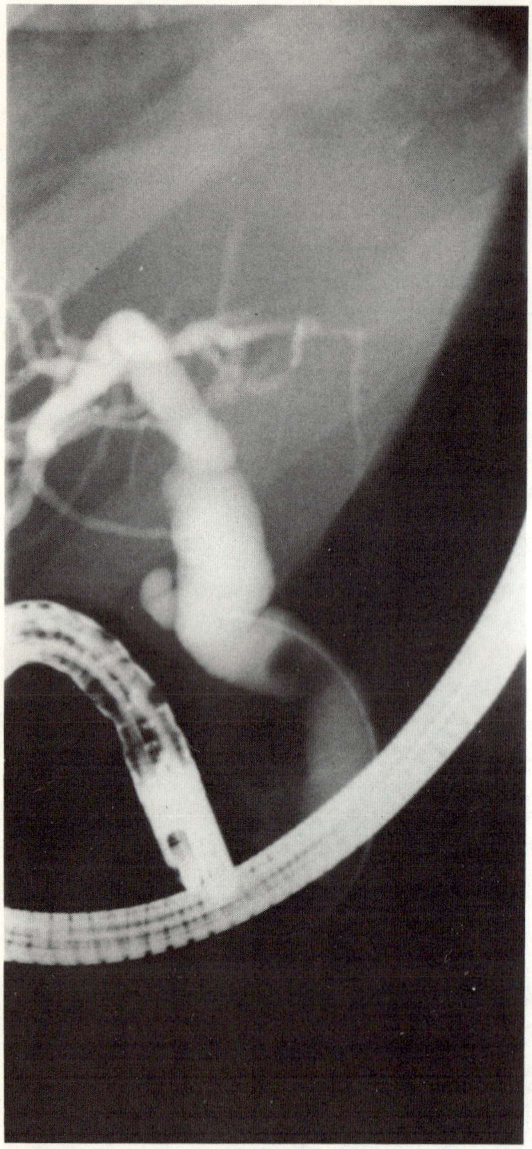

Figure 31-6. An endoscopic retrograde cholangiogram demonstrating a stone on the common bile duct. (Courtesy of S. Iyer, M.D., SUNY Health Science Center, Brooklyn, NY.)

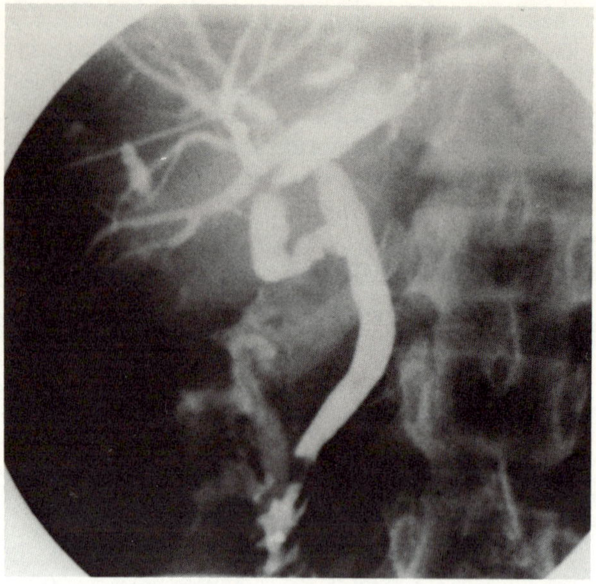

Figure 31-7. A percutaneous transhepatic cholangiogram demonstrating a stone in the common bile duct. (Courtesy of R. De Silva, M.D., SUNY Health Science Center, Brooklyn, NY.)

ter choledochoduodenostomy than after simple t-tube drainage substantiate the advantage of permanent duct decompression.

When stones are found on operative cholangiogram, the common duct should be opened through a longitudinal dochotomy. Stones are removed in the usual manner with irrigation, stone forceps, and Fogarty type balloon catheters. A small red rubber catheter or Bakes dilator is passed into the duodenum to assure patency of the ampulla. If there is a question of residual or impacted stones, choledochoscopy may be helpful. Simple t-tube drainage is acceptable if there are a small number of stones in a normal size, patent ductal system. Otherwise, enteric drainage is indicated. Both choledochoduodenostomy and transduodenal sphincteroplasty are acceptable drainage procedures. Most often, choledochoduodenostomy is the quickest and technically easiest procedure to perform, especially in the presence of a markedly dilated duct. In the presence of a stone impacted in the ampulla, a transduodenal sphincteroplasty may be the procedure of choice.

The management of CBD stones in the absence of a gallbladder is considerably different. The development of endoscopic sphincterotomy and stone extraction has markedly decreased the need for reoperation for retained or recurrent CBD stones (41).

Results

Choledochotomy is necessary in 20% to 40% of elderly patients undergoing cholecystectomy. The addition of choledochotomy is reported to increase operative mortality from 0% to 3% for cholecystectomy alone to 4% to 7% (13, 18). However, in a recent prospective study of biliary surgery in patients over age 65 years, the mortality for elective surgery was only 0.8% in spite of a 36% incidence of CBD exploration (19). The mortality after elective choledochotomy appears to be related to the method of managing the duct. Lygidakis (32) reported a 4.3% mortality for choledochoduodenostomy and a 17.5% mortality for simple t-tube drainage. Although confirmation of this excessively high mortality for t-tube drainage is not available, Moesgaard et al. (54) corroborate the safety and efficacy of choledochoduodenostomy. The overall mortality for the elderly patients in this series was 4%. The use of choledochoduodenostomy in the setting of emergency cholecystectomy is less strongly supported. Although Lygidakis (32) reported a 3.9% mortality for choledochoduodenostomy and a 26.4% mortality for simple t-tube drainage in this setting, the nature of the emergencies and the status of those patients undergoing choledochoduodenostomy was not clear from the data. It is therefore difficult to recommend choledochoduodenostomy in the emergency setting at this time.

Acute Cholangitis

Acute cholangitis is principally a disease of the elderly. It is characterized by extrahepatic biliary obstruction with overgrowth of bacteria in stagnant bile and elevated intraductal pressures. This elevation of pressure allows for reflux of bacteria and bacterial toxins into the systemic circulation, thus producing the clinical syndrome of acute cholangitis. The obstruction in acute cholangitis is usually partial and is most often associated with benign pathology, such as common duct stones and benign strictures. Malignant strictures and complete obstruction are also associated with cholangitis but less frequently (55–59).

The term "acute cholangitis" is used to describe a broad spectrum of clinical and pathological conditions. These range from "cholangitis," a mild systemic illness with infected bile, to "acute suppurative cholangitis" with severe sepsis and pus under pressure in the bile ducts. Unfortunately, clinical presentation and pathologic findings do not always correlate.

The clinical presentation of "cholangitis" is very variable. Charcot's Triad of intermittent fever and chills, jaundice, and right upper quadrant pain is *not* present in as many as 30% to 40% of cases (57, 58). Reynold's Pentad (Charcot's Triad, central nervous system depression, and shock) has been used to identify patients with "acute suppurative cholangitis," but it, too, is unreliable. Often in the elderly, mild systemic sepsis may lead to confusion and hypotension. Therefore, the presence of Reynold's Pentad does not correlate well with the severity of the disease or with the presence of pus in the CBD. Physical examination is likewise variable. Mild right upper quadrant tenderness is common, but signs of peritonitis and active intra-abdominal sepsis are less frequent (58).

Diagnosis

The diagnosis of acute cholangitis can be difficult. Fever is usually present, although frequently low grade (57, 58). White blood cell (WBC) counts are also frequently elevated, but these elevations are usually modest. They have been reported as less than 10,000/mm^3 in 35% of cases and greater than 14,000/mm^3 in only 24% of cases (57). A marked shift to the left on differential is often present when WBC counts are less than 10,000/mm^3. Alkaline phosphatase is elevated in over 90% of cases. Serum bilirubin is usually elevated, but in approximately half of cases, this elevation is less than 5 mg/dl. Other liver function tests are also frequently abnormal (57, 58).

The initial radiographic study of choice is sonography. It is the best study to demonstrate stones in the gallbladder and dilated intrahepatic and extrahepatic ducts (52). While it is also used to identify masses in the head of the pancreas and masses or abscesses in the liver, it is less useful in this regard than computed tomographic scanning. Other diagnostic studies, including percutaneous transhepatic cholangiography (PTC) and endoscopic retrograde cholangiopancreatography (ERCP), are excellent for imaging the biliary tree (60) and may be used therapeutically as well.

Treatment

There is some confusion in the literature about the treatment of acute cholangitis, primarily because of the variability in the severity of the illness. Unfortunately, the clinical picture does not always correlate with the findings at operation, and the distinction between "cholangitis" and "acute suppurative cholangitis" may be difficult to make.

There is general agreement that for most patients who present without shock and with only mildly elevated fever, WBC's, and bilirubin, medical management is appropriate. This consists of hydration, restricted oral intake, and broad-spectrum intravenous antibiotics (56, 59, 61). Blood cultures should be obtained before initiating antibiotic therapy (62). Marked clinical improvement is expected in 12 to 24 hours. This approach to mild illness is the same regardless of age. However, as with any other source of intra-abdominal sepsis in the elderly, the presenting clinical picture can be deceiving. It is therefore necessary to consider every elderly patient with suspected cholangitis as a potential candidate for biliary decompression as well. Failure to improve rapidly on antibiotic therapy is an indication for urgent duct decompression.

In the past, surgery was the only available method for biliary decompression. The risk of operation under general anesthesia in elderly septic patients was high. Operative decompression therefore was reserved for those patients who failed antibiotic therapy or who presented in unremitting shock and were suspected to have pus under pressure in the bile ducts.

Now, however, several methods of nonoperative biliary drainage have become available. The first of these is percutaneous transhepatic drainage (PTD), using a skinny needle technique (63). Under local anesthesia, a catheter can be introduced with fluoroscopic guidance into the dilated intrahepatic bile ducts and advanced into the common duct. Pressure in the ducts is then relieved by establishing drainage of infected bile to the outside. When sepsis is controlled, cholangiography can be performed through the same catheter to delineate the anatomy and etiology of the obstruction.

An alternative to PTD is sphincterotomy or drainage via endoscopic retrograde cannulation of the papilla of Vater (64, 65). Under direct vision through a side viewing endoscope, a cannula is introduced into the distal common duct, and decompression is accomplished by sphincterotomy and/or tube drainage. Drainage tubes can be left as indwelling stents or can be brought out through the nose. Cholangiography through the nasobiliary cannula can be performed once sepsis is controlled.

While there are strong advocates of both procedures, there is some suggestion that endoscopic drainage is associated with fewer complications (66, 67). However, many surgeons feel that PTC gives more useful anatomical information than does endoscopic cholangiography. Both procedures require skilled physicians familiar with the use of these techniques.

Even in patients who respond to antibiotics without decompression, the cause of the cholangitis must be sought. Visualization of the biliary tract either by PTC or ERCP will delineate the abnormality and allow for planned operative intervention with preoperative knowledge of the biliary anatomy. Both procedures should be performed while the patient is on antibiotic coverage, and a plan for urgent biliary drainage should be available since these methods of imaging the biliary tract are themselves causes of cholangitis. The choice of definitive operation for cholangitis depends on the etiologic finding on cholangiography.

Patients who come to early emergent operative decompression are usually those who can least well tolerate the intervention but who will not survive without it. At operation the duct should be opened, and manipulation should be minimal to avoid further bacteremia. External drainage with a large bore t-tube is usually all that the patient's condition will allow. Concomitant cholecystostomy may be necessary if stones are found in the gallbladder. Cholecystostomy alone is not sufficient treatment for cholangitis (56).

Results

The outcome of surgery for cholangitis depends on the setting of the operation and the severity of the disease. In the series by Boey and Way (56), emergency surgery for cholangitis carried an operative mortality of 40% in patients with a mean age of 62. Malignant obstruction accounted for 50% of emergency operations and choledocholithiasis for 20%. However, only 15% of all cases of cholangitis required emergency surgery. The overall mortality for all types of cholangitis was 16%; 36% for acute suppurative cases, and 10% for nonsuppurative cases. These data are confirmed by other series (55, 58). When shock is present and decompression is not rapidly established, mortality is 100% (55). It should be noted that these series do not address the issue of acute cholangitis in the elderly specifically. However, as with any acute surgical disease, mortality in the elderly can be expected to be even higher than in these reports.

Gallstone Ileus

The term gallstone ileus is used to describe the bowel obstruction caused by a large gallstone impacted in the small intestine. The stone enters the intestinal lumen through a cholecystoenteric fistula. The site of this fistula is usually the duodenum (90% of cases) although fistulae to the colon, jejunum, and stomach have been reported (68).

Gallstone ileus is a disease of the elderly, with mean reported age of 70 years (69). Approximately 85% of patients are female. Gallstone ileus is a relatively unusual cause of small bowel obstruction. It is estimated to be responsible for approximately 1% to 2% of cases but can be implicated in 25% of cases in patients over age 65. The incidence is even higher in those elderly patients who have had no prior surgery. An excellent review of the literature on gallstone ileus can be found elsewhere (68).

Diagnosis

The clinical presentation of gallstone ileus is that of small bowel obstruction with no particularly distinguishing features. A history of gallstones may or may not be present (70). Rapid diagnosis requires an awareness of the possibility of gallstone ileus in an elderly patient with small bowel obstruction, particularly when there is no history of previous surgery. A flat plate of the abdomen is often diagnostic. In addition to the pattern of air filled bowel loops typical of small bowel obstruction, air in the biliary tree may be visualized (Fig. 31-8). It is reported that in 50% of cases, biliary air can be identified preoperatively (68). Retrospective review will frequently identify biliary air that was unnoticed before the diagnosis of gallstone ileus was made at operation (71). In approximately 20% of cases, the obstructing gallstone contains enough calcium to allow visualization on the plain abdominal film. Upper gastrointestinal barium studies may demonstrate contrast in the bile ducts or may actually outline the obstructing stone (70). The correct preoperative diagnosis is made in approximately half of all cases (71).

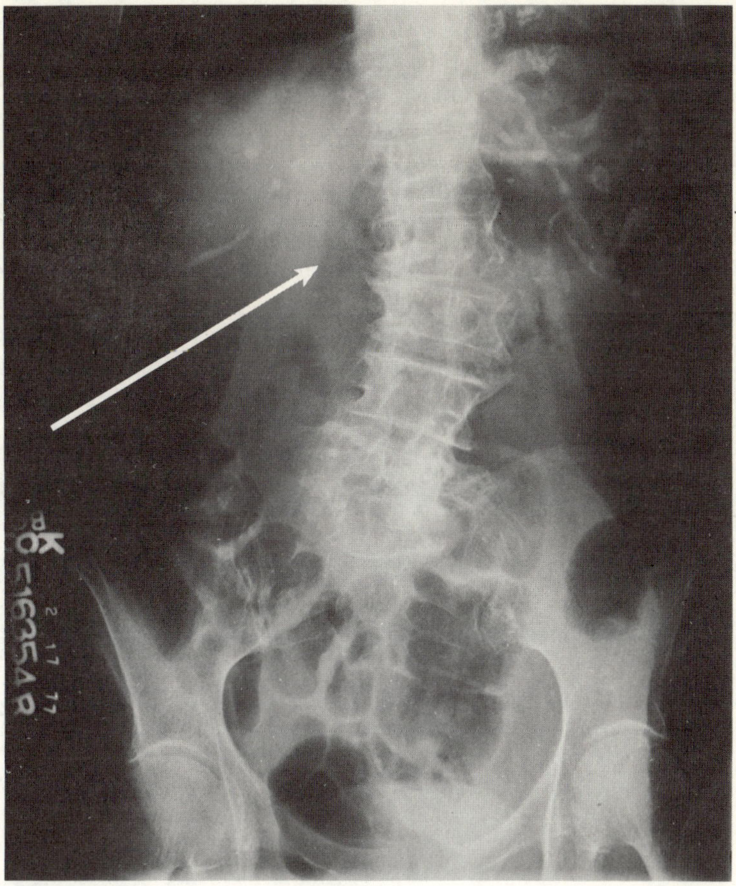

Figure 31-8. A flat plate of the abdomen showing air within the biliary tree in the right upper quadrant. (Courtesy of R. De Silva, M.D., SUNY Health Science Center, Brooklyn, NY.)

Treatment

The treatment for gallstone ileus is early relief of the small bowel obstruction by operative removal of the obstructing stone. Preoperative hydration and nasogastric decompression are routine. At operation, the stone is removed by making an enterotomy proximal to the point of obstruction and extruding the stone. The entire length of the small bowel should be carefully examined to determine the presence or absence of additional stones. Multiple stones can be found in as many as 10% of cases (68).

Disagreement exists as to whether or not cholecystectomy and closure of the fistula should be performed at the same time as relief of the bowel obstruction. Proponents claim that cholecystectomy reduces the risk of recurrent stones and decreases the need for interval cholecystectomy. Opponents state that the rate of recurrence is only 4%, and the mortality from recurrence is also low (68). Therefore, the risk of a prolonged and often technically difficult operation to remove the gallbladder in a compromised elderly patient is not justified. The palpation of additional stones in the gallbladder may be an indication for cholecystectomy in this acute setting.

The need for interval cholecystectomy after simple relief of the small bowel obstruction must be individualized since the risk of recurrence of the complications of gallbladder disease is relatively low. Interval cholecystectomy is by no means mandatory in the elderly. Careful follow-up and surveillance, however, are extremely important (68).

Results

Over the past several decades, overall mortality from gallstone ileus has been reported to be 20% (68). Recent improvements in preoperative preparation and intraoperative monitoring have decreased the mortality to 10% to 15% (69). The causes of death do not vary significantly from the causes of death from other complications of biliary tract disease. They include intra-abdominal sepsis as well as cardiac, pulmonary, and renal compromise.

Incidental Cholecystectomy

The presence of previously undetected gallstones at the time of laparotomy for nonbiliary pathology is a common finding in elderly patients. While there may be a reluctance to perform an additional procedure on patients already at higher risk for postoperative complications, the benefits of incidental cholecystectomy appear to outweigh the risks. Schreiber et al. (72) reviewed their experience with the management of incidentally discovered cholelithiasis at the time of other major abdominal surgery in patients over 60 years of age. The indications for abdominal exploration are shown in Table 31-7. The addition of cholecystectomy did not alter the mortality or morbidity expected from the primary procedure alone.

The incidence of acute cholecystitis in the postoperative period increases after age 50 years, particularly in those patients with stones (73). The diagnosis is often obscured by the symptoms normally associated with recent abdominal surgery. Delays and errors in diagnosis can lead to perforation and disseminated intra-abdominal sepsis. Incidental cholecystectomy is therefore recommended unless it is technically hazardous or the patient is too unstable to tolerate the additional operative time.

Operative Management of Gastric Disorders

Duodenal Ulcer Disease

Confusion exists about the significance of duodenal ulcer disease in the elderly. While it is recognized that gastric ulcer can be severe in this age group, duodenal ulcer is not readily recognized as a serious problem. It has been stated that peptic ulcer disease develops most frequently in the active middle years of life. Over the past several decades it has become more apparent that not only does duodenal ulcer disease also occur in the elderly, but when it does it is more likely to be accompanied by serious complications or death (74–79). In a recent study by Permutt and Cello (74) hospitalized elderly (>60 years) and younger (<60 years) patients with duodenal ulcer were compared. One-third of the patients in this study were over 60 years of age. Older patients were found to have a significantly higher mortality rate than younger patients, with 50% of the mortality being directly attributed to complications of the ulcer disease (Table 31-8).

Table 31-7. Indications for primary abdominal procedures association with incidental cholecystectomy

Surgical indication	Number of cases
Carcinoma of colon	12
Diverticular disease of colon	2
Sigmoid volvulus	2
Peptic ulcer disease	10
Carcinoma of stomach	3
Aortic aneurysm	3
Small bowel obstruction	2
Carcinoma of pancreas	1
Hiatus hernia	3
Trauma	1
Other	5
Total	44

Reprinted, with permission, from Schreiber H, Macon WL, and Walter JP. 1978. Incidental cholecystectomy during major abdominal surgery in the elderly. *Am J Surg* 135:196–198.

Duodenal ulcer may be present for many years or, as in over half the cases, may present de novo in old age (75). When ulcer disease does present for the first time in the elderly, it tends to be virulent. Fenyo (7) reported that in half of elderly patients with a complication of duodenal ulcer disease, there was no prior history of ulcer.

In general, there is a clear age-related increase in the frequency of duodenal ulcer complications. Levrat et al. (75) demonstated that by age 75 to 79, 76% of ulcer patients had an acute complication. It has been suggested that nonsteroidal anti-inflammatory drugs (NSAID) may be responsible in part for the increased frequency of duodenal ulcer complications in this age group (80). Watson et al. (79) reported that 40% of elderly patients who presented with bleeding and 30% of those with perforation were using NSAID. Permutt and Cello (74) reported a similar incidence of bleeding and perforation in the elderly but could not demonstrate a significant difference between the younger and older patients in the use of NSAID. The role of these drugs in the etiology and high rate of complications of duodenal ulcer in the elderly is still unclear.

The lack of awareness of the significance of duodenal ulcer in the elderly is compounded by the peculiarity of clinical presentation in this age group. Epigastric pain, which is relieved by eating or antacids and is the hallmark of peptic disease in young patients, is often absent. Clinch et al. (81) reported that 35% of patients over 60 with duodenal ulcer had no abdominal pain compared to only 8% of patients between 20 and 50 years old. Older patients

Table 31-8. Comparison of patients >60 and <60 with duodenal ulcer

	<60 years (%)		>60 years (%)	
Overall mortality	2/114	(2)	8/54	(15)
Ulcer mortality	0/2	(0)	4/8	(50)[a]
Rebleeding	21/114	(18)	22/54	(41)[a]
Total blood tranfused	2.6 ± 0.3		4.5 ± 1.1[b]	

[a] $p<.01$ by chi square.
[b] $p<.05$ by *t*-test.
Adapted from Permutt RP, and Cello JP. 1982. Duodenal ulcer disease in the hospitalized elderly patient. *Dig Dis Sci* 27:1–6.

presented instead with hematemesis and melena, unexplained anemia, anorexia, and weight loss, and nausea and vomiting. In patients with unexplained anemia, secondary complications such as angina, congestive heart failure, and changes in mental status can be the presenting complaints. The diagnosis of duodenal ulcer disease is therefore often not made until a major complication has occurred.

Indications for Surgery, Treatment, and Outcome

The indications for surgery in duodenal ulcer disease in the elderly have changed over time (Table 31-9) There has been a decrease in the number of operations performed for intractability and obstruction. This decline is attributed to the wisespread use of H_2-receptor antagonists. While bleeding is the most common complication and was the most common indication for surgery in the past (82, 83), perforation now appears to have surpassed bleeding as the leading cause of operation for duodenal ulcer in the elderly (34, 79).

Bleeding. While the incidence of bleeding from gastric ulcer does increase with age, the majority of bleeding ulcers, even in patients over age 70, are duodenal in location (84). In as many as half the cases of bleeding in this age group, there is no prior history of ulcer symptoms (78). In one surgical series, 80% of fatal massive hemorrhages occurred in patients in whom bleeding was the first sign of ulcer disease (76). Recurrent bleeding is approximately twice as likely in the elderly as in the young (Table 31-8). Permutt and Cello (74) reported rebleeding rates of 40% for patients over age 60 and 18% for those younger than 60. These figures are confirmed by Hoare et al. (85) who reported a 44% rebleeding rate for elderly patients compared to 20% for younger patients.

Mortality rates for bleeding duodenal ulcer correlate with the amount of blood transfused. Kaplan et al. (83) reported an operative mortality of 7.5% if fewer than 3 liters of blood were transfused. This mortality increased to 26% for 3 to 5 liters and to 35% for more than 5 liters. It has also been demonstrated that the amount of transfusion required to control bleeding duodenal ulcers increases from approximately 2 to 3 units in patients less than 60 years of age to 4 to 6 units in patients over 60 (74, 79) (Table 31-8). It had been thought in the past that atherosclerotic changes in the arteries supplying the duodenum limited the ability of the vessels in ulcers in this location to contract and stop bleeding. However, pathologic studies do *not* confirm this hypothesis (86).

It is important to try to identify those elderly patients at risk for persistent or recurrent bleeding and to operate on them before massive blood replacement becomes necessary. Criteria have been suggested that will identify those patients in need of early operative intervention. These are: overt hematemesis, shock at presentation, hemoglobin less than 9 g at presentation or an initial blood replacement requirement of 1,500 cc (78). Hypotension in association with bleeding duodenal ulcer in patients over 70 has been associated with a mortality rate in excess of 45% (84). Rebleeding on the same admission, a second episode of hemorrhage, and demonstration of a visible bleeding vessel at endoscopy are also viewed as operative indications.

Special consideration must be given to elderly patients with coronary artery disease. There is a general reluctance to operate on these patients because of the fear of precipitating a perioperative myocardial infarction. However, the stress of massive hemorrhage and hypovolemia is also capable of initiating significant cardiac ischemia. Prolonged attempt at medical control of the hemorrhage with multiple transfusions leaves the patient at even higher risk of death if this approach fails (84).

The diagnosis of bleeding duodenal ulcer can usually be established rapidly by gastroduodenal endoscopy. Unfortunately, the rate of spontaneous cessation of hemorrhage in the elderly is lower than in younger patients. Watson et al. (79) reported that 50% of elderly patients who presented with bleeding required surgery. Therefore preparation for possible surgery should be part of the initial management.

The surgical treatment of bleeding duodenal ulcer is directed toward controlling the hemorrhage and limiting

Table 31-9. Indications for surgery for duodenal ulcer

Indication	1940–1955 Cutler (82)	1956–1969 Kaplan (83)	1975–1980 Watson (79)	1977–1980 Permutt (74)
Bleeding (%)	23	49	40	44
Perforation (%)	20	16	42	50
Obstruction (%)	23	24	7	6
Intractability (%)	34	11	12	0
Number of cases	176	185	101	18

Adapted from Permutt RP, and Cello JP. 1982. Duodenal ulcer disease in the hospitalized elderly patient. *Dig Dis Sci* 27:1–6.

rebleeding. The most common procedure performed is suture ligation of the ulcer and truncal vagotomy with a drainage procedure, usually pyloroplasty. This is the procedure of choice in 78% to 85% of cases (79, 83). Partial gastrectomy (i.e., antrectomy) and truncal vagotomy are performed in approximately 15% of cases. The choice of operation is in large part dependent on technical considerations and the overall condition of the patient. When there is a large ulcer or when there is severe scarring of the bulb, a standard Heineke-Mikulicz pyloroplasty may be difficult. Alternative drainage procedures or antrectomy must accompany truncal vagotomy in this setting.

The overall operative mortality for bleeding duodenal ulcer in the elderly varies from 10% to 18% in the recent literature (79, 83, 84). It is unclear whether the mortality for each of the individual procedures differs significantly. Kaplan et al. (83) reported the mortality for vagotomy and drainage and for partial gastrectomy to be 18% and 14% respectively. However, it is unclear from these data whether bleeding gastric ulcers are included as well. In Watson's series (79), where only duodenal ulcers are included, the majority of cases were treated by vagotomy and pyloroplasty. The overall operative mortality in this study was 10%. Other authors suggest a lower mortality for vagotomy and pyloroplasty than for resection (87).

It is of particular interest that the non-operative management of bleeding ulcers in Watson's series (79) was associated with twice the mortality of operative therapy (20% versus 10%) (Table 31-10). Other series support this considerably higher mortality for non-operative versus operative treatment (84).

The long-term follow-up of elderly patients treated for bleeding duodenal ulcer is difficult to determine from the literature. While some reports suggest that rebleeding occurs less often with antrectomy and vagotomy (83) in this age group, there are no clear data to support this contention. The risk of resection with all the associated postgastrectomy complications must be weighed against the speculative long-term protection against rebleeding in these patients who tolerate postoperative complications poorly.

Perforation. Perforation is the second most common presentation of duodenal ulcer in the elderly and is the most common recent indication for surgery (Table 31-9). Data from the United Kingdom indicate a recent rise in duodenal ulcer perforations in the elderly, particular in women (88). Once the diagnosis is established, perforated duodenal ulcer is clearly a surgical disease in the elderly.

In younger patients, the diagnosis of perforated duodenal ulcer is usually made on the basis of history and physical exam. This diagnosis is confirmed by the demonstration of free air under the diaphragm on an upright chest X-ray or left lateral decubitis abdominal film. Unfortunately, in the elderly, the diagnosis is often delayed and occasionally made only at post mortem examination. The major reasons for the delays and errors in diagnosis include the vague nature of symptoms and the seemingly benign physical examination. Severe abdominal pain followed shortly by the development of peritoneal signs is often absent. Instead, there may be a longer history of vague abdominal pain, and the abdomen may be soft and only minimally tender. In a retrospective study of elderly patients with a discharge or post mortem diagnosis of perforated duodenal ulcer, Coleman and Denham (89) found that 37% of the patients were not even suspected of having a surgical illness at the time of admission and were therefore placed on medical services. In one-quarter of these elderly patients, the diagnosis was not made within the first 24 hours of admission. The differences in the presenting signs and symptoms of medical and surgical admissions are seen in Table 31-11. All of the patients admitted to surgery had severe abdominal pain, but in nearly 80% of medical admissions or 30% of the total number, severe pain was not a significant complaint. In one-quarter of the surgical patients and nearly half of the total number, guarding was absent, and in over 40% of all patients, rigidity was also absent. This mild presentation of abdominal signs and symptoms has been confirmed by other authors (7).

The absence of radiographically demonstrated intraperitoneal free air may also be misleading. It has been

Table 31-10. Surgical versus nonsurgical management of duodenal ulcer in the elderly

		Surgical		Nonsurgical	
	# of Patient (%)	# Cases (%)	Mortality	# Cases (%)	Mortality
Bleeding	81 (50%)	41 (51)	10%	40 (49)	20%
Perforation	47 (29%)	43 (92)	21%	4 (8)	100%
Obstruction	8 (5%)	7 (88)	0	1 (12)	0
Intractability	27 (16%)	12 (45)	0	15 (55)	0

Adapted from Watson RJ, Hooper TL, and Ingram G. 1985. Duodenal ulcer disease in the elderly: A retrospective study. *Age Ageing* 14:225–229.

Table 31-11. Symptoms and signs of perforated ulcer

	Surgical Cases %	Medical Cases %	Total
Number of patients	24	14	38
Severe abdominal pain	24 (100)	3 (21)	27 (71)
Nausea and vomiting	0 (0)	6 (43)	6 (16)
Guarding	18 (75)	3 (21)	21 (55)
Rigidity	19 (79)	3 (21)	22 (58)

Adapted from Coleman JA, and Denham MJ. 1980. Perforation of peptic ulceration in the elderly. *Age Ageing* 9:251–257.

reported that in 25% to 50% of elderly patients with perforated duodenal ulcer, no X-ray evidence of pneumoperitoneum can be found (7, 78, 90).

Paracentesis may be useful in clarifying the diagnosis of perforated viscus in the elderly with atypical abdominal pain. The presence of bilious peritoneal fluid with a high amylase content can confirm the diagnosis. However, a high index of suspicion is necessary to establish the diagnosis of perforated duodenal ulcer rapidly in many older patients.

The choice of procedure for perforated duodenal ulcer in the elderly depends on the amount of inflammation and contamination found at surgery and the overall condition of the patient. If there is considerable soilage and inflammation, or if the patient is unstable, simple omentopexy and thorough irrigation of the abdomen is usually the procedure of choice. If there is little spillage and a small perforation with a pliable duodenum, then truncal vagotomy and pyloroplasty can be accomplished quickly and safely. The latter procedure is preferable when there is a history of duodenal ulcer disease in the past. Unfortunately, in patients with a positive prior history, the duodenum is often deformed or scarred, making pyloroplasty difficult. Therefore, a simple plication maybe warranted even in this setting. Studies indicate that in younger patients, the addition of proximal gastric or parietal cell vagotomy to omentopexy decreases the chance of recurrence without significantly increasing operative mortality or morbidity (91). No similar data exist in the elderly, in whom the addition of one or more hours to the operative time may be prohibitive.

The outcome of surgery in elderly patients with perforated duodenal ulcer depends in part on the length of time from perforation to operation. In one series, the operative mortality for patients operated on after 12 hours from the time of perforation was twice that of those undergoing surgery in the initial 12 hours (77). The overall surgical mortality for perforated duodenal ulcer in the elderly is reported from 21% to 32% (7, 77, 79, 89, 92), although mortality rates as low as 11% have been reported (83).

The choice of procedure does appear to influence the operative mortality. Kaplan et al. (83) reported operative mortality for vagotomy and drainage to be 25% versus 16% for simple omentopexy or plication. The results of this study are confused by the inclusion of perforated gastric ulcers in the data. However, the higher mortality for other than simple plication is also suggested by Stanfford et al. (77) who reported a doubling of operative mortality for the few patients who underwent additional procedures.

It should be noted that there appears to be little if any place for "conservative" or nonoperative management of perforated duodenal ulcer in the elderly. Reported mortality for this mode of therapy is 100% (79, 89). Normal mechanisms that wall off perforations in younger patients appear not to function well in the elderly. Therefore, uncontrolled intra-abdominal sepsis ensues if perforations are not closed surgically.

Obstruction. Obstruction has recently become a less common indication for surgery in elderly patients with duodenal ulcer (Table 31-8). This is in part attributed to the use of H_2-receptor antagonists. Since patients with obstruction usually have a long history of ulcer disease, recent changes in therapy may be effective in controlling the progression of the disease. In addition, there has been an increase in the use of total parenteral nutrition in these debilitated, dehydrated, and undernourished patients. This allows time for healing and resolution of acute inflamation and edema with subsequent relief of many partial or near total obstructions.

When obstruction is persistent in spite of nasogastric decompression, total parenteral nutrition and H_2-receptor antagonist therapy, then surgery is indicated. Preoperative endoscopy and biopsy is important to rule out the diagnosis of antral cancer as the cause of obstruction since the incidence of gastric malignancies increases with age. (See Gastric Cancer.) The procedure of choice is antrectomy and truncal vagotomy (78). This procedure can be accomplished under elective conditions in a well-nourished, well-prepared patient. The stomach should be adequately decompressed for a long enough period of time to allow it to regain its normal size and tone. Perioperative antibiotics and preoperative gastric lavage are recommended to decrease bacterial concentrations in the obstructed lumen. If resection is technically difficult and duodenal stump closure appears tenuous, then truncal vagotomy and gastrojejunostomy is an acceptable although infrequently needed alternative.

Operative mortality for outlet obstruction secondary to duodenal ulcer has been reported to be approximately 10% (77, 83). However, mortality rates as low as 0% have recently been reported (79).

Intractability. Persistence of symptoms in the elderly in spite of medical therapy is unusual and has become an uncommon indication for surgery (74, 78, 79, 83). Entities other than routine duodenal ulcer must be considered when pain is the outstanding feature of the disease. Ulcer penetration posteriorly into the pancreas or superiorly into the liver or biliary tract, or giant ulceration with destruction of a large portion of the bulb may be responsible. While unusual in this age group, Zollinger-Ellison syndrome must also be considered (90).

However, nonhealing ulcers may be present without significant pain in the elderly (81). Therefore, careful surveillance for nonhealing is warranted in these patients. Once the diagnosis of duodenal ulcer disease is established, repeat UGI series or endoscopy can be justified to assure healing and prevent complication in those patients with absent or atypical pain. Nonhealing, frequent exacerbations, or inability of the patient to comply with medical therapy may be viewed as relative indications for surgery in this age group.

Valid data exist about the choice of procedure for chronic duodenal ulcer in the general population. Koo et al. (93) in a prospective randomized trial, compared proximal gastric vagotomy (PGV), truncal vagotomy with drainage, and truncal vagotomy with antrectomy for the treatment of chronic duodenal ulcer. When recurrence was excluded, functional assessment (i.e., presence of unwanted side effects) showed the best outcome with PGV. However, when recurrence was considered, PGV lost the advantage. Vagotomy and antrectomy was clearly better in minimizing recurrence. Unfortunately, no similar data exist about the treatment of chronic duodenal ulcer in the elderly. In fact, patients over age 70 were specifically excluded from the study by Koo et al. (93). However, the consideration of recurrence versus side effects is particularly important in this age group. While definitive data do not exist, the fear of recurrence and reoperation seems to be a more important factor than the occurrence of side effects. Therefore, at present, vagotomy and antrectomy appear to be the procedures of choice in the elderly (78). In cases where resection is technically hazardous, either vagotomy and drainage or PGV may be used, depending on the individual surgeon's experience and expertise.

Overall mortality for elective procedures for intractability varies from 0% to 5% (79, 83). This is consistent with the approximately 3% mortality associated with all elective gastric surgery in other series (76).

Giant Duodenal Ulcer

Giant duodenal ulcer is a relatively unusual entity. It is defined as a duodenal ulcer that is either greater than 2 cm in diameter or has destroyed the majority of the bulb (90). It is of interest because it occurs primarily in elderly males with no prior history of ulcer disease (94). Although abdominal pain predominates, it is usually atypical in character (94, 95). It can simulate the pain of biliary tract disease or pancreatitis because of penetration into these adjacent organs. Nausea and vomiting occur in a large majority of cases and marked weight loss is also common (94). Bleeding is often the major presenting feature (94–96) but is usually not massive (90, 95).

The diagnosis of giant ulcer is made on upper gastrointestinal (UGI) series. A rigid, unchanging bulb is usually the predominant finding. There maybe nodularity in the floor of the ulcer, resembling a tumor (94, 95). There also may be the appearance of an ulcer within an ulcer. Giant duodenal ulcers were frequently missed in the past, because they were mistaken for a severely deformed duodenal cap (95). Recent recognition of this entity has made this error less frequent (Fig. 31-9).

Some reports suggest that with the use of H_2 antagonists and intensive antacid therapy, giant duodenal ulcers may heal without surgical intervention. However, follow-up is short (2 to 21 months) (96) and reccurrence rates are high. At present, because of their size and propensity to lead to complications, surgery is the usual treatment of choice (94). Medical therapy with H_2 blockers and total parenteral nutrition is useful in the preoperative preparation of these often ill and malnourished patients.

Antrectomy and truncal vagotomy with exclusion of the ulcer is the usual procedure (94). If there is doubt about closure of the duodenal stump, a lateral de-

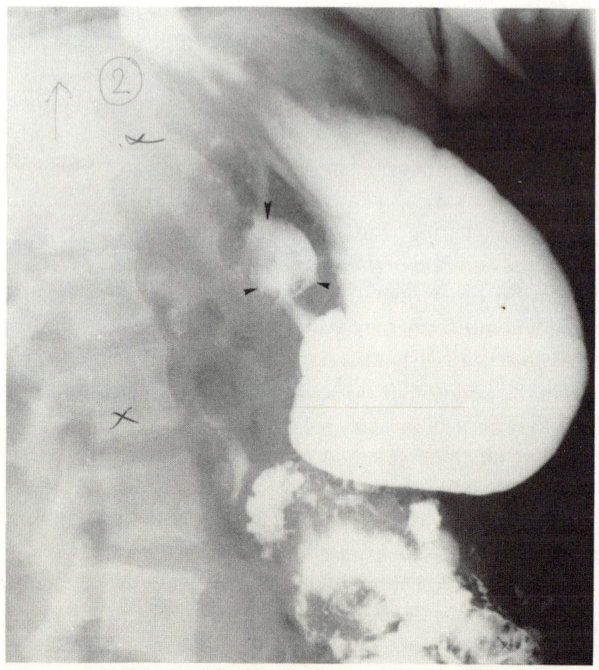

Figure 31-9. Arrows indicate a giant duodenal ulcer. (Courtesy of S. Iyer, M.D., SUNY Health Science Center, Brooklyn, NY.)

compressing tube duodenostomy may be necessary. Occasionally, resection is impossible because of the size of the inflammatory mass. In this circumstance, vagotomy and gastrojejunostomy is the procedure of choice.

Results of surgical management have improved over the years. Recent overall mortality for all ages is reported to be 7% (94). Most deaths occur in patients who are operated upon emergently.

Gastric Ulcer

Although duodenal ulcers are more common than gastric ulcers in the elderly, two out of three deaths from ulcer disease in this age group are related to those ulcers arising in the stomach (75). Recently, the incidence of duodenal ulcer disease has decreased, while the overall incidence of gastric ulcer has remained unchanged. The percentage of patients over age 60 with gastric ulcer, however, has increased approximately 20% (97). The natural history of gastric ulcer is that of a chronic disease characterized by healing and exacerbation. Recurrence rates for a medically managed gastric ulcer are high and range from 40% to 75% (75, 98, 99).

The clinical presentation of gastric ulcer is even more misleading than its duodenal counterpart. Pain may or may not be present. When present, it may easily be mistaken for pain of biliary, pancreatic, or cardiac origin. The location of gastric ulcer in the elderly tends to be more proximal on the lesser curve, approaching the esophagogastric junction in approximately 2 times the overall frequency (over 40% of cases) (99). Dysphagia may therefore be the presenting symptom. Moderate to severe weight loss can be present with no specific abdominal complaints at all. Anemia from chronic blood loss may cause malaise, congestive heart failure, or mental status changes, which further confound the diagnosis.

Diagnosis

The diagnosis of gastric ulcer is usually made by upper gastrointestinal (UGI) series. The frequent location of these gastric ulcers high on the posterior wall of the stomach may make detection somewhat more difficult (Fig. 31-10). Erect lateral and oblique films may be helpful in detecting ulcers in this location (99). Once the presence of the ulcer is established, it becomes necessary to determine whether the ulcer is benign or malignant. In approximately 70% to 80% of cases, the appearance of the ulcer on contrast studies will allow this distinction (100). More recent studies suggest a 93% to 97% accuracy for detecting malignancy on UGI series in some hands (101). In most circumstances however, gastroduodenal endoscopy with multiple biopsies and cytology is essential to confirm the diagnosis of benign versus malignant ulcer, particularly in the elderly (90, 98, 102). The combination of benign radiographic appearance and negative biopsies and cytology is accurate in 95% to 99% of cases (98, 101, 102). In the remaining 1% to 5% of cases, the ulcers are malignant in spite of the benign finding. Therefore careful monitoring of healing with repeat UGI series and/or endoscopy is mandatory.

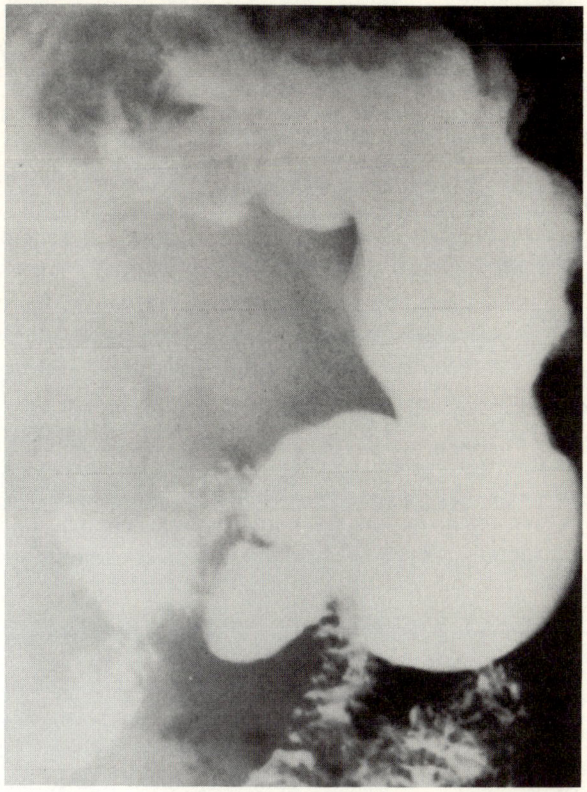

Figure 31-10. Upper gastrointestinal series showing a gastric ulcer high on the lesser curvature of the stomach. This ulcer has the typical appearance of a "Geratric Ulcer". (Reprinted, with permission, from Amberg JR, and Zboralske FF. 1966. Gastric ulcers after 70. *Am J Roentgenology* 96: 393–399.) (99).

Indications for Surgery, Treatment, and Outcome

The diagnosis of gastric ulcer carries a much higher likelihood of surgery than does duodenal ulcer. The results of medical management in general are not nearly as good as similar management for duodenal ulcer. Successful healing of gastric ulcer on medical management has been defined as a 50% reduction in size in 3 weeks, 90% in 6 weeks, and 100% in 12 weeks. In a large Veterans Administration cooperative study of gastric ulcer (103), 42% of patients who healed according to the above protocol suffered a recurrence within 2 years. Of those patients who healed more slowly, 62% had a recurrence in the same time period. Amberg et al. (99) reported considerably slower rates of healing for gastric ulcers in patients over

70. It would seem, therefore, that elderly patients are at a higher risk of recurrence. The poor outcome for medical management in the elderly is confirmed by Amberg et al. (99), who reported a 39% mortality from ulcer disease in patients over age 70 treated medically. In a recent study by Adkin (100), only 36% of patients of all ages were considered successes of medical management. Of those who came to surgery as failures of medical management, 35% required emergency procedures. These authors emphasize the need to be aggressive in managing gastric ulcers in the elderly who tolerate emergency surgery so poorly.

The recommended treatment for uncomplicated gastric ulcer in the elderly is therefore a closely monitored course of medical management followed by surgery if healing is not complete within 6 to 12 weeks, if symptoms persist, or if recurrence or a complication occurs. When a "giant gastric ulcer" (>3 cm) is present, complications are so frequent and healing so slow, that even earlier surgical intervention is often indicated (90). The objective of planned elective surgery is to minimize the development of complications such as bleeding and perforation.

The selection of operation for gastric ulcer disease depends on the location of the ulcer and the presence or absence of evidence of duodenal or prepyloric ulcer. For ulcers in the body of the stomach without evidence of duodenal or prepyloric ulcer, distal gastric resection to include the ulcer, without vagotomy, is the treatment of choice (98, 100). Vagotomy is added if there is evidence of duodenal or prepyloric ulcers. Recurrence rates of 0% to 5% (98) are reported for gastric ulcer treated by distal resection.

Ulcers at or near the esophagogastric junction present a special problem. Although they too can usually be excised in continuity with a distal resection, occasionally this is not technically feasible. In such cases, local excision with vagotomy and pyloroplasty may be necessary. This option is less satisfactory than resection because of a higher recurrence rate but may be unavoidable (98, 100).

The overall mortality for emergency surgery for gastric ulcer in the elderly is reported to approach 30% (82, 83, 99, 104). Elective mortality varies from 2% to 9% (76, 82, 104), but a 0% mortality has been reported when nonhealing ulcer is the indication for surgery (83).

Bleeding. Initial hemorrhage from gastric ulcer tends to be massive, and recurrent bleeding is frequent. Most deaths from hemorrhage occur in patients with symptoms for 4 weeks or less (105). As with duodenal ulcers, mortality increases with the severity of the hemorrhage. Jensen et al. (105) reported the operative mortality in all ages to be 4% when the presenting symptom was hematemesis or melena. This mortality increased to 15% if shock was initially present. The nonoperative mortality for patients in shock, however, was over three times as great (48%).

The surgical treatment of choice for bleeding gastric ulcer is also resection (83, 84). For distal ulcers, distal resection to include the ulcer is adequate. Vagotomy is added if there is evidence of duodenal or prepyloric ulcer. For bleeding sites closer to the esophagogastric junction, either local excision of the ulcer, or biopsy and oversewing the bleeding point combined with vagotomy and pyloroplasty is usually satisfactory.

The overall mortality reported by Jensen et al. (105) for surgically treated bleeding gastric ulcer in patients over 60 years was 14% compared to 26% for those treated medically. Although the operative mortality for bleeding gastric ulcer reported in other studies was somewhat higher, ranging from 20% to 26% (77, 83, 84), the mortality for nonoperative cases was still twice that of operative cases (84). Early surgical intervention for bleeding gastric ulcers in the elderly should therefore be encouraged.

Perforation. Perforation is an ominous complication of gastric ulcers in the elderly. Kaplan et al. (83) reported a mortality rate of 57% for perforated gastric ulcers, compared to 11% for perforated duodenal ulcers. The operative procedures for perforation vary from biopsy and simple closure to resection. The choice depends on the overall condition of the patient, the length of time from perforation and the amount of contamination found at operation.

Gastric Cancer

While the incidence of gastric cancer in the Western world in general is declining, the risk in the elderly has remained basically unchanged (106, 107). The peak incidence is in the seventh decade, with 60% to 95% of cases occurring in patients over age 60 (108, 109).

The changes in the gastric mucosa that occur with aging are frequently found in association with gastric cancer. The nature of this association, however, is somewhat controversial. While most authors agree that atrophic gastritis is a premalignant lesion (90, 106, 110, 111), others believe that the gastric atrophy found in 80% to 90% of the elderly is not (107, 112). Although achlorhydria is found in 75% of patients with gastric cancer (113), the usual decrease in acid secreting ability that accompanies aging is not thought to be a precursor of malignancy (90). There is agreement, however, that intestinal metaplasia, the autoimmune gastritis associated with pernicious anemia, and adenomatous polyps are all precancerous conditions.

The iatrogenic gastritis associated with Billroth II

reconstructions for benign ulcer disease has also been implicated in the development of gastric malignancies. While there are data that suggest a causative relationship (113), recent studies fail to confirm this conclusion (114, 115).

Pathology

The majority of gastric cancers are the ulcerative type, with the diffuse, superficial, and polypoid varieties each accounting for about 10% of cases (107).

Histologically, gastric cancers in the elderly are predominantly the "intestinal type" with differentiated glandular elements, as opposed to the diffuse or infiltrative, less differentiated type found in younger patients. These tumors are generally slow growing and have a high incidence of synchronous lesions. In general, these types of lesions have a better prognosis than diffuse tumors (110).

A thorough review of the TNM classification of gastric cancer is found elsewhere (116). Briefly, Stage I and II disease is confined to the stomach with no nodal, contiguous organ, or distant spread. Stage III has contiguous spread but is resectable and/or has positive nodes. Stage IV is unresectable and/or has distant metastasis.

Diagnosis

Unfortunately, gastric malignancies are difficult to diagnose in the early stages when the tumors are resectable. In a study by Coluccia et al. (108), none of the 139 elderly patients studied was found to have Stage I tumors at the time of diagnosis, and 60% were found to have Stage IV disease. Only one-half of the elderly patients in this study were resectable at the time of laparotomy.

The symptoms of gastric cancers are often vague and nonspecific, particularly in the elderly. Upper abdominal discomfort can easily be confused with biliary tract disease and other intestinal disorders. Symptoms such as fatigue and general malaise, and signs of congestive heart failure secondary to blood loss may be most prominent. In one series (117), two-thirds of patients admitted with gastric cancer had different diagnoses at the time of admission. In one-third, anemia was the stated reason for hospitalization.

Early detection of gastric cancers in the elderly can only be accomplished if there is a high index of suspicion in patients with any upper GI complaints. Careful physical examination can reveal evidence of metastasis to supraclavicular, axillary, or umbilical lymph nodes. Rectal exam may reveal tumor in the cul de sac (Blumer's shelf), and pelvic exam may disclose ovarian metastasis (Krukenberg tumors). A large palpable epigastric mass is suggestive, although not confirmatory of contiguous organ involvement. Barium UGI series is the usual first study. Demonstration of a gastric ulcer on UGI should be followed immediately by endoscopic evaluation with multiple biopsies and brushings, because of the higher incidence of malignant ulcers in the elderly (107). The demonstration of healing by contrast radiography does not eliminate the possibility of malignancy (118), and endoscopic follow-up is recommended. Once the diagnosis of gastric cancer is established, the extent of the disease should be determined. Computed tomographic scanning of the abdomen may be useful to identify metastasis to the liver and gross nodal involvement outside the region of the tumor. It should not, however, be used to confirm contiguous spread or to determine resectability (119).

Treatment

The treatment of adenocarcinoma of the stomach in the absence of gross metastatic disease is surgical, especially when bleeding or obstructive symptoms are present. Many elderly patients with gastric malignancies are nutritionally impaired. Nutritional status must be assessed, and a period of hyperalimentation preoperatively may be necessary to minimize the pulmonary and wound complications associated with malnutrition in this age group (120). A complete bowel prep is necessary to facilitate colon resection should there be direct extension of the tumor into the colon or mesocolon. Major gastric resections may be lengthy and involve large fluid shifts intraoperatively. Therefore, central monitoring via Swan-Ganz catheter is nearly always indicated.

The location of the tumor plays a large role in the decision making for surgical management of gastric cancer. Distal tumors, even those extending beyond the confines of the gastric wall, should be excised along with the regional nodes and a portion of the involved adjacent organs. Distal gastric resection is usually tolerated quite well.

Lesions at or close to the esophagogastric junction, on the other hand, present greater operative risk. Often thoracotomy is necessary to facilitate resection of proximal gastric tumors. Therefore, careful preoperative evaluation of pulmonary status is essential. Total gastrecotomy for proximal gastric adenocarconima is a formidable surgical stress and is associated with many debilitating postoperative complications even in younger patients. It is therefore only recommended for those elderly patients with few other disorders in whom the chance of cure is worth the significant risk of operative mortality and morbidity. Age alone does not preclude total gastrectomy. Palliation of proximal lesions has been difficult in the past, but recent utilization of endoscopic laser therapy is promising, particularly for bleeding tumors (121). In the presence of gross metastatic disease, palliation by partial gastric resection, if technically feasible, is preferable to simple gastrojejunal bypass procedures.

Results

The results of surgery on elderly patients with gastric carcinoma are interesting. The majority of tumors in the elderly are in the middle or lower third of the stomach and are therefore amenable to partial gastrectomy when resectable (108). Unfortunately, as with younger patients, only about one half of tumors are resectable (108, 122). Coluccia et al. (108) compared operative mortality for total gastrectomy and partial gastrectomy in patients greater or less than age 65 with gastric cancer. Surprisingly, mortality for total gastrectomy was not different between the two age groups. The operative mortality for partial gastrectomy and total gastrectomy in the elderly patients was approximately the same (12.2% versus 10.5%). However, operative mortality for partial gastrectomy for younger patients was signficantly less than for the elderly (0% versus 12.2%).

Even more interesting is the survival data by year following resection (Table 31-12). While 1-year survival was lower in patients greater than age 65 (57% versus 72%), 5-year survival was higher (23% versus 11%). In patients greater than age 65 with Stage II disease, two-thirds survived 5 years compared to only 10% of the younger patients. No patient younger than age 65 with Stage IV disease survived 3 years. However, there were several patients older than 65 with similar disease who were alive at 5 years. Data from this and other studies (117) confirm that not only can resection for gastric carcinoma in the elderly be accomplished with acceptable mortality, but in fact long-term survival in those patients appears to be at least as good if not better than in younger patients with comparable disease.

Late Complications of Gastric Resection

The late complications of gastric resection in the elderly are similar to those in younger patients and are reviewed elsewhere (98). Two of these complications, however, are of particular importance because they can be serious when unrecognized but are treatable when identified early.

Table 31-12. Survival after surgery for gastric cancer

Alive (%) at 1 yr / at 5 yr	Stage of tumor at operation I	II	III	IV	Total
<65 years	100	100	65	50	72
	43	10	8	0	11
>65 years	—	100	41	50	57
		67	7	10	23

Adapted from Coluccia C, et al. 1987. Gastric cancer in the elderly: Results of surgical treatment. *Int Surg* 72:4–10.

Nutrition

While data in this area is limited, there do seem to be significant nutritional differences between elderly patients with gastric resection and without. Mellström and Rundgren (123) longitudinally studied elderly men between the ages of 70 and 75 with partial gastrectomy and compared them to nonoperated age-matched controls. They found a progressive decline in weight between age 70 and 75 in operated patients as compared to controls. Energy intake between the two groups did not differ, indicating an impairment in utilization rather than supply. Bone mineral content was found to be lower, and bone fracture rates were higher among operated subjects as well. Anemia from the deficiency of iron or vitamin B_{12} was also found more frequently in the patients with partial gastrectomy than in unoperated subjects. Careful surveillance for nutritional defects should therefore continue long after the initial postoperative period.

Bezoars

Concretions of various ingested materials in the stomach or small intestines are termed Bezoars. Phytobezoar containing fruit and vegetable matter occur in elderly patients post gastrectomy, as well as in some elderly patients with intact gastrointestinal tracts. Several factors contribute to the development of these phytobezoars. Edentulous elderly patients are unable to properly chew and grind fibrous food products. Large pieces of fibrous matter, therefore, enter the stomach virtually unaltered. Once in the stomach, the relative absence of acid further impairs the breakdown of these materials. In patients with partial gastrectomy, the lack of mixing and propulsive actions of the antrum allow the undigested fibrous matter to accumulate. These pieces of matter become adherent and form large proteinaceous masses or concretions. The presence of such bezoars may cause obstruction or local irritation and bleeding.

Citrus fruit and pulpy vegetables are most often the offending agents. Segments of unchewed, undigested orange for example, can get impacted in the distal ileum and present as small bowel obstruction. In general, however, the patients with phytobezoars are relatively asymptomatic in spite of the large size these masses may reach (Fig. 31-11).

The treatment of phytobezoars is dissolution and extraction of the mass either chemically with commercially

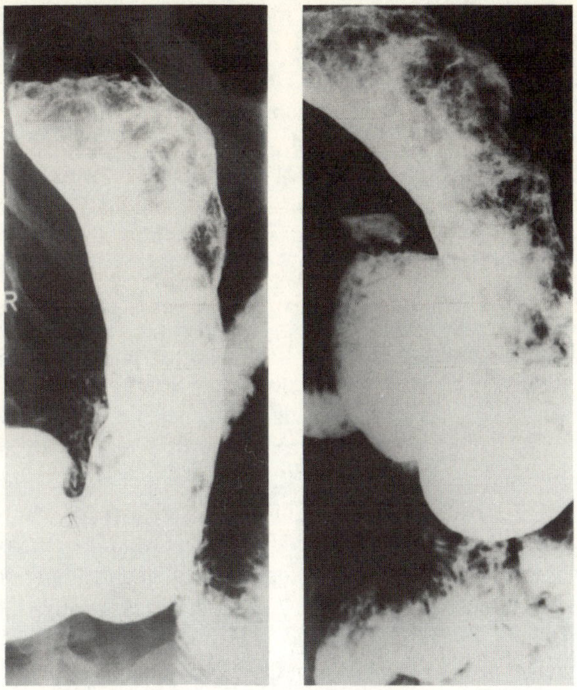

Figure 31-11. Upper gastrointestinal series showing a large bezoar occupying most of the fundus and body of the stomach. (Courtesy of A. Samin, M.D., SUNY Health Science Center, Brooklyn, NY.)

available enzymes, or mechanically via the endoscope (90). Operative removal may become necessary if endoscopic removal fails or if the bezoar has entered the small bowel. Bethanecal (a parasympathomimetic) and metaclopramide (an antidopaminergic) have been used to stimulate gastric motility and prevent the reaccumulation of these bezoars.

Operative Management of Colonic Disorders

Lower Gastrointestinal Bleeding

Lower GI bleeding is a relatively common problem in elderly patients. Over the past few years, improvements in technique, including fiberoptic endoscopy and selective angiography, have made it possible to precisely identify the site of bleeding in many cases. These modalities have also provided new options for either temporary or permanent control of the hemorrhage.

The causes of lower GI bleeding in the elderly are significantly different from those in younger patients. In children, Meckel's diverticulum, polyps, and inflammatory bowel disease are common. In adults less than 60 years of age, diverticulosis is probably the most common cause of bleeding, followed by polyps, inflammatory bowel disease, and malignancies (124).

Etiology

As the ability to make an accurate diagnosis in lower GI bleeding in the elderly has been refined, the theories about its etiology have changed. In the 1920s, neoplasms were considered the most common cause of bleeding, and diverticular bleeding was considered rare. However, this changed by the 1940s and 1950s, as reports of bleeding from diverticula increased. By the 1960s, there was a clear distinction between the relatively frequent occurrence of bleeding from diverticulosis and rare bleeding resulting from diverticulitis (124). During this period, any significant episode of lower GI bleeding without a discernible cause was attributed to a diverticulosis. In 1960, Margulis, Heinbecker, and Bernard (125) first demonstrated colonic angiodysplasia angiographically. Since then this entity has been recognized to have a prominent role in lower GI bleeding in elderly patients. At present, there is controversy over which of these disorders is most frequent. In some elderly patients, a definitive bleeding source cannot be identified. In these cases, the hemorrhage is often attributed to diverticulosis without sufficient evidence. In 1979, Boley et al. (126) reviewed 99 patients with major lower GI bleeding. Forty-three were discharged with a diagnosis of bleeding diverticulosis, but only 18% met strict angiographic diagnostic criteria. Boley et al. (126, 127) and Baum et al. (128) have suggested that angiodysplasia is at least as important as diverticulosis as a cause of lower GI bleeding in older patients.

The major difficulty in definitively identifying the source of massive lower GI hemorrhage in the elderly is that both diverticula and angiodysplasia are common incidental findings in this age group. Boley et al. (129) have demonstrated that approximately 25% of normal patients over the age of 60 years have right colonic angiodysplasia. It is also estimated that up to 50% of elderly patients have diverticula coli (124). Therefore, unless extravasation of contrast agent is demonstrated angiographically, or bleeding is seen at colonoscopy, the exact etiology of the hemorrhage may remain obscure. Postoperatively, injection of contrast into the feeding artery of a resected specimen of colon under fluoroscopy may demonstrate a bleeding site. Alternatively, immediate injection of the arterial supply with a silicone rubber derivative and dissection of the vascular structures may reveal angiodysplasia. Finally, Hagihara (130) has suggested that manual compression from both sides of the specimen may be helpful in demonstrating an erosion at the bleeding site especially in diverticular hemorrhage.

Pathology

Angiodysplasia is a degenerative lesion that almost always occurs in the right colon. Also known as arteriovenous malformation, vascular ectasia, and angioma, it represents a condition that is distinct from congenital colonic vascular malformations. These lesions are seen in patients over the age of 60, are not associated with angiomatous lesions of the skin or other viscera, almost always occur in the proximal colon, are less than 5 mm in diameter, and are difficult to visualize macroscopically (124).

Histologically, these lesions consist of dilated submucosal veins with subsequent dilatation of the venules and capillaries of the mucosa. The submuscosal venous dilatation is often very impressive. In its final stage, the mucosa may become replaced with a maze of dilated vessels. Boley (129) has postulated that there is degenerative low-grade submucosal venous obstruction, producing increased pressure within the veins and later within the venules and capillaries. As the capillaries dilate, there is loss of pre-capillary sphincters and arteriovenous communications develop, producing increased flow (Fig. 31-12). Arterial changes occur very late in the process. These lesions occur more commonly in the right colon because of the greater tension in the wall of the bowel in this location.

Diverticula occur primarily in the sigmoid colon but can be found throughout the large bowel. Diverticular bleeding is, however, much more likely to occur from the right side of the colon, doing so in 50% to 80% of patients (124). Left-sided diverticula are the result of intermittent increases in intraluminal pressure, while right-sided diverticula are associated with connective tissue abnormalities and weakened support of the vascular network. It is this lack of support that is thought to predispose right-sided diverticula to bleed.

Clinical Presentation

The nature of the bleeding from angiodysplasia, at least initially, is usually more venous than arterial. The common presentation of bleeding from these lesions is low grade, though about 10% to 15% will present with an acute serious hemorrhage (124). Bowden et al. (131) reported a 20% incidence of orthostasis or hypotension in patients proven to have angiodysplasia. Over 60% had required multiple admissions for bleeding, and the duration of bleeding ranged up to 23 years. Occasionally, the bleeding is occult, and the presenting sign may be a guaiac positive stool or iron deficiency anemia. Boley et al. (124) reported these findings in approximately 15% of cases. In addition, the quantity of bleeding may vary, so that patients may bleed briskly once and then have only occasional losses in the stool later. This pattern reflects the various zones of pressure present in these arteriovenous malformations.

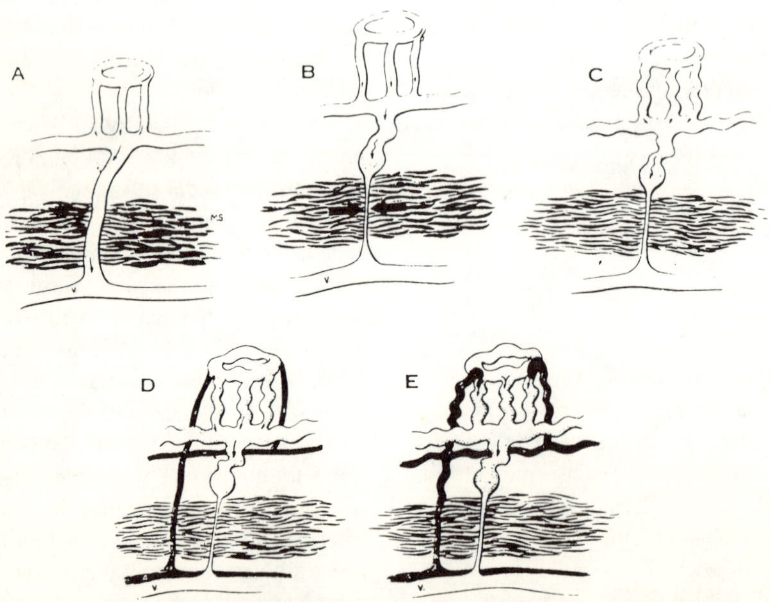

Figure 31-12. A diagrammatic illustration of the proposed concept of the development of cecal vascular ectasia. A, Normal state of the vein perforating the muscular layers. B, With muscular contraction or increased intraluminal pressure, the vein becomes partially obstructed. C, After repeated episodes over many years, the submucosal vein becomes dilated and tortuous. D, Later the veins and venules draining into the submucosal vein become similarly involved. E, Ultimately, the capillary ring becomes dilated, the precapillary sphincter becomes incompetent, and a small arteriovenous communication appears. (Reprinted, with permission, from Boley SJ, et al. 1977. On the nature and etiology of vascular ectasis of the colon. *Gastroenterology* 72: 650–660.) (134).

There has been an increased association reported between valvular heart disease and GI bleeding, and in particular between bleeding from angiodysplasia and calcific aortic stenosis (132). Boley et al. (124) reported a 25% incidence, although others have reported no such association. While aortic stenosis may predispose to the development of angiodysplasia, Boley has postulated that the low perfusion pressure produced by aortic stenosis may instead cause ischemia of the thinned out mucosal layer overlying the angiodysplasia, producing an increased chance of hemorrhage.

In contrast, diverticular bleeds are caused by an erosion into an artery in the base of a diverticulum. Thus, the bleeding is usually more impressive than that seen with angiodysplasia. Diverticular hemorrhage stops spontoneously in 75% of patients when the bleeding artery thromboses (124). In addition, it is less likely to recur than is the bleeding from angiodysplasia. It is postulated that once a diverticular bleeding site thromboses, it cannot bleed again, and recurrent bleeding represents bleeding from another diverticulum. Simultaneous bleeding from multiple diverticula is rare (124, 126).

Diagnosis

The diagnostic approach to lower GI bleeding depends on what has occurred and whether or not the bleeding seems to be active. However, all patients with bleeding suspected to be from a lower GI source should have a nasogastric tube placed and gastric aspiration performed as the initial test. Bilious effluent containing no blood virtually proves that the source of the hemorrhage is not in the upper GI tract. The absence of bile in the aspirate, however, only rules out an esophogeal or gastric bleeding source. Upper GI endoscopy should be performed to rule out bleeding from the duodenum before proceeding with a diagnostic workup for a colonic source. A BUN level over 30 mg/dl is reported to occur in two-thirds of patients with a major upper GI hemorrhage and is suggestive of bleeding proximal to the colon. Proctoscopy should be performed early to rule out rectal bleeding and a coagulation profile performed to rule out a coagulopathy (124).

Patients who have had a recent episode(s) of bleeding that has stopped should be evaluated with colonoscopy. Boley (124) has asserted that no patient, with the possible exception of a young patient with a bleeding pattern suggestive of hemorrhoids, is adequately studied by anything less than total colonoscopy. Rigid sigmoidoscopy is uncomfortable, and even flexible sigmoidoscopy does not visualize the right side of the colon where most bleeding originates in older patients. In addition, colonoscopy has the potential advantage of treating some of the causes of bleeding either by polypectomy or coagulation. If colonoscopy is not revealing, a barium enema should be performed. It is an accurate method of determining mass lesions, which may be missed by colonoscopy, especially if there was any residual blood at the time of endoscopy. It should, however, be delayed until after the danger of recurrent bleeding has passed.

Colonoscopy also has a role in acute hemorrhage. Forde (133) recently reported a series of 25 patients who underwent colonoscopy while actively bleeding. The procedure was successful in 23 of the 25 patients and was diagnostic in 80%. It aborted a planned operation in four patients and limited the resection in seven others. It was noncontributory only in the two patients in whom it was technically unsatisfactory. There was one complication, perforation of an actively bleeding diverticulum. There were some technical modifications in performing the colonoscopy in this study. Clots were fragmented using a Water-Pik attached to one of the channels of the colonoscope. The instrument was passed by areas of pooled liquid blood by changing the patient's position. Visual inspection of the colon was performed during withdrawal of the scope after it had been inserted to the maximum length possible. Other authors have also reported good success using colonoscopy as the initial diagnostic study. In the series by Bowden et al. (131), eleven of the seventeen patients with angiodysplasia underwent colonoscopy. It was diagnostic in five patients and suggestive in three others. There were no complications. Boley et al. (127), however, reported obtaining an accurate diagnosis by using acute colonoscopic evaluation in only two of eleven patients who were bleeding from angiodysplasia. They also caution that angiodysplasia must be identified on the initial inspection of the colon with the colonoscope, as minor endoscopic trauma to the mucosa may produce an appearance similar to that of an angiodysplastic lesion.

Radionuclide scanning is indicated in those patients who do not have a bleeding source identified at colonoscopy or in whom colonoscopy is unsuccessful. Both technetium-99m sulfur colloid and technetium-99m labeled red cells should be used, as they are complementary. Sulfur colloid scanning is sensitive and may detect bleeding as subtle as 0.1 ml/min. However, the agent is concentrated in the liver and spleen, and therefore is not useful for locating an upper abdominal site. Furthermore, the agent is relatively rapidly cleared by the body so that if the patient is not bleeding at the exact time of scanning, the examination will be futile. Labeled red blood cells remain active for up to 24 hours, permitting serial scanning if necessary (124, 132).

If the combination of colonoscopy and technetium scanning is negative and the bleeding continues, selective angiography is indicated. In the vast majority of patients who come to angiography, a right-sided lesion is expected. Therefore, superior mesenteric arterial injection should be the initial study performed. If this is negative, the inferior mesenteric artery should be studied next, followed by the celiac axis.

Angiography may detect bleeding rates as low as 0.5 ml/minute and has been successful in detecting the source of bleeding in about two-thirds of patients with massive lower GI hemorrhage. It is most useful in those patients with diverticular bleeds, demonstrating the site in up to 75% of cases (124). Angiography should be considered positive when contrast material is seen to extravasate and pool in a diverticulum.

Extravasation is seen in far fewer patients bleeding from angiodysplasia (10% to 20% of cases). Boley et al. have described angiographic signs to diagnosis angiodysplasia even in the absence of extravasation. These include the appearance of a densely opacified vein, a slowly filling tortuous vein, a vascular tuft, or an early filling vein. The densely opacified vein corresponds to the dilated submucosal vein and is present in 90% of cases. A vascular tuft is seen in about 70% of patients, and an early filling vein, the latest sign, is seen about half the time. Extravasation without any of the above signs is strong evidence against bleeding from angiodysplasia and favors a diverticular source (129, 134, 135).

Barium enema has an extremely limited role in the emergency evaluation of the bleeding patient. It is an anatomic but not a functional exam. Lesions seen, i.e., polyps or diverticula, may not necessarily be the source of bleeding. Furthermore, opacification of the colon with barium will greatly limit the utility of further diagnostic tests such as colonoscopy and angiography. Barium enema should therefore be delayed until bleeding has stopped (132).

Treatment and Results

The initial therapy of lower GI bleeding is resuscitation and stabilization. This is especially important in elderly patients in whom hypoperfusion and emergency surgery are poorly tolerated. Fortunately, most patients can be at least temporarily stabilized and undergo the appropriate diagnostic exams as outlined above.

Recently, endoscopic techniques have gained importance as therapeutic as well as diagnostic tools. Facility with colonoscopic polypectomy has allowed even large polyps to be removed without inordinate complications. Endoscopic electrocoagulation is now available to manage angiodysplasia. Various other methods, including argon and Nd-YAG lasers, endoscopic sclerosis, and monopolar and bipolar electrocoagulation are gaining popularity (129, 136). Each method has advantages, but none of them has emerged as clearly superior to the others. The rate of rebleeding following endoscopic ablation of angiodysplastic lesions is not well documented. There is also a relative paucity of data correlating endoscopic and histologic appearances of these lesions. Question also exists as to the management of asymptomatic angiodysplasias seen on endoscopy. At present, routine ablation of these lesions is not recommended.

Similarly, angiographic methods can be used therapeutically as well as diagnostically. Transcatheter embolization has been described using gelfoam or autologous blood clot. However, complications, including colonic infarction and late strictures, have been reported (137–139). Vasopressin infusion, administered either selectively or peripherally, has had more promising results. Hemorrhage has been controlled in up to 80% of patients in whom extravasation was angiographically demonstrated (129). When bleeding is from the left colon, peripheral infusion is as effective as selective infusion and probably safer. Boley (124, 129) has reported sigmoid infarction and lower extremity ischemia as a result of selective infusion of vasopressin into the inferior mesenteric artery. When bleeding is from the right colon, selective arterial infusion is more effective.

Surgical resection remains the treatment of choice in almost all patients with a documented source of colonic bleeding. Exceptions are those patients who are prohibitive surgical risks or who have lesions identified that can be managed non-operatively by endoscopic ablation.

The majority of elderly patients with major hemorrhage who have a bleeding site identified definitively have a right-sided lesion. In these patients, right hemicolectomy is the treatment of choice. The presence of diverticula in the left colon is not an indication for resection unless bleeding has been demonstrated from the left colon. Patients who have bled from angiodysplasia should also undergo right hemicolectomy. Although these lesions are almost always multiple, they rarely occur in the left colon, and right hemicolectomy should therefore be curative. Patients who have documented angiodysplasia and chronic blood loss, but have not had an acute hemorrhage, should also undergo elective right hemicolectomy. Eighty to ninety percent of patients will not rebleed following surgery, and not all who do rebleed require reoperation (124, 129). Segmental resection is the treatment of choice for patients with proven diverticular bleeding. Rates of subsequent rebleeding are low.

Subtotal colectomy is a procedure that should rarely be necessary. If the diagnosis is pursued aggressively, the site of bleeding will be identified in the majority of cases. Emergency subtotal colectomy carries an operative mortality between 15% and 50%, and there are reports of disabling postoperative diarrhea in up to 16% of elderly patients (129). Subtotal colectomy should be reserved for those patients who continue to bleed without an identifiable source despite all diagnostic tests, or for those who bleed at a rate precluding any diagnostic workup (129). Intraoperative endoscopy has recently been described as an additional diagnostic maneuver in such patients, but its role at present is unproven (130).

Colon Cancer

Carcinoma of the colon is the second most common malignancy in the United States and accounts for next to the largest number of cancer deaths in men and women (140, 141). In the elderly, colon cancer is the most common malignancy with the exception of carcinoma of the prostate (142).

Risk Factors

Age is clearly the leading risk factor in the development of carcinoma of the colon. While there are reports of colon cancer in patients in their twenties and thirties, risk begins around 40 years of age. At 50 years, the risk sharply increases and doubles each decade until age 80 (Table 31-13) (140).

Hereditary factors also contribute. There is an increased risk of colon cancer in primary relatives of patients with this disease and in patients with familial polyposis, ulcerative colitis, or a history of adenomatous colonic polyps.

Recently, new emphasis has been placed on dietary risk factors for colon cancer. Fried foods and foods high in animal fat have been implicated in the emergence of this disease. Japanese people, whose diet consists of very little animal fat, have an increase in the incidence of colon cancer when they move to Western countries and change their dietary habits. It is postulated that an increase in dietary animal fat produces changes in bacterial fecal flora, intestinal bile acids, and colonic cholesterol content. The increase in fecal secondary bile acids is associated with an increased incidence of colon cancer (4).

Fiber content may also play a role in the pathogenesis of colon cancer. Diets deficient in fiber increase colonic transit time, thus increasing the time carcinogens are in contact with the colonic mucosa.

Table 31-13. Annual age-specific incidence of colorectal cancer per 100,000 population (1973–1976)

	Colon		Rectum	
Age group	Males	Females	Males	Females
0	0.0	0.0	0.0	0.0
1–4	0.0	0.0	0.0	0.0
5–9	0.0	0.4	0.0	0.0
10–14	0.6	0.2	0.0	0.0
15–19	0.3	1.6	0.0	0.0
20–24	1.0	0.6	0.0	0.0
25–29	1.6	1.5	0.0	0.2
30–34	2.5	2.5	1.1	0.9
35–39	3.9	3.8	3.2	3.6
40–44	6.2	8.0	4.4	5.4
45–49	14.3	14.2	8.0	12.4
50–54	20.8	29.3	19.3	23.5
55–59	37.1	44.9	25.2	45.7
60–64	60.6	55.2	38.3	66.9
65–69	80.9	78.2	41.8	102.7
70–74	132.5	119.4	62.6	139.0
75–79	204.1	142.1	89.9	182.2
80–84	223.0	216.0	96.4	171.6
85+	239.2	209.8	141.6	225.8

Reprinted, with permission, from Brocklehurst JC. 1985. Colonic diseases. *Clin Gastroenterol* 14:725–747.

Diagnosis

While the signs of colon cancer are not different in elderly patients, i.e., bleeding, weight loss, or evidence of obstruction, the presenting complaints of the elderly may be surprisingly different from those offered by younger patients. Apathy, loss of vigor, or changes in mental status secondary to iron deficiency may be the only symptoms. Changes in bowel habits and constipation are such common chronic complaints in the geriatric populations that they are frequently ignored by both the patient and the physician. The diagnosis of colon cancer in the elderly is often not made, therefore, until a major complication has occurred. Waldron et al. (143) reported that 58% of the 522 patients over the age of 70 years with colon cancer presented as emergencies.

The major difficulty in the early detection of colonic malignancy is the lack of a reliable and specific screening test. Determination of fecal occult blood is one of the easiest available examinations. However, polyps or malignancies may bleed unevenly resulting in unreliable stool guaiac testing. In a 1983 study of the utility of stool guaiac, only 37% of the patient population actually completed the test. Two percent were positive for blood. In 50% of the positive tests, the bleeding was from a neoplastic lesion. While this represented a 3.6 times greater detection rate than in the control group, it does point out some of the limitations of this form of testing (144).

Rigid sigmoidoscopy has been utilized in the past to detect distal colonic and rectal tumors. Recently, flexible sigmoidoscopy has beome more popular because of its ability to detect more proximal lesions. A Memorial Sloan Kettering study demonstrated that patients over the age of 70 with positive occult fecal blood had a significant incidence of colon cancers and/or adenomas. Flexible sigmoidoscopy doubled the yield of detection by picking up additional lesions in patients with negative stool guaiac tests (141). In another recent study, where colonoscopy was routinely employed, it was found that two-thirds of patients with Duke's A and B colon cancer had negative tests for fecal occult blood (Fig. 31-13) (145). The routine

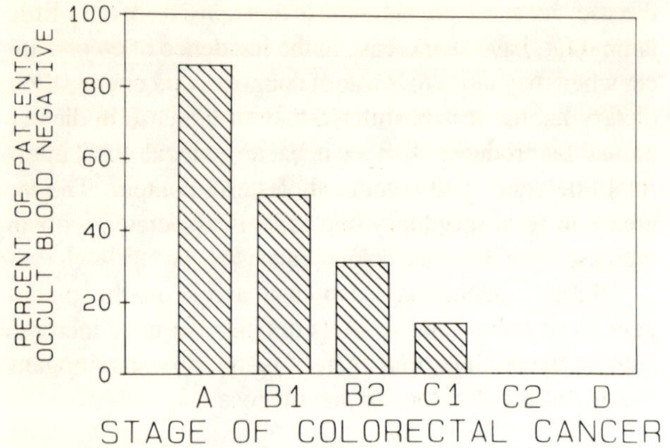

Figure 31-13. This graph depicts the percent of patients with negative stool occult blood tests according to the stage of the colorectal tumor found. These results indicate that testing stool for occult blood detects few early colorectal cancers. (Reprinted, with permission, from Longo WE, Ballantyne GH, and Modlin IM. 1988. Colonoscopic detection of early colorectal cancers: Impact of a surgical endoscopy service. *Ann Surg* 207: 174.) (145).

use of endoscopic procedures can, therefore, be expected to significantly increase the detection of early colon cancer in the elderly.

Barium enema has also been used as a screening test for colon cancer. Some data suggest, however, that colonoscopy is more helpful. In 1988, Bongiorno (106) studied 80 elderly patients who had polyps discovered on routine barium enema. All patients subsequently underwent colonoscopy, and endoscopic confirmation of these polyps was found in only 60 of the 80 patients. In addition, 24 patients had other polypoid masses discovered with colonoscopy that were not identified with barium enema. It is particularly interesting that 65% of patients thought that the barium enema was more uncomfortable than colonoscopy, while only 15% thought colonoscopy was more uncomfortable. The other 20% thought the two exams were equally uncomfortable.

At present, the National Cancer Institute recommends yearly stool guaiac testing in every person over the age of 50 years. The American College of Surgeons also recommends routine endoscopic examinations every 3 to 5 years in patients over age 50, even when stool guaiac tests are negative. Screening should be performed even more often in patients who have had a previous history of colon cancer or in those in high risk groups (141).

Treatment and Results

Colectomy for carcinoma is a serious intra-abdominal operation, requiring a significant amount of physiologic reserve. Although there is concern that elderly patients may not have the reserve necesasary to tolerate optimal surgical treatment, data do not support this concern. In 1988, Irvin (146) reviewed 306 patients with adenocarcinoma of the colon and rectum. There were 171 patients over the age of 70 and 135 under 70 years. There was no difference in tumor location or Duke's classification between the two groups. When actuarial survival curves were used, there was also no difference in the perioperative mortality between the two groups (8).

Most other studies support the concept that elective resection may be safely performed for colon cancer in the elderly. Perioperative mortality rates vary from 2% to 8%. Mortality is primarily due to coexisting cardiac disease (2, 147, 148).

As with other abdominal conditions, elderly patients with colon cancer tend to present late in the course of the disease. Frequently, medical attention is not sought until obstruction or perforation has occurred. Webbes (147) has reported that a significant number of elderly patients have such advanced disease at the time of presentation, that curative resection is often not possible (9). Unfortunately, when elderly patients undergo emergency operation, the mortality rate rises sharply. Waldron et al. (143) reported a mortality of between 10% and 18% for elective operations. When operation was carried out as an emergency, the mortality increased to 19% in the patients less than 70 years and 38% in patient over 70 years. It is interesting that this rapid increase in mortality may not be due to an increase in complications. Cohen et al. (148) demonstrated the same incidence of complications in emergency and elective surgery for colon cancer in geriatric patients. However, the death rate from these complications was 68% in those operated on emergently versus 28% in those operated on electively.

Diverticulitis

Diverticulitis, inflammation in the outpouchings of the left colon, is primarily a disease of the elderly. It is estimated that 30% of patients over age 60 years and 40% of patients over age 80 have diverticula (149). While most patients with diverticulosis are asymptomatic, diverticulitis must always be included in the differential diagnosis in any elderly patient complaining of abdominal pain.

Etiology

Colon diverticula are acquired herniations of colonic mucosa through the muscle coat. The region between the longitudinal teniae and the circular muscle represents an area of relative muscular weakness. This area is further weakened by the segmental blood vessels that perforate through on either side of the colon. The herniation is caused by repetitive intermittent increases in the intracolonic pressure.

The predominant risk factor for the development of diverticula is a low-residue diet common in most Western countries. Diverticular disease is largely unknown in countries where the diet consists of unrefined sugars, grains, and natural fibers. Animal studies have shown that rats fed a low-residue diet will develop diverticula (149). Painter (150) has postulated that a low-residue diet increases nonpropulsive colonic motility. The increased activity of the circular muscle then predisposes to segmental high pressure zones in the weakest area of the bowel where the arteries perforate.

Aging may play a role as well in the formation of diverticula. While it is possible that the dietary factors simply take time to become manifest, approximately 10% of elderly patients with colonic diverticula have diverticula in other hollow viscera as well. Obesity, fatty atrophy causing muscle wall degeneration, muscle atrophy, and constipation have all been postulated to play a part in the development of this entity. While it is possible that these conditions do play a small role, they are no longer considered primary factors in the development of these diverticula (149).

Clinical Presentation

As with many abdominal disorders in the elderly, the symptoms of diverticulitis may be relatively nonspecific. The workup is complicated by the fact that diverticula may be present but not responsible for the acute illness. As a result, many elderly patients hospitalized with this disorder have had undiagnosed symptoms for years.

Abdominal pain is the most common presenting complaint occurring in 70% to 80% of patients with diverticulitis (151, 152). It is usually moderate to severe, may be colicky in nature and is most often in the suprapubic area or left lower quadrant. A change in bowel habits is also quite common—either constipation, diarrhea, or both. There may be a considerable amount of abdominal distention, because colonic spasm secondary to the inflammation produces intermittent and/or complete bowel obstruction. Nausea, vomiting, and heartburn occur in about 25% of patients (153). In 15% to 20% of cases, bleeding may also occur in the presence of acute inflammation (151–153).

Occasionally, patients with diverticulitis will present with one of the complications of the disease. Colovesical fistula is a relatively common complication, especially in males. It may also occur in women after hysterectomy, because the uterus is no longer present to act as a barrier between the sigmoid colon and bladder. The most dramatic presenting symptom is pneumaturia, although pyuria or recurrent urinary tract infections may be the only evidence of the fistula. Mitty (152) reported a 2.5% incidence of pneumaturia and a similar incidence of pyuria as the presenting symptom in diverticulitis. Rectovaginal fistulae may also occur and was the presenting finding in approximately 2% of the cases in this study. Occasionally, the inflamed diverticulum will perforate and seal, forming a pericolic collection. Pale (154) reported the presence of a left lower quadrant mass in 20% of patients. In the series by Mitty (152), there was 1.7% incidence of a painless abdominal mass at presentation.

Diagnosis

The differential diagnosis of diverticulitis may be extremely difficult. The colicky nature of the pain may be suggestive of renal calculi. In addition, a spastic colon may present in an identical manner with crampy pain, constipation, and bloating. It is most important however, to differentiate between diverticulitis and colon cancer. Both diseases most often occur in the same age group and colonic location. The symptoms may be identical as well. Although colonoscopy and barium enema are often useful in distinguishing diverticulitis from colon cancer, they, too, are sometimes inconclusive. While findings such as external mass effect and colonic spasm may be suggestive of diverticulitis, stricture and obstruction may be easily confused with carcinoma. Therefore, patients with longstanding chronic disease should undergo elective resection.

When diverticulitis is acute, many diagnostic studies may be difficult to obtain or interpret. Plain films of the abdomen are usually nonspecific, and pneumoperitoneum is seldom demonstrated even if perforation has occurred. Colonoscopy or flexible sigmoidoscopy, while useful in the diagnosis of chronic diverticulitis, are contraindicated when acute inflammation is suspected. Computerized tomographic (CT) scanning has been reported to be an excellent study for the diagnosis of acute diverticulitis (155). The demonstration of a pericolic phlegmon or fluid collection in the region of the sigmoid colon, among other findings, is highly suggestive of acute diverticulitis (Fig. 31-14). The water-soluble contrast agent gastrograffin, used by enema, either in combination with CT or by routine technique, may be helpful in cases where CT alone is equivocal. Contrast enema using barium is contraindicated when there is a possibility of perforation.

Treatment and Results

When the diagnosis of acute diverticulitis is made in an elderly patient, hospitalization is advised. Although younger patients may be treated successfully at home, older patients must be carefully observed. The limited ability of such patients to compensate for infection may quickly lead to fulminant septic shock. Fortunately, many patients will respond to conservative measures. These include restricted oral intake, intravenous hydration, and

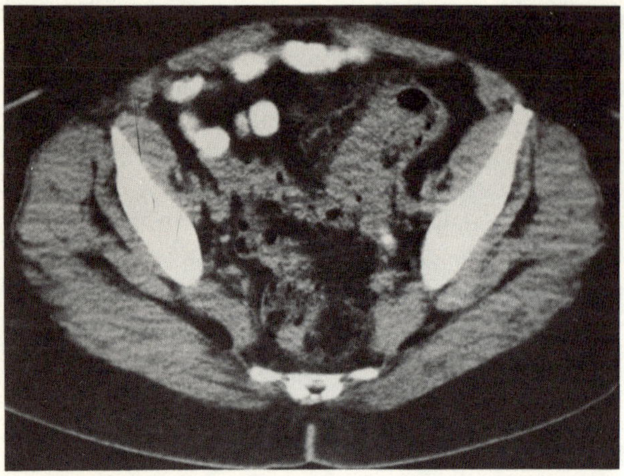

Figure 31-14. Computed tomogram showing an inflammatory mass surrounding the sigmoid colon in the left lower quadrant. This appearance is indicative of acute diverticulitis. (Courtesy of A. Cantor, M.D., SUNY Health Science Center, Brooklyn, NY.)

parenteral antibiotics. Those patients who fail to improve or who develop an acute complication such as pelvic abscess or rupture with peritonitis must be explored.

Operative therapy as an emergency should be designed to eradicate sepsis and divert the colonic stream. In the past, staged surgical treatment with diverting colostomy and drainage as the first stage had been advocated. Colostomy and drainage, however, leaves the affected segment of colon in situ and increases the possibility of chronic complications, especially fistulae. In cases where there is a large inflammatory mass in a poorly compensated patient, colostomy and drainage is still the quickest and safest procedure. Recently, however, initial resection with creation of an end colostomy and mucus fistula or blind rectal pouch (Hartman's Procedure) has become the operation of choice in most cases. In 1987, Finlay et al. (156) reviewed 78 patients who underwent emergency surgical procedures for diverticulitis. In those patients treated with colostomy and drainage, over half were left with permanent colostomies, and many developed fistulae. In those treated with resection, only 16% required permanent colostomies, and fistulae were significantly less common. There was, however, no difference in mortality between the two groups.

When patients do respond to conservative therapy, it is tempting not to operate at all once the acute attack has resolved. The chance of recurrence and subsequent emergency surgery is real, however, and elective treatment must be considered. Clearly, the safest way to operate on patients with diverticulitis is electively. Resection in this setting is a one stage procedure and almost never requires a colostomy. Boyd et al. (2) reported a mortality of only 3.4% for elective resection. The mortality in this study for emergency procedures was 17%. Other studies report an emergency mortality of 20% to 30% (156).

Pseudo-obstruction of the Colon

Pseudo-obstruction of the colon is a condition that has only recently become recognized as a specific disease entity. As recently as 1979 (157), textbooks of surgery referred to it as psychogenic and/or idiopathic megacolon and thought it was mainly restricted to institutionalized psychotic patients.

The syndrome of colonic pseudo-obstruction was originally reported by Sir Heneage Ogilvie in 1948 (158). He described two patients who developed functional colonic obstruction associated with diffuse abdominal malignancy involving the periaortic area. He postulated that the tumor had infiltrated the celiac plexus, producing splanchnic nerve destruction. Since then, this functional colonic obstruction has been given various names, including Ogilvie's Syndrome, Colonic Ileus, Idiopathic Large Bowel Obstruction, and Large Intestinal Colic.

Etiology

Colonic pseudo-obstruction is the final common pathway of a multiplicity of problems (159). It is commonly seen in patients suffering from orthopedic problems, especially fractures. Any trauma, however minor, as well as any condition that requires prolonged bed rest, is associated with a relatively high incidence of pseudo-obstruction. All metabolic abnormalities may produce the syndrome, although hypokalemia and hypovolemia are the most common. Uremia and diabetes are likewise common causes of colonic ileus (Table 31-14).

Clinical Presentation

While pseudo-obstruction of the colon is still most often diagnosed in elderly hospitalized patients, it is now being

Table 31-14. Illnesses associate with pseudo-obstruction

Associated illness	Number of patients
None	5
Spinal surgery	3
Spinal injury	1
Rectroperitoneal hematoma	1
Orthopedic surgery	2
Cerebrovascular events	3
Diabetic ketoacidosis	1
Myxedema	1
Neuropsychiatric drugs	2
Total	19

Adapted from Bullock PR, and Thomas WE. 1984. Acute pseudoobstruction of the colon. *Ann R Coll Surg Engl* 63:327.

seen more often in younger patients as well. The typical presenting symptom is abdominal distention. While a few patients complain of crampy abdominal pain, most do not, and the absence of pain is often striking. Rarely, the abdominal distention is great enough to produce shortness of breath. Constipation and/or obstipation are the rule although occasionally patients have diarrhea. Nausea and vomiting are usually surprisingly absent, occurring in only about 20% of patients in a recent review. Most patients tolerate a full diet up to the time of diagnosis (159, 160).

It may be extremely difficult to differentiate between colonic ileus and other potentially catastrophic intra-abdominal conditions. In general, the diagnosis is made by history and physical exam and is corroborated by plain film of the abdomen. These should demonstrate a distended colon from cecum to rectum without any air-fluid levels (Fig. 31-15). Occasionally, however, one may see an abrupt end to the colonic air similar to that seen with a mechanical obstruction. This "cut off sign" usually occurs at either the splenic flexure or in the sigmoid and is thought to be secondary to kinking of the colon from gaseous distention. Serial radiographs may show this cut off progressing distally (159).

It is crucial to be able to differentiate between colonic ileus and mechanical colon obstruction. Mechanical colonic obstruction secondary to mass lesions or strictures more often presents with nausea, vomiting, and crampy abdominal pain. The X-ray picture should confirm the diagnosis. If any question remains, colonoscopic evaluation will definitively differentiate between functional and mechanical obstruction.

Cecal or sigmoid volvulus may also mimic pseudo-obstruction. In general, both conditions present with symptoms more similar to those of a mechanical obstruction. The characteristic X-ray picture of cecal volvulus should confirm that diagnosis (Fig. 31-16). The radiographic differentiation of sigmoid volvulus versus pseudo-obstruction may be more difficult since the involved segment of sigmoid in a volvulus may look similar to the highly distended sigmoid in pseudo-obstruction (Fig. 31-17). Sigmoidoscopy is invaluable in these cases.

Occasionally, acute gastric dilatation will present with abdominal distention that mimics colonic ileus. The diagnosis should be easily made by physical exam and/or plain films of the abdomen.

Treatment and Results

While the care of patients with colonic pseudo-obstruction must be individualized, a few general principles govern the management of the majority of these patients. Non-operative therapy is the initial treatment of choice. This includes withholding oral intake or nasogastric de-

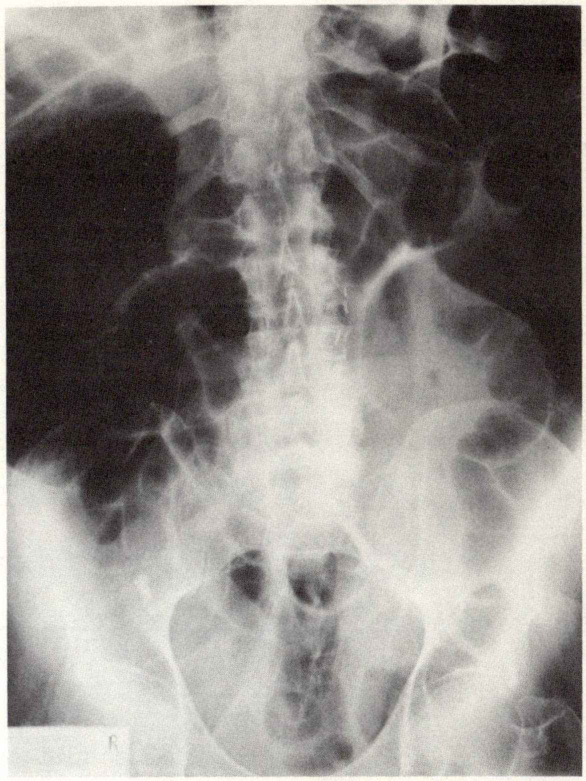

Figure 31-15. Flat plate of the abdomen showing the massive colonic distention found in patients with pseudo-obstruction.

compression, and ultravenous hydration. Rectal tubes are often useful. In approximately 85% of patients with an easily identifiable cause of pseudo-obstruction (i.e., electrolyte abnormalities), the ileus tends to resolve spontaneously once the cause is corrected (161). However, the rate of spontaneous resolution drops to about 33% in patients with idiopathic colonic ileus, and approximately 25% of patients die while being observed, usually from the underlying disease (159).

Surgical decompression was the only option for failed expectant therapy until 1977 when Kukora and Dent (162) described colonoscopic decompression for colonic ileus. They successfully decompressed eight of nine patients colonoscopically. Two of the eight recurred but were successfully decompressed with a second endoscopic procedure. Since them, colonoscopy has become accepted as an excellent therapeutic as well as diagnostic maneuver in the management of colonic pseudo-obstruction. Colonoscopic placement of a proximal rectal tube is also helpful in hastening colonic decompression.

Most authors report a 50% to 90% success rate with colonoscopic decompression (161–166). In a recent review, Nano et al. (161) treated 25 patients with colonic ileus. Seventeen required colonoscopic decompression, seven with endoscopic placement of a rectal tube. Four

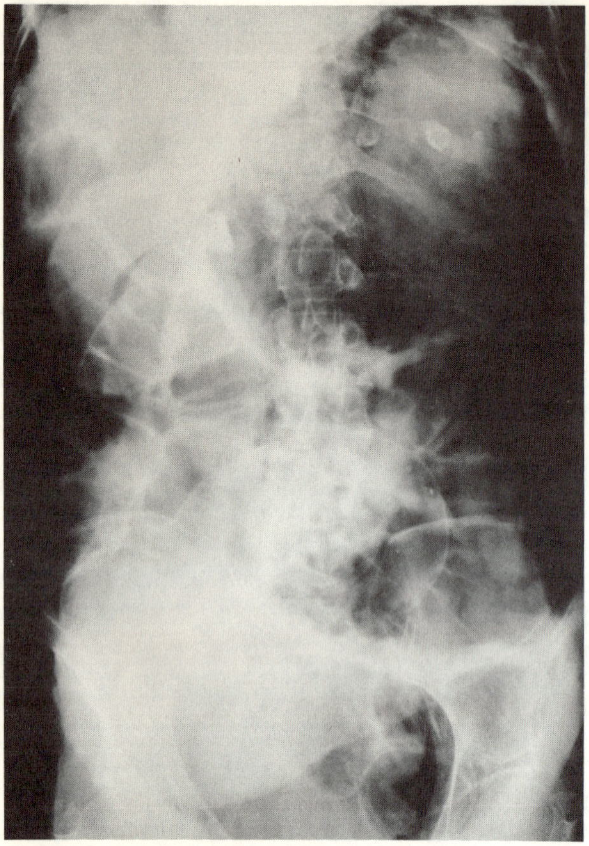

Figure 31-16. Cecal volvulus. (Courtesy of R. De Silva, SUNY Health Science Center, Brooklyn, NY.)

patients failed. Of the 13 patients who were successfully decompressed initially, three recurred. These results are consistent with the 20% recurrence quoted by other authors (162–166). While colonoscopy has the potential to worsen colonic distention and cause colonic perforation, the complication rate in skilled hands is extremely low (167). This mode of decompression should therefore be routinely employed in patients who fail expectant therapy.

Surgical management should be reserved for those patients who present with or develop peritonitis while being observed. In general, the mechanism for this peritonitis is cecal ischemia followed by infarction and perforation. The cecum is the most likely site for ischemia because of its distensibility and the thinness of its wall relative to the remainder of the colon. The critical diameter at which point cecal ischemia becomes a risk is unclear. Most texts quote a cecal diameter of 9 to 12 cm as an indication for decompression, but there does not seem to be any hard data to support these recommendations (168, 169). In fact, there have been reports of patients with cecal diameters up to 25 cm that have been successfully treated non-operatively. It seems that serial films to chart the progression of cecal size may be more valuable than a single determination (170).

Any surgical intervention in the presence of pseudo-obstruction can be hazardous and technically challenging. Creation of a decompressing loop colotomy is the standard procedure. Frequently, colotomy and partial decompression, with all the attendant risks of opening an unprepared bowel, is necessary to facilitate the formation of the stoma. Simple cecostomy would appear to be a viable alternative, although it, too, is not without risk. Under local anesthesia, exposure is often poor, and differentiating cecum from redundant sigmoid may be very difficult. Cecostomy under general anesthesia is also a significant operative insult and is associated with a mortality of 40% (162, 171). The high mortality associated with operative procedures for pseudo-obstruction is due primarily to the debilitated condition of most patients with this disorder. Therefore, an aggressive attempt at nonoperative management is nearly always indicated.

Volvulus

Colonic volvulus has been recognized as an entity since ancient times. While it is an uncommon cause of intestinal obstruction in general, it is the third most common cause of colonic obstruction in the United States after malignancies and diverticular disease. In the so-called "volvulus belt" of Africa, India, and Iran, it is very common and accounts for over one-half of colonic obstructions (172).

Etiology

The exact etiology of volvulus of the colon remains unclear. In 1849, Rokitansky (173) first observed that a long, floppy colonic mesentery was necessary for colonic volvulus to occur. Later, Treves (174) observed that a long colonic loop with a mesocolon that is narrow at its parietal attachment brings the limbs of the loop close together, allowing a volvulus to occur. In a cadaver study, Wolfer et al. (175) also demonstrated that in 37% of cases, the cecum is mobile enough to allow a volvulus to occur.

The clear-cut geographic predisposition to the development of colonic volvulus is thought to be due to dietary variations. Many authors have suggested that a high vegetable fiber diet is an important etiologic factor (176–179). Chronic intake of coarse vegetable fiber leads to the development of a long redundant colon (176). In the United States, chronic constipation is thought to be responsible for the development of long redundant colonic loops and subsequent volvulus (178, 179). In addition, chronic dependence on laxatives is common in patients with this disorder. It is possible that excessive laxative use may damage mesenteric nerves, producing disordered colonic motility, megacolon, and volvulus (173).

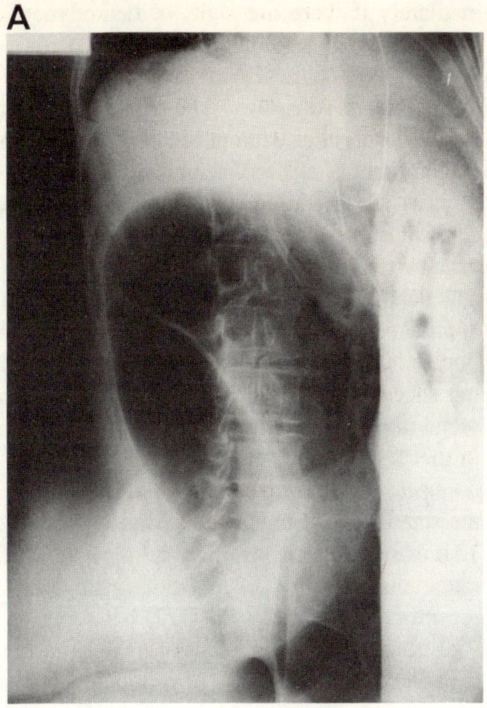

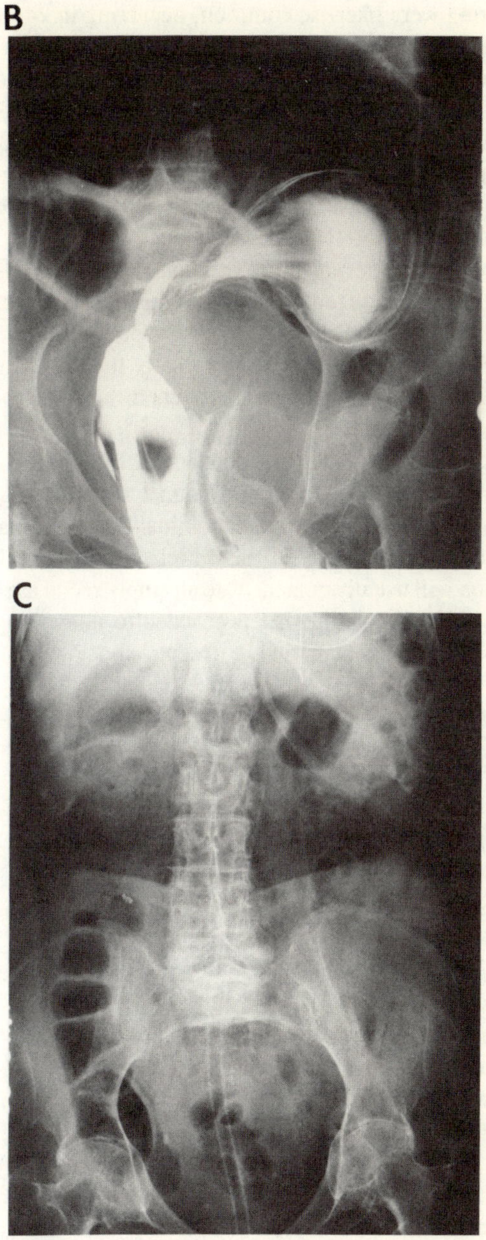

Figure 31-17. Sigmoid volvulus. A, Plain film of the abdomen showing the bent inner tube appearance of sigmoid volvulus. B, Barium enema demonstrating the point of torsion of the colon. C, Plain film after successful decompression showing the rectal tube in place. (Courtesy of R. De Silva, M.D., SUNY Health Science Center, Brooklyn, NY.)

In Western countries, volvulus tends to occur in older debilitated patients who are often institutionalized. Mangiante et al. (172) reported the presence of neuropsychiatric disease in 71% of patients with sigmoid volvulus. Prolonged inactivity, chronic debilitation, and psychotropic drugs together produce alterations in colonic motility with subsequent constipation and volvulus.

Previous abdominal operation may predispose to colonic volvulus as well. Ballantyne (176) reported that 68% of patients with volvulus had undergone previous abdominal surgery. In another review, Ballantyne et al. (178) postulated that adhesions at the base of the mesocolon may provide a narrow point around which a redundant colon may twist. Another possible etiologic process is recurrent mesosigmoiditis. Treves first postulated that constipation caused local peritonitis and inflammatory adhesion at the base of the mesocolon (174–176). While this has not been discussed in the American literature, it has been reported in India and may play a role in the development of volvulus (176).

Clinical Presentation and Diagnosis

Classically, patients with volvulus present with abdominal pain and distention. In a recent series from Denmark (180), 100% of the 26 patients had abdominal distention and 24 of the 26 complained of abdominal pain. Nausea and vomiting were likewise common, occurring in 24 of the 26 patients. This acute distention and pain is often superimposed on a chronic picture of recurrent or chronic constipation. Many patients give a history of similar episodes in the past. Ballantyne (176) reported a 44% incidence of prior similar problems in patients with sigmoid volvulus. Mangiante et al. (172) reported a 33% incidence of previous attacks thought to be volvulus.

As patients suffering from volvulus are usually elderly and institutionalized, they often present late in the course of the illness. The duration of symptoms and the degree of vascular compromise caused by the volvulus are the determinants of the patient's condition on presentation.

Physical findings likewise depend on the duration and severity of the volvulus. Abdominal distention is present in nearly every patient. Abdominal tenderness is variable, as is the character of the bowel sounds. Rectal examination will usually demonstrate an empty rectal ampulla (179). If the volvulus has proceeded to infarction, signs of peritonitis, dehydration, and septic shock will be present.

Colonic volvulus must be differentiated from mechanical colonic obstruction caused by malignancy or diverticulitis. The other common entity that mimics volvulus is pseudo-obstruction. Both may present with remarkable distention and relatively little pain until infarction or perforation occurs.

The diagnosis of volvulus can be confirmed by plain films of the abdomen. The "coffee bean" or "bird's beak" like appearance of a distended loop of bowel is suggestive of cecal volvulus (Fig. 31-16). In cases of sigmoid volvulus, the bowel loop may resemble a "bent inner tube" or "horseshoe" (Fig. 31-17A). Classically, the convex surface of the distended loop is pointed away from the area of tension (179). Unfortunately, plain films are not always sufficient to confirm the diganosis. Ballantyne et al. (178) reported diagnostic plain films in 38% of cases with cecal volvulus and 37% of cases with sigmoid volvulus. Other authors have reported a 50% to 62% rate of diagnosis by plain abdominal X-ray (172, 180, 181).

If plain films are inconclusive, a barium enema may help elucidate the pathology, especially in the case of a suspected sigmoid volvulus (Fig. 31-17B). In addition, barium enema has been reported to accomplish detorsion of sigmoid volvulus in 3% to 5% of cases (179).

Treatment and Results

While the specific treatment of colonic volvulus depends on the evaluation of the colonic pathology, certain general principles exist. The initial care of all patients should be resuscitation and stabilization. Surgery should follow immediately if there are signs of hemodynamic collapse, septic shock, or obvious peritonitis.

Sigmoid volvulus. The treatment of patients with sigmoid volvulus without signs of colonic infarction or perforation has changed with time. Early in the 20th century, as anesthetic and surgical technique became more sophisticated, early operative intervention for volvulus became the rule (182). The significant rate of recurrence and death following nonoperative therapy justified this approach. However, in 1947, Brunsgaard (183) revolutionized the treatment of sigmoid volvulus by demonstrating successful acute decompression by proctoscopy and rectal tube insertion in 123 of 148 patients. The mortality in this series was 14%. Since then, an initial attempt at nonoperative therapy for sigmoid volvulus has become the standard of care. In 1982, Ballantyne (182) reviewed 12 previous American series and reported a 75% success rate in nonoperative reduction of sigmoid volvulus. More recently, Mangiante et al. (172) has reported success in 95% of cases. Most authors stress the importance of rectal tube placement at the time of sigmoidoscopic detorsion to prevent immediate recurrence.

Colonoscopy has become popular as well in the acute management of sigmoid volvulus, and recent series have demonstrated its efficacy (184–186). Perhaps most impressive was a report by Arigbabu et al. (187) of 100% successful acute reductions of sigmoid volvulus in a series of 83 patients. The total mortality in this series was 2.1%.

Acute endoscopic treatment of sigmoid volvulus allows for nonemergent operation but is not by itself definitive treatment. Recurrence rates following endoscopic treatment range from 18% to 35% in most series (182, 188). In 1967 Hines et al. (189) reported a 90% recurrence rate when nonoperative treatment alone was used. It must also be emphasized that if there is any question regarding colonic viability at the time of endoscopic detorsion, attempts should immediately be abandoned and the patient prepared for emergency laparatomy. Successful initial endoscopic treatment must be documented radiographically, and any patient who is not successfully decompressed must be explored (Fig. 31-17C).

The operative management of volvulus depends on the viability of the bowel at exploration. There is general agreement that nonviable colon must be resected, and the bowel ends managed by colostomy and mucus fistula or blind distal pouch. However, there is no clear-cut consensus of opinion about the operative approach to viable colon at the time of emergency operation. Several options exist, the simplest of which is detorsion. However, recurrence rates with this procedure alone are unacceptably high, and it is therefore not usually advised. Other options include detorsion coupled with elective resection at 1 to 2 weeks, tube sigmoidostomy, sigmoidopexy, and extraperitonealization of the sigmoid loop (179–182). Recently, Hellman and Cramer (190) have described a technique of mesh fixation of the mesentery as definitive therapy.

Most authors advocate elective resection either with primary anastomosis or permanent colostomy if nonoperative reduction is accomplished (172, 176, 182). Both Mangiante et al. (172) and Parhlman et al. (191) underscore the importance of an initial attempt at nonoperative therapy, reporting a significantly higher mortality in those patients who require emergency surgery. In addition, Bak and Boley (192) have demonstrated that elective resection can be accomplished safely even in elderly patients and do not feel that age alone should be a criteria for adopting a nonoperative approach.

The most important determinant for survival is the viability of the colon at the time of presentation. The mortality rate when infarcted colon is present is approximately 40%. This drops to 5% to 10% in those patients who are first decompressed nonsurgically and later undergo elective operation. The overall mortality for sigmoid volvulus is approximately 15%.

Cecal volvulus. Because of the lack of proximity of cecal volvulus to the rectum, non-operative detorsion has not been available until recently. The success with colonoscopic decompression of sigmoid volvulus has led to some enthusiasm for application of the same approach to cecal volvulus. However, at present, the utility of this technique is unproven (193). It is perhaps a reasonable option during the period of resuscitation, but definitive treatment should not be delayed. At present, the treatment of cecal volvulus is surgical. The appropriate operation once detorsion has been accomplished remains unclear. The various surgical options include detorsion alone, detorsion and cecopexy, and detorsion followed by cecostomy or right hemicolectomy. Simple detorsion carries a recurrence rate of 5% to 10% and a subsequent mortality of 33% (178, 179). It is therefore not recommended. There is however, little agreement beyond that. Ballantyne et al. (182) reported no recurrences in a series of 11 patients using detorsion and cecopexy (simple suturing of the cecum to the lateral peritoneal reflection). This technique avoids opening unprepared bowel and should decrease the incidence of postoperative infection. Others, however, have reported 25% to 35% incidence of recurrence following cecopexy (191). Todd and Forde (194) advocate cecostomy, reporting no recurrences in 31 cases.

Resection is certainly the most definitive treatment but is the largest physiologic insult. Morris et al. (195) reported a series of 10 debilitated patients who presented with cecal volvulus. All were operated on within 12 hours of emergency department admission. Three of the four patients with viable colon who were treated with right hemicolectomy died. The authors made a plea for a more conservative operation in this setting. Parhlman et al. (191) however, reported that in 33 patients with cecal volvulus, the mortality with resection was 14% compared to 21% with cecopexy or cecostomy.

As with sigmoid volvulus, the mortality rate depends on colonic viability. When the colon is viable at operation, the mortality is 12% to 15%. This increases to 30% to 40% once infarction has occurred. The overall mortality for cecal volvulus is 15% to 25% (178, 179, 194).

Rectal Prolapse

Rectal prolapse is a relatively uncommon although often disabling condition. Although it was first recognized as early as 1500 BC, the exact etiology and therapy remain controversial (196).

Classifications and Etiology

Although a number of classification systems exist, a good deal of confusion still surrounds the description of rectal prolapse. It is important to differentiate among these clinical disorders as the therapy of each is markedly different.

The least debilitating form of this disorder is mucosal prolapse. It is due to a loosening or breakdown of the connective tissue between the submucosa and the muscular layers of the bowel wall that results in prolapse of the mucosa alone. It is generally considered to be a completely separate entity from true rectal prolapse.

Internal rectal prolapse refers to a prolapse of the full thickness of the wall of the distal sigmoid colon and rectum into the rectal lumen, but not out of the anal opening. Other names sometimes used to describe this condition are first degree rectal prolapse, hidden prolapse, and concealed procidentia. While some authors feel that internal prolapse predisposed to true prolapse in the majority of cases, others disagree. Estimates of the incidence of the progression of this form of prolapse vary from 2% to 100% (196).

True rectal prolapse, also called complete prolapse, procidentia, and overt rectal prolapse, refers to a circumferential prolapse of the rectum through the anal orifice. The most common etiologies are congenital predisposition, trauma, iatrogenic injury, and chronic constipation. Some authors feel that multiparity is a possible etiology, but this is not universally accepted. Pelvic fractures are associated with an increased incidence of rectal prolapse, but the exact explanation for this relationship is unclear. Certain pelvic operations are also associated with an increased incidence. These include hysterectomy, rectal pull-through procedures, and low anterior resection. Chronic constipation is thought to predispose to the development of rectal prolapse as well. High intra-abdominal pressure due to repeated straining, combined with lax attachments of the rectum, allows the rectosigmoid to intussuscept into the rectum and prolapse.

The theory of intussusception as an underlying mechanism of rectal prolapse has not always been accepted. Initially, Moschowitz (197) postulated a pelvic sliding hernia mechanism, in which the pouch of Douglas formed the hernia sac. Increased intra-abdominal pressure pushed the hernia sac and the anterior wall of the rectum into the rectal lumen. Eventually, intra-abdominal contents would herniate through this space and then through the levator muscle, producing rectal prolapse. Supporting this theory were observations that there was usually a deep retrovaginal or retrovessical pouch with a redundant rectosigmoid and absence of normal rectal fixation in these patients. In addition, lax pelvic muscles and poor sphincter tone were also common (196).

Recently, rectosigmoid intussusception has become generally accepted as the cause of rectal prolapse. Broden and Snellman (198), utilizing cineradiography, demonstated circumferential rectosigmoid intussusception, with a lead point at 6 to 8 cm from the anal verge in patients with complete prolapse.

Incontinence is a relatively common condition that occurs coincidentally with rectal prolapse. Internal rectal sphincter dysfunction and persistent rectal distention from constipation and straining may predispose to the loss of continence. Initially this condition may be reversed by simple correction of the prolapse (196). Schlinlkert et al. (199) suggest that the incontinence may be related to a combination of internal sphincter dysfunction and decreased rectal inhibitory reflex (4). Others suggest that prolapse and incontinence may be two different manifestations of pelvic denervation. Patients without complete neuropathy may develop prolapse as a result of straining. Those with complete neuropathy will develop significant incontinence as well (192).

Clinical Presentation

Rectal prolapse is a relatively uncommon disease affecting women far more often than men. The incidence increases with age, peaking in the sixth and seventh decades.

The usual presenting complaint is the prolapse itself. Initially, it may appear only with defecation, but later any manuever that increases intra-abdominal pressure may produce the prolapse. Eventually, even such simple things as standing in an erect position may cause the prolapse to appear.

Other symptoms may be present or even predominate early in the course of the disorder. Changes in bowel regulation, rectal or pelvic pain, a sensation of incomplete evacuation, and tenesmus all may occur in various combinations. Persistent rectal prolapse may produce a mucoid rectal discharge and/or rectal bleeding.

Some symptoms are present in virtually all patients, but the prolapse itself may not be obvious at the time of examination. Usually it is easily produced by asking the patient to bear down or strain. The prolapsed portion of the rectum is usually edematous and thickened. The perineum may be excoriated and inflamed from the mucoid rectal discharge and/or fecal incontinence.

In patients with internal rectal prolapse, the disorder may be more difficult to detect. They will usually complain of incomplete evacuation, pelvic pressure or fullness, or incontinence. In 30% of patients the examiner will be able to palpate the edge of the intussuscepting bowel on rectal exam. Sigmoidoscopy may reveal the leading edge, although one may see only proctitis with thickened, erythematous mucosa (196).

Solitary ulcer of the rectum syndrome is a condition that has been associated with rectal prolapse, but the exact relationship is unclear. This condition consists of a single or multiple ulcers that are found on the anterior rectal wall usually at 4 to 12 cm from the anal verge. They are shallow ulcers with a greyish white base and a characteristic histologic appearance. Various series have estimated that rectal prolapse occurs in between 25% and 100% of patients with these ulcers (196).

Colitis cystica profunda is a syndrome consisting of firm nodules on the anterior rectal wall with overlying edematous mucosa. These nodules are found 6 to 12 cm from the anus. They may coexist with solitary rectal ulcers and may actually represent the healing phase of these lesions. While one author reported that none of his patients with Colitis Cystica Profunda had rectal prolapse, others have reported an incidence of up to 57% (196). It is postulated that both of these lesions are produced by the repeated trauma that occurs when the anterior rectal wall first begins to intussuscept into the distal rectum and lies against the puborectalis band.

Diagnosis

The evaluation of patients with suspected or proven complete rectal prolapse is straightforward. Rectal exam will identify the prolapse in many cases. It may also reveal a patulous anus, predicting incontinence. One must also evaluate both resting anal tone as well as voluntary anal contraction. In women, a pelvic exam is necessary to evaluate the possibility of coincident uterine prolapse.

Proctosigmoidoscopy is essential in all patients with demonstrated or suspected rectal prolapse. Occasionally the intussusception producing rectal prolapse may have an anatomic lead point such as a malignancy or a polyp. The usual protoscopic appearance in rectal prolapse is an 8 to 10 cm length of reddened and swollen rectal mucosa; however, the exam may be surprisingly normal. Barium enema and/or colonoscopy should be performed to rule out concomitant colonic pathology and to confirm the diagnosis.

Although not available in many centers, cinedefacography is the definitive test for internal rectal prolapse. It is absolutely indicated in all patients with solitary ulcer of the rectum syndrome or Colitis Cystica Profunda. If a history of constipation is present, a fecal transit time may be helpful to quantitate a possible etiologic role. Anal manometry and pelvic nerve conduction studies are investigational and, while helpful, are probably not necessary in the workup of patients with rectal prolapse.

Treatment and Results

Nonoperative methods of treating rectal prolapse such as perineal muscle excercises or strapping the buttocks with tape are largely ineffective. They should be reserved for patients who are too ill to survive even a minor operative procedure or for those who refuse surgery. While the indication for surgery is debatable in those patients with infrequent episodes of prolapse, repeated espisodes should be considered an absolute indication for surgical correction. It is possible for the prolapsed rectum to become so edematous that it cannot be reduced into the anus and infarction may occur. While the relationship between the development of incontinence and the presence of prolapse is unclear, most authors feel that a causal relationship does exist. The longer the prolapse exists, the greater is the chance that incontinence will occur. If nonoperative therapy is chosen, periodic re-evaluation with anal manometry is necessary to detect the development of incontinence as early as possible.

Once the decision to operate has been made, there are a large number of possible surgical options. They can be divided into intra-abdominal or perineal procedures. Numerous studies have discussed the various options, yet there are few that actually compare the different operative techniques. Most series contain a relatively small number of patients and follow-up periods vary greatly. Some authors feel that the majority of recurrence occurs within the first 2 to 3 years after operation, but all agree that late failures do occur. As rectal prolapse is a disease of the elderly, many patients die of unrelated causes or are lost to follow-up. Thus, the best surgical option remains controversial.

Abdominal approach. In general, intra-abdominal procedures are effective for the treatment of rectal prolapse. The disadvantage of this approach is that it exposes the patient to the risks of general anesthesia and to all the potential complications associated with laparotomy. The various types of intra-abdominal operations available include sacral slings, posterior rectopexy, and colon resection. Pelvic floor repairs have generally been abandoned.

The pelvic sling operation or anterior rectopexy was popularized by Ripstein (200). In this operation, the rectum is mobilized and then fixed to the sacrum with a circumferential sling made of some foreign material (Fig. 31-18). Originally, Ripstein reported using a 360° sling made of Teflon. Later, he and others changed to Marlex mesh because Teflon was so inert that it produced little reaction and was prone to stretch. Marlex, however, had the opposite problem of being too reactive and occasionally caused colonic kinking or small bowel obstruction. Most recently, McMahan and Ripstein (201) have reported the use of a 5 × 10 cm piece of Goretex that is wrapped around the rectum, leaving a 3 to 4 cm strip of the anterior wall unbound. This allows some distention and prevents postoperative fecal impaction, which was one of the more common complications in Ripstein's early data. Utilizing this approach, McMahan and Ripstein (201) have treated 23 patients. There were no recurrences and no postoperative incontinence, although the follow-up ranged from only 3 to 30 months, with a mean of 16 months. Others have reported recurrence rates of approximately 0% to 4% following various types of Ripstein procedures (202). Most series have reported a mortality rate less than 2%, but complication rates have been reported to approach 17%. These generally include fecal impaction, bleeding, stricture, pelvic abscess, and impotence (196, 197).

The Ripstein approach has now been modified further. In 1984, Heitama et al. (203) described a method of treating rectal prolapse using a "double peritoneal sling" constructed from parietal pelvic peritoneum. In this series, there were no complications and no recurrences in 14 patients, although the length to follow-up was not specified. Beltran de Heredia (204) has reported using a complete peritoneal wrap combined with a "hammock-like" suspensory hook. No recurrences were reported in a follow-up period of 1 to 6 years, although three patients died during that period.

Posterior rectopexy, the Wells procedure (205) involves fixing the rectum posteriorly to the sacrum. Most commonly, this involves inserting some reactive material, usually an Ivalon sponge, and allowing the subsequent inflammatory reaction to fix the rectum to the sacrum. As the rectum is not encircled, the problems of stricture and fecal impaction should not occur. Operative mortality is

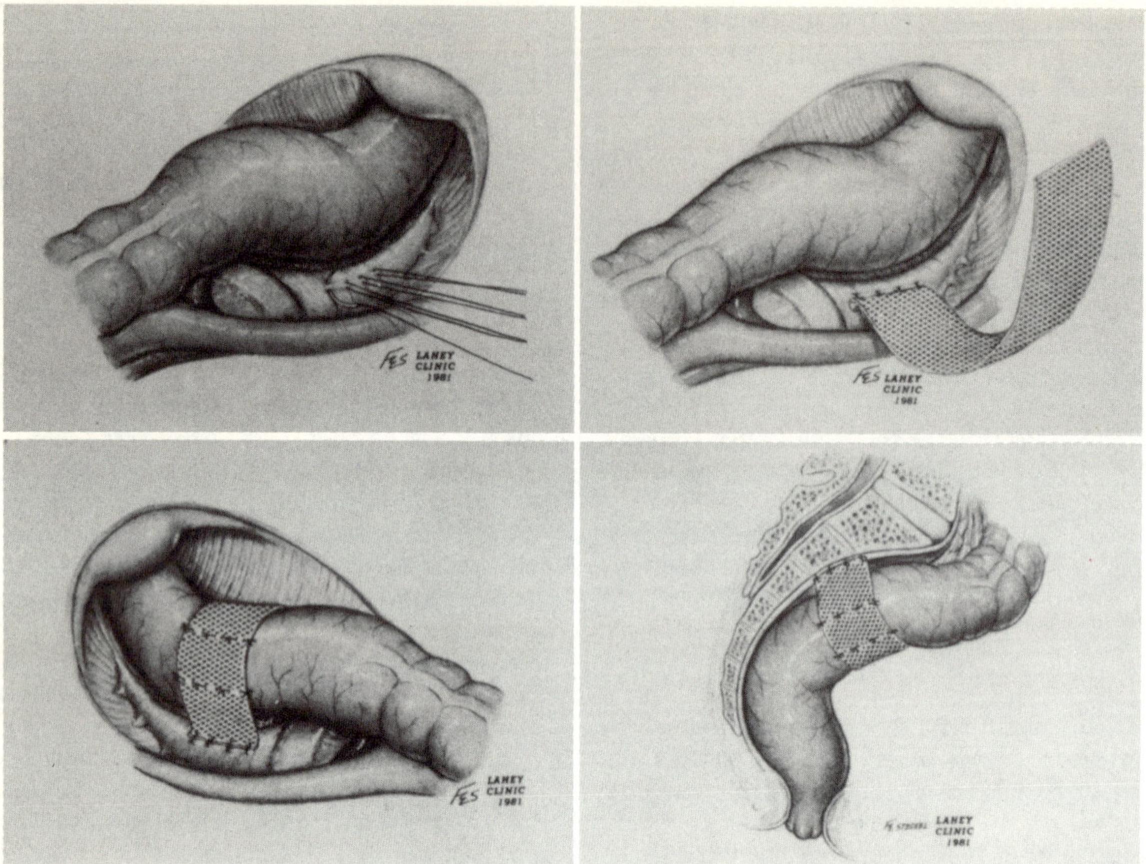

Figure 31-18. The presacral sling repair for rectal prolapse. *Top left,* The rectum is mobilized and heavy nylon sutures are placed in the periosteum of the sacrum. *Top right,* The appropriate length of mesh is secured in place. *Bottom left,* While cephalad tension is being maintained, the mesh is brought to the left side of the sacrum and secured in place. *Bottom right,* Lateral view of the rectum showing satisfactory placement of the sling. (Reprinted, with permission, from Roberts PL, et al. 1988. Ripstein procedure, Lahey Clinic experience 1963–1985. *Arch Surg* 123: 554–557.) (278).

generally under 2% to 3%, but the recurrence rates vary up to 10% (196, 205–207). This high rate of recurrence may be due to inadequate scarring or fragmentation of the sponge. In addition, pelvic sepsis may occur, which requires removal of the foreign body. Often, the prolapse does not recur, even after the sponge is removed. Lake et al. (208) reported four cases of postoperative sponge related pelvic sepsis, all due to *Staphylococcus aureus*. Perioperative antibiotic coverage that includes antistaphylococcal therapy may therefore decrease the incidence of this complication.

Others have decribed simple posterior rectopexy, fixing the rectum to the sacrum with nonabsorbable sutures (209–211). This procedure may be combined with resection. Carter (209) and Graham et al. (210) reported a 0% mortality in 46 patients treated by this method. Neither series reported any recurrences although the follow-up period was variable. Between 72% and 80% of patients in the series by Carter (209) and Graham et al. (210) subjectively described their operative result as good or excellent.

Simple resection was first described in 1955 by Muir (212), who felt that fibrosis from colonic mobilization at the level of the anastomosis would effectively fix the rectum to the sacrum. Schlinlkert et al. (199) reviewed 113 patients treated with resection. The recurrence rate was 9%, and there was one perioperative death. However, there was a 30% rate of major complications, half of which were related to the anastomosis.

Lahaut's operation is an additional intra-abdominal option that avoids the potential dangers of foreign materials and of opening the bowel. In this procedure, the rectum is mobilized and fixed by implanting it outside the abdomen into the posterior rectus sheath. Although this technique was first described in 1956 (213), there are few series describing the results of its use. In 1984, Mortensen et al. (214) published the results of 34 patients treated in this manner. Although the follow-up period is unspecified, no late recurrences were reported. One patient, died, however, and one recurred in the recovery room, requiring immediate reoperation.

Perineal approach. While good results are reported with abdominal procedures, perineal operations, performed under regional anesthesia, are an attractive alternative in elderly debilitated patients. One such operation is perineal rectosigmoidectomy (Altemeier's procedure) (215). In this operation, the affected segment of rectum is first fully prolapsed through the anal orifice. An incision is then made into the outer layer of the prolapsed bowel. The inner layer is visualized and the mesorectum controlled and divided. The segment is then divided, and an anastomosis is fashioned between the distal rectum and anal mucosa. This is a technically easy operation and in Altemeier's hands had a low recurrence rate (215). However, the recurrence rates have varied widely in other series (196, 216). One significant side effect of the procedure is that almost all patients have some degree of postoperative incontinence. This typically lasts up to 2 months. Prasad et al. (216) reported no recurrence in a series of 25 patients treated by perineal resection combined with posterior rectopexy. In addition, 22 of the 25 patients eventually regained continence postoperatively. Bennett et al. (217) have described a stapler modification of this procedure, using an EEA stapler for the anastomosis. They likewise reported a low incidence of lasting postoperative incontinence.

The Delorme's operation is another perineal procedure. It involves mucosal stripping of the prolapsed segment and then using the bowel wall to form a plug in the supralevator space to prevent futher episodes. While some authors perform the procedure under general anesthesia, others utilize regional blocks with sedation. Mortality is low, but recurrence rates vary from 2% to 34% (196). Monson et al. (218) have modified the technique by stripping additional mucosa and increasing the size of the supralevator plug. The reported recurrence rate in this series was 8%.

The technique of anal encircling was first described by Thiersch (219). In the original description, silver wires were placed around the anus at the level of the sphincters. Because of the relatively high rate of complications, others have modified his approach utilizing different materials. Most recently, Larach and Vasquez (220) reported good results using a silastic mesh implant, as have Earnshaw and Hopkinson (221) using silicone rubber sutures. Rogers et al. (222) report similar results with postanal repair, using intersphincteric Ivalon sponge placement.

There are few studies directly comparing these various methods of treating rectal prolapse. In addition, the lack of uniform long-term follow-up makes the results reported in the literature difficult to interpret. At present, it would seem that an intra-abdominal procedure is the best choice to treat patients who are fit to undergo general anesthesia. Posterior rectopexy with or without resection has been demonstrated repeatedly to achieve good results and avoid the potential dangers of foreign material. Resection, if performed, should be carried out at a convenient level as low anastomoses seems to carry a high complication rate. For those who cannot undergo a general anesthetic, perineal rectosigmoidectomy is a good choice. As procedures continue to be modified, new options may emerge.

Stercoral Ulceration and Perforation

Stercoral ulceration of the colon was first described by Berry in 1894 (223). While there have been a number of recent reports concerning this topic, there still is considerable debate about the exact incidence, etiology, and optimal treatment. It is generally regarded to be a relatively rare entity. However, there remains some disagreement even about the number of cases that exist in the literature.

Etiology

Strictly speaking, stercoral ulceration is caused by ischemic pressure necrosis of the colonic mucosa and muscularis caused by a fecolith or by excessive distension. Consequently, an ulcer or an area of ischemia must be present with varying degrees of reactive acute and chronic inflammation. It is important to differentiate this from other types of colonic ulceration and perforation. Spontaneous perforation of the colon is a disease entity that may be confused with stercoral perforation. This usually involves a longitudinal or transverse tear in the colonic wall with macroscopically normal edges and no histologic evidence of inflammation (224, 225). In 1981, Gekas and Shuster (225) reported one case of stercoral perforation and reviewed all the existing cases to date. In only 38 of the 63 reported cases were the strict criteria for stercoral perforation met.

This confusion makes even the determination of the etiologic factors difficult. Maull et al. (226) asserted that constipation is an almost constant feature in these patients. Bed rest and poor bowel habits tend to decrease colonic mucous production, forming concretions that serve as the nidus for stercoral ulceration. Yet in the series by Gekas (225), only 22 of the 38 patients had constipation. Antacids and/or phenothiazines, also thought to predispose to constipation and stercoral ulceration (227), were used by only six patients in this study. In addition, Selye et al. (228) have reported that stercoral ulceration is much more likely to occur in the presence of vasoconstriction in a rat model, but no human data exists to support this. Finally, there are scattered reports of stercoral perforation secondary to narcotic use, pneumatosis cystoides intestinales causing obstruction, and scleroderma, but these are extremely rare (229–231).

The overwhelming majority of stercoral perforations occur on the antimesenteric aspect of the rectosigmoid, although there was a recent case report of perforation in the transverse colon (232). This is probably due to the presence of hard fecal material in the narrow sigmoid lumen, and to the pressure of surrounding pelvic structures that limits rectal distensibility (225, 226). Avinoah et al (233) also suggest that the rectosigmoid is most at jeopardy because chronic constipation may cause abnormal sigmoid motor activity, oversegmentation, and a sudden increase in intracolonic pressure. However, there was no pathologic confirmation for this in the seven patients reported. A similar explanation is possible for the etiologic mechanism of spontaneous perforation of the colon as well.

Clinical Presentation

Stercoral ulceration is a disease of elderly often debilitated patients. It may be discovered incidentally at the time of sigmoidoscopy or colonoscopy. While no definitive treatment of the ulceration is necessary, measures to avoid further constipation and fecal impaction should be routine. Biopsy of the ulcers should be taken to exclude the possibility of coincident malignancy. Bleeding from stercoral ulceration may occur in as many as 30% of cases (226). It is rarely severe enough to be life threatening and to require operative intervention.

The presenting symptom of stercoral perforation is almost always severe lower abdominal pain. This disorder should be in the differential diagnosis of any elderly patient with chronic constipation who develops acute symptoms. Approximately 50% of patients have peritonitis mandating operation on initial presentation, although elderly patients tend to present late in the course of the disease (225, 226). Consequently, some will present with septic shock or cardiovascular collapse. Free air is present on an upright chest or abdominal film in about 25% of cases, although there is one case report of stercoral perforation presenting as pneumomediastinum (234). A huge rectosigmoid full of stool may also be seen on abdominal X-ray (Fig. 31-19).

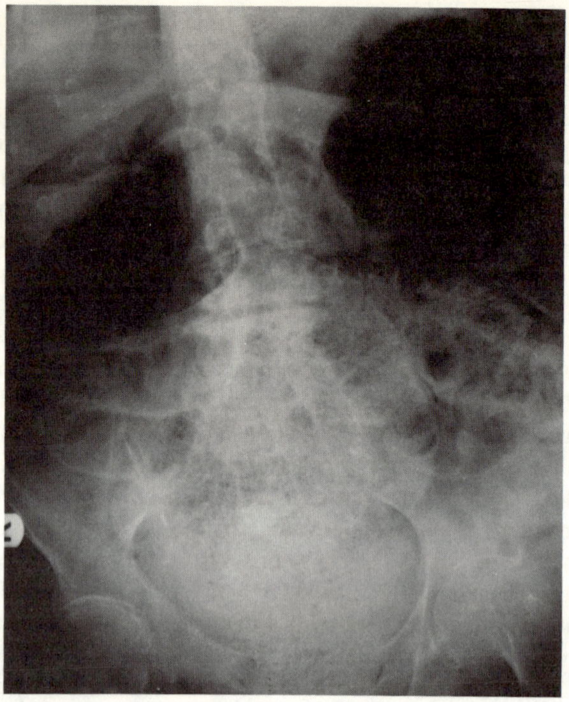

Figure 31-19. Stercoral perforation. Note the grossly distended rectum filled with feces in the mid-abdomen. At operation, multiple ischemic perforations of the rectum from massive overdistension were found.

Treatment and Results

Treatment of stercoral perforation is surgical. Gekas et al. (225) cited exteriorization of the perforation as the most common operation performed and felt it was the best option. Maull et al. (226), however, feel that exteriorization is often technically impossible because of the extent of affected colon and therefore favor resection and colostomy. This is supported by Guyton et al. (235) who reported an operative mortality of 23% for resection with end colostomy, 71% for exteriorization as a loop colostomy, and 44% for plication with proximal colostomy.

Overall mortality for stercoral perforation approaches 50% in most reports (225, 226, 235). This high mortality is most likely due to the delayed presentation and the underlying debilitation of the patients affected by this process.

Appendicitis

Acute appendicitis is the most common acute surgical condition in the abdomen. While it occurs most commonly in the second and third decades of life, it has a second peak in elderly males. Appendicitis requiring appendectomy comprises about 2% to 10% of total cases reported in recent reviews of operative procedures in the geriatric population (236–238). Diagnosed and treated early, it is a relatively simple problem even in aged patients. However, the morbidity and mortality in the elderly rises sharply when acute appendicitis is complicated by perforation and/or pelvic abscess.

Clinical Presentation

It is a common perception that appendicitis is a different disease in the elderly patient and that the signs and symptoms are not the same as they are in younger patients. Perhaps it would be more accurate to say that the presentation of appendicitis in the elderly is not as dramatic as it is in younger patients. Delays in seeking medical attention are therefore common. Lau et al. (236) reported the presence of symptoms for more than 24 hours in 65% of elderly patients. Vorhes (237) compared time from onset of symptoms to operation in 1,018 cases of appendicitis. Ninety-five percent of those patients under the age of 55 were operated on within 48 hours, while only 75% of those over age 55 years were similarly treated. This delay was most pronounced in elderly females, of whom 13% were not operated on until after the 5th day. Occasionally, vague symptoms may be present for weeks before the patient seeks medical attention. In these cases, periappendiceal abcess maybe the presenting finding (Fig. 31-20).

The clinical symptoms and signs of appendicitis in the elderly are subtle, and the diagnosis is often in question at the time of admission. In one series 80% of patients over the age of 55 years proven to have appendicitis were admitted with a diagnosis of abdominal pain. Almost all elderly patients with appendicitis describe some abdominal pain, although it is often nonspecific. In 1978, Owens and Hamit (238) reviewed 68 patients between the ages of 65 to 99 years who underwent appendectomy for acute appendicitis. Ninety-two percent had abdominal pain listed as their chief complaint, and all patients admitted to pain when specifically questioned. Nausea and vomiting were likewise very common.

Like the symptoms of appendicitis in the elderly, the physical findings may be subtle. Although right lower quadrant tenderness has been reported in as many as 80% to 90% of cases (238–240), in one series local tenderness was absent in 25% to 33% of patients (239). Rebound tenderness, while common in young patients, is relatively rare in the elderly, occurring in only 40% to 50% of patients (238–239).

Fever and leukocytosis are traditionally thought to be nonspecific and frequently absent in infectious processes in the elderly. A white blood cell count over 10,000 is absent in only 5% to 20% of elderly patients with appendicitis, but fever may be absent in nearly 25% of patients (238–239).

With careful attention to subtle historical and physi-

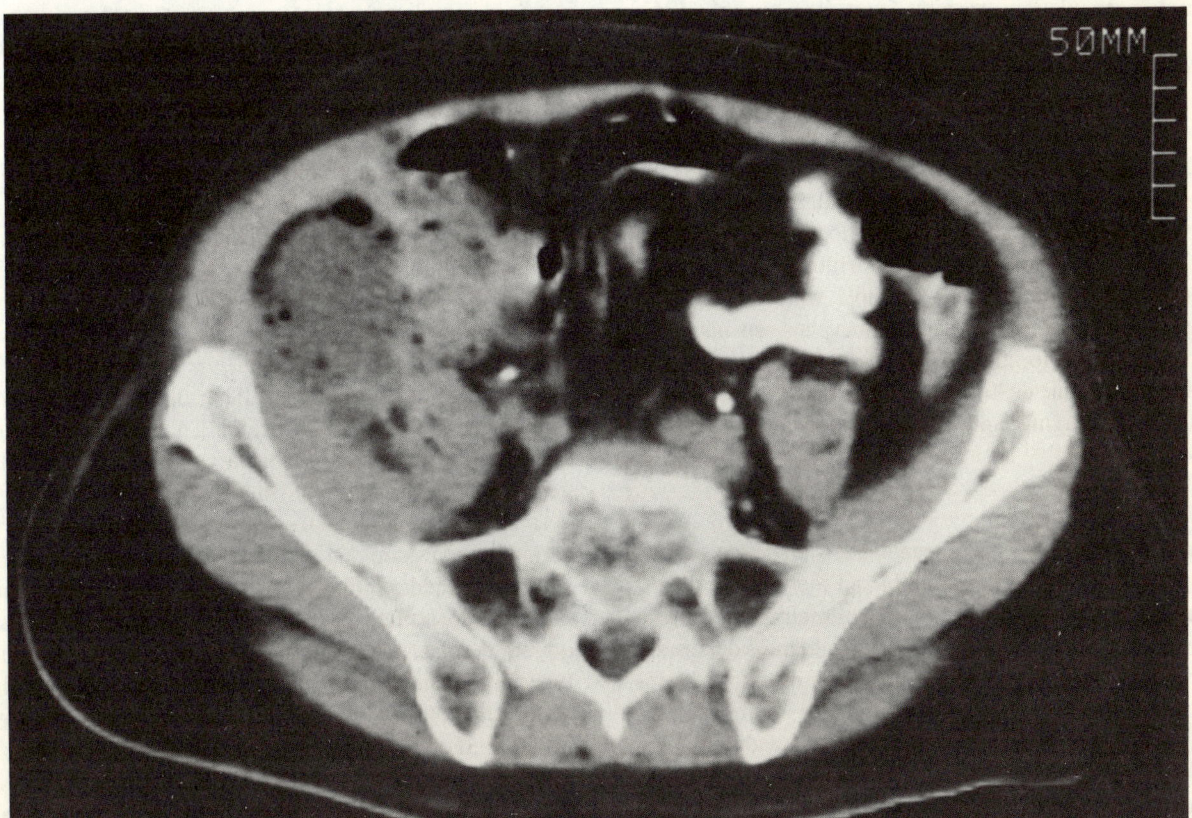

Figure 31-20. Computed tomogram showing a right lower quadrant mass, consistent with a periappendiceal abscess.

cal findings, a correct diagnosis of appendicitis can be made preoperatively in the majority of cases. In a review of 104 patients over the age 65 with acute appendicitis, Lau et al. (236) found that eighty-four patients had a history and physical examination thought to be indicative of appendicitis. Sixteen patients presented with diffuse pain and widespread peritonitis. While the diagnosis was not clear, there were clear-cut indications for laparotomy. Only four patients presented with truly atypical history. All four had no abdominal pain but instead described constipation and abdominal distention. At operation, all four patients had acute appendicitis with perforation. In another study, Hall and Wright (241) reported that the correct diagnosis of appendicitis was made preoperatively in 88% of elderly patients. Misdiagnosis does occur, however. Yusuf and Dunn (242) reported that small bowel obstruction was the most common diagnostic error.

Treatment

In some elderly patients with appendicitis, the operative approach is the same as in younger patients. However, if the diagnosis is not clear or if symptoms have been present for a prolonged period of time, a lower midline laparotomy incision is appropriate. The incidence of perforation at the time of appendectomy is strikingly higher in the geriatric population, varying from 60% to 75% (241, 243). Pus in the peritoneal cavity is often present in spite of the absence of rebound tenderness or other signs of peritonitis on physical exam.

While delay in operation almost certainly contributes to the alarming incidence of perforation in elderly patients, it is not the sole explanation. Hall and Wright (241) reported a 66% incidence of perforation in spite of the fact that 68% of patients were in the operating room within 8 hours of hospital admission and 86% within 24 hours of the onset of symptoms. Theories to explain this increased incidence of perforation include decreased inflammatory defenses, chronic destructive changes in the appendix associated with aging, and impaired appendicial blood supply (243).

Results

There is no question that appendicitis is associated with a significantly increased morbidity and mortality in the elderly patient population. Operative mortality ranges from 0% to 10% (236, 237, 239, 240). While most deaths are directly attributable to other underlying diseases, the increased rate of perforation and infectious complications certainly plays some role in taxing the already compromised physiologic resources of these patients. The presence of associated medical problems significantly increases the risk of death. This may explain the increased mortality rate as age increases, even in those patients over 65 years. Owens and Hamit (238) reported a 5% mortality in patients 65 to 75 years and a 24% mortality in those 75 to 99 years.

The incidence of serious complications is approximately 20% to 35%. Wound infection accounts for 50% to 65% of complications, followed by pulmonary and cardiac problems. Pelvic abscesses account for a surprisingly small percentage of postoperative complications and occur in 0% to 10% of patients (239, 241).

Operative Management of Abdominal Wall Hernia

Abdominal wall hernias are estimated to occur in 13/1000 men over the age of 65 years (244). The incidence of hernia in women is approximately one-eighth to one-fourth that of men. Often these hernias have been present and neglected for many years (average of 10 to 20 years) (245). Some hernias have been present for as long as 50 to 60 years (246, 247). They are therefore frequently large and have destroyed much of the normal surrounding tissues usually used for repair. In the elective setting, repair of these hernias can be challenging but is usually accomplished with low operative mortality and morbidity. Unfortunately, prolonged neglect also leads to a high incidence of complications, including bowel dysfunction with constipation and impaction, incarceration, bowel obstruction, and intestinal necrosis. Bowel obstruction and strangulation from incarceration account for approximately 10% of emergency abdominal operations in the elderly in most studies (248), although a frequency as high as 30% has been reported (249). Incarcerated hernia is also responsible for over one-third of cases of bowel obstruction in this age group (250).

Etiology and Distribution

The etiologies of abdominal wall hernias in the young and in the aged are somewhat different. Although hernias of congenital origin, so common in youth, do occur in the geriatric population as well, the significance of acquired hernias increases markedly with aging. Increased intra-abdominal pressure due to longstanding constipation and straining, bladder outlet obstruction, chronic cough, and kyphoscoliosis predispose to the development of these acquired hernias. The relative frequency of the various types of hernias therefore changes with aging as well. The distribution of groin hernias from two large series is seen in Table 31-15. Indirect inguinal hernia, seen in nearly 90% of cases in young men, decreases to approximately 50% to 60% in older men. Direct hernias increase, totaling approximately 35% of cases in men. The high incidence of direct hernia in women in Nehme's (245) series

Table 31-15. Distribution of groin hernias

	Ponka (246) 1938–1970		Nehm (245) 1970–1981	
Type of hernia	Number of patients %		Number of patients %	
	Men	Women	Men	Women
Indirect	110 (61)	13 (26)	734 (47)	51 (24)
Direct	27 (15)	0 (0)	506 (33)	112 (54)
Femoral	23 (13)	37 (74)	186 (12)	41 (20)
Other	20 (11)	0 (0)	121 (8)	4 (2)
Total	180	50	1547	208

is not corroborated elsewhere, but data regarding inguinal hernias in elderly women are scarce. While older studies reported a 3:1 predominance of femoral to indirect hernias in elderly women, Nehme's and other larger studies (251) show a majority of hernias are inguinal in both men and women. Femoral hernia, however, is more common in elderly women than men. Indirect sliding hernias are also common, accounting for approximately 10% of all groin hernias by the eighth decade of life (252).

Approximately 15% to 30% of herniorrhaphies in the elderly are performed emergently for incarceration (245, 253). The distribution of incarcerated hernias is shown in Table 31-16. As seen from the study by Fenyo (248), there is a preponderance of incarcerated femoral hernias in females, while in males the majority of incarcerated hernias are inguinal.

Umbilical hernia, while less common, accounts for approximately 10% of hernias presenting as bowel obstruction. The presence of this type of hernia is not an uncommon finding in elderly patients with cirrhosis (248, 250, 254).

An additional type of hernia of special concern in the elderly is the occult herniation through the obturator canal. While this hernia is rare, it occurs primarily in elderly women and can present a unique diagnostic challenge (see "Obturator Hernia").

Also of special interest is the giant scrotal hernia in which resides a large portion of the abdominal contents. Reduction of the contents of such hernias into the peritoneal cavity at the time of hernia repair may be difficult because the organs have "forfeited the right of domicile." Forced reduction can impair diaphragmatic function and cause respiratory distress.

Diagnosis

The diagnosis of most abdominal wall hernias is usually clear. Over 70% of patients with groin hernias complain of a groin or scrotal mass and pain in the inguinal area. Many patients have been aware of the hernia for years and have been using a truss unsuccessfully to control the symptoms. Many have also severely limited their activities in order to avoid discomfort from the hernia. Hernias in the femoral location can be more difficult to diagnose. Pain may be ill localized, and the hernia sac itself may not be easily appreciated. Unfortunately, femoral hernias in the elderly are frequently not diagnosed until incarceration has occurred (246).

As with most surgical conditions in the elderly, the presence of coexisting pathology is high, with cardiovascular and pulmonary disorders predominating. In one large series, 75% of patients had one disorder, 50% had two, and 15% had three additional illnesses (1). In another large study, Nehme (245) reports that prostatic enlargement or a history of prostatectomy was present in 82% of 1,292 elderly men evaluated for groin hernia repair. Diverticulosis coli and colon cancer are also frequent findings.

When the diagnosis of primary abdominal wall hernia is made, operative repair should be considered. Elective hernia surgery can be accomplished safely regardless of the patient's age. However, in the emergency setting, mortality rates increase 5- to 10-fold. Therefore, after a careful search is made for correctable causes of increased intra-abdominal pressure, elective herniorrhaphy should be considered. Only in cases where the overall life expectancy of the patient is short due to other disease processes should elective hernia repair be denied.

Table 31-16. Distribution of incarcerated hernias

	Fenyo, 1974 (248)		Green, 1969 (250)	Nehme, 1983 (245)
Type of hernia	Number of patients			
	Men	Women	Both	Both
Indirect	19 (73)	8 (18)	57 (54)	143 (60)
Direct				35 (14)
Femoral	4 (15)	22 (50)	26 (25)	41 (17)
Umbilical	1 (4)	7 (16)	10 (9)	0
Ventral	2 (8)	7 (16)	8 (7)	0
Other	0	0	5 (5)	23 (9)
Total	26	44	106	242

Elective Herniorrhaphy

The operative management of abdominal wall hernias in the elderly depends somewhat on the location and nature of that specific type of hernia. However, some general principles do apply.

Prior to surgery, a detailed history concentrating on respiratory, urologic, and gastrointestinal symptoms should be obtained. On physical examination, particular attention should be paid to any signs of pulmonary infection or chronic bronchitis. Abdominal exam should include a careful search for masses or intra-abdominal fluid. A thorough rectal exam for masses, prostatic enlargement, and occult stool hemoglobin should be routine.

If an abnormality is identified, a complete workup should be performed prior to herniorrhaphy. This may include chest X-ray and sputum cultures, urologic evaluation with cystoscopy, and barium enema or colonoscopy as indicated. Many surgeons feel that either barium enema or colonoscopy should be routine in the preoperative evaluation of these elderly patients because of the high incidence of false negative stool guaiac found with early colon tumors (245).

Anesthesia

The surgical morbidity and mortality from elective herniorrhaphy can be minimized by avoiding anesthetic technique that places stress on cardiac, pulmonary, and renal reserves. Both general and spinal anesthesia are associated with a significant incidence of related perioperative complications. For example, Guillen and Aldrete (255) reported that in men over 70 years of age undergoing inguinal herniorrhaphy, there was a 49% and 36% incidence of hypotension with spinal and inhaled anesthetic respectively. Young (256) recently reported a significantly higher incidence of complications, particularly urinary and respiratory, in older patients receiving spinal and general anesthesia when compared with those receiving local field block (Table 31-17). Job et al. (257) found similar results when epidural was compared to general and local anesthesia. In a randomized trial of local versus general anesthesia in all age patients, Teasdale et al. (258) found a significantly higher percentage of patients were able to ambulate and pass urine at 6 hours after surgery when local anesthetic was used. This early ambulation is a particularly important factor in decreasing postoperative pulmonary complications in elderly patients (120).

It seems therefore that local anesthesia is associated with few, if any, additional stresses on organ reserves in the elderly and is therefore the ideal anesthetic method for elective hernia repair in this age group. The only potential limitation to the use of local anesthesia is patient compliance. Several studies have demonstrated that satisfaction with this technique is high. Approximately 85% of patients surveyed stated they would choose local anesthesia again if they required further hernia surgery (255). In the demented patient, however, or in those who are unable to lie still and cooperate for other reasons, local anesthesia may not be satisfactory.

Table 31-17. Complications versus type of anesthesia in patients over age 65 years

Complication	Local ($n=45$)	Spinal ($n=44$)	General ($n=39$)
Urinary	9 (20)[a]	20 (45)[b]	12 (31)[b]
Respiratory	2 (4)	10 (23)	8 (21)
Wound hematoma	2 (4)	5 (11)	12 (31)
Wound infection	0	2 (5)	0
Total	13	37	32

[a]% in each anesthetic group.

[b]$p<.05$ local versus spinal; local versus general.

Adapted from Young DV. 1987. Comparison of local, spinal, and general anesthesia for inguinal herniorrhaphy. *Am J Surg* 120:760–763.

Nearly painless herniorrhaphy under local anesthesia can be accomplished in the elderly if the neuroanatomy of the inguinal region is understood. Although detailed descriptions of neuoranatomy and field block of the inguinal area can be found elsewhere (259), a brief review will be helpful here. Figure 31-21 shows the neural supply to the lower abdominal wall and inguinal area. Ponka (260) describes a seven-step procedure for local anesthesia based on the nerve supply shown. *Step 1:* Skin anesthesia is first obtained by raising an intradermal wheal not more than 2 com above the anterior superior iliac spine. *Step 2:* The ilioinguinal and iliohypogastric nerves are blocked by injection of the local anesthetic deep to the external oblique muscle and fascia at this level (Fig. 31-22). *Step 3:* Further subcutaneous injection is made toward the umbilicus, toward the anterior superior spine and obliquely parallel to the inguinal ligament in the line where the incision is to be placed. *Step 4:* After the skin and subcutaneous tissues are open, injection under the external oblique aponeurosis anesthetizes free nerve endings in the fascia. *Step 5:* Injection at the base of the cord blocks the genital branch of the genitofemoral nerve and anesthetizes the peritoneum at the internal ring. *Step 6:* Anesthetic is then injected directly into the area of the pubic tubercle and Cooper's ligaments. *Step 7:* With the sac open, under direct vision, the peritoneum is injected. If the sac is large, direct instillation of dilute anesthetic agent into the peritoneal cavity may be necessary.

The choice of anesthetic agent is variable (244, 246, 261, 262), although the use of epinephrine is discouraged in patients with evidence of heart disease or hypertension.

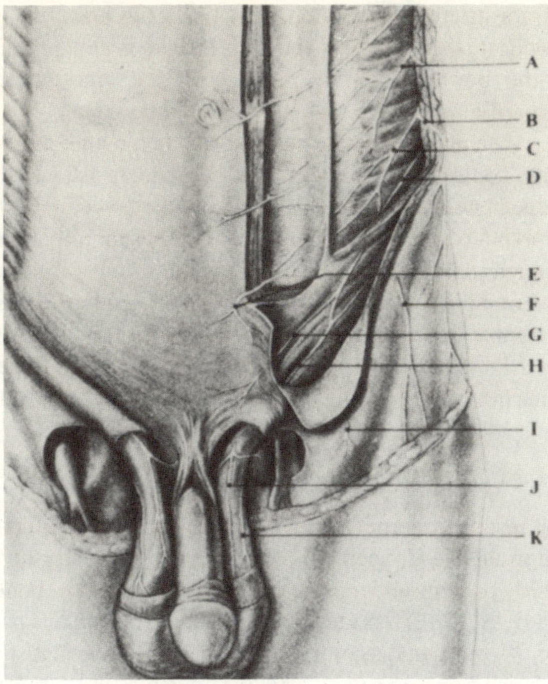

Figure 31-21. The nerve supply to the inguinal region. A, Eleventh thoracic nerve. B, Lateral branch of the twelfth thoracic nerve. C, Anterior branch of the twelfth thoracic nerve. D, Iliohypogastric nerve. E, Twelfth thoracic nerve (anterior branch). F, Lateral femoral cutaneous nerve. G, Iliohypogastric nerve (anterior branch). H, Ilioinguinal nerve. I, Femoral branches of the genitofemoral (lumboinguinal nerve). J, The anterior scrotal (ilioinguinal nerve). K, Genital branch of the genitofemoral nerve. (Reprinted, with permission, from, Lichtenstein, IL, et al. 1988. Pain after hernia surgery. *Contemp Surg* 33: 18–22.) (279).

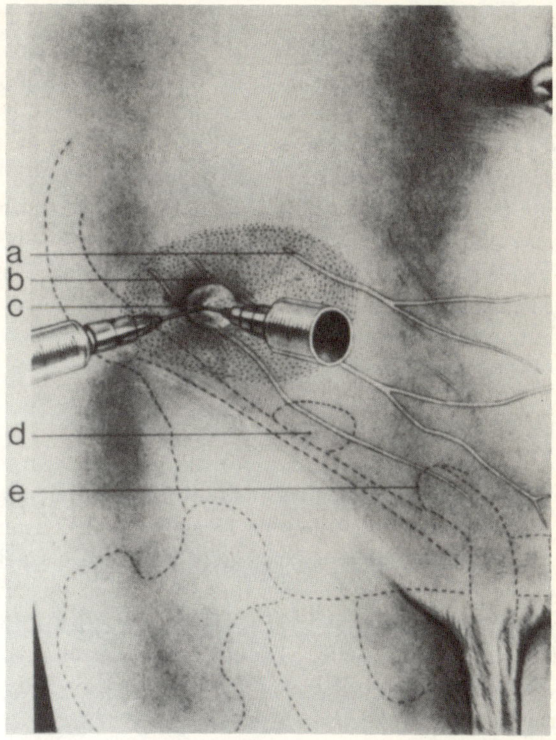

Figure 31-22. Ilioinguinal and iliohypogastric nerve block. A, Twelfth thoracic nerve. B, Iliohypogastric nerve. C, Ilioinguinal nerve. D, Internal ring. E, External ring. (Reprinted, with permission, from Lichtenstein IL, et al. 1988. Montllor, MM: Pain after hernia surgery. *Contemp Surg* 33: 18–22.) (279).

Some authors routinely avoid anesthetic agents with epinephrine in all elderly patients.

Operative Techniques

There is no one correct choice of hernia repair that has received universal acceptance in the elderly. Table 31-18 shows the distribution of repairs from two studies (244, 245). Other series confirm the use of Bassini and McVay for indirect hernias and McVay and Shouldice for direct and femoral hernias (257). While new techniques have been proposed (263) and others strongly advocated (264), there are no compelling data comparing the recurrence rates for different types of hernia repair in older patients. It is therefore generally accepted that careful attention to technical details, including careful tissue manipulation and hemostasis, are more important than specific techniques of repair. It should be emphasized that caution must always be exerted when entering and dissecting a hernia sac in the elderly because of the high incidence of sliding hernias.

For recurrent hernias where the anatomy is distorted or for large and complicated defects where there is little tissue for repair, the use of synthetic materials has proven valuable. These materials can used to replace the inguinal floor, either as a patch sutured in place through a standard groin incision, or as a barrier placed in a preperitoneal manner. In the latter approach, the preperitoneal space posterior to the inguinal floor is entered by dividing the rectus sheath and retracting the muscle laterally. A direct hernia sac can then be easily reduced, and an indirect component identified and ligated. The mesh can then be laid in place behind the inguinal floor to prevent future

Table 31-18. Methods of groin hernia repair

	Nehme, 1983 (245)	Deysine, 1987 (244)
Technique	Number of patients (%)	Number of patients (%)
Bassini	342 (27)	83 (38)
McVay	630 (49)	21 (10)
Shouldice	234 (18)	114 (52)
Other	73 (6)	0
Total	1,279	218

herniation (265, 266). Excellent results have been reported in a large series from France, using prosthetic materials either as a patch or in a preperitoneal position (267). Although this series studied patients of all ages, the use of prosthetics is recommended particularly for older patients with large sliding hernias or recurrences. While these techniques are not often required, they should be kept in mind for these complicated circumstances. When multiple recurrences have occurred, sacrifice of the cord structures and orchiectomy may be necessary to obtain a secure repair.

Emergency Herniorrhaphy

In elderly patients, it is often difficult to distinguish infarcted from viable incarcerated bowel in a hernia sac. Symptoms and signs of acute local inflammation and systemic sepsis are often muted or absent. Delays in treatment are therefore common and unfortunately, devastating. Williams and Hale (247) reported that in all elderly patients who died after emergency herniorraphy, bowel obstruction had been present for at least 3 days prior to treatment.

It is therefore important to recognize an incarcerated hernia quickly and to aggressively prepare the patient for emergency exploration and repair. Attempted nonoperative reduction should be avoided. En masse reduction of unrecognized necrotic bowel may not be immediately apparent because of the benign response of the elderly to intra-abdominal sepsis.

Preoperatively, fluid and electrolyte balance must be restored. Large fluid losses into the obstructed bowel lumen may be unrecognized without central monitoring. Therefore either central venous or Swan-Ganz catheters should be used to assess losses accurately and to guide rapid replacement. Nasogastric decompression is essential to avoid aspiration at the time of induction of anesthesia. Broad-spectrum antibiotic coverage should be started immediately, since the extent of bowel necrosis is not always obvious.

Some authors suggest that local anesthesia can be used successfully for incarcerated hernias (246). However, effective local anesthesia often requires considerable supplemental sedation. These medications can easily cause mental obtundation in an inadequately hydrated, obstructed, and possibly septic older patient. Manipulation of the hernia sac and tension on the mesentery may cause pain and vomiting, which, in an obtunded patient, can result in massive aspiration. We therefore prefer general anesthesia with endotracheal tube control of the airway for emergency cases.

The hernia is approached directly and the sac opened and explored. All contaminated fluid is removed before the constricting ring is opened. Once the bowel is released, it is assessed for viability. If there is any question of the bowel status, it is resected and anastomosed primarily.

If en mass reduction has occurred before the sac contents could be inspected, the peritoneum should be opened enough to allow inspection of the bowel until the incarcerated portion is identified. If this cannot be done through the inguinal incision, a short lower midline laparotomy should be performed. The consequence of unrecognized necrotic bowel in the abdomen far outweighs the risk of the additional incision and exploration. Repair of the hernia can usually then be performed expeditiously.

Results of Operative Treatment

The results of hernia surgery in the elderly are excellent. Tingwald and Cooperman (253) reported no deaths in 44 elderly patients undergoing elective herniorrhaphy. Ponka and Brush (246) reported only 1 death in 200 patients over age 70 years undergoing herniorrhaphy. Their statistics included approximately 10% incarcerated and strangulated femoral hernias. In the large series by Nehme (245), elective mortality was 1.3%.

Emergency herniorrhaphy in most series is associated with much higher mortality. Table 31-19 shows elective and emergency mortality from several series. Mortality in the emergency setting rises to 7.5% to 22%.

Operative mortality from herniorrhaphy is usually related to preexisting disease. Cardiovascular and pulmonary causes are most frequent. In emergency cases, sepsis becomes a significant cause of death as well, although cardiovascular causes are still most common in these cases (245, 247).

Urinary retention and wound complication are the most common minor complications, and each occur in approximately 10% of patients (253). As mentioned previously, when general anesthesia is used pulmonary complications are common and also occur in approximately 10% of patients. Most wound infections occur in cases with strangulated bowel. Complication rates in emergency cases rise to approximately 50% (247, 253) (Table 31-19).

Although Ponka (246) reported a 2% hernia recurrence rate for elderly patients followed from 6 months to 22 years, convincing data regarding long-term recurrence rates of inguinal hernia in the elderly are sparse. There is little reason, however, to suspect that recurrence would be any greater than that in younger patients, particularly when predisposing factors are controlled preoperatively.

The long-term outlook for patients with elective hernia repair is also good. One large Danish (268) study showed crude survival for patients over 70 years old at 30

Table 31-19. Comparison of results of herniorraphy in the elderly

	Williams & Hale, 1966 (247)	Tingwald & Cooperman, 1982 (253)	Nehme, 1983 (245)	Deysine, 1987 (244)
Age of patients	>60	>70	>65	>65
Elective operation				
Number of cases	222	44	1044	234
Complications	59 (26.5)[a]	8 (18)	273 (26)	3 (1.2)
Death	4 (1.8)	—	14 (1.3)	—
Emergent operation				
Number of cases	48	18	235	7
Complications	25 (52)	10 (55.5)	131 (55.7)	—
Deaths	6 (12.5)	4 (22.2)	18 (7.6)	1 (14)

[a]Number in parenthesis indicate %.

Adapted from Deysine M, Grimson R, and Soroff HS. 1987. Herniorrhaphy in the elderly. Benefits of a clinic for the treatment of external abdominal wall hernias. *Am J Surg* 153:387–391.

days, 1 year, and 10 years after elective herniorrahaphy to be 99.4%, 98.4%, and 76.1% respectively. When hernia repair was performed as an emergency, however, survivals at 30 days, 1 year, and 10 years fell to 86.2%, 81.1%, and 30.5%. This data may in part indicate that emergency herniorrhaphy is performed in overall poorer risk patients. The reluctance to subject these patients, who are already at increased risk, to elective surgery exposes them to the even greater risk of emergency operation.

Elective herniorrhaphy in the elderly can be performed safely, particularly under local anesthesia, with a low risk of operative mortality and only minor morbidity. Once incarceration occurs, operative mortality and morbidity soars. Therefore, early elective surgical correction of hernias should be encouraged to both improve the quality of life and decrease the risks associated with emergency repair.

Obturator Hernia

Herniation of the bowel through the obturator canal is a rare condition first described by Pierre Roland Arrand de Ronsile in 1724. The first successful repair was performed by Henry Obre in 1851 (269). The herniation occurs between the suprapubic ramus and the obturator membrane at the point in the obturator foramen where the neurovascular bundle leaves the pelvis. Small bowel, particularly distal ileum, is present in the sac in the majority of cases. Richter's type hernias involving only one portion of the bowel wall are not infrequent (270). In a 1980 review, Temple and Miller (271) found fewer than 550 reported cases in the literature, with a female to male ratio of 9:1.

The etiology of herniation through the obturator canal is thought to be a combination of factors including relaxation of the pelvic musculature with aging and multiparity, loss of fat in the obturator canal, and increased intra-abdominal pressure. The typical patient, therefore, is a frail, poorly nourished multiparous female in the 7th or 8th decade of life with a history of chronic pulmonary disease or chronic constipation.

Diagnosis

In the majority of cases, the presenting symptoms are those of bowel obstruction. Previous episodes of similar symptoms frequently have occurred and resolved spontaneously. Pain along the medial aspect of the thigh radiating to the knee, known as the Howship-Romberg sign, is present in approximately 50% of cases (270, 272). The pain is caused by the pressure of the hernia sac contents on the obturator nerve. This pain is exacerbated by extension, abduction, and internal rotation of the hip. Pressure on the nerve can also cause the absence of the adductor reflex. This is known as the Hannington-Kiff sign and may occur even in the absence of a positive Howship-Romberg sign (273). In nearly 20% of cases, a mass may be felt lateral to the abductor longus tendon in the proximal medial thigh. In another 10% to 20% of cases, rectal or vaginal exam may reveal a lateral mass (274).

Abdominal X-rays are usually nonspecific, showing a pattern of partial or complete small bowel obstruction. A gas shadow in the region of the obturator foramen may be present but is not usually easy to discern. Other radiographic techniques have been used to demonstrate the presence of obturator hernias. Computed tomography has been reported to demonstrate the presence of such hernias, although its usefulness has not been well studied (275). Herniography in which contrast is injected into the peritoneal cavity has also been reported to be helpful in establishing the presence of an obturator hernia (Fig. 31-23) (276).

The absence of external manifestations of obturator

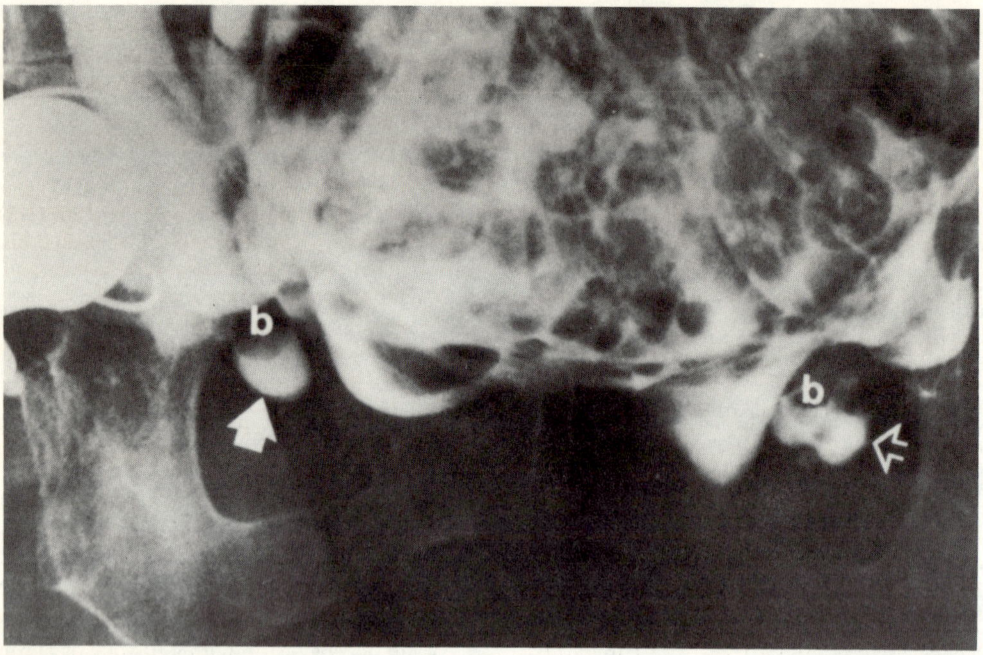

Figure 31-23. Herniography showing intraperitoneal contrast agent in bilateral obturator hernia sacs. (Reprinted, with permission, from Persson NH, Bergqvist D, and Edberg O. 1987. Obturator hernia–clinical significance of radiologic diagnosis. *Acta Chir Scand* 153: 361–364.) (276).

hernia often makes the diagnosis obscure. The correct diagnosis is made preoperatively in fewer than one-third of cases, and long preoperative delays are still common (273).

Treatment

The treatment of obturator hernia consists of operative reduction of the hernia contents and repair of the defect. The vast majority of obturator hernias are diagnosed at the time of incarceration. Patients are usually being treated for bowel obstruction of uncertain etiology. For this reason, exploratory laparotomy is the most common procedure. This approach allows for thorough examination of the incarcerated loop to assure viability and perform resection if necessary. It also affords excellent exposure of the obturator ring and facilitates secure repair without injury to the obturator vessels and nerve. Repair can usually be accomplished by primary closure of the defect with nonabsorbable sutures. In some cases, synthetic mesh may be necessary to obliterate the defect securely. The use of the bladder as a patch to cover the defect has been suggested in cases where bowel resection is necessary, and the use of synthetic materials is not advisable (274). Other approaches, such as the Cheatle-Henry retropubic approach or the inguinal approach, are reserved for those cases where the diagnosis is made preoperatively and the possibility of strangulation is low (269).

Results

The mortality for obturator hernia in the past had been reported to range from 12% to 70%. More recently, mortality has fallen, but is still formidable at 10% to 20%. Preoperative delays of 2 to 7 days are common, and, therefore, strangulated bowel is often present at the time of exploration and repair. Resection is required in approximately 50% of cases (271). A high index of suspicion in frail elderly females with signs and symptoms of small bowel obstruction or intermittent bouts of obstipation and vomiting is essential for the early diagnosis of obturator hernia. The presence of the Howship-Romberg sign in this setting is pathognomonic for incarceration. Its absence, however, should not delay other attempts to establish diagnosis, including computed tomography and laparotomy.

References

1. Wilder RJ, and Fishbein RH. 1961. Operative experience with patients over 80 years of age. *Surg Gynecol Obstet* 113:205–212.
2. Boyd BJ, Bradford B, and Watne AL. 1980. Operative risk factors of colon resection in the elderly. *Ann Surg* 192:743–746.
3. Janzon L, Ryden CL, and Zederfeldt B. 1982. Acute abdomen in the surgical emergency room. Who is taken care of when for what? *Acta Chir Scand* 148:141–148.

4. Reiss R, Deutsch AA, and Nudelman L. 1987. Abdominal surgery in elderly patients: Statistical analysis of clinical factors prognostic of mortality in 1000 cases. *Mt Sinai J Med* 54:135–140.
5. Ponka JL, Welborn KJ, and Brush BE. 1963. Acute abdominal pain in aged patients: An analysis of 200 cases. *J Am Geriatr Soc* 11:993–1007.
6. Greenburg GA, et al. 1981. Mortality and gastrointestinal surgery in the aged. Elective vs emergency procedures. *Arch Surg* 116:788–791.
7. Fenyo G. 1974. Diagnostic problems of acute abdominal diseases in the aged. *Acta Chir Scand* 140:396–405.
8. Fenyo G. 1982. Acute abdominal disease in the elderly. Experience from two series in Stockhom. *Am J Surg* 143:751–754.
9. Crump C. 1931. The incidence of gallstones and gallbladder diseases. *Surg Gynecol Obstet* 53:447–455.
10. Newman HF, and Northup DJ. 1959. Autopsy incidence of gallstones. *Int Abst Surg* 109:1–13.
11. Pigott JP, and Williams GB. 1988. Cholecystectomy in the elderly. *Am J Surg* 155:408–410.
12. Margiotta SJ, et al. 1988. Cholecystectomy in the elderly. *Am J Surg* 156:509–512.
13. Smith N, and Martin MH. 1987. Gallbladder surgery in patients over 60: Is there an increased risk? *South Med J* 80:472–474.
14. Huber DF, Martin EW, and Cooperman M. 1983. Cholecystectomy in elderly patients. *Am J Surg* 146:719–722.
15. Sullivan DM, Hood RT, and Griffen WO. 1982. Biliary tract surgery in the elderly. *Am J Surg* 143:218–220.
16. Reiss R, Deutsh AA, and Eliashiv A. 1983. Decision-making process in abdominal surgery in the geriatric patient. *World J Surg* 7:522–526.
17. Gallbladder Survey Committee, Ohio Chapter, American College of Surgeons. 1970. 28,621 Cholecystectomies in Ohio. Result of a survey in Ohio Hospitals. *Am J Surg* 119:714–717.
18. McSherry CK, and Glenn F. 1980. The incidence and causes of death following surgery for nonmalignant biliary tract disease. *Ann Surg* 191:271–275.
19. Houghton PWJ, Jenkinson LR, and Donaldson LA. 1985. Cholecystectomy in the elderly—a prospective study. *Br J Surg* 72:220–222.
20. Harness JK, Strodel WE, and Talsma SE. 1986. Symptomatic biliary tract disease in the elderly patient. *Am Surg* 8:442–445.
21. Schoenfield LJ, and Lachin JM. 1981. The Steering Committee, The National Cooperative Gallstone Study Group. Chenodiol (Chenodeoxycholic acid) for dissolution of gallstones: The national co-operative gallstone study: A controlled trial of efficacy and safety. *Ann Intern Med* 95:257–282.
22. Bouchier LAD. 1983. Gallstone dissolving agents. *Br Med J* 286:778–780.
23. Thistle JL, et al. 1989. Dissolution of cholesterol gallbladder stones by methyltert-butyl ether administered by percutaneous transhepatic catheter. *N Engl J Med* 320:633–639.
24. Sackmann M, et al. 1987. Extracorporeal shock wave lithotripsy of gallbladder stones: Results of 101 treatments. *Gastroenterology* 92:1608.
25. Wenckhert A, and Robertson B. 1966. The natural course of gallstone disease. *Gastroenterology* 50:376–381.
26. Lund J. 1960. Surgical indications in cholelithiasis prophylactic cholecystectomy elucidated on the basis of long-term followup on 526 nonoperated cases. *Ann Surg* 151:153–162.
27. Gracie WA, and Ransohoff DF. 1982. The natural history of silent gallstones. *N Engl J Med* 307:798–800.
28. McSherry CK, et al. 1985. The natural history of diagnosed gallstone disease in symptomatic and asymptomatic patients. *Ann Surg* 202:59–63.
29. Roslyn J, and Busuttil RW. 1979. Perforation of the gallbladder: A frequently mismanaged condition. *Am J Surg* 137:307–312.
30. Berk RN, and Leopold GR. 1978. The present status of imaging of the gallbladder. *Invest Radiol* 13:477–489.
31. Herman RE. Spectrum of billiary stone disease. *Am J Surg* In press.
32. Lygidakis NJ. 1983. Operative risk factors of cholecystectomy—choledochotomy in the elderly. *Surg Gynecol Obstet* 157:15–19.
33. Morrow DJ, Thompson J, and Wilson SE. 1978. Acute cholecystitis in the elderly. A surgical emergency. *Arch Surg* 113:1149–1152.
34. Pellegrini CA, and Way LW. 1987. Acute cholecystitis. In *Surgery of the Gallbladder and Bile Ducts,* Eds., LW Way and CA Pellegrini. Philadelphia: WB Saunders.
35. Matolo NM, LaMorte WW, and Wolfe BM. 1981. Acute and chronic cholecystitis. *Surg Clin North Am* 61:875–883.
36. Brandt LJ. 1984. Gallbladder and biliary tree. In *Gastrointestinal Disorders of the Elderly,* Ed., LJ Brandt. New York: Raven Press.
37. Laing FC, et al. Ultrasonic evaluation of patients with acute right upper quadrant pain. *Radiology* 140:449–455.
38. Weissman HS, et al. 1979. Rapid and accurate diagnosis of acute cholecystitis with ^{99m}Tc-HIDA cholescintigraphy. *Am J Roentgenol* 132:523–528.
39. Herman RE, and Martin JC. 1969. Biliary disease and advancing age. *Geriatrics* 24:139–145.
40. Siegel JH. 1981. Endoscopic papillotomy in the treatment of biliary tract disease: 258 procedures and results. *Dig Dis Sci* 26:1057.
41. Mee AS, et al. 1983. Nonoperative removal of bile duct stones by duodenoscopic sphincterotomy in the elderly. *Br Med J* 283:521–523.
42. Klimberg S, Hawkins I, and Vogel S. 1987. Percutaneous cholecystostomy for acute cholecystitis in high-risk patients. *Am J Surg* 153:125–128.
43. Glenn F. 1981. Surgical management of acute cholecystostomy in patients 65 years of age and older. *Ann Surg* 193:56–59.
44. DenBesten L. 1987. Choledocholithiasis. In *Surgery of the Gallbladder and Bile Ducts,* Eds., LW Way and CA Pellegrini. Philadelphia: WB Saunders.
45. Glenn F, and McSherry CK. 1975. Calculus biliary tract disease. *Curr Prob Surg* June: 1–38.
46. Gaines RD. 1977. Surgery for gallbladder disease in the elderly. *Geriatrics* 32:71–74.
47. Bernhoft RA, et al. 1984. Composition and morpohologic and clinical features of common duct stones. *Am J Surg* 148:77–85.

48. Maki T. 1966. Pathogenesis of calcium bilirubinate gallstones: Role of E. Coli, beta-glucoronidase and coagulation by inorganic ions, polyelectrolytes and agitation. *Ann Surg* 164:90–100.
49. Lygidakis NJ. 1981. Choledochoduodenostomy in calculus biliary tract disease. *Br J Surg* 68:762–675.
50. Cronan JJ. 1987. The imaging of choledocholithiasis. *Semin Ultrasound* 8:75–84.
51. Chardavoyne R, et al. 1987. Comparison of intraoperative ultrasonography and cholangiography in detection of small common bile duct stones. *Ann Surg* 206:53–55.
52. Taylor KJW, and Rosenfield AT. 1977. Grey-Scale: Ultrasonography in the differential diagnosis of jaundice. *Arch Surg* 112:820–825.
53. Baron RL, et al. 1982. A prospective comparison of the evaluation of biliary obstruction using computed tomography and ultrasonography. *Radiology* 160:91–98.
54. Moesgaard F, et al. Protective choledochoduodenostomy in multiple common duct stones in the aged. *Surg Gynecol Obstet* 154:232–234.
55. Pitt HA, and Longmire WP Jr. 1971. Suppurative cholangitis. In *Critical Surgical Illnesses,* ed. 2, Ed., JM Hardy. Philadelphia: WB Saunders.
56. Boey JH, and Way LW. 1980. Acute cholangitis. *Ann Surg* 191:264–269.
57. Thompson JE, Tompkins RK, and Longmire WP Jr. Factors in management of acute cholangitis. *Ann Surg* 195:137–145.
58. Saharia PC, and Cameron JL. 1976. Clinical management of acute cholangitis. *Surg Gynecol Obstet* 142:369–372.
59. Saik RP, et al. 1975. Spectrum of cholangitis. *Am J Surg* 130:143–150.
60. Elias E, et al. 1976. A randomized trial of percutaneous transhepatic cholangiography with Chiba needle versus endoscopic retrograde cholangiography for bile duct visualization in jaundice. *Gastroneterology* 71:439–443.
61. Pitt HA, and Cameron JL. 1987. Acute cholangitis. In *Surgery of the Gallbladder and Bile Ducts,* Eds., LW Way and CA Pellegrini. Philadelphia: WB Saunders.
62. Norman DC, and Yoshikawa T. 1983. Intraabdominal infections in the elderly. *J Am Geriatr Soc* 31:677–684.
63. Kadir S, et al. Percutaneous biliary drainage in the management of biliary sepsis. *Am J Radiol* 138:25–27.
64. Delmotte JS, et al. 1982. Initial duodenoscopic sphincterotomy in patients with acute cholangitis or pancreatitis complicating biliary stones. *Gastroenterology* 82:1042.
65. Marks WM, et al. 1984. Endoscopic retrograde biliary drainage. *Radiology* 152:357–360.
66. Stanley J, et al. 1988. Biliary decompression: An institutional comparison of percutaneous and endoscopic methods. *Radiology* 168:328–330.
67. Mueller PR. 1988. Interventional radiology of the biliary tract: A decade of progress. *Radiology* 168:328–330.
68. Way LW. 1987. Gallstone ileus. In *Surgery of the Gallbladder and Bile Ducts,* Eds., LW Way and CA Pellegrini. Philadelphia: WB Saunders.
69. Kurtz RJ, et al. 1985. Patterns of gallstone ileus over a 45 year period. *Am J Gastroenterol* 80:95–98.
70. Raf L., and Spangen L. 1971. Gallstone ileus. *Acta Chir Scand* 137:655–675.
71. Kurtz RJ, Aeimann TM, and Kurtz AB. 1983. Gallstone ileus: A diagnostic problem. *Am J Surg* 146:314–317.
72. Schreiber H, Macon WL, and Walter JP. 1978. Incidental cholecystectomy during major abdominal surgery in the elderly. *Am J Surg* 135:196–198.
73. Bell GA, and Holubitsky IB. 1969. Acute cholecystitis following unrelated surgery. *Can Med Assoc J* 101:94–96.
74. Permutt RP, and Cello JP. 1982. Duodenal ulcer disease in the hospitalized elderly patient. *Dig Dis Sci* 27:1–6.
75. Levrat M, et al. 1966. Peptic ulcer in patients over 60. *Am J Dig Dis* 2:279–285.
76. Brooks JR, and Eraklis AJ. 1964. Factors affecting the mortality from peptic ulcer. The bleeding ulcer and ulcer in the aged. *N Engl J Med* 271:803–809.
77. Stanfford CE, Joergenson EJ, and Murray GC. 1956. Complications of peptic ulcer in the aged. *Calif Med* 84:92–94.
78. Narayanan M, and Steinheber FU. 1976. The changing face of peptic ulcer in the elderly. *Med Clin North Am* 60:1159–1172.
79. Watson RJ, Hooper TL, and Ingram G. 1985. Duodenal ulcer disease in the elderly: A retrospective study. *Age Ageing* 14:225–229.
80. Griffin MR, Ray WA, and Schaffner W. 1988. Nonsteroidal drug use and death from peptic ulcer in elderly persons. *Ann Intern Med* 109:359–363.
81. Clinch D, Banejee AK, and Ostick G. 1985. Absence of abdominal pain in elderly patients with peptic ulcer. *Age Ageing* 13:120–123.
82. Cutler CW. 1958. Clinical patterns of peptic ulcer after sixty. *Surg Gynecol Obstet* 107:23–30.
83. Kaplan MS, et al. 1972. Surgical management of peptic ulcer disease in the aged patient. *Arch Surg* 104:667–671.
84. Meyer KA, and Kozoll DD. 1964. Emergency treatment in massively bleeding geriatric ulcer patients. *Geriatrics* 19:812–823.
85. Hoare AM, Bradby GVH, and Hawkins CF. 1979. Cimetidine in bleeding peptic ulcer. *Lancet* 2:671–673.
86. Rachlin L, and Ceide-Echevarria A. 1973. Bleeding duodenal ulcer in elderly patients. *Am Surgeon* 39:174–176.
87. Klug TS, Zollinger RM, and Ellensohn J. 1963. A long-term evaluation of two conservative surgical procedures for duodenal ulcer. *Am J Surg* 105:370–374.
88. Walt R, et al. 1986. Rising frequency of ulcer perforation in elderly people in the United Kingdom. *Lancet* 489–492.
89. Coleman JA, and Denham MJ. 1980. Perforation of peptic ulceration in the elderly. *Age Ageing* 9:251–257.
90. Brandt, LJ. 1984. The stomach. In *Gastrointestinal Disorders in the Elderly,* Ed., LJ Brandt. p. 101. New York: Raven Press.
91. Boey J, et al. 1982. Immediate definitive surgery for perforated duodenal ulcers. *Ann Surg* 196:338–344.
92. Blake R, and Lynn J. 1976. Emergency abdominal surgery in the aged. *Br J Surg* 63:956–960.
93. Koo J, et al. 1983. Proximal gastric vagotomy, truncal vagotomy with drainage, and truncal vagotomy with antrectomy for chronic duodenal ulcer. *Ann Surg* 197:265–271.
94. Nussbaum MS, and Schusterman MA. 1985. Management of giant duodenal ulcer. *Am J Surg* 149:357–361.

95. Lumsden K, Maclarnon JC, and Dawson J. 1970. Giant duodenal ulcer. *Gut* 11:592–599.
96. Jaszewski R, Crane SA, and Cid AA. 1983. Giant duodenal ulcers. Successful healing with medical therapy. *Dig Dis Sci* 28:486–489.
97. Elashoff JD, and Grossman MI. 1980. Trends in hospital admissions and death rates for peptic ulcer in the United States from 1970–1978. *Gastroenterology* 78:280–285.
98. Jordan PH Jr. 1987. Gastric ulcer. In *Surgery of the Stomach, Duodenum and Small Intestine,* Eds., WH Scott and JL Sawyers. Boston: Blackwell Scientific Publications.
99. Amberg JR, and Zboralske FF. 1966. Gastric ulcers after 70. *Am J Roentgenol* 96:393–399.
100. Adkin RB, et al. 1985. The management of gastric ulcers: A current review. *Ann Surg* 201:741–751.
101. Lewis JH. 1983. Treatment of gastric ulcer; what is old and what is new? *Arch Intern Med* 143:264–273.
102. Shackelford RT, and Zuidema, GD. 1981. Gastric and duodenal ulcers. In *Surgery of the Alimentary Tract,* ed. 2, Eds., RI Shackelford and GD Zuidema, vol. 2. Philadelphia: WB Saunders.
103. Sun DCH, and Stempien SJ. 1971. Site and size of the ulcer as determinants of outcome. Veterans administration cooperative study on gastric ulcer. *Gastroenterology* 61:576–584.
104. Kraus M, Mendeloff G, and Condon RE. 1976. Prognosis of gastric ulcers. Twenty five year follow up. *Ann Surg* 184:471–476.
105. Jensen HE, et al. 1972. Bleeding gastric ulcer. Surgical and nonsurgical treatment of 225 patients. *Scand J Gastroenterol* 7:535–540.
106. Bongiorno CP. 1988. Appropriate prevention and detection of gastrointestinal neoplasms in the elderly. *Clin Geriatr Med* 4:223–233.
107. Keppen M. 1987. Upper gastrointestinal malignancies in the elderly. *Clin Geriatr Med* 3:637–648.
108. Coluccia C, et al. 1987. Gastric cancer in the elderly: Results of surgical treatment. *Int Surg* 72:4–10.
109. Yukiyoski E, Hirokawak, and Yamashiro M. 1987. Multiple gastric cancers in the aged with special reference to intramucosal cancers. *Cancer* 59:560–565.
110. Correa P. 1985. Clinical implications of recent developments in gastric cancer pathology and epidemiology. *Semin Oncol* 12:2–10.
111. Morson BC, and Jass JR. 1985. *Precancerous Lesions of the Gastrointestinal Tract.* London: Bailliere Tindal.
112. MacDonald JS, Cohn I, and Gunderson LL. 1986. Cancer of the stomach. In *Cancer Principles and Practice of Oncology,* Eds., VT Devita, S Hellman, and SA Rosenberg. Philadelphia: JB Lippincott.
113. Scott HW, Longmire WP, and Gray GF. 1986. Carcinoma of the stomach. In *Surgery of the Stomach, Duodenum and Small Intestine,* Eds., HW Scott and JL Sawyers. Boston: Blackwell Scientific Publications.
114. Schafer LW, et al. 1983. The risk of carcinoma after surgical treatment for benign ulcer disease. *N Engl J Med* 309:1210–1213.
115. Fischer AB, Graem N, and Jensen OM. 1983. Risk of gastric cancer after Billroth II resection for duodenal ulcer. *Br J Surg* 70:552–554.
116. Kennedy BJ. 1970. TNM classification for stomach cancer. *Cancer* 26:971–983.
117. Edelman DS, Russin DJ, and Wallack MK. 1987. Gastric cancer in the elderly. *Am Surg* 53:170–173.
118. Kirsh IE. 1971. Radiological aspects of cancer after apparent healing. *Gastroenterology* 61:606–627.
119. Dehn TCB, et al. 1981. The preoperative assessment of advanced gastric cancer by computed tomography. *Br J Surg* 71:413–417.
120. Rosenthal RA, and Andersen DK. 1985. Surgery in the elderly. In *Principles of Geriatric Medicine,* Eds., R Andres, EL Bierman, and WR Hazzard. New York: McGraw-Hill.
121. Fleischer D, and Sivak MV. 1984. Endoscopic ND: YAG laser therapy as palliative treatment for advanced adenocarcinoma of the gastric cardia. *Gastroenterology* 87:815–820.
122. Cady B, Ramsden DA, and Choe DS. 1976. Treatment of gastric cancer. *Surg Clin North Am* 56:599–605.
123. Mellström D, and Rundgren A. 1982. Long-term effects of partial gastrectomy in elderly men. A longitudinal population study of men between 70 and 75 years of age. *Scand J Gastroenterology* 17:433–439.
124. Boley SJ, Brandt LJ, and Frank MS. 1981. Severe lower intestinal bleeding. Diagnosis and treatment. *Clin Gastroenterol* 10:65–91.
125. Margulis AR, Heinbecker D, and Bernard HR. 1960. Operative mesenteric arteriography in the search for the site of bleeding in unexplained gastrointestinal bleeding. *Surgery* 48:534.
126. Boley SJ, et al. Lower intestinal bleeding in the elderly. *Am J Surg* 137:57–63.
127. Boley SJ, et al. 1979. Vascular ectasias of the colon. *Surg, Gynecol, Obstet* 149:353–359.
128. Baum S, Athanasoulus CA, and Waltman AC. 1977. Angiodysplasia of the right colon: A cause for gastrointestinal bleeding. *Am J Roentgenology* 129:789.
129. Boley SJ, and Brandt LJ. 1986. Vascular ectasias of the colon—1986. *Dig Dis Sci* 31 (supplement):26s–42s.
130. Hagihara PF, Chariara VP, and Guflin WO. 1977. Arteriovenous malformation of the colon. *Am J Surg* 133:681–687.
131. Bowden TA, Hawks WH, and Mansberger AR. 1982. Intestinal vascular ectasias: A new look at an old disease. *South Med J* 75:1310–1317.
132. Avotine KV, and Wanah DE. 1985. Colonic bleeding in the elderly. *Clin Geriatr Med* 2:33–44.
133. Forde KF. 1977. Colonoscopy in acute rectal bleeding. *Gastrointest Endosc* 27:650–660.
134. Boley SJ, et al. 1977. On the nature and etiology of vascular ectasias of the colon. *Gastroenterology* 72:650–660.
135. Sprayrogen S, and Boley SJ. 1970. Vascular ectasias of the right colon. *J Am Med Assoc* 239:962–964.
136. Brandt LD, and Boley SJ. 1984. The role of colonoscopy in the diagnosis and management of lower intestinal bleeding. *Scand J Gastroenterology 19* (supplement) 102:61–70.
137. Sniderman KW, Franklin J, and Sos TA. 1978. Successful transcather embolization of a bleeding cecal vascular ectasia. *Am J Roentgenol* 131:157–159.
138. Matalo NM, and Link DP. 1979. Selective embolization for control of gastrointestinal hemorrhage. *Am J Surg* 138:840–844.
139. Mitty HA, Efrenudes S, and Keller RJ. 1979. Colonic

stricture after transcatheter embolization for diverticular bleeding. *Am J Roentgenology* 133:519–521.

140. Weilaw B. 1987. Colorectal cancer. *Clin Geriatr Med* 3:625–635.

141. List ND. 1987. Perspectives in cancer screening in the elderly. *Clin Geriatr Med* 3:433–445.

142. Brocklehurst JC. 1985. Colonic diseases. *Clin Gastroenterol* 14:725–747.

143. Waldron RD, et al. 1988. Emergency presentation and mortality from colorectal cancer in the elderly. *Br J Surg* 73:214–216.

144. Hardcastle T. 1983. Controlled trial of fecal occult blood testing in the detection of colorectal cancer. *Lancet* 1:1–4.

145. Longo WE, Ballantyne GH, and Modlin IM. 1988. Colonoscopic detection of early colorectal cancers: Impact of a surgical endoscopy service. *Ann Surg* 207:174.

146. Irvin TT. 1988. Prognosis of colorectal cancer in the elderly. *Br J Surg* 75:419–421.

147. Webbes TH. 1985. Carcinoma of the colon and rectum in geriatric patients. *Age Ageing* 14:321–326.

148. Cohen JP, et al. 1978. Carcinoma of the large bowel in patients aged 70 years and older. *Aust NZ J Surg* 48:405–408.

149. Berman PM, and Kirsner JB. 1972. Diverticular disease of the colon in the elderly. *Geriatrics* 27:70–75.

150. Painter WS. 1969. Diverticular disease of the colon. The disease of the century. *Lancet* 2:586–588.

151. Brocklehurst JC. 1980. Disorders of the lower bowel in old age. *Geriatrics* 35:47–54.

152. Mitty WF, Befelen D, and Grossi C. 1971. Surgical management of diverticulitis in the elderly. *Am Fam Phys* 3:94–98.

153. Colcock BP. 1968. Diverticulitis in the elderly. *Geriatrics* 23:122–127.

154. Pale JG. 1969. Natural history of diverticular disease of the colon. *Br Med J* 4:639–645.

155. Hulnick DH, et al. 1984. Computed tomography in the evaluation of diverticulitis. *Radiology* 152:491–495.

156. Finlay IG, and Carter DC. 1987. A comparison of emergency resection and staged management in perforated diverticular disease. *Dis Colon Rectum* 30:929–933.

157. Storer EH, Goldberg SM, and Nivatvong S. 1979. Colon, rectum and anus. *Principles of Surgery,* ed. 3, Ed., S. Schwartz. New York: McGraw-Hill.

158. Ogilvie H. 1948. Large intestine colic due to sympathetic deprivation: A new clinical syndrome. *Br J Med* 2:671–673.

159. Bullock PR, and Thomas WE. 1984. Acute pseudoobstruction of the colon. *Ann R Coll Surg Engl* 66:327.

160. Fausel CJ, and Groff JS. 1985. Nonoperative management of acute idiopathic colonic pseudoobstruction. *West J Med* 143:50–54.

161. Nano D, et al. 1987. Colonoscopic therapy of acute pseudoobstruction of the colon. *Am J Gastroenterology* 82:145–148.

162. Kukora JS, and Dent DT. 1977. Colonoscopic decompression of massive non-obstructed cecal dilatation. *Arch Surg* 112:512–517.

163. Wann G, Garbiwa A, and Luchelt P. 1982. Ogilvie Syndrome: Review of the literature and four additional cases. *Dis Colon Rectum* 25:157–166.

164. Bode WE, Beart RW, and Spence RT. 1984. Colonoscopic decompression for acute pseudoobstruction of the colon. *Am J Surg* 147:243–245.

165. Strodd WE, Nostrant TT, and Eckhavder PE. 1983. Therapeutic and diagnostic colonoscopy in non-obstructive colonic dilation. *Ann Surg* 197:416–421.

166. Nivatvong S, Verbeuler PB, and Tong DJ. 1982. Colonoscopic decompression of acute pseudoobstruction of the colon. *Ann Surg* 196:598–600.

167. Geechoed G. 1985. Colonic pseudoobstruction in surgical patients. *Am J Surg* 149:258–265.

168. Addison NU. 1983. Pseudoobstruction of the large bowel. *J R Soc Med* 76:252–255.

169. Bachulis BL, and Smith WE. 1978. Pseudoobstruction of the colon. *Am J Surg* 136:66–72.

170. Baker DA, et al. 1979. Colonic ileus: Indication for prompt decompression. *JAMA* 241:263–264.

171. Martin FM, Robinson AM, and Thompson WR. 1988. Therapeutic colonoscopy in the treatment of colonic pseudoobstruction. *Am Surg* 54:519–522.

172. Mangiante EC, et al. 1989. Sigmoid volvulus: A four decade experience. *Am Surg* 55:41–44.

173. Rokitansky KE, (Sieveking E, Translator). 1849–1854. *A Manual of Pathologic Anatomy.* London: Sydehan Society.

174. Treves F. 1894. *Intestinal Obstruction, Its Varieties with Their Pathology Diagnosis and Treatment.* Philadelphia: Henry Lea and Company.

175. Wolfer JA, Beaton LE, and Anton BJ. 1942. Volvulus of the cecum: Anatomical factors in its etiology—Report of a case. *Surg, Gynecol, Obstet* 74:882–894.

176. Ballantyne GH. 1982. Review of sigmoid volvulus: Clinical patterns and pathogenesis. *Dis Colon Rectum* 25:823–830.

177. Andersen DA. 1968. Volvulus of the sigmoid colon. *Br Med J* 196:765.

178. Ballantyne GH, et al. 1985. Volvulus of the colon: Incidence and mortality. *Ann Surg* 202:83–92.

179. Avots-Avotens KU, and Waugh DE. 1982. Colon volvulus and the geriatric patients. *Surg Clin North Am* 62:249–260.

180. Hjortrup A, et al. 1987. Volvulus of the cecum. *Danish Med Bull* 34:331.

181. Arnold AJ, and Nance FC. 1973. Volvulus of the sigmoid colon. *Ann Surg* 177:527–531.

182. Ballantyne UH. 1982. Review of sigmoid volvulus: History and results of treatment. *Dis Colon Rectum* 25:494–501.

183. Brunsgaard C. 1947. Volvulus of the sigmoid colon and its treatment. *Surgery* 22:466–478.

184. Starting JP. 1979. Initial treatment of sigmoid volvulus by colonoscopy. *Ann Surg* 190:36–39.

185. Ghazi A, Shinya H, and Wolff WI. 1976. Treatment of volvulus of the colon by colonoscopy. *Ann Surg* 183:263–265.

186. Defelice G. 1986. Sigmoid volvulus treated by colonoscopy. *Gastrointest Endosc* 32:244–245.

187. Arigbabu AO, Badejo OA, and Akinola AO. 1985. Colonoscopy in the emergency treatment of colonic volvulus in Nigeria. *Dis Colon Rectum* 28:795–798.

188. Sutcliffe MML. 1968. Volvulus of the sigmoid colon. *Br J Surg* 55:903–910.

189. Hines JR, Guerkink RE, and Bass RT. 1967. Recurrence

and mortality rates in sigmoid volvulus. *Surg Gynecol Obstet* 124:567–570.
190. Hellman AA, and Cramer WO. 1988. Mesh fixation of the mesentery for treatment of volvulus and recurrent stomal prolapse. *Surg Gynecol Obstet* 167:249–250.
191. Parhlman L, et al. 1989. Volvulus of the colon: A review of 93 cases and current aspects of treatment. *Acta Chir Scand* 155:53–56.
192. Bak MD, and Boley SJ. 1986. Sigmoid volvulus in elderly patients. *Am J Surg* 151:71–75.
193. Andersen MJ, Okike W, and Spencer RJ. 1978. The colonscope in cecal volvulus. *Dis Colon Rectum* 21:71.
194. Todd GJ, and Forde KA. 1979. Volvulus of the cecum: Choice of operation. *Am J Surg* 138:632–634.
195. Morris AM, Eisenstat J, and Hall GM. 1982. Management of cecal volvulus in debilitated patients. *South Med J* 75:1069–1071.
196. Lowry AC, and Goldberg SM. 1987. Rectal prolapse gastroenterology. *Surg Clin North Am* 16:47–70.
197. Moschowitz AU. 1912. The pathogenesis, anatomy, and care of prolapse of the rectum. *Surg Gynecol Obstet* 15:7.
198. Broden B, and Snellman B. 1968. Procidental of the rectum studied by cineradiography: A contribution to the discussion of causative mechanism. *Dis Colon Rectum* 11:330.
199. Schlinlkert R, et al. 1985. Anterior resection for complete prolapse. *Dis Colon Rectum* 28:409–412.
200. Ripstein CB. 1965. Surgical care of massive rectal prolapse. *Dis Colon Rectum* 8:34–48.
201. McMahan JD, and Ripstein CB. 1987. Rectal prolapse: An update on the rectal sling. *Am Surg* 53:37–40.
202. Holstrom B, Broden A, and Dolk A. 1986. Result of the Ripstein operation in the treatment of rectal prolapse and internal rectal procidentiam. *Dis Colon Rectum* 29:845–848.
203. Heitama HF, et al. 1984. The treatment of complete rectal prolapse by transabdominal posterior rectopexy. *Neth J Surg* 36:73–76.
204. Beltran de Heredia JM. 1983. A new surgical procedure for treatment of complete rectal prolapse: Preliminary report. *Int Surg* 68:161–162.
205. Atkinson KG, and Taylor DC. 1984. Wells procedure for complete rectal prolapse. *Dis Colon Rectum* 27:96–98.
206. Andersen JR, Wilson BG, and Parks TG. 1984. Complete rectal prolapse—the results of Ivalon sponge rectopexy. *Postgrad Med J* 60:411–414.
207. Mann CV, and Hoffman C. 1988. Complete rectal prolapse: The anatomical and functional results of treatment by an extended abdominal rectopexy. *Br J Surg* 75:34–37.
208. Lake SA, Hancock BD, and Lewis AAM. 1989. Management of pelvic sepsis after Ivalon rectopexy. *Dis Colon Rectum* 27:589–590.
209. Carter AE. 1983. Rectosaral suture fixation for complete rectal prolapse. *Br J Surg* 70:522–523.
210. Graham W, Clegg JR, and Taylor V. 1984. Complete rectal prolapse: Repair by simple technique. *Ann R Coll Surg Engl* 66:87–89.
211. Loygue J, et al. 1984. Rectopexy to the promontory for the treatment of rectal prolapse. Report of 257 cases. *Dis Colon Rectum* 27:356–359.
212. Muir EG. 1955. Rectal prolapse. *Proc R Soc Med* 48:33–44.
213. Lahaut J. 1956. Cure radicale des grandes prolapsus de rectum. *J Chir* 72:565.
214. Mortensen W, Vallacott KD, and Wilson NG. 1984. Lahaut's operation for rectal prolapse. *Ann R Coll Surg Engl* 66:17–18.
215. Altemeier WA, and Culbertson WR. 1965. Technique for perineal repair of rectal prolapse. *Surgery* 58:758–764.
216. Prasad ML, et al. 1986. Perineal proctectomy, posterior rectopexy, and postanal levator repair for the treatment of rectal prolapse. *Dis Colon Rectum* 29:547–552.
217. Bennett BH, and Gealhoed GW. 1985. A stapler modification of the Altmeier procedure for rectal prolapse. *Am Surg* 51:116–120.
218. Monson JR, et al. 1986. Delorme's operation, the first choice in complete rectal prolapse? *Ann R Coll Surg Engl* 68:143–146.
219. Goligher JC. 1984. Rectal prolapse. In *Surgery of the Anus, Rectum and Colon,* ed. 5, Ed., JC Goligher. London: Baillier Tindall.
220. Larach SW, and Vazquez B. 1986. Modified Thiersch procedure with Silastic mesh implant: A simple solution for fecal incontinence and severe prolapse. *South Med J* 79:307–309.
221. Earnshaw JJ, and Hopkinson BD. 1987. Late results of silicon? Perineal suture for rectal prolapse. *Dis Colon Rectum* 30:86–88.
222. Rogers J, and Jeffrey PJ. 1987. Posterior repair and intersphincteric Ivalon sponge rectopexy for the treatment of rectal prolapse. *Br J Surg* 74:384–386.
223. Berry J. 1984. Dilatation and rupture of the sigmoid flexure. *Br Med J* 1:301.
224. Berger DL, and Shaw RE. 1961. Spontaneous rupture of the colon. *Br Med J* 1:1422–1425.
225. Gekas D, and Shuster MM. 1981. Stercoral perforation of the colon: Case report and review of the literature. *Gastroenterology* 80:1054–1058.
226. Maull KI, Kinning WK, and Kay S. 1982. Stercoral ulceration. *Am Surg* 48:20–24.
227. Welch JP, Schweizer RJ, Bartus S. 1980. Management of antacid impactions in hemodialysis and renal transplant patients. *Am J Surg* 139:561–568.
228. Selye H, Winindy G, and Gavviani A. 1966. Production and prevention of stercoral ulcers in the rat. *Am J Pathol* 48:299–303.
229. Stunger MD, Greenfield S, McIrvine AJ. 1987. Stercoral perforation of the colon following postoperative analgesia. *J R Soc Med* 80:115–116.
230. Meikle G. 1965. A case of pneumatosis coli: Pneumatosis cystoides intestinales of the sigmoid colon causing intestinal obstruction, stercorals ulcer and perforation. *J R Coll Surg Edinb* 11:65–67.
231. Robinson JC, and Teidellbaum SL. 1974. Stercoral ulceration and perforation of the sclerodermatous colon: Report of two cases and review of the literature. *Dis Colon Rectum* 17:622–632.
232. Lui RC, et al. 1988. Stercoral perforation of the colon: Report of a new location. *Am J Gastroenterol* 83:457–459.
233. Avinoah E. 1987. Sigmoid perforation in patients with chronic constipation. *J Clin Gastroenterol* 9:62–64.
234. Strutinsky W, and Orron D. 1987. Stercoral perforation of the descending colon appearing radiographically as pneumomediastinum. *Mt Sinai J Med* 54:436–439.

235. Guyton DP, Evans D, and Schreibe H. 1985. Stercoral perforation of the colon: Concepts of operative management. *Am Surg* 51:520–522.
236. Lau WY, et al. 1985. Acute appendicitis in the elderly. *Surg Gynecol Obstet* 161:157–160.
237. Vorhes CE. 1987. Appendicitis in the elderly. The case for better diagnosis. *Geriatrics* 42:89–92.
238. Owens RJ, and Hamit HF. 1978. Appendicitis in the elderly. *Ann Surg* 187:392–396.
239. Goldberg IS. 1955. Acute appendicitis in the aged. *Geriatrics* 10:324–328.
240. Yushikaura TT. 1983. Intra-abdominal infection in the elderly. *J Am Geriatr Soc* 31:677–684.
241. Hall A, and Wright T. 1976. Acute appendicitis in the geriatric patient. *Am Surg* 42:147–150.
242. Yusuf MR, and Dunn E. 1979. Appendicitis in the elderly. Learn to discern the UNtypical picture. *Geriatrics* 34:73–79.
243. Money V. 1970. Appendicitis in elderly patients. *Br Med J* 3:177.
244. Deysine M, Grimson R, and Soroff HS. 1987. Herniorrhaphy in the elderly. Benefits of a clinic for the treatment of external abdominal well hernias. *Am J Surg* 153:387–391.
245. Nehme AE. 1983. Groin hernias in elderly patients. Management and prognosis. *Am J Surg* 146:257–260.
246. Ponka JL, and Brush BE. 1974. Experiences with the repair of groin hernia in 200 patients aged 70 or older. *J Am Geriatr Soc* 22:18–24.
247. Williams JS, and Hale HW. 1966. The advisability of inguinal herniorrhaphy in the elderly. *Surg Gynecol Obstet* 122:100–104.
248. Fenyo G. 1974. Diagnostic problems of acute abdominal diseases in the aged. *Acta Chir Scand* 140:396–405.
249. Blake R, and Lynn J. 1976. Emergency abdominal surgery in the aged. *Br J Surg* 63:956–960.
250. Green WW. 1969. Bowel obstruction in the aged patient. A review of 300 cases. *Am J Surg* 118:541–545.
251. Glassow F. 1963. Inguinal hernia in the female. *Surg Gynecol Obstet* 116:701–704.
252. Ryan EA. 1956. An analysis of 313 consecutive cases of indirect sliding inguinal hernias. *Surg Gynecol Obstet* 102:45–58.
253. Tingwald GR, and Cooperman M. 1982. Inguinal and femoral hernia repair in geriatric patients. *Surg Gynecol Obstet* 154:704–706.
254. Pescovitz MD. 1983. Umbilical hernia repair in patients with cirrhosis. No evidence for increased incidence of variceal bleeding. *Ann Surg* 199:325–327.
255. Guillen J, and Aldrete JA. 1970. Anesthetic factors influencing morbidity and mortality of elderly patients undergoing inguinal herniorrhaphy. *Am J Surg* 120:760–763.
256. Young DV. 1987. Comparison of local, spinal, and general anesthesia for inguinal herniorrhaphy. *Am J Surg* 153:560–563.
257. Job CA, et al. 1979. Inguinal hernia repair. Comparison of local, epidural, and general anesthesia. *NY State J Med* 79:1730–1733.
258. Teasdale C, et al. 1982. Aspects of treatment. A randomized controlled trial to compare local with general anesthesia for short stay inguinal hernia repair. *Ann R Coll Surg Engl* 64:238–242.
259. Raj PP. 1985. *Handbook of Regional Anesthesia.* New York: Churchill Livingstone.
260. Ponka JL. 1963. Seven steps to local anesthesia for inguinal or femoral hernia repair. *Surg Gynecol Obstet* 117:115–120.
261. Glassow WF. 1984. Inguinal hernia repair using local anesthesia. *Ann R Coll Surg Engl* 66:382–387.
262. Earle AS. 1960. Local anesthesia for inguinal herniorrhaphy. *Am J Surg* 100:782–786.
263 Nano M. 1983. Technique for inguinal hernia repair in the elderly patient. *Am J Surg* 146:373–375.
264. Glassow F. 1976. Short-stay surgery (Shouldice technique) for repair of inguinal hernia. *Ann R Coll Surg Engl* 58:133–139.
265. Rosenthal D, and Walters MJ. 1986. Preperitoneal synthetic mesh placement for recurrent hernias of the groin. *Surg Gynecol Obstet* 163:285–286.
266. Read RC. 1988. Preperitoneal herniorrhaphy. *Contemp Surg* 33:13–16.
267. Stoppa RE, et al. 1986. Prosthetic repair in the treatment of groin hernias. *Int Surg* 71:154–158.
268. Anderson BM, and Ostberg J. Long-term prognosis in geriatric surgery: 2–17 year followup of 7922 patients. *Am J Geriatr Surg* 20:255–258.
269. Gumbs MA, Pandya SG, and Kim YH. 1986. Obturator hernia. *NY State J Med* 86:150–151.
270. Gray GW, et al. 1974. Strangulated obturator hernia. *Surgery* 75:20–27.
271. Temple TF, and Miller RE. 1980. Incarcerated obturator hernia: Two case reports and review of the literature. *J Natl Med Assoc* 72:513–515.
272. Bachir JS. 1984. Obturator hernia. *Wisc Med J* 83:23–26.
273. Hershman MJ, Reilly DT, and Swift RL. 1986. Strangulated obturator hernia: Delayed diagnosis still the rule. *J R Coll Surg Edinb* 31:282–283.
274. Bragg WD, Weaver WL, and Hoover EL. 1989. Obturator hernias: A case report and literature review of a potentially lethal disorder. *Contemp Surg* 34:24–27.
275. Cubillo E. 1983. Obturator hernia diagnosed by computed tomography. *Am J Radiol* 140:735–736.
276. Persson NH, Bergqvist D, and Edberg O. 1987. Obturator hernia—clinical significance of radiologic diagnosis. *Acta Chir Scand* 153:361–364.
277. Hatfield PM, and Wise RE. 1976. *Radiology of the Gallbladder and Bile Ducts.* Baltimore, MD: Williams & Wilkins.
278. Roberts PL, et al. 1988. Ripstein procedure, Lahey Clinic experience 1963–1985. *Arch Surg* 123:554–557.
279. Lichtenstein IL, et al. 1988. Pain after hernia surgery. *Contemp Surg* 33:18–22.

32

Vascular Surgery in the Elderly

Robert G. Atnip

The discipline of vascular surgery is concerned with the management of all disease of the veins, arteries, and lymphatics, but in practical terms, atherosclerosis overshadows all other disorders seen by the vascular surgeon. Atherosclerosis is a degenerative disease of arteries, that is, it is a disease of aging. As such, it is the leading cause of mortality among all ages greater than 40 in Western civilization and exacts a nearly immeasurable toll in disability and premature death. Because it is a systemic disease, it is often the cause of dysfunction of multiple organ systems, with a predilection for vital organs, such as the brain, heart, and kidney. By its very nature, it is often accompanied by other disorders such as diabetes mellitus, hypertension, and blood lipid dyscrasias, all of which act in concert, if not synergistically, to accelerate organ failure and death.

The clinical spectrum of atherosclerosis encompasses patients who span a wide range of both chronologic and physiologic age. Because the population of individuals in the United States over 70 years old is steadily increasing, vascular surgeons are encountering growing numbers in this older age group with symptomatic arterial disease. Optimal management of these patients is based on a risk-benefit equation that is not fundamentally different from that encountered in other contexts. In essence, the risks conferred by the natural history of the disease must be compared to the risks of therapy. In addition, however, rational care of the elderly patient requires understanding of the influence of age on the course of the disease, on the prognosis of concomitant diseases, and on the patient's response to therapy.

Unfortunately, the information that the surgeon needs to make fully informed decisions is not always available. Individual patients may not behave according to statistical dictates. The management of each patient will therefore always require the exercise of clinical judgment, which must incorporate concern for the quality as well as the preservation of life. The goals of the surgeon are not only to prolong life, but also to preserve function and forestall disability.

It is the purpose of this chapter to establish what little organized information is available regarding the management of vascular diseases in the elderly, and to propose rational guidelines for optimal care of this burgeoning element of our society. Consideration will be given to both arterial and venous disorders, but the emphasis must naturally be placed on the clinical syndromes related to atherosclerosis.

Pathogenesis of Atherosclerosis

Although its cause is unknown, a large body of information is available regarding the pathologic evolution of atherosclerosis. It is a disease of the arterial intima, affecting large and medium-sized arteries almost exclusively. Atherosclerotic plaque is thought to begin as a localized mound-like thickening of the intima, which slowly expands in both surface area and thickness, gradually encroaching on the lumen of the artery and creating increasing resistance to blood flow. Though plaques may remain "simple" in morphology, they often undergo further degenerative changes such as hemorrhage within the lipid core of the plaque, ulceration of the overlying endothelium, and heterotopic calcification, and are then referred to as "complex" plaques.

A compelling body of experimental evidence would indicate that the development of the atherosclerotic plaque is a "response-to-injury" of the arterial wall (1) (Fig. 32-1). The agents that are capable of initiating the response are multiple, but the best known are cholesterol and low-density lipoprotein (2). Whatever the noxious stimulus, the final common pathway proposed by this theory is injury to the endothelium, with loss of the barrier function of that cellular monolayer, allowing entry of both molecular and cellular elements of the blood into the subendothelial connective tissue of the intima. According to the "response-to-injury" hypothesis, the process is reversible in this early stage, and healing of intima ensues if the injurious agent is removed. However, in the face of repetitive or continuous endothelial injury, the process evolves. The platelet, the blood monocyte, the endothelial cell, and the arterial smooth muscle cell are all thought to play a role in the subsequent cellular proliferation that occurs within the intima. All of these cells release mitogens, recruit inflammatory cells, and cause alterations in the intercellular matrix of the arterial wall (3). Cells within the early lesion then accumulate lipid, leading to the formation of a mature atherosclerotic plaque, with a lipid core and a fibrous, cellular envelope.

Arterial Occlusion

Arterial stenosis or occlusion is the most common clinical presentation of atherosclerosis. Most atherosclerotic plaques are eccentric, and there is evidence that affected arteries may undergo eccentric dilatation as a means of compensation for the encroachment of the plaque (4). Furthermore, the plaque must expand to occupy 75% of the luminal cross-sectional area before there will be a significant reduction in flow. Thus, atherosclerosis has generally progressed to an advanced stage by the time it produces

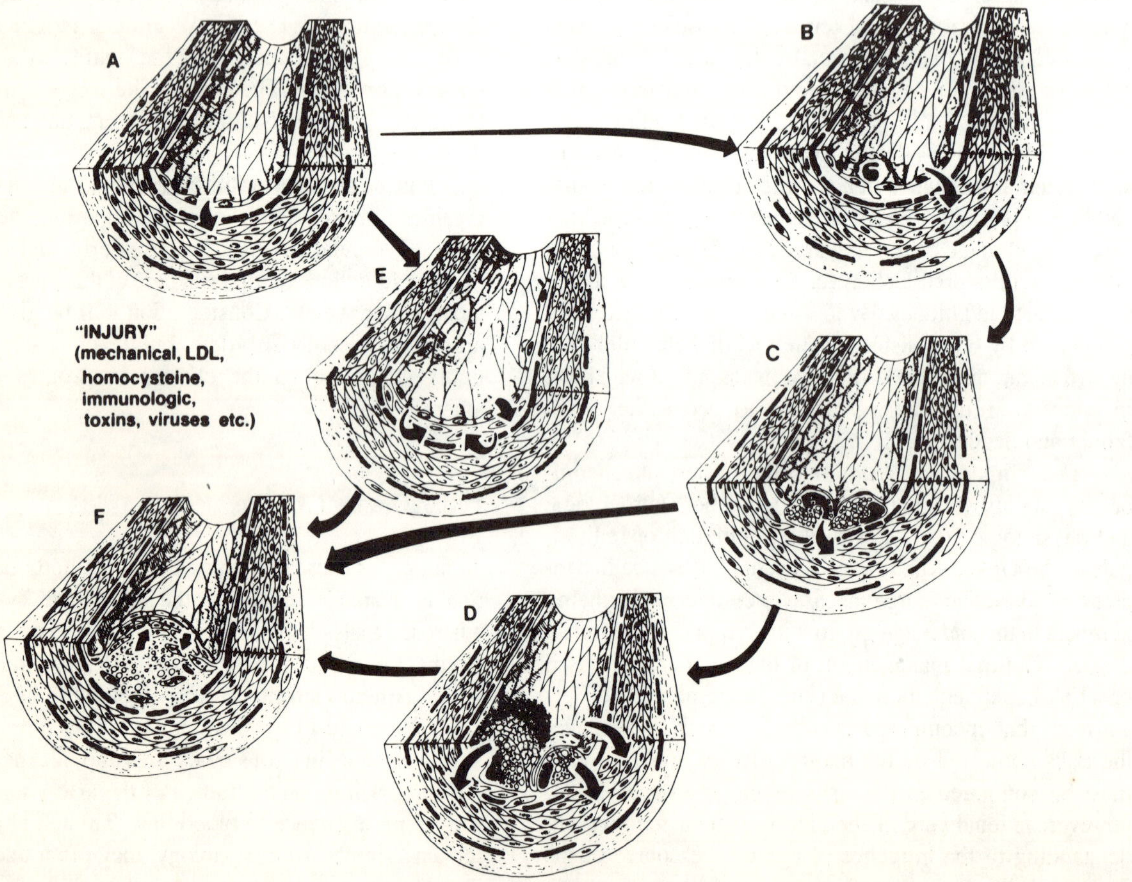

Figure 32-1. The Response-to-Injury Hypothesis. Advanced intimal proliferative lesions of atherosclerosis may occur by at least two pathways. In the clockwise sequence from *A* to *F,* intimal injury promotes monocyte attachment (*B*) and migration through the intima (*C*) with release of both monocyte- and endothelial-derived growth factors, and formation of a fatty streak. Platelet aggregation at lesion sites causes further cellular proliferation (*D*), as the lesion evolves into a fibrous plaque (*F*). In the second mechanism depicted by sequence *A-E-F* above, intimal injury leads directly to increased endothelial turnover (*E*), with secondary recruitment of smooth muscle cells from the media and formation of a proliferative lesion (*F*). (Reprinted with permission from Ross, R. 1986. The pathogenesis of atherosclerosis—an update. *N Engl J Med* 314: 488.)

symptoms of flow reduction. However, plaques may also produce symptoms through ulceration or intraplaque hemorrhage. Ulceration occurs when the endothelium and fibrous cap overlying some part of the plaque break down, exposing the lipid core to the bloodstream. Atheromatous debris may embolize to the distal arterial bed directly or may cause thrombosis at the site of the ulcer, leading either to local arterial occlusion or distal embolism. In a similar fashion, acute hemorrhage within the plaque (the cause of which is not well understood) can lead to sudden expansion or rupture of the plaque, again associated with local thrombosis or distal embolization. It is a useful generalization that slow expansion of atherosclerotic plaque leads to the syndromes of chronic organ ischemia, whereas plaque complications such as ulceration and hemorrhage result in more acute ischemic symptoms.

Atherosclerotic Aneurysms

In addition to arterial occlusion, atherosclerosis can result in the formation of degenerative aneurysms. The pathogenesis of aneurysm formation is very different from that of progressive arterial occlusion, although there is no recognizable morphologic difference in the atherosclerotic plaque of the two lesions. Aneurysms result from the progressive loss of collagen and elastin from the arterial wall. Increased collagenase and elastase activity has been well documented in aneurysm wall, but the exact cellular or humoral stimulus for this has not been defined (5,6). Aneurysms occur in a familial pattern more often than can be explained by the presence of atherosclerosis alone, and this observation has led to the supposition that deficiencies of collagen cross-linking enzymes may be responsible for aneurysm formation, at least in some circumstances (7).

Atherosclerotic aneurysms occur most commonly in the distal abdominal aorta, perhaps due to alterations in the lamellar architecture, or sparsity of vasa vasora in this segment (8). They may, however, occur in any segment of the aorta or in any other artery, commonly including the iliac, femoral, and popliteal arteries. As many as one half of patients with peripheral aneurysms will have concomitant aortic aneurysms.

It cannot be overemphasized that atherosclerosis is a complex, systemic disease. Patients may differ according to location, presentation, and rate of progression of the disease, but rarely is the pathologic process confined to a single arterial bed. This concept of multicentricity has readily apparent implications, as regards both the immediate and ultimate morbidity and mortality of patients with vascular disease. Although this chapter is organized according to specific syndromes of arterial disease, the approach of the clinician must be unified and not compartmentalized. And although age does not correlate absolutely with the severity of atherosclerosis, it correlates strongly with loss of organ reserve. Elderly patients must thus be treated with particular cognizance of the diffuse nature of their disease.

Preoperative Evaluation of the Elderly Patient

A general approach to preoperative evaluation has been described in detail in earlier chapters. For the elderly patient in need of arterial reconstruction, specific attention must be focused on the cardiovascular system, recognizing that myocardial ischemia accounts for the majority of perioperative and postoperative deaths among patients with peripheral vascular disease.

Preoperative evaluation begins with a thorough history and physical examination, but the absence of any history of cardiopulmonary symptoms may be deceiving in a patient who is sedentary or unable to exercise because of lower limb ischemia or general debility. Similarly, the routine electrocardiogram is a static and not a functional test, and has a correspondingly limited ability to predict the response of the myocardium to the stress of major surgery.

The need to define perioperative risk more precisely has led to the development of three diagnostic approaches for vascular surgical patients with known or suspected coronary artery disease. These are graded exercise treadmill testing, coronary arteriography, and dipyridamole-thallium imaging.

Graded treadmill exercise according to standard protocols should be employed for patients who have the capacity to exercise to the requisite heart rate. The test is *not* contraindicated in patients with asymptomatic aortic aneurysms. Patients with negative tests require no further evaluation, whereas those with equivocal or positive tests should be considered for coronary arteriography.

Cardiac catheterization and coronary arteriography are clearly indicated for patients with severe or unstable myocardial ischemia. Some vascular surgeons have advocated liberal use of this procedure for preoperative screening of all vascular surgical patients, particularly those in need of carotid artery or aortic operations, with the contention that agressive myocardial revascularization will reduce not only perioperative but also long-term mortality (9, 10). However, the validity of this approach remains unproven. Most cardiologists remain reluctant to advise coronary arteriography for patients without objective evidence of myocardial ischemia. The disadvantages of the procedure as a screening test include its risk and expense, and its inability to predict the functional response of the myocardial circulation to stress.

At present, it appears that the most promising approach is that of dipyridamole-thallium imaging, in which exercise is mimicked by the maximal vasodilatory effects of intravenous dipyridamole (Persantine®). There is compelling evidence that this procedure accurately identifies patients with reversible myocardial ischemia who are at greatest risk for perioperative myocardial events (11–13). Intravenous dipyridamole is expected to be approved and available for general use in the near future.

The management of patients with significant coronary artery disease (CAD) identified by preoperative screening remains the subject of debate. In an elderly population, the value of "prophylactic" coronary bypass surgery in prolonging life has not been demonstrated, and elderly patients generally experience higher perioperative morbidity and mortality from cardiac surgery. Acceptable indications for coronary bypass should be discussed among vascular and cardiac surgeons within each institution, and patients managed accordingly (14).

An additional issue that often arises during the preoperative evaluation of the elderly patient is that of the asymptomatic carotid bruit. Although noninvasive evaluation of the carotid arteries is warranted in such circumstances, the presence of a cervical bruit per se is not a risk factor for perioperative stroke after general or peripheral vascular operations (15). Those patients found to have significant carotid atherosclerosis should be managed according to the guidelines outlined in the following section.

Cerebrovascular Disease

Stroke is the second most common cause of death in patients over 70, and a much feared cause of major debility among the elderly population (16). Two-thirds of cerebral infarcts are believed to be the result of extracranial atherosclerotic occlusive disease, located principally at the bifurcations of the cervical carotid arteries (17). The association between carotid bifurcation atheroma and cervical bruit has become widely recognized, with a resultant steady increase in the number of patients being referred to vascular surgeons for evaluation of neck bruits.

Symptoms

For optimal management, patients with carotid atherosclerosis should be classified as either symptomatic or asymptomatic, based on the presence or absence of any history of cerebral ischemic events (Table 32-1). Such events may be classified as either amaurosis fugax, transient ischemic attack (TIA), residual ischemic neurologic deficit (RIND), or completed stroke. Amaurosis fugax, or transient monocular blindness, is defined as transient loss of vision in one eye, resolving in less than 24 hours, usually much sooner. A transient ischemic attack is a hemispheric neurologic deficit that resolves completely within 24 hours. A deficit that lasts more than 24 hours, but resolves within a few days, is classified as a RIND. Deficits that are permanent, or resolve over a period of weeks to months, are considered to be completed strokes. The vast majority of these events are thought to be the result of thromboemboli from carotid atheromata, but decreased cerebral blood flow may play a role in some patients (18). The determinants of regional cerebral blood flow and cerebral ischemia are poorly understood, and do not lend themselves to simplistic explanations.

Table 32-1. Frequency of symptoms in TIA

Distribution	Patients (%)
Carotid	
Paresis	61
Paresthesia	57
Monocular visual	32
Facial paresthesia	30
Facial paresis	22
Vertebrobasilar	
Binocular visual	57
Vertigo	50
Paresthesia	40
Diplopia	38
Ataxia	33
Paresis	33

Data from Canadian Cooperative Study Group: A randomized trial of aspirin and sulfinpyrazone in threatened stroke. *N Engl J Med* 299:53, 1978.

The classic symptoms of anterior cerebral hemispheric ischemia are contralateral motor and/or sensory deficits, often accompanied by speech difficulties. Deficits involving the face and hands are common because of the large areas of cerebral cortex devoted to these structures. Posterior or vertebrobasilar ischemic symptoms include diplopia, vertigo, ataxia, syncope, and drop attacks. A thorough history must be obtained to determine whether symptoms are truly consistent with focal cerebral ischemia. Because selection of proper therapy is dependent on accurate interpretation of the history, a neurologist should be consulted if there is doubt as to the source of the symptoms.

Diagnostic Evaluation

Patients with suspected extracranial carotid disease, whether symptomatic or not, should undergo noninvasive testing as the initial diagnostic procedure. The best currently available modality is the Duplex scan, which combines B-mode ultrasonic imaging of the carotid bifurcation with Doppler velocity spectral analysis. If performed by properly trained personnel, the test is highly accurate, easily repeatable, and provides both anatomic and hemodynamic information (19). Because of this latter feature, Duplex scanning is complementary to angiography, and it is the author's practice to obtain the test even in symptomatic patients who are slated to undergo angiography. Conversely, Duplex scanning may miss minimal lesions and shallow ulcerations capable of causing cerebral emboli, and thus a "normal" Duplex scan cannot suplant arteriography in the symptomatic patient.

Management of Symptomatic Patients

Patients with symptomatic carotid bifurcation atheroma face a substantial risk of stroke if untreated. The risk of stroke within two years after the onset of transient ischemic attacks is about 20%. A patient who has had a nonfatal stroke faces a 25% risk of suffering another stroke. The medical treatment options that are currently available—antiplatelet therapy and warfarin anticoagulation—have not been shown to reduce the incidence of stroke in these patients. On the other hand, carotid endarterectomy, in competent hands, can be performed with a combined perioperative mortality and stroke morbidity of 5% or less, and a late stroke incidence of 2% to 3% per year, clearly superior to the natural history of the disease or the best medical therapy.* It is thus the author's general opinion that carotid endarterectomy is the treatment of choice for patients with symptomatic carotid atherosclerosis. Furthermore, the data given in the following paragraph would seem to indicate that age per se is *not* a contraindication to operation.

There are no prospective studies comparing the morbidity and mortality of carotid endarterectomy in patients of different ages. However, in a retrospective study of nearly 20,000 major vascular procedures from the Cleveland Vascular Registry, carotid endarterectomy was the most commonly performed operation and carried no higher morbidity and mortality in the 3,259 patients over 75 years old. It was, in fact, the only procedure for which risk did not increase with age (20). Similar findings emerged in a study of 77 carotid endarterectomies performed in patients over 75 at the University of Rochester (21). In another report of 45 carotid endarterectomies in 42 patients aged 80 to 97, there was only one postoperative stroke and one cardiac death (22).

In a nonrandomized, retrospective comparison of 90 octogenarians who were treated surgically and 82 who were treated medically for cerebrovascular disease, there were 5 postoperative strokes (a rate of 6%), but the cumulative stroke incidence was significantly lower in the operated group (23). Of significance, these authors noted a fivefold higher incidence of *intracranial* vascular disease in their elderly study population compared to an unmatched younger population, and it was in those patients with intracranial disease that most of the perioperative and late strokes occurred.

It is not possible to conclude from the available data that *all* elderly patients with symptomatic carotid atheroma should undergo endarterectomy, and many physicians and surgeons will remain convinced that patients over 75 or 80 are "too old" for the operation. Dogmatism in either direction is imprudent. The total surgical risk should be assessed in each patient, with particular regard to cardiopulmonary factors. It is well recognized that coronary artery disease, and not stroke, is the leading cause of death in both operated and unoperated patients with carotid atherosclerosis. Patients with uncorrectable coronary disease or ischemic cardiomyopathies are thus unlikely to see any long-term benefit of carotid endarterectomy. The same might be true of patients with other advanced diseases. The best data would indicate, however, that a patient should not be denied operation on the basis of age alone.

Management of Asymptomatic Patients

Considerable therapeutic uncertainty faces the clinician in regard to the management of patients with asymptomatic carotid stenosis. The indications for endarterectomy in the asymptomatic patient are the subject of intense controversy among surgeons and neurologists, and two large randomized prospective trials are underway to determine whether these patients should be treated medically or surgically. Unfortunately, the issue has been clouded by conflicting data from a number of biased and poorly designed studies. Although it is impossible in this context to explore fully the arguments for and against surgery, an effort will be made to summarize them.

Although there has been a confounding lack of uniformity among the patient populations studied and the diagnostic methods used, most recent reports would indicate that, in general, patients with asymptomatic carotid stenosis face a low risk of subsequent stroke, probably less than 5% per year. However, there is suggestive evidence from two studies that certain subgroups may be at three-to-fourfold higher risk (24, 25). In each of these studies, large numbers of patients were followed prospectively with serial Duplex scans. The stroke risk was greatest in those patients with greater than 80% unilateral stenosis, severe bilateral carotid stenosis, severe stenosis and contralateral carotid occlusion, and carotid stenosis that progressed from less than 80% to greater than 80%.

*For an excellent review of the natural history and results of treatment of cerebrovascular disease, the reader is referred to Bernstein (48).

Furthermore, up to two-thirds of the strokes in these subgroups occurred without antecedent transient ischemic attacks. This latter fact lies at the crux of the argument that asymptomatic carotid stenosis should be treated by endarterectomy.

Carotid endarterectomy is a successful and appropriate therapy for asymptomatic stenosis only if it reduces the cumulative stroke risk of the affected patients. To accomplish this, it must be performed with a combined perioperative mortality and stroke morbidity of less than 5%. Proponents of "prophylactic" endarterectomy point out that experienced vascular surgeons are capable of achieving such results. Opponents claim that these optimal surgical results cannot be achieved on a national basis, and point to community-wide statistics from large metropolitan areas that reveal distressingly high perioperative morbidity and mortality.* Carefully conducted multicenter trials are needed to answer the question; however, it is most disturbing that the issue is moving out of the scientific arena, as large insurance carriers in several states have decided to withhold reimbursement for prophylactic carotid endarterectomy.

Because of this escalating controversy, it is the author's opinion that elderly patients with asymptomatic carotid stenosis should be advised to undergo endarterectomy only for well-defined indications. All of these patients should undergo an initial Duplex scan. Patients with severe bilateral disease as defined above should be evaluated as operative candidates. Patients with unilateral disease, even if severe, should be placed on antiplatelet therapy and followed with serial Duplex scans every 3 to 6 months. Those with documented disease progression should be considered for operation. The ultimate decision to proceed with endarterectomy will depend on the patient's general medical condition and his own desires. The surgeon must be willing to constantly re-evaluate the indications for surgery as new information becomes available.

Operative and Postoperative Management

The techniques of carotid endarterectomy are amply described in other texts and will not be reviewed here. There is no evidence that decisions to employ shunts or patch angioplasty should be made differently in elderly patients than in younger ones.

All patients who have undergone carotid endarterectomy must be followed with periodic postoperative Duplex scans, both to assess the status of the unoperated vessel, and to detect recurrent carotid stenosis, a potential cause of late stroke. Although some degree of recurrent stenosis may be detected in as many as 25% of patients, severe restenosis requiring reoperation occurs in 5% or less of cases (26).

Role of Arteriography

Clarification must be made regarding the optimal utilization of carotid arteriography in the management of cerebrovascular disease. The arterigogram has three functions: to serve as a "road map" for surgery, to define the extent of intracranial disease, and to define the patterns of collateral circulation in patients with severe carotid stenosis or occlusion. As an invasive procedure, angiography should be performed only after the decision to operate has been made on the basis of the patient's history and/or Duplex scan. A patient who is not a candidate for carotid endarterectomy should not be subjected to carotid angiography. Only rarely, in a patient with ambiguous symptoms or an equivocal Duplex scan, is arteriography needed to determine whether there is sufficient carotid bifurcation disease to explain the patient's symptoms.

When arteriography is indicated, the desired information can generally be obtained by digital imaging techniques, with injection of contrast into the aortic arch (Fig. 32-2). Selective carotid injections are occasionally needed for better resolution, but the digital modality allows this to be done with small volumes of contrast. Digital imaging, the availability of nonionic contrast media, the use of smaller catheters, and the Seldinger technique have combined to make carotid angiography an extremely low-risk procedure. Studies can often be done in the outpatient setting, even in elderly patients.

Intra-*arterial* digital angiography should not be confused with intra*venous* digital imaging. This latter technique was at one time acclaimed as a valuable screening procedure for carotid stenosis, but requires large volumes of contrast and gives unacceptably poor resolution in elderly patients. In essence, it has no place in the management of carotid disease.

Brachiocephalic Occlusive Disease

Atherosclerotic occlusive disease of the innominate, subclavian, and common carotid arteries is common in elderly patients, but due to the abundant collateral networks of the brain and upper extremities, it is rare for such lesions to cause clinically significant symptoms (27, 28). In most large centers, the number of operations for proximal disease of the aortic arch branches is only a small fraction of the number for carotid bifurcation atheroma. In elderly

*For an enlightening discussion of the controversy surrounding prophylactic carotid endarterectomy, see Archie, JP, Jr, and Batson, RC, 1984. Advocates in vascular controversies. *Surgery* 95:739–746.

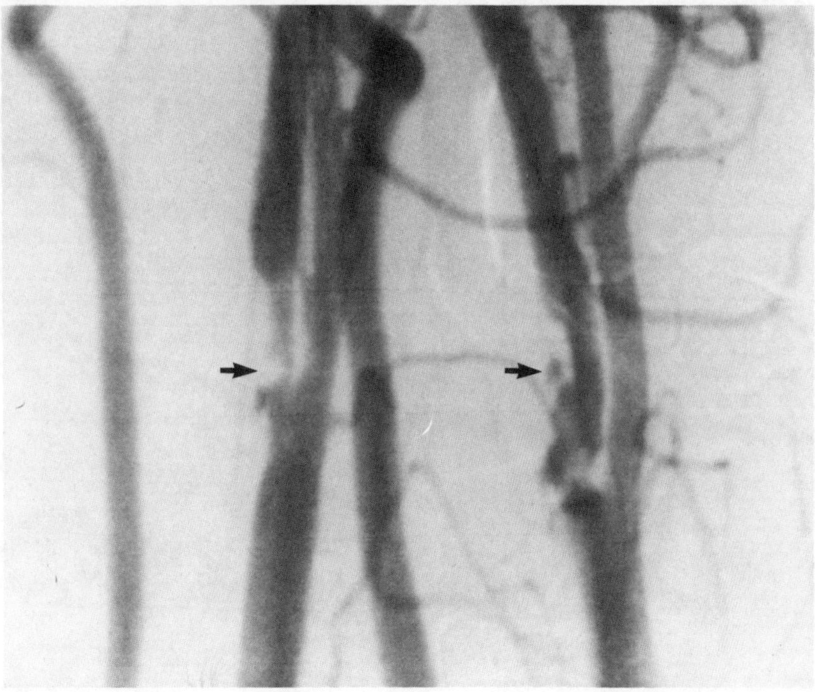

Figure 32-2. Intra-arterial digital subtraction angiogram of the cervical carotid arteries revealing severe bilateral ulcerative lesions (*arrows*). Note the quality and resolution of the images.

patients, giant cell arteritis must always be considered in the diagnosis of cerebral and upper extremity ischemia.

Cerebral Symptoms

The single most common site of atherosclerotic disease in these vessels is the origin of the left subclavian artery, followed in decreasing frequency by the right subclavian, the innominate, and the carotids (29). Correspondingly, the best-known symptom complex is that known as the "subclavian steal" syndrome, in which severe stenosis or occlusion of the proximal subclavian artery creates a gradient for reversal of flow in the vertebral artery, precipitating symptoms of posterior fossa ischemia (vertigo, ataxia, diplopia), classically after arm exercise. However, radiographically demonstrable reversal of vertebral flow occurs in many patients who have no symptoms (Fig. 32-3), and some patients with classic symptoms do not have reversal of flow. These observations have created considerable confusion in the use of the term "subclavian steal." Such poor correlation between pathologic anatomy and symptoms is typical of brachiocephalic occlusive disease.

Patients with lesions of the aortic arch branches may also exhibit symptoms of hemispheric cerebral ischemia. Frequently such patients will be found to have concomitant disease at the carotid bifurcations, and carotid endarterectomy alone has been reported to relieve symptoms (27, 30). Most vascular surgeons would thus agree that symptomatic patients with simultaneous stenoses of the proximal common carotid and carotid bifurcation should undergo standard carotid endarterectomy prior to or in conjunction with more proximal reconstruction.

Upper Extremity Symptoms

Upper extremity ischemic symptoms are uncommon, even with severe stenosis or occlusion of the innominate or subclavian arteries. Some patients may notice mild to moderate arm claudication or easy fatigability, but resting ischemia is extremely uncommon. Resting ischemic symptoms are usually manifested as digital ischemia or ulceration, which may be due to reduction in total arm blood flow, but is more commonly embolic in origin. Distal emboli cause cyanotic, ulcerated fingertip lesions very similar to the "blue toe" syndrome of lower extremity atheroembolic disease. Arm claudication does not generally warrant brachiocephalic reconstruction unless it is disabling. In contrast, peripheral embolization is a harbinger of ischemic limb loss, and is thus a compelling indication for arteriography and vascular repair.

Surgical Management

There are two surgical approaches to management of symptomatic brachiocephalic occlusive disease: the direct

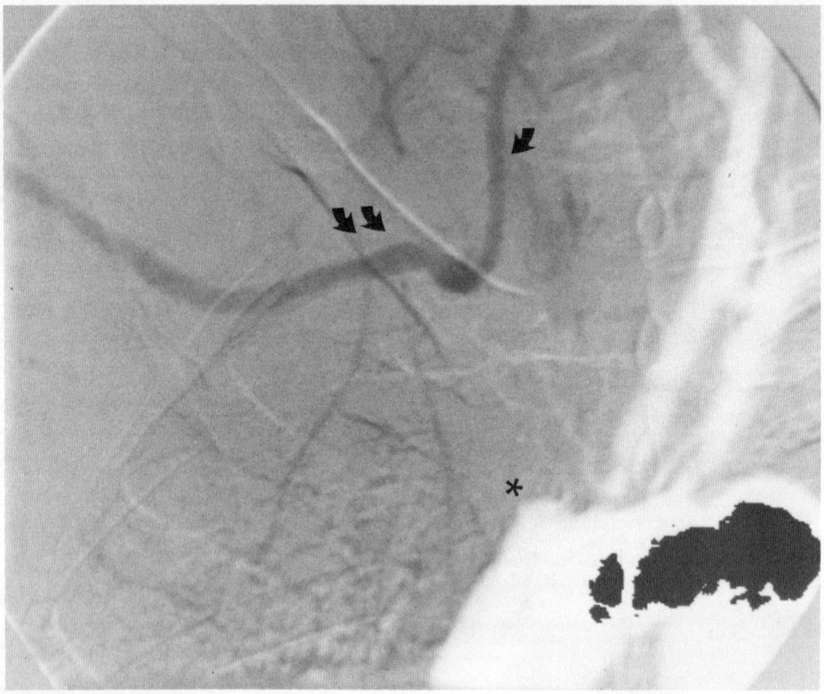

Figure 32-3. "Subclavian steal." The right vertebral artery (*arrow*) fills retrograde to reconstitute the right subclavian artery (*double arrow*). The innominate artery is occluded at its origin (*asterisk*). The patient had no symptoms.

or transthoracic approach, and the extrathoracic or extra-anatomic approach.

The innominate and left common carotid arteries are accessible through a median sternotomy incision; the proximal left subclavian is best exposed through a high left thoracotomy. When approached in this fashion, endarterectomy or anatomic bypass of these vessels can be readily accomplished by the experienced surgeon. Alternatively, if the disease is confined to one subclavian or carotid vessel, reconstruction can be carried out by "extra-anatomic" bypass or transposition, using the ipsilateral uninvolved artery as the inflow. Such procedures are performed through a neck or supraclavicular incision, without entry into the mediastinum or thorax. The carotid-subclavian bypass is the most commonly employed example of this technique (Figs. 32-4 and 32-5).

If the disease is in the innominate artery or involves multiple vessels, the surgeon will generally be forced to use a trans-sternal approach. Endarterectomy and anatomic bypass are, in fact, more durable procedures than extra-anatomic bypass, but they also carry a substantially higher risk of technical complications and cardiac death, particularly in poor-risk patients. For these reasons, the extrathoracic approach is much preferred in the elderly patient (31–34).

Lower Extremity Ischemia

Atherosclerosis of the arteries supplying the lower extremities is extremely common. Although many patients with disease of the lower extremity vessels have only minor symptoms, a substantial number of them will develop limb-threatening ischemia and ultimately face major amputation. The vast majority of leg amputations for ischemia are performed in patients over 60 years old, individuals for whom the loss of limb has grave physical, psychologic, and social implications (35, 36).

Lower extremity ischemia may be the result of either acute or chronic arterial occlusion. Because the pathophysiology, evaluation, treatment, and prognosis of these two entities differ substantially, each will be discussed separately.

Acute Arterial Occlusion

Acute arterial occlusion is the result of either embolism or thrombosis of a pre-existent arterial lesion, usually an atherosclerotic plaque. In reference to the lower extremities, it may involve any artery from the aorta to the digital vessels. The abrupt decrease in perfusion to the affected vascular bed generally results in profound isch-

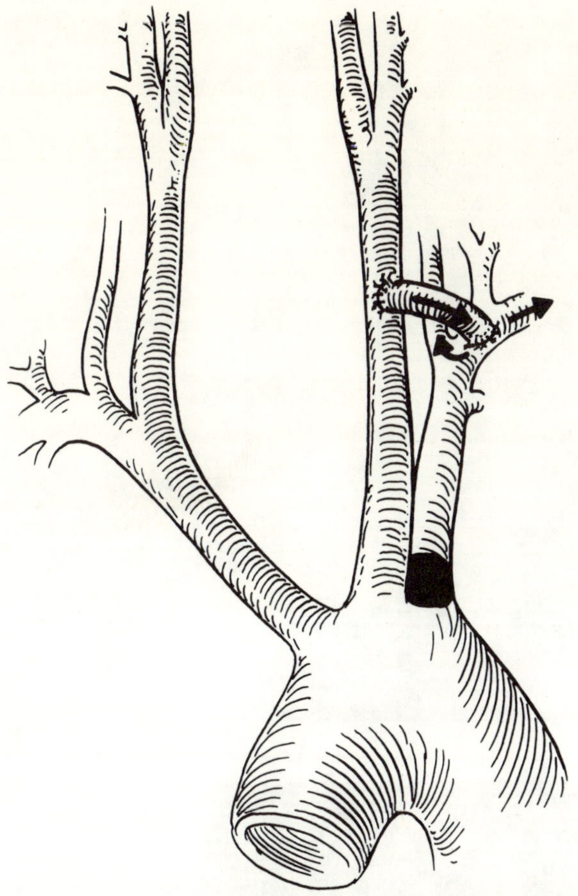

Figure 32-4. Carotid-subclavian bypass in a patient with occlusion of the left subclavian artery. Arrows illustrate direction of flow through the graft and vertebral artery. (Reprinted with permission from Moore, WS, and Quinones-Baldrich, WJ. 1983. Extracranial cerebrovascular disease. In *Vascular Surgery: A Comprehensive Review,* Ed., WS Moore. Orlando, FL: Grune & Stratton. Inc.)

emia, leading to the classical clinical syndrome of the "Five P's"—pain, pallor, paralysis, pulselessness, and paresthesias (Table 32-2). If adequate perfusion is not restored within a few hours, there is a high probability of subsequent tissue necrosis and limb loss.

Embolism

Eighty-five to ninety percent of emboli to the arteries supplying the lower limbs arise from the heart, primarily in patients with chronic atrial fibrillation (37). Noncardiac sources of emboli include aortic aneurysms and severe atheromatous plaques. Atherosclerotic heart disease has replaced rheumatic heart disease as the most common underlying cardiac pathology in these patients, and thus the average age of patients with arterial embolism has increased from 50 years to nearly 70 years old (37).

The diagnosis of embolism is suggested in a patient with acute arterial occlusion who has atrial fibrillation, gives no prior history of chronic ischemic symptoms such as claudication, and has a normal vascular exam in the unaffected limb. However, these criteria are not absolutely reliable in differentiating embolism from thrombosis, and in confusing cases, arteriography should be employed (38).

Surgical management of arterial embolism was greatly simplified by the introduction of the Fogarty embolectomy catheter in 1963, enabling the surgeon to perform embolectomy under local anesthesia in many cases. Yet in spite of technical improvements and advances in critical care medicine, there has been virtually no change over the past few decades in the 25% to 30% postoperative mortality associated with major arterial embolectomy. This figure reflects in part the severity of the underlying disease, but is also a result of the profound systemic metabolic changes that may be produced by reperfusion of severely ischemic limbs (39).

Optimal management of embolic arterial occlusion is based on the severity and duration of the ischemia. Severity is judged primarily by the neurologic status of the limb, but also by cutaneous findings such as pallor, mottling, cyanosis, or frank gangrene. The more profound the motor and sensory neurologic deficit, the greater the urgency to restore perfusion to the limb. On the other hand, advanced cutaneous changes signify that the ischemia is both severe and longstanding, and portend a poor prognosis for limb salvage. Limb swelling, muscle turgor, and rigor are additional adverse prognostic signs. Attempts to salvage such limbs are seldom justified in elderly or poor-risk patients, who are likely to die from rhabdomyolysis and its attendant complications. In these patients, primary amputation is the treatment of choice.

Therapy for limb salvage is indicated in patients whose ischemia has not produced irreversible neurologic or myocutaneous injury. Although 6 hours is often quoted as the tolerable limit of skeletal muscle to warm ischemia (40), clinical decisions should be based on assessment of the individual patient according to the signs listed in the preceding paragraph.

The author believes that prompt embolectomy remains the treatment of choice for embolic arterial occlusion associated with severe ischemia. Patients with lesser degrees of ischemia are also candidates for embolectomy, but anticoagulation with heparin alone has yielded favorable results in this group, particularly those who are deemed poor operative risks (41). Intra-arterial infusion of thrombolytic agents represents another alternative in patients for whom time is not of the essence and in whom there is no contraindication to the use of these drugs. However, thrombolytic therapy does carry a higher risk of

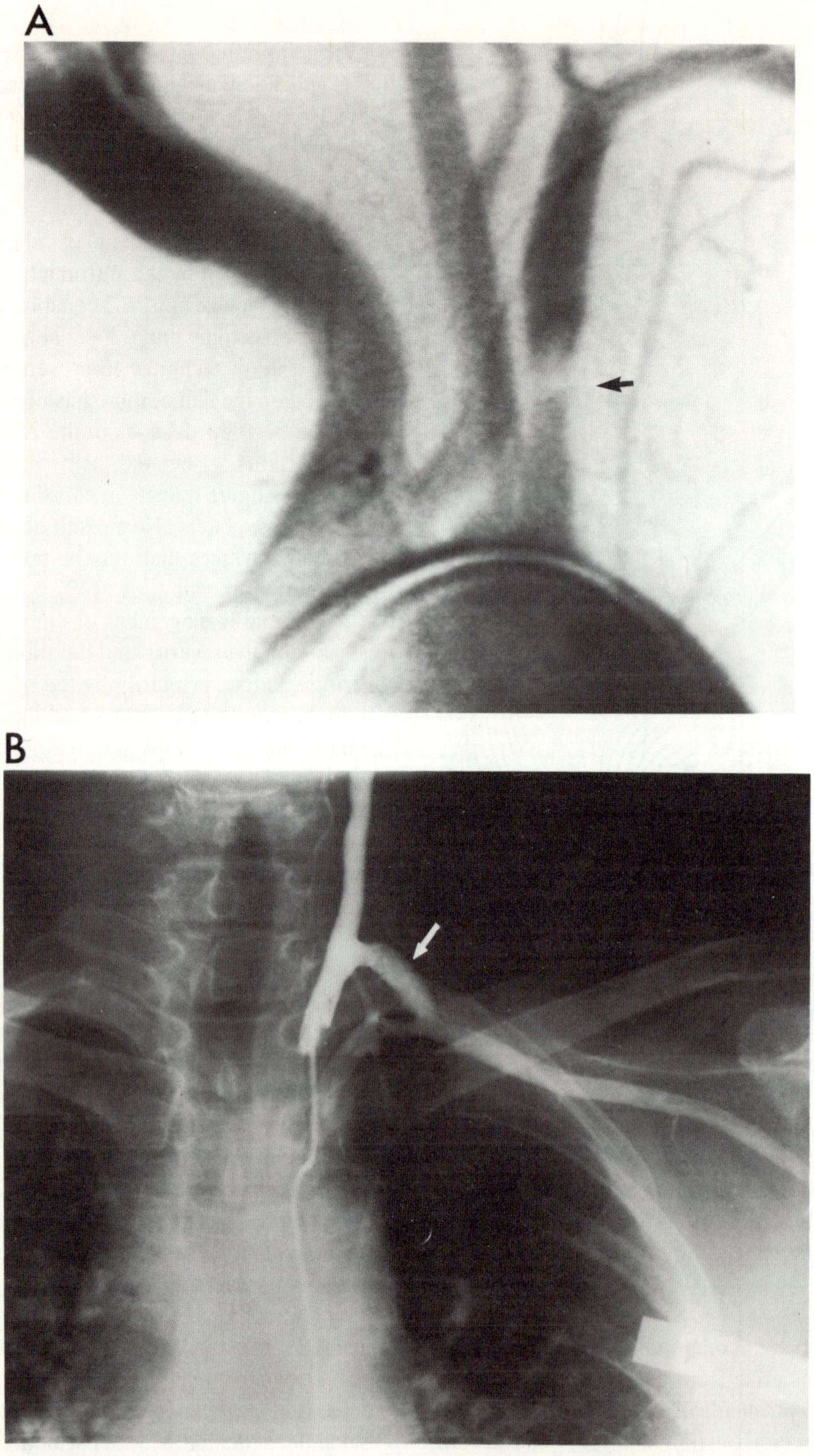

Figure 32-5. *A*, Digital angiogram depicting severe left subclavian artery stenosis (*arrow*) in a patient with emboli to the left hand. *B*, Postoperative arteriogram showing Dacron carotid-subclavian graft (*arrow*).

major bleeding complications in older patients (42, 43). Limited success and a substantial incidence of bleeding complications have dampened the enthusiasm of many vascular surgeons for the use of thrombolytic drugs (44).

All patients who have had major arterial embolism must be anticoagulated for life unless there are compelling contraindications. It has been well documented that recurrent emboli to the limbs and vital organs cause a dra-

Table 32-2. Acute arterial occlusion

Symptoms and signs
Pain
Paresthesias
Paralysis
Pallor
Pulselessness

matic increase in morbidity and mortality in patients who are not permanently anticoagulated (45).

Thrombosis

Acute arterial thrombosis may be due to trauma, aneurysm, or atherosclerotic plaque. The diagnosis is suggested on the basis of history and physical exam, but differentiation from embolism may be difficult on clinical grounds alone. The clinician should make liberal use of angiography to differentiate these two causes of acute arterial occlusion and to choose the proper therapy.

Unlike embolism, arterial thrombosis generally cannot be managed by clot extraction alone, since the underlying arterial lesion will tend to cause rethrombosis. Arterial reconstruction by graft replacement or bypass is the definitive treatment and should be considered for all patients who are acceptable operative risks and have reversible ischemia. The timing of operation is dictated by the severity and duration of ischemia, based on the same criteria used in cases of embolism. Patients who do not require immediate operation, and those who are prohibitive operative risks, should be anticoagulated with heparin. This drug should be used as adjunctive therapy to prevent propagation of clots in patients who undergo operation. Direct intra-arterial infusion of fibrinolytic agents may be effective in selected patients, either alone or in conjunction with percutaneous angioplasty. Endovascular technologies will also find a role in the management of acute arterial thrombosis.

In most series, the mortality of acute arterial thrombosis is lower than that of embolism, but it is of note that the data from the Cleveland Vascular Registry demonstrated a mortality of 25% to 30% for patients over 75 who suffered acute arterial occlusion, regardless of cause (20). The metabolic complications of prolonged ischemia and reperfusion figure prominently in the lethality of this condition in elderly patients. It had been the author's experience that the diagnosis of limb ischemia is usually delayed in older patients, especially those who are institutionalized. By the time the patient is brought to medical attention, amputation is frequently the only reasonable alternative.

Amputation is more commonly required for acute arterial thrombosis than for embolism, reflecting the more diffuse arterial disease associated with acute thrombosis. In addition, both early and long-term results of emergency arterial reconstruction are generally poorer than the results of elective bypass procedures (38). There are several intuitively obvious explanations for this disparity, but clearly the need for emergency operation implies the presence of severe ischemia, which *a priori* confers a poorer prognosis.

Chronic Lower Extremity Ischemia

Arterial occlusion that develops gradually is tolerated much better than that which occurs suddenly. Because of collateral circulation, adequate resting perfusion is maintained to the distal extremity in the vast majority of patients with single-segment chronic occlusive disease. Many of these patients will have no symptoms at all; however, in some, the collateral bed will be unable to meet the perfusion requirements of exercise, and exertional muscular ischemia will develop, manifested as *intermittent claudication*. In patients with multisegmental occlusion or poor collateral development, perfusion may be compromised to the extent that resting ischemia occurs. *Ischemic rest pain* will develop, and may progress to *ischemic ulceration* or *gangrene*.

Intermittent claudication is a remarkably benign symptom, in that 80% of claudicants will never progress to resting ischemia if risk factors such as cigarette smoking are eliminated. With exercise, which stimulates collateral formation, some may even improve. Only 5% to 8% of claudicants ultimately require amputation; thus, claudication is not considered a limb-threatening disorder (46).

In contrast, patients who present with ischemic rest pain, ulceration, or gangrene face a 40% chance of major amputation within a year after onset, and for many, the risk is immediate. Because of this very significant difference in natural history, resting ischemia is considered an absolute indication for arterial reconstruction, whereas surgery is indicated for claudication only it if is progressive or disabling (47).

It has been repeatedly shown that patients with symptoms of chronic lower extremity ischemia are more likely to die of myocardial infarction than to suffer limb loss. This statement, although an inescapable reminder of the diffuse nature of atherosclerosis, should nonetheless not be viewed as an argument against surgery for limb salvage. Survival cannot be accurately predicted in individual patients, and the physical and psychological debility resulting from limb loss warrant reasonable efforts to prevent it; however, limb can never take precedence over life. In high-risk patients, including the elderly, surgery for limb ischemia must be undertaken for only the strictest indications.

Diagnosis

A careful history and physical exam will suggest the diagnosis of arterial insufficiency, but confirmation that symptoms are truly ischemic in origin requires noninvasive physiologic testing. Resting perfusion may be accurately assessed using a combination of segmental Doppler pressures and segmental air plethysmography, often referred to as pulse volume recordings or PVRs (Fig. 32-6). The clinician can obtain systolic ankle pressures with only a standard blood pressure cuff and a Doppler flow probe. Elderly and diabetic patients with arterial medial calcinosis may have falsely elevated segmental pressures, and in such patients, plethysmography will more accurately reflect diminished perfusion. Toe pressures and perfusion at sites of ulcers can be assessed with infrared photoplethysmography (PPG) probes. Extensive discussion of all these techniques and their interpretation can be found in Bernstein (48). Duplex scanning is becoming an increasingly useful tool as well, in the evaluation of the lower limb arteries.

Patients whose primary complaint is exertional limb pain must be evaluated both at rest and after treadmill exercise (Fig. 32-7). A significant fall in ankle pressure will occur after exercise in those patients with arterial insufficiency.

The role of arteriography in the evaluation of chronic lower extremity ischemia is misunderstood by many clinicians. Arteriography provides anatomic information that is essential to the planning of arterial operations, but the angiographic findings correlate only qualitatively with blood flow and with the severity of limb ischemia. Angiography is a static test that does not answer the dynamic question of whether blood flow is adequate. It should be employed only if reduced perfusion has already been demonstrated by physiologic testing. Arteriography can help determine whether arterial reconstruction is technically feasible but arteriographic findings must never be

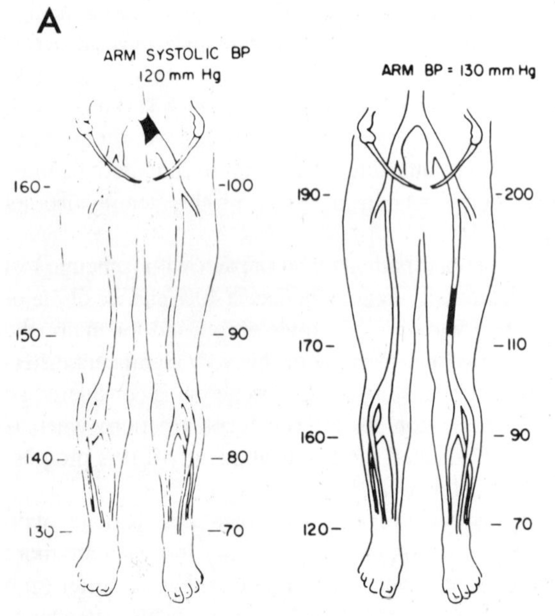

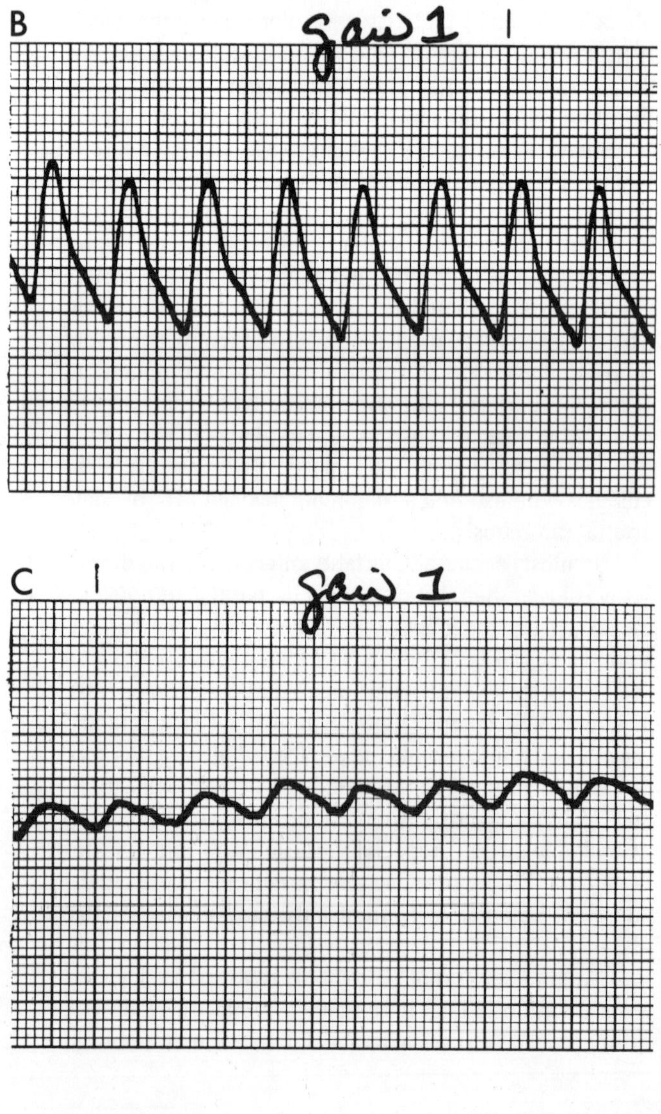

Figure 32-6. Segmental arterial pressures and plethysmography. *A*, Representative segmental pressures in patients with hypothetical iliac and femoral occlusions. *B*, A normal pulse volume recording with good amplitude and brisk upstroke. *C*, An abnormal pulse volume recording with poor amplitude and sine-wave configuration indicative of moderate to severe arterial obstruction.

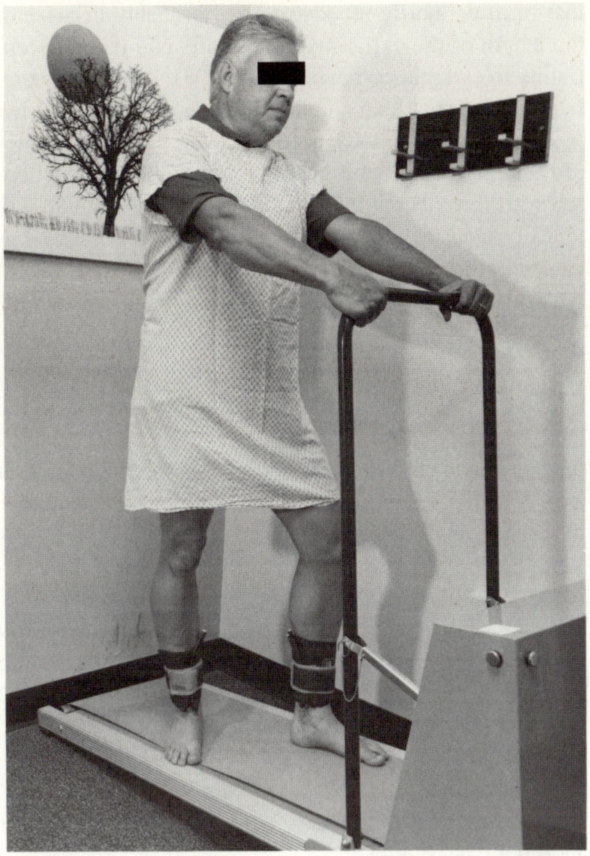

Figure 32-7. A standard treadmill for evaluating patients with exertional lower limb symptoms. Segmental pressures are obtained before and after exercise.

interpreted outside of the clinical context. Angiography, which is both invasive and expensive, is generally not indicated until the need for surgery has already been established in a patient who is an acceptable operative risk.

High-quality arteriography is a prerequisite to successful vascular surgery. It is mandatory that the surgeon work in close conjunction with the vascular radiologist to ensure that each study is complete.

Methods of Reconstruction

Although lower extremity atherosclerosis is occasionally diffuse, it tends more often to be segmental. It is useful clinically to classify patients according to this segmental distribution of the disease. Four "patterns" of disease have been identified—aortoiliac, femoropopliteal, popliteal-tibial, and combined. The pattern of disease generally defines the treatment options that are available.

Aortoiliac occlusive disease. Occlusive disease of the distal aorta and iliac arteries most commonly produces intermittent claudication of the thighs and buttocks. In the male, infrarenal aortic occlusion produces the LeRiche syndrome of claudication, impotence, and atrophy of the leg muscles (Fig. 32-8). Ischemic ulceration and gangrene are uncommon in the absence of associated distal occlusive disease.

Reconstructive options are listed in Table 32-3. Aortoiliac endarterectomy should only be employed in patients with well-localized disease in the aorta and common iliac arteries. It is technically demanding, but has a major advantage in avoiding the use of prosthetic graft and the attendant risk of infection (49).

Percutaneous transluminal angioplasty has proven to be a safe, effective and durable method of relieving discrete segmental stenoses of the iliac vessels (50). Newer technologies such as laser angioplasty and percutaneous atherectomy may eventually complement the use of percutaneous angioplasty for more extensive aortoiliac disease.

At present, however, endarterectomy and angioplasty are applicable to only a minority of patients. The majority have such extensive disease that ischemia can only be alleviated by prosthetic bypass. Such reconstructions can be accomplished either by direct or extra-anatomic methods.

Direct reconstruction for aortoiliac occlusive disease is generally accomplished by aortobifemoral bypass, using either Dacron or PTFE (expanded polytetrafluoro-

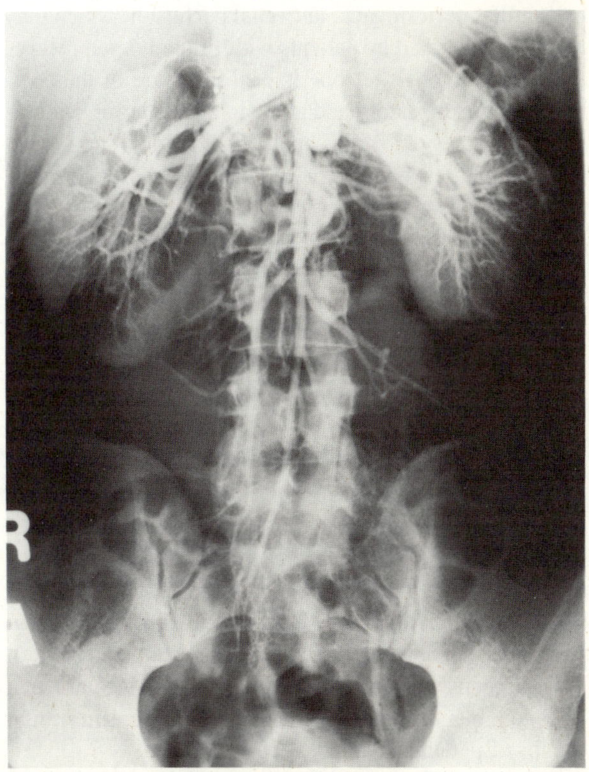

Figure 32-8. Atherosclerotic chronic occlusion of the infrarenal aorta in a patient with Leriche syndrome.

Table 32-3. Aortoiliac occlusive disease

Reconstructive options
1. Aortoiliac endarterectomy
2. Aortofemoral bypass
3. Percutaneous angioplasty
4. Extra-anatomic bypass

ethylene) prosthesis. Dacron has been in use for 25 to 30 years and has proven durability, whereas a substantial long-term experience with PTFE is only now being accumulated. Nonetheless, each material is considered acceptable, and selection of prosthesis is usually based on personal preference. The long-term patency of aortobifemoral bypass is excellent, ranging from 70% to 80% at 10 years in virtually all large series, with operative mortality rates of 2% to 5%.

Patients with aortoiliac occlusive disease are younger on the average than those with either aneurysms or femoropopliteal disease (51), and little comparative information is available regarding the risks of aortobifemoral bypass in the elderly. Existing data would support the general impression that there is a substantial added risk with increasing age (20, 51, 52). Not surprisingly, this parallels the age-associated risk of aortic surgery for aneurysms, as discussed later in this chapter. Aortic cross-clamping is know to initiate changes in hemodynamics, myocardial performance, and renal perfusion, which may be poorly tolerated by patients with limited organ reserve (53, 54). Although retroperitoneal exposure of the aorta may reduce respiratory and gastrointestinal complications of aortic surgery (55), this approach does not alter the hemodynamic response to aortic clamping. In contrast, techniques designed to reduce aortic cross-clamp time appear to improve outcome in high-risk patients (56).

Most surgeons remain hesitant to perform direct aortic reconstruction in elderly patients, and rely instead on extra-anatomic procedures such as axillofemoral and femorofemoral bypass. These operations are generally considered to be safer methods of aortoiliac bypass, because they do not require entry into the body cavities or clamping of the aorta. Paradoxically, most series of extra-anatomic aortic reconstructions have had significantly *higher* mortality rates than those of aortofemoral bypass, but this fact merely underscores the poor condition of patients for whom the extra-anatomic approach is chosen. Because of convincing evidence that extra-anatomic bypass is less durable than aortofemoral bypass (see below), few surgeons will offer it to their good-risk patients. Thus, comparative studies of the two operations in similar groups of patients have not been performed.

The chief disadvantage of axillofemoral and femorofemoral bypass is that tong-term patency is poorer than that of direct aortic reconstruction, probably because of the length of the extra-anatomic grafts and their susceptibility to external compression (57, 58). Axillobifemoral bypass performs better than unilateral axillofemoral bypass in this regard, undoubtedly due to higher flow rates (59). Regardless of the geometry of the reconstruction, repeated thrombectomy may be required to maintain extended patency. Nevertheless, extra-anatomic bypass is currently the preferred operation for the high-risk patient with severe aortoiliac disease, including many patients who are elderly.

Femoropopliteal occlusive disease. Atherosclerotic occlusion of the femoral and popliteal arteries is the most common cause of lower extremity ischemic symptoms. Isolated chronic occlusion of the superficial femoral artery, while quite common, seldom results in limb-threatening ischemia. Rest pain and tissue loss may supervene, however, it there is concomitant disease of the common femoral, profunda femoris, or popliteal arteries.

Table 32-4 lists the reconstructive options for arterial disease at these levels. Endarterectomy has not proven to be either highly successful or durable below the inguinal ligament. Endovascular technologies hold some promise for selected patients, but do not yet have established long-term durability (60). Most patients with advanced infrainguinal occlusive disease will require arterial bypass for relief of ischemia.

Femoropopliteal bypass. In patients with chronic occlusion of the superficial femoral artery, patency of the popliteal artery is often preserved by collateral flow through the profunda femoris to the geniculate branches of the popliteal artery. Femoropopliteal bypass procedures have been in use for almost 40 years and have a well-established record of favorable long-term patency and limb salvage.

Much has been written about the influence of factors such as site of distal anastomosis and patency of tibial vessels on the outcome of femoropopliteal reconstruction. Although these elements must be taken into account, the variable that has the greatest effect on patency and limb salvage is the type of conduit used for the bypass. In this regard, autogenous saphenous vein provides results that are far superior to any prosthetic material and is une-

Table 32-4. Femoropopliteal occlusive disease

Reconstructive options
1. Femoropopliteal bypass
2. Endarterectomy
3. Isolated popliteal segment bypass
4. Femorotibial bypass
5. Profundaplasty
6. Percutaneous angioplasty

quivocally the conduit of choice for any infrainguinal arterial reconstruction. At the femoropopliteal level, there is no convincing evidence that *in situ* or "nonreversed" configurations of the vein yield better results than reversed vein grafts. In the absence of technical error, autogenous vein grafts offer 5-year patency and limb salvage rates of 75% to 80% (61). The utility of these procedures in elderly patients is discussed further in the next section.

Popliteal-tibial disease. Because single-segment arterial disease seldom produces resting ischemia in the leg and because elderly patients are generally not considered for operation in the *absence* of resting ischemia, it follows that most older patients who come to arterial reconstruction will have multisegmental disease. The most common pattern encountered is combined femoropopliteal and tibial disease. Also commonly found, especially among diabetic patients, is extensive occlusion of the tibial and peroneal arteries in the face of minimally diseased proximal vessels. Such patients may have advanced ischemic lesions of the feet, but yet have palpable popliteal pulses. In the author's experience, elderly patients with tibial vessel occlusive disease, either alone or in combination with femoropopliteal disease, are comprising a steadily growing part of vascular surgical practice. In general, the surgeon has only two options for the treatment of such patients: amputation, or bypass to a tibial or pedal artery.

The feasibility of distal bypass in the leg is largely the result of the development of the *in situ* saphenous vein bypass (62). Although some authors claim that reversed vein grafts are equally successful for distal bypass (63), the *in situ* method has become the standard technique, with very high vein utilization rates and excellent patency and limb salvage rates documented by numerous authors.

The highly favorable performance of autogenous vein, particularly for very distal bypasses, derives from its intact endothelial lining and associated fibrinolytic capabilities, which allow the vein to resist thrombosis, even at low flow rates. These properties allow the technique to be applied to patients whose only patent recipient vessels are the arteries of the foot. Grafts to the dorsalis pedis artery and posterior tibial artery or even to their first order branches are technically feasible, and, in the author's experience, highly successful for limb salvage. Other authors have had similarly favorable results with bypasses at and beyond the ankle, provided that autogenous vein was available as the conduit (64).

The utility of distal bypass in older patients is affirmed by several reports in the literature. In Buchbinder's series just cited, the authors achieved an 80% limb salvage rate at 2 years in 47 patients, about half of whom were 70 or older, with *no* postoperative deaths. Scher and colleagues (65) performed 156 femoropopliteal and femorotibial bypasses for limb salvage in a group of patients over 80 years old, with a life-table limb salvage rate of 74% at 2 years. Their perioperatvie mortality was only 6%, and among the group of late deaths, 76% had intact limbs. The data from the Cleveland Vascular Registry showed a similar operative mortality of 6.7% in older patients undergoing lower extremity bypass and an overall amputation rate equal to that of younger patients (6.4% versus 6.6%) (20). Comparable results were also obtained by Edwards et al. (22) and Hines (66). In all series, both early and late deaths were generally due to cardiac or cerebral ischemia.

In the absence of saphenous vein, prosthetic conduits such as PTFE may be used for distal bypasses, but with a much lower chance of favorable outcome. Buchbinder found that 53% of distal PTFE grafts were patent at 1 year, but none at 2 years. The Montefiore group, who have been vocal advocates of PTFE, admit its poor performance for distal bypass (65). Nonetheless, these authors argue that an attempt at limb salvage using a prosthetic conduit may be appropriate in patients with limited life expectancy.

It is thus apparent that bypass grafts to tibial arteries are a valuable means of limb salvage in elderly patients, particularly if the *in situ* autogenous vein can be used. Early mortality is somewhat increased in these patients compared to their younger cohorts, but still remains acceptably low. The vast majority of patients treated by arterial reconstruction will retain their limbs until death.

Combined aortoiliac and infrainguinal occlusive disease. Patients with combined proximal and distal occlusive disease will have either severe claudication or resting ischemia. Surgical treatment of these patients is predicated upon repair of the aortoiliac or "inflow" lesion, with selective management of "outflow" disease. Simultaneous distal reconstruction should be considered in two circumstances: in the presence of extensive ischemic necrosis in the foot and in the patient with a severely diseased or poorly developed profunda femoris. In the first case, the maximum possible perfusion must be restored to the foot to enable healing of an ischemic lesion or a distal amputation. In the second case, collateral perfusion of the distal extremity will be inadequate, and there will be a higher incidence of aortofemoral graft limb thrombosis secondary to inadequate "outflow" (67, 68). Most surgeons have found that only a small minority of patients will require combined reconstruction; however, Rutherford and colleagues (69) have recently presented evidence that untreated distal occlusive disease may cause hemodynamic failure of the aortofemoral graft in more patients than previously recognized.

Most aortobifemoral bypass procedures include patch angioplasty of the orifice of the profunda femoris, although it has not been shown that there is any benefit to this unless the profunda orifice is severely stenotic (69). The role of profundaplasty alone in the management of limb ischemia is limited to those patients with focal stenoses of the proximal profunda, well-developed profunda-geniculate collaterals, and minimally diseased popliteal and tibial arteries.

Lumbar sympathectomy. Ablation of the lumbar sympathetic trunks was at one time the only procedure available for the treatment of limb ischemia and is still advocated by some for patients who do not have reconstructible arterial anatomy. In recent years, percutaneous sympathetic ablation by chemical means has found favor as a nonoperative means of sympathectomy. Some surgeons employ sympathectomy as an adjunct to arterial reconstruction. The value of sympathectomy remains a subject of debate, although the weight of the evidence indicates that it provides no lasting benefit in terms of relief of ischemic symptoms or avoidance of amputation (70).

Amputation for Advanced Lower Extremity Ischemia

There are about 30,000 to 50,000 major lower extremity amputations performed yearly in the United States, and close to 90% of these are done because of arteriosclerosis and/or diabetes mellitus. The mean age of these patients is 62, and a significant proportion of them are over 70 years old (Fig. 32-9). Ninety percent of lower extremity amputations are performed because of ischemic necrosis of the foot or of a prior amputation site (36, 71). The monetary cost of amputation in the elderly far exceeds the cost of successful arterial reconstruction (72).

There are four issues that pertain to the performance of amputations in the elderly. These are the choice of amputation level, the likelihood of rehabilitation, the operative risk, and the long-term survival. All are adversely affected by increasing age (Fig. 32-10), a fact that serves to emphasize that amputation is by no means an expeditious solution to severe limb ischemia in the elderly.

Choice of Level

Choice of amputation level is made on the basis of demonstration of adequate arterial perfusion at the chosen level, balanced against the goal of maintaining maximal limb length. A number of clinical and laboratory parameters have been proposed to predict the probability of healing of amputations, but all have significant limitations. Discussion of these methods is beyond the scope of this text but may be found in standard sources. In general, the combination of clinical examination and segmental Doppler pressure studies, including toe plethysmography, will allow a rational decision about amputation level to be made. Amputation at a given level should not be performed if there is dependent rubor, cellulitis, or ischemic necrosis at that level. Within those confines, however, efforts should be made to preserve as much of the limb as possible, particularly as regards the knee joint. The premise that a popliteal pulse must be present for healing of a

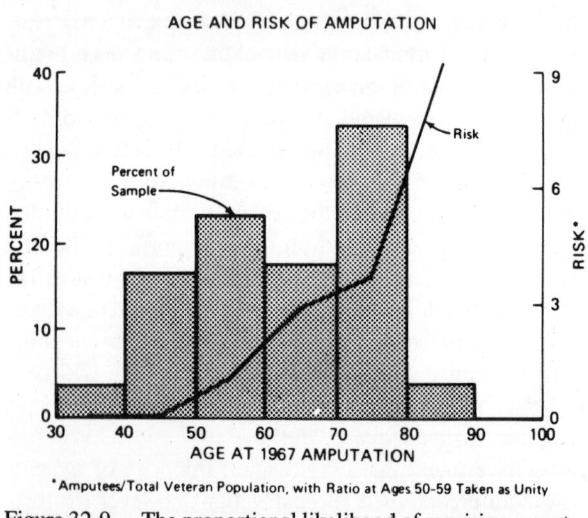

Figure 32-9. The proportional likelihood of requiring amputation increases rapidly in elderly patients. Note the large proportion of patients in the 70- to 80-year age category. (Reprinted with permission from Kihn, RB, et al. 1972. The geriatric amputee. *Ann Surg* 176: 306. Copyright by J.B. Lippincott Co.)

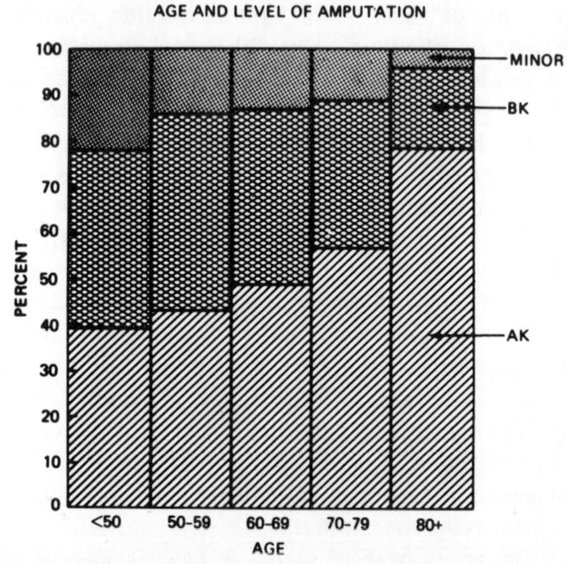

Figure 32-10. Influence of age on amputation level. Elderly patients are more likely to require higher levels of amputation. (Reprinted with permission from Kihn, RB, et al. 1972. The geriatric amputee. *Ann Surg* 176: 306. Copyright by J.B. Lippincott Co.)

below-knee amputation is not valid, as it has been shown that such amputations will heal in up to 75% of patients without a palpable popliteal pulse (36).

Success of Rehabilitation

The preservation of limb length has direct bearing on the success of rehabilitation, because the energy expenditure of walking rises dramatically as the ankle and knee joints are lost. Most authors agree that this effect is magnified in the elderly, resulting in a lower rate of rehabilitation of elderly amputees, particularly those who have undergone above-knee amputation (36, 71, 73). Furthermore, as many as one-third of patients who learn to used a prosthesis will subsequently discard it. Nonetheless, the elderly amputee should not be denied the opportunity for rehabilitation on the basis of age alone. In the absence of dementia and other debilitating illness, many elderly amputees *can* be successfully rehabilitated (74, 75).

Operative Risk

The goal of maintaining limb length must be weighed against the risk of repetitive operations, should the initial procedure fail. Patients are generally chosen for amputation because the risk of vascular reconstruction is deemed too high; however, amputation itself carries a significant mortality risk in patients with advanced atherosclerosis. In the collected Veterans Administration experience, the overall perioperative mortality for major limb amputation was 11%, but rose to 17% among patients over 70 years old (36). Similar figures were reported by Couch and associates (73), and in both series, mortality rose when repeat amputation was necessary.

Malone and colleagues (71) have reported substantially lower mortality among amputees in whom immediate postoperative prostheses and early ambulation were employed. Unfortunately, the expense and logistics of this method have prevented it from being widely adopted.

Long-Term Survival

The long-term prognosis for elderly amputees remains poor, even under the best of circumstances. Patients who have lost one limb face a 5% to 10% per year risk of losing the other limb, and those who come to bilateral amputation are unlikely to maintain independence or be able to walk again. Even more ominous is the fact that in all major series, the 2-year survival rate after bilateral amputation is less than 50%, and decreases steadily with age at time of amputation. As expected, the causes of late death are coronary and cerebral vascular disease and malignancy.

In summary, lower limb amputation in the elderly is a poor alternative to vascular reconstruction and should be reserved for those patients with unreconstructible vascular disease and those who are very poor operative risks. When amputation is necessary, objective criteria must be used to determine the level at which healing is likely to occur. Reasonable effort should be made to spare the knee joint in patients who were ambulating preoperatively and are considered candidates for rehabilitation.

Arterial Aneurysms

True aneurysms result from degeneration of the collagen and elastin framework of the arterial wall. A few result from trauma, infection, or known connective tissue disorders such as Marfan's and Ehlers-Danlos syndromes. The overwhelming majority of aneurysms in older patients are attributed to atherosclerosis, but the exact etiology and pathogenesis are not really known. A familial tendency has been observed, but this holds true for atherosclerosis in general.

The most common sites of aneurysm formation are the infrarenal abdominal aorta and common iliac arteries (Fig. 32-11). Aneurysms involving the suprarenal aorta comprise fewer than five percent of abdominal aneurysms. Peripheral arterial aneurysms are most likely to be found in the femoral and popliteal arteries and are often accompanied by simultaneous aortic aneurysms.

Aortic Aneurysms

Aneurysms of the aorta become increasingly prone to rupture as their maximal diameter increases, with the risk rising rapidly at diameters greater than 5.5 to 6.0 cm (Fig. 32-12). The vast majority of aneurysms cause no symptoms prior to rupture, and most are discovered incidentally on physical exam or during diagnostic tests for unrelated conditions. A few present with acute thrombosis or distal embolization of atheromatous material. In contrast, peripheral aneurysms seldom become large enough to rupture and present most commonly with acute thrombosis, distal embolization, or compression of adjacent veins and nerves.

The median age of patients with aortic aneurysmal disease exceeds that of patients with aortic occlusive disease by nearly a decade (Fig. 32-13). The peak incidence of aneurysmal disease is in the seventh decade consistent with its presumed degenerative origin. Hypertension, coronary artery disease, and chronic obstructive pulmonary disease are common among patients with atherosclerotic aneurysms. Nonetheless, natural history studies have shown that about two-thirds of patients with untreated aortic aneurysms will die of aneurysm rupture, and only one-third will die of coexistent diseases (76). This fact in and of itself justifies resection and graft repair

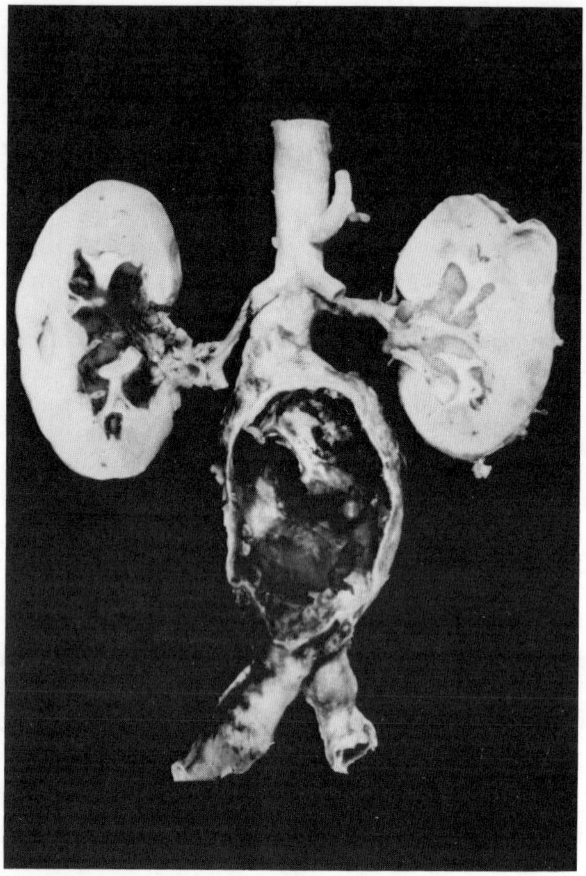

Figure 32-11. Pathology specimen of atherosclerotic infrarenal aortic aneurysm, opened anteriorly to show thrombus and atheromatous debris within. (Reprinted with permission from the Wellcome Museum of Pathology, Royal College of Surgeons of England, Gower Medical Publishing, London.)

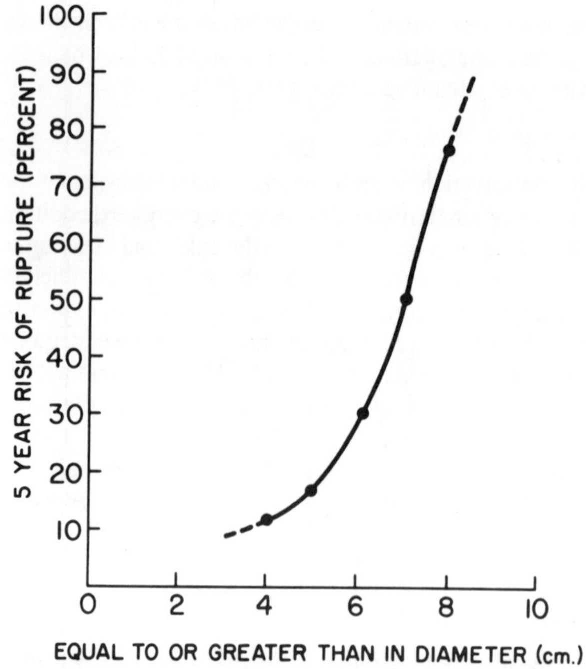

Figure 32-12. Risk of rupture of aortic aneurysm according to maximal diameter. (Reprinted with permission from Rutherford, RB. 1984. *Vascular Surgery,* ed. 2. Philadelphia: W.B. Saunders Co.)

as the treatment of choice for these patients. Survival of patients treated surgically is superior to the results of any other therapeutic course (76) (Fig. 32-14).

The currently accepted indications for aortic aneurysm repair are listed in Table 32-5. Aneurysms less than 5 cm in diameter have a low (though not zero) incidence of rupture and are generally not repaired unless symptomatic. Patients with small aneurysms should be followed by periodic examination with B-mode ultrasound, which is an accurate, reproducible, and noninvasive means of assessing aneurysm diameter.

The mortality rate for elective aortic aneurysm repair is less than 5% in virtually all reported series, a figure which is exceeded 5 to 10-fold in repair of ruptured aneurysms. Nonetheless, vascular surgeons continue to debate whether elective aneurysm repair should be performed in elderly and other "high-risk" patients.

There is no question that the risk of elective aneurysm repair is increased in patients over 75 years old. In the collective review from Cleveland, an 11.3% mortality rate was reported for elective operation in older age groups (20). Edwards and coworkers (22) achieved a 12% elective mortality rate among octogenarians with aortic aneurysms. However, these figures are still *well* below the mortality for patients with ruptured aneurysms. Furthermore, O'Donnell and colleagues (77) and Hollier and associates (78) reported mortality of only 4.7% and 5.7%, respectively, for high-risk and elderly patients undergoing repair of nonruptured aneurysms. Again, in O'Donnell's series, the mortality of operation for ruptured aneurysm in patients over 80 was 74%, and half of nonoperated patients died of aneurysm rupture. An additional striking finding of this study was that the late survival of patients who had undergone successful aneurysm repair was parallel to that of the general population. These data provide strong support for elective repair of large aneurysms in the elderly population.

Those who contend that aneurysm repair in the elderly carries excessive risk have advocated various "nonresective" procedures, whose goal is to produce aneurysm thrombosis and thereby prevent rupture. Among the methods attempted have been intraluminal wiring, external wrapping, and ligation, all combined with extra-anatomic bypass to maintain perfusion to the legs. Although these techniques can be accomplished with low

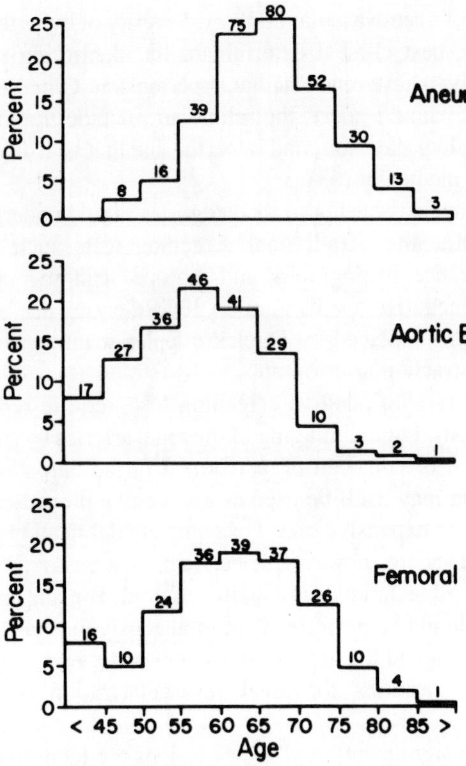

Figure 32-13. Age distribution of patients with vascular diseases. Note the greater median age of patients with aneurysmal disease. (Reprinted with permission from Burnham, SJ, Johnson, G, and Gurri, JA. 1982. Mortality risks for survivors of vascular reconstructive problems. *Surgery* 92: 1072–1076. Copyright by C.V. Mosby Co.)

operative morbidity and mortality, the nonresective approach has invariably been complicated by inability to produce aneurysm thrombosis in some patients, late rupture in spite of thrombosis in others, and the need for secondary procedures to maintain axillofemoral graft patency. Death from late aneurysm rupture has occurred in as many as 30% of patients treated in this fashion, leaving considerable doubt as to the propriety of nonresective treatment. (The arguments for and against nonresective treatment have been well summarized by Karmody et al. [79] and Inahara et al. [49]).

The author believes that elective repair with prosthetic graft is the *optimal* treatment for abdominal aortic aneurysms that are larger than 5.5 to 6.0 cm maximal diameter or are expanding. The elderly or high-risk patient should be urged to undergo elective repair, unless another disease process exists that severely curtails life expectancy.

Coronary artery disease is common among patients with aortic aneurysmal disease, and is the most common cause of postoperative death. Patients with severe coronary disease as identified by exercise testing or radionuclide myocardial scans should be considered for preoperative coronary arteriography and myocardial revascularization (10). In patients over 70, however, the risk of coronary artery bypass must be carefully assessed before choosing this aggressive approach.

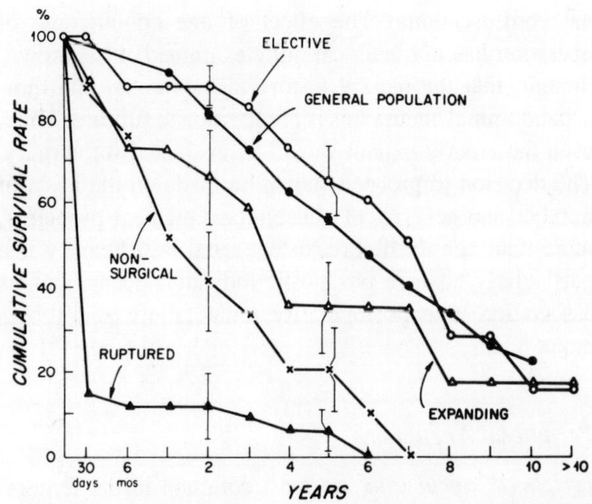

Figure 32-14. Cumulative survival rates of patients with aortic aneurysms according to method of treatment and timing of operation. The survival of patients after elective repair is far superior to that of untreated patients. (Reprinted with permission from O'Donnell, TF, et al. 1976. Is 80 years too old for aneurysmectomy? *Arch Surg* 111: 1250–1257. Copyright by the American Medical Association.)

Suprarenal Aortic Aneurysms

Approximately 5% of atherosclerotic aortic aneurysms involve the *suprarenal* as well as the infrarenal aorta, and some of these involve the lower thoracic aorta as well. The techniques used for repairing such aneurysms have been described extensively by Crawford, who has accumulated the largest experience with these patients (80). The morbidity and mortality of suprarenal aneurysm repair are higher than for infrarenal aneurysm repair, due to a number of factors, including increased blood loss and a higher incidence of myocardial ischemia, renal failure, and spi-

Table 32-5. Abdominal aortic aneurysm

Indications for repair
1. Maximal diameter > 5.5 cm
2. Increase in diameter > 0.5 cm/yr
3. Acute abdominal or back pain
4. Rupture
5. Thrombosis
6. Peripheral embolization
7. Aortocaval fistula

nal cord ischemia. The effect of age on outcome of operation has not been carefully examined. It is known, though, that the natural history of suprarenal and thoracoabdominal aneurysms is progression to rupture. Thus, even the elderly patient should be evaluated for surgery. The decision to proceed should be made on the basis of number and severity of concomitant medical problems, more than age itself. Preexistent renal insufficiency is a particularly adverse prognostic indicator, because of its association with postoperative renal failure and subsequent death.

Peripheral Aneurysms

Peripheral aneurysms are most common in the femoral and popliteal arteries. Unlike aortic aneurysms, the greatest risk of peripheral aneurysms is thrombosis and acute limb ischemia, not rupture. Other significant complications are distal embolization and compression of adjacent veins or nerves. Because all of these conditions are difficult to treat once they have occurred, most surgeons advocate elective prophylactic operation for femoral and popliteal aneurysms greater than 2 cm in diameter. Femoral aneurysms are amenable to direct excision with graft replacement. Popliteal aneurysms are treated by proximal and distal ligation and femoropopliteal bypass. The risk of these procedures in older patients is no different when they are done for aneurysmal disease than for occlusive disease, as described above (81, 82).

Other Aneurysms

Visceral artery aneurysms are rare, and little is known about their incidence of rupture. It *is* known, however, that rupture of these aneurysms is often fatal because of hemorrhage into the free peritoneal cavity. Symptoms rarely occur prior to rupture. Thus, visceral aneurysms of greater than 2.0 to 2.5 cm diameter should be resected electively in patients without prohibitive operative risk.

Renovascular Disorders

Renovascular Hypertension

Significant occlusive lesions of the renal arteries produce renin-mediated hypertension. Fibromuscular dysplasia accounts for about 30% of renovascular hypertension, but is rare in the elderly. The remaining 70% of cases are the result of atherosclerosis. Although most of these patients are under 70 years of age, severe hypertension (diastolic >115 mm Hg) in a patient over 70 should provoke strong suspicion of a renovascular etiology. Severity of hypertension is the best clinical determinant for identifying patients likely to have renovascular hypertension. Other features that should alert the clinician include rapidly worsening hypertension, and hypertension that is difficult to control medically (83).

Patients in these high-risk categories should undergo further screening. Traditional screening tests such as rapid-sequence pyelography and isotope scanning can give false-negative results in up to 30% of cases, and are rapidly being replaced by Duplex doppler scanning and digital subtraction arteriography.

Patients with positive screening tests require renal arteriography. Digital imaging of the renal arteries by aortic injection is safe, can be performed in the outpatient setting, and may itself be used as a screening procedure, albeit a more expensive one. For complete delineation of the arterial lesions, however, selective renal arteriography with standard techniques is usually required. Biplane aortography should be performed simultaneously to evaluate both the aorta and the hepatic and splenic arteries as possible donor arteries for renal revascularization (Fig. 32-15).

When significant renal artery lesions are identified, selective renal vein renin assays are needed to confirm a renovascular basis for hypertension. Criteria for performing and interpreting these studies have been described (84). Surgical cure or improvement of hypertension are highly likely in patients with demonstrable renin hypersecretion.

Renal Insufficiency

In addition to causing hypertension, renal artery stenosis or occlusion can in some circumstances result in deterioration of renal function. However, it is axiomatic that *unilateral* renal arterial disease does not cause renal insufficiency unless there is concomitant *bilateral* renal parenchymal disease (nephrosclerosis). Because virtually all patients with severe renal atherosclerosis have some degree of coexisting nephrosclerosis, renal artery reconstruction may stabilize renal function, but rarely results in restoration of a normal serum urea nitrogen or creatinine. Dean has proposed several criteria for selecting those patients with renal artery occlusion who are likely to benefit from arterial reconstruction (85).

Methods of Reconstruction

Renal revascularization may be accomplished by either endarterectomy or bypass. If the latter is chosen, aortorenal bypass is the preferred technique, and good results may be obtained with either saphenous vein or prosthetic

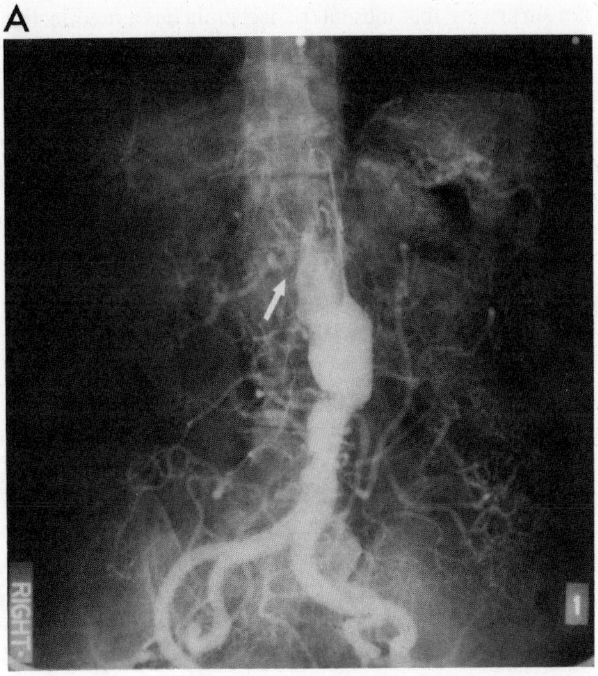

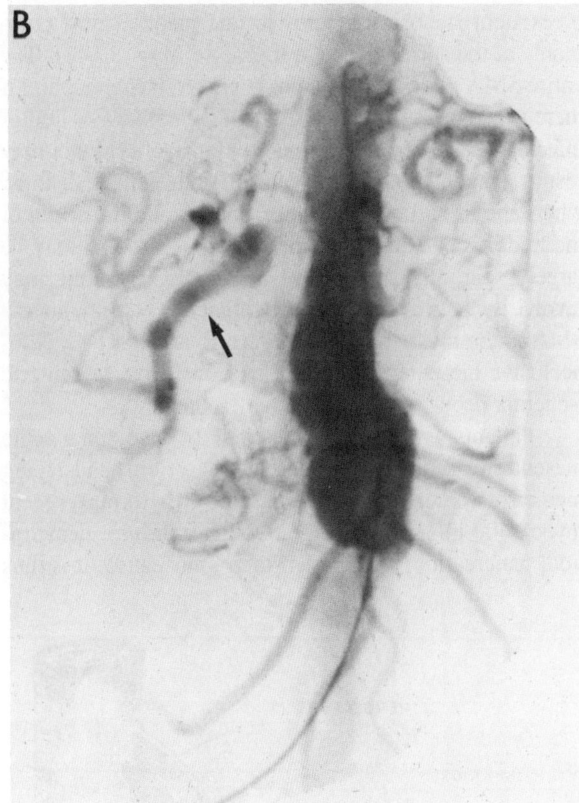

Figure 32-15. A, Preoperative arteriogram of patient with renovascular hypertension, severe right renal artery stenosis (*arrow*), and aneurysmal aorta. B, Postoperative arteriogram in the same patient, demonstrating patent hepatorenal saphenous vein graft (*arrow*).

conduit. Severe aneurysmal or occlusive disease of the aorta must often be repaired simultaneously unless an alternate source of inflow is available. Both the hepatic and splenic arteries have been used for this purpose with good results, providing that the celiac axis is widely patent (86).

Elderly patients who have hypertension or renal insufficiency of a renovascular etiology generally have diffuse atherosclerosis and face a correspondingly higher operative risk for renal artery reconstruction, particularly if combined aortic and renal artery procedures are required or if there is moderate to marked elevation of serum creatinine (87, 88). Nonetheless, the morbidity of poorly controlled hypertension is well known, and there is evidence that loss of renal function is accelerated in patients with renovascular hypertension who are treated medically (89). Because there has been no direct comparison of surgical versus medical management of renovascular diseases in the elderly, the role of surgery remains undefined. Each case must be approached individually, with a systematic evaluation as described in detail in the references cited above. Selected elderly patients with poorly controlled hypertension or severe bilateral renal artery stenosis associated with renal insufficiency may be offered surgical therapy with the expectation of a highly satisfactory outcome.

Mesenteric Ischemia

There are four major clinical syndromes of mesenteric ischemia—acute mesenteric ischemia, ischemic colitis, postoperative colon ischemia and chronic mesenteric ischemia. Each is a distinct clinical entity, and each may occur in the elderly patient with vascular disease. As opposed to other major arterial disorders, the symptoms and signs of mesenteric ischemia are often nonspecific, and the diagnosis is thus often delayed, with catastrophic consequences. This can only be avoided if the diagnosis of mesenteric ischemia is included in the differential of every patient with abdominal pain.

Acute Mesenteric Ischemia

Acute mesenteric ischemia results from thromboembolic occlusion of the mesenteric arterial circulation, or from nonocclusive hypoperfusion due to low cardiac output or splanchnic vasoconstriction. The distribution of ischemia is that of the superior mesenteric artery, including the small bowel and variable amounts of the colon proximal to the splenic flexure. Isolated colonic ischemia is a separate entity that usually develops in the distribution of the inferior mesenteric artery (see below).

Thrombosis of the SMA usually occurs at the site of

preexistent stenosing atherosclerotic plaque, most commonly at the aortic orifice of the vessel (Fig. 32-16). The entire SMA distribution is thus rendered ischemic, and if there is coexisting severe disease of the celiac axis and/or inferior mesenteric artery, more extensive ischemia may result. In contrast, emboli tend to lodge more distally, where the SMA begins to taper, just beyond the origin of the middle colic artery. In these cases, the colon may be largely spared. Nonocclusive mesenteric ischemia may involve the entire GI tract from stomach to rectum, but the SMA is the most commonly affected vascular bed. Nonocclusive mesenteric ischemia and occlusive mesenteric ischemia occur with nearly equal frequency.

Patients who are at greatest risk of developing acute mesenteric ischemia are those with serious underlying medical disorders, especially cardiac arrhythmias, recent myocardial infarction, congestive heart failure, dehydration, pancreatitis, or hypertension of any cause. It is thus not surprising that mesenteric ischemia has a predilection for older patients. Boley and colleagues (90) noted that more than half of their patients were over age 70. In Ottinger's series, the median age was 70 (91). Crawford and coworkers found that two-thirds of their patients were over 60 (92). In all of these series, there was a preponderance of women over men.

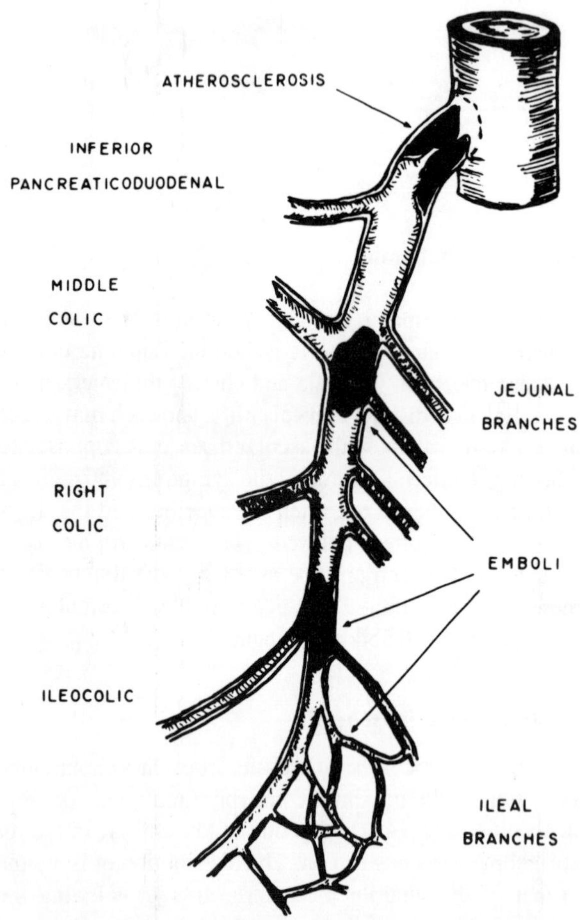

Figure 32-16. Sites of occlusion of the superior mesenteric artery by thrombosis or embolism. (Reprinted with permission from Boley, SJ, and Veith, FJ. 1983. Acute mesenteric ischemia. In *Textbook of Surgery*, Ed., JD Hardy. Philadelphia: J.B. Lippincott Co.)

Clinical Features

The clinical findings of acute mesenteric ischemia are highly variable, accounting for the fact that the diagnosis is frequently delayed or missed altogether. Abdominal pain is virtually always present in patients with occlusive ischemia but may be absent in those with the nonocclusive syndrome. The location and severity of the pain may also be quite variable. The severity is often said to be out of proportion to the physical findings, which tend to be meager, at least early in the course. Signs of peritonitis usually indicate that intestinal infarction has already occurred. When present, pain is often accompanied by diarrhea, which in many patients will be guaiac-positive or grossly bloody. Leukocytosis, acidosis, and amylasemia are often, but not invariably, present.

Diagnosis and Treatment

The diagnosis of acute mesenteric ischemia can be definitively established only by angiography or surgical exploration. The most widely accepted diagnostic and therapeutic plan is that proposed by Boley and colleagues (90) and displayed in algorithmic form in Figure 32-17. Aortography and selective SMA angiography are used to establish the diagnosis and direct therapy. Direct infusion of vasodilators such as papaverine or priscoline into the SMA via percutaneous catheter is used as the primary treatment of nonocclusive ischemia (Fig. 32-18), and as an adjunct to the management of embolectomy or thrombectomy. Patients with peritonitis or other signs of intestinal infarction must undergo laparotomy, but revascularization should be undertaken before a final decision about intestinal viability is made. Second-look laparotomies are generally advisable. With this approach, Boley has reported a 54% mortality, with preservation of most of the small bowel in survivors, compared to the 80% to 90% mortality rate associated with traditional therapy employing operation but no vasodilators. An aggressive approach to acute mesenteric ischemia is thus clearly warranted, but mortality remains high in this generally poor-risk group of patients.

Acute Ischemic Colitis

The left side of the colon is supplied by the inferior mesenteric artery (IMA), with contributions from the left

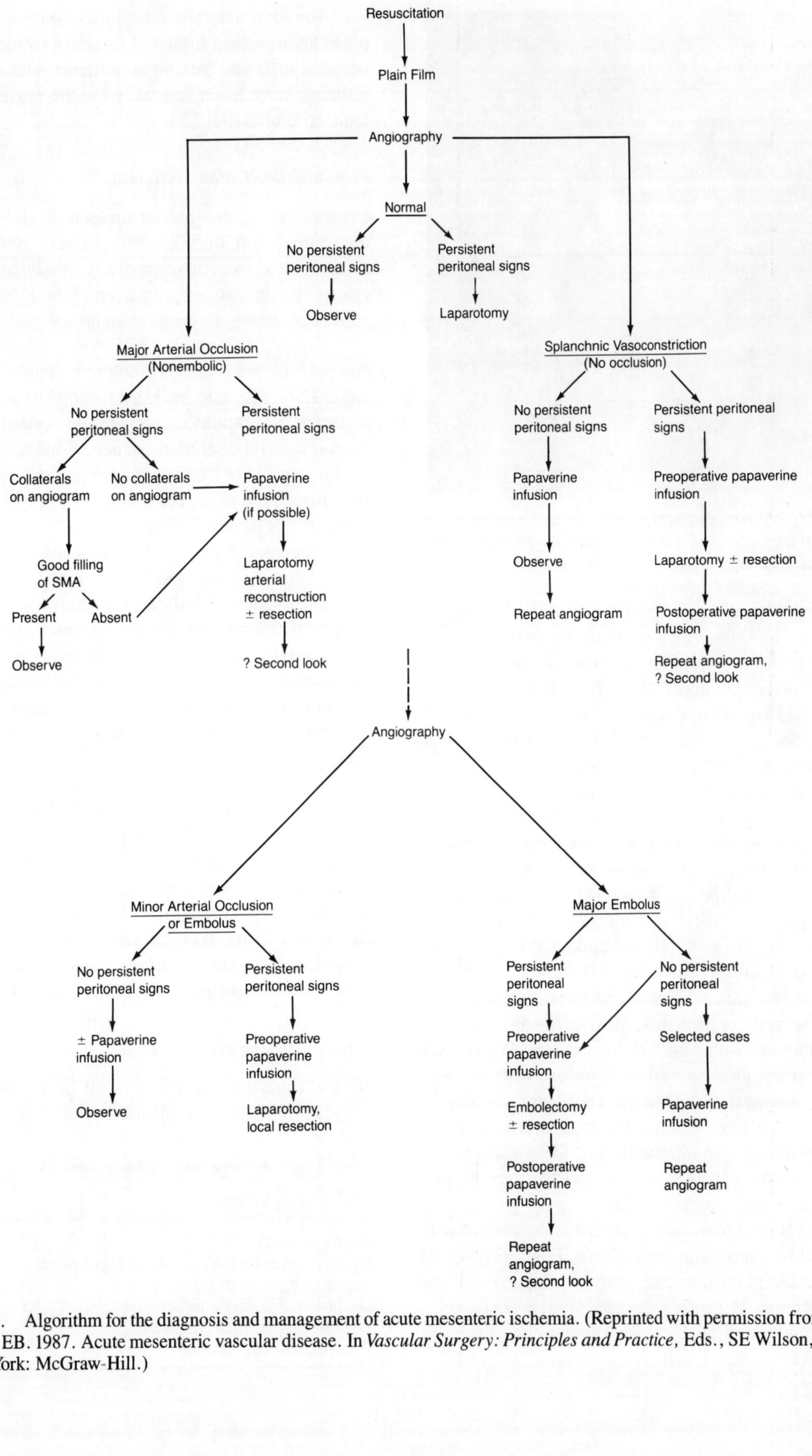

Figure 32-17. Algorithm for the diagnosis and management of acute mesenteric ischemia. (Reprinted with permission from Boley, SJ, and Borden, EB. 1987. Acute mesenteric vascular disease. In *Vascular Surgery: Principles and Practice*, Eds., SE Wilson, FJ Veith, et al. © New York: McGraw-Hill.)

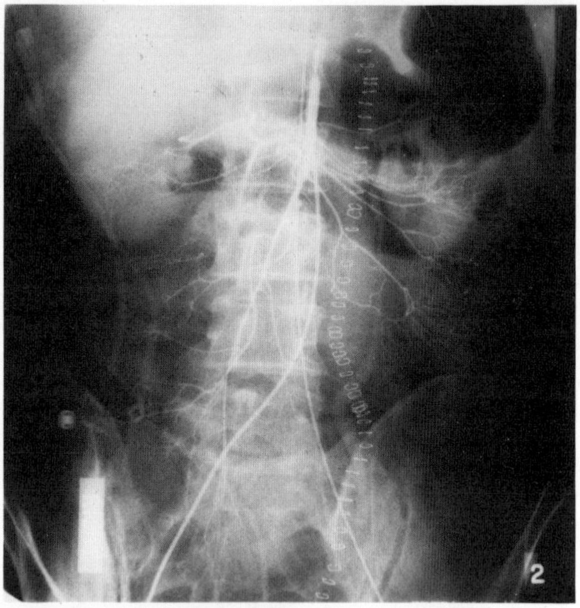

Figure 32-18. Superior mesenteric arteriogram demonstrating the marked attenuation of the vessel and its distal branches characteristic of nonocclusive mesenteric ischemia.

branch of the middle colic artery, and from the internal iliac artery. The IMA orifice is frequently found to be occluded in patients with atherosclerosis of the infrarenal aorta, and collateral anastomoses from the middle colic and internal iliac vessels are often not well developed. The left colon is thus the part of the colon that is most prone to arterial insufficiency. Paradoxically, major vascular occlusion can usually *not* be identified in cases of acute colon ischemia, and the exact etiology in individual cases is often obscure. Although younger patients may be affected, the elderly and those with severe cardiac and other concomitant illnesses remain at the highest risk (93, 94).

As with acute mesenteric ischemia, there are no classic clinical findings. Left-sided abdominal pain and bloody diarrhea are common. Tenderness varies according to the severity of ischemia. Mild ischemia may affect only the mucosa, with a mild clinical course. With severe ischemia, transmural necrosis will ensue, with resultant peritonitis and systemic toxicity. The diagnosis may be confirmed by barium enema, showing mucosal edema ("thumb-printing") or intramural air. Colonoscopy will also establish the presence of ischemia but must be performed only with extreme caution.

Cases of mild to moderate severity may resolve with only bowel rest and intravenous fluids. Frank peritonitis, or a worsening clinical course, mandates laparotomy and bowel resection. Because a discrete arterial occlusion is seldom identified, arterial reconstruction plays little role in treatment.

The morbidity and mortality of colonic necrosis and perforation remain high and can only be reduced by earlier diagnosis and treatment. Patients with only mucosal ischemia have lower mortality but are at risk for late colonic strictures (93, 95).

Postoperative Colon Ischemia

Compromise of the inferior mesenteric artery or internal iliac circulation during aortic surgery may precipitate acute colonic ischemia, generally involving the sigmoid colon. The incidence varies from 2% to 15% of infrarenal aortic operations, depending on how vigorously the diagnosis is sought. A number of factors predispose to the occurrence of postoperative colon ischemia, as listed in Table 32-6. The surgeon must be cognizant of patients at high risk, but should assess sigmoid perfusion at the end of *every* aortic operation, either by assessment of IMA stump pressure or Doppler interrogation of mesocolic vessels. Inspection of the colon alone is misleading and unreliable unless ischemia is severe.

When perfusion is judged to be insufficient by objective methods, reimplantation or bypass of the inferior mesenteric artery is indicated. Prevention is preferable to treatment of established colon ischemia, particularly because the diagnosis may be difficult to make in the postoperative period. Bloody rectal discharge is frequent but not invariable. Hypotension, metabolic acidosis, oliguria, abdominal distention, or virtually any form of early postoperative instability should bring the diagnosis of colon ischemia to mind, and persistence of these states without other explanation is an indication for sigmoidoscopy. As with other forms of colon ischemia, mucosal ischemia alone may be managed expectantly. Transmural ischemia requires prompt laparotomy and resection, but the rate of septic complications and death remains high. Monitoring of intraluminal colonic pH has recently been proposed as a more accurate means of early detection of ischemia, both during and after operation (96).

Chronic Mesenteric Ischemia

Normal digestive processes result in a substantial postprandial increase in splanchnic blood flow, primarily

Table 32-6. Postoperative colon ischemia

Predisposing factors
Ruptured aneurysm
Patent inferior mesenteric artery (IMA)
Improper ligation of IMA
Occlusion of superior mesenteric artery
Loss of internal iliac collaterals
Perioperative hypotension

through the superior mesenteric artery. When occlusive disease of the visceral arteries interferes with this adaptive response, the syndrome of chronic mesenteric ischemia, or *intestinal angina*, may result. Because of the collateral pathways within the mesenteric circulation, it is generally agreed that intestinal angina does not occur unless more than one of the three major arteries (celiac, SMA, IMA) is severely diseased or occluded.

The syndrome is most common among patients in the sixth and seventh decades, but does occur in older patients as well. The usual symptoms are postprandial abdominal pain and weight loss, and the diagnosis should be reconsidered if these complaints are not present. Nonetheless, intestinal angina should be considered in any patient with chronic debilitating abdominal pain of unexplained origin. A diagnosis of chronic mesenteric ischemia requires biplane abdominal aortography to confirm mesenteric vascular occlusion. Although Duplex scanning is being evaluated as an adjunctive diagnostic tool, its usefulness has not yet been defined.

Mesenteric revascularization is the only effective treatment for intestinal angina. In large series, transaortic endarterectomy and antegrade bypass from the aorta have proven to be the most durable operations. Prosthetic conduit seems to function better than vein in this location. If operation is undertaken, both celiac and SMA should be repaired for optimal results (78, 97).

Specific information regarding the risk of mesenteric vascular repair in elderly patients is not available. However, the operations do require partial or complete aortic clamping and may thus be accompanied by major hemodynamic alterations. In general, surgery should be reserved for patients with well documented disease and debilitating symptoms.

Venous Diseases

The six recognized syndromes of venous disease include acute deep vein thrombosis (DVT), recurrent deep vein thrombosis, pulmonary embolism, the post-phlebitic syndrome, superficial thrombophlebitis, and varicose veins. The principles of diagnosis and management of these disorders are no different for elderly patients than for any other patient population, and the reader is referred to standard textbooks for a review of those fundamentals.

In spite of the fact that venous diseases are very common, few clinicians have developed a rational approach to their management As a result, many patients have been treated improperly, or even dismissed as hopeless. It is thus worthwhile to re-emphasize the salient features of diagnosis and therapy.

Acute Venous Disease

It is of paramount importance that the diagnosis of deep vein thrombosis or pulmonary embolism *never* be made without objective documentation. Clinical diagnosis has been repeatedly shown to be *unreliable*. Venous Doppler evaluation, impedance plethysmography (IPG), and phleborheography (PRG) are all highly accurate diagnostic tests for clinically significant DVT, when performed by experienced personnel. Contrast venography is the current standard of diagnosis and should be employed without hesitation when noninvasive studies are equivocal.

With regard to pulmonary embolism, treatment with heparin may be initiated on the basis of radionuclide ventilation/perfusion lung scan if unequivocally positive or negative, but pulmonary arteriography should be obtained if there is *any* doubt as to the interpretation of the lung scan. Patients who are to undergo thrombolytic therapy, vena caval interruption, or operative embolectomy *must* undergo pulmonary arteriography to verify the diagnosis.

The vast majority of patients with acute venous thrombosis or pulmonary embolism can be managed with heparin alone, but adjunctive measures are occasionally required. The role of thrombolytic therapy is evolving as newer, more specific agents such as tissue plasminogen activator are being evaluated. Venous thrombectomy has been largely abandoned as a routine therapeutic modality but is the treatment of choice for patients with limb-threatening massive iliofemoral venous thrombosis (*phlegmasia cerulea dolens*). Similarly, pulmonary embolectomy is not required for most patients with pulmonary emboli but may represent the only hope for survival in patients with massive emboli and cardiovascular collapse.

Chronic Venous Disease

Patients with chronic venous disorders should also undergo objective evaluation with either IPG or PRG to document the degree of venous obstruction and/or reflux and to obtain a baseline for future comparison.

The pathophysiology of the post-phlebitic syndrome, i.e., chronic limb edema, fatigue, stasis dermatitis, pain, and ulceration, is *venous hypertension*. No form of treatment that fails to combat venous hypertension can possibly succeed in alleviating the patient's complaints. A carefully prescribed and managed program of elastic compression is *highly* effective in counteracting venous hypertension and providing relief of symptoms. Various types of elastic compressive bandages facilitate healing of venous ulcers, while graded compression stockings are utilized for patients without active ulcers. Proprietary type "support hose" and T.E.D. anti-embolism stockings do *not* provide adequate compression and are ineffective in the treatment of chronic venous disease.

Patients with severe and extensive venous stasis ulceration usually require hospital management with bedrest, leg elevation, and debridement. Noninvasive arterial studies should be performed to identify any element of coexistent arterial insufficiency. Skin grafts should only be applied once ulcers are clean and granulating. After healing has been achieved, elastic stockings are worn to prevent recurrence.

Surgery for Venous Disorders

A variety of surgical procedures has been proposed for the management of "intractable" venous disease. These range from vein stripping and ligation of venous perforators to vein valve transplantation, transposition, or venous bypass operations. Ligation or injection sclerotherapy of venous perforators may be a very useful adjunct to elastic compression in patients with recurrent ulcers. The use of venous reconstructive surgery has not achieved widespread acceptance. Some centers have reported favorable results, but there continues to be debate as to the efficacy of these procedures over and above elastic compression therapy (98–100).

Summary

Vascular diseases, particularly peripheral atherosclerosis, are prevalent among the aged. The limited organ reserve of aged patients compounds the pathologic effects of vascular insufficiency and complicates its management. The morbidity and mortality of most forms of major arterial reconstruction increase as patients reach and exceed age 70. Nonetheless, for many older individuals, vascular surgery provides highly effective palliation against death and disability, and significantly forestalls the loss of physical and physiologic integrity that accompanies senescence. The vascular surgeon must assume the responsibility of choosing the most appropriate therapy for each individual patient.

References

1. Ross, R, 1986. The pathogenesis of atherosclerosis—an update. *N Engl J Med* 314:488–497.
2. Goldstein, JL, and Brown, MS, 1977. The low-density lipoprotein pathway and its relation to atherosclerosis. *Annu Rev Biochem* 46:897–930.
3. Ross, R, et al. 1984. The role of endothelial injury and macrophage interactions in atherosclerosis. *Circulation* 70(Suppl 3):11177–11182.
4. Glagov, S, et al. 1987. Compensatory enlargement of human atherosclerotic coronary arteries. *N Engl J Med* 316:1371–1375.
5. Busuttil, RW, et al. 1982. Elastase activity: The role of elastase in aortic aneurysm formation. *J Surg Res* 32:214–217.
6. Busuttil, RW, Zam-Zam, AM, and Machleder, HI. 1980. Collagenase activity of the human aorta. *Arch Surg* 115:1373–1378.
7. Tilson, MD, and Davis, G. 1983. Deficiencies of copper and a compound with ion—exchange characteristics of pyridinoline in skin from patients with abdominal aortic aneurysms. *Surgery* 94:134–141.
8. Zatina, MA, et al. 1984. Role of medial lamellar architecture in the pathogenesis of aortic aneurysms. *J Vasc Surg* 1:442–448.
9. Hertzer, NR, et al. 1979. Routine coronary angiography prior to elective aortic reconstruction: Results of selective myocardial revascularization in patients with peripheral vascular disease. *Arch Surg* 114:1336–1344.
10. Hertzer, NR, et al. 1984. Coronary artery disease in peripheral vascular patients. A classification of 1000 coronary angiograms and results of surgical management. *Ann Surg* 199:223–233.
11. Boucher, CA, et al. 1985. Determination of cardiac risk by dipyridamole-thallium imaging before peripheral vascular surgery. *N Engl J Med* 312:389–394.
12. Cutler, BS, and Leppo, JA. 1987. Dipyridamole thallium 201 scintigraphy to detect coronary artery disease before abdominal aortic surgery. *J Vasc Surg* 5:91–100.
13. Cutler, BS. 1986. Prevention of cardiac complications in peripheral vascular surgery. *Surg Clin North Am* 66:281–292.
14. Reigel, MM, et al. 1987. Late survival in abdominal aortic aneurysm patients: The role of selective myocardial revascularization on the basis of clinical symptoms. *J Vasc Surg* 5:222–227.
15. Ropper, AH, Wechsler, LR, and Wilson, LS. 1982. Carotid bruit and the risk of stroke in elective surgery. *N Engl J Med* 307:1388–1390.
16. *A Guide to the National Institute of Neurologic and Communicative Disorders and Stroke*. U.S. Department of Health and Human Services, Public Health Service, National Institutes of Health, Sep 30, 1984.
17. Easton, JD, et al. 1983. Diagnosis and management of ischemic stroke. *Curr Probl Cardiol* 8(5):1–76.
18. Moore, WS, and Hall, AD. 1970. Importance of emboli from the carotid bifurcation in the pathogenesis of cerebral ischemic attacks. *Arch Surg* 101:708–716.
19. Sumner, DS, Moore, DJ, and Miles RD. 1985. Doppler ultrasonic arteriography and flow velocity analysis in carotid artery disease. *In Noninvasive Diagnostic Techniques in Vascular Disease*, Ed., EF Bernstein, pp. 349-366. St. Louis: C.V. Mosby Co.
20. Plecha, FR, et al. 1985. The early results of vascular surgery in patients 75 years of age and older: An analysis of 3259 cases. *J Vasc Surg* 2:769–774.
21. Ouriel, K, et al. 1986. Carotid endarterectomy in the elderly patient. *Surg Gynecol Obstet* 162:334–336.
22. Edwards, WH, Mulherin, JL, and Rogers, DM. 1982.

Vascular reconstruction in the octogenarian. *South Med J* 75:648–652.
23. Rosenthal, D, et al. 1986. Carotid endarterectomy in the octogenarian: Is it appropriate? *J Vasc Surg* 3:782–786.
24. Chambers, BR, and Norris, JW. 1986. Outcome in patients with asymptomatic neck bruits. *N Engl J Med* 315:860–865.
25. Roederer, GO, et al. 1984. The natural history of carotid arterial disease in asymptomatic patients with cervical bruits. *Stroke* 15:605–613.
26. Zierler, RE, et al. 1982. Carotid artery stenosis following endarterectomy. *Arch Surg* 117:1408–1415.
27. Blaisdell, WF, Clauss, RH, and Galbraith, JG. 1969. Joint study of extracranial arterial occlusion: IV: A review of surgical considerations. *JAMA* 209:1889–1895.
28. Fields, WS, and Lemak, NA. 1972. Joint study of extracranial arterial occlusion. VII. "Subclavian steal": a review of 168 cases. *JAMA* 222:1139–1143.
29. Crawford, ES, et al. 1962. Thrombo-obliterative disease of the great vessels arising from the aortic arch. *J Thorac Cardiovasc Surg* 43:38–53.
30. Hewitt, RL, Weichert, RF, and Drapanas, T. 1970. Centrifugal cerebral ischemia. *Arch Surg* 101:155–160.
31. Crawford, ES, Stowe, CL, and Powers, RW, Jr. 1983. Occlusion of the innominate, common carotid, and subclavian arteries: Long term results of surgical treatment. *Surgery* 94:781–791.
32. Vogt, DP, et al. 1982. Brachiocephalic arterial reconstruction. *Ann Surg* 196:541–552.
33. Wylie, EW, and Effeney, DJ. 1979. Surgery of the aortic arch branches and vertebral arteries. *Surg Clin N Am* 59:669–680.
34. Brewster, DC, et al. 1985. Innominate artery lesions; Problems encountered and lessons learned. *J Vasc Surg* 2:99–112.
35. Otteman, MG, and Stahlgren, LH. 1965. Evaluation of factors which influence mortality and morbidity following major lower extremity amputations for arteriosclerosis. *Surg Gynecol Obstet* 120:1217–1220.
36. Kihn, RB, Warren, R, and Beebe, GW. 1972. The "geriatric" amputee. *Ann Surg* 176:306–314.
37. Abbott, WM, et al. 1982. Arterial embolism: A 44 year perspective. *Am J Surg* 143:460–464.
38. Cambria, RP, and Abbott, WM. 1984. Acute arterial thrombosis of the lower extremity. *Arch Surg* 119:784–787.
39. Haimovici, H. 1979. Muscular, renal, and metabolic complications of acute arterial occlusions: Myonephropathic-metabolic syndrome. *Surgery* 85:461–468.
40. Harris, K, et al. 1986. Metabolic response of skeletal muscle to ischemia. *Am J Physiol* 250:H213–H220.
41. Blaisdell, WF, Steele, M, and Allen, RE. 1978. Management of acute lower extremity arterial ischemia due to embolism and thrombosis. *Surgery* 84:822–834.
42. Hess, H, et al. 1982. Local low-dose thrombolytic therapy of peripheral arterial occlusion. *N Engl J Med* 307:1627–1630.
43. Rush, DS, et al. 1983. Selective infusion of streptokinase for arterial thrombosis. *Surgery* 93:828–833.
44. Ricotta, JJ, Green, RM, and DeWeese, JA. 1987. Use and limitations of thrombolytic therapy in the treatment of peripheral arterial ischemia: Results of a multi-institutional questionnaire. *J Vasc Surg* 6:45–50.
45. Elliott, JP, et al. 1980. Arterial embolization: Problems of source, multiplicity, recurrence, and delayed treatment. *Surgery* 88:833–845.
46. Boyd, AM. 1962. Natural course of arteriosclerosis of the lower extremities. *Proc R Soc Med* 53: 591–593.
47. Juergens, JC, Barker, NW, and Hines, EA. 1960. Arteriosclerosis obliterans: Review of 520 cases with special reference to pathogenic and prognostic factors. *Circulation* 21:188–195.
48. Bernstein, EF. 1985. The clinical spectrum of ischemic cerebrovascular disease. *In Noninvasive Diagnostic Techniques in Vascular Disease*, Ed., EF Bernstein, pp. 301–315. St. Louis: The C.V. Mosby Co.
49. Inahara, T, et al. 1985. The contrary position to the nonresective treatment for abdominal aortic aneurysm. *J Vasc Surg* 2:42–48.
50. Waltman, AC. et al. 1982. Transluminal angioplasty of the iliac and femoropopliteal arteries. Current status. *Arch Surg* 117:1218–1221.
51. Burnham, SJ, Johnson, G, Jr, and Gurri, JA. 1982. Mortality risks for survivors of vascular reconstructive procedures. *Surgery* 92:1072–1076.
52. Ziffren, SE, and Hartford, CE. 1972. Comparative mortality for various surgical operations in older versus younger age groups. *J Am Geriatr Soc* 20:485–489.
53. Attia, RR, Murphy, JD, and Snider, M. 1976. Myocardial ischemia due to infrarenal aortic cross-clamping during aortic surgery in patients with severe coronary artery disease. *Circulation* 53:961–965.
54. Berkowitz, HD, and Shetty, S. 1974. Renin release and renal cortical ischemia following aortic cross-clamping. *Arch Surg* 109: 612–617.
55. Williams, GM, et al. 1980. The extended retroperitoneal approach for treatment of extensive atherosclerosis of the aorta and renal vessels. *Surgery* 88:846–854.
56. Purdy, RT, et al. 1986. Reduced aortic cross-clamp time in high-risk patients with abdominal aortic aneurysm. *J Vasc Surg* 3:320–823.
57. Plecha, FR, and Plecha, FM. 1984. Femorofemoral bypass grafts: Ten year experience. *J Vasc Surg* 1:555–561.
58. Burrell, MJ, et al. 1982. Axillofemoral bypass: A ten-year review. *Ann Surg* 195:796–798.
59. Logerfo, FW, et al. 1977. A comparison of the late patency rates of axillo-bilateral femoral and axillo-unilateral femoral grafts. *Surgery* 81:33–40.
60. Sanborn, TA, et al. 1987. Human percutaneous and intraoperative laser thermal angioplasty: Initial clinical results as an adjunct to balloon angioplasty. *J Vasc Surg* 5:83–90.
61. Veith, FJ, et al. 1984. Femoral-popliteal-tibial occlusive disease. In *Vascular Surgery: A Comprehensive Review,* Ed., WS Moore, pp. 389–412. New York: Grune & Stratton.
62. Leather, RP, and Karmody, AM. 1986. In-situ saphenous vein arterial bypass for the treatment of limb ischemia. *Adv Surg* 19:175–219.
63. Taylor, IM, Phinney, ES, and Porter, JM. 1986. Present status of reversed vein bypass for lower extremity revascularization. *J Vasc Surg* 3:288–297.
64. Buchbinder, D, et al. 1985. Ankle bypass: Should we go the distance? *Am J Surg* 150:216–219.
65. Scher, LA, et al. 1986. Limb salvage in octogenarians and nonagenarians. *Surgery* 99:160–165.

66. Hines, GL. 1983. Limb salvage in octogenarians—a 4 year review. *Vasc Surg* July/Aug: 220–224.
67. Royster, TS, Lynn, R, and Mulcare, RJ. 1976. Combined aortoiliac and femoro-popliteal occlusive disease. *Surg Gynecol Obstet* 144:143–149.
68. Brewster, DC, and Darling, RC. 1978. Optimal methods of aortoiliac reconstruction. *Surgery* 84:739–748.
69. Rutherford, RB, et al. 1986. Serial hemodynamic assessment of aortobifemoral bypass. *J Vasc Surg* 4:428–435.
70. Lange, DA, et al. 1987. Lumbar sympathectomy. *In Vascular Surgery*, Eds., SE Wilson, et al. pp. 437-443. New York: McGraw-Hill Book Co.
71. Malone, JM, et al. 1979. Therapeutic and economic impact of modern amputation program. *Ann Surg* 189:798–802.
72. Mackey, WC, et al. 1986. The costs of surgery for limb-threatening ischemia. *Surgery* 99:26–35.
73. Couch, NP, et al. 1977. Natural history of the leg amputee. *Am J Surg* 133:469–473.
74. Reyes, RL, Leahey, EB, and Leahey, EB, Jr. 1977. Elderly patients with lower extremity amputations: Three-year study in a rehabilitation setting. *Arch Phys Med Rehab* 58:116–123.
75. Anderson, AD, et al. 1967. The use of lower extremity prosthetic limbs by elderly patients. *Arch Phys Med Rehab* 48:533–538.
76. Szilagyi, DE, et al. 1966. Contribution of abdominal aortic aneurysmectomy to prolongation of life. *Ann Surg* 164:678–699.
77. O'Donnell, TF, Jr, Darling, RC, and Linton, RR. 1976. Is 80 years too old for aneurysmectomy? *Arch Surg* 111:1250–1257.
78. Hollier, LH, et al. 1981. Surgical management of chronic intestinal ischemia: A reappraisal. *Surgery* 90:940–946.
79. Karmody, AM, et al. 1983. The current position of non-resective treatment for abdominal aortic aneurysm. *Surgery* 94:591–597.
80. Crawford ES, et al. 1986. Thoracoabdominal aortic aneurysms: Preoperative and intraoperative factors determining immediate and long term results of operations in 605 patients. *J Vasc Surg*, 3:389–404.
81. Graham, L, et al. 1980. The clinical significance of arteriosclerotic femoral artery aneurysms. *Arch Surg* 115:502–507.
82. Queral, LA, et al. 1979. Management of peripheral arterial aneurysms. *Surg Clin N Am* 59:693–706.
83. Simon, N, et al. 1972. Clinical characteristics of renovascular hypertension. *JAMA* 220:1209–1218.
84. Whelton, PK, et al. 1977. Renal vein renin activity: A prospective study of sampling techniques and methods of interpretation. *Johns Hopkins Med J* 141:112–118.
85. Dean, RH, et al. 1985. Retrieval of renal function by revascularization. *Ann Surg* 202:367–375.
86. Moncure, AC, et al. 1986. The use of the hepatic and splenic arteries for renal revascularization. *J Vasc Surg* 3:196–203.
87. Hallett, JW, et al. 1987. Renovascular operations in patients with chronic renal insufficiency. *J Vasc Surg* 4:622–627.
88. Dean, RH, et al. 1984. Aortic and renal vascular disease: Factors affecting the value of combined procedures. *Ann Surg* 200:336–343.
89. Dean, RH, et al. 1981. Renovascular hypertension. *Arch Surg* 116:1408–1415.
90. Boley, SJ, et al. 1977. Initial results from an aggressive roentgenological and surgical approach to acute mesenteric ischemia. *Surgery* 82:848–855.
91. Ottinger, LW. 1978. The surgical management of acute occlusion of the superior mesenteric artery. *Ann Surg* 188:721–731.
92. Crawford, ES, et al. 1977. Celiac axis, superior mesenteric artery, and inferior mesenteric artery occlusion: Surgical considerations. *Surgery* 82:856–866.
93. O'Connell, TX, Kadell, B, and Tompkins, RK. 1976. Ischemia of the colon. *Surg Gynec Obstet* 142:337–342.
94. Cogbill, CL, et al. 1977. Ischemic colitis. *Am Surg* 43:137–143.
95. Boley, SJ, et al. 1963. Reversible vascular occlusion of the colon. *Surg Gynecol Obstet* 116:53–60.
96. Fiddian-Green, RG, Amelin, PM, Herrmann, JB. et al: Prediction of the development of sigmoid ischemia on the day of aortic operations. Indirect measurements of intramural pH in the colon. *Arch Surg* 121:654-660, 1986.
97. Stoney, RJ, Reilly, LM, and Ehrenfeld, WK. 1987. Chronic mesenteric ischemia and surgery for chronic visceral ischemia. *In Vascular Surgery: Principles and Practice,* Eds, SE Wilson, et al. pp. 672-684. New York: McGraw-Hill Co.
98. Halliday, JP, Harris, JP, and May, J. 1985. Femoro-femoral crossover grafts: A long-term follow-up study. In *Surgery of the Veins,* Eds., JJ Bergan and JST Yao. Orlando, FL: Grune & Stratton.
99. Gruss, JD. 1985. The saphenopopliteal bypass for chronic venous insufficiency. In *Surgery of the Veins,* Eds., JJ Bergan and JST Yao. Orlando, FL: Grune & Stratton.
100. Kistner, RL. 1985. Venous valve surgery. In *Surgery of the Veins,* Eds., JJ Bergan and JST Yao. Orlando, FL: Grune & Stratton.

33

Transplantation Surgery in the Elderly

Harold C. Yang, Francis L. Delmonico, and Paul S. Russell

Although the evolution of transplantation as a field of medicine has been rapid, its application to the care of the elderly has been limited. A shortage of donors has contributed to the preferential allocation of organs to recipients from age groups with the potential for more extended survival. Nevertheless, perhaps no group of patients may come to realize the benefit of organ replacement as much as the elderly, particularly since more of our population today is reaching older age. The opportunity to utilize organ transplantation to extend the productive life of an elderly patient by several years, by perhaps even a decade, has been enhanced as a result of increased experience and success in organ transplantation among all age groups. This chapter will examine the historical aspects and the current practice of organ transplantation as they pertain to renal and extrarenal allograft recipients, with a special focus upon the elderly.

Renal Transplantation

The Health Care Financing Administration (HCFA) estimated in 1984 that 50% of patients with end-stage renal disease were older than 55; yet these patients only represented 10% of those receiving kidney transplants (1). An explanation for this disproportionate distribution of kidneys was that the elderly patient presented too high a risk for transplantation. Indeed, data from both the United States and European registries from 1966 to 1978 showed that while the survival rate at 3 years was equivalent for patients under the age of 34 treated with transplantation or dialysis, survival was substantially worse for the elderly patient over 55 after cadaveric transplantation as compared to dialysis treatment. One- and 3-year survival rates for patients on chronic hemodialysis were 82% and 55%, respectively, but only 60% and 45% for those receiving kidney transplants (2).

Recent data from many centers suggest that transplantation can now be performed safely in the older patient (3–8). In fact, adjusted mortality rates for this age group are no worse than those for younger patients undergoing transplantation. Much of this improvement in the outcome for the older patient can be attributed to cyclosporine. Judicious administration of newer antirejection measures such as OKT3 monoclonal antibody has also contributed to better allograft survival.

Immunosuppression

Historical Aspects

Although Mathieu Jaboulay reported the first human kidney transplant as early as 1906, it was the application of chemical immunosuppression that ushered in the modern era of transplantation. Prednisone was introduced in the late 1950s and azathioprine in the early 1960s. In the two decades that followed, prednisone, azathioprine, and antilymphocyte sera were used in various combinations to produce long-term function in patients undergoing kidney transplantation.

In 1976 Borel et al. (9, 10) demonstrated the in vivo and in vitro immunosuppressive activity of cyclosporine. After its efficacy for whole organs was shown in animal systems, the first clinical trials using cyclosporine were performed by Calne et al. (11) in 1979. It was introduced into the United States for widespread use in January 1984.

The method of fusing lymphocytes and myeloma cells to create hybridomas was established by Kohler and Milstein (12) in 1975. This technique has produced a number of monoclonal antibodies, including OKT3, which is specifically directed against the T3 receptor of all lymphocytes. This agent was first introduced at the Massachusetts General Hospital in 1980 (13). The advantages of monoclonal preparations such as OKT3 include their relative specificity and uniformity. In contrast, antilymphocyte sera are polyclonal and are more broadly reactive against components of the immune system and even against variable numbers of antigens present on other tissues. This lack of specificity results in the higher incidence of infection accompanying treatment of rejection reactions with these polyclonal agents as compared to OKT3.

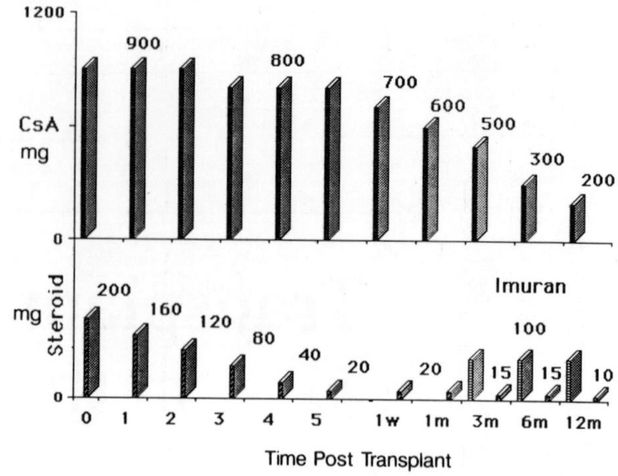

Figure 33-1. Treatment protocol for kidney transplantation from non-HLA-identical donor. CsA, Cyclosporin A.

Current Protocols

Because of the excellent outcome achieved routinely with HLA-identical, living, related renal transplants (95%), cyclosporine has not been routinely administered to these allograft recipients. Instead, azathioprine (Imuran) and prednisone have been the mainstay of immunosuppression (Table 33-1). Azathioprine is begun at 5 mg/kg/day and then is maintained indefinitely at a dose of 1.5 to 2.0 mg/kg/day. This dose is altered, however, if a white blood cell count of less than 3,000/cm^3 is observed.

All other renal allograft recipients are treated with cyclosporin A (CSA) and prednisone, as detailed in Figure 33-1. This group of patients includes recipients of renal allografts from cadaver donors, from living unrelated donors, and from living related donors who are haploidentical in their HLA match (Table 33-1). In the Massachusetts General Hospital protocol, Imuran is not added initially to the regimen of cyclosporine and prednisone except under one of the following circumstances: a preservation injury to the allograft immediately after transplantation (acute tubular necrosis [ATN]) or cyclosporine toxicity, both of which necessitate reduction or discontinuation of cyclosporine; acute allograft rejection; and after a second renal allograft when the primary transplant has failed because of rejection (Table 33-1). However, in many centers throughout the world, a triple drug regimen of cyclosporine, prednisone, and Imuran is given routinely from the outset after transplantation. The rationale for delaying the introduction of Imuran in our own protocol arises from a desire to avoid leukopenia until a reduced dose of cyclosporine is achieved.

Table 33-1. Massachusetts General Hospital renal transplantation immunosuppressive regimen

Circumstance	Regimen
HLA identical donor	Imuran + prednisone
Haploidentical donor	CsA + prednisone
Cadaver donor	CsA + prednisone
Living unrelated donor	CsA + prednisone
ATN	Add Imuran
CsA toxicity	Add Imuran
Rejection	Add Imuran
Second transplant	Add Imuran

CsA, Cyclosporin A.

The initial cyclosporine dose is 12 mg/kg/day. During the first week after transplantation, the cyclosporine dose is tapered to maintain a plasma level of 50–100 ng/ml by radioimmunoassay (Fig. 33-1). The steroid dosage is initiated at a level of 200 mg/day and tapered rapidly to 20 mg/day by the 5th day after transplantation. Thereafter the prednisone is continued at 15 mg/day from the 3rd to 12th month after transplantation (14), when it is reduced to a baseline maintenance dosage of 10 mg/day (Fig. 33-1).

If oliguric ATN occurs immediately after transplantation, cyclosporine is withdrawn temporarily. Antithymocyte globulin (ATG) is begun at 10 to 15 mg/kg/day and continued until dialysis is no longer required (Fig. 33-2). With the resolution of the ATN, cyclosporine is reinstituted at 6 mg/kg/day. Imuran is also added to the protocol because of the reduced dosage of cyclosporine.

Because of a frequent incidence of ATN at some centers, cyclosporine has been withheld until 5 to 7 days after transplantation (15, 16). During this period the renal allograft has an opportunity to recover from the ischemic injury, without the potential hazard of concomitant cyclosporine nephrotoxicity.

Renal allograft rejection is routinely treated with intravenous methylprednisolone, using a bolus dose of 500 mg. Rejection is determined by several factors including fever, reduced urine output, and a rising serum creatinine

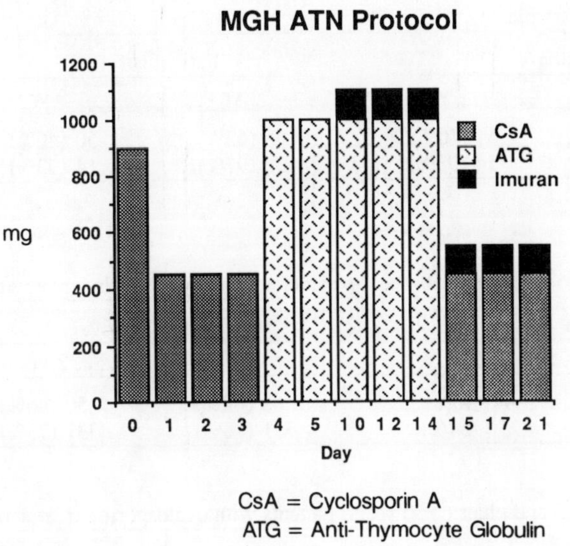

Figure 33-2. Treatment protocol for post-transplantation oliguric ATN.

level; however, renal allograft dysfunction may also occur as a result of cyclosporine toxicity. Thus, a biopsy of the allograft is necessary before instituting more potent therapy such as OKT3 (17), which is usually given for 10 to 14 days (Fig. 33-3).

Comparative Outcome in the Elderly

From the inception of the transplantation program at the Massachusetts General Hospital in 1963 to December 1983, when prednisone and azathioprine were used in combination with antilymphocyte serum of local origin and later with a very similar material prepared by the Upjohn Company, ATGAM, for immunosuppression, graft function and patient survival rates among the elderly at 1 year were only 48% and 62%, respectively. This survival rate for older recipients of kidney transplants was inferior to that reported for age-matched patients treated with hemodialysis. It was also evident during the same time period that the results in younger patients were significantly better.

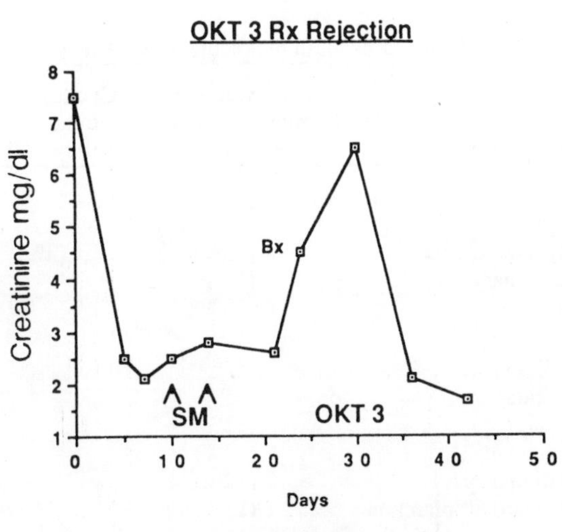

Figure 33-3. Treatment of renal allograft rejection and response.

A change in our results with transplantation in the elderly occurred with the institution of cyclosporine treatment in January 1984. There has been a significant increase in graft function and patient survival rates in those treated with more recently devised regimens (Table 33-2). This improvement does not just represent a refinement in medical care over two decades: in 1983 the 1-year survival rate for patients over 50 receiving a kidney transplant was still only 58.3% at our institution.

It is always difficult to compare patient populations from different historical periods. The currently used immunosuppressive program will be characterized as using cyclosporine and the previously employed programs as being without cyclosporine. Although the introduction of cyclosporine has been a major component of the more recently introduced treatment program, it would be an oversimplification to attribute the improvements noted by us and others to this single agent exclusively. A better perspective of the beneficial effect of cyclosporine can be obtained by comparing patients above and below the age of 50 from the same time period. Without cyclosporine there was a significant difference in both graft function and patient survival rates between younger and older patients, as illustrated in Table 33-3. With the use of cyclosporine, a statistical difference cannot be appreciated between the two groups (Table 33-4).

In a recent review the yearly mortality rates for patients aged 55 to 65 and those over 65 treated with dialysis were 20% and 35%, respectively (1). The more recent experience with cyclosporine would suggest that transplantation is a favorable alternative to dialysis therapy.

What accounts for the improved outcomes of transplantation in the elderly? Eliminating death as a cause of graft failure has had a substantial impact. Prior to the use of cyclosporine, half of the kidney allografts lost during the first year at the Massachusetts General Hospital were attributable to death in this older age group. It was still the leading cause for graft failure in the second year (Table 33-5). Now patients over the age of 50, like their younger counterparts, lose their transplanted kidneys most often because of rejection.

Transplant surgeons have learned that immunosuppression represents a balance between inadequate treatment, which results in rejection, and overtreatment, which leads to infection. There are cases, however, in

Table 33-2. Outcome of kidney transplantation in patients over 50 years old

Immunosuppression	n	Graft function 1 yr	Graft function 2 yr	Patient survival 1 yr	Patient survival 2 yr
No cyclosporine	109	52 (48%)	44 (40%)	68 (62%)	50 (46%)
Cyclosporine	37	33 (89%)	14 (93%)[a]	36 (97%)	14 (93%)[a]

[a]Actuarial, $n = 15$.

Table 33-3. Outcome of kidney transplantation in younger (<50 years) and older (>50 years) patients without cyclosporine treatment

Immunosuppression	n	Graft function 1 yr	Graft function 2 yr	Patient survival 1 yr	Patient survival 2 yr
>50 years old	109	52 (48%)	44 (40%)	68 (62%)	50 (46%)
<50 years old	451	285 (63%)	256 (57%)	351 (78%)	337 (75%)

Table 33-4. Outcome of kidney transplantation in younger (<50 years) and older (>50 years) patients with cyclosporine treatment

Immunosuppression	n	Graft function 1 yr	Graft function 2 yr	Patient survival 1 yr	Patient survival 2 yr
>50 years old	37	38 (89%)	14 (93%)[a]	36 (97%)	14 (93%)[a]
<50 years old	167	138 (83%)	45 (78%)[b]	155 (93%)	52 (90%)[b]

[a]Actuarial, $n = 15$.
[b]Actuarial, $n = 58$.

which enough immunosuppression cannot be given to prevent rejection without leading to overwhelming infection. Before cyclosporine was available overwhelming infection was the primary cause of death in the elderly recipient during the first year. It was not unusual for transplant centers to report patients in this age group dying of sepsis with functioning allografts. Remarkably, at 2 years, sepsis was still the leading cause of graft failure in this age group (Table 33-6). Cyclosporine has virtually eliminated sepsis as a primary cause of graft failure within the first year. This has improved graft function substantially.

With aging there is a gradual reduction in immune system responsiveness. Prior to the use of cyclosporine, the number of rejection episodes experienced by older and younger patients was indistinguishable. With cyclosporine, however, older patients clearly have fewer rejections than younger ones (Table 33-7). When rejection episodes do occur, nearly 60% are treated successfully with first-line immunosuppression, i.e., steroids alone. Another 30% require the addition of OKT3 or antilymphocyte serum with an overall salvage rate of 86%. These data illustrate that there is an increase in the number of successfully treated rejections with less immunosuppression.

The recent experience of others with cyclosporine would tend to confirm our observation that renal trans-

Table 33-5. Cause of graft failure in the elderly patient

Cause	Noncyclosporine 1 yr (n = 57)	Noncyclosporine 2 yr (n = 8)	Cyclosporine 2 yr (n = 4)
Death	27 (47%)	6 (75%)	1 (25%)
Rejection	26 (46%)	1 (13%)	3 (75%)
Technical	3 (5%)		
Peritransplant abscess	1 (2%)		
Recurrent disease		1 (13%)	

Table 33-6. Cause of death in recipients over 50 years old

Cause of death	Nonconventional Immunosuppression (n = 109)	Cyclosporine treatment (n = 37)
One year		
Sepsis	23 (56%)	
Myocardial infarction	8 (20%)	1 (3%)
Pulmonary embolus	2 (5%)	
Other	8 (20%)	—
Total	41	1
Two years		
Sepsis	3 (33%)	0
Unknown	2 (22%)	
Malignancy	2 (22%)	
Myocardial infarction	1 (11%)	
Dialysis dementia	1 (11%)	—
Total	9	0

Table 33-7. Rejection episodes and treatment in recipients greater than 50 years old

	No Cyclosporine (n = 109)	Cyclosporine Treatment (n = 37)
Total number of rejection episodes	62 (57%)	14 (38%)
Successful treatment with:		
Steroids alone	16 (26%)	8 (57%)
Steroids + OKT3 and/or ATG	8 (13%)	4 (29%)
Overall allograft salvage rate	39%	86%

plantation can be performed safely in the older patient. In the United States, Fryd et al. (5) from the University of Minnesota, Shah et al. (8) from the University of Cincinnati, and Pirsch et al. (6) from the University of Wisconsin have reported individually that graft function and patient survival rates have improved in the cyclosporine-treated elderly recipient of a kidney transplant (Table 33-8). Early data from the HCFA, which encompassed the collective experience of renal transplantation in the United States, also showed this beneficial effect: from 1982 to 1983 patient survival and graft function rates at 1 year were 83% and 67%, respectively, in cyclosporine-treated recipients of kidney transplants aged 55 to 65 (1). The corresponding mortality rates for dialysis treatment in this age group were worse, at 20%. The 1-year graft function rates in recipients aged 35 to 55 were only slightly better, at 73%. The European experience with cyclosporine in elderly patients is as promising as that of United States (Table 33-8) (4, 7).

Liver Transplantation

Liver transplantation has become a well-accepted method of treatment for patients with end-stage liver failure. A routine protocol of immunosuppression for liver allograft recipients is displayed in Figure 33-4. A triple drug regimen of cyclosporine, Imuran, and prednisone begins immediately after transplantation. In contrast to renal allograft recipients, liver transplant patients receive cyclosporine intravenously until they are able to take it orally. Rejection of a liver allograft is recognized by elevations in the serum bilirubin and the serum transaminase level (SGOT). Intravenous methylprednisolone is administered at least twice before the institution of OKT3 therapy. A liver allograft biopsy is routinely performed prior to the institution of OKT3, and a characteristic pattern of mononuclear cell infiltration is observed.

The course of a 68-year-old male who underwent liver transplantation at Massachusetts General Hospital because of hepatocellular carcinoma is illustrated in Figure 33-5. This patient experienced an episode of acute rejection, for which he received intravenous methylprednisolone and OKT3 therapy. After the rejection episode the patient then experienced liver allograft dysfunction. On this occasion, however, a biopsy of the allograft revealed cytomegalic viral hepatitis. His doses of immunosuppressive agents were reduced. The hepatitis resolved with these measures, and, more than 6 months after transplantation, the patient continues to do well. This patient's course illustrates the need for biopsy to determine the cause of liver allograft dysfunction. It also demonstrates that a patient 68 years of age may achieve a successful outcome despite two severe episodes of dysfunction, either of which might have been life threatening.

The outcome of liver transplantation at the Massachusetts General Hospital has continued to improve in recent years. As is illustrated in Figure 33-6, the percentage of patients surviving at 36 months has improved during the past 3 years when compared to the entire series, which originated in 1983. Until recently, data pertaining

Table 33-8. Outcome in cyclosporine-treated elderly patients receiving cadaveric kidney transplants

Period	Authors (institution)	Patient number	Age (yr)	Patient survival at 1 yr	Graft function at 1 yr
1979–84	Fryd et al. (5) (Univ. of Minnesota)	24	50–70	96%	83%
1982–84	Krakauer et al. (1) (HCFA)	198	>55	83%	67%
1980–85	Ringden et al. (7) (Huddinge Hospital, Sweden)	29	55–71	86%	72%
1983–85	Brynger et al. (4) (Sahlgren's Hospital, Sweden)	51	55–60	86%	70%
1984–86	Shah et al. (8) (Univ. of Cincinnati)	26	50–64	82%	65%
1985–88	Pirsch et al. (6) (Univ. of Wisconsin)	36	60–73	92%	78%

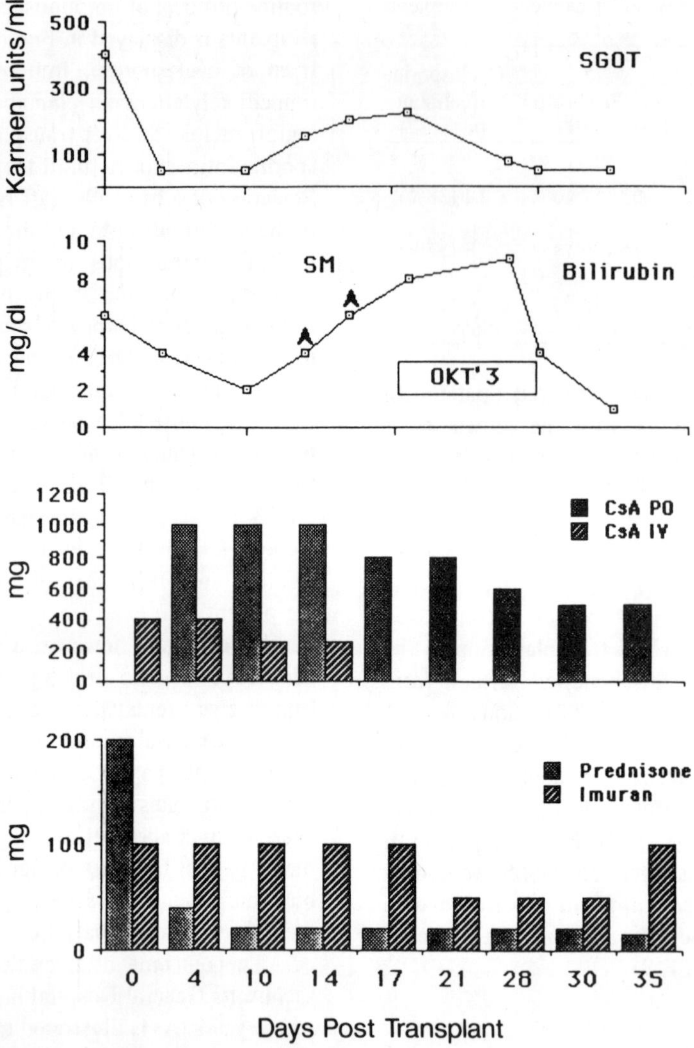

Figure 33-4. Immunosuppression protocol for liver allograft recipients.

to the outcome of liver transplantation in the elderly have not been available. At the Massachusetts General Hospital, 23 of the 69 patients who have undergone liver transplantation were more than 50 years old. Six of these patients were 60 years of age or older. The causes of liver failure for this older age group were predominantly cirrhosis and hepatocellular carcinoma (Table 33-9). Three of these patients have died, one of them within one month after transplantation; however, the other two patients did not die until 13 months and 22 months after transplantation, of lymphoma and pneumocystic pneumonia. Nevertheless, analysis of this older age group reveals that these patients fared surprisingly well when compared to all other age groups (Fig. 33-7). In a letter to the editor of the *New England Journal of Medicine*, Starzl et al. (18) showed that patient survival after liver transplantation was the same for recipients above and below the age of 50.

Heart Transplantation

To date nearly 7,000 heart transplants have been performed worldwide. The increasing success of heart transplantation is underscored by the proliferation of heart transplant centers throughout the world and by the most recent data, which reveal an actuarial 5-year survival rate of 73% (19). Once again, older age patients have fared quite well. In fact, the best survival rates are currently found in a group between 55 and 68 years of age: 78% at 5 years after transplantation. The Registry for the International Society for Heart Transplantation concludes that donor availability remains the biggest obstacle to permitting more heart transplants throughout the country and particularly in this older age group.

In an individual report from St. Louis University, Miller et al. (20) compared the results of heart transplan-

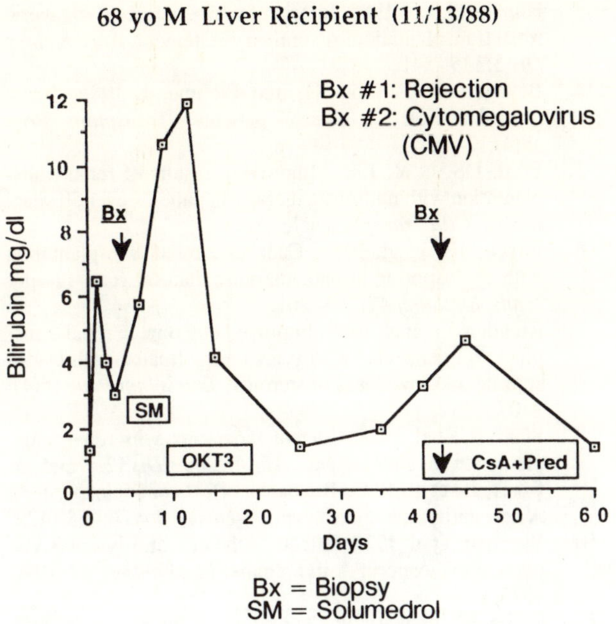

Figure 33-5. Course of a 68-year-old male liver transplant recipient.

tation in patients over and under the age of 55. Despite the fact that the elderly patients were actually sicker preoperatively (as determined by their NATCO status), their length of stay postoperatively in the intensive care unit and in the hospital was no longer than their younger counterparts. All (100%) of the recipients over 55 had survived, although the average follow-up was short (10.4 months).

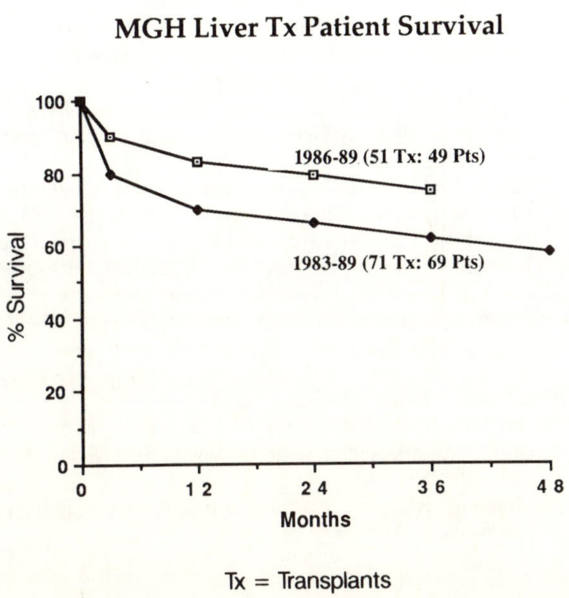

Figure 33-6. Outcome of liver transplantation at Massachusetts General Hospital. Pts, Patients.

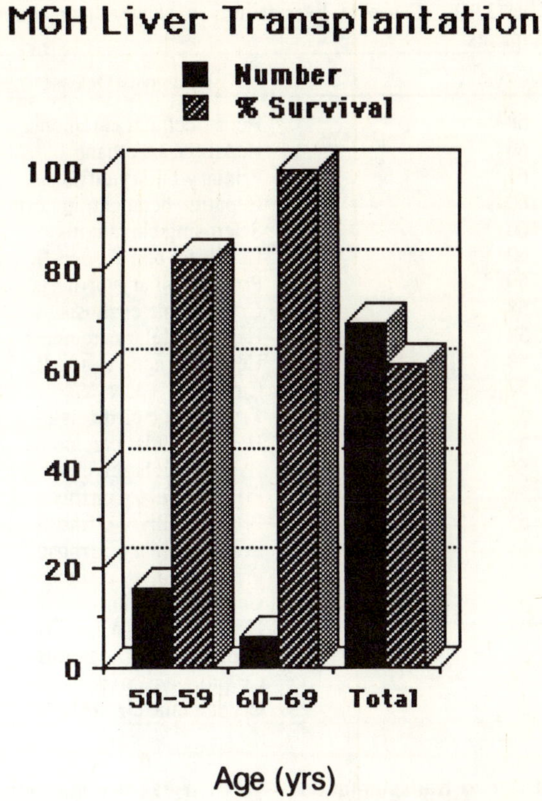

Figure 33-7. Outcome of liver transplantation in different age groups.

A report by Olivari et al. (21) from the University of Minnesota confirmed the findings above. Again, graft function and patient survival rates were no different for 34 and 23 heart recipients less than and greater than age 55, respectively. In a comparison of complications, there was no difference in the number of rejections and neurologic events, i.e., strokes and seizures. However, the incidence of infection, steroid-induced diabetes, and osteoporosis appeared to be higher among the elderly. In this vein Gay et al. (22), from the University of Utah, have described using prophylactic OKT3 in the hope of discontinuing steroids in recipients of heart transplants. An opportunity to discontinue steroids in this age group would help obviate the complications reported by the University of Minnesota.

Conclusion

In 1971 Simmons et al. (23) labeled the patient over 45 as a "high" risk for transplantation. This classification was justified by their early experience, in which the mortality rate was 60% at 1 year for elderly recipients of a kidney transplant. Today, with the improvement and judicious administration of immunosuppression, age is no longer a

Table 33-9. Cause of liver failure in elderly liver allograft recipients

Age (yr)	Diagnosis/Disease
68	Hepatocellular carcinoma
66	Hepatitis, halothane
61	Primary biliary cirrhosis
60	Hepatitis hemochromatosis
60	Sclerosing cholangitis
60	Hepatitis, non-A, non-B, s/p
59	Primary biliary cirrhosis
58	Cryptogenic cirrhosis
58	Hepatocellular carcinoma
58	Hepatitis, non-A, non-B
57	Cirrhosis
57	Cryptogenic cirrhosis
56	Hepatocellular carcinoma
56	Hepatocellular carcinoma
56	Primary biliary cirrhosis
55	Primary biliary cirrhosis
55	Primary biliary cirrhosis
55	Primary biliary cirrhosis
54	Cirrhosis, Laennec's
51	Hepatitis, non-A, non-B
50	Hepatitis, non-A, non-B
50	Cryptogenic cirrhosis
50	Cryptogenic cirrhosis

barrier to transplantation. Age then has become only a relative contraindication to transplantation. For the potential elderly recipients of kidney or liver transplants, good results can be obtained in the absence of concomitant medical problems each as severe coronary artery disease. In general, patients should be ambulatory and not comatose. There should be no evidence of untreated foci of infection. Renal, heart, and liver transplantation can be performed safely in patients over the age of 50. The largest obstacle remains the shortage of organ donors. Fifty percent of those with end-stage cardiac disease die waiting for an available donor. Waiting lists for kidney transplantation continue to expand as the demand for donors outweighs supply. As more of our elderly population comes to dialysis, this shortage will be more acutely experienced.

References

1. Krakauer, H, et al. 1985. The current experience with cyclosporine in the United States: Recipient age considerations. *Transplant Proc* 17:2808–2810.
2. Kjellstrand, CM, et al. 1980. Cadaver transplantation versus hemodialysis. *Trans Am Soc Artif Intern Organs* 26: 611–624.
3. Hunsicker, LG. 1985. Impact of cyclosporine on cadaveric renal transplantation: A summary statement. *Am J Kidney Dis* 5:335–341.
4. Brynger, H, Persson, H, and Blohme, I. 1986. Renal transplantation in elderly patients. *Transplant Proc* 18(4):12–13.
5. Fryd, DS, et al. 1987. Improving results of renal transplantation with multidrug therapy in patients over 50 years of age. *Clin Transplant* 1:75–80.
6. Pirsch, JD, et al. 1989. Cadaveric renal transplantation with cyclosporine in patients more than 60 years of age. *Transplantation* 47:259–261.
7. Ringden, O, et al. 1983. Improved outcome in renal transplant recipients above 55 years of age treated with cyclosporine and low doses of steroids. *Transplant Proc* 15(4): 2507–2512.
8. Shah, B, et al. 1988. Current experience with renal transplantation in older patients. *Am J Kidney Dis* 12:516–523.
9. Borel, JF, et al. 1976. Biological effects of cyclosporin A: A new antilymphocytic agent. *Agents Actions* 6:468–475.
10. Borel, JF, et al. 1977. Effects of the new anti-lymphocytic peptide cyclosporin A in animals. *Immunology* 32:1017–1025.
11. Calne, RY, et al. 1979. Cyclosporin A initially as the only immunosuppressant in 34 recipients of cadaveric organs: 32 kidneys, 2 pancreases, and 2 livers. *Lancet* :1033–1036.
12. Kohler, G, and Milstein, C. 1975. Continuous cultures of fused cells secreting antibody of predefined specificity. *Nature* 256:491–495.
13. Cosimi, AB, et al. 1981. Treatment of acute renal allograft rejection with OKT3 monoclonal antibody. *Transplantation* 32:535–539.
14. Shield, CF III, Cosimi, AB, and Tolkoff-Rubin, N. 1983. Antithymocyte globulin as the primary treatment for renal allograft rejection. *Transplantation* 36:587–589.
15. Deierhoi, MH, Sollinger, HW, and Kalayoglu, M. 1987. Quadruple immunosuppression in 305 consecutive cadaver renal allografts. *Clin Transplant* 1:71–75.
16. Sommer, BG, Henry, M, and Ferguson, RM. 1987. Sequential antilymphoblast globulin and cyclosporine for renal transplantation. *Transplantation* 43:85–90.
17. Thistlethwaite, JR Jr, et al. 1984. Evolving use of OKT3 monoclonal antibody for treatment of renal allograft rejection. *Transplantation* 38:695–701.
18. Starzl, TE, et al. 1987. Liver transplantation in older patients (letter to the editor). *N Engl J Med* 316:484–485.
19. Fragomeni, CS, and Kaye, MP. 1988. The Registry of the International Society for Heart Transplantation: Fifth Official Report—1988. *J Heart Transplant* 7:249–253.
20. Miller, LW, et al. 1988. Heart transplantation in patients over age fifty-five years. *J Heart Transplant* 7:254–257.
21. Olivari, MT, et al. 1987. Heart transplantation in elderly patients. *J Heart Transplant* 7:258–264.
22. Gay, WA Jr, et al. 1988. OKT3 monoclonal antibody in cardiac transplantation: Experience with 102 patients. *Ann Surg* 208:287–290.
23. Simmons, RL, et al. 1971. Renal transplantation in high-risk patients. *Arch Surg* 103:290–298.

34

Pressure Sores in the Elderly

Zeno N. Chicarilli

A pressure sore describes an ulcerative lesion that develops over a part of the body subjected to prolonged and/or excessive compressive and shear forces. They most commonly occur in an area where a bony prominence underlies a relatively thin subcutaneous-cutaneous padding. Although frequently referred to as "decubitus ulcers," this term should be applied only to those sites where ulceration is incurred from a supine, prone, or lateral position. Decubitus is derived from the Latin *decumber* meaning to lie down and is therefore an inaccurate adjective for ulcers that develop in the sitting position.

The key factors that provide for avoidance of pressure ulcerations include the sensory input of discomfort followed by a voluntary motor execution to alter one's position and alleviate the noxious stimulus. These actions are such an integral part of our daily living that we accept them as second nature. We continually alter compressive weight-bearing forces by shifting our weight while standing or sitting and adjusting our position when lying down, mitigating their injurious nature. It is only when these conscious and subconscious safeguards become impaired that the destructive consequences of unmitigated pressure become evident. The geriatric patient represents a subpopulation that is at high risk for pressure ulceration by virtue of failing organ systems, which may compromise protective mechanisms. Sensory input and motor response may be impaired by a sensitive response to sedative and pain medication, cerebrovascular accident, coma, spinal or lower extremity fractures, and general debility. Therefore, it is not uncommon that an elderly patient admitted with a diagnosis of myocardial infarction, pneumonia, or a fractured hip may incur the additional diagnosis of a sacral pressure sore during his hospitalization due to the imposed or obligate immobility.

Although the implication of a pressure sore may seem trivial compared to the underlying disease, the sore's inherent morbidity remains significant. The overall estimated incidence of pressure sore development during hospitalization is around 3% to 4% or about 43 per 100,000 population (1, 2). The incidence of pressure sores in those patients with spinal cord injury is even higher, ranging from 25% to 85% (3, 4). A mortality rate of 7% to 8% has been attributed to pressure ulceration management and its complications (4).

The sophisticated medical care available today has served to increase the geriatric population base that is at high risk to developing pressure sores. A Connecticut Governors Commission estimated that from 1980 to the year 2000, the projected growth of the state's elderly population (over 65) would be around 41%, while that of the general population would be only 9%. They also estimate a 31% increase in acute care hospital days consumed by the elderly (5). When one realizes that each pressure ulceration costs on the average between $20,000 to $25,000 to heal, the present and future economic burden is self evident and dictates a policy aimed at prevention (2).

Etiopathogenesis

Pressure sores have been a well-recognized entity throughout history with early cited references dating back to the biblical periods, including their demonstration in autopsies performed on Egyptian mummies (6).

Many of the early works on the etiopathogenesis of pressure sores rightfully implicated pressure as the major causal factor. In 1852, Brown-Sequard described the development of ulcers in paraplegic mammals and birds secondary to the effect of continued pressure in the presence of moisture (urine and feces) (7). From his animal studies, he postulated that these sores heal as quickly in paraplegics as they do in normal animals and that by alleviating continual compression forces and maintaining good hygiene in the cord-transected animals, these ulcers could be avoided. Additional reinforcement for this pressure-induced theory was given by Paget in 1873, who described the process similar to what we know today as an ischemic insult based on anoxic tissue necrosis. He also pointed out the fact that this process is accelerated in those individuals who are old or debilitated (8).

Despite these reputable works, the late 19th and early 20th century outlook on pressure sore prevention and treatment was dismal owing to their inevitability as espoused by Charcot's neuropathic theory (9). According to Charcot, injury to the central nervous system released an intrinsic neurotrophic factor regulating nutrition and effecting a decrease in tissue tolerance to pressure resulting in eventual ulceration. This pessimistic viewpoint found similar proponents as late as 1940, when Munro indicated tissue tolerance to pressure was lowered through abnormal cutaneous vascular reflexes secondary to autonomic dysfunction below the level of cord injury (10). He also felt aggressive surgical treatment was unjustified since intrinsic factors would eventuate in recurrent ulceration. Charcot's neuropathic theory was never proven and although autonomic dysfunction does occur following spinal cord injury as stated by Munro, its precise role in the development of pressure sores remains enigmatic.

After 1940, the theory came full circle and once again concentrated on the main issue of pressure in producing these ulcerations. Groth, applying pressure to the gluteal muscle region of rabbits, was able to experimentally reproduce pressure sores found in man. The damage to local tissues was dependent on an inverse relationship between the magnitude of applied force and the duration of its application. Pressures ranging from 23 to 143 mm Hg over varying time periods produced both clinical and microscopic changes, with greater destruction occurring from the higher pressures and/or prolonged application. Clinically, early changes were limited to erythema and swelling, which would eventually lead to hemorrhagic necrotic foci. Microscopically, capillary hemorrhage and waxy degeneration of the gluteal muscles was seen followed by scar replacement. Another important observation derived from this study was the fact that those animals with greater muscle mass demonstrated more tolerance to applied pressure than those with less padding. Second, the destructive process increases in magnitude from the skin surface to the underlying bony process like a cone, due to a greater force generated adjacent to the focal bony process (11) (Fig. 34-1). This feature has led to the view that skin changes seen in pressure sores represent only the "tip of the iceberg," with greater destruction occurring in the subjacent undermined tissues (adipose, muscle) overlying the bone. Another explanation to this differential destructive process has always cited a greater susceptibility to pressure of the adipose and muscle tissues than skin. However, Groth's impressions were subsequently confirmed by simultaneous external and internal pressure sensor measurements, demonstrating higher generated forces beneath the skin surface (12). Groth also noted that the damage created by pressure served as a "locus minorum" in septicemic animals, resulting in local infection with abscess production and greater tissue destruction. These observations remain valid today despite Groth's failure to appreciate ischemia as the mechanism by which pressure produces tissue necrosis (11).

In a classic experiment, Husain applied pressure to a rat's limb with a pneumatic cuff. He showed similar pathologic changes after applying 600 mm Hg for 1 hour or 100 mm Hg for 2 hours. However, with 100 mm Hg over a 6-hour period, these changes were much more severe, leading him to believe the time factor was more important than pressure intensity. In this same study, he evaluated the effect of vitamin C deficiency on guinea pigs developing pressure sores. He found normal guinea pigs developed changes with 200 mm Hg after 2 hours, whereas scorbutic guinea pigs were much more sensitive, showing similar changes with 50 mm Hg after only 1 hour. He also reproduced Groth's work on bacteremic localization to incipient pressure sores enhancing patho-

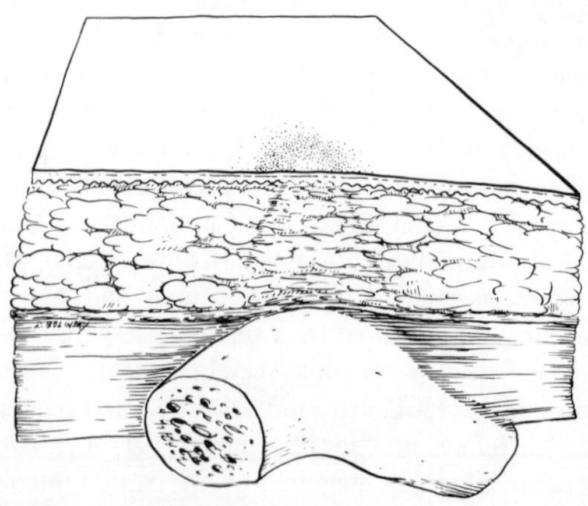

Figure 34-1. Cross-section of developing pressure sore demonstrating early changes, which are most pronounced in the subcutaneous tissues. Morphologically, the zone of injury resembles a cone with its apex at the skin and the wider base located adjacent to the bony pressure point.

logic changes and concurred with his morphologic pressure cone descriptions (13).

The pressure and time to produce histologic changes, either reversible or irreversible, and that which produces actual ulceration were evaluated by Kosiak through the application of pressure to the trochanteric and ischial regions of mongrel dogs. He demonstrated microscopic irreversible changes with 70 mm Hg applied for 2 hours constantly, which could be avoided by intermittent relief every 5 minutes. The minimum pressure to produce an overt ulcer was 150 mm Hg over at least 9 hours (15). Dinsdale performed a similar study on paraplegic swine to delineate the absolute constant pressure necessary to produce ulceration, as well as the effect of repetitive pressure application and shear (friction) forces. In those swine receiving continuous pressure for 3 hours, a minimum force of 480 mm Hg was necessary to produce ulceration; however, when friction was added, ulceration was noted with only 240 mm Hg. Dinsdale concluded that with continuous pressure friction became a significant factor in ulceration when the pressure was less than 500 mm Hg. With repetitive application of pressure, which is more common in daily living, the force required to produce ulceration was much less, occurring at 290 mm Hg for pressure alone and with as little as 45 mm Hg when friction was also applied. The duration of these repetitive forces was one and a half hours with a 1-hour rest. The exact mechanism by which shear forces accelerated ulceration was not readily evident and isotope clearance studies did not implicate increased ischemia (4). This study was the first to demonstrate ulceration with a force as low as 45 mm Hg, although this still represents a pressure well above the accepted range of capillary perfusion pressure, which is 16 to 33 mm Hg (15). Therefore, it appears that any force exceeding capillary perfusion pressure is capable of producing pressure sores, given the additional factors of friction, repetition, and prolonged application.

Lindan and co-workers have studied the normal forces applied to the body surfaces during sitting, supine, and prone positions, mapping out the areas most susceptible to point pressure. The significance of this study lies in the fact that despite surfaces that were considerably padded compared to standard beds and chairs, most pressure measurements taken over bony prominences (40 to 100 mm Hg) were well in excess of capillary perfusion pressure. During sitting, ischial pressures were noted to be higher when the feet were supported (80 to 100 mm Hg), than if left to hang freely (60 mm Hg), whereby the posterior thigh equally shared pressure distribution (60 mm Hg) (16). Kosiak demonstrated even higher pressures over the ischial region during sitting, ranging from 150 to 500 mm Hg, which correlated to a varied surface padding (17) (Fig. 34-2).

Although pressure sores can develop almost anywhere on the body, they are most frequently found over bony processes, which naturally generate higher pressure

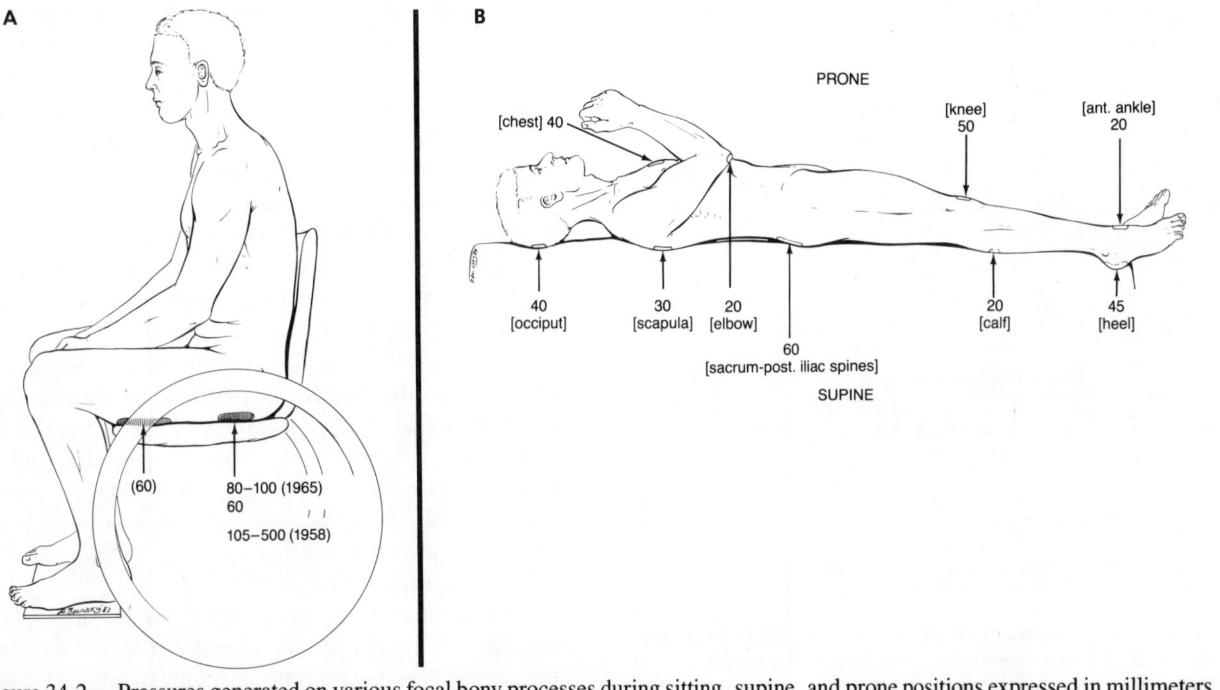

Figure 34-2. Pressures generated on various focal bony processes during sitting, supine, and prone positions expressed in millimeters of mercury (mm Hg). Note higher pressures in ischial region during sitting when feet are supported compared to hanging freely ( ). See text for explanation. Data from Lindan et al. (16) and Kosiak et al. (17).

during surface contact. Sixty-five percent of these ulcerations develop in the pelvic region and about 30 percent in the lower extremity. The upper body is less frequently affected (18–21) (Fig. 34-3).

Patient Risk Profile

Petersen and Bittman (20) studied a pressure sore population and found that 63% of patients developed their ulcerations while in the hospital. A breakdown of this group revealed that 53% occurred in bedridden patients, 37% in wheelchair patients, and 10% in ambulatory patients. Realizing that certain patients are at greater risk for developing pressure sores upon entering the hospital or during convalescence should alert health care professionals to institute additional measures for their prevention. High-risk factors that affect the incidence of pressure sore development are listed in Table 34-1.

Neurologic deficits can be transient or permanent, but either may place the patient at risk for pressure ulceration. Those patients with permanent deficits, however, must make pressure avoidance a part of their everyday life. Altered consciousness may result from alcohol or drug overdose, head trauma, cerebrovascular accident, surgical or postsurgical sedation. Without adequate sensory input, artificial means must be employed to periodically relieve pressure points and maintain adequate circulation. Paraplegia and quadriplegia, resulting from spinal cord trauma, tumors, or demyelinating diseases, represent a continuing challenge, and this patient population is the most widely studied group at risk for pressure sores. The psychologic impact of these chronic conditions upon the patient often creates periods of depression during which their motivation to avoid prolonged pressure fluctuates. The pressure sore incidence in this group has been reported to be from 44% to 86% (22, 23).

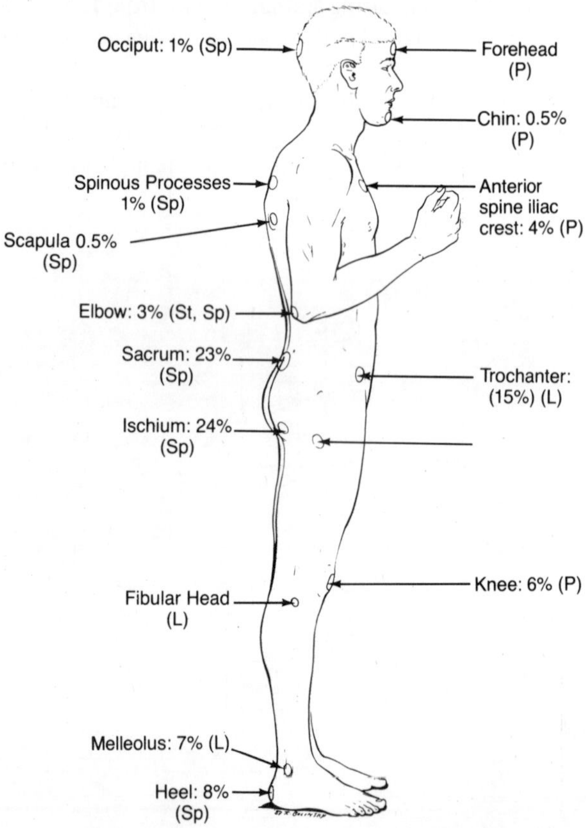

Figure 34-3. Frequency of pressure sore development according to site. ( ) indicates the body position which predisposes to that particular pressure sore: (L)–lateral, (P)–prone, (Sp)–supine, and (St)–sitting. Modified from Agris and Spira (21) and Linder and Upton (2).

Table 34-1. Systemic risk factors

Systemic risk factors
1. Neurologic deficit
2. Geriatric age group
3. Malnutrition
4. Immobilization
5. Debilitating medical disease

The geriatric age group also presents a significant susceptibility to pressure sores for various reasons, and in one study, 71% of the patients with pressure sores were over 70 years of age (24). Nutritional deficiency and loss of body mass combine to increase the force applied to bony prominences through loss of adipose padding. Muscle atrophy and lack of mobility and ambulation often prolong their duration spent in one particular position. Multisystem failure in the elderly—including fractures, cancer, cerebrovascular, coronary, and peripheral vascular disease—may impose further sedentary activity and lower tissue resiliency to pressure. Once a pressure sore develops, these same predisposing factors create additional risks for the development of pressure sores in other sites while trying to alleviate pressure from the primary ulcer. For an established ulcer wound, repair proceeds at a slower rate in the geriatric population, prolonging both conservative and surgical measures of correction and increasing the morbidity risk. Therefore, in this patient population with high rates of immobility, body wasting, associated debilitating diseases, and urinary or fecal incontinence, intensive nursing care is a prerequisite for avoiding pressure ulceration (25).

Malnutrition also plays a critical role in the development and subsequent healing of pressure sores. As demonstrated by Husain (13) experimentally, scorbutic guinea pigs developed pressure ulceration at lower forces over a shorter period of time than normal guinea pigs. It is also known that recently healed wounds will lose tensile strength when a scorbutic state is induced, since ongoing scar metabolism results in removal of normal collagen and its replacement by immature and poorly polymerized collagen molecules. Contraction of open wounds is similarly impaired. Starvation sufficient to produce a 20% weight loss through inadequate calorie and protein intake produces a similar impairment of wound healing. Negative nitrogen balance results in catabolism of body stores and lean body mass leading to body wasting. The end result can be much the same as the geriatric patient who loses padding over bony prominences and lacks sufficient energy to remain mobile and avoid prolonged pressure. The additional morbidity associated with the nutritionally catabolic patient, particularly infection, may lead to further immobility and longer hospitalization, accentuating the predisposition to skin breakdown. Nutritional assessment should include a visceral protein evaluation of serum albumin and transferrin levels and immune competency testing as determined by delayed hypersensitivity to various antigens. If indicated, nitrogen balance studies should be performed to guide corrective therapy. Adequate nutritional repletion can usually be carried out by the enteral route, with total parenteral alimentation reserved for patients with nonfunctioning gastrointestinal tracts or excessive metabolic demands.

Immobilization for whatever reason places the patient at jeopardy to pressure ulceration, even when forces applied are relatively low. This situation is common in patients with multisystem trauma, hip and lower extremity fractures, extensive burns requiring grafting to the trunk, pulmonary insufficiency necessitating prolonged ventilatory support, and in critically ill patients who receive multisystem support and monitoring. The critical factor in avoiding pressure sores in this population is good nursing care, along with specialized body support systems designed to minimize pressure and shear forces.

The last group of patients at risk are those with various medical problems that are commonly associated with individuals who are prone to debility and, as such, subsequent ulceration. These include cancer, cardiovascular diseases, diabetes, high-dose steroid therapy, and hepatic and renal insufficiency. Malnutrition and prolonged immobilization are frequent co-factors in this group when pressure sores develop during hospitalization. The effect of aggressive care during the hospital course of these patients can reduce the incidence of breakdown from 30% to 3% (25–27).

The local factors responsible for pressure sores are outlined in Table 34-2, with unrelieved pressure being the primary cause. Shear forces have already been mentioned as a significant secondary problem, which increases a patient's susceptibility to pressure ulceration and is a common problem when transferring patients from a bed to a stretcher or chair. Shear forces are also generated in the pelvic region when raising a patient's bed from a supine to a sitting position. Additional shear is applied if the patient repetitively "slides down" from this sitting position and is pulled up without actually lifting the patient out of contact with the bed during repositioning. Contusions may also result in initial blistering and skin breakdown that is subsequently more susceptible to pressure forces, particularly if these minor wounds become infected. Poor hygiene and infection often go together in aiding pressure sore development. Patients with urinary and/or fecal incontinence may develop maceration of the nearby tissues that are kept in contact with soiled linens. These relatively minor wounds may then become superficially infected, which in combination with additional pressure and shear forces, increases susceptibility to further breakdown and overt ulceration. Certainly, the surface characteristics and texture of the sleeping and sitting supports can be another significant factor to either enhance or minimize the absolute pressures applied to the body as well as their distribution.

Table 34-2. Local factors causing pressure sores

Reconstructive options
Primary
1. Pressure
Secondary
1. Local tissue injury
a. Shear
b. Contusion
c. Maceration
2. Poor hygiene
a. Incontinence
a. Soiled linen
3. Infection
4. Body support surface

By knowing which patients are at high risk for pressure ulceration during hospitalization, appropriate measures can be instituted to alter the local factors responsible for producing pressure sores. An awareness of the clinical course of pressure sores is also necessary to know when simple protective measures must be supplemented by aggressive local care or surgical management.

Clinical Pathology

The incipient pressure sore is characterized by erythema of the involved skin secondary to a hyperemic response. Alleviation of pressure at this point will completely reverse the injury. However, continued pressure will lead to swelling and induration, which are indicative of a destructive process, whereby capillary extravasation of inflammatory cells and local hemorrhage lead to scar deposition in the subdermal tissues (e.g., adipose). This ischemic event may be accompanied by superficial epidermal and dermal ulceration. Microscopically, the pathologic morphology of the pressure cone (Fig. 34-1) becomes evident with greater changes occurring in the more pressure sensitive tissues adjacent to the bony prominence (e.g., adipose, muscle). In order of ischemic pressure sensitivity, nerves, adipose, and muscle undergo degeneration much more rapidly than dermis, fascia, and bone. The injury to local nerves at this point serves to decrease the painful sensory input of pressure and therefore the patient's awareness of ongoing injury is diminished. Induration of local adipose and muscle serves to decrease the supple padding, allowing a greater transmission of force from bone to skin. At this point in the production of a pressure sore, prolonged pressure relief, local skin care, and topical antibacterials for those with skin breakdown to prevent infection is often sufficient to prevent progression and allow for recovery.

The third step in pressure sore development involves full-thickness cutaneous necrosis with variable injury to the subcutaneous adipose layer. If caught early in its course, some of the fatty tissues may recover, although they are predominantly replaced by connective tissue scar. Healing by secondary intention with contraction of the granulating wound and epithelialization may proceed over a protracted course with appropriate debridement, pressure avoidance, and topical wound hygiene. In larger and deeper wounds with more extensive undermining—whereby fascia, muscle, or even bone is exposed following debridement—surgical closure is often indicated to expedite wound healing and provide a more stable coverage. An important consideration in the decision process at this point is whether or not the underlying etiology leading to pressure ulceration is transient or permanent. In the patient who develops a pressure sore postoperatively due to temporary complications requiring enforced bedrest, which will be resolved following adequate treatment, a point for conservative management can be upheld. On the other hand, if a patient with paraplegia develops a deep ulceration and will be at lifelong risk, a stronger case for surgical intervention would be considered to provide a new padding to the susceptible pressure point instead of secondary healing scar tissue.

The fourth phase of pressure ulceration involves extension of the necrotic process to tissues often not in direct line with the pressure point as well as the bony process itself. Muscle is usually not present directly over bony weight-bearing processes and therefore its involvement by necrosis often signifies a lateral undermining extension of the pressure sore. This degree of involvement indicates a large area of necrosis. Despite the fact that the skin ulceration may only appear as a 2 to 3 cm eschar, the underlying cavity may be 2 to 4 times this size. In addition, since the muscles take origin or insert on the bony process that produces the focal pressure, this bone is often affected by a periostitis or localized osteitis. Further progression may lead to overt osteomyelitis or extension into adjacent bursal sacs or synovial joints. If this occurs with an intact eschar to prevent drainage and a systemic infection seeds this area or extends from the eschar itself, a closed abscess cavity may develop with associated symptoms and signs of sepsis, requiring immediate drainage. More commonly, the collections found beneath these eschars consist of liquefied necrotic fat and nonviable muscle. Adequate escharectomy and debridement of the cavity with good wound toilet and topical antibacterials will usually avoid infection of these pressure ulcerations by either systemic or local contamination. Once opened and allowed to drain, it is extremely unusual for pressure sores to produce sepsis except in extremely debilitated or immunosuppressed patients. In most patients with "open" pressure sores and sepsis, the source is found elsewhere, most commonly the urinary tract or a pulmonary focus. Nevertheless, pressure sores that reach this degree of destruction necessitate surgical debridement and closure since spontaneous healing is rarely achieved within a reasonable period, if at all.

Several staging systems have been devised to classify pressure sores and relate their progression to the appropriate treatment modality (Table 34-3) (25, 28, 29).

Prevention

Avoidance of pressure ulceration begins with three basic principles: basic skin care, alternation of weight-bearing forces, and weight dispersion devices (30).

For those patients deemed to be at high risk, good skin care is an absolute necessity from the start. This must be initiated by the physician and nursing staff during the hospitalization period and continued by the patient or a family member following discharge, unless the predisposing factor(s) is transient. It is mandatory that the staff or the patient periodically check all surfaces at risk for pressure injury. Mirrors with long handles are available for self-inspection of the sacral and ischial areas by the patient. Early signs of redness or progressive blistering and induration should be agressively relieved of pressure with the additional use of topical antibacterials for areas of skin breakdown. The skin should be kept clean and dry by washing with a mild soap and drying with a towel at least once a day. For those areas subject to moisture accumulation (perspiration, urinary or fecal soilage), this must be

Table 34-3. Pressure sore stages

Campbell, 1959 (28)	Edberg et al., 1973 (29)	Daniel et al., 1979 (25)
1. Erythrema—reversible	Hyperemia (< min.) —reversible with pressure of 1 hr	Erythema or induration
2. Redness, swelling, induration ± blistering —reversible with prolonged pressure relief and hygiene	Ischemia (2–6 hr) —reversible with minimum 36-hr pressure relief	Superficial ulceration into dermis
3. Skin destruction and fat exposure —if small: reversible	Necrosis (>6 hr) —not relieved over a set period of pressure relief	Ulceration into subcutaneous tissue
4. Necrosis of skin and fat to fascia or muscle —trial of conservative management —usually surgery indicated	Ulceration —within 2 weeks necrotic eschar will ulcerate	Deep ulceration extending through muscle to bone
5. Skin, fat, muscle necrosis —surgery indicated		Extensive ulceration along bursae, into joints, or body cavities (e.g., rectum, vagina)
6. Bony periostitis, osteitis —surgery indicated		
7. Osteomyelitis, septic arthritis —surgery indicated		

repeated as often as necessary during the day to avoid maceration and localized infection. Strong astringents (e.g., alcohol) are to be avoided so as not to excessively dry out the skin and predispose to cracking. If dry, fragile skin is a problem, a lanolin-moisturizing cream should be gently massaged onto the area to restore surface lubrication. This surface lubrication will also aid in reducing shear (friction) forces. On the other hand, in areas that tend to frequently remain moist, a fine talcum powder lightly and evenly applied will aid in the absorption of excess fluid accumulation. Bed linens and body clothing must be changed as indicated to maintain a dry contact surface, relatively free of wrinkles. Avoidance of constricting garments, particularly those with circumferential elastics, is important, and this also applies to urinary and fecal collecting systems, which should be preferably pinned to clothing. If prolonged dressings are required, Montgomery straps should be utilized instead of repeated taping, which can quickly lead to blistering and maceration.

Despite excellent skin care, the basic dictum of pressure relief consciousness is mandatory. Ungar (30) has recommended that while lying in bed, turning to alternate weight-bearing surfaces should be carried out on a regular schedule of at least every 2 to 4 hours. Initially, these positions involved left lateral, supine, and right lateral with certain patients being turned prone. Positions midway between lateral and supine may also be used and are more comfortable than going to a prone position. Use of pillows and foam supports, as well as sheepskin, can help to more evenly distribute weighted surfaces over a broader area and provide a contact that reduces shear. When sitting, patients with poor mobility or paraplegia must be taught or assisted to lift themselves free of contact for 10 seconds every 10 minutes. These frequent pressure relief measures must be individualized and periodically reassessed since some patients over a period of time will be able to sleep through an entire night without a position change, if adequately positioned and padded. In addition, sitting patients may demonstrate that position changes are necessary only on half-hour or hourly intervals, which greatly reduces the stress on patient and staff alike. It is also important that during position changes in bed or transfer to chairs or stretchers the patient be lifted out of contact with the surface during movement so that dragging shear forces are avoided.

Pressure dispersion devices begin with proper placement of pillows and supports beneath the patient to distribute the patient's weight as evenly as possible over a broad area. These supports must necessarily taper smoothly and evenly to avoid sharp pressure points themselves. Therefore, local pressure relief measures with cut out foam rings and cloth doughnuts are contraindicated since they sharply redistribute the weight-bearing area to a new localized pressure point. This is commonly seen with heel rings to avoid pressure over the calcaneus. They often lead to pressure ulceration over the achilles tendon. Sheepskin heel and elbow pads or foam "space" boots provide a better alternative to minimize shear and pressure to these areas. While sitting, foam cutouts to alleviate an ischial pressure point may risk coccygeal or contralateral ischial injury. Here viscoelastic gel pads and, to a lesser extent, air pillow cushions are more effective in an attempt to distribute a more even pressure gradient (31, 32). This latter principle of trying to completely redistribute pressure-bearing areas has led to the frequent use of total body support mattresses (e.g., spenco and water mattresses) in the bedridden or immobilized patient as a routine preventive measure (33). However, none of these devices can create an environment whereby the applied pressure is less than capillary perfusion pressure and the need for periodic position change is still necessary (34).

A body dispersion device of practical use and routine availability that has consistently demonstrated an ability to maintain surface pressures below that of capillary perfusion is the air-fluidized bed (e.g., Clinitron®) (13). Originally designed and utilized for the treatment of major burn patients, this bed can maintain contact pressures in the reclining patient below 32 mm Hg, eliminating frequent turning other than that for basic skin care and linen changes (35, 36). The principle of air fluidization provides a flotation environment by forcing warm filtered air through a tank of glass beads. These beads take on the property of a fluid medium, which is actually dry and bacteriocidal (37). Since the patient floats on this device, the shear forces from friction are also reduced. The disadvantages of this unit involve its weight and bulky size, making bed movement and patient mobilization difficult. Sitting the patient upright is possible with a foam backrest but this reduces the bed's effectiveness significantly and is awkward. Patients with severe pulmonary disease may have difficult with ventilatory excursions since they are actually lying within the flotation medium and prone positioning is not possible. An alternative total pressure relief system, which allows upright sitting of the patient and prone positioning, incorporates adjustable continuous segmental air pillow support, termed low air loss (e.g., Howmedica Mediscus®). This bed system has also demonstrated effective pressure reduction below that of capillary pressure over all body points and has worked well for those patients where pulmonary considerations and prone positioning make air-fluidized support inappropriate (38–41). A similar low air loss chair has recently been brought into clinical use (Howmedica Dermarest®) but its effectiveness awaits further trials (Table 34-4).

For those patients with spasticity or contractures, positioning and adequate pressure dispersion may be an impossible task. Pharmacologic treatment with diazepam or dantrolene sodium should be initiated for spasticity. If this is refractory to medical management and represents the main source of continued pressure ulceration, neurosurgical treatment by cordotomy or rhizotomy may be necessary (42). Similarly, if contractures are the cause of persistent pressure and skin breakdown despite good skin care and attempts at pressure relief, surgical tenotomy may allow better positioning and more even pressure distribution.

Table 34-4. Support surface pressures (maximum recordings in mm Hg)

1.	Air-fluidized bed	30 (mean 18–25)
2.	Low-air-loss bed	32 (mean 18–25)
3.	Feather pillows on foam	36
4.	Water-bed	58
5.	Foam mattress	68
6.	Sprung mattress	164
7.	Operating table	140–>260

Data tables modified from Scales (40) and Krouskop et al. (41).

It is mandatory for the staff or patient to periodically check all surfaces at risk for pressure injury. This can be done during each turning period or at specifically scheduled times. Early signs of redness or progressive blistering and induration should be agressively relieved of pressure with the additional use of topical treatment to areas of skin breakdown.

Treatment

Once a pressure sore is recognized and its stage of development assessed, the treatment can be divided into either conservative (debridement and topical care) or aggressive (debridement and surgical closure). This division of appropriate care is usually based on whether the ulcer is superficial or deep, the inciting cause temporary or permanent, and the patient's age and overall medical condition. The ideal candidate for conservative management would be an elderly patient who develops a sacral pressure sore, with or without exposed presacral fascia, following prolonged bedrest for a myocardial infarction and congestive heart failure. In this case, surgery is contraindicated for a minimum of 3 to 6 months; the inciting cause of the ulceration is transient, which should allow for excellent avoidance of continued unremitting pressure. On the other hand, a young otherwise healthy paraplegic patient with a large ischial pressure sore and associated cavity with exposed ischial bone would be considered a candidate for surgical closure to avoid an unnecessarily long period for secondary healing to occur and to provide a new surface of composite healthy tissue to resist a lifelong application of undue pressures. In between these extremes, experience and judgement will dictate whether a trial of conservative therapy is indicated prior to resorting to definitive surgical closure to expedite convalescence.

Conservative Management

Conservative management must reiterate those principles utilized in prevention several fold in order to avoid a second pressure sore, while relieving applied pressures to an area of existing damage. Therefore, good basic skin care, alternating positions, and weight dispersion devices become even more important. As discussed by Campbell (28) and Edberg (29), Stage I hyperemic pressure damage is usually reversed by pressure relief of at least 1 hour and should be closely observed with foreshortened subsequent periods of pressure application for an additional 24 hours. Stage II ischemia with the addition of swelling and induration should have a minimum of 36 hours pressure relief and then abbreviated pressure application and close follow-up should be continued until the induration softens. If blistering occurs, the exposed moist dermis should be protected from dessication and contamination from excretory waste by synthetic semipermeable barriers (e.g., Tegaderm®, Op site®) with or without the use of a topical antibacterial. Detection and reversal of pressure sore development is most easily achieved at these stages prior to exposure of ischemic adipose tissue. Therefore, if despite aggressive local care and pressure relief induration or blistering progresses or a new site of pressure injury develops in a nonambulatory patient, a more sophisticated pressure dispersion device should be employed in the form of a low-air-loss (Mediscus®) or air-fluidized (Clinitron®) bed.

Once the patient's disease process enters Stage III with overt necrosis and subsequent ulceration, the principles of wound care must incorporate adequate surgical debridement to remove nonviable tissue, which can serve as a medium for bacterial proliferation and additional tissue damage. Although all wounds will demonstrate a variety of microbial flora on swab culture, the quantitation of this bacterial proliferation allows a distinction between mere colonization and tissue infection. Robson (43) has shown that bacterial tissue concentrations greater than 10^5 per gram, constitute a wound infection and are associated with decreased wound healing. Concentrations in excess of 10^9 are often associated with systemic sepsis. Many organisms have been associated with pressure sores usually as a mixed flora. Daltrey (44) found that *Proteus mirabilis, Pseudomonas aeruginosa,* and *Bacteroides* species were more commonly associated with necrotic and enlarging sores. To minimize the deleterious effects of bacterial overgrowth in necrotic pressure ulcerations, numerous topical agents have been employed from enzymatic debridement to antibacterials and hyperbaric oxygen (46). None of these have demonstrated any magical result in obtaining faster closure of wounds beyond the effect of reducing bacterial growth to acceptable levels ($<10^5$/gram tissue). Therefore, when a topical agent is selected as an adjunct to surgical debridement, the choice should be based on proven antibacterial efficiency. This should take into consideration ease of application, antibacterial spectrum, and ability to penetrate necrotic eschar. The most widely used and effective in this regard have been silver sulfadiazine (Silvadene®) and mafenide (Sulfamyalon®). Providone iodine and Dakin's solution are second line choices (43, 46). Silver sulfadiazine cream applied in sufficient quantity provides a 24-hour duration of broad spectrum activity with a moderate tissue penetration and minimal side effects. Therefore, only one dressing change per day is necessary. Although mafenide has greater tissue penetration, this is usually unnecessary when adequate tissue debridement has been provided surgically. In addition, twice daily dressing changes are necessary since its duration of action is only 12 hours. Malfenide may also produce discomfort and pain when applied to partial-thickness areas of skin injury. Povidone-iodine and Dakin's solution have poorly documented ability to penetrate eschar and much shorter durations of action (4 to 6 hours). Their utilization as a wet to dry gauze saturated dressing every 6 hours is most successful in a wound that needs minimal or cautious debridement (e.g., relatively clean granulating ulcer or vital structures at the base).

It is axiomatic that despite the title of "conservative management," surgical debridement, whether at the bedsise or in the operating room, is an integral part of ulcerations with necrotic tissue. This is particularly evident when systemic sepsis develops secondary to an infected pressure sore. Survivial is predicated upon appropriate systemic antibiotic coverage and timely surgical debridement. In one study of pressure sore sepsis, mortality was reduced from 85% with antibiotic treatment alone to 28% when surgical debridement was also performed (47).

Once an ulcer in this more advanced stage is considered clean with bacterial counts less than 10^5 per gram and viable granulation tissue is present, a period of conservative observation for secondary healing may ensue. During this time, attention should be directed toward maximizing the nutritional status and improving coexisting medical conditions. Depending on the depth, size, and location of the ulceration, this process may extend for several months (48). Failed closure of a pressure sore may not in itself be an indication for surgical closure, and this principle also applies to higher grade ulcerations (e.g., $\geqslant$Grade IV). If the reason for poor healing is negative nutritional balance, poorly controlled diabetes or anemia, surgery may also be likely to fail with additional morbidity and even mortality attendant to the surgical procedure. As already mentioned, the medical condition(s) of the patient may serve as a contraindication to surgery despite a high-grade ulceration, which would otherwise be typically selected for surgical closure. Therefore, despite our technical desire to complete a therapeutic program that provides the patient with a healed ulcer, in some cases, a more prudent and medically sound approach may desirably fall short of this objective. Once this wound has been stabilized in size through preventive education and is bacteriologically clean (<10^5 organisms) through daily dressings, the patient may be followed *ad infinitum* or, if medical conditions improve, reconsidered as a surgical candidate.

For those patients without medical contraindications to surgery, a recalcitrant Stage III and most all Stage IV or greater deep ulcerations are considered candidates for surgical closure, once wound hygiene has been achieved by conservative treatment.

Surgical Management

The surgical management of pressure sores dates back to 1938, when Davis (49) recommended advancement flap closure of unstable scarred lumbosacral wounds. Following World War II (1945–1947), a substantial experience with pressure sores in paraplegics found its way into the literature. Those early publications dealt with excision and primary closure (50, 51), excision and advancement or rotation flap closure (51, 52), and excision with split-thickness skin grafts (51). With these various surgical procedures, healing could be achieved in about 70% to 85% of patients (51, 53–55), although the skin grafts were noted to be less durable and more prone to recurrences (55). During this same period, it became evident that a surgical reduction of any offending bony prominence (e.g. trochanter, ischium, etc.) should be an integral part of the wound excision, while the addition of muscle flaps to the wound closure as padding for the remaining underlying bone would further reduce the likelihood of recurrent pressure ulceration (56, 57). These basic principles of complete pressure sore excision, including extensions of the bursal sac, reduction of bony projections, and coverage with healthy tissues—preferably utilizing flaps (skin, fat ± muscle)—are still valid today (Fig. 34-4).

A decade later in 1956, Conway and Griffith (48) reviewed 1000 cases of pressure sores in paraplegics and concluded that surgery was the most satisfactory form of treatment for necrotic deep pressure sores to obtain healing and decrease recurrence. They found five key principles to surgical success: (*a*) excision of the ulcer, peripheral scar, adjacent bursa, and soft tissue calcifications; (*b*) radical bone reduction or removal; (*c*) utilization of fascia or muscle flaps to cover bony stumps and obliterate dead space; (*d*) composite skin-fat regional flap coverage of the ulcer without tension, placing suture lines outside the area of the original pressure sore; and (*e*) split-thickness skin graft closure of the flap donor site if necessary. Using this method, they obtained closure of sacral, trochanteric, and ischial pressure sores in 84%, 86%, and 97% respectively with a recurrence rate of 11%, 6%, and 3% over a 6-month to five-year follow-up period.

The major recent advances in pressure sore surgery have come from a better understanding of cutaneous (58–60), muscle (61, 62), and musculocutaneous (62–64) flap physiology and blood supply. This has led to a greater number of available local and regional flaps to provide reliable composite closure.

Despite early work demonstrating a high sensitivity of muscle to pressure with resultant ischemic necrosis (14), others have shown that muscle can effectively pad the site of pressure, absorbing and dispersing its injurious effects on the skin, even though these benefits may diminish over a period of time (65, 66). The reason for this loss of protection afforded by muscle include atrophy following flap transfer and replacement by fibrosis subsequent to repeated ischemia-producing pressure episodes. Nevertheless, the transfer of muscle or musculocutaneous flaps can provide several immediate advantages including: (*a*) tissue bulk to obliterate the "dead space" of resected pressure sore cavities, (*b*) transfer of large blocks of tissue that remain well vascularized on relatively narrow pedicles, and (*c*) an apparent greater ability to clear a given bacterial innoculum than random cutaneous flaps (67). This latter point should be clarified, in that axial cutaneous (61) and fasciocutaneous (68) flaps may be just as resistant to bacterial infection and possess similar bacterial clearance capability as musculocutaneous flaps (69).

The guidelines of sugical closure today are much the same as those espoused by Conway and Griffith in 1956. One must also realize that large flaps are usually necessary when recurrence is a posibility to allow for their reelevation and repeated usage. If a small flap has been designed and inset into a pressure sore and a recurrent ulceration develops, the prior flap may be inadequate to resurface this new wound, and one must immediately seek another source for flap coverage. On the other hand, if a very large flap is advanced, upon re-ulceration, the remainder may be re-elevated and used repeatedly. This foresighted principle will preserve reconstructive options at any subsequent surgery. In keeping with this same philosophy, when a flap is chosen several others should also be outlined. This allows the surgeon to maximize the size of the particular flap chosen, while forcing him to give mental and visual consideration to alternative choices, should the primary flap fail. One last operative dictum is to place the patient into a position that will place maximum tension on the local tissues undergoing repair. It is from this position that a tension-free closure must be accomplished to ensure ultimate success. The classic example of this can be made with an ischial pressure sore. If the patient is placed prone and flat on the operating table it will falsely lure the surgeon into assuming that a "small" primary closure should suffice. However, if the table is flexed into a jack-knife position, simulating sitting, the tension will be readily apparent and dispel the fallacy of such reconstructive attempts. It will also demonstrate the true tension that will be applied to any flap brought into the damaged area, allowing for its adequate size estimation and necessary tissue release (undermining, backcuts at the pedicle base, and skin grafting of donor sites too tight for primary closure). One must always remember that a pressure sore destroys local tissue, resulting in a need to borrow from adjacent areas. If at the time of surgery this fact no longer seems valid, check the patient's position and place any nearby joint through its maximum range to avoid unexpected postoperative tension on the repair site and unnecessary contractures from the prolonged immobilization needed to minimize this tension.

Given the fact that a pressure sore may develop anywhere on the body and that a myriad of surgical closure techniques are available to accomplish healing of the wound, a selection of the more common sites of ulcer development and the favored techniques for closure of each are presented.

Ischium

The ischium is one of the most common sites of pressure sore development due to the excessive forces applied to this area during sitting (*see* Figs. 34-2 and 34-3). For the elderly patient recovering from an illness with limited ambulation or those patients with infirmities that severely curtail ambulation, sitting may be the only alternative to bedrest. Due to the early pressure-sensitive damage to cutaneous nerves, pain is rarely a complaint, and the sore's obscure location makes direct self observation impossible without the use of mirrors. Therefore, this area should be routinely inspected. If a pressure sore develops, there are several choices available for repair following excision.

Excision is accomplished with the patient in a prone position on the operating table with the hips maximally flexed (jack-knife). This recreates the natural tension applied to this area during sitting and displays the true diameter of the cutaneous defect. The bursal sac, which is a pseudosac of condensed collagen scar or granulation tissue, should be completely excised or debrided to minimize the bacterial contamination of the wound and create fresh surgical surfaces that will more readily adhere following would closure. To aid in this complete debridement, the bursal sac and its peripheral and deep extensions can be topically coated with a colored dye. A gauze sponge moistened with gentian violet is packed into the wound to completely mark the ulcer surface. Following excision, the dyed tissue should have been removed. If any remains, it should be removed prior to closure. The outline of the cutaneous excision is dependent on several factors. First, any tissue that is necrotic or ischemic with discoloration and induration from pressure sore scar deposition must be removed. Second, if there is a significant peripheral extension of the bursal sac, creating a thin tenuous flap of skin and fat, the viability and durability of this tissue must be assessed following complete debridement of the ulcer cavity (including the undersurface of this tissue). This assessment must also take into consideration adjacent incisions for flap elevation and closure of the ulcer, which may further compromise its viability. If a decision is made to retain this tissue, a primary or secondary muscle flap will often need to be designed to obliterate the dead space of the cavity. On the other hand, if it is to be sacrificed during debridement, the dimensions of the cutaneous flap must be sufficient to close this additional skin deficit. The third decision determining the amount of peripheral skin excision is based on the geometric flap design. A rotation flap usually demands a circular defect, whereas rectangular advancement or transposition flaps require a triangular or squared defect for proper insetting.

Excision of the cutaneous margin and bursal sac will then leave a raw crater at the base of which is the ischial tuberosity. In most cases, it is sufficient to perform a partial ostectomy with a sharp osteome, removing diseased bone and flattening the offending pressure point. Although recurrences have been reportedly higher with partial ostectomy, the complications are considerably less than with total ischiectomy. This latter more aggressive approach also necessitates a contralateral total ischiectomy to prevent uneven sitting and pressure ulceration on the opposite ischium (49). Following bilateral total ischiectomy, weight-bearing pressure is transferred to the pubic rami, perineum, and proximal femur, which can result in perineal ulcers, urethral diverticulae, and fistulae (Fig. 34-5) (70, 71). Therefore, most ischial pressure sores are managed by a conservative partial ischiectomy unless recurrent ulcerations become problematic and resistant to customary treatment.

Closure of ischial wounds requires some form of a flap. Split- and full-thickness skin grafts are inadequate for ischial wounds due to the direct application of repetitive high compressive and shear forces. Although a graft may initially "take" over the raw surface, including the cancellous portion of ischial bone, it is doomed to failure due to mobility and inadequate padding.

The simplest flap closure is direct advancement of the adjacent tissues following elliptical excision of the pressure sore, allowing for a primary closure directly overlying the ischium (72). This may be suitable for small pressure sores in a patient who has been temporarily incapacitated and in whom no future predisposing factors are

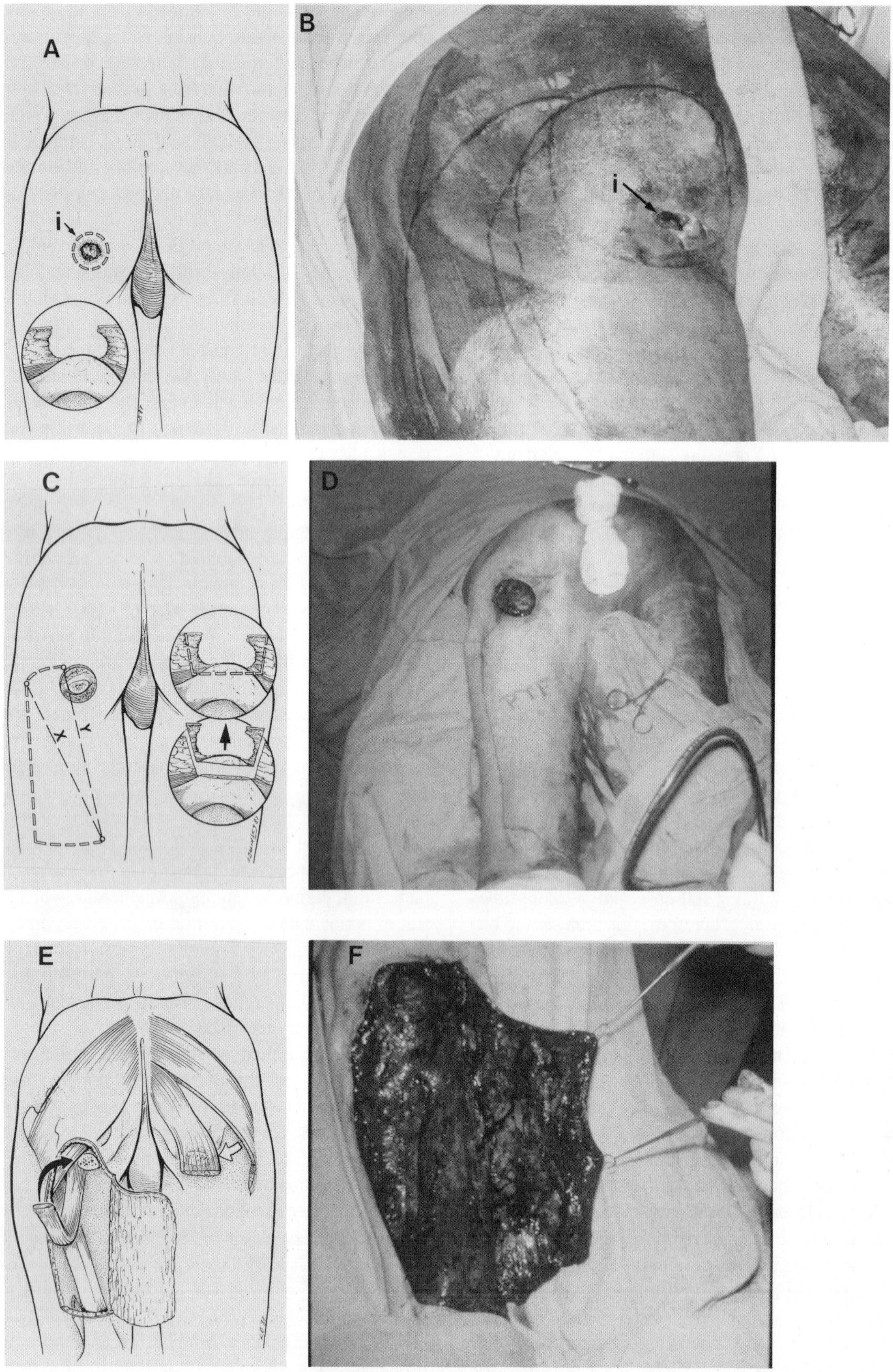
A
i
B
i
C
D
E
F

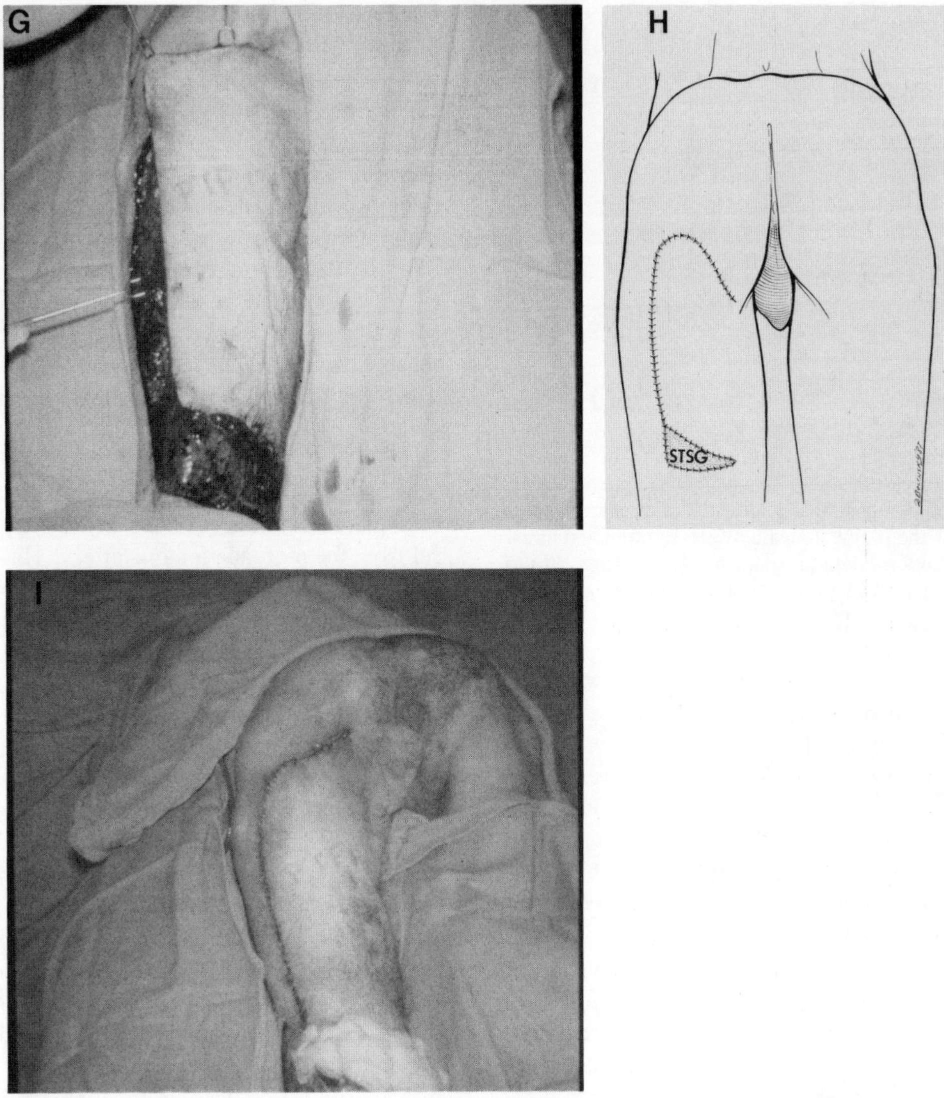

Figure 34-4. Schematic drawing and clinical case demonstrating excision and closure of an ischial pressure sore, utilizing a random medially based posterior thigh advancement flap (PTF) with or without an independent myoplasty. *A, B,* Ischial cutaneous ulceration (i) deep to which is a wider undermined cavity containing a variable amount of necrotic debris. Inset demonstrates undermining on cross-section. *C, D,* Excision of the ulcer must include all recesses of the undermining cavity and ostectomy to reduce the offending bony projection. Skin resection is limited to necrotic and scarred tissues adjacent to the ulcer. If during excision of a widely undermined ulcer the overlying skin is devascularized, it should be removed and reconstructed with healthy tissue. Therefore, flap design is finalized after complete ulcer excision. Inset demonstrates excision of ulcer crater with a narrow "V", but with a widely undermined ulcer this excision should resemble an inverted "V" following the conical configuration of the ulcer cavity, allowing for preservation of uninvolved overlying skin, which remains viable following excision. The PTF is based on a broad medial pedicle with its arc of rotation limited by the medial aspect of the caudal transverse incision (rotation point-RP). A line from this point to the superolateral aspect of the flap (X) should equal a similar line extending to the superolateral aspect of the excised ulcer (Y) to ensure adequate flap length. This general principle applies to all pedicle flaps. *E, F,* The flap is elevated superficial to the muscle fascia. If a deep ulcer cavity is present, an independent myoplasty can be added for bulk using either the biceps or gluteal muscles. In the ambulatory patient, only the inferior gluteal muscle should be used to avoid a functional deficit. Alternatively, the cephalad portion of the PTF may be de-epithelialized and turned under itself for additional bulk. *G,* Adequate flap advancement is demonstrated. However, if initial flap design proved erroneous in estimating appropriate length, the rotation point can be moved cephalad by a judicious back-cut incision into the medial base of the flap taking care not to devascularize the flap. This maneuver adds effective length to the flap at the expense of its broad medial base. *H, I,* Completed flap transfer and insetting with skin graft (STSG) and tie over cotton dressing applied to inferior donor site.

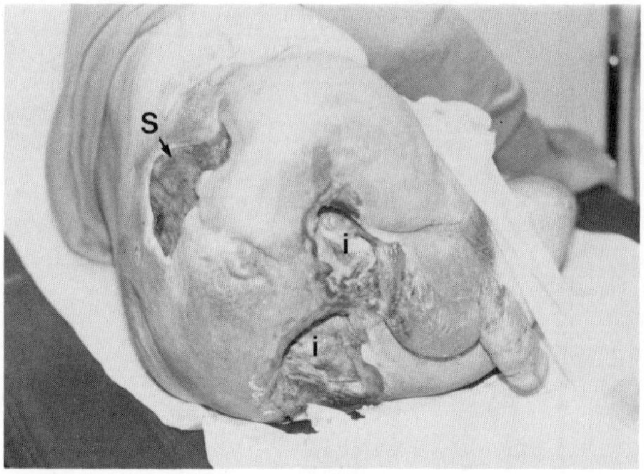

Figure 34-5. Bilateral amputee with recurrent bilateral ischial (i) and sacral (S) pressure sores. This patient had previous total ischiectomies and demonstrates confluence of the ischial pressure sores across the perineal area between scrotum and anus. Pressure in this area resulted in complete necrosis from skin to the pubic ramus, including a segment of the intervening urethra.

readily anticipated (Fig. 34-6). The major drawback of this procedure involves placement of the suture line directly between the forces of applied pressure and the underlying bone. The scar itself is considered the weak point of any closure and here the flaps actually lie to either side of the major pressure axis. This is usually not a problem with someone who will subsequently be either fully ambulatory or completely bedridden, where the repair will not be unduly stressed. The second problem involves larger pressure sores requiring extensive elliptical excision and mobilization of adjacent tissues, thereby compromising adjacent flap territories, which offer more reliable tension free closure and optimal suture line placement for the ischial region.

The most commonly used cutaneous flap for the ischial pressure sore that has withstood the test of time is the *random medially based posterior thigh advancement flap* (Fig. 34-4) (48). This is designed as a large modified rectangle over the posterior thigh, extending from the ischium to within one hand's-breadth of the popliteal fossa. This inferior limit avoids placing a skin graft over the hamstring tendons, which become prominent at this level. The flap is elevated in a plane superficial to the deep fascia of the posterior thigh muscles from lateral to medial, preserving a random vascular supply at the broad medial flap base. If additional advancement is needed, an oblique backcut may be made at the inferior base. Following advancement of the flap, the donor defect is closed with a split-thickness skin graft. The donor site may be partially closed from its lateral inferior aspect with a V-Y technique to minimize the area to be grafted. Alternatively, the entire flap may be designed more in the shape of a large oval so that advancement is complemented by rotation, which can allow for a primary closure of the donor site. This later principle is usually only possible with smaller ulcers. Large drains are used to apply suction to the ulcer cavity and flap dead space. If bulk is needed to obliterate a deep cavity in the ischial region, the posterior thigh flap may be de-epithelialized superiorly and turned under itself and into the cavity.

Alternatively, a second flap of muscle can be utilized to obliterate the cavity and subsequently can be covered by the posterior thigh flap. The most commonly used muscles are the biceps femoris and the gluteus maximus. The bicep femoris should only be used in nonambulatory patients, for its division results in a functional deficit that is significant. The biceps may be divided inferiorly and reflected superiorly, maintaining its vascular integrity through preservation of its most superior perforating vessel from the profunda femoris artery. This vessel usually enters the biceps about 10 cm below the ischium. Therefore, division of the biceps should be low enough to allow transposition of its distal end to the ischium without elevating the proximal 10 cm of the muscle (62). For ambulatory patients, the gluteus maximus muscle is preferable to avoid a functional deficit. Although gluteus maximus function is necessary for normal gait leg swing, its double vascular supply from the superior and inferior gluteal vessels allows a reliable transfer of either the superior or inferior half, preserving the other for functional gait. For the ischium, the inferior half of the gluteus maximus muscle may be transferred based on the medial origin of its inferior gluteal vessels, detaching and transferring its trochanteric insertion (73), or it may be based laterally on its secondary blood supply from the medial and lateral femoral circumflex arterial arcade, transposing its detached origin from the sacroiliac region (74). In addition to the random posterior thigh flap, cutaneous coverage can be obtained with a *random gluteal rotation (advancement) flap* (Fig. 34-7). This flap is outlined in a semicircular area over the buttock and elevated superficial to the gluteal muscle fascia. With larger sores, it may be necessary to skin graft the donor defect to avoid tension.

An axial fasciocutaneous flap, which has been reliably utilized in the ischial region, is the *gluteal thigh flap* (75). This flap is based on the inferior gluteal vessels and includes the posterior femoral cutaneous nerve for sensation. Flap design over the posterior thigh extends from the mid-gluteal region to within 8 cm of the popliteal fossa, and its central axis is midway between the trochanteric and ischial tuberosities, with a point of rotation marked 5 cm above the ischium (Fig. 34-8). A flap 15 cm in width and 34 cm in length may be raised, but primary closure of the donor site is difficult when the width is greater than 12 cm. The flap is elevated from distal to proximal by sharp

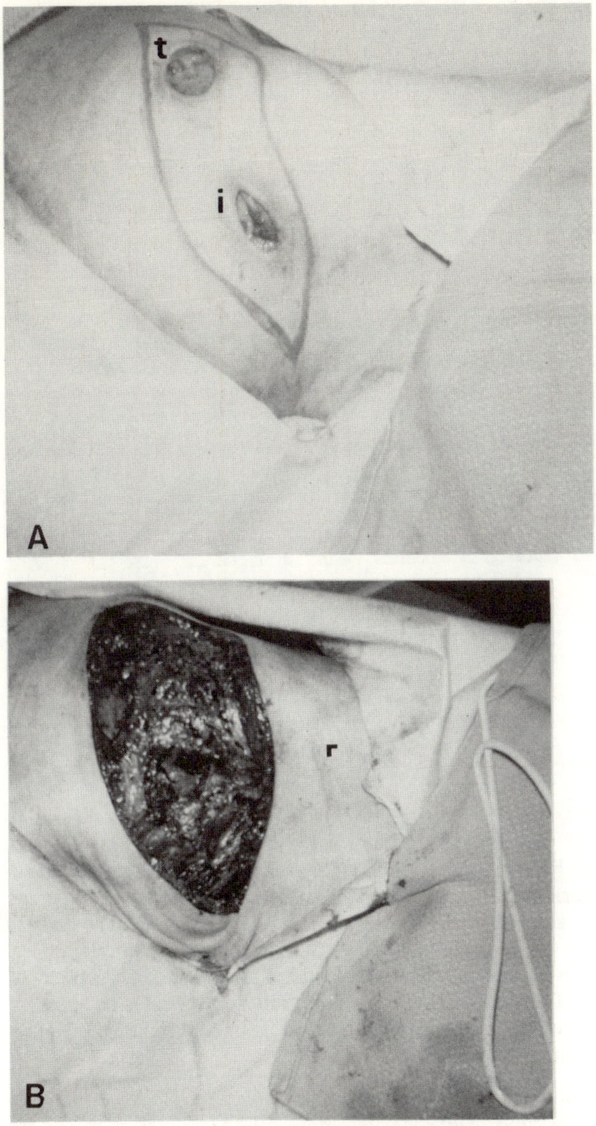

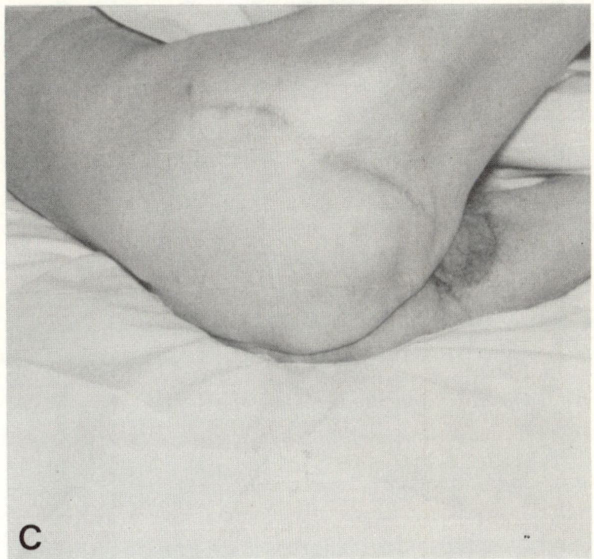

Figure 34-6. *A,* Right trochanteric (t) and ischial (i) pressure sores in elderly ambulatory patient following complicated course of pneumonia. Elliptical excision outlined to include both ulcers. *B,* Excisional defect. *C,* Primary closure accomplished with advancement flaps.

dissection over the hamstring muscles, taking care to avoid injury to the sciatic nerve above the superolateral border of the biceps femoris muscle. At the inferior edge of the gluteus, continued elevation of the flap must include the inferior gluteus maximus since the vessels run beneath this muscle to their origin from between the piriformis and superior gemellus muscles (which is the absolute rotation point of this axial flap). Its axial pedicle allows elevation on a narrow stalk of tissue with the skin transposed as a complete island, and its arc allows coverage to the ischial, trochanteric, and even sacral regions. This flap allows greater mobility due to its axial blood supply and has retained sensory innervation; these are definite advantages over the random posterior thigh flap. However, it is somewhat more difficult to design and inset a large flap, which can be re-elevated and advanced should a recurrence develop. As for bulk, its thickness is similar to a posterior thigh flap and requires deepithelialized burying of its tip or myoplasty as an adjunctive measure for deep cavities. To provide a bulk of tissue for deep cavities and cutaneous coverage in one flap, the myocutaneous reconstructions mentioned below are preferable.

The *gluteus maximus myocutaneous flap* allows for transfer of muscle bulk and cutaneous cover in one flap on an axial vascular pedicle (76–78). This may be elevated as an island for greater mobility, utilizing only the inferior half of the muscle (on the inferior gluteal vessels) to preserve gait function of the superior gluteus maximus. The skin paddle is outlined over the distal aspect of the inferior gluteus maximus muscle proximal to its trochanteric insertion (Fig. 34-9). Following excision of the ischial ul-

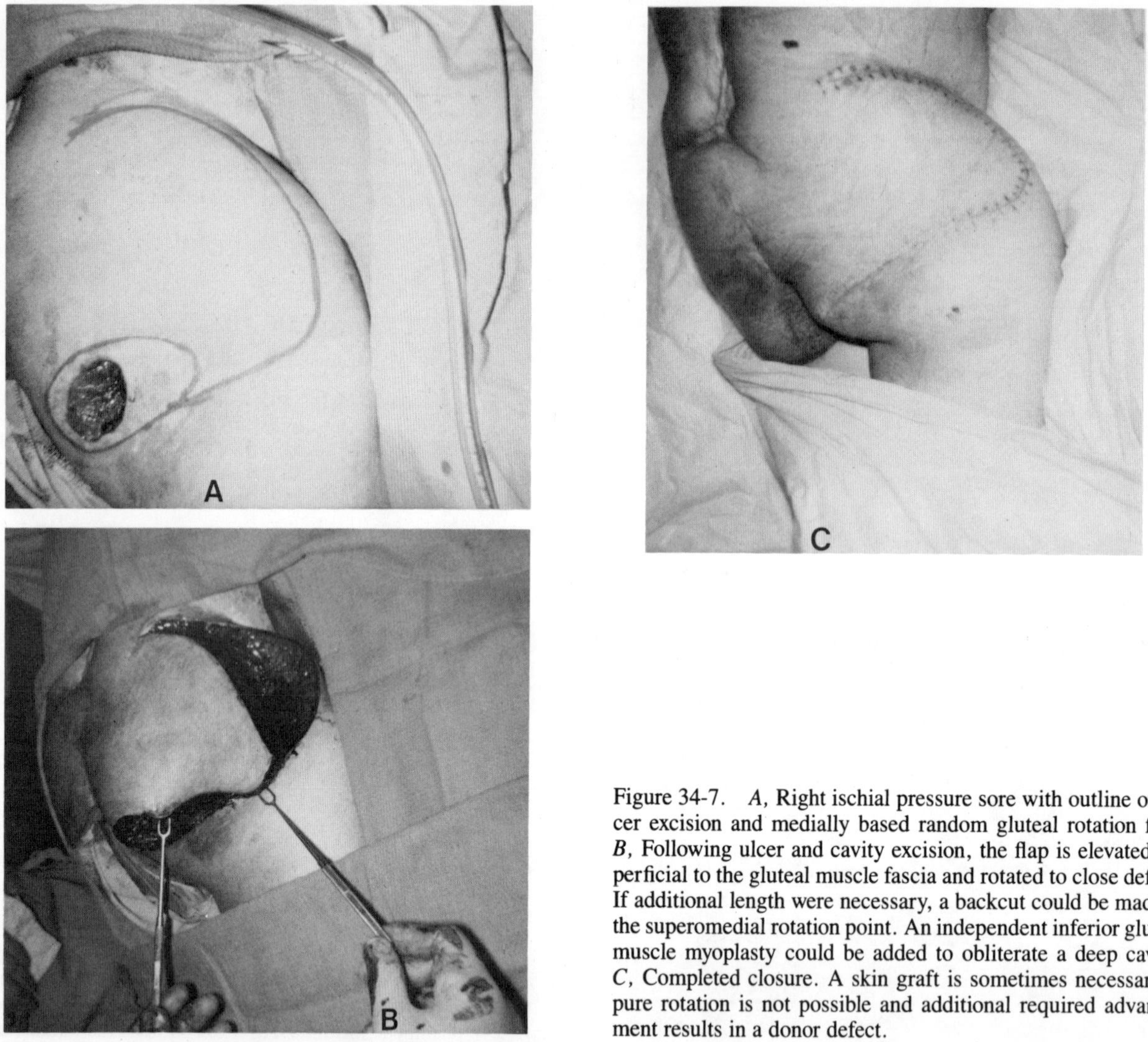

Figure 34-7. *A,* Right ischial pressure sore with outline of ulcer excision and medially based random gluteal rotation flap. *B,* Following ulcer and cavity excision, the flap is elevated superficial to the gluteal muscle fascia and rotated to close defect. If additional length were necessary, a backcut could be made at the superomedial rotation point. An independent inferior gluteal muscle myoplasty could be added to obliterate a deep cavity. *C,* Completed closure. A skin graft is sometimes necessary if pure rotation is not possible and additional required advancement results in a donor defect.

cer, the cutaneous paddle is incised circumferentially down to the muscle fascia. Absorbable sutures are used to tack the skin paddle dermis to the muscle fascia, in order to protect the fine myocutaneous vasculature from damaging shear forces during subsequent flap manipulation. The adjacent buttock skin is sharply elevated from the proximal gluteal muscle fascia. The inferior gluteal muscle with overlying skin paddle is then elevated from its distal and inferior aspects to visualize and include the inferior gluteal vessels. A muscle-splitting incision to separate the inferior and superior gluteal muscles completes the flap elevation. The flap is then transposed to the ischial cavity with primary closure of the donor site.

The *V-Y hamstring myocutaneous flap* is another useful axial flap for closure of ischial ulcers with deep craters (79, 80). Advancement is made possible by outlining a triangular skin paddle over the posterior thigh with its base superiorly measuring slightly greater than the width of the ischial ulcer defect. The length of the flap should include about two-thirds of the posterior thigh to allow for re-advancement should that become necessary (Fig. 34-10). Following excision of the ulcer crater, the skin paddle is similarly incised down through to the underlying muscle fascia. The flap may be advanced significantly with this skin release alone for moderate-sized defects, preserving the integrity of the underlying hamstrings, which are essential in an ambulatory patient. For those nonambulatory paraplegics, the flap may be elevated and advanced further, as originally described, on the biceps femoris, semitendinosis, and semimembranosus muscles. Distally, these muscle tendons are identified and transected with muscle elevation proceeding proximally to within 10 cm of the ischium, where the most superior segmental profunda femoris perforators enter these mus-

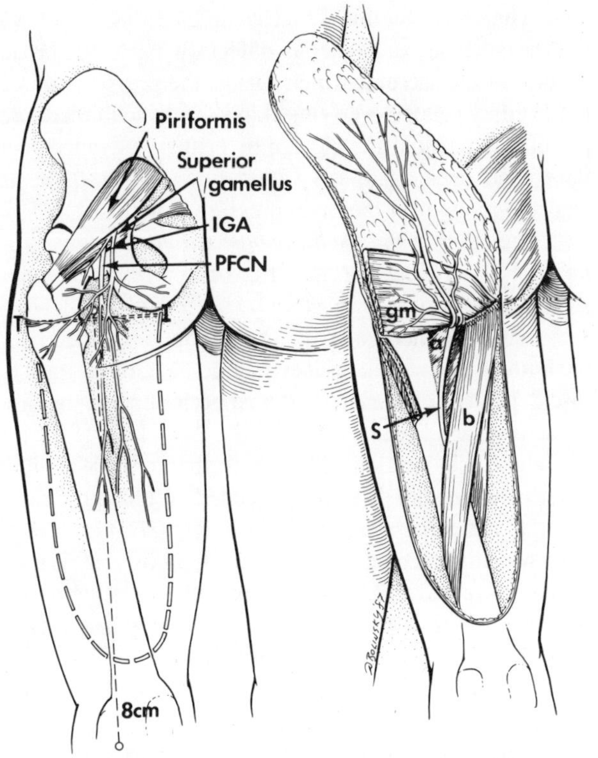

Figure 34-8. Schematic of gluteal thigh flap. *A*, This flap is based on the inferior gluteal vessels (IGA) and includes the posterior femoral cutaneous nerve (PFCN) for sensibility. The central flap axis is determined by a perpendicular line dropped from the midpoint between the trochanter (T) and ischium (I) with a length extending to within 8 cm of the popliteal fossa. The effective rotation point is limited by the inferior gluteal vascular pedicle, which is approximately 5 cm above the ischial tuberosity. *B*, The flap is elevated in the thin fatty layer deep to the fascia lata and superficial to the hamstring muscle fascia, taking care not to injure the sciatic nerve (S) located between the long head of the biceps (b) and adductor (a). Superiorly, additional pedicle length is gained by dissecting the vascular leash under the gluteus maximus (gm) to its origin between the pirifomis and superior gamellus muscles. (Modified from Hurwitz, DJ, et al. 1981. The gluteal thigh flap: A reliable sensate flap for the closure of buttock and perineal wounds. *Plast Reconstr Surg* 68: 521) (Ref. 75).

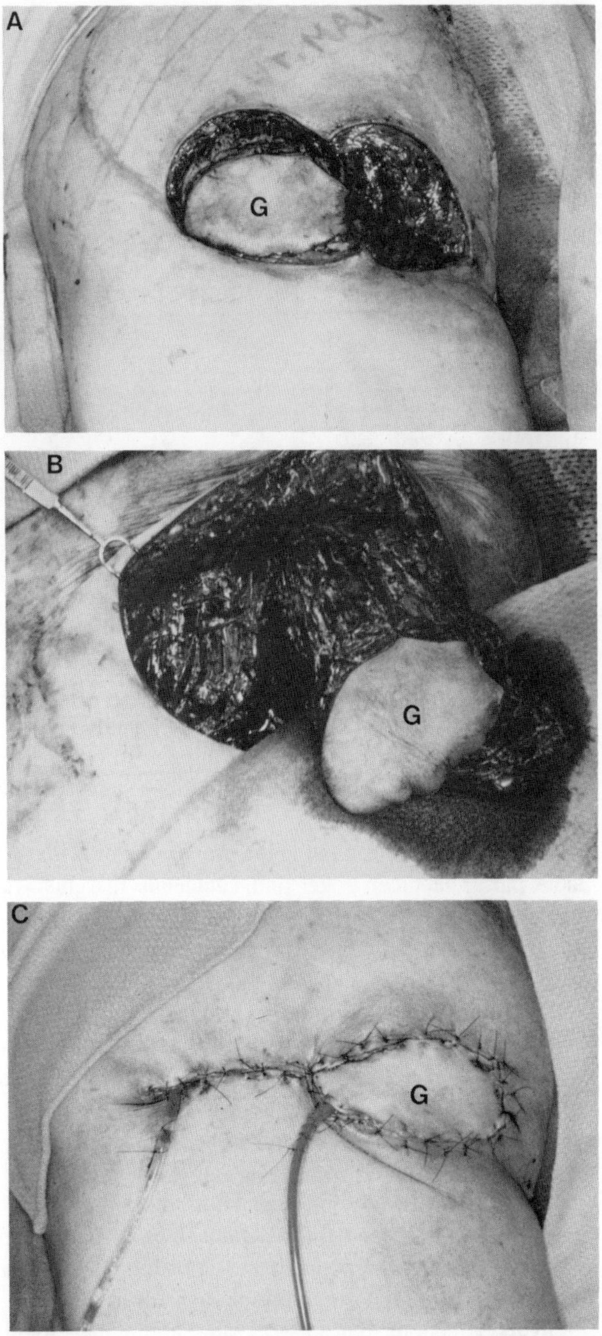

Figure 34-9. *A*, Left ischial ulcer excision completed and skin paddle of an inferior gluteus maximus myocutaneous flap (G) designed over distal aspect of muscle and incised down to muscle fascia. *B*, Myocutaneous flap has been separated from the superior gluteal muscle to the left by a muscle splitting incision and transposed to the ischial defect. *C*, Flap insetting completed with donor site closed primarily.

cles. These flap muscles may be carefully elevated proximal to this point if care is taken to preserve these delicate vascular pedicles. The flap is then moved cephalad to obliterate the ischial crater with a primary closure of the donor site (V-Y technique).

Other less commonly used myocutaneous flaps for the ischial pressure sore include the island gracilis myocutaneous (81) and extended tensor fascia late myocutaneous flap (82, 83) (Fig. 34-19).

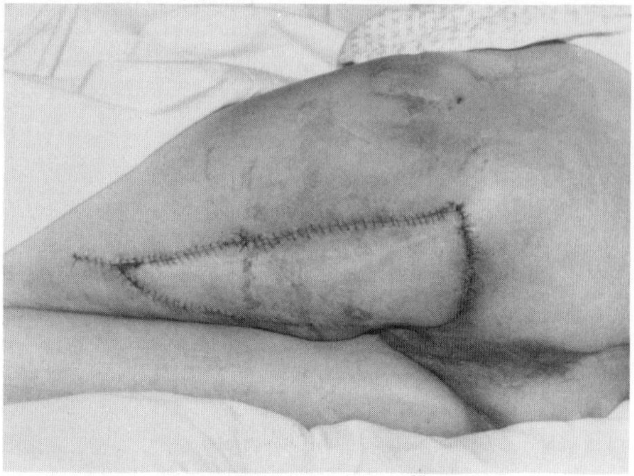

Figure 34-10. V-Y hamstring myocutaneous flap: completed advancement and insetting of the flap.

Sacrum

The sacrum is another area extremely susceptible to pressure ulceration due to its prominent location, mainly with the bedridden, recumbent patient, but also to a lesser extent with semi-sitting positions. The additional effects of shear are notable for patients requiring repositioning in a bed or recliner, whereby they are slid into a semi-upright position without lifting.

Excision is carried out in the prone position with the table flat. The ulcer crater and cutaneous margins are treated in a similar fashion as outlined with ischial ulcers, and the sacral prominence may be shaved with a sharp osteotome.

Unlike ischial ulcers, the superficial sacral ulcer may be covered with a reversed dermal graft and/or a split-thickness skin graft (84). This is particularly true for the sacral ulcer, which, following topical treatment, presents with a clean granulating bed and no peripheral undermining. Here graft "take" without further excision or partial sacrectomy may be accomplished with a minimum of surgical intervention, and the resultant closure is usually more stable than if the wound were to heal by spontaneous epithelialization. The durability of such coverage is certainly more tenuous than a flap closure, but for the patient with concomitant medical problems in whom subsequent independent ambulation is anticipated, this procedure poses a lesser surgical risk than extensive flap dissection and often provides sufficient wear capacity.

For ulcers that require excision and partial sacrectomy, especially in patients with poor ambulatory capacities, a skin graft may succeed in temporarily closing the wound, but its long-term reliability is considerably less than with flap repair (85).

Although primary advancement flap closure is possible in small sacral pressure sores, its use is limited in this area. The reason for this is that sacral ulcers often present with a rather large cutaneous defect owing to the broad surface of the sacrum, which acts as the pressure source to the thinly padded overlying skin. It is difficult therefore to obtain a tension-free closure by primary advancement flaps, and once again the suture line of scar tissue is placed directly over the main pressure axis (54).

The *inferior and medially based random gluteal rotation (+ advancement) flap* has been a reliable reconstructive technique for most sacral ulcers (48). Following excision of the ulcer, a semicircular flap is outlined over the buttock and elevated superficial to the gluteus muscle fascia, preserving the larger gluteal perforators to the skin in the parasacral region (Fig. 34-11). A backcut of the inferolateral skin incision will allow further reach of the flap in a cephalomedial direction if needed. With a pure rotation flap the donor site is closed directly (*see* Fig. 34-7), but when advancement is also utilized, a skin graft is necessary to avoid tension. For extremely large sacral wounds, bilateral opposing gluteal flaps may be utilized. This is a reliable random flap and is often sufficient for sacral closure without adjunctive myoplasty, since sacral ulcers rarely present with deep cavities.

The *transverse lumbosacral flap* is based on the intercostal and lumbar perforating vessels, which through vascular communications in the subdermal plexus allow for flap elevation across the midline (86). The flap width is outlined from the sacral ulcer to the lower thoracic or first lumbar vertebrae. Its distal margin may lie 2 to 5 cm lateral to the sacrospinalis muscle and is elevated over the lumbar fascia to the contralateral sacrospinalis muscle (Fig. 34-12). At the lateral border of this muscle, the perforators enter the base and must be preserved. A flap base width-to-length ratio of 1:1.5 is generally considered safe. The flap is then transposed to the sacral defect with the addition of a small backcut superolaterally, if necessary, and the donor defect skin grafted. Although the proximal one-third of this flap is considered axial, the distal two-thirds represents a random extension.

The axial *gluteal thigh flap* has already been described under ischial pressure sores, and it is a useful potential sensate flap for the sacral region (75). For two reasons, it should not be considered a primary repair for the sacrum when local gluteal tissues are available and adequate. First, its elevation will disrupt one of the primary areas for ischial repairs should this later become a problem. Second, it must traverse the gluteal area medially to be inset, thus disrupting this area as well. However, if a sacral and ischial pressure sore present concomitantly, it would be an excellent choice for simultaneous closure of both defects.

The *superior gluteus muscle flap* (73, 87, 88) may be utilized to close most moderate-sized sacral pressure

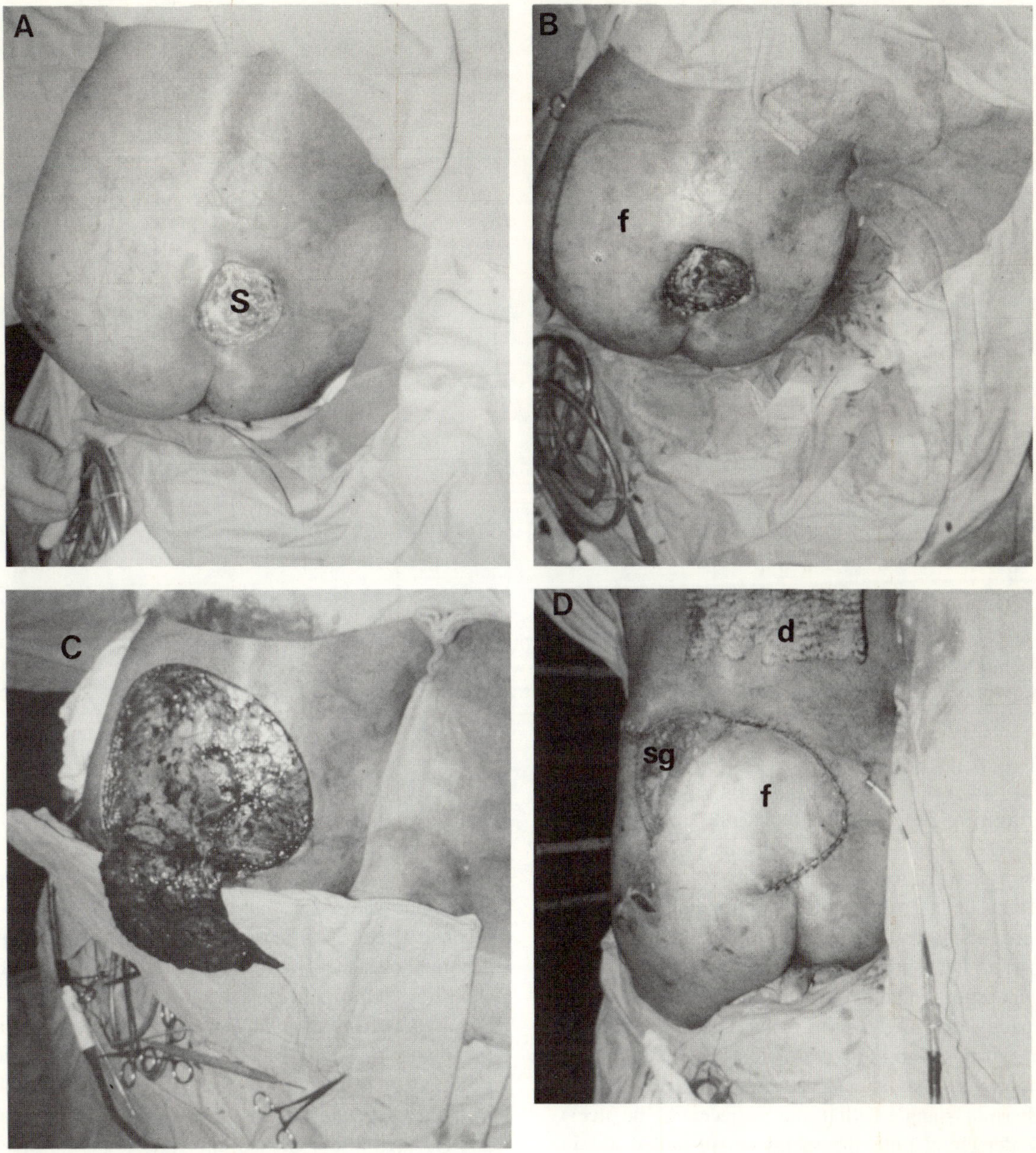

Figure 34-11. *A,* Sacral ulcer. *B,* Following excision of the ulcer, a random gluteal rotation advancement flap (f) is designed. *C,* The flap is elevated superficial to the gluteal muscle fascia. *D,* Insetting of the flap is completed with a skin graft (sg) applied to the flap donor site. The skin graft donor site (d) was taken from the lower back.

sores. This flap adds padding, and a split-thickness skin graft is applied for cutaneous resurfacing. Exposure to the muscle may be gained through a similar incision utilized for the random gluteal rotation flap, so that this flap is preserved if needed for a recurrence. A more direct approach employs a simple inferolateral incision from either side of the ulcer, directly over the superior gluteal muscle, elevating skin flaps above and below for exposure (Fig. 34-13, *A* and *B*). The superior gluteus maximus is split in the direction of its fibers from the inferior gluteus maximus muscle, detached distally from the trochanteric insertion and elevated proximally to be based on the superior gluteal vessels, which exit between the gluteus minimus and piriformis muscles about 4 cm from the posterior midline. This vessel is about 3 cm in diameter and branches to supply the gluteus maximus dorsally and then continues laterally to the minimus and medius muscles. The separation of the superior gluteus maximus at its cephalad margin from the gluteus medius often requires a sharp dissection since there is no true areolar plane, unlike its lower half,

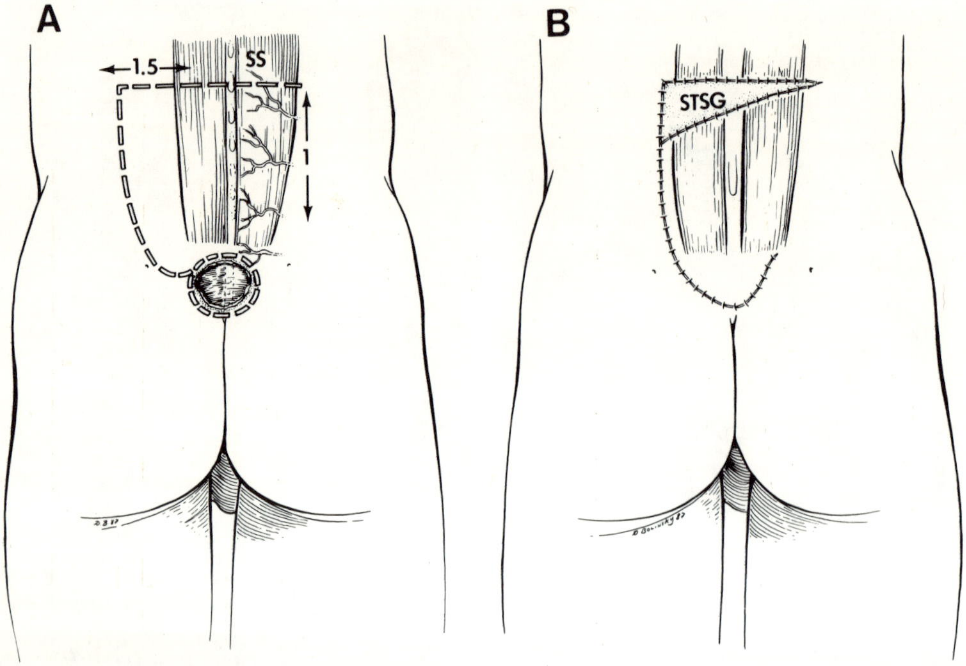

Figure 34-12. *A*, Schematic drawing of sacral ulcer and outline of a transverse lumbosacral flap based on lumbosacral perforators, which lie immediately lateral to the sacrospinalis muscle (ss). Base-width dimensions are 1:1.5 with the proximal one-third axial and the distal two-thirds randomly extended across the midline. *B*, Flap transposition is completed and a split-thickness skin graft (STSG) applied to the donor defect.

which is more easily elevated from the gluteus minimus and piriformis. The superior gluteal muscle flap is then turned over on itself at the base (or rotated), and its distal insertion is sutured to the sacral defect margins. The exposure incision is closed primarily and a split skin graft is placed over the remaining exposed muscle. Alternatively, the superior gluteus may be transferred as a *myocutaneous unit* by incorporating the overlying adipose and skin as an island paddle designed over its distal muscle belly, which is then transposed to the sacral defect (76, 89, 90). The skin island may also be designed over the proximal muscle belly (as a triangle with its base adjacent to the ulcer), and by detaching both the sacral origin and distal insertion, a 6 cm medial slide of the muscle can provide closure of smaller ulcers. This latter procedure can be performed bilaterally to increase coverage size up to 10 cm (77, 90–92) (Fig. 34-13, *C* and *D*). With either myocutaneous flap, the donor site can usually be closed primarily, by either direct advancement or V-Y techniques, respectively. The myocutaneous flap technique is useful for the patient who will be in a recumbent position for prolonged periods since it transfers more padding, having a full complement of muscle, adipose, and skin. Its use, however, consumes both a muscle and cutaneous flap, which could otherwise serve as two reconstructive procedures should the first attempt later fail. In addition, readvancement of the myocutaneous flap is limited in this region. Therefore, myocutaneous flaps in this area should be reserved for difficult cases in well-motivated or cared-for patients.

The *intercostal or sensory island flap* is a sophisticated innervated flap that allows sensory transfer to the reconstructed sacral region (93, 94). This flap is usually designed over the T9–10 interspace as far ventral as possible to maximize pedicle length and allow reach of the skin paddle from its pivot point located lateral to the sacrospinatus muscles (Fig. 34-14). The ventral island of skin may be as large as 18 × 12.5 cm and is limited more by ability to primarily close the wound. The flap is incised and elevated to the chosen interspace, and the incision is then continued dorsally, taking extreme care to identify and preserve in the subcutaneous pedicle the lateral cutaneous nerve branch, which is identified at the midaxillary line and traced into the flap. The rib superior to the interspace is removed subperiosteally, and the entire intercostal contents are dissected away from the pleura, including the periosteum with the underlying adherent neurovascular bundle. The island flap is tunnelled to the sacral defect and inset, while the donor site is closed primarily with a chest tube in place. This flap is extremely useful when local tissues have been exhausted and possesses the unique ability to transfer sensation to the sacral area of paraplegics, if their sensory level is below this donor site. This flap may also be transferred as an axial free flap by

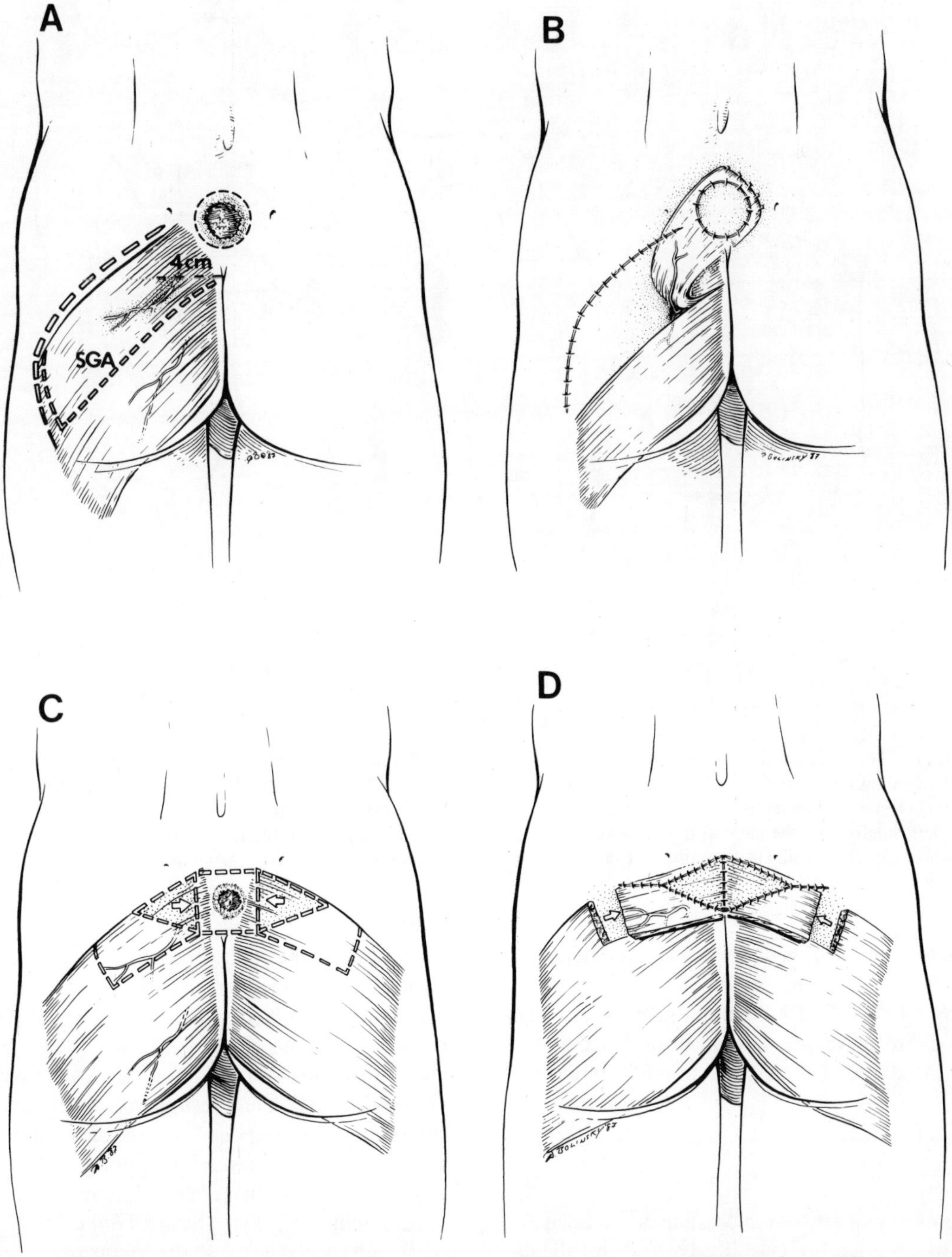

Figure 34-13. *A,* The superior gluteal muscle can be elevated on the superior gluteal vessels (SGA) to within 4 cm of the midline. *B,* The muscle is then turned on itself to resurface the excised sacral ulcer and a split-thickness skin graft applied for cutaneous coverage. The access incision is then closed primarily. Alternatively, a skin paddle may be designed over the distal aspect of either the superior or inferior gluteal muscle and elevation performed to the respective vascular pedicle. The proximal muscle is then sectioned, preserving the vascular leash and the flap rotated one hundred and eighty degrees to resurface the sacrum. The donor site can usually be closed primarily. *C,* The V-Y sliding gluteal myocutaneous flap may be used unilaterally for small defects (≤6 cm) or bilaterally for medium defects (6–10 cm). A triangular skin paddle is outlined over the superior gluteal muscle with its base adjacent to the ulcer. The superior gluteal muscle is then divided distally and proximally as well as separated from the inferior muscle, while preserving the superior vascular pedicle. *D,* The myocutaneous unit is then moved medially to provide sacral coverage and the donor site closed primarily as a V-Y.

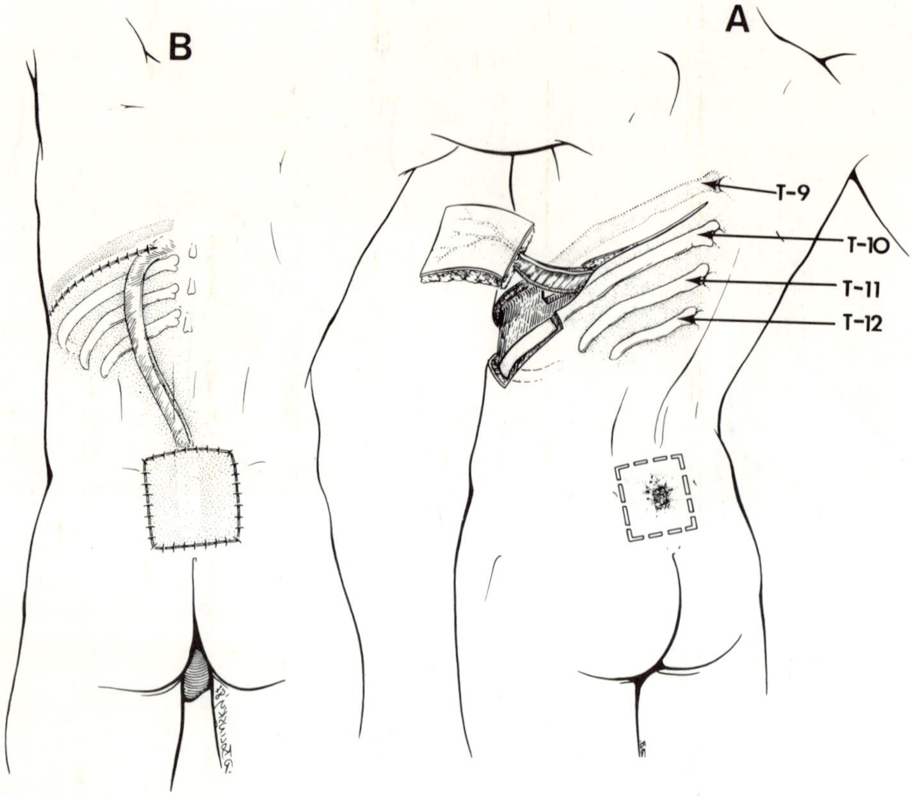

Figure 34-14. *A,* The intercostal sensory flap is an axial unit based on the intercostal neurovascular pedicle, usually T9, 10. This sophisticated flap allows for transfer of sensation to the sacral area in paraplegics whose sensory deficit is caudal to the flap pedicle. The skin paddle is centered over the chosen intercostal interspace as far ventral as possible to maximize pedicle length. The superior rib is removed subperiosteally, and the intervening contents of the interspace are elevated from the pleura to the pedicle base lateral to the sacrospinatus muscle. *B,* The flap is then tunneled subcutaneously to the sacral ulcer and inset, while the donor site is closed primarily over a chest tube.

microvascular technique if necessary. Any axial flap possessing an adequate vascular pedicle may be transferred as a free flap for closure of difficult pressure sores when other methods are unavailable or inadequate based on the obliterative needs of the ulcer cavity (95, 96) (Fig. 34-15).

Trochanter

Third in frequency of pressure ulceration is the trochanteric area, which often becomes involved when patients remain for a prolonged period in the lateral decubitus position to minimize or avoid supine pressures. The pressure ulcer excision and ostectomy are performed with the patient lying on the contralateral side and the ipsilateral leg draped free to allow hip flexion during surgery. Following flap transfer, the hip can then be manipulated to assess tension on the flap with extension as well as flexion.

The trochanteric region is similar to the ischium when it comes to skin grafting and is usually poorly tolerated except as a temporary biological dressing. The reason for this is in the nature of the underlying bony surface, which for the trochanter and ischium presents as a localized projection, generating high pressures with significant peripheral undermining and sizable cavities. On the other hand, the sacrum presents a broader surface area with less projection and results in a larger cutaneous ulceration but less peripheral subcutaneous destruction on the average. The necessary osteotomy is therefore also greater with the trochanter and ischium.

The *anteriorly based random lateral thigh flap* (97) is designed and executed on the lateral aspect of the thigh with the same dimensions and technique as for the ischial random posterior thigh flap. This flap provides a reliable coverage with the ability of future advancement should a recurrence occur (Fig. 34-16). For these reasons, it is much safer then the random bipedicle flap (48) which is more tenuous in its transfer, places a suture line and donor site graft close to the area of pressure, and cannot be reutilized.

The second workhorse of trochanteric ulcer reconstruction is the *tensor fascia lata (TFL) myocutaneous*

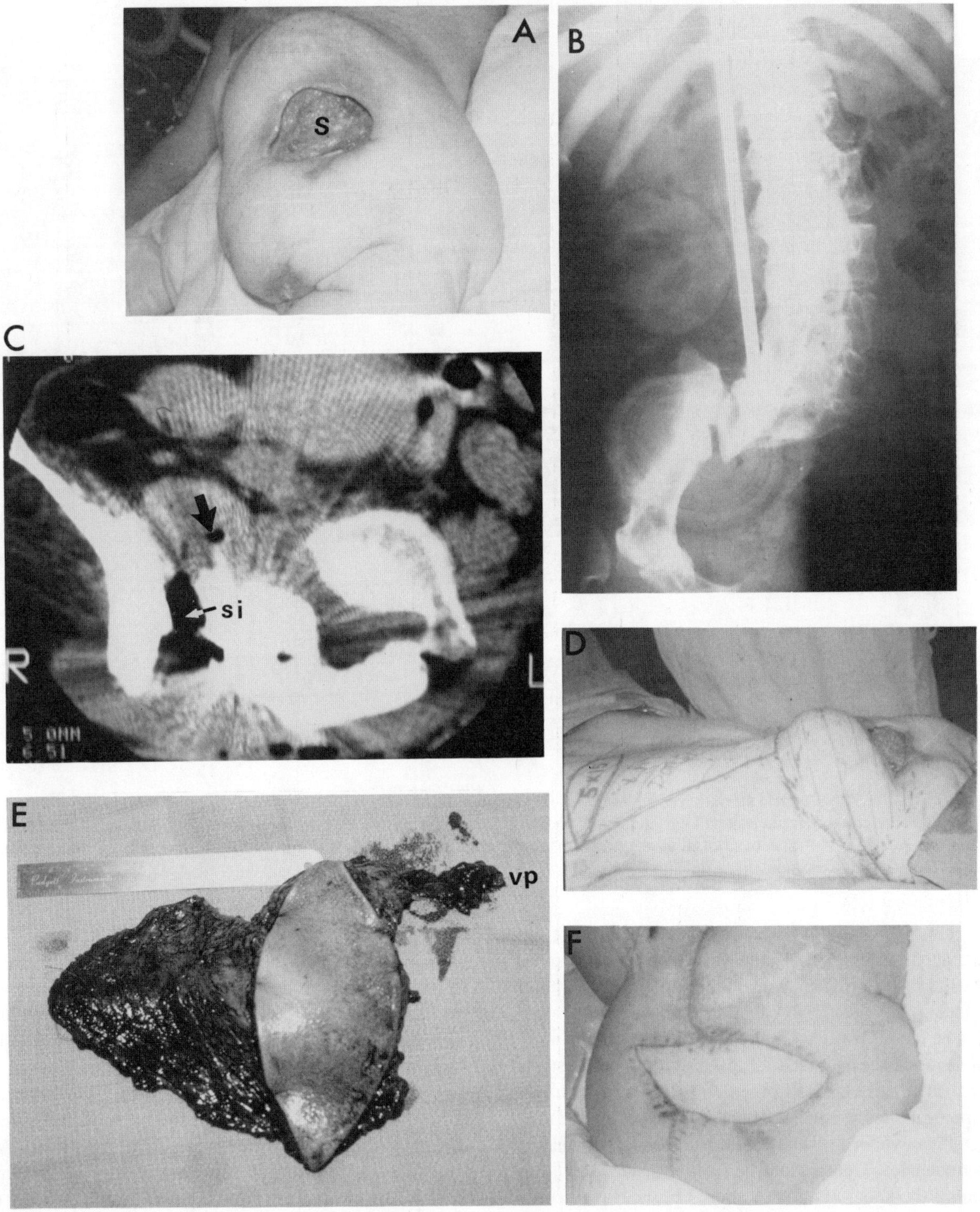

Figure 34-15. *A*, Complex pressure sores may demand tissue coverage beyond that which is available locally. This patient presented with a large multiply recurrent sacral pressure sore (5) having had a previous left hemi-pelvectomy for osteomyelitis. *B*, A Harrington rod was exposed in the depth of the wound and necessitated removal. Erosion of lumbosacral spine had produced a spinal CSF leak. *C*, Body CT scanning demonstrated a cavity extending through the right sacroiliac joint (si) with air present in the right psoas muscle retroperitoneally (*solid black arrowhead*). Appropriate debridement would subsequently require a sizable and reliably well vascularized flap to obliterate this cavity and seal the CSF leak. *D*, Following treatment of the cavity, including resection of the SI joint and debridement of the intra-psoas cavity, a left latissimus dorsi myocutaneous flap was outlined and elevated on its thoracodorsal vascular pedicle. *E*, This was transferred as a free flap to the sacral defect, anastomosing the donor vascular pedicle (vp) to the superior gluteal vessels. The muscle provided sufficient bulk to reach the retroperitoneal cavity and adequately sealed the CSF leak. The skin paddle secured a watertight closure. *F*, Completed insetting of the flap with primary healing.

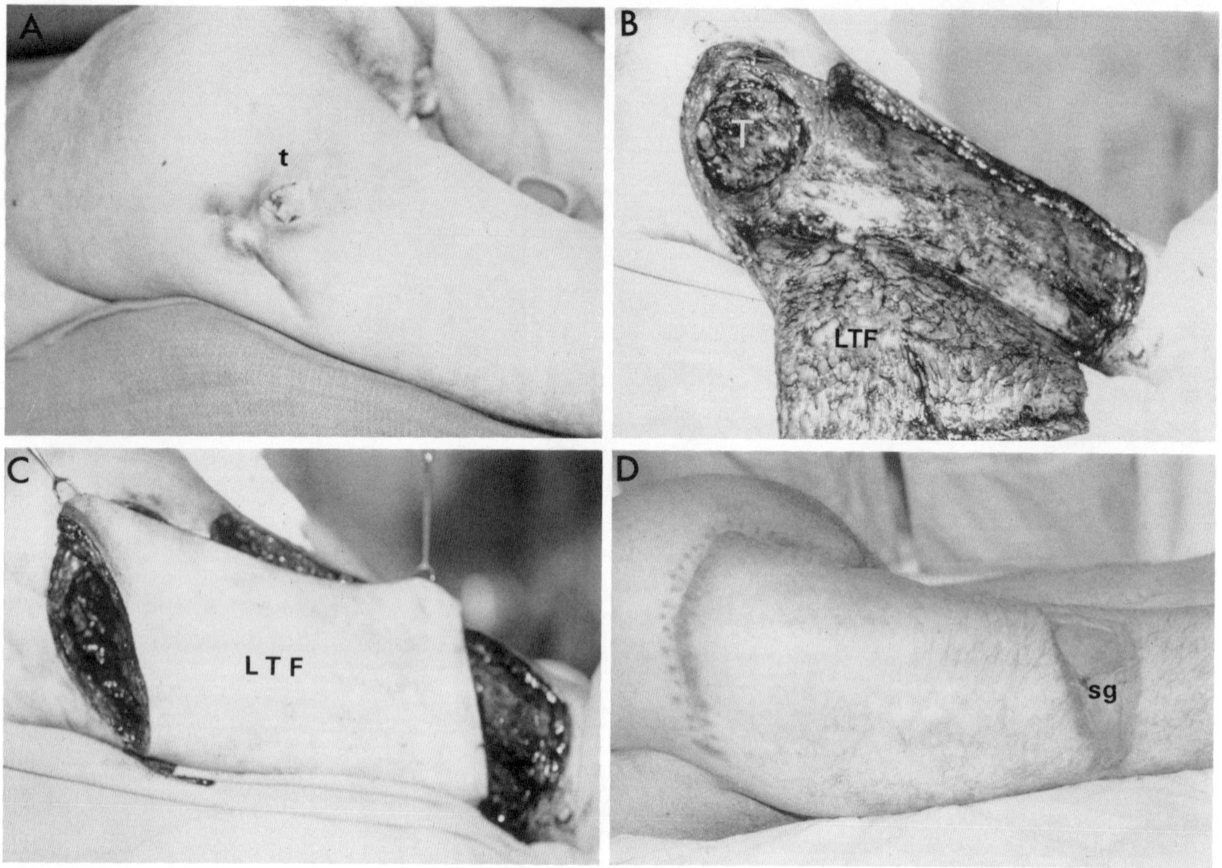

Figure 34-16. *A,* Trochanteric ulceration (t) with surrounding indurated unstable scar. *B,* Following complete ulcer excision including ostectomy of the prominent trochanter (T), a lateral thigh flap (LTF) randomly based on a broad anterior pedicle is elevated superficial to the muscle fascia. *C,* Advancement of thigh flap to cover trochanteric defect. *D,* Final healing with a split-thickness skin graft (sg) utilized to resurface the caudal donor defect.

flap (82). This flap possesses the potential to transfer an innervated sensory skin paddle with inclusion of the cutaneous branch of T12 proximally and the lateral femoral cutaneous nerve distally. A single dominant vascular pedicle, the lateral femoral circumflex artery, enters its anterior deep surface about 8 to 10 cm below the anterior superior iliac spine. Outline of the flap anteriorly is done by dropping a line from the anterior superior iliac spine to the lateral condyle of the tibia, and the posterior boundary is the trochanter. The flap may be safely extended to within 8 cm of the knee, although a short TFL is usually sufficient for the trochanteric region (Fig. 34-17). Elevation is performed from distal to proximal incising through skin and underlying tensor fascia. The dissection is continued until tension free transposition can be performed. If desired, the flap may be completely isolated as an island on its vascular pedicle and rotated 90° to the trochanteric defect, avoiding a "dog-ear" posterosuperiorly. This requires direct identification and dissection of the vascular pedicle (Fig. 34-18). The donor site is closed by either primary closure if narrow or, more commonly, a split skin graft. No ambulatory deficit is noted following its transfer. Today, this flap dominates the clinical literature for trochanteric reconstruction due to its superior reliability. Although several variations have been described, the straightforward transposition TFL Flap is the most common utilization (98–103). The extended TFL has been utilized to reconstruct ipsilateral trochanteric and ischial ulcers simultaneously with a single flap (Fig. 34-19). Attention to detail, careful handling of the tissues, and tension-free closure are imperative to ensure survival of the distal flap, which closes the ischial ulcer.

The *distally based gluteus maximus muscle flap* as described for ischial pressure sores was initially utilized as a muscle turnover flap for trochanteric ulcers using a split skin graft cover (74). This flap, based on the cruciate anastomosis near the distal insertion, derives its vascular inflow from the inferior gluteal and transverse branches of the medial and lateral femoral circumflex vessels, which need not be visualized during transfer of the inferior glu-

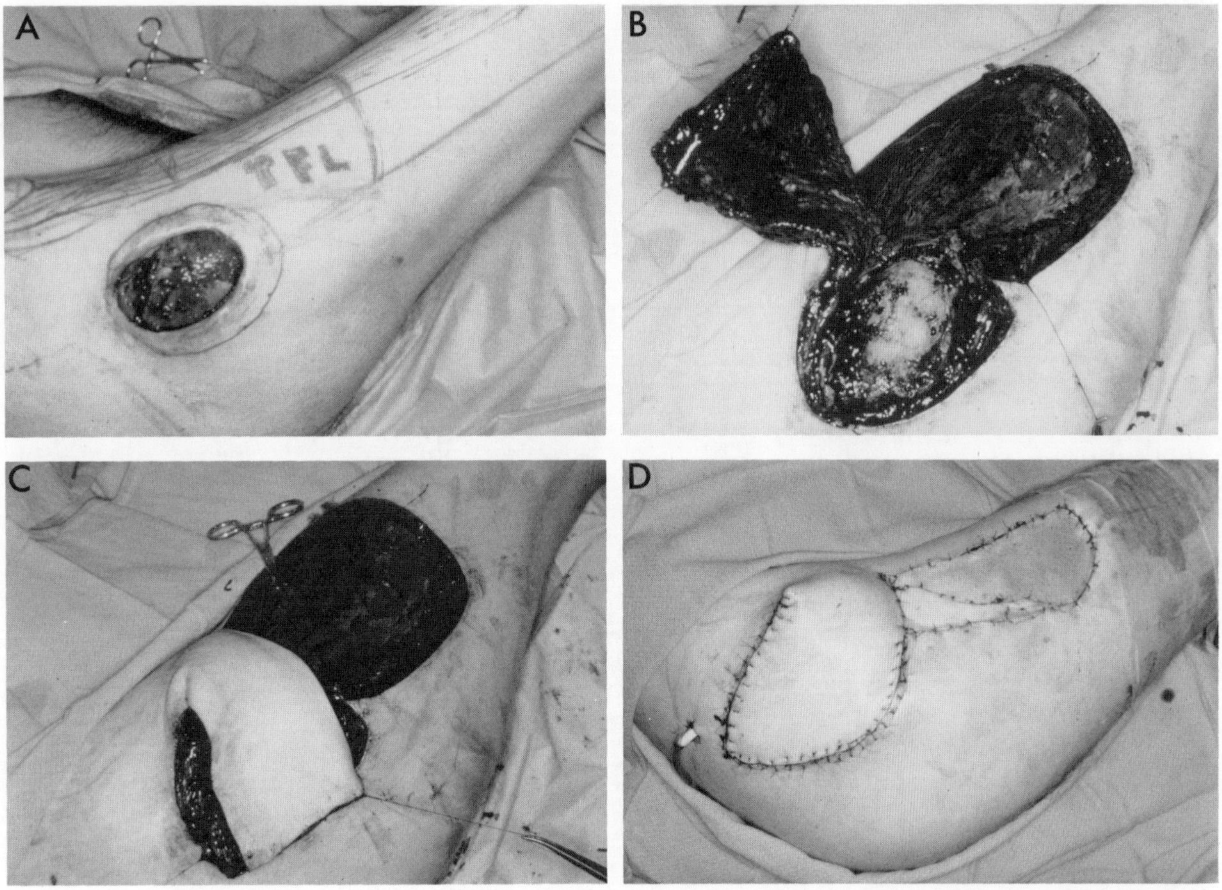

Figure 34-17. *A,* Large trochanteric ulcer with outline of a wide short tensor fascia lata (TFL) pedicle flap. *B, C,* Ulcer excised and flap elevated permitting tension free transposition. *D,* TFL inset complete and donor site skin grafted. Note "dog-ear" at posterosuperior flap base.

teus maximus. The sacral attachment is divided and the pedicle of the inferior gluteal vessels ligated, allowing mobilization of the proximal muscle belly toward the trochanter for coverage. A skin graft is then applied and the donor site incision closed primarily.

The *gluteal thigh flap* (75) is another secondary consideration for the trochanteric area in ambulatory patients; it provides reliable sensate coverage. For non-ambulatory patients, the *vastus lateralis myoplasty* (104, 105) or *myocutaneous flap* (106–108) and the *gluteus medius-tensor fascia latae flap* (109) may be utilized to reconstruct a trochanteric ulcer. These possess additional bulk to fill deep cavities, including those with intra-articular involvement of the hip. However, they result in functional gait disturbances and should be avoided in the ambulatory patient. In those ambulatory patients where excess bulk is needed to obliterate a deep cavity, (with or without joint involvement) where the TFL and/or inferior gluteal are inadequate, a free flap myoplasty is indicated (Fig. 34-20).

Before leaving the three major areas of ulceration—the ischium, sacrum, and trochanter—mention of the non-ambulatory, paraplegic pressure sore patient should include the *lower extremity fillet flap* (110–112). As an alternative to free flap transfers, which often necessitate a violation and scarring of the upper torso, the lower extremity may be sacrificed skeletally, preserving its abundant soft tissue for bulk muscle padding and cutaneous coverage. Amputations may also improve the patient's transferring capacity from bed to chair by decreasing weight and eliminating a spastic or flaccid extremity. This may allow easier lifting of the rump to minimize shearing forces created when the patient drags his or her body during these maneuvers (113). Even more radical and rarely used is the hemicorpectomy for intractable life-threatening decubitus ulcers (114, 115). These procedures are formidable and should be reserved for those crippled patients with multiple recurrent recalcitrant ulcerations often complicated by deep-seated osteomyelitis, not amenable to improved local care and regional flap closure.

An additional conservative measure, which can be taken both prior to and following any surgical procedure is the use of a circumferential body support jacket, which

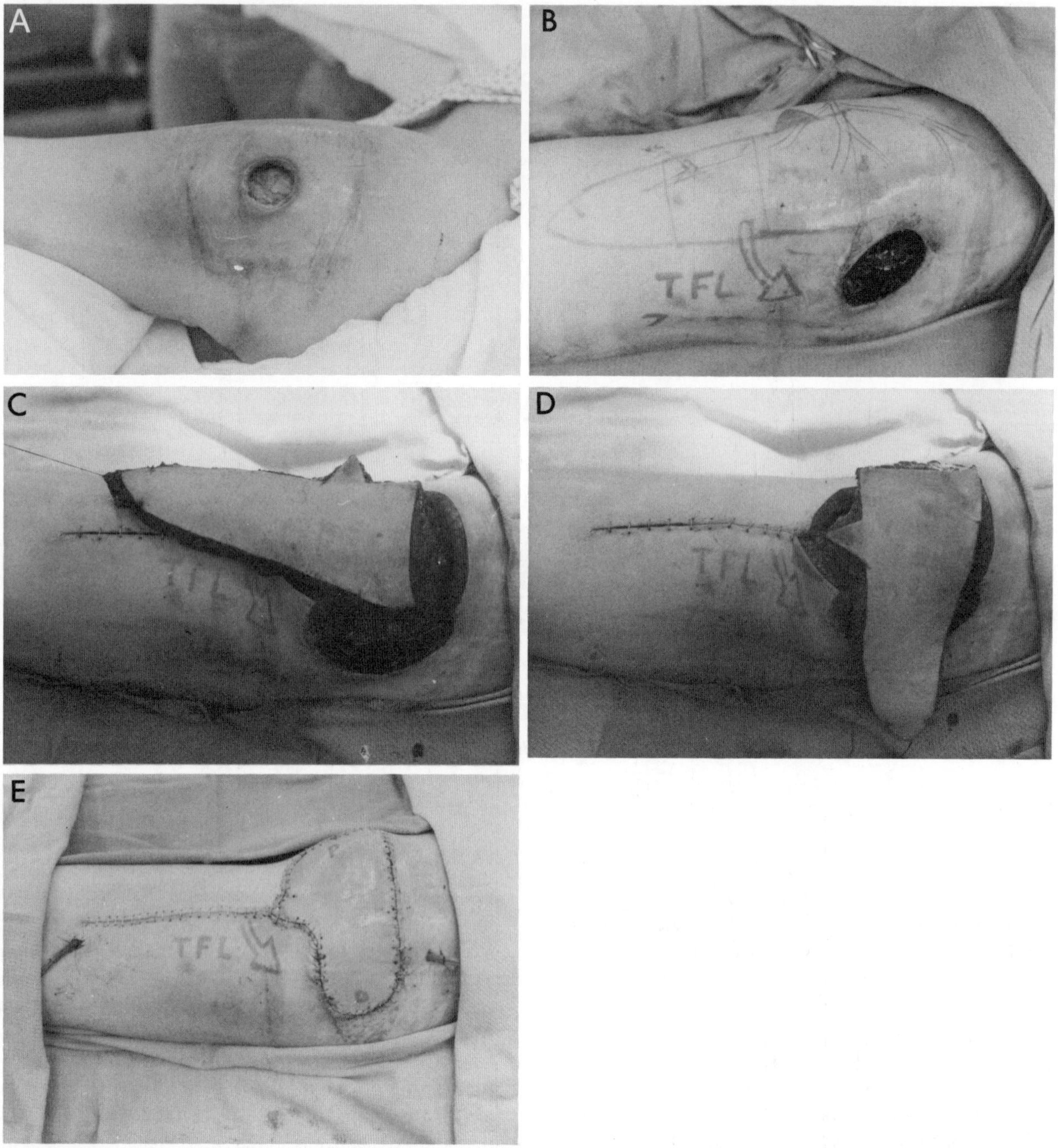

Figure 34-18. *A,* Recurrent trochanteric ulcer previously repaired with small rhomboid flap (note incisional scar anteriorly). *B,* Outline of tensor fascia lata (TFL) flap with lateral femoral circumflex artery drawn in anteriorly demonstrating its three branches. *C,* TFL is elevated as a complete island flap isolated on its vascular pedicle. *D,* Ninety degree rotation allows for precise insetting and eliminates superior "dog-ear". The small "dart" included on the anterior border of the flap aids primary closure of the superior donor site where tension is present. *E,* Completed primary closure of ulcer cavity and donor site. The entire flap was utilized with the distal tip (D) having been de-epithelialized and turned under to add padding directly over the ostectomized trochanter.

transfers the weight bearing of sitting to the sensate upper thoracic cage region. This jacket is a padded, individually molded, one-piece unit that can attach to a wheelchair or car seat, allowing the patient to sense the pressure of sitting in the chest area, while the anesthetic rump is maintained out of contact from the sitting surface (Fig. 34-21). The upper torso discomfort forces the patient to frequently change positions, unlike a spinal cord patient who, experiencing no discomfort while sitting in contact with a chair surface, may remain immobile for hours. The

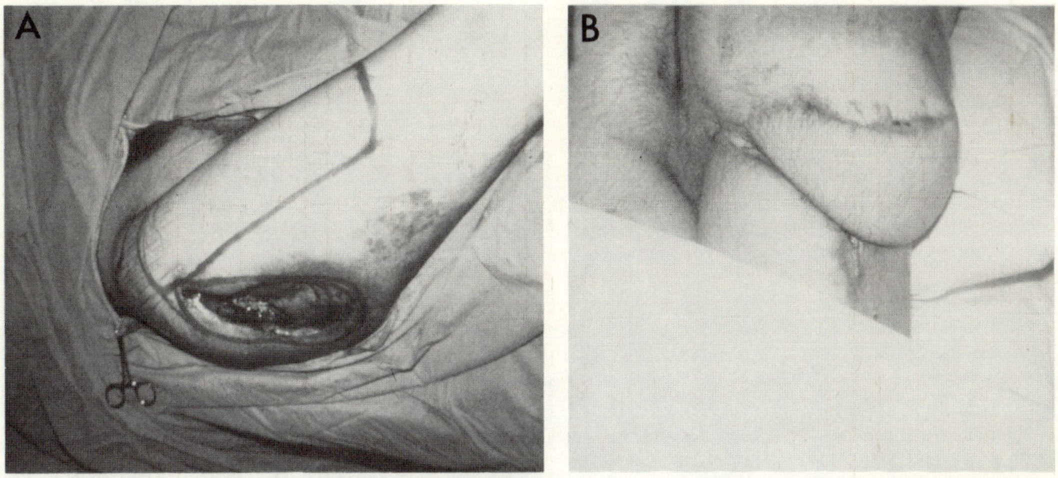

Figure 34-19. *A*, Combined trochanteric and ischial pressure sore with outline of extended tensor fascia lata (TFL) flap for simultaneous coverage. *B*, TFL transposed providing primary healing of both sites with the donor site skin grafted.

major drawbacks of this device are poor patient compliance and limited pulmonary reserve in the elderly (116).

Heel and Achilles

Ulcerations over the heel and Achilles region account for approximately 8% of pressure sores. These result from prolonged pressure exerted on the calcaneus or Achilles region following enforced bedrest, lengthy surgery, or cast application to this region when careful attention to intermittent relief or sufficient padding is ignored. In the elderly population and particularly in those with peripheral vascular disease and/or diabetes, ulcerations may develop despite attentive inspection and local precautions. A vascular evaluation in this group, including noninvasive Doppler pressure studies as a minimum, is often helpful to determine whether a vascular bypass or angioplasty would enhance wound-healing capabilities. Pressure ulcers in this region rarely have deep or extensive peripheral undermining and therefore ulcer debridement is relatively straightforward with sacrifice of as little normal tissue as possible. Treatment of the underlying bony or tendinous surface is limited to removal of necrotic or infected tissues with no attempt to minimize their prominence since this would result in a functional disability.

Reconstructions of the heel and Achilles area may be accomplished with split-thickness skin grafts if a vascularized soft tissue covering remains over the calcaneus and Achilles tendon (117–119). If a paratenon is absent, a graft will not reliably take on the avascular Achilles tendon, and although a skin graft may survive on a bare or decorticated calcaneus, it will not provide sufficient tissue to avoid recurrent breakdown during weight-bearing ambulation. These factors are therefore an indication for flap reconstruction.

There are several local myoplasty techniques for transfer to the heel area, including *abductor hallucis* (120), *abductor digiti minimi* (120), and *flexor digitorum brevis (FDB)* (121–122). The first two flaps are limited in size and reach although they may be useful for very small defects. Conversely, the flexor digitorum brevis is much more substantial and can be used even for posterior heel defects when raised as an island on its most posterior vascular pedicle. The FDB is approached through a midline plantar incision and exposed beneath the plantar fascia (Fig. 34–22). Its distal tendinous insertions are transected and elevation begins distally from the quadratus plantae muscle. The medial and lateral plantar vessels course deep on either side of the FDB muscle (between FDB and the adjacent abductors). The medial plantar vessels give off branches at the mid-muscle belly and may be divided, while the lateral plantar vessels give off a branch to the proximal muscle belly as they course from medial to lateral deep to the FDB and superficial to the quadratus. This branch must be preserved. The flap may then be turned over on itself or the proximal origin divided from the calcaneus and the entire muscle rotated 180 degrees. Slight additional freedom may be gained by transecting the lateral plantar vessels distal to the FDB branch and dividing the abductor hallucis to mobilize the proximal plantar vascular pedicle. Alternatively, to gain additional posterior reach, the calcaneus may be reduced in height by surgical partial ostectomy. The flap is then covered with a skin graft after transposition and the donor site closed primarily. The flexor digitorum brevis has also been described as a myocutaneous flap (123–124), but this has been overshadowed by the medial plantar fascial flap described below when innervated skin transfer is desired; the latter minimizes the donor defect depression.

The *medial plantar fascial flap* has become a utility

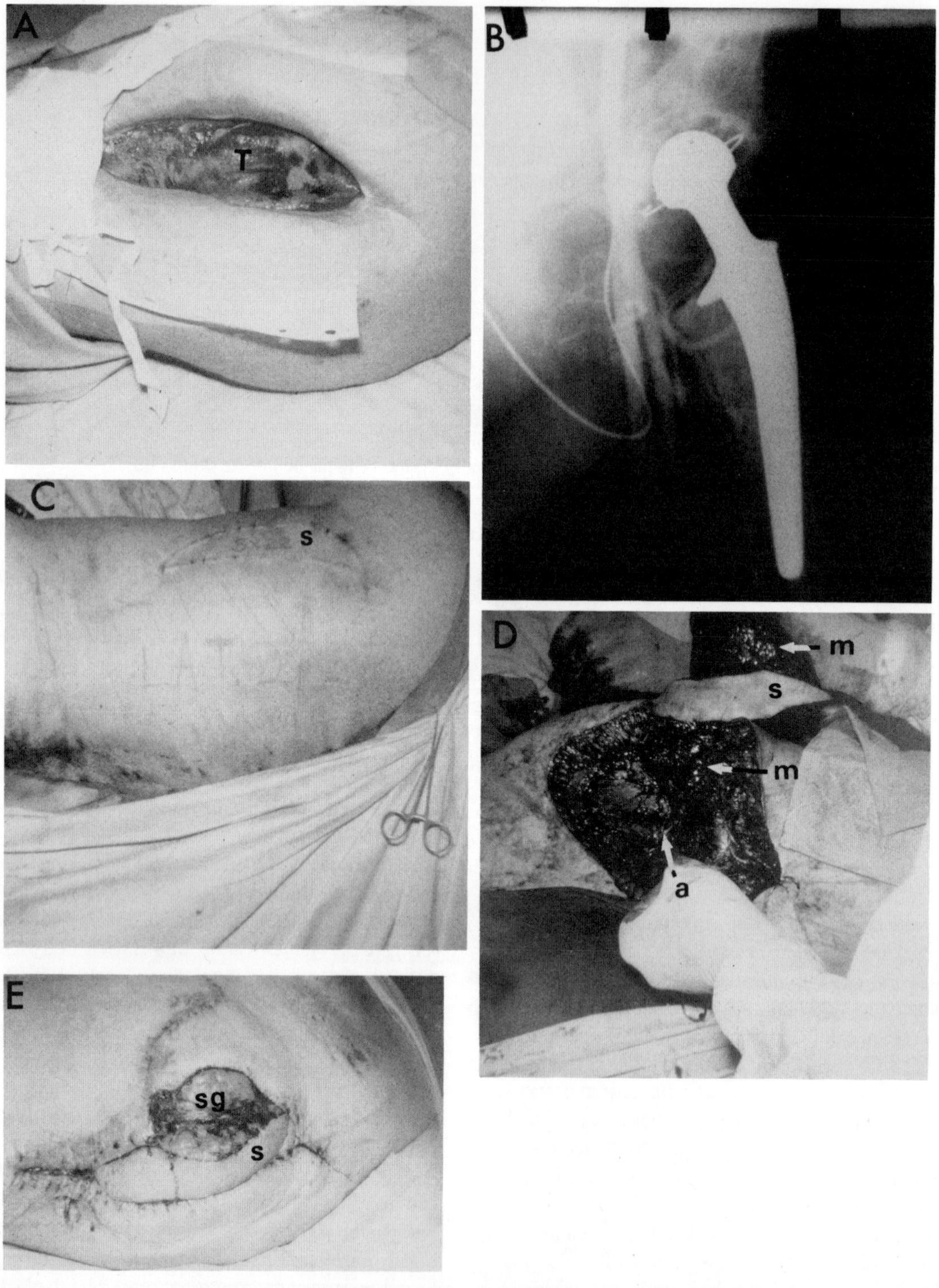

Figure 34-20. *A,* Complex left trochanteric ulcer (T) involving previously reconstructed prosthetic left hip joint at its depth. *B,* Arteriogram demonstrates patent lateral femoral circumflex vessel branching from the femoral artery. Prosthesis was removed and a girdlestone operation performed. *C,* A left latissimus dorsi myocutaneous flap was outlined with a 5 × 22 cm skin paddle (s). *D,* The entire muscle (m) was elevated with the small attached skin paddle (s) on its thoracodorsal vascular pedicle (a). The flap was detached and transferred to the trochanteric wound. *E,* The free flap was anastomosed to the lateral femoral circumflex vessels and the muscle used to obliterate the hip cavity. A skin graft (sg) was necessary to resurface a portion of the muscle to avoid tension on the closure.

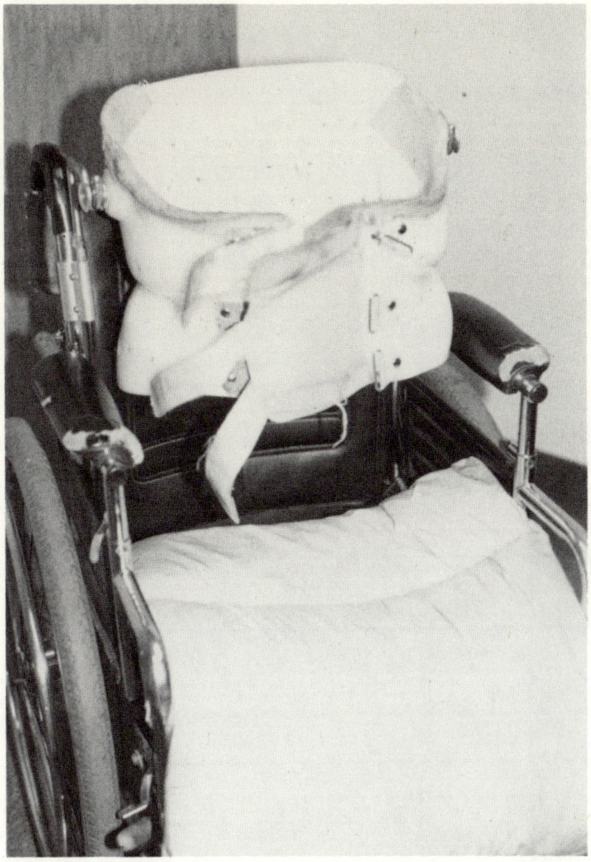

Figure 34-21. Custom molded body support jacket suspended on back of wheelchair by metal hooks, which accept rings attached to side of jacket. Similar metal hooks can be installed on car seat.

flap in heel reconstruction (125–127). It possesses a reliable vascular pedicle (medial and/or lateral plantar vessels) along with neurosensory capability by maintaining the cutaneous sensory twigs within the flap while separating them from their main nerve trunks with an intraneural dissection. The flap is outlined over the nonweight-bearing instep of the foot (Fig. 34-23), although extension to the immediate lateral border is possible as long as the head and base of the fifth metatarsal are avoided. Following incision of the cutaneous paddle outline through skin and plantar fascia, the elevation is begun from distal to proximal. Incorporation of either or both plantar vessels within the flap necessitates their distal division. The dorsal blood supply of the foot must be intact to remove both plantar vessels, and this should be checked with an arteriogram preoperatively. The fine cutaneous nerves are maintained in the flap and dissected intraneurally from their respective medial and lateral plantar trunks to lengthen the pedicle. Elevation is continued over the abductor and flexor digitorum brevis muscles until adequate pedicle length for transposition is obtained. The flap may be elevated as a complete island of skin and the pedicle dissected through the abductor hallucis and tarsal tunnel, all the way back to the posterior tibial artery if necessary. Following transposition, the donor site is skin grafted. This flap may also be elongated with interposition vein grafts to its pedicle or transferred as a free flap to the contralateral foot.

Additional anatomic cadaver studies and their clinical application have further elucidated the plantar circulation, demonstrating local plantar flap transfers based on medial and lateral subcutaneous pedicles without the need for subfascial dissections while still preserving sensory innervation (128, 129).

Microvascular *free flap* reconstruction of the heel and achilles region offers the ability to transfer any axial flap, with vessels of adequate size for anastomosis, to cover this region when local tissues are inadequate and recipient vessels are available. An arteriogram is useful to assess the recipient vasculature, particularly in elderly patients who often have concomitant vascular disease. Various asensate as well as potential sensory transfers have been successfully performed for soft tissue deficits in this region (130–136) (Fig. 34-24). To provide sensory input to tissue reconstuctions, various techniques are available involving sensory nerve transfers (137).

Other commonly employed flaps for this region include the lateral calcaneal artery flap (138, 139) (Fig. 34-25), dorsalis pedis artery flap (140), and local muscle turnover flaps [e.g., peroneus muscles] (62) (Fig. 34-26).

Malleolus

Despite the frequency of malleolar ulcerations (7%) from pressure application and their tendency to recur in those patients with underlying vascular disease, treatment is often much simpler than with the aforementioned areas. This fact is due to the lack of direct pressure in this region with normal ambulation, sitting, and supine bedrest. Ulcers here tend to be superficial with little undermining, and debridement is limited to removing necrotic debris. Bony manipulation is reserved for those cases with overt infection, which is uncommon.

Following debridement, the majority of cases will accept a split-thickness skin graft, and this is often sufficient even when placed directly on the periosteum, bare or decorticated bone. For those unusual cases where a graft is inadequate, with poor take or recurrent ulceration or if intra-articular exposure occurs, a flap coverage is indicated.

Local segmental muscle flap transfer with a skin graft for cutaneous coverage is the most common technique utilized in this area. The muscle flaps that have adequate reach to this region include the peroneus brevis, extensor digitorum brevis, abductor hallucis, and abductor

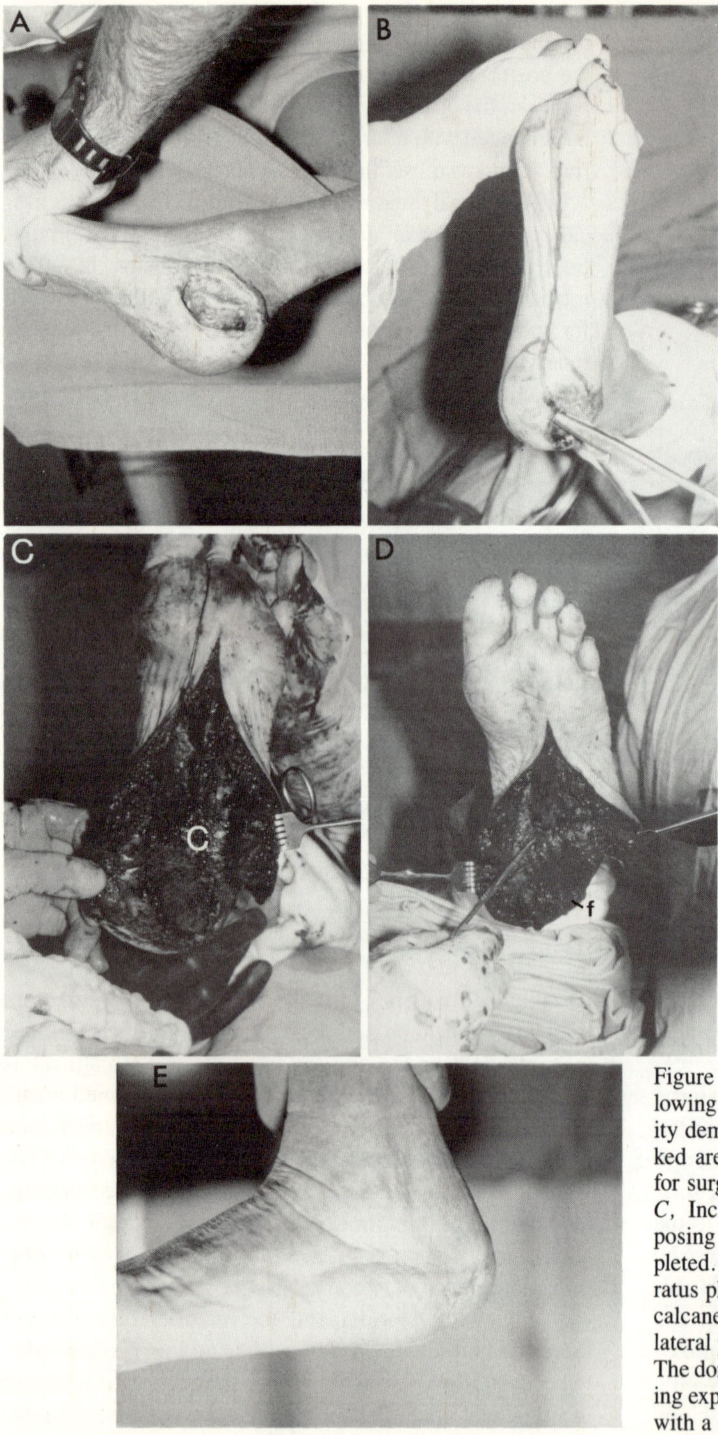

Figure 34-22. *A,* Lateral calcaneal ulceration following hip surgery. *B,* Extent of undermining of cavity demonstrated by inserted scissors and circular inked area over heel. Midline plantar incision marked for surgical access to flexor digitorum brevis (FDB). *C,* Incision taken down through plantar fascia exposing FDB. Partial calcaneal ostectomy (*C*) completed. *D,* FDB (f) has been elevated from the quadratus plantae and turned posteriorly on itself to cover calcaneal defect. The hemostat on the left points to the lateral plantar vascular bundle at the base of the flap. The donor incision is closed primarily and the remaining exposed muscle over the lateral calcaneus covered with a skin graft. *E,* Healed wound.

digiti minimi (62). The flexor digitorum brevis has the potential for reaching the malleolar area if elevated completely on its posterior tibial trunk origin.

The cutaneous flaps which allow coverage to the malleolar region include the dorsalis pedis (140), lateral calcaneal artery (139), medial plantar instep (elevated on its posterior tibial trunk), and reverse anterior tibial artery flap (141). Beyond this small armamentarium, one must resort to microvascular free tissue transfer as outlined under heel and achilles reconstructions.

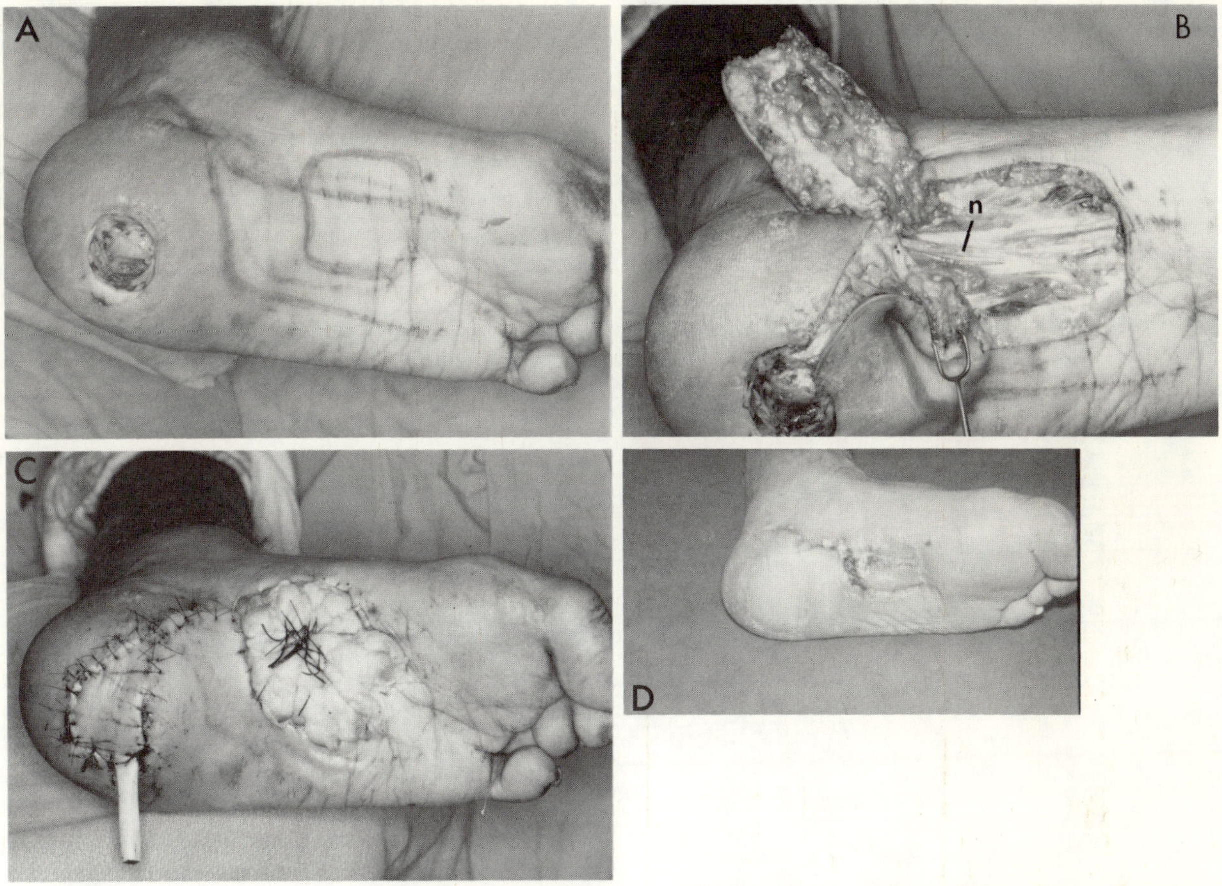

Figure 34-23. *A*, Plantar calcaneal ulceration. Medial plantar fasciocutaneous neurovascular island flap outlined over nonweight-bearing instep. *B*, Flap elevated on medial plantar vessels. Cutaneous nerve fibrils were maintained to flap by intraneural dissection from medial plantar nerve (*n*) whose main trunk was preserved for sensation to the medial distal foot. *C*, Flap transferred and inset to calcaneal defect and a split skin graft was applied to the donor instep. *D*, Healed wound and donor site.

Knee

Ulcerations about the knee frequently occur over the patellar region but may also develop over the lateral fibular head and to a lesser extent medial tibial condyle. These pressure sores tend to be superficial and often close spontaneously with appropriate local care or the addition of a split-thickness skin graft. Ulcerations on the lateral or medial aspects may be amenable to primary closure when small. When bone is exposed, debridement is usually kept to a minimum and flap closure is again indicated for those larger ulcerations that fail to demonstrate granulation and contraction. Intra-articular exposure, whether impending or overt, should also be treated with a flap reconstruction.

The workhorse and most popular flap presently utilized for wounds about the knee is the gastrocnemius muscle with an overlying skin graft or as a myocutaneous flap (142–146). The medial gastrocnemius allows coverage of the medial knee and patella regions, while the lateral gastrocnemius is suitable for the lateral knee. A skin paddle can be outlined over the medial muscle belly and the fascia distally to within 5 cm of the malleolus. The incisions are developed down to and through the muscle fascia, elevating the gastrocnemius muscle and its fascia distally from the soleus underneath. The tendon is divided from the achilles and the flap freed proximally to its vascular pedicle (respective sural arteries). Transposition can be facilitated by dissection of the flap as an island on the sural vascular pedicle if additional length is needed. The donor site may be closed primarily if muscle alone is utilized or if a narrow cutaneous paddle is taken (Fig. 34-27), otherwise a skin graft is necessary. No functional deficit occurs during ambulation even with utilization of both gastrocnemius muscles as long as the soleus remains intact. When bulk is unnecessary, a fasciocutaneous flap may be utilized based on similar vascular territories in-

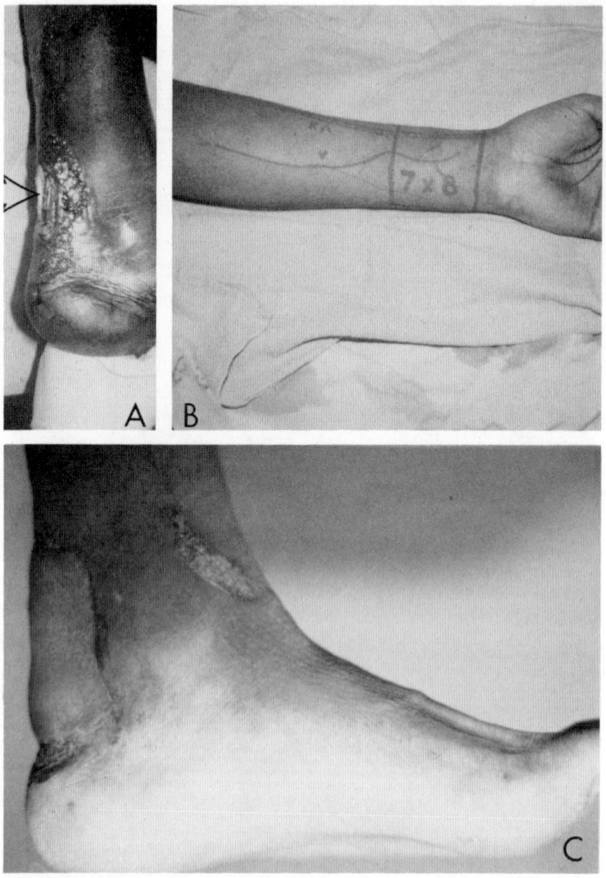

Figure 34-24. *A*, Exposed bare Achilles tendon (*open arrow*) following breakdown of unstable skin graft. *B*, A free radial forearm fasciocutaneous neurovascular flap was harvested from the left forearm based on the radial artery (RA) and a cutaneous vein (V). The skin paddle measures 7 × 8 cm. *C*, The flap was anastomosed to the posterior tibial artery and a vena comitantes. The medial antebrachial cutaneous nerve of the flap was repaired to the sural nerve to achieve protective sensation. Note coverage of the Achilles area without excessive bulk. The donor site on the forearm is covered with a skin graft.

cluding the muscle fascia but leaving the muscle undisturbed (68, 147).

While other local muscles of the thigh have been used as turndown flaps based on their distal segmental vascular pedicles, most are associated with functional deficits in ambulatory patients. Recently, a clinical report on a distally based vastus lateralis muscle flap for knee coverage in five ambulatory patients demonstrated good wound coverage with minimal to no functional deficit (148). The blood supply is based on the superior lateral geniculate artery. If local flaps are unavailable, one must turn to microvascular free tissue transfer to accomplish closure of large avascular wounds about the knee.

Purposely absent in a discussion concerning closure of lower extremity wounds in the elderly patient is the utilization of staged cross leg flaps. These transfers require prolonged immobilization (approximately 3 weeks) of both lower extremities, while a flap developed from one leg is attached to the other, allowing for the recipient leg to develop a circulatory ingrowth into the flap. The flap is detached from the contralateral leg when a viable circulation has been established from the recipient leg. This type of reconstruction is contraindicated in patients over 40 years of age due to the high incidence of thrombophlebitis, lower extremity contractures, and additional pressure sore development. The advent of muscle and myocutaneous flaps as well as microvascular transfers has similarly proven more reliable with less complications even for patients under 40 years of age, relegating cross leg flaps to a position of historical interest only for the contemporary reconstructive surgeon.

Postoperative Care

For most patients following pressure sore surgery, grafts and flaps are protected for a minimum of 3 weeks and often 6 weeks for grafts that are required to accept weight-bearing forces. This is most easily accomplished in an air-fluidized or low-air-loss bed system. Weighted pressure is then gradually increased to assess graft and flap tolerance until full weight bearing is accomplished.

Closed suction drains placed in flap recipient and donor sites are left in place until their discharge is less than 20 ml over a 24-hour period to minimize hematoma and seroma accumulation. Suction drains also help to eliminate dead space by improving flap coaptation to the recipient bed. Infection and wound dehiscence are greater problems following premature drain removal and subsequent seroma accumulation than are prolonged drain usage and so called "retrograde" bacterial drain contamination. Sutures are usually removed after 2 weeks.

Nutrition should be maintained postoperatively to optimize wound healing, and for those patients with sacral and ischial repairs, a low-residue diet is helpful for the first week to minimize fecal contamination. Constipating regimens and diversion colostomy are rarely needed when good preoperative bowel preparation is combined with a low-residue diet. Urinary diversion for incontinent patients may be accomplished with a closed drainage system, which in males can be easily converted to a condom catheter. Further protection to the suture lines can be derived from the use of petrolatum-based antibiotic ointments, which afford a water-insoluble barrier.

Attention to pulmonary toilet with incentive spirometry and respiratory therapy is indicated in these patients due to prolonged immobility, and in high-risk groups, prophylaxis for deep venous thrombosis with subcutaneous heparin should be employed. In keeping with the

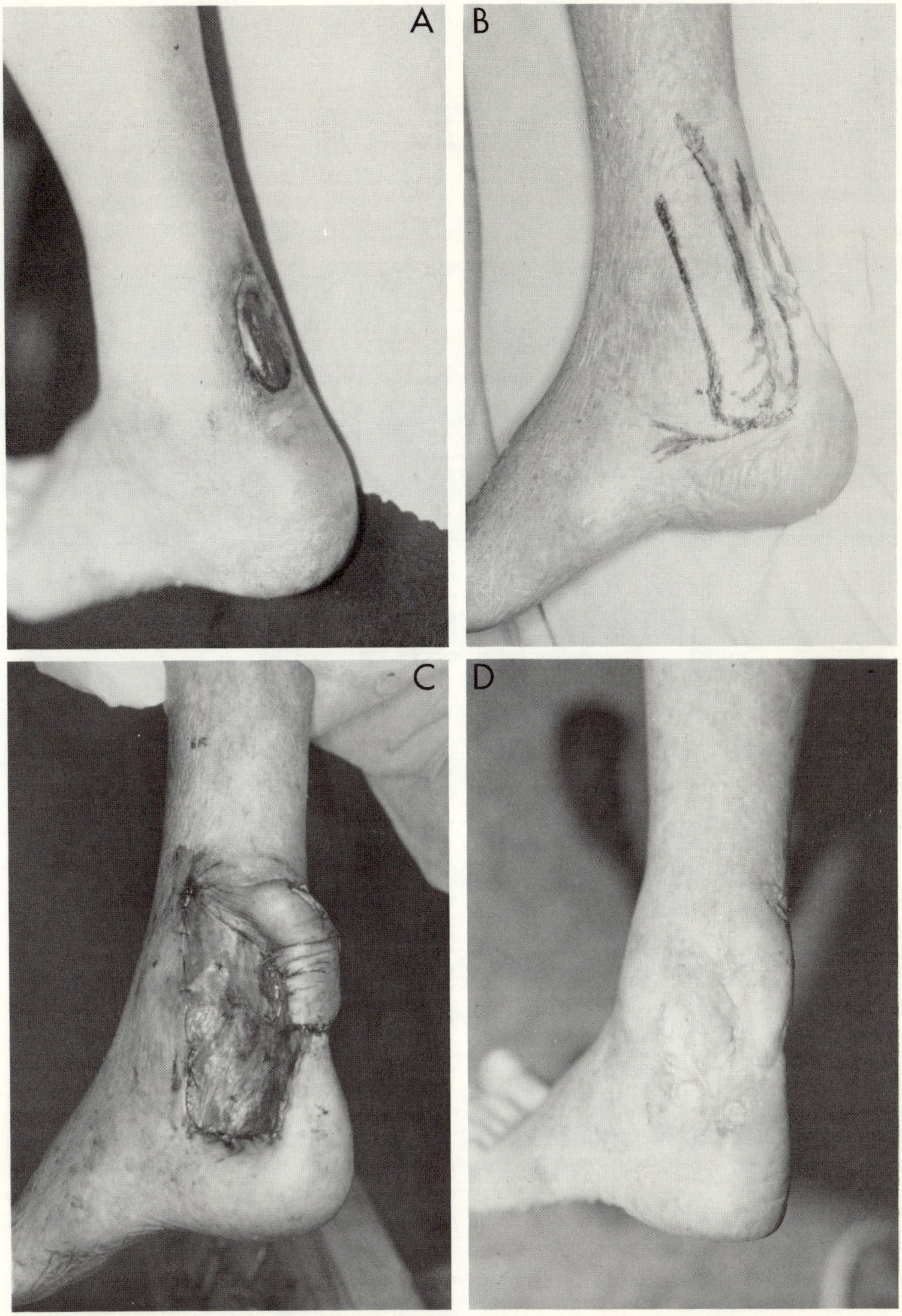

Figure 34-25. *A*, Exposed Achilles tendon. *B*, Outline of a lateral calcaneal artery flap. The presence of the lateral calcaneal artery (a terminal branch of the peroneal artery) should be checked by doppler and facilitates tracing its course. *C*, The flap is elevated from distal to proximal superficial to the flexor retinaculum and transposed posteriorly without tension. The donor site is skin grafted. *D*, Healed wound provides stable coverage.

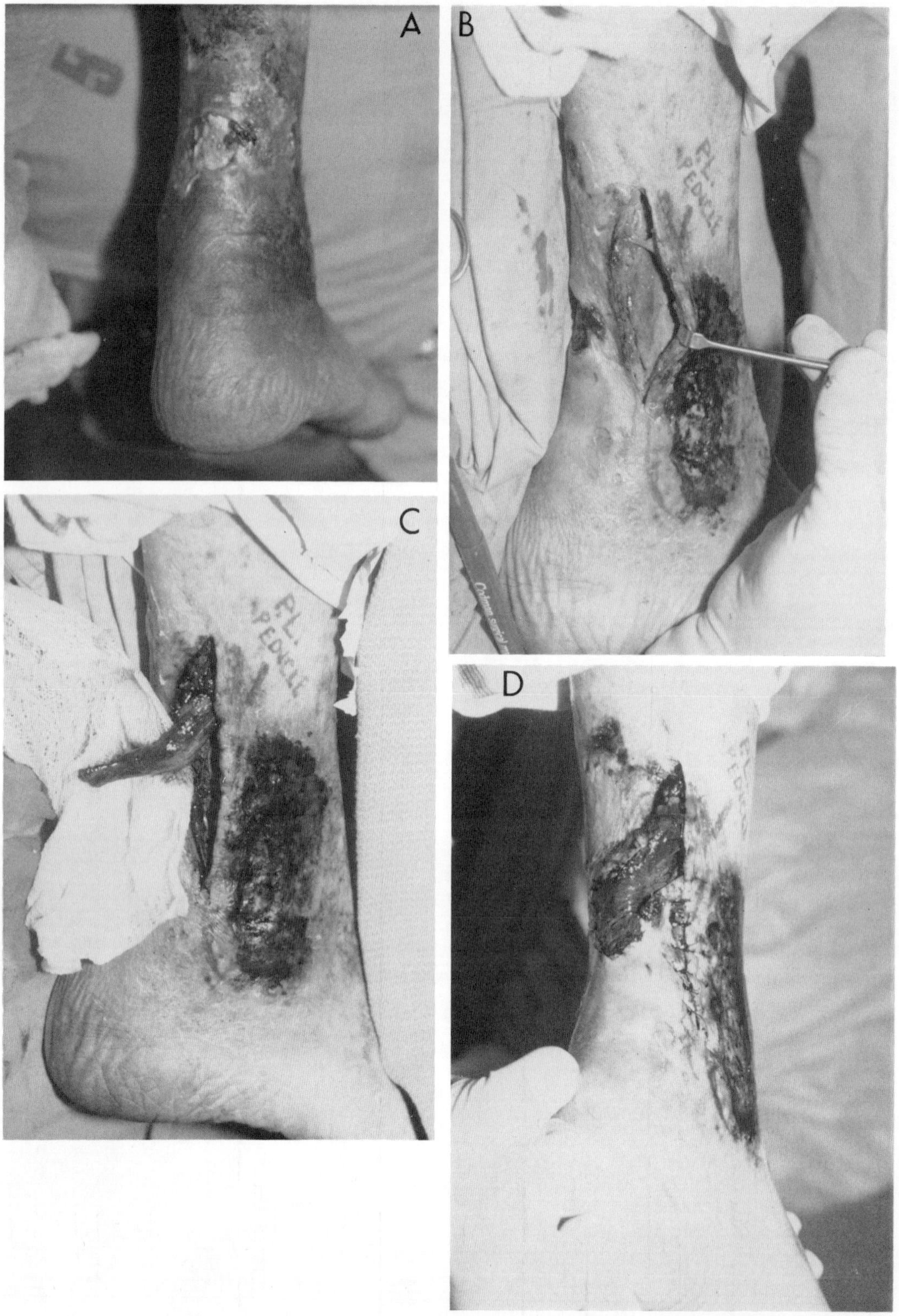

Figure 34-26. *A*, Exposed Achilles tendon with poor quality surrounding skin precluding a local cutaneous flap. *B*, A vertical incision exposes the peroneus longus muscle (PL). *C*, The PL is transected distally and elevated proximally, identifying and preserving one of its segmental vascular pedicles once adequate length is obtained for tension free transfer. *D*, The muscle is inset and a skin graft used for coverage.

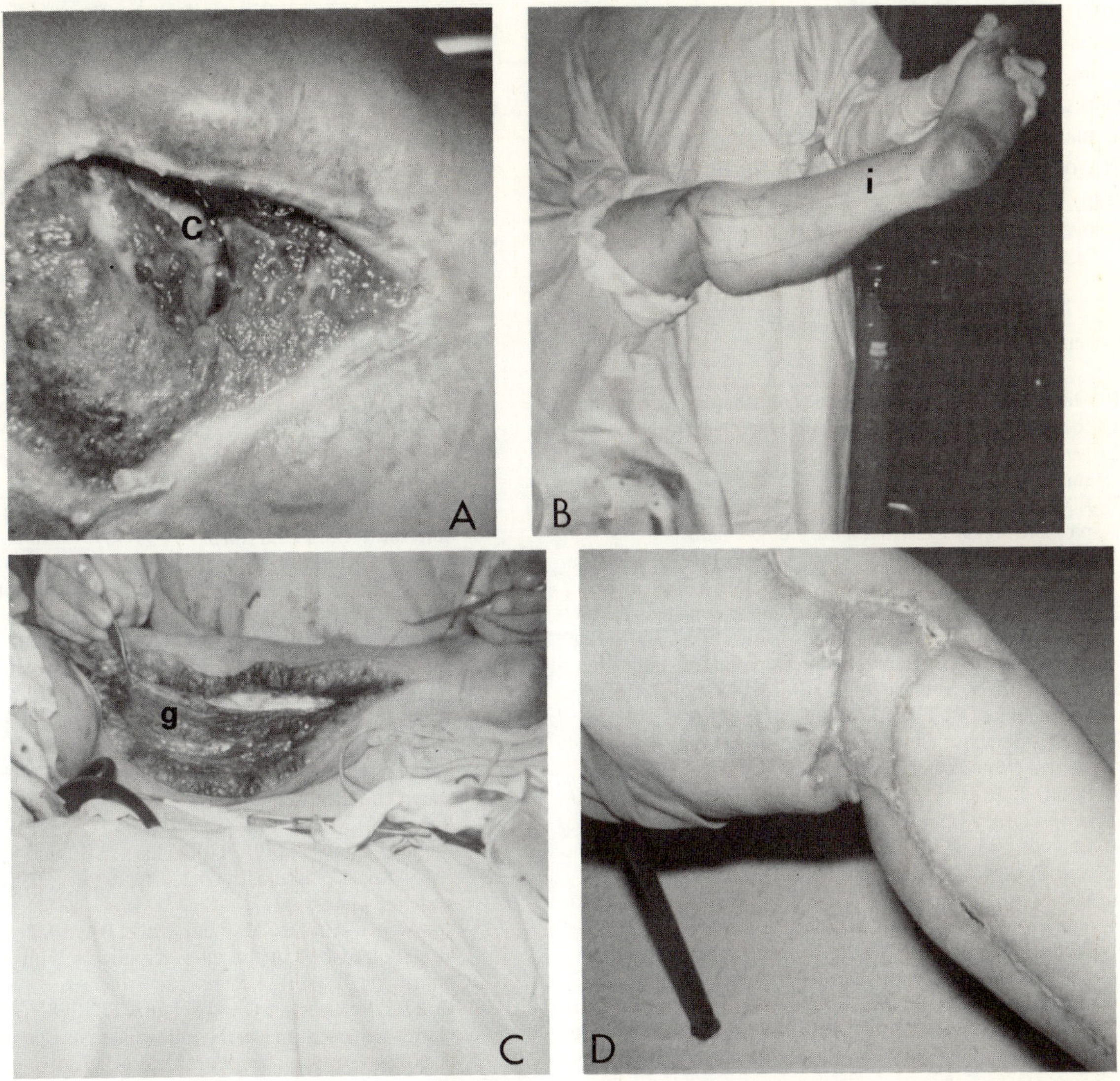

Figure 34-27. *A,* Large ulceration on medial knee, which exposes the femoral articular cartilage (C) at its base. *B,* The medial gastrocnemius is shaded in and its posterior midline outlined. The access incision (i) is marked near the anterior border of the muscle and posterior to the tibia. *C,* Exposure of the muscle (g) with forceps holding its anterior edge. The muscle is freed from the underlying soleus with blunt dissection and then released from its achilles insertion. Sharp division in the posterior midline separates the muscle from its lateral counterpart and allows cephalad transposition to cover the knee. *D,* A skin graft is placed over the exposed muscle and the donor incision is closed primarily.

prime objective for closure of pressure ulcerations, close observation for any incipient new pressure sores should be routine.

Conclusions

The present status of pressure sores continues to be a formidable problem for the geriatric patient. Coupled with the increasing geriatric population, this malady places increasing strains on the medical profession from both a preventive and therapeutic standpoint. Given the economic and manpower resources available, prevention will provide the most efficient utilization. Nevertheless, once a pressure sore develops, recent innovative weight dispersion devices and improved surgical procedures have provided an alternative to living with an open sore that requires continual cleansing and dressing changes. The persistence of these ulcerations with the need for constant attention and care, restricted activities, and at times narcotic-dependent pain can produce a psychological drain that may lead to further physical debilitation. An additional consideration is the risk of carcinoma development in chronically draining wounds which have a much more fulminant prognosis than de novo squamous cell carcinoma of the skin (149–153). It therefore behooves the treating physician to delineate those patients at high risk for pressure ulceration and institute appropriate preventive measures early during their hospital course. Similarly, once an ulceration develops, timely conservative therapy or aggressive surgical reconstruction should be employed to hasten recovery and minimize morbidity.

References

1. Manley, MT. 1978. Incidence, contributory factors, and cost of pressure sores. *South Afr Med J* 53:217.
2. Linder, MR, and Upton, J. 1983. The prevention of pressure sores. *Surg Rounds* 2:42.
3. El-Toraei, I, and Chung, B. 1977. The management of pressure sores. *J Dermatol Surg Oncol* 3:507.
4. Dinsdale, SM. 1974. Decubitus ulcers: Role of pressure and friction in causation. *Arch Phys Med Rehab* 55:147.
5. Connecticut Governor's Commission on Private and Public Responsibilities for Financing Long Term Care for the Elderly, 1987. Connecticut State Department Publication.
6. Thompson, S, and Rowling, J. 1961. Pathological changes in mummies. *Proc R Soc Med* 54:409.
7. Brown-Sequard, CE. 1853. *Experimental Researches Applied to Physiology and Pathology.* New York: H. Balliere.
8. Paget, J. 1873. Clinical lecture on bedsores. *Students J Hosp Gazette (Lond)* 1:144.
9. Charcot, JM. 1879. *Lectures on the Diseases of the Nervous System.* Philadelphia: Henry C. Lea.
10. Munro, D. 1940. Care of the back following spinal cord injuries: consideration of bedsores. *N Engl J Med* 223:391.
11. Groth, KE. 1942. Klinsische beobachtungen und experimentalle studien uben die enstehung des dekubitus. *Acta Chir Scand* 87 [suppl 76]:1–209.
12. Khanh, M Le, et al. 1984. An in-depth look at pressure sores using monolithic silicon pressure sensors. *Plast Reconstr Surg* 6:745.
13. Husain, T. 1953. An experimental study of some pressure effects on tissues, with reference to the bedsore problem. *J Pathol Bacteriol* 66:347.
14. Kosiak, M.1959. Etiology and pathology of ischemic ulcers. *Arch Phys Med Rehab* 40:62.
15. McLennan, CE, McLennan, MT, Landis, EM. 1942. The effect of external pressure on the vascular volume of the forearm and its relation to capillary blood pressure and venous pressures. *J Clin Invest* 21:319.
16. Lindan, O, Greenway, RM, and Piazza, JM. 1965. Pressure distribution on the surface of the human body: I. Evaluation in lying and sitting positions using a "bed of springs and nails." *Arch Phys Med Rehab* 46:378.
17. Kosiak, M, et al. 1958. Evaluation of pressure as a factor in production of ischemic ulcers. *Univ Minn Med Bull* 29:206–220.
18. Yeoman, MP, and Hardy, AG. 1954. The pathology and treatment of pressure sores in paraplegics. *Br J Plast Surg* 7:179.
19. Dansereau, JG, and Conway, H. 1964. Closure of decubiti in paraplegics. Report on 2000 cases. *Plast Reconstr Surg* 33:474.
20. Petersen, NC, and Bittman S. 1971. The epidemiology of pressure sores. *Scand J Plast Reconstr Surg* 5:62.
21. Agris, J, and Spira, M. 1979. Pressure ulcers: Prevention and treatment. *Clinical Symposia CIBA* 31:1–32.
22. Harding, RL. 1961. An analysis of one hundred rehabilitated paraplegics. *Plast Reconstr Surg* 27:235.
23. Conrad, RW, and Whitesides, ES. 1954. Traumatic paraplegia: A classification and fifteen year follow up. *South Med J* 47:350.
24. Barbenel, JC, et al. 1977. Incidence of pressure sores in the greater Glasgow health board area. *Lancet* 2:548.
25. Daniel, RK, Hall, EJ, and MacLeod, MK. 1979. Pressure sores: A re-appraisal. *Ann Plast Surg* 3:53.
26. Petersen, NC. 1976. The development of pressure sores during hospitalization. In *Bedsore Biomechanics,* Eds., RM Kennedi, and JM Cowden. Baltimore: University Park Press, 219.
27. Gerson, LW. 1975. The incidence of pressure sores in active treatment hospitals. *Int J Nurs Stud* 12:201.
28. Campbell, RM. 1959. The surgical management of pressure sores. *Surg Clin North Am* 39:509.
29. Edberg, EL, Cerny, K, and Stauffer, ES. 1973. Prevention and treatment of pressure sores. *Phys Ther* 53:246.
30. Ungar, GH. 1971. The care of the skin in paraplegia. *Practitioner* 206:507.
31. Spence, W, et al. 1967. Gel support for prevention of decubitus ulcers. *Arch Phys Med Rehab* 28:283.
32. Walden, R, et al. 1971. Inoperable pressure sores. *NY State J Med* 71:657.
33. Siegel, RJ, Vistnes, LM, and Laub, DR. 1973. Use of the waterbed for prevention of pressure sores. *Plast Reconstr Surg* 36:31.
34. Redfern, SJ, Jeneid, PA, Gillianharn, ME, and Lunn, HF. 1973. Local pressures with ten types of patient-support systems. *Lancet* 1:277.
35. Newson, TW, Johns, LA, and Pruitt, BA. 1972. Use of an air fluidized bed in the care of patients with extensive burns. *Am J Surg* 124:52.
36. Dolezal, R, Cohen, M, and Schultz, RC. 1985. The use of clinitron therapy unit in the immediate postoperative care of pressure ulcers. *Ann Plast Surg* 14:33.
37. Shanbaugh, RJ, Hargest, TS, and Wright, FA. 1973. Further studies on the bacteriocidal effect of the air fluidized bed. *Ann Surg* 39:253.
38. Scales, JT, et al. 1974. The prevention and treatment of pressure sores using air-support systems. *Paraplegia* 12:118.
39. Leeder, CJ. 1979. Use of low air loss bed system. *Scand J Plast Surg* 13:159.
40. Scales, JT. 1982 (June). Pressure sore prevention. *Care Sci Pract.*
41. Krouskop, T, Williams, R, and Krebs, M. 1984 (Nov.). The effectiveness of air flotation beds. *Care Sci Pract.*
42. Reuler, JB, and Cooney, TG. 1981. The pressure sores: Pathophysiology and principles of management. *Ann Intern Med* 94:661.
43. Robson, MC, Krizek, TJ, and Heggars, JP. 1973 (March). Biology of surgical infection. *Curr Probl Surg* pp. 16–20, 36–42,49–53.
44. Daltrey, DC, Rhodes, B, and Chattwood, JG. 1981. Investigation into the microbial flora of healing and non-healing decubitus ulcers. *J Clin Pathol* 34:701.
45. Morgan, JE. 1975. Topical therapy of pressure ulcers. *Surg Gynecol Obstet* 141:945, 1975.

46. Kucan, JO, et al. 1981. Comparison of silver sulfadiazine, povidone-iodine, and physiologic saline in the treatment of chronic pressure sores. *J Am Geriatr Soc* 29:232.
47. Galpin, JE, et al. 1976. Sepsis associated with decubitus ulcers. *Am J Med* 61:346.
48. Conway, H, and Griffith, BH. 1956. Plastic surgery for closure of decubitus ulcers in patients with paraplegia. Based on experience with 1000 cases. *Am J Surg* 91:946.
49. Davis, JS. 1938. The operative treatment of scars following bedsores. *Surgery* 3:1.
50. Lamon, JC, and Alexander, E. 1945. Secondary closure of decubitus ulcers with the aid of penicillin. *JAMA* 127:396.
51. Barker, DE. 1945. The surgical treatment of decubitis ulcers. *JAMA* 129:160.
52. White, JC, Hudson, HW, and Kennard, HE. 1945. The treatment of bedsores by total excision with plastic closure. *US Naval Med Bull* 45:454.
53. Barker, DE, Elkins, C, and Poer, D. 1946. Methods of closure of decubitus ulcers in paralysed patients. *Ann Surg* 123:523.
54. White, JC, and Hamm, WG. 1946. Primary closure of bedsores by plastic surgery. *Ann Surg* 124:1136.
55. Barker, DE. 1947. Late results in surgery for decubitus ulcers. *Am J Surg* 74:180.
56. Croce, EJ, and Beakes, CHC. 1947. Operative treatment of decubitus ulcer. *N Engl J Med* 237:141.
57. Kostrubala, JC, and Greeley, PW. 1947. The problem of decubitus ulcers in paraplegics. *Plast Reconstr Surg* 2:403.
58. Milton, SH. 1970. Pedicled skin flap—The fallacy of the length-width ratio. *Br J Surg* 57:502.
59. Milton, SH. 1966. Experimental studies on island flaps: The surviving length. *Plast Reconstr Surg* 48:574.
60. MacGregor, IA, and Morgan, G. 1973. Axial and random pattern flaps. *Br J Plast Surg* 26:202.
61. Ger, R. 1972. Surgical management of ulcerative lesions in the leg. *Curr Probl Surg* 10:1.
62. Mathes, SJ, and Nahai, F. 1979. *Clinical Atlas of Muscle and Musculocutaneous Flaps*. St. Louis: CV Mosby Co.
63. McCraw, JB, and Dibbell, DG. 1977. Experimental definition of independent myocutaneous vascular territories. *Plast Reconstr Surg* 60:212.
64. McCraw, JB, Dibbell, DG, and Carraway, JH. 1977. Clinical definition of independent myocutaneous vascular territories. *Plast Reconstr Surg* 60:341.
65. Nola, GT, and Vistnes, LM. 1980. Differential response of skin and muscle in the experimental production of pressure sores. *Plast Reconstr Surg* 66:728.
66. Daniel, RK. 1982. Muscle coverage of pressure points. The role of myocutaneous flaps. *Ann Plast Surg* 8:446.
67. Chang, N, and Mathes, SJ. 1982. Comparison of the effect of bacterial innoculation in musculocutaneous and random pattern flaps. *Plast Reconstr Surg* 70:1.
68. Tolhurst, DE, Haeseker, B, and Zeeman, RJ. 1983. The development of the fasciocutaneous flap and its clinical applications. *Plast Reconstr Surg* 71:597.
69. Masem, M, et al. 1987 (Oct.). Comparative bacterial clearances of muscle and subcutaneous tissues with and without dead bone. Surgical Forum Presented at ACS, San Francisco.
70. Bors, E, and Comarr, E. 1958. Perineal urethral diverticulum complication of removal of ischium. *JAMA* 168:2000.
71. Karaca, AR, Binns, JH, and Blumenthal, FS. 1978. Complications of total ischiectomy for the treatment of ischial pressure sores. *Plast Reconstr Surg* 62:96.
72. Arregui, J, et al. 1965. Long term evaluation of ischiectomy in the treatment of pressure sores. *Plast Reconstr Surg* 36:383.
73. Ger, R, and Levine, SA. 1976. The management of decubitus ulcers by muscle transposition—An eight-year review. *Plast Reconstr Surg* 58:419.
74. Becker, H. 1979. The distally based gluteus maximus muscle flap. *Plast Reconstr Surg* 63:653.
75. Hurwitz, DJ, Swartz, DM, and Mathes, SJ. 1981. The gluteal thigh flap: A reliable sensate flap for the closure of buttock and perineal wounds. *Plast Reconstr Surg* 68:521.
76. Minami, RT, Mills, R, and Pardoe, R. 1977. Gluteus maximus myocutaneous flaps for repair of pressure sores. *Plast Reconstr Surg* 60:242.
77. Scheflan, M, Nahai, F, and Bostwick, J. 1981. Gluteus maximus island musculocutaneous flap for closure of sacral and ischial ulcers. *Plast Reconstr Surg* 68:533.
78. Stevensen, TR, et al. 1987. The gluteus maximus musculocutaneous island flap: Refinements in design and application. *Plast Reconstr Surg* 79:761.
79. Hurteau, JE, et al. 1981. V-Y advancement of hamstring musculocutaneous flap for coverage of ischial pressure sores. *Plast Reconstr Surg* 68:539.
80. Tobin, GR, et al. 1981. The biceps femoris myocutaneous advancement flap: A useful modification for ischial pressure ulcer reconstruction. *Ann Plast Surg* 6:396.
81. Wingate, GB, and Friedland, JA. 1978. Repair of ischial pressure ulcers with gracilis myocutaneous island flaps. *Plast Reconstr Surg* 62:245.
82. Nahai, F, et al. 1978. The tensor fascia lata musculocutaneous flap. *Ann Plast Surg* 1:372.
83. Krupp, S, Kuhn, W, and Zaech, GA. 1983. The use of innervated flaps for closure of ischial pressure sores. *Paraplegia* 21:119.
84. Wesser, DR, and Kahn, S. 1967. The reversed dermis graft in the repair of decubitus ulcers. *Plast Reconstr Surg* 40:252.
85. Gibbon, JH, and Freeman, LW. 1946. The primary closure of decubitus ulcers. *Ann Surg* 6:1148.
86. Hill, HL, Brown, RG, and Jurkiewisc, MJ. 1978. The transverse lumbosacral back flap. *Plast Reconstr Surg* 62:177.
87. Ger, R. 1971. The surgical management of decubitus ulcers. *Surgery* 69:106.
88. Stallings, JO, Delgado, JP, and Converse, JM. 1974. Turnover island flap of gluteus maximus muscle for the repair of sacral decubitus ulcer. *Plast Reconstr Surg* 54:52.
89. Maruyama, Y, et al. 1980. A gluteus maximus myocutaneous island flap for the repair of sacral decubitus ulcer. *Br J Plast Surg* 33:150.
90. Parry, SW, and Mathes, SJ. 1982. Bilateral gluteus maximus myocutaneous advancement flaps: Sacral coverage for ambulatory patients. *Ann Plast Surg* 8:443.
91. Ramirez, OM, Orlando, JC, and Hurwitz, DJ. 1984. The sliding gluteus maximus myocutaneous flap: Its relevance in ambulatory patients. *Plast Reconstr Surg* 74:68.
92. Ramirez, OM, Hurwitz, DJ, and Futrell, JW. 1984. The expansive gluteus maximus flap. *Plast Reconstr Surg* 74:757.
93. Dibble, DG. 1974. Use of a Long Island flap to bring sensation to the sacral area of young paraplegics. *Plast Reconstr Surg* 54:220.

94. Daniel, RK, Kerrigan, CL, and Gard, DA. 1978. The great potential of the intercostal flap for torso reconstruction. *Plast Reconstr Surg* 61:653.
95. Bostwick, J, et al. 1979. Sixty latissimus dorsi flaps. *Plast Reconstr Surg* 63:31.
96. Nahai, F, and Hagerty, R. 1986. One stage microvascular transfer for a latissimus flap to the sacrum using vein grafts. *Plast Reconstr Surg* 77:312.
97. Vasconez, LD, Schneider, WJ, and Jurkiewisc, MJ. 1977. Pressure sores. *Curr Probl Surg* 24:23.
98. Hill, HL, Nahai, F, and Vasconez, LO. 1978. The tensor fascia lata myocutaneous free flap. *Plast Reconstr Surg* 61:517.
99. Nahai, F, Hill, HL, and Hester, TR. 1979. Experiences with the tensor fascia lata flap. *Plast Reconstr Surg* 63:788.
100. Dibble, DG, McCraw, JB, and Edstrom, LE. 1979. Providing useful and protective sensibility to the sitting area in patients with meningomyelocele. *Plast Reconstr Surg* 64:796.
101. Schulman, NH. 1980. Primary closure of trochanteric decubitus ulcers: The bipedicle tensor fascia lata musculocutaneous flap. *Plast Reconstr Surg* 66:740.
102. Lewis, VL, Jr., Cunningham, BL, and Hugo, NE. 1981. The tensor fascia lata V-Y retroposition flap. *Ann Plast Surg* 6:34.
103. Cochran, JH, Jr., Edstrom, LE, and Dibbell, DG. 1981. Usefulness of the innervated tensor fascia lata flap in paraplegic patients. *Ann Plast Surg* 7:286.
104. Minami, RT, Hentz, VR, and Vistnes, LM. 1977. Use of vastus lateralis muscle flap for repair of trochanteric pressure sores. *Plast Reconstr Surg* 60:364.
105. Dowden, RV, and McCraw, JB. 1980. The vastus lateralis muscle flap. Technique and applications. *Ann Plast Surg* 4:396.
106. Boret, JL, et al. 1982. The vastus lateralis musculocutaneous flap in the repair of trochanteric pressure sores. Technique and indications. *Plast Reconstr Surg* 69:830.
107. Hauben, DJ, et al. 1983. The use of vastus lateralis musculocutaneous flap for the repair of trochanteric pressure sores. *Ann Plast Surg* 10:359.
108. Drimmer, MA, and Krasna, MJ. 1987. The vastus lateralis myocutaneous flap. *Plast Reconstr Surg* 79:560.
109. Little, JW, and Lyons, JR. 1983. The gluteus medius tensor fascia latae flap. *Plast Reconstr Surg* 71:366.
110. Weeks, PM, and Brower, TD. 1968. Island flap coverage of extensive decubitus ulcers. *Plast Reconstr Surg* 42:433.
111. Royer, J, Pickrell, K, Georgiade, N, et al. 1969. Total thigh flaps for extensive decubitus ulcers. A 16-year review of 41 total thigh flaps. *Plast Reconstr Surg* 44:109.
112. Chen, H, et al. 1986. Coverage of multiple extensive pressure sores with a single filleted lower leg myocutaneous free flap. *Plast Reconstr Surg* 78:396.
113. Chase, RA, and White, WL. 1959. Bilateral amputation in rehabilitation of paraplegics. *Plast Reconstr Surg* 24:445.
114. Aust, JB, and Absolon, KB. 1962. A successful lumbosacral amputation, hemicorpectomy. *Surgery* 52:756.
115. Pearlman, NW, et al. 1976. Hemicorpectomy for intractable decubitus ulcers. *Arch Surg* 111:1139.
116. Ariyan, S, and Chicarilli, Z. 1987. A suspensory jacket permitting long term sitting in paraplegic patients. *Plast Reconstr Surg* 79:284.
117. Maqueira, NO. 1974. An innervated full-thickness skin graft to restore sensibility to finger tips and heels. *Plast Reconstr Surg* 53:568.
118. Lister, GB. 1978. Use of an innervated skin graft to provide sensation to the reconstructed heel. *Plast Reconstr Surg* 62:157. 1978.
119. Woltering, EA, et al. 1979. Split thickness skin grafting of the plantar surface of the foot after wide excision of neoplasms of the skin. *Surg Gynecol Obstet* 149:229.
120. Ger, R. 1975. The surgical management of ulcers of the heel. *Surg Gynecol Obstet* 140:909.
121. Mathes, SJ, McCraw, JB, and Vasconez, LO. 1974. Muscle transposition flaps for coverage of lower extremity defects. *Surg Clin North Am* 54:1337.
122. Bostwick, J. 1976. Reconstruction of the heel pad by muscle transposition and split skin graft. *Surg Gynecol Obstet* 143:973.
123. Hartrampf, CR, Scheflan, M, and Bostwick, , J, III. 1980. The flexor digitorum brevis muscle island pedicle flap. A new dimension in heel reconstruction. *Plast Reconstr Surg* 66:264.
124. Ikuta, Y, et al. 1984. Reconstruction of the heel pad by flexer digitorum brevis musculocutaneous flap transfer. *Plast Reconstr Surg* 74:86.
125. Reiffel, RS, and McCarthy, JG. 1980. Coverage of heel and sole defects: A new subfascial arterialized flap. *Plast Reconstr Surg* 66:250.
126. Harrison, DH, and Morgan, BDG. 1981. The instep island flap to resurface plantar defects. *Br J Plast Surg* 34:315.
127. Morrison, WA, et al. 1983. The instep of the foot as a fasciocutaneous island and as a free flap for heel defects. *Plast Reconstr Surg* 72:56.
128. Hildalgo, DA, and Shaw, WW. 1986. Anatomic basis of plantar flap design. *Plast Reconstr Surg* 78:627.
129. Shaw, WW, and Hildago, DA. 1986. Anatomic basis of plantar flap design: Clinical applications. *Plast Reconstr Surg* 78:637.
130. Rigg, BM. 1975. Transfer of a free groin flap to the heel by microvascular anastomoses. *Plast Reconstr Surg* 55:36.
131. May, JW, Jr, Hall, MJ, and Simon, SR. 1985. Free microvascular muscle flaps with skin graft reconstruction of extensive defects of the foot. A clinical and gait analysis study. *Plast Reconstr Surg* 75:627.
132. Chicarilli, Z, Ariyan, S, and Cuono, C. 1986. Versatility of the free radical forearm flap for head and neck, lower extremity reconstructions. *J Microsurg* 2:221.
133. Chicarilli, ZN, and Price, GJ. 1986. Complete plantar foot coverage with the free neurosensory radial forearm flap. *Plast Reconstr Surg* 78:94.
134. Stevenson, TR, and Mathes, SJ. 1986. Management of foot injuries with free muscle flaps. *Plast Reconstr Surg* 78:665.
135. Colen, LB. 1987. Limb salvage in the patient with severe peripheral vascular disease: The role of microsurgical free tissue transfer. *Plast Reconstr Surg* 79:389.
136. Stevensen, TR, Greene, TL, and Kling, TF, Jr. 1987. Heel reconstruction with the deep circumflex iliac artery osteocutaneous flap. *Plast Reconstr Surg* 79:982.
137. Chang, KN, DeArmond, SJ, and Buncke, HJ. 1986. Sensory reinnervation in microsurgical reconstruction of the heel. *Plast Reconstr Surg* 78:652.
138. Grabb, WC, and Argenta, LC. 1981. The lateral calcaneal

artery skin flap (The lateral calcaneal artery, lesser saphaneous vein, and sural nerve skin flap). *Plast Reconstr Surg* 68:723.

139. Gang, RK. 1987. Reconstruction of soft tissue deficit of the posterior heel with a lateral calcaneal artery island flap. *Plast Reconstr Surg* 79:415.
140. Caffee, HH, and Hoefflin, SM. 1979. The extended dorsalis pedis flap. *Plast Reconstr Surg* 64:807.
141. Rocha, JFR, et al. 1987. The anterior tibial artery flap: Anatomic study and clinical application. *Plast Reconstr Surg* 79:396.
142. McCraw, JB, Fishman, JH, and Sharzer, LA. 1978. The versatile gastrocnemius myocutaneous flap. *Plast Reconstr Surg* 62:15.
143. Feldman, JJ, Cohen, BE, and May, JW, Jr. 1978. The medial gastrocnemius myocutaneous flap. *Plast Reconstr Surg* 61:531.
144. Arnold, PG, and Mixter, RC. 1983. Making the most of the gastrocnemius muscles. *Plast Reconstr Surg* 72:38.
145. Nahai, F, and Mathes, SJ. 1984. Musculocutaneous flap or muscle flap and skin graft. *Ann Plast Surg*. 12:199.
146. Krull, SS, and Marcadis, A. 1987. Aesthetic considerations of the medial gastrocnemius myocutaneous flap. *Plast Reconst Surg* 79:67.
147. Ponten, B. 1981. The fasciocutaneous flap: Its use in soft tissue defects of the lower leg. *Br J Plast Surg* 34:215.
148. Swartz, WM, et al. 1987. Distally based vastus lateralis muscle flap coverage of wounds about the knee. *Plast Reconstr Surg* 80:255.
149. Marjolin, JN. 1828. Ulcere. *Dictionaire Medecine T* 21:31.
150. Fitzgerald, RH, Jr, Brewer, NS, and Dahlin, DC. 1976. Squamous cell carcinoma complicating chronic osteomyelitis. *J Bone Joint Surg* 58:1146.
151. Novick, M, Gard, DA, Hardy, S, et al. 1977. Burn scar carcinoma: A review and analysis of 46 cases. *J Trauma* 17:809.
152. Mustoe, T, et al. 1986. Carcinoma in chronic pressure sores: A fulminant disease process. *Plast Reconstr Surg* 77:116.
153. Chicarilli, Z. 1987. Follicular occlusion triad: Hidradentis suppurativa, acne conglobata, and dissecting cellulitis of the scalp. *Ann Plast Surg* 18:230.

35

Neurosurgery in the Elderly

Lawrence F. Borges and Kevin Kiwak

Of all the age-related changes, those in the nervous system are of paramount importance and are often used by our society to define aging. One need only to consider the portrayal of an elderly person by an actor walking slowly with a stoop and shuffling gait, speaking softly with a soft, quivering voice, trying to steady tremulous hands, and exhibiting poor recall of recent events—to realize the extent to which our concepts of aging and nervous system decline are inter-related. The neurological changes most consistently associated with aging have been studied by Critchley (1) and include presbyopia, presbycusis (especially for high tones), diminished sense of smell, reduced motor activity, slowed reaction time, small pupils with reduced pupillary reflexes, limited upward gaze, reduced vibratory perception, impaired coordination, reduced perception, and reduced or absent Achilles tendon reflexes. Pathologic changes are also found consistently within the aged brain. These include decreased brain weight, loss of neurons, increased gliosis, accumulation of lipofuschin pigments within neurons, senile plaques, deposits of amyloid, and thickening and hyalinization of small blood vessels (2, 3). Although the pathologic changes of the aged brain are well described, the precise clinical change that occurs from each morphological change remains poorly understood. These changes and correlations are discussed more fully in Chapter 12.

Despite the pathologic alterations in the nervous system caused by aging, the span of neurosurgical disorders that afflict the elderly is similar to that seen in younger patients. However, certain neurosurgical problems are unusually common in the elderly, and other disorders require special consideration for their proper management. Therefore, this chapter focuses on these two categories of neurosurgical disease.

Since alterations in the normal neurologic examination are a part of the aging process, the identification of neurosurgically treatable disease can be a difficult task (4,5). The initial recognition of such potentially treatable disease usually falls to the patient's family doctor or internist. Guidelines to assist in separating the neurologic changes of aging from those suggesting more serious nervous system pathology are given in Chapters 12 and 13. When significant neurological dysfunction is recognized in an elderly patient, a complete medical, endocrine, and neurologic evaluation is indicated. The neurologic evaluation of the elderly is aided by the availability of computerized axial tomographic (CT) scanning and magnetic resonance scanning, which is available in most large cities and often obviates the need for more dangerous, invasive evaluation such as pneumoencephalography, angiography, and myelography.

Occasionally, some physicians will exhibit a reluctance to refer elderly patients for neurosurgical intervention, fearful that their advanced age makes them poor candidates for a neurosurgical procedure. On the Neurosurgical Service at the Massachusetts General Hospital we have not found advanced age, per se, to be a significant factor for predicting outcome following neurosurgical procedures. Any patient, elderly or young, may have accumulated enough dysfunction in certain organ systems (i.e., poor pulmonary function, cardiac ischemia, etc.) to be considered at high risk for tolerating the systemic stress of surgery. However, in the absence of such identifiable risk factors, advanced age should not be a deterrent to surgical intervention. It must be recognized that advanceed age does result in physiologic changes in the kidney (Chapter 7) and in the liver (Chapter 8), which alter the metabolism of many drugs. Therefore, special considerations need to be used when selecting the anesthetic for the long procedures often required in neurosurgery (Chapter 22). Since a clear sensorium is desirable after neurosurgical procedures to facilitate clinical evaluation, special consideration should also be given to postoperative analgesics and anticonvulsants. While dosing with narcotic analgesics every 3 to 4 hours is appropriate in younger patients, a longer dosing interval (i.e., every 6 to 8 hours) is often preferred in the elderly. Following craniotomy, we routinely use Codeine 30 mg every 6 to 8 hours for analgesia if Tylenol is insufficient. Anticonvulsant levels should be monitored closely in the elderly, especially after surgery. Clinically apparent phenytoin toxicity can occur at serum levels in the upper therapeutic range and are manifested by altered sensorium, vomiting, ataxia, and nystagmus. Such symptoms in the postoperative patient may mimic the symptoms of cerebral edema and lead to unnecessary concern and diagnostic studies.

Neoplasms

The incidence of intracranial neoplasms increases throughout most of adulthood. Some clinical studies have shown that the incidence peaks between 50 and 60 years of age (6, 7), while other studies (8) have found a continuing increase in the incidence of brain tumor beyond age 60. Studies that include autopsy data suggest that the occurrence of intracranial neoplasm continues to increase beyond 60 years of age (9, 10). This would suggest that many brain tumors are not diagnosed during life in elderly patients. Most studies demonstrate that the incidence of meningioma and metastatic tumors is higher in patients over 70 years of age than in young patients (8, 9, 11).

Intracranial tumors may come to medical attention because of the development of neurologic symptoms or they may be found incidentally on a CT scan performed for another reason. The neurologic symptoms will vary with the location of the tumor. Increased intracranial pressure, which causes headaches and vomiting in young adults, may present insidiously in the elderly (12, 13). Symptoms such as apathy, lethargy, confusion, increasing immobility, and incontinence are seen commonly in elderly patients with increased intracranial pressure. These symptoms are common to many disorders and therefore can be misinterpreted by physicians. Intracranial tumors can also present with dementia (14), hemiplegia (15), and seizures (16) in elderly patients.

The diagnostic evaluation of the elderly patient with a suspected intracranial neoplasm does not differ from the evaluation recommended in younger patients. Usually a head CT scan with and without intravenous contrast infusion is performed to delineate the abnormality and allow the formulation of a differential diagnosis. Certain tumors (i.e., some meningiomas and acoustic neuromas) have such a characteristic appearance on CT scan that the physician can make a reliable histologic diagnosis from the CT scan alone. Other neoplasms may require biopsy before a firm diagnosis can be made. Angiography is reserved for those lesions in which precise knowledge of the vascular anatomy may obviate a diagnostic biopsy or is necessary for planning surgical intervention. Angiography carries greater risk in the elderly than in younger patients, because of the presence of atheromatous lesions in the extracranial vessels in a high percentage of elderly patients.

The management of symptomatic intracranial neoplasms in elderly patients is identical to their management in younger patients. This management includes stereotactic biopsy, surgical resection, radiation therapy, and chemotherapy. Deciding which modality to employ in an individual patient is based on the details of the lesion and not on the patient's age. Corticosteroids are administered during the perioperative period and as needed during radiation therapy. Some investigators have found a higher complication rate from corticosteroids in elderly patients than is found in younger patients (17). Therefore, steroids should be stopped as soon as practical. Surgery for intracranial neoplasm has been performed satisfactorily on patients in their nineties at the Massachusetts General Hospital without a higher complication rate in such patients as compared with younger patients (18). A higher complication rate, however, has been observed by other investigators (19).

One special problem in the elderly is the management of intracranial neoplasms discovered incidentally. The proliferation of CT scanners has allowed most patients to have ready access to these valuable diagnostic instruments. As the use of CT scanning increases, previously unrecognized intracranial pathology is being found before it has become symptomatic. Thus, an elderly patient may undergo a CT scan for the evaluation of dizziness and be found to have a small frontal meningioma, which is unrelated to the presenting symptom. Our approach has been to follow such patients clinically and with repeat CT scans. We have recommended surgery only in those patients who develop symptoms directly related to the intracranial tumor or in whom the tumor enlarges on repeated CT scanning. We have observed many meningiomas in elderly females that do not enlarge or become symptomatic over several years followup.

Pain

The management of pain transcends many different medical specialties. The neurosurgeon is often consulted for two pain disorders in the elderly: trigeminal neuralgia and postherpetic neuralgia.

Trigeminal neuralgia, originally described in 1677 (20) is a syndrome of paroxysmal, lancinating pain in the trigeminal nerve distribution that is triggered by certain stimuli (i.e., light touch, chewing, facial movements, speaking, etc.). More than 70% of patients afflicted with this problem are older than 50 years of age, and the disorder has been seen in patients in the 9th decade of life (21). The severity of the facial pain precludes satisfactory nutrition and patients can become dehydrated and lose considerable weight. The disorder is more common in women than in men (2:1). The clinical presentation of this disorder is so characteristic that the diagnosis is usually made from the history. Often the history must be told by a family member or written by the patient, as the severe pain precludes conversation. In most patients with trigeminal neuralgia, the etiology will remain unknown. However, a small number of patients will harbor a neoplasm or vascular abnormality that irritates the trigeminal nerve. Therefore, patients are advised to undergo CT scans on initial presentation to assess for these problems.

Trigeminal neuralgia is a disorder that remits and recurs. Initial treatment of this problem is pharmacologic and utilizes either phenytoin or carbamazepine. We prefer to begin with carbamazepine (100 mg four times a day) and increase the dose until pain relief is achieved or toxicity occurs (22). Phenytoin is prescribed at 100 mg, 3 times a day. Both of these drugs may cause hematologic and hepatic dysfunction and appropriate blood studies must be monitored. Once pain relief is achieved, drug therapy is continued for 2 to 3 weeks and then gradually tapered. It is reinstituted if pain recurs. Other medications, such as clonazepoin and baclofen, have also been reported to be of some value in trigeminal neuralgia, but their precise role in the management of these patients is uncertain.

Patients who fail to improve with pharmacologic treatment or who cannot tolerate the drug side effects are considered for surgical therapy. While many surgical procedures have been tried for trigeminal neuralgia, three remain in frequent use today: percutaneous trigeminal radiofrequency thermocoagulation, percutaneous glycerol rhizotomy, and microvascular decompression (23–25). The selection of one procedure over another is determined by the experience of the surgeon and the precise details of the patient's pain distribution. In most elderly patients, percutaneous trigeminal radiofrequency thermocoagulation is preferred. Although this procedure will cause facial numbness, most patients find this an acceptable tradeoff for pain relief.

Postherpetic neuralgia is a debilitating syndrome that is defined as the persistence of pain after an episode of herpes zoster neuralgia and is most prevalent in individuals older than 60 years. An excellent and thorough review of this problem has been published recently (26). Many pharmacologic and anesthetic treatment approaches have been tried. Neurosurgeons have lesioned virtually all levels of the nociceptive pathways in these patients with generally disappointing results. More recently Nashold has expanded his technique of dorsal root entry zone thermocoagulation to these patients with encouraging results (27). A novel approach to this problem has been reported recently by Bernstein et al. (28). They treated 14 patients with postherpetic neuralgia with the topical application of capsaicin, a naturally occurring substance found in some plants, which is toxic to substance P containing neurons and axons. Seventy-five percent of the treated patients reported substantial pain relief. While these observations need to be corroborated by other investigators, they represent a major potential advance in the management of this difficult problem.

Head Injury

Traumatic injury to the central nervous system can occur at any age in life. In fact, most epidemiologic studies point out that the incidence of head injury is greatest in teenagers and young adults and declines considerably in older adults. The etiology of head injury also changes during adulthood. While most head injuries in teenagers and young adults occur secondary to high velocity motor vehicle accidents, those in the elderly are usually the result of low velocity falls. Despite this epidemiologic data, elderly patients fare more poorly after head injury than do younger individuals. Howard et al. (29) have recently reported a 75% mortality in elderly individuals with acute subdural hematoma. This mortality is higher than the mortality observed in younger patients that present with comparable Glasgow Coma Scores. Of particular interest is that many of these elderly patients presented with a history of a relatively minor head injury. Since minor head injuries can have major consequences in the elderly, clinicians should have a lower threshold for admitting these patients to the hospital and for obtaining CT scans of the head. The subsequent management of identified abnormalities does not differ from their management in younger patients.

The acute subdural hematoma deserves further special mention in elderly patients. Classically, subdural hematomas are caused by venous bleeding in the subdural space. As people age, the cortical arteries over the surface of the brain hemispheres become more adherent to the undersurface of the dura. These adhesions can result in cortical artery rupture with head trauma and are probably the cause of arterial subdural hematomas. Arterial subdural hematomas are found more commonly in elderly patients and cause rapid loss of neurologic function because of the high pressure of the bleeding source. They have a poor prognosis.

Subacute and chronic subdural hematomas represent the other extreme of bleeding in the subdural space. Subacute hematomas develop between 3 days and 3 weeks after injury, while chronic hematomas develop longer than 3 weeks after injury. Chronic subdural hematoma occurs primarily in patients older than 50 years and may occur bilaterally. Because of the long time span between injury and symptomatic hematoma, many patients will not recall a specific injury event (30). It has been hypothesized that an injury event occurs, leading to some bleeding in the subdural space. As the hematoma liquifies, it becomes enveloped between a membrane separating it from the brain and the dura. This membrane becomes vascularized with friable blood vessels. Enlargement of these hematomas is postulated to occur by repeated hemorrhages from the friable vessels within the subdural membrane (31).

The symptoms and signs of chronic subdural hematoma are variable and apt to be confused with other problems of the elderly, particularly dementia. The diagnosis can usually be established by CT scan. However, the chronic subdural hematoma may appear isodense with brain. Full delineation of the extent of the hematoma may require intravenous infusion of iodine-containing contrast prior to CT scanning.

Chronic subdural hematomas can be managed conservatively or with surgery. Small chronic subdural hematomas that produce minimal symptoms may be followed clinically and by CT scans. Hematomas that are large, cause significant symptoms, or enlarge on follow-up scans are treated surgically. Since the chronic subdural hematoma is a liquid collection, it can usually be evacuated through burr holes. Our approach has been to place two burr holes over the hematoma and wash out the blood with warm normal saline. Postoperatively, the patient is kept flat in bed for 2 days. We have a low recurrence rate with this management and have seldom had to resort to craniotomy. Other investigators have had a similar experience (32).

Normal Pressure Hydrocephalus

Described initially by Hakim and Adams in 1965, normal pressure hydrocephalus (NPH) is a syndrome comprised of mild impairment of memory with slowness of thought and action, difficulty with gait, urinary incontinence, normal CSF pressure, and large cerebral ventricles. The syndrome may follow certain disorders, most commonly subarachnoid hemorrhage, or may occur in an idiopathic form, without preceding central nervous system pathology. NPH following a specific event can occur at any age, but the mean age for the idiopathic disorder that afflicts men and women equally is 68 years (33). The idiopathic syndrome has assumed particular importance for elderly patients because it represents a treatable form of dementia.

Treatment for NPH is straightforward and involves placing a ventriculoatrial or ventriculoperitoneal shunt to lower cerebrospinal fluid pressure. Unfortunately, only 41% of patients with idiopathic NPH have responded to shunt surgery (34). The experience with this problem at the Massachusetts General Hospital has been reviewed recently (35). Significant gait difficulty on presentation or the full triad of dementia, ataxia, and incontinence were associated with improvement after shunting. Most patients who presented with dementia initially, or in whom dementia was the most prominent symptom, failed to improve after shunting. A CT scan with periventricular low density and/or small sulci along with expansion of the entire ventricular system was also strongly associated with a good outcome after shunting.

Vascular Disease

Cerebrovascular disease is a common problem in elderly individuals. The annual incidence rates increase from 6 per 100,000 at 40 years old to 1,000 per 100,000 at 85 years old. The mortality rates from cerebrovascular disease are also age dependent, being substantially higher in elderly individuals (36). Cerebrovascular disease can result from many different pathologic processes. In this section, three specific etiologies of stroke will be discussed: extracranial arterial occlusive disease, intracerebral hemorrhage, and subarachnoid hemorrhage.

Elderly patients presenting with evidence of extracranial arterial occlusive disease are evaluated in the same manner as younger patients. After a thorough history and physical examination, initial evaluation includes noninvasive studies of the carotid arteries (37). Patients found to have evidence of significant stenosis (residual lumen less than 2 mm) on noninvasive testing are usually studied further with full angiography or digital subtraction angiography. The risks of angiography, including the possible nephrotoxicity of the contrast agent, are higher in elderly patients. Therefore, we prefer to limit these investigations as much as possible.

Many controversies exist regarding the management

of extracranial arterial occlusive disease and the role of carotoid endarterectomy in the management of this problem. A recent thoughtful review of this area has been given by Conomy (38). At present, a large clinical trial is underway that may provide the data on which to base future recommendations. Presently management decisions should be related more to the presence or absence of concomitant coronary artery disease and be less concerned with the patient's precise age. Myocardial infarction is clearly the major source of morbidity and mortality in these patients.

Intracerebral hemorrhage is the third most frequent cause of stroke in the elderly. Arterial hypertension is implicated frequently as the cause of these hemorrhages (39). In patients older than 65 years, however, amyloid angiopathy may equal hypertension as a causative factor (40). Amyloid deposition has been observed in the brain of 60% of individuals older than 90 years (41). Amyloid angiopathy is important to the clinician because it is often associated with multiple and recurrent brain hemorrhages.

The clinical syndrome of brain hemorrhage is one of abrupt onset and rapid evolution of symptoms and signs over minutes to hours. No warning or prodromal symptoms occur to herald the catastrophe. Patients presenting with such a catastrophic neurologic event are evaluated by CT scan, which gives a precise delineation of the extent of the hemorrhage.

The management of intracerebral hemorrhage is based on the location of the hemorrhage and the neurologic condition of the patient. The details of this management have been reviewed recently (42).

The other significant neurovascular problem in the elderly is the management of cerebral aneurysms and subarachnoid hemorrhage. While the peak incidence of subarachnoid hemorrhage from aneurysm is between 50 and 54 years old (43), aneurysmal subarachnoid hemorrhage continues as a significant problem in later adult life (44). Age influences the natural history of this problem. Elderly patients have a higher early mortality after subarachnoid hemorrhage than do younger patients. In many series, the mortality has been greater than 50% for patients older than 60 years (45–47). Increased age is also associated with a higher mortality from conservative treatment of ruptured aneurysm (47, 48).

Since the mortality of this problem is substantial if untreated or treated only by conservative care, many neurosurgeons have managed these patients surgically. While most reports contain relatively small series of patients, the outcome from surgical management is more encouraging. Of particular importance is the observation that indirect procedures (i.e., carotid ligation) carry a higher mortality and morbidity than do direct procedures (i.e., craniotomy). The Cooperative Study (48) demonstrated a 60% mortality in patients older than 60 years who underwent carotid ligation following subarachnoid hemorrhage. Indeed Martindale and Garfield (49) also observed a significant mortality following carotid ligation, which led them to conclude that elderly patients should not be referred to tertiary centers for neurosurgical treatment of this problem. Other surgeons have observed that direct craniotomy for aneurysm clipping carries a higher morbidity and mortality in elderly patients compared to younger patients. Nevertheless, this morbidity and mortality is low enough that craniotomy is the accepted management approach in most neurosurgical centers (50–53). Unless elderly patients with subarachnoid hemorrhage have a major medical contraindication to surgery, they are not managed any differently than younger patients at our institution. In recent years, we have also been using early surgical intervention (within 48 hours of the subarachnoid hemorrhage) in these patients without a significant increase in morbidity or mortality.

A special problem confronting the neurosurgeon is what to recommend when an aneurysm is discovered incidentally in an elderly individual. Of most importance in this regard is that aneurysms can develop and enlarge in elderly individuals (18, 54). Aneurysms that measure greater than 10 mm are more likely to rupture than smaller aneurysms (55). Since subarachnoid hemorrhage has a much higher morbidity and mortality than craniotomy for clipping of unruptured aneurysms, elective aneurysm clipping is preferrrd.

Spine

Degenerative changes in the spine appear to be one of the unavoidable pathologic changes of aging. After 60 years of age, it is rare to find a completely normal spine on radiographic investigation (56, 57). Despite these observable changes, many elderly individuals never experience significant symptoms of spinal disease. This fact must be recognized by the physician so that complaints of pain in the back or extremities are investigated in a serious manner, rather than assumed to be secondary to "spinal arthritis." The differential diagnosis of back and extremity pain is substantial, and the same careful investigations usually used in younger patients must also be applied to the elderly.

One of the most common spine problems in the general population is that of degenerative disc disease and disc herniation. Many individuals older than 20 years will have some evidence of degenerative change in the intervertebral discs that can be seen with magnetic resonance imaging (MRI). The incidence of this change, believed to be secondary to a loss of water from the disc, increases with age. It is of some interest, therefore, that the clinical problem of disc herniation is primarily a problem of young adulthood. True herniation of degenerated fragments of disc (in either the cervical or lumbar spine) into the epidural space is an unusual problem in elderly individuals. Furthermore, when it does occur, the herniation occurs at levels higher than those usually seen in younger patients. In the lumbar spine disc herniations at L_2–L_3 and L_3–L_4 and in the cervical spine at C_3–C_4 are more common in elderly individuals than in younger patients. The reason for this difference is unknown. Presumably these higher segments of the cervical and lumbar spine retain more mobility than the lower segments with aging and, therefore, are more prone to rupture in later life. Disc herniation at these unusual levels can be a difficult diagnostic problem. A disc herniation at C_3–C_4 almost never presents with radicular pain. Rather, a subtle myelopathy develops, characterized most by stiffness of the fingers and inability to use the hands for activities requiring fine motor coordination. Disc herniation in the upper lumbar spine usually presents with radicular pain, but the pain referral is to the anterior thighs or the entire leg and is often rather vague. Clear alterations in reflexes are not always found. Once recognized, these problems then require surgical intervention.

Stenosis, or narrowing of the spinal canal, can occur congenitally or develop as the result of osteoarthritic changes in the spine. This condition is most commonly known as spondylosis and occurs primarily in the cervical and lumbar spine. Often spondylosis becomes symptomatic because osteoarthritic changes occur in a congenitally narrowed spinal canal and compress the neural elements. Symptomatic stenosis is encountered more commonly in the elderly population than in younger individuals. These topics have been reviewed well in previous monographs and chapters related specifically to this problem (58, 59). Cervical spondylosis presents as cervical myelopathy. Radicular pain or neck pain are not always present. The presenting complaint will often center on a change in the patient's gait. The gait becomes more stiff, uncertain, or may become wide based. On examination, signs of motor and long tract dysfunction usually predominate. Wasting and weakness of hand intrinsic muscles, hyperactive reflexes, clonus, and the Babinski sign are observed commonly. This predominance of motor signs can sometimes raise the suspicion of motor system disease (amyotrophic lateral sclerosis). Careful sensory testing will usually reveal some evidence of sensory dysfunction. Patients suspected of having symptomatic cervical spondylosis are studied initially with an MRI scan. This allows an immediate delineation of where the spinal cord is compressed. As more experience with MR imaging is gained, myelography is being used less for the evaluation of this problem. The only treatment for this problem is surgical decompression of the compressed spinal cord. The decision to recommend surgery will depend on the severity of the problem and its temporal progression weighed against the medical condition of the patient. Decompression can be accomplished by a posterior approach (laminectomy) or an anterior approach (anterior resection of osteophytes or vertebral bodies). Selecting which approach will best suit an individual patient is a topic of debate at present and requires significant experience on the part of the surgeon.

Lumbar stenosis presents as a different syndrome. The typical situation is a patient who is comfortable when lying or sitting, but who develops radicular pain in one or both legs with ambulation. The symptoms can predominate in one leg despite the radiographic changes appearing symmetrical. As the symptoms worsen, the patient will be able to walk for shorter distances before experiencing pain. Sitting down when the pain develops will lead to resolution of symptoms. Hence the term "neurogenic claudication" is often applied to this problem. In contrast to cervical spondylosis, patients with lumbar stenosis often have a normal neurologic examination at rest. It is possible to provoke abnormalities (i.e., weakness, reflex changes) by having the patients ambulate until pain occurs. Although MRI may also be useful in the evaluation of this problem in the future, myelography and postmyelogram CT scanning are primarily relied upon to identify the areas of stenosis. CT scanning is also useful in identifying pars defects that may cause degenerative spondylolisthesis. Most of these patients will be very symptomatic when referred to a surgeon. The only satisfactory treatment is surgical decompression. This decompression is performed posteriorly and must be planned to include lateral recess decompression. Laminectomy alone, without lateral recess decompression, is not nearly as effective in relieving symptoms. An important management decision is how to handle the degenerative spondylolisthesis that may be present. Typically this is found at L_4–L_5 (60). Traditionally, intertransverse process fusion after decompression has been recommended to prevent further slippage and recurrent nerve root compression in selected patients (61). Internal instrumentation including pedicle screws and plate fixation are now being advocated by some authors (62). This technique allows reduction of the spondylolisthesis. However, this procedure requires a very experienced spine surgeon and may not be necessary in all situations. Further study of this area is needed.

Conclusion

Although aging produces many pathologic changes in the nervous system, the spectrum of neurosurgical disorders is remarkably similar throughout life. Treatment decisions are best made by considering the pathologic process leading to the patient's symptoms and the functional capacity of the patient on presentation.

References

1. Critchley, M. 1956. Neurologic changes in the aged. *J Chronic Dis* 3:459–463.
2. Kokmen, E, et al. 1977. Neurologic manifestations of aging. *J Gerontol* 32:411–420.
3. Ball, MJ. 1977. Neuronal loss, neurofibrillary tangles and granulovacuolar degeneration in the hippocampus with aging and dementia. *Acta Neuropath* 27:111–118.
4. Jenkyn, LR, et al. 1985. Neurologic signs in senescence. *Arch Neurol* 42:1154–1157.
5. Katzman, R, and Terry, RD. 1983. *The Neurology of Aging*. Philadelphia: FA Davis.
6. Schoenberg, BS, Christine, BW, and Whisnant, JP. 1976. The descriptive epidemiology of primary intracranial neoplasms: The Connecticut experience. *Am J Epidemiol* 104:499–510.
7. Cohen, A, and Modau, B. 1968. Some epidemiologic aspects of neoplastic diseases in Israeli immigrant population. *Cancer* 22:1323–1328.
8. Percy, AK, et al. 1972. Neoplasms of the central nervous system. *Neurology* 22:40–48.
9. Schoenberg, BS, Christine, BW, and Whisnant, JP. 1978. The resolution of discrepancies in the reported incidence of primary brain tumor. *Neurology* 28:817–823.
10. Guomundsson, KR. 1970. A survey of tumors of the central nervous system in Iceland during the 10 year period 1954–1963. *Acta Neurologica Scand* 46:538–552.
11. Moersch, FP, Craig, WM, and Kernohan, JW. 1941. Tumors of brain in aged patients. *Arch Neurol Psychiatr* 45:235–245.
12. Friedman, H, and Odom, GL. 1972. Brain tumors in the elderly. *Geriatrics* 27:105–110.
13. Cooney, LM, and Solitaire, GB. 1974. *Mod Geriatr* 4:234–237.
14. Hurwitz, LJ, and Swallow, M. 1971. An introduction to the neurology of aging. *Geront Clin* 13:97–113.
15. Knox, EW, and Adams, GF. 1969. The hemiplegic onset of brain tumors. *Geront Clin* 11:1–12.
16. Caird, FI. 1982. *Neurological Disorders in the Elderly.* Boston: Wright.
17. Thomas, TPL. 1984. The complications of systemic corticosteroid therapy in the elderly. *Gerontology* 30:60–65.
18. Borges, LF. Unpublished observations.
19. Awad, IA, et al. Intracranial meningiomas in the aged. Presented at the American Association of Neurological Surgeons, May, 1987.
20. Stookey, B, and Ransohoff, J. 1959. Trigeminal Neuralgia: Its History And Treatment. Springfield, IL: Charles C Thomas.
21. Wilkins, RH. 1985. Trigeminal neuralgia: Introduction. In *Neurosurgery,* Eds., RH Wilkins and SS Rengachary. New York: McGraw-Hill.
22. Wilkins, RH. 1979. Tic doloreaux. *Contemp Neurosurg* 1:1–6.
23. Nugent, RG. 1985. Trigeminal neuralgia: Treatment by percutaneous electrocoagulation. In *Neurosurgery,* Eds., RH Wilkins and SS Rengachary. New York: McGraw-Hill.
24. Lunsford DL. 1985. Trigeminal neuralgia: Treatment by glycerol rhizotomy. In *Neurosurgery,* Eds., RH Wilkins and SS Rengachary. New York: McGraw Hill.
25. Janetta, PJ. 1985. Trigeminal neuralgia: Treatment by microvascular decompression. In *Neurosurgery,* Eds., RH Wilkins and SS Rengachary. New York: McGraw Hill.
26. Portenoy, RK, Duma, C, and Foley, KM. 1986. Acute herpetic and postherpetic neuralgia: clinical review and current management. *Ann Neurol* 20:651–664.
27. Friedman, AH, and Nashold, BS. 1984. Drez lesions for postherpetic neuralgia. *Neurosurgery* 15:969–970.
28. Bernstein, JR, et al. 1987. Treatment of chronic postherpetic neuralgia with topical capsaicin. *J Am Acad Dermat* 17:93–96.
29. Howard, MA, Dacey, RG, and Winn, HR. Acute subdural hematomas in the elderly. Presented at the American Association of Neurological Surgeons Meeting, May, 1987.
30. Fogelholm, R, and Waltimo, O. 1975. Epidemiology of chronic subdural hematoma. *Acta Neurochir* 32:247–250.
31. Ito, H, Komai, T, and Yamamoto, S. 1978. Fibrinolytic enzyme in the lining walls of chronic subdural hematoma. *J Neurosurg* 48:197–200.
32. Cameron, MM. 1978. Chronic subdural hematoma: A review of 114 cases. *J Neurol Neurosurg Psychiat* 41: 834–839.
33. Black, P McL. 1980. Idiopathic normal pressure hydrocephalus: Results of shunting in 62 patients. *J Neurosurg* 52:371:377.
34. Katzman, R. 1977. Normal pressure hydrocephalus. In *Dementia,* ed. 2. Ed., LE Wells. Philadelphia: FA Davis.
35. Black, P McL, Ojemann, RG, and Tzouras, A. 1984. CSF shunts for dementia, incontinence and gait disturbance. *Clin Neurosurg* 32:632–651.
36. Kurtzke, JF. 1985. Epidemiology of cerebrovascular disease. In *Cerebrovascular Survey Report*. Eds., RH McDowell and LR Caplan. National Institute of Neurological and Communicative Disorders and Stroke.
37. Garcia, JH, and Geer, JC. 1985. Carotid artery atherosclerotic disease pathology and detection. In *Cerebrovascular Survey Report,* Eds., FH McDowell and LR Caplan. National Institute of Neurological and Communicative Disorders and Stroke.
38. Conomy, JP. 1986. The future of carotid endarterectomy: A neurologist's point of view. *Clin Neurosurg* 34:123–133.
39. Mohr, JP, Caplan LR, Melski JW, Goldstein RJ, et al. 1978. The Harvard Cooperative Stroke Registry: A prospective registry. *Neurology* 28:754–762.
40. Okazaki, H, and Whisnant, JP. 1983. Clinical pathology of hypertensive hemorrhage intracerebral hemorrhage. In *Hypertensive Intracerebral Hemorrhage,* Eds., M Mizukami, et al. New York: Raven Press.
41. Vinters, HV, and Gilbert, JJ. 1983. Cerebral amyloid angiopathy: Incidence and complications in the aging brain II. Distribution of amyloid vascular changes. *Stroke* 14: 924–928.
42. Borges, LF. 1988. Management of nontraumatic brain hemorrhage. In *Neurological and Neurosurgical Intensive Care,* Eds., AH Ropper and SK Kennedy. Rockville, MD: Aspen Publishers.

43. Skultety, FM, and Nishioka, H. 1966. Report on the cooperative study of intracranial surgery in the treatment of aneurysm. *J Neurosurg* 25:683–704.
44. Walton, JN. 1956. *Subarachnoid Hemorrhage*. Edinburgh: Livingstone.
45. Richardson, AE. 1975. The natural history of patients with intracranial aneurysm after rupture. *Prog Brain Res* 30:269–273.
46. McKissock, W, Paine, KW, and Walsh, LS. 1960. An analysis of the results of treatment of ruptured aneurysms. *J Neurosurg* 12:762–776.
47. Keller, AZ. 1970. Hypertension, age, and residence in the survival with subarachnoid hemorrhage. *Am J Epidemiol* 91:139–143.
48. Skultety, FM, and Nishioka, H. 1966. Report on the cooperative study of intracranial surgery in the treatment of aneurysm. *J Neurosurg* 25:683–704.
49. Martindale, BV, and Garfield, J. 1978. Subarachnoid hemorrhage above the age of 59: Are intracranial investigations justified? *Br Med J* 1:465–466.
50. Hugosson, R. 1973. Intracranial arterial aneurysms: Considerations on the upper age limit for surgical treatment. *Acta Neurochir* 28:157–164.
51. Sengupta, RP, Lassman, LP, and Hankinson, J. 1978. Scope of surgery for intracranial aneurysms in the elderly: A preliminary report. *Br Med J* 1:246–247.
52. Fein, JM. 1982. Aneurysms in geriatric patients. In *Clinical Management of Intracranial Aneurysms,* Eds., CN Hopkins and DM Long. New York: Raven Press.
53. Amacher, AC, et al. 1977. How the old tolerate intracranial surgery for aneurysms. *Neurosurgery* 1:242–244.
54. Dacey, RG, Pitkethly, D, and Winn, HR. 1985. Enlargement of an intracranial aneurysm in the eighth decade of life. *J Neurosurg* 62:600–602.
55. Dell, S. 1982. Asymptomatic cerebral aneurysm: Assessment of its risk of rupture. *Neurosurgery* 10:162–165.
56. Lawrence, JS. 1969. Disc degeneration: Its frequency and relationship to symptoms. *Ann Rheum Dis* 28:121–137.
57. Lawrence, JS. 1977. *Rheumatism in population*. London: Heinemann Medical.
58. Bailey, RW, et al. 1983. *The Cervical Spine*. Philadelphia: JB Lippincott.
59. Weinstein, PR, Ehric, G, and Wilson, LB. 1977. Lumbar Spondylosis: Diagnosis, Management and Surgical Treatment. Chicago: Year Book Publishers.
60. Rosenberg, MI. 1975. Degenerative spondylolisthesis. *J Bone Joint Surg* 51A:467–471.
61. Wisneski, RJ, and Rothman, RH. 1975. Posterior intertransverse fusion: Indications, pathomechanics and results. *Journal of Bone & Joint Surg* 51A:467–471.
62. Hsu, K, et al. 1987. Internal fixation with pedicle screws. In *Lumbar Spine Surgery,* Eds., AH White, RR Rothman, and CD Ray. St. Louis: CV Mosby.

36

Orthopaedic Surgery in the Elderly

Joseph D. Zuckerman and Jeffrey M. Spivak

Orthopaedic surgery in the elderly has grown tremendously over the past 30 years. Many musculoskeletal conditions and injuries are now amenable to surgical management. The effect of this has been to significantly improve the "quality" of life of many patients and the "quantity" of life for some. Advances in medical and anesthetic management techniques have enabled many elderly patients to successfully undergo orthopaedic surgical procedures that may have been contraindicated in the past because of associated medical problems.

This chapter discusses the orthopaedic surgical procedures most commonly performed in the elderly. For each procedure, indications and contraindications, specific preoperative considerations, some technical aspects of the procedure, the anticipated outcomes, and potential complications are discussed.

Spectrum of Orthopaedic Surgery

There are hundreds if not a few thousand orthopaedic procedures that may be used to treat musculoskeletal problems in the elderly. It is well beyond the scope of this chapter to discuss all of these procedures; however, in an effort to present an appropriately focused discussion we have surveyed the 1987 operating room records for the Hospital for Joint Diseases. The Hospital for Joint Diseases is a 200-bed orthopaedic institute caring specifically for musculoskeletal problems. In 1987, 8,600 orthopaedic procedures were performed—approximately 2,150 or 25% of these procedures were performed in patients over the age of 60. The most common procedures are listed in Table 36-1. In the pages that follow, the procedures most commonly performed in patients over the age of 60 at the Hospital for Joint Diseases are discussed.

Total Joint Replacement

The development of total joint replacement has dramatically improved the treatment of patients with severe disabling arthritis (323, 324). This is particularly true for the geriatric patient because of the increasing incidence of arthritis of the major joints that occurs with age. The number of joint replacements performed each year reflects in large part the varying incidence of symptomatic arthritis of the joints. It is most commonly performed for the hip and knee (23, 141, 167, 252, 272). It is here, in the major weight-bearing joints of the lower extremity, where it probably has its greatest effect because of the potential to return a patient to independent ambulation. However, total joint replacement of the shoulder (6, 62, 187, 214), although performed less commonly, can be equally important in restoring an independent level of function to the geriatric patient.

Total Hip Replacement

Preoperative Considerations

All patients should undergo a comprehensive preoperative medical evaluation to identify specific problems that may impact on their ability to undergo surgery. For total hip replacements specific areas of concern include a history of thromboembolic disease, urinary retention, bleeding dyscrasias, or occult infections. Postoperative throm-

Table 36-1. Orthopaedic surgery in the elderly, Hospital for Joint Diseases—1987

	Number of procedures	Average age (years)
Total joint replacement	725	70.2
Hip		
Primary	416	
Revision	38	
Knee		
Primary	242	
Revision	9	
Shoulder/elbow	20	
Total fractures	404	
Hip	188	79.8
Misc. lower extremity	95	68.7
Proximal humerus	34	75.8
Misc. upper extremity	87	68.6
Total spine	112	
Laminectomy	99	68.1
Biopsy	13	70.4
Total arthroscopy	257	
Knee	235	
Shoulder	22	65.3
Total miscellaneous	183	
Rotator cuff repairs	27	66.6
Carpal tunnel release	83	70.8
Forefoot reconstruction	73	66.1

boembolic complications are of significant concern following total hip replacement (145). Prophylactic anticoagulation using aspirin, Dextran, or similar medications is routinely utilized. However, patients with a history of thrombophlebitis or pulmonary emboli are at increased risk for postoperative thromboembolic complications. These patients require more specific treatment postoperatively with Coumadin, with close monitoring of prothrombin time. Urinary retention occurs relatively frequently in men after total hip replacement. This usually requires short-term use of an indwelling urinary catheter which increases the risk of urinary tract infection. Postoperative urinary retention in men usually reflects the presence of benign prostatic hypertrophy. Normal urinary function usually returns as the patient is mobilized out of bed. However, in some situations postoperative urinary retention does not resolve, and a transurethral resection of the prostate is necessary. This usually occurs in patients who have a history of urinary frequency and nocturia preoperatively. Instrumentation of the genital urinary tract, either with a urinary catheter or for a transurethral prostatic resection, carries a risk of bacteremia with hematogenous seeding of the hip implant. Therefore, it is best to identify significant benign prostatic hypertrophy preoperatively to avoid any potential problems caused by postoperative urinary retention. All patients should also be questioned about the use of aspirin or other nonsteroidal anti-inflammatory medications since these medications are known to interfere with platelet function. They should be stopped at least 10 days before surgery to avoid the risk of increased surgical blood loss. Lastly, a thorough evaluation should be made for remote sources of infection. This should include close inspection of the teeth and gums as well as the feet. A seemingly innocuous carbuncle or furuncle can be a source of bacteremia that infects a newly implanted hip replacement. Surgery should be postponed until all sources of infection are eradicated.

Surgical Technique

The vast majority of total hip replacements are performed in a "clean air" environment to minimize the risk of infection. This may include the use of a laminar flow system, investing gowns and hoods with personal exhaust, or overhead ultraviolet light. Prophylactic antibiotics are used routinely. For patients without penicillin allergy, a cephalosporin is the antibiotic of choice and is continued for 48 hours after surgery. For patients with penicillin allergy, Vancomycin is used for the same duration. Studies have shown that clean air environments and prophylactic antibiotics significantly decrease the incidence of postoperative wound infection.

The procedure can be performed through various surgical approaches. The choice of approach is determined by the presence of previous incisions, surgeon's preference, and the need for additional procedures (bone graft, release of soft tissue contracture, correction of deformity). Anterior and anterolateral approaches are generally performed with the patient in a supine position. The posterolateral approach is performed with the patient in the lateral position. The lateral approach can be performed with the patient in either the supine or lateral position. Elective osteotomy of the greater trochanter was initially used for all hip replacements. However, currently it is not routinely performed for primary hip replacement. Rather, it is reserved for situations where additional exposure is necessary (obese patients, severe deformity, ankylosed hips, revisions). Surgical approaches that approach the hip through the anterior capsule generally preserve the posterior supporting structures. Those that approach the hip through the posterior capsule generally preserve the anterior supporting structures. This is important in determining the appropriate postoperative positions to prevent instability.

After exposure of the hip joint, the femoral head is dislocated, either anteriorly or posteriorly depending upon the approach utilized. The femoral head is removed by performing an osteotomy of the femoral neck. The level of the osteotomy is determined preoperatively by evaluation of leg length discrepancy. In most primary cases, the osteotomy is performed approximately 1½ cm above the lesser trochanter. Removal of the femoral head allows the proximal femur to be displaced anteriorly or posteriorly to expose the acetabulum. The acetabulum is prepared using reamers that remove the remaining articular cartilage, with care taken to preserve the supporting subchondral bone. The appropriate size of the acetabular component is determined by trial implants. The acetabulum is prepared for cementing by making 10 to 15⅛ inch drill holes approximately 5 mm in depth. This provides additional area for cement intrusion to firmly anchor the prosthesis. Prior to cementing, the acetabulum and the component must be free of any soft tissue or bony debris that would interfere with cement fixation. The component should be completely dry prior to cementing. Methylmethacrylate is mixed and packed into the acetabulum, usually with special instruments for pressurization. The component is placed with care to assure proper position of approximately 45 degrees abduction and 10 to 15 degrees anteversion. The component is held firmly in position, while excess cement is removed and the cement is allowed to set completely. When the acetabulum is completed, attention is turned to the preparation of the femoral canal.

The femoral canal must be prepared to accept a prosthesis with an intermedullary stem. This requires entering the femoral canal centrally and enlarging the canal using a series of reamers and rasps until the appropriate fit is obtained. The appropriately fitting prosthesis should leave room for a 2- to 3-mm cement mantle. Trial femoral components are used to perform a trial reduction to assess stability and leg length. When a component of appropriate stem size and neck length is chosen, final canal preparations are made. Any loose cancellous bone is removed. An intramedullary plug is placed approximately 1½ to 2 cm distal to the tip of the prosthesis to enhance cement pressurization and prevent excessive distal placement of the cement. After thorough irrigation and drying of the canal, cement is introduced, usually by manual injection with a large bore syringe, and then pressurized. The prosthesis is inserted with care taken to maintain the component in a central or slight valgus position with 10 to 15 degrees of anteversion. The prosthesis is held firmly in place and any excess cement is removed. When the cement has set completely, the hip is then reduced and once again range of motion, stability, and leg length are assessed. Newer modular designs allow alteration of the head and neck component if soft-tissue tension or leg length is not acceptable. If the trochanter has been osteotomized, it is reattached securely, using a two- or three-wire technique. Deep suction drains are placed, and the wound is closed in layers.

Postoperative management will vary somewhat based upon the surgical approach used, presence of trochanteric osteotomy, and surgeon's preference. In general, intravenous antibiotics are continued for 48 hours. Thromboembolic prophylaxis (aspirin, Dextran, Coumadin) is continued during most of the hospitalization until the patient is actively ambulating. Anti-embolic stockings are also commonly used. The major portion of the postoperative management is directed at rehabilitation for ambulation training and hip muscle strengthening. This program begins on the 2nd or 3rd postoperative day with the patient getting out of bed to a chair and progressing to ambulation with assistive devices. Patients are instructed in positioning precautions to avoid dislocation of the prosthesis. This depends upon the surgical approach used. Approaches in which the hip is dislocated posteriorly are unstable in flexion/adduction/internal rotation. Approaches in which the hip is dislocated anteriorly are unstable in extension/abduction/external rotation. Patients are also instructed in hip abductor strengthening exercises to improve gait. At the time of discharge, patients are generally able to ambulate independently with a walker or crutches. They usually progress to a cane 6 weeks after surgery and are able to ambulate independently 4 to 6 weeks later. This will vary from one patient to another depending upon the extent of coexisting orthopaedic problems.

Complications

The most serious complication following total hip replacement is infection (72, 140, 258, 297). Fortunately, the use of "clean air" operating rooms, minimizing operating room traffic, prophylactic antibiotics, and our appreciation for the importance of proper handling of soft tissues have combined to keep the deep infection rate at less than 1%. Infections can be present early in the postoperative period (acute), or later (subacute), or long after the surgery (delayed). Most late infections represent hematogenous seeding from distant sites of infection (urinary tract, dental abscesses, skin infections). This emphasizes the importance of prompt treatment of any suspected infection and the use of prophylactic antibiotics for any urologic or dental procedures. Treatment of deep infection generally requires surgical debridement combined with intravenous antibiotics (235). Debridement may include only soft-tissue debridement if the infection is acute and the components are not loose. However, debridement may require removal of the components and cement if there is loosening or the infection involves the bone/cement interface. Reimplantation of a new hip replacement may be possible after eradication of the infection. This generally requires at least 3 to 12 months delay depending on the virulence of the causal organism.

Thromboembolic complications—thrombophlebitis and pulmonary embolism—occur relatively frequently following total hip replacement (72, 145). However, the incidence has decreased significantly with the use of prophylactic measures. Prophylactic measures include early ambulation, use of compression stockings, and anticoagulants (aspirin, Dextran, Coumadin).

Postoperative dislocations occur in about 1% to 3% of primary total hip replacements (171). Most dislocations occur within the first 6 weeks following surgery. When treated with bracing or casting to maintain the hip in a stable position while the pseudocapsule forms, most of these dislocations do not recur. Recurrent dislocations are often the result of component malposition, nonunion, and proximal migration of the greater trochanter following a transtrochanteric approach, and failure to restore proper soft-tissue tension. In these cases, revision surgery may be necessary to prevent further episodes of dislocation.

Other complications include neurovascular injury (192) and heterotopic bone formation (40). Neurovascular injury is very uncommon. Sciatic or femoral nerve palsies have been reported in 1% to 2% of primary total hip replacements (192). Most represent partial deficits and spontaneous recovery occurs in the majority of cases. Vascular injuries involving the femoral vessels or pelvic vessels are quite rare and occur in about 0.1% of cases. Heterotopic bone formation is common following total hip replacement, however, significant symptoms associated with heterotopic bone is very infrequent (40). Those at high risk include men with osteoarthritis and extensive osteophyte formation and patients with ankylosing spondylitis. In these patients, prophylactic measures (diphosphinates, low dose irradiation) should be considered.

Outcomes

Patients undergoing primary total hip replacement can expect satisfactory pain relief in over 95% of cases (23, 252, 296, 323). With adequate pain relief, ambulation and overall function improves as does the overall quality of life. The best results are in patients with osteoarthritis (Fig. 36-1). Patients with rheumatoid arthritis have equivalent rates of pain relief but functional improvement is less than in osteoarthritis because of the polyarticular nature of the disease. With longer term follow-up, mechanical loosening of the components becomes more problematic (Fig. 36-2). In general, 10 years following total hip replacement symptomatic loosening may be present in 10% to 15% of cases (128, 156, 225). Femoral component loosening has been a problem, encountered earlier in the course of follow-up as opposed to acetabular loosening. However, it tends to stabilize while acetabular loosening has been shown to become more significant with follow-up beyond 10 years (156). It is important to keep in mind that series with 10- to 15-year follow-up reported in the 1980s were performed in the early and middle 1970s, and represent the surgical techniques utilized at those times. It is anticipated that current advances in technique—improvements in the design of acetabular and femoral components, optimization of cement technique, and ap-

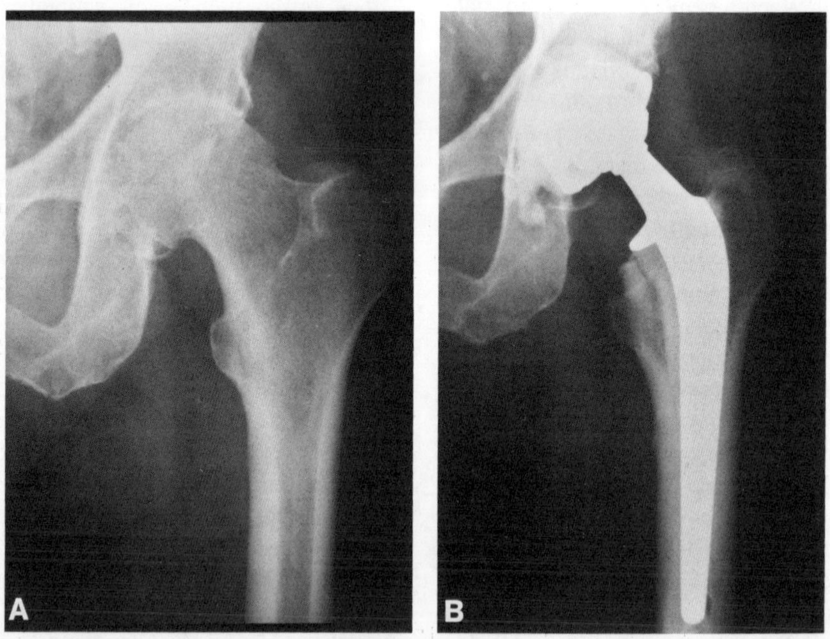

Figure 36-1. 76-year-old male with advanced osteoarthritis of the left hip (*A*). There is complete loss of the joint space superiorly with sclerotic changes of the acetabulum and femoral head. There is mild flattening of the supior portion of the femoral head. In addition, there is a medial osteophyte, which results in some lateral subluxation of the femoral head. A cemented total hip replacement was performed (*B*) with excellent relief of pain and improvement of overall function.

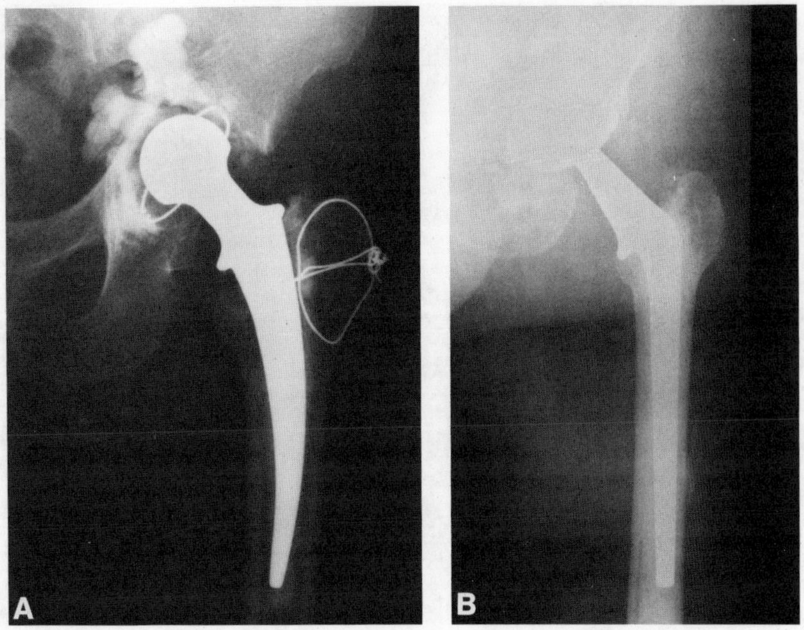

Figure 36-2. 72-year-old male, 8 years following left cemented total hip replacement (*A*). Radiographs show loosening of the acetabulum component and the femoral component. Revision surgery was performed (*B*) including replacement of the acetabular and femoral prostheses. The patient had a 2-cm leg length discrepancy, which was able to be corrected at the time of surgery.

preciation for proper bone preparation and prosthesis placement—will significantly decrease the incidence of mechanical loosening reported in the 1990s (129).

Revision Total Hip Replacement

Revision total hip replacement represents one of the most challenging areas of orthopaedic surgery (Fig. 36-2). Revisions are most commonly performed for mechanical loosening and less commonly for infection. The difficult problems encountered—significant bone loss, difficult cement removal, broken prostheses, femoral canal perforation or fracture, difficulties with trochanteric reattachment—make it relatively easy to understand why the results of revision surgery do not approach those of primary total hip replacement (156, 225). Revision hip surgery is well beyond the scope of this chapter. However, it is important to note that complications are more likely following revision surgery including infection, dislocation, neurovascular injury, and mechanical loosening (156, 225).

Uncemented Total Hip Replacement

Problems with mechanical loosening of cemented primary total hip replacement have led to the development of femoral and acetabular components that do not rely on cement for fixation, but rather rely on biological fixation (Fig. 36-3). Two basic forms of noncemented fixation have been used—macro-interlock and micro-interlock. Macro-interlock refers to opposition between surrounding bone and macro irregularities on the surface of the prosthesis (128). Micro-interlock refers to bony or fibrous ingrowth into small pores on the surface of the prosthesis. Recently fixation of acetabular components of either type has been augmented by screw fixation. Use of noncemented components has had two main areas of application: (*a*) in younger patients because these patients have the highest incidence of mechanical loosening; and (*b*) in revision hip replacement because of the high incidence of early mechanical loosening of cemented prostheses. The next 10 years will provide important information about the long-term results of these prostheses compared to conventional cemented total hip replacement.

Total Knee Replacement

Total knee replacement has become the treatment of choice for almost all cases of advanced arthritis of the knee (112, 141, 272) (Fig. 36-4). Indications for total knee replacement are severe pain and functional disability in association with advanced degenerative arthritis that has been refractory to non-operative measures. The pain is usually severe enough to limit ambulation to only a few blocks. Assistive devices are often necessary, and the pain can interfere with sleep. Simple activities of daily living (putting on shoes and socks, getting up from a chair) are difficult and in some cases impossible. Osteoarthritis is the most common underlying cause in elderly patients un-

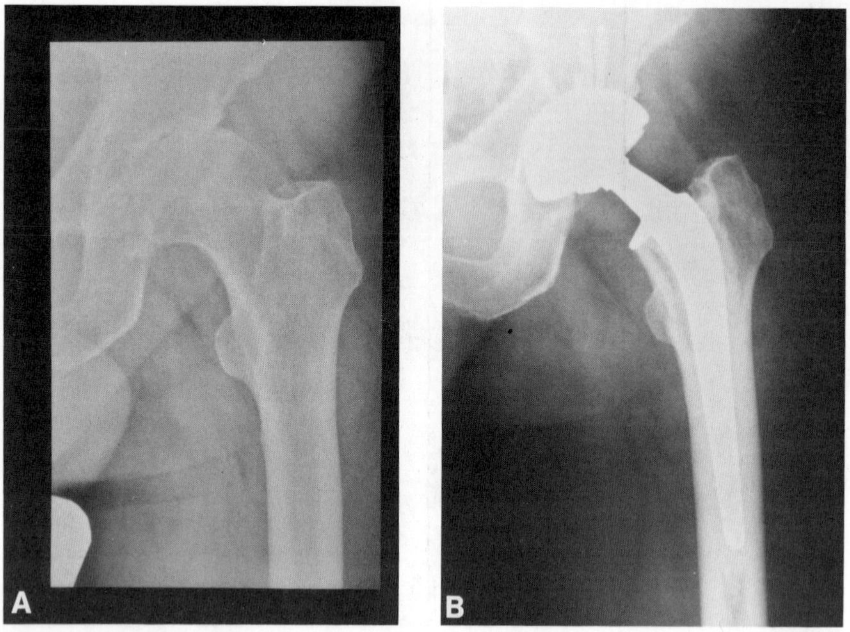

Figure 36-3. 64-year-old male with severe left hip pain secondary to osteoarthritis (*A*). Because of the patient's age, a noncemented acetabular component was used in combination with a cemented femoral component (*B*).

dergoing total knee replacement (141). However, rheumatoid arthritis (Fig. 36-4), post-traumatic arthritis, and osteonecrosis of the femoral condyles are also frequently encountered (167, 176, 272).

Contraindications include the presence of active sepsis, either within the joint or elsewhere in the body. Ancient sepsis is a concern and should be thoroughly evaluated (bone scan, Indium scan, aspiration) before proceeding with surgery, but in and of itself is not an absolute contraindication. Loss of muscular function about the knee (quadriceps) is also a contraindication, because in these cases the functional outcome is anticipated to be

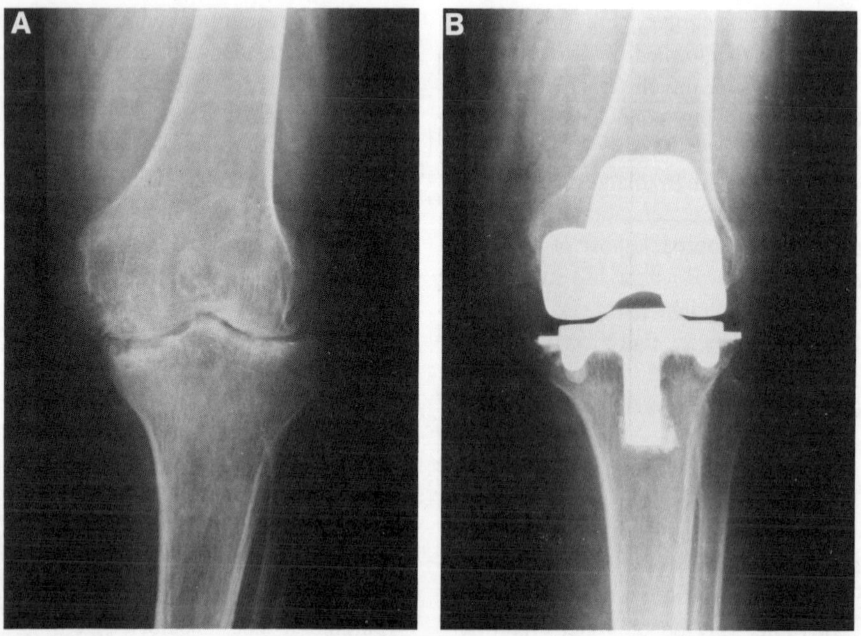

Figure 36-4. 78-year-old female with rheumatoid arthritis of the left knee (*A*). Radiograph shows complete loss of joint space with erosive changes evident on both the femoral and tibial sides. There is mild lateral tibial subluxation, as well. A total knee replacement was performed (*B*) with excellent relief of pain and improvement of function.

poor, and an arthrodesis would be preferable. Neuropathic arthropathy is also a contraindication because of poor bone quality. Specific problems including extensive bone loss, marked instability, or ankylosis significantly increase the technical difficulty of the surgery but arc not contraindications.

Preoperative Considerations

The preoperative considerations for patients undergoing total knee replacement are similar to those described for total hip replacement. A comprehensive medical evaluation is essential; previous problems with thromboembolic disease, bleeding disorders, occult infection, and urinary retention all require specific attention. Of particular concern in patients undergoing total knee replacement is the vascular status of the involved lower extremity. Arterial insufficiency may have an important impact on the surgery, especially in terms of intraoperative use of tourniquet and wound healing. Any patient with diminished or absent distal pulses or skin changes consistent with vascular insufficiency should undergo a vascular evaluation. The decision to proceed with surgery can then be made in consultation with the vascular specialist. In some cases, proceeding with surgery without the use of tourniquet is recommended. However, if there are concerns about satisfactory wound healing, surgery should not be undertaken, and consideration should be given to vascular reconstruction.

Surgical Technique

Although most total knee replacements are performed using some type of "clean air" measures (ultraviolet light, investing gowns and hoods with personal exhaust), the use of laminar flow operating rooms is not recommended. One study has shown an increased incidence of infection with laminar flow compared to the use of standard operating room environment (251). This probably resulted from the position of the surgeons with respect to the operative site and the direction of the laminar flow. Preoperative prophylactic antibiotics started immediately preoperatively and continued for 24 to 48 hours after surgery has become a standard part of treatment.

Most surgeons perform total knee replacement using a tourniquet, but its use is not mandatory. However, it is specifically advantageous when components are cemented in place to maintain a dry bone/cement interface to enhance fixation. Duration of tourniquet use should be as short as possible, preferably not to exceed 1½ to 2 hours. A midline incision is used with specific avoidance of development of excessive skin flaps. This decreases the risk of postoperative skin slough or healing problems. A limited medial flap is developed to facilitate the medial parapatellar capsulotomy. This extends proximally into the quadriceps tendon (junction of the medial one-third and lateral two-thirds) and distally to the tibial tubercle just medial to the patellar tendon. Intra-articular adhesions should be released to allow eversion of thc patclla with the knee flexed to 90 degrees. This must be performed carefully with adequate releases to prevent compromise of the patella tendon insertion at the tibial tubercle.

The main principles of total knee replacement include: (*a*) proper ligament and soft tissue balancing to correct deformity, (*b*) resection of diseascd articular surfaces with preservation of subchondral bone, (*c*) restoration of physiologic valgus alignment, and (*d*) restoration of proper patella tracking. To accomplish these goals, it is essential to have a clear understanding of the deformities present. Most osteoarthritic knees present with a varus (bow leg) deformity. This generally requires some release of the medial supporting structures. If a valgus (knock knee) deformity is present, release of the lateral structures will be necessary. Flexion deformities can usually be corrected by release of the cruciate ligaments and/or posterior capsule. Extension contractures may require lengthening of the quadriceps mechanism. Correction of deformities must be performed carefully such that the deformity is corrected, but stability is maintained. Extensive bone loss may be present in knees with severe long-standing deformities, those with post-traumatic arthritis (i.e., following tibial plateau fracture), or with osteonecrosis of the femoral condyles. The problem can be worsened by excessive bone resection in an effort to correct deformity. In these cases, bone grafting, filling of defects with bone cement, or use of custom prostheses may be necessary.

Virtually all total knee replacement systems currently available utilize a series of mechanical alignment jigs to assist in performing the proper bony resection and choosing the appropriate size components. Although these systems all differ somewhat from each other they all strive for essentially the same goals. The proximal tibial surface should be resected perpendicular to the longitudinal axis of the tibia in the anteroposterior view and with a slight (5-degree) posterior slope on the lateral view. The distal femur should be resected with a 5- to 8-degree valgus alignment in the anteroposterior view. On the lateral view, it should be parallel to the longitudinal axis of the femur with care taken to avoid notching of the anterior cortex. Resection of the posterior one-third of the patella is also performed. Excessive patella resection increases the risk of fracture and may compromise patellar component fixation.

After completion of soft tissue balancing and resection of the articular surfaces, trial components are placed. Alignment, stability and range of motion are assessed and any necessary changes can be made. Patellar tracking requires specific attention. If the patella subluxes or dislocates laterally with flexion, a lateral retinacular release should be performed. This decreases the laterally displacing force on the patella and allows correction of tracking. At this point, the bony surfaces are prepared for cementing. A pulsating lavage system is commonly used to remove debris from the surfaces and allow better cement fixation. The tibia is usually cemented first, followed by the femoral component. A separate batch of bone cement is used. The patella component can be cemented at the same time as either the tibial or femoral component. Currently available systems utilize a modular tibial component. This consists of a polyethylene insert of varying thickness and a metal tray. After the metal tray is cemented in place the thickness of the polyethylene component can be changed for correct soft tissue tensioning.

When the cement has completely hardened and the components are securely fixed, the wound should be carefully inspected for cement debris. If a tourniquet has been used is should be deflated prior to closure to achieve satisfactory hemostasis. Deep closed suction drainage should also be used. The most important aspect of closure is secure repair of the quadriceps tendon and medial capsular incision. Range of motion should be performed after this closure to assess the security of the repair. Closure should be completed in layers. The knee is usually placed in a well-padded splint in extension.

Postoperative regimens will vary based upon the specific procedures performed and the surgeon's preference. In general, patients can begin ambulating 2 to 3 days after surgery. Range of motion exercises are begun 3 to 4 days after surgery. Partial weight bearing or weight bearing as tolerated is allowed. Use of continuous passive motion machines have become an important adjunct to the postoperative rehabilitation program to regain range of motion. Patients are usually discharged 10 to 14 days after surgery. At that time, they are ambulating independently with a walker or crutches and have 90 degrees of knee flexion. They usually progress to a cane within 4 to 6 weeks after surgery and independent ambulation 4 to 6 weeks later, depending on the extent of coexisting musculoskeletal problems.

Complications

The most significant complication following total knee replacement is deep infection (193, 201, 235). Fortunately, infection rates for primary total knee replacement have been reported in the range of 1% to 3% (251). Some of these reflect late infection from hematogenous spread, for which patients with rheumatoid arthritis are at increased risk. The low rate of infection reflects in part the use of perioperative prophylactic antibiotics, specific "clean air" measures, and appreciation for meticulous soft tissue handling. Deep infections that occur early in the postoperative period can usually be treated by surgical debridement of soft tissues and intravenous antibiotics. If this approach is unsuccessful, removal of the prosthesis and cement will be necessary. Delayed or late infections generally require removal of the prosthesis and intravenous antibiotics (235). Reinsertion of components should be delayed for 6 weeks and can be considered if the infection has been successfully eradicated. In some cases, inadequate soft tissue, residual infection, or loss of quadriceps mechanism may necessitate arthrodesis. This is often difficult to obtain but, once successful, provides acceptable function. Resection arthroplasty is another option following component removal for infection. However, although patients maintain some degree of range of motion, instability is often a problem that requires bracing and can compromise function.

Thrombophlebitis has not proven to be as much of a problem following total knee replacement as it is after total hip replacement (289). Although venography has shown calf thrombi to be relatively common, the incidence of clinical thrombophlebitis or pulmonary embolism is very small. This probably reflects in part the use of prophylactic thromboembolic measures. Vascular injury is very uncommon and when present usually involves the popliteal vessels. Neurologic injury (other than tourniquet associated) is also very uncommon (242). The most common problem encountered is peroneal nerve palsy after correction of excessive valgus deformity. Patellar instability is also uncommon and when present may represent inadequate soft-tissue releases or component malposition. If recurrent problems develop, additional surgery to correct the underlying cause may be necessary (193).

Outcomes

Primary total knee replacement using currently available techniques and prostheses has been reported to provide over 90% good or excellent results (112, 141, 167, 260, 272). Significant improvements can be expected in terms of pain relief, ambulation, and overall function. Longer follow-up studies have shown minimal deterioration over time. In general, results deteriorate at a rate of approximately 1% per year. This usually reflects problems with component loosening. However, this is becoming less of a problem as our appreciation for the principles of total knee replacement have increased. The rate of loosening increases in association with component malposition and poor cement fixation techniques. It is anticipated that the revision rates for prostheses currently being implanted will be even less than previously reported because of the improved techniques and prostheses available.

Revision Total Knee Replacement

Revision total knee replacement presents some specific technical problems that make it a very challenging area of orthopaedic surgery. It has all of the difficulties encountered in revision hip surgery as well as others related to the anatomic location of the knee. Specifically, exposure is often a problem because of significant scarring of the quadriceps mechanism. A quadriceps tenotomy may be necessary or, less desirable, a tibial tubercle osteotomy, to obtain adequate exposure. Removal of prosthesis and cement must be done carefully to avoid excessive loss of bone stock. Standard prosthesis may not be suitable for some revision cases. When ligament stability has been compromised, a more constrained prosthetic design may be necessary. If bone stock is deficient, a custom prosthesis may be necessary. In addition, components with long intramedullary stems may also be necessary to obtain adequate cement fixation. The results of revision surgery are generally not as satisfactory as primary knee replacement in terms of pain relief and range of motion (119, 234). The complication rate is higher as well. However, significant improvement can be anticipated although not as gratifying as in primary knee replacements for either the surgeon or the patient.

Total Shoulder Replacement

Total shoulder replacement (Fig. 36-5) is performed much less frequently than total hip or knee replacement. This reflects in part the lower incidence of symptomatic glenohumeral arthritis as compared to hip and knee arthritis. In addition, arthritis of the joints of the upper extremity tend to be better tolerated than for the lower extremity because of their relative "non-weight-bearing" function. Nonetheless, advanced arthritis of the glenohumeral joint associated with significant pain and functional limitation can be treated quite successfully by prosthetic replacement (6, 18, 62, 187, 214). Over the past 20 years many different designs have been utilized with varying success. At the present time it is generally accepted that a nonconstrained design is preferred. The most commonly used implant is the Neer total shoulder replacement (214).

Indications

The indications for total shoulder replacement are significant pain and functional disability associated with advanced glenohumeral arthritis that is no longer responsive to nonoperative measures. The timing of surgery is important. A successful shoulder replacement is highly dependent on the integrity of the surrounding soft tissues. Advanced disease resulting in extensive soft-tissue contracture and rotator cuff loss can compromise the results of surgery. Therefore, the timing of surgery should be considered not only in terms of the severity of symptoms but also in the context of the condition of the soft tissues.

Total shoulder replacement is most commonly performed for osteoarthritis (Fig. 36-5) and rheumatoid arthritis. Other less common indications include post-traumatic arthritis, nonrheumatoid inflammatory arthritis, arthritis of recurrent dislocations, osteonecrosis of the humeral head, and cuff tear arthropathy.

Contraindications to total shoulder replacement include the presence of active sepsis either involving the glenohumeral joint or in the periarticular area (subacromial space, acromioclavicular joint), neuropathic joint, or paralysis of the shoulder musculature that includes both the rotator cuff and deltoid. Severe loss of glenoid bone stock is a contraindication to total shoulder replacement but may be an indication for proximal humeral hemiarthroplasty. Massive rotator cuff tears will compromise the results of total shoulder replacement but in and of itself is not an absolute contraindication.

Preoperative Considerations

Total shoulder replacement represents a major surgical procedure and requires a comprehensive preoperative medical evaluation. When evaluating the significance of cardiopulmonary problems it is important to remember that this procedure can be performed under regional anesthesia in the form of an interscalene block. This approach provides adequate anesthesia with decreased risk of cardiopulmonary complications. Any history of bleeding disorders also requires evaluation. Anticoagulants or nonsteroidal anti-inflammatories should be discontinued long enough in advance of surgery to prevent any bleeding problems. Patients with glenohumeral arthritis often have arthritic involvement of the lower extremity as well. It is important to fully evaluate the extent of lower extremity involvement before undertaking total shoulder replacement. If advanced hip or knee arthritis is present such that a total hip or total knee replacement would be necessary in the near future, it would probably be best to postpone the shoulder replacement until the lower extremity surgery is completed. Although the use of crutches would be difficult following lower extremity joint replacement because of the painful shoulder, this is preferable to the necessity of using crutches or a walker shortly after total shoulder replacement because of lower extremity joint replacement. In general, use of crutches or a walker should be postponed for 3 to 6 months following total shoulder replacement. In some cases, it is preferable to avoid their use altogether because of the compromised nature of the soft tissues. This is a decision that needs to be made on an individual basis for each patient.

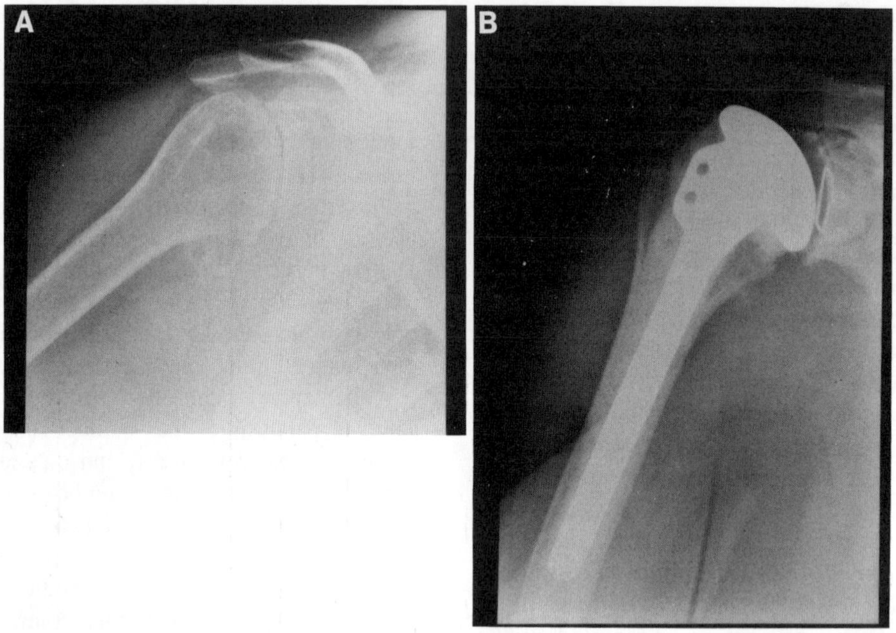

Figure 36-5. 70-year-old female with advanced osteoarthritis of the right glenohumeral joint (*A*). Radiographs show complete loss of joint space with flattening of the humeral head and peripheral osteophyte formation. There is some decrease in the subacromial space noted. A total shoulder replacement was performed (*B*) with resurfacing of the glenoid and insertion of a proximal humeral prosthesis. The patient had good pain relief and improvement in range of motion and overall function.

Surgical Technique

Prophylactic perioperative antibiotics should be utilized. The most common regimen includes providing the first dose just prior to surgery and then every 6 or 8 hours for 48 hours following surgery. Proper positioning of the patient is essential to perform this surgery. The "beach chair" position is most commonly utilized with the head of the operating table elevated to 30 to 45 degrees. The patient should be moved to the side so the humerus can be placed in extension with the arm perpendicular to the floor. A folded sheet should be placed behind the scapula to enhance glenoid exposure. Different surgical approaches have been utilized in the past, but at present most agree that an extended deltopectoral incision without detachment of the deltoid from its clavicular or acromial origin is preferred. The cephalic vein marks the deltopectoral interval. It should be preserved if possible and is usually retracted laterally. As the deltopectoral interval is developed, the clavipectoral fascia is exposed and divided parallel to the muscles of the conjoined tendon that arise from the coracoid process. The proximal portion of the humerus can then be visualized and landmarks identified. In some patients the coracoacromial ligament is excised to facilitate exposure or as a treatment for underlying impingement syndrome. In rheumatoid patients, it is generally preserved because it acts as a constraint to superior subluxation and further compromise of the rotator cuff. At this point, adhesions within the subacromial space can be released by passing a blunt flat elevator along the outside of the rotator cuff muscles. The joint is entered by a vertical incision in the subscapularis tendon and the underlying capsule approximately 1 to 2 cm medial to the lesser tuberosity. In patients with a significant internal rotation contracture, a "Z" lengthening of the subscapularis should be performed by separating it from the underlying capsule and dividing the capsule medial to the subscapularis tenotomy.

The humerus should be externally rotated to facilitate dislocation of the humeral head anteriorly. This usually requires release of the capsule from the inferior portion of the humeral neck. Osteotomy of the humeral head should be performed so that the humeral component will be in 30 to 45 degrees of retroversion. Care must be taken to avoid excessive humeral head resection since this will lead to instability and rotator cuff dysfunction. At this point, prior to preparation of the glenoid, the joint and periarticular area should be carefully inspected. Any additional procedures should be performed at this point as will be discussed. Retraction of the proximal humerus posteriorly facilitates exposure of the glenoid. The glenoid is prepared by first removing all remaining articular cartilage. Care should be taken to preserve the subchondral bone. The boundaries of the glenoid must be clearly visualized to permit accurate placement of the component. A trough is made that is centered over the glenoid neck. This is deepened to accept the keel of the glenoid component and bone cement. Care must be taken to shape the face of the glenoid so that the glenoid component lies flat without a tendency for "rocking." After the trough is irrigated and dried, the glenoid component is cemented in place.

The arm is then extended and externally rotated. The humeral canal is prepared to receive the humeral component, and a trial component is inserted. Range of motion and stability are tested, and adjustments in humeral retroversion or soft tissue tension are made. In most cases the humeral component can be "press fit" without cement. However, if bone stock is deficient or of poor quality, cement fixation should be used. The subscapularis is then repaired as is the rotator interval for additional stability. Deep suction drains are used, and the wound is closed in layers. A sling with Ace bandages is used for Velpeau type immobilization.

Frequently, additional procedures may be necessary during total shoulder replacement. For example, most rheumatoid patients undergo synovectomy and bursectomy. Rotator cuff tears should be repaired to provide optimal function and maintain stability. These are most commonly encountered in rheumatoid patients. When chronic impingement is present, anterior acromioplasty, coracoacromial ligament excision, and rotator cuff repair will be required. Symptomatic acromioclavicular joint arthritis should be treated by resection of the lateral clavicle. Whenever possible, the need for these additional procedures should be determined preoperatively.

Postoperatively, the patient is encouraged to ambulate as soon after surgery as possible. Intravenous antibiotics are continued for 48 hours after surgery. A supervised rehabilitation program is essential for a successful surgical result. Exercises are usually begun on the 1st or 2nd postoperative day. The specific rehabilitation program utilized should be individualized based upon the findings at surgery and the need for additional procedures. In general, a sling is worn for 3 weeks following surgery, or 6 to 8 weeks if a rotator cuff repair is performed.

Complications

Complications following nonconstrained total shoulder replacement include infection, nerve injury, instability, and component loosening (62, 214). The incidence of deep infection is consistently less then 1%. When deep infection develops (either early or late), surgical management is indicated for soft tissue debridement with or without removal of prosthetic components. Intravenous antibiotics should be utilized as well. The principles for reinsertion of prosthetic components are the same as outlined previously. However, care must be taken to preserve the soft tissues. Nerve injury is also uncommon. The axillary nerve is most commonly involved and usually represents a neuropraxia, which improves or resolves over time. Postoperative instability may develop as a result of component malposition, inadequate restoration of soft-tissue tension, or muscle weakness. Fortunately, the incidence is also quite low. Treatment depends on the underlying cause, which should be carefully evaluated before considering revision surgery. Postoperative rotator cuff tears cause significant loss of function; instability may become a problem as well. This often requires additional surgery for rotator cuff repair to improve shoulder function. Component loosening has been an area of controversy. Most large series of nonconstrained total shoulder replacements have reported a very high incidence of glenoid radiolucent lines at the bone/cement interface. These have ranged from 30% to 89% (18, 62, 214). This is of concern because of the association with component loosening. However, the glenoid revision rate has ranged from 0% to 11% for the same series reported (18, 62, 214). Disparity between the incidence of glenoid radiolucent lines and symptomatic loosening is not well understood. Longer follow-up studies, thus far, have not shown a significant increase in the need for glenoid revision. Humeral component loosening has been an insignificant problem. It appears that "press fit" components do not develop problems with loosening with any greater frequency than cemented components.

Outcomes

The results of total shoulder replacement are dependent in large part on the underlying diagnosis. In general, over 90% of all patients achieve satisfactory pain relief (6, 18, 62, 214). However, functional improvements as determined by postoperative range of motion is directly related to the integrity and function of the rotator cuff. Consequently, patients with osteoarthritis obtain better range of motion than patients with rheumatoid arthritis. Improvement in range of motion may also be limited in patients with post-traumatic osteoarthritis because of the significant scarring and tuberosity malalignment that may be present. Certainly the pain relief possible after total shoulder replacement is comparable to that reported for total hip and total knee replacements. However, the importance of the soft tissues in achieving functional improvement cannot be overemphasized.

Fractures

Fractures in the elderly constitute a major health care problem which, in many cases, requires surgical management. Specific fractures occur with significant frequency in the elderly and these primarily include hip, proximal humeral, and distal radius fractures. These are osteoporosis associated fractures, characterized by an increasing incidence with older age and a predominance in females. They occur primarily in areas of cancellous bone. These fractures will be discussed in detail. Fractures about the elbow and knee are much less common in the elderly and will not be discussed.

Hip Fractures

By current estimates over 270,000 hip fractures occur each year in the United States, the vast majority of which are in patients over 65 years. Since almost all of these fractures are treated surgically, hip fracture surgery represents the most common orthopaedic procedure performed in the elderly. It is estimated that by the year 2040 the number of hip fractures occurring annually will double, making hip fracture surgery even more significant in the future.

The problem of hip fractures in the elderly has been studied extensively, particularly with respect to risk factors and mortality. Age remains an important risk factor. The incidence of hip fractures increases with advancing age beyond age 50, possibly even doubling with each additional decade after age 50 (75). Hip fractures occur more commonly in females by a ratio of at least 2:1 (71, 75, 195). Elderly white females are at highest risk, while black males are at the lowest risk (31, 88, 95). Hip fractures also occur more commonly in urban than in rural populations (75, 195). This may reflect a higher concentration of institutionalized elderly patients, a higher incidence of alcohol and tobacco consumption, and a more sedentary life-style in the urban populations. Institutionalized patients also have a higher incidence of hip fracture (109, 150, 299), probably related to dementia, other comorbid conditions, and use of psychotropic medications. Increased risk has also been identified in patients with previous fractures (hip or other fractures) (35, 98, 194), those taking psychotropic medication (237), patients with Alzheimers type dementia (42) and those on low calcium diets (134, 189).

Mortality following hip fracture remains one of the most important aspects of the problem. Recent studies that focused on elderly hip fracture patients treated operatively in the 1980s found a 1-year mortality rate of approximately 25% (264, 309). This is significantly greater than the anticipated mortality for an age- and sex-matched population who have not sustained hip fractures (160, 313). Most authors agree that the highest risk of mortality occurs within the first 6 months following fracture. Generally, after 1-year mortality rates approach those for an age- and sex-matched non-hip fracture population.

Many studies have attempted to identify those factors that contribute to the increased mortality rates. Although it is difficult to isolate any one specific factor from other contributing factors, some important information has been identified. Factors that increase mortality risk include significant comorbid medical conditions (105, 264, 309), male sex (113, 196), underlying cognitive disorders (199, 270), institutionalized pre-fracture living environment (75, 135), poor pre-fracture mobility (22, 56, 113), and the presence of postoperative complications (2, 73, 86, 264). Factors not necessarily associated with increased mortality include age (160, 309), fracture type (77, 147, 264, 309), and timing of surgical treatment (28, 104, 160, 264). The difficulty in the interpretation of these data rests on the difficulty in isolating one specific factor; i.e., is age important by itself or is it primarily a reflection of the greater medical comorbidities present in older patients? This area will require clarification in the future. It is an important area to be studied because identification of risk factors may lead to more effective treatment approaches.

Fracture Types

Fractures of the proximal femur are generally classified according to their anatomic location into femoral neck, intertrochanteric, and subtrochanteric fractures (Fig. 36-6). Based upon our experience with over 500 hip fractures in patients over age 65, more than 95% are femoral neck or intertrochanteric fractures. These fractures occur with just about equal frequency (106). The remaining small

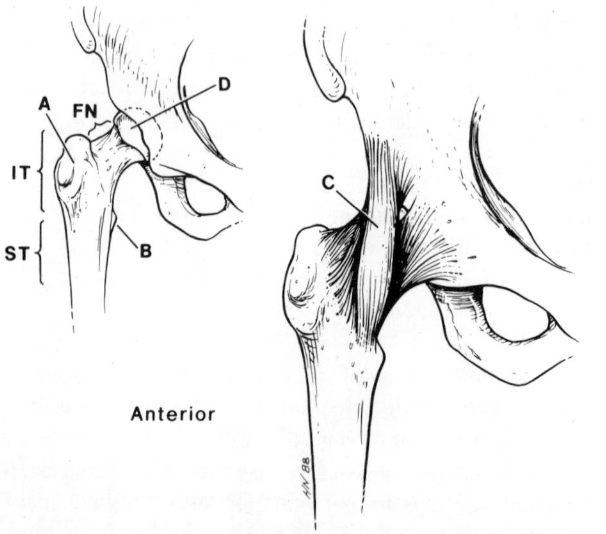

Figure 36-6. Anterior anatomy of the hip. Note that the hip joint capsule extends to the intertrochanteric line anteriorly and to the midportion of the femoral neck posteriorly. **A,** Greater trochanter; **B,** lesser trochanter; **C,** joint capsule; **D,** femoral head; **FN,** femoral neck; **IT,** intertrochanteric region; **ST,** subtrochanteric region.

percentage are subtrochanteric fractures, which occur more commonly in younger patients sustaining high-energy injuries. Therefore, our discussion will focus on femoral neck and intertrochanteric fractures.

Femoral Neck Fractures

Fractures of the femoral neck are intracapsular fractures that occur in the proximal femur in an area beginning inferior to the articular surface of the femoral head and ending just superior to the intertrochanteric region. The majority of these fractures occur as a result of a simple fall. These are low-energy injuries that result in a fracture in part because of the inability of the osteoporotic bone of the proximal femur to withstand the relatively low stresses involved.

The intracapsular location of the fracture has important implications on fracture healing and the development of femoral head osteonecrosis. The blood supply for the femoral head arises from the medial and lateral femoral circumflex arteries, which enter the posterior and anterior portions of the femoral neck respectively (Fig. 36-7). They form an extracapsular arterial ring at the base of the femoral neck and give rise to ascending cervical arteries, which traverse the neck proximally and form an intracapsular ring at the junction of the femoral head and neck.

This blood supply is distally based. Therefore, displaced femoral neck fractures may result in disruption of the blood supply, resulting in significant risk for osteonecrosis and nonunion. These are the two complications that have resulted in displaced femoral neck fractures being referred to as the "unsolved fracture".

Different classification systems have been used for femoral neck fractures (78, 107, 224). The most popular one is the Garden classification (Fig. 36-8), which divides these fractures into four types based upon the degree of displacement. Type I is an incomplete, impacted fracture; Type II is a complete fracture without displacement; Type III is a complete fracture with partial displacement; and Type IV is a complete fracture with total displacement of the fragments. Radiographically, it is often difficult to differentiate the four different types. Therefore, a simpler system has evolved in which Types I and II are considered nondisplaced fractures and, Types III and IV are displaced fractures. As noted, the degree of displacement has important implications on the development of healing complications.

Clinical Evaluation

The clinical presentation of femoral neck fractures in the elderly is dependent primarily upon the type of fracture. Patients with nondisplaced or impacted fractures may have only minimal pain at the extremes of motion and remain ambulatory with mild discomfort. However, there may be significant symptoms associated with this that preclude ambulation. Displaced fractures are generally much more symptomatic at presentation. The patients are unable to stand or ambulate, and the affected lower extremity may be externally rotated and shortened. Any motion of the hip will also be painful. Standard radiographic examination of the hip includes an anteroposterior view of the pelvis and a cross table lateral view. The AP view of

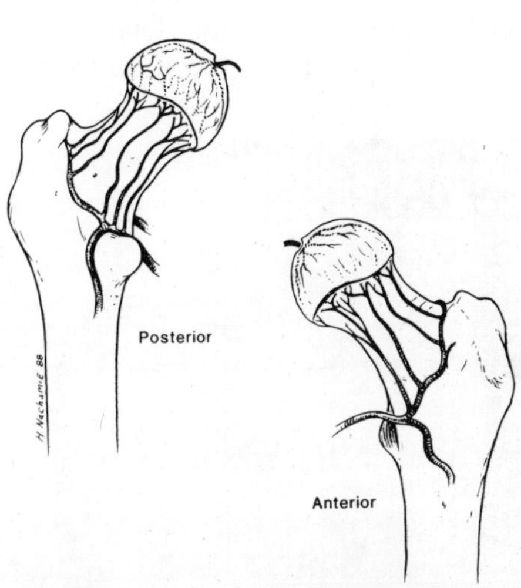

Figure 36-7. The blood supply to the femoral head (see text). It is important to note that the blood supply to the femoral head traverses the femoral neck in a distal-to-proximal direction. Therefore, femoral neck fractures that disrupt the ascending cervical arteries deprive the femoral head of its blood supply.

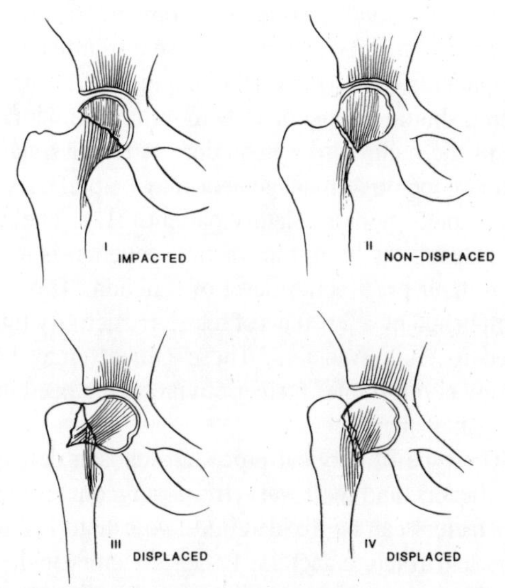

Figure 36-8. Garden classification of femoral neck fractures (see text). It is important to recognize that Type I (impacted) and Type II are nondisplaced fractures, while Type III and Type IV are displaced fractures. It is usually difficult to differentiate Type III and Type IV fractures.

the pelvis allows comparison with the uninvolved side, which may be helpful in identifying nondisplaced or impacted fractures. This standard radiographic evaluation will easily identify all displaced fractures. However, in difficult to identify nondisplaced or impacted fractures, an internal rotation view of the hip may be helpful. This is taken with the lower extremity internally rotated approximately 15 degrees. By correcting for anatomic anteversion, this view permits visualization of the entire femoral neck. When a femoral neck fracture is suspected but standard radiographs do not show a fracture, a technetium bone scan should be obtained. This is a sensitive indicator of an unrecognized femoral neck fracture (94). It is important to maintain a very high index of suspicion for femoral neck fracture in all elderly patients with hip pain following even a trivial injury to the hip.

Treatment

All patients with femoral neck fractures should be admitted and maintained on strict bed rest. Whereas light skin traction has been utilized in the past, we generally prefer to maintain the leg in a position of comfort, which is usually slight hip flexion and external rotation supported by pillows. All patients should undergo prompt medical evaluation in preparation for surgical management of the fracture.

There is general agreement that surgical management is the treatment of choice for almost all femoral neck fractures. There are some exceptions to this general rule. For example, patients with severe medical problems resulting in significant risk of perioperative mortality can be considered for nonoperative management. However, prolonged bed rest and traction also pose a significant risk to these patients. Therefore, if nonoperative treatment is chosen it should consist of early mobilization with acceptance of the malunion or nonunion. Another situation in which nonoperative management may be preferred is for the demented, nonambulatory patient (312). The goal in these patients, as in all hip fracture patients, is to return them to their pre-fracture level of function. This may be accomplished by a few days of restricted activity followed by bed to chair transfers. These patients may be surprisingly comfortable, further obviating the need for surgical management.

The type of surgical procedure chosen depends on many factors and will vary from surgeon to surgeon. These factors can be divided into two categories: patient factors and fracture factors. Patients factors include the patient's age, ambulatory ability, functional status, mental status, ability to participate in a rehabilitation program, and associated medical problems. Fracture factors include the amount of displacement, osteoporosis, comminution, and the age of the fracture. All of these factors are important. However, in the treatment of femoral neck fractures the most important differences in treatment approach are determined by fracture displacement. Therefore, we will discuss the treatment options by considering nondisplaced and displaced femoral neck fractures separately.

Nondisplaced Fractures

Nondisplaced fractures include garden Type I and Type II fractures. Impacted fractures (Type I) are inherently stable because of the impaction at the fracture site. In the past, there has been some support for nonoperative management of these fractures. However, problems with late displacement and healing complications (24, 25, 136) have led to support for operative management. Nondisplaced fractures that are nonimpacted (Type II) do not have the inherent stability of impacted fractures and carry a very high risk of displacement. Therefore, internal fixation is the treatment of choice.

Impacted and nondisplaced femoral neck fractures should undergo in situ internal fixation using multiple pins or screws (Fig. 36-9). Sliding hip screw devices have also been used, but the results have been inferior to multiple pins (287). There are many screws and pins available, and acceptable results have been reported with many different devices. However, we prefer to use cannulated screws or 6.5 mm. cancellous screws (54, 282, 292) because of the improved lag effect provided by the outside thread diameter and the relatively short length of threads. The optimal number of screws or pins to be used for internal fixation has not been determined (291). We prefer to use three screws placed in parallel on both the AP and lateral views of the proximal femur. Screws should be inserted under fluoroscopic control. However, it is essential to obtain permanent AP and lateral radiographs prior to

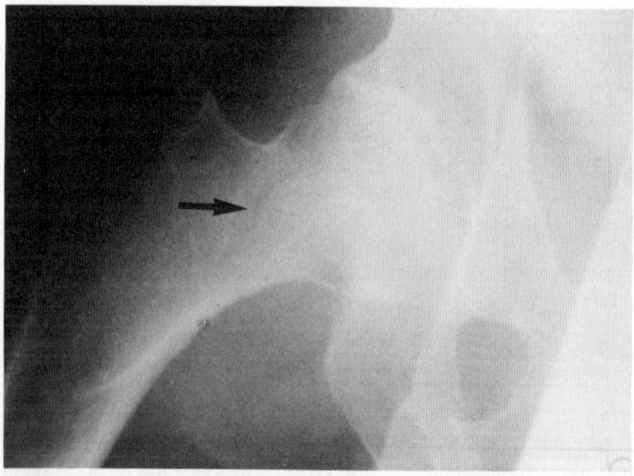

Figure 36-9. Nondisplaced femoral neck fracture in a 62-year-old female treated by internal fixation with 6.5-mm AO cancellous screws.

completion of the surgery. The fluoroscopic views are often inadequate for determining the true alignment of the fracture fragments and the position of the screws.

Postoperative management is directed at early mobilization of the patient since one of the primary reasons for surgical management is to prevent the complications of prolonged recumbency. The patient should be out of bed and sitting in a chair at bedside on the first postoperative day. Ambulation should follow the next day. Weight bearing is allowed as tolerated with assistive devices as needed. This is an important aspect of the postoperative rehabilitation program. There does not appear to be any advantage to restricted weight bearing following internal fixation of these fractures (9). There is, however, a distinct disadvantage to limiting weight bearing because of the difficulty elderly patients have in ambulation with these restrictions.

Displaced Fractures

Whereas virtually all patients with displaced femoral neck fractures should be treated by internal fixation, such is not the case for displaced femoral neck fractures in the elderly. The relatively high risk of nonunion and osteonecrosis has led to the development and popularity of primary prosthetic replacement as a treatment option. Since both symptomatic nonunion and osteonecrosis following internal fixation are treated by prosthetic replacement, primary prosthetic replacement has been advocated for these high risk fractures as a means of decreasing the need for reoperation. In reality, the choice of internal fixation versus prosthetic replacement may be difficult. It should be based upon a careful consideration of the patient's age, fracture comminution, bone quality, age of the fracture, and associated medical conditions. Based upon these factors, we will outline the treatment approach that we favor.

For displaced fractures in active, healthy patients under the chronological age of 70, we feel that treatment by anatomic reduction and internal fixation is preferred over primary prosthetic replacement (Fig. 36-10). We will also consider internal fixation for selected active and healthy patients between the ages of 70 and 75, if good bone quality is present and an acceptable reduction with secure fixation can be obtained. We treat this fracture as an urgent situation with rapid medical stabilization and surgical treatment whenever possible within 24 hours of admission. Treatment consists of a closed reduction of the fracture under fluoroscopic control. This is the most important and often the most difficult step in treatment. Closed reduction can be performed by flexing the hip to 45 degrees and externally rotating the femur to disengage the fracture fragments. Traction should then be applied as the leg is internally rotated and brought into full extension. Traction is maintained by placing the extremity in the foot holder of the fracture table. Anterior-posterior (AP) and lateral views should be obtained. If an obvious malreduction is present, the maneuver should be repeated. We will attempt a gentle closed reduction up to three times defore deciding to reevaluate our treatment options.

Permanent radiographs should be obtained to evaluate the reduction. Careful evaluation of these radiographs is essential to proceed with an appropriate treatment. This evaluation should be directed at determining the adequacy of the reduction as well as the presence and extent of comminution of the posterior portion of the femoral neck. This is important because it will compromise the security of the reduction as well as fixation. Therefore, if significant posterior comminution is present that would ultimately compromise internal fixation, a primary prosthetic replacement should be performed.

If the reduction is acceptable and posterior comminution is not significant, then internal fixation should be performed using multiple screws or pins as described previously. If the reduction is unacceptable without significant posterior comminution, then another closed reduction can be attempted. If an adequate reduction cannot be obtained, then a decision has to be made as to whether to proceed with open reduction and internal fixation or primary prosthetic replacement. This is based upon a careful assessment of the patient and fracture factors as described. If the reduction is unacceptable and there is significant posterior comminution, then primary prosthetic replacement is indicated. If the post-reduction radiographs show an acceptable reduction but there is significant posterior comminution, then internal fixation can be considered if the bone quality is sufficient to allow secure internal fixation. Even in this situation, the risk of fixation failure is greater because of the posterior comminution, but the increased risk may be acceptable based upon a careful evaluation of the patient and fracture factors listed. However, if bone quality is poor, then primary prosthetic replacement is preferred.

Postoperative management has been a source of controversy. Some have recommended restricted weight bearing until the fracture has healed (78, 149, 217, 231), while others have shown that unguarded weight bearing can be started immediately without detrimental effects (1, 9, 48, 106, 114, 200). Biomechanical data have shown that non-weight-bearing ambulation places significant stresses across the hip as a result of muscular contraction at the hip and knee (232, 248, 249). Therefore, attempts at unloading the hip by non-weight-bearing ambulation are not realistic. In addition, geriatric patients have great difficulty ambulating under these conditions. Therefore, for our geriatric patients we encourage weight bearing as

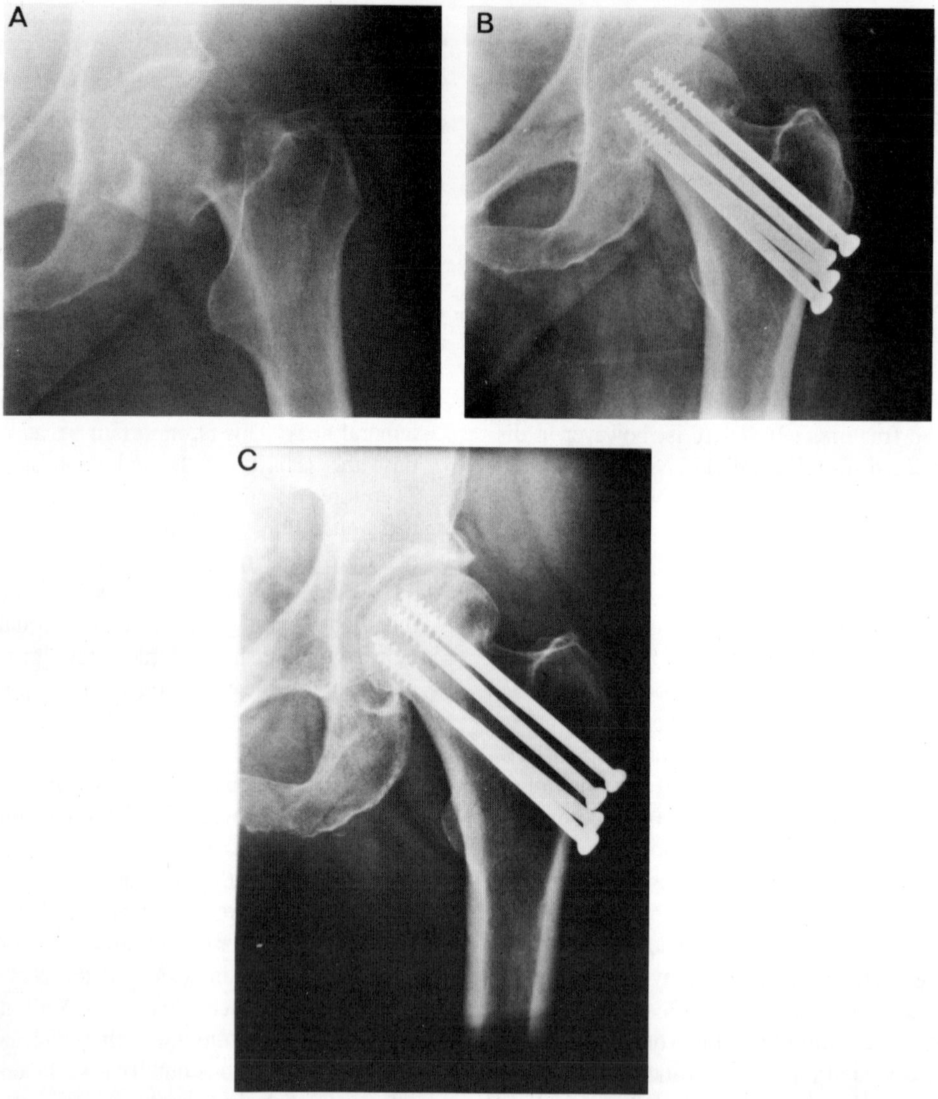

Figure 36-10. 60-year-old female sustained a displaced femoral neck fracture from a fall (*A*). A closed reduction was successful and internal fixation was performed using 6.5-mm AO cancellous screws (*B*). The fracture healed but 18 months after surgery osteonecrosis with collapse is evident (*C*). This patient required total hip arthroplasty because of progressively worsening hip pain.

tolerated for virtually all femoral neck fractures. We believe that an adequate reduction and secure internal fixation are the mainstays of treatment, and guarded weight bearing postoperatively will have little effect on the ultimate outcome of treatment.

Primary Prosthetic Replacement

Since the introduction of the Austin-Moore prosthesis in the early 1950s, primary prosthetic replacement for displaced femoral neck fractures has undergone an important evolution both in terms of indications and prosthetic design. At one time primary prosthetic replacement was felt to be the answer to the "unsolved fracture." At present, this is certainly not the case. However, primary prosthetic replacment does have an important place in the management of displaced femoral neck fractures in the elderly. The earliest prostheses utilized for the management of acute femoral neck fractures were the Austin-Moore and the Thompson prostheses (Figs. 36-11 and 36-12). These were hemiarthroplasties that replaced the femoral head but did not provide any resurfacing of the acetabulum. One of the problems noted with the use of these hemiarthroplasties was pain, which was frequently caused by progressive acetabular erosion, sometimes leading to protrusio acetabulae (46, 53, 162, 250, 274, 310). Therefore, bipolar endoprostheses were designed (Figs. 36-13 and 36-14). These consist of a smaller size femoral head, which articulates via a snap fit with a polyethylene liner

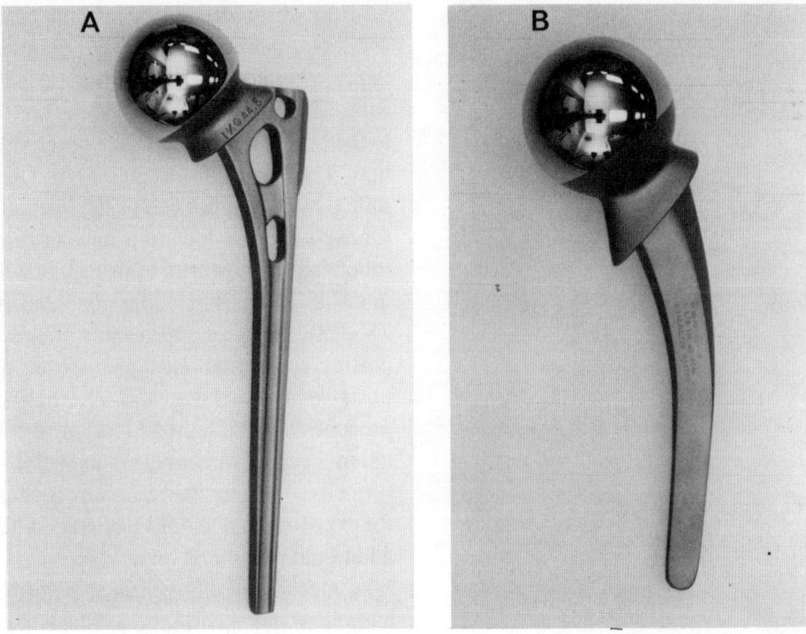

Figure 36-11. Austin-Moore endoprosthesis with a fenestrated straight stem (*A*). Thompson endoprosthesis provided a longer neck compared to the Austin-Moore design (*B*).

(inner bearing) of a metal acetabular shell, which in turn articulates within the anatomic acetabulum (outer bearing) by a suction fit. These prostheses allow motion between the prosthetic femoral head and the polyethylene liner as well as between the metallic shell and acetabular cartilage. By allowing motion at the inner bearing surface, it has the theoretical advantage of causing less acetabular wear, thereby overcoming one of the problems

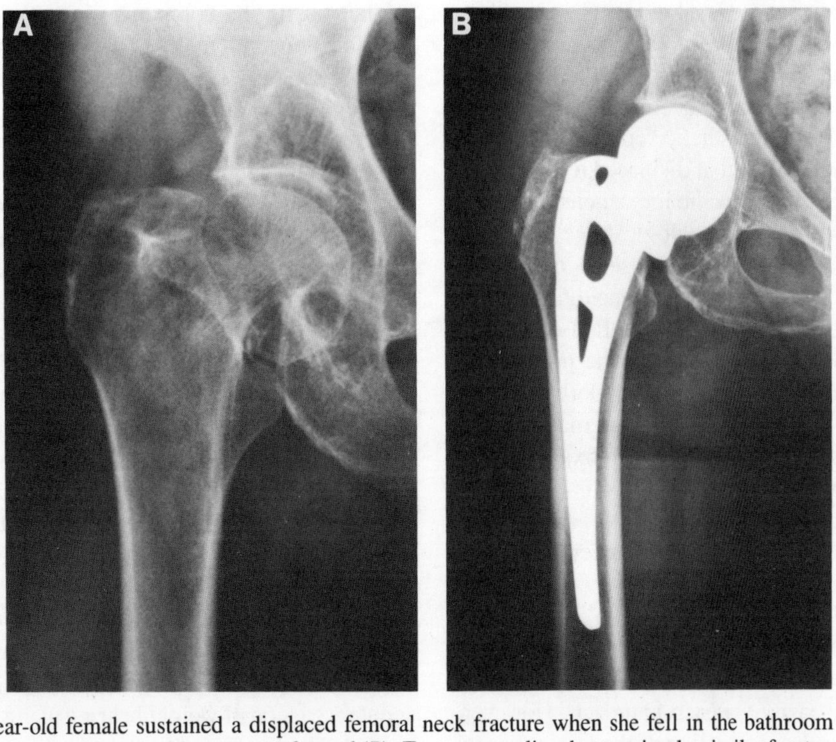

Figure 36-12. 84-year-old female sustained a displaced femoral neck fracture when she fell in the bathroom in her home (*A*). An uncemented Austin-Moore hemiarthroplasty was performed (*B*). Two years earlier she sustained a similar fracture of the left hip treated with a hemiarthroplasty.

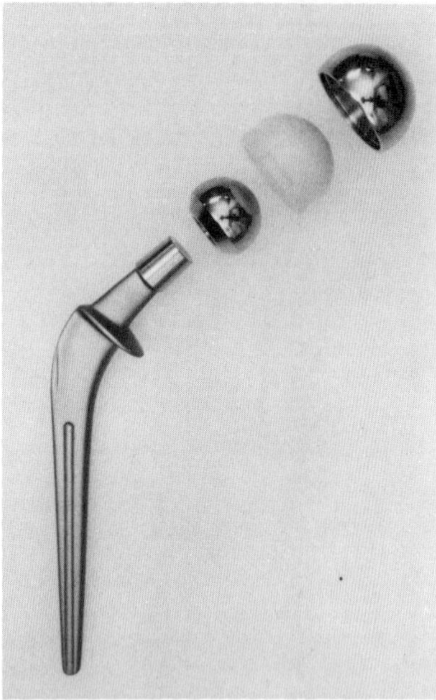

Figure 36-13. Bipolar endoprosthesis consisting of modular femoral stem with femoral head component; femoral head articulates with the polyethylene liner by a "snap-fit," which is captured by the metal acetabular shell; the shell articulates with the acetabulum by a "suction-fit".

with unipolar designs. Over the last ten years, bipolar endoprostheses have been used extensively, and the results have been quite satisfactory (37, 84, 133, 168, 170, 300). In most centers, bipolar prostheses have become the implant of choice for the treatment of displaced femoral neck fractures requiring prosthetic replacement.

We feel that primary prosthetic replacement has an important place in the treatment of displaced femoral neck fractures in the elderly. Our specific indications for its use include: (*a*) patients whose chronological age is greater than 75 years, regardless of activity level or general health; (*b*) selected patients whose chronological age is less than 75 years after careful consideration of activity level and general medical condition; (*c*) the presence of significant comminution of the posterior portion of the femoral neck, which precludes secure internal fixation; and (*d*) a high subcapital fracture in which fixation of the proximal fragment would be tenuous. Of course, these indications should be considered as guidelines, and it is important to consider all relevant factors in deciding on the ultimate treatment choice.

Different surgical approaches can be used for insertion of the prosthesis including anterior, lateral, and posterior approaches. Insertion of the prosthesis can be performed relatively easily via each approach. However, in the anterior approach, preparation of the femoral canal is more difficult unless special offset instruments are available. Some studies have shown an increased incidence of infection using the posterior approach (138, 318). This probably relates to the proximity of the incision to the peroneal area and the potential for fecal contamination. The position of stability for the prosthesis is determined by which portion of the hip joint capsule is incised for exposure. Dislocations have occurred more frequently following the posterior approach in which the prosthesis is unstable in flexion, adduction, and internal rotation (7, 76, 318). Anterior approaches preserve the posterior supporting structures and are stable in this position but are unstable in extension and external rotation. Lateral approaches are stable in adduction, flexion, and internal rotation because an anterior capsulotomy is usually performed. Transtrochanteric approaches are not necessary for exposure and should be avoided because of the risk of additional complications.

A few specific technical points concerning surgical technique for prosthetic replacement should be mentioned. At the Hospital for Joint Diseases, a posterior surgical approach is preferred for most patients. This approach can be performed in the lateral decubitus position with a limited amount of blood loss. A posterior capsulotomy is performed, and care is taken to preserve the entire acetabular labrum. A cemented bipolar prosthesis is most commonly utilized. The sizing of the acetabular shell is an important step in obtaining the proper "suction fit." Undersizing the component increases the probability of dislocation and may increase central acetabular wear. Using an oversized component will limit outerbearing motion and possibly increase peripheral acetabular wear. Most bipolar endoprostheses currently available are of a modular design, which permits accurate restoration of soft tissue tension. To enhance posterior stability, the capsule should be repaired and the short external rotators reattached to the drill holes in the posterior portion of the greater trochanter. We prefer an anterior "iliofemoral approach" or a direct lateral approach for patients with dementia or fecal incontinence. It should also be considered for patients who are expected to be nonambulators after surgery. These approaches place the incision away from the perineal area, provide enhanced stability in patients who are unable to follow position precautions, and reduce the risk of dislocation in patients whose activity will be restricted to bed to chair transfers by health care personnel.

Postoperatively, patients are mobilized out of bed and into a bedside chair on the first postoperative day. An abduction pillow is used while in bed. Ambulation without restriction of weight bearing using assistive devices as needed is started on the second postoperative day. Patients

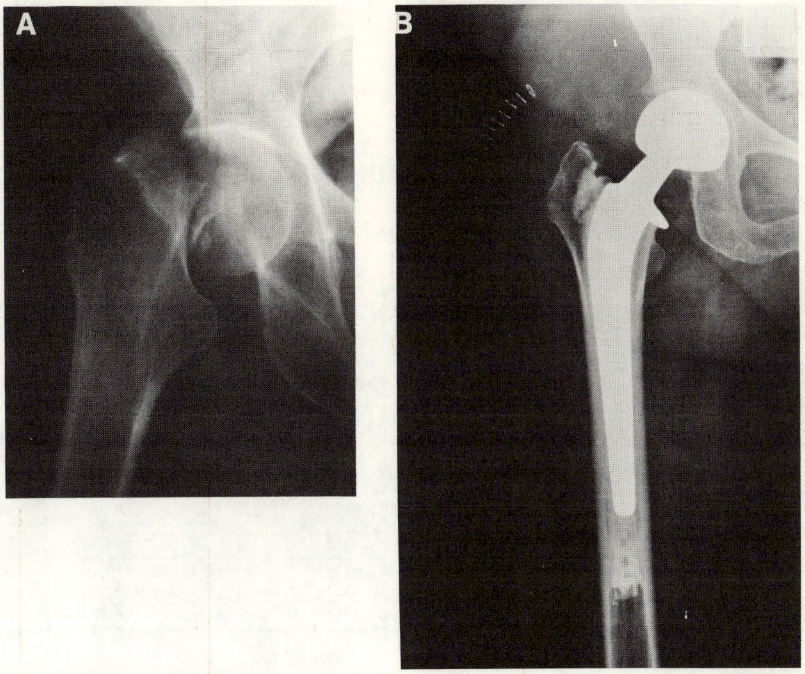

Figure 36-14. 81-year-old male sustained a displaced femoral neck fracture after being knocked down by a bicycle messenger (*A*). A cemented bipolar hemiarthroplasty was performed the following day (*B*).

are carefully instructed in positioning precautions depending upon the surgical approach used.

Special Situations

Elderly patients with Parkinson's disease who sustain femoral neck fractures present a difficult challenge to the physicians responsible for their care. Morbidity and mortality rates are much higher than for hip fracture patients without Parkinson's disease (70, 78, 92, 245). Different authors have reported widely varying results with both internal fixation and prosthetic replacement (70, 139, 245, 276). In deciding upon an appropriate treatment plan, it is essential to consider the status of the disease. Parkinson's disease is a movement disorder whose clinical manifestations can range from mild tremors without significant functional limitations to complete incapacitation with severe contractures. The response to medical treatment is also important since well-controlled disease should not alter the choice of treatment. In addition, fracture and patient factors must also be considered. Therefore, for patients with Parkinson's disease, it is essential to evaluate each case individually rather than attempt to employ a unidimensional approach. We prefer the following guidelines. Patients with nondisplaced or impacted fractures should be treated with multiple screw fixation and early mobilization regardless of age. Patients with displaced femoral neck fractures, who are relatively young and active and whose disease is well-controlled, should be treated by anatomic reduction and internal fixation, using the approach previously described. Older patients with displaced fractures and those patients with poorly controlled disease and significant loss of function should be treated by primary prosthetic replacement.

Elderly patients with Paget's disease present with two types of femoral neck fractures: incomplete or fissure fractures and complete fractures. We will address the specific problem of complete fractures, which for the most part represent displaced fractures. Different reports have documented the increased incidence of healing complications following internal fixation of femoral neck fractures in Paget's disease (83, 198, 216, 283, 306). Reports of treatment with prosthetic replacement reported both satisfactory (83) and unsatisfactory results (19, 216). We feel that primary prosthetic replacement is the treatment of choice for complete femoral neck fractures in Paget's disease (Fig. 36-15). The question to be answered is whether an endoprosthesis or total hip replacement is preferred. To make the proper choice, it is important to determine the presence and severity of pre-fracture hip symptoms as well as the extent of Pagetoid involvement in the acetabulum. If there is no history of preexisting symptoms and acetabular involvement is minimal, then a heiarthroplasty should be performed. We prefer a cemented bipolar endoprosthesis. However, when significant pre-fracture symp-

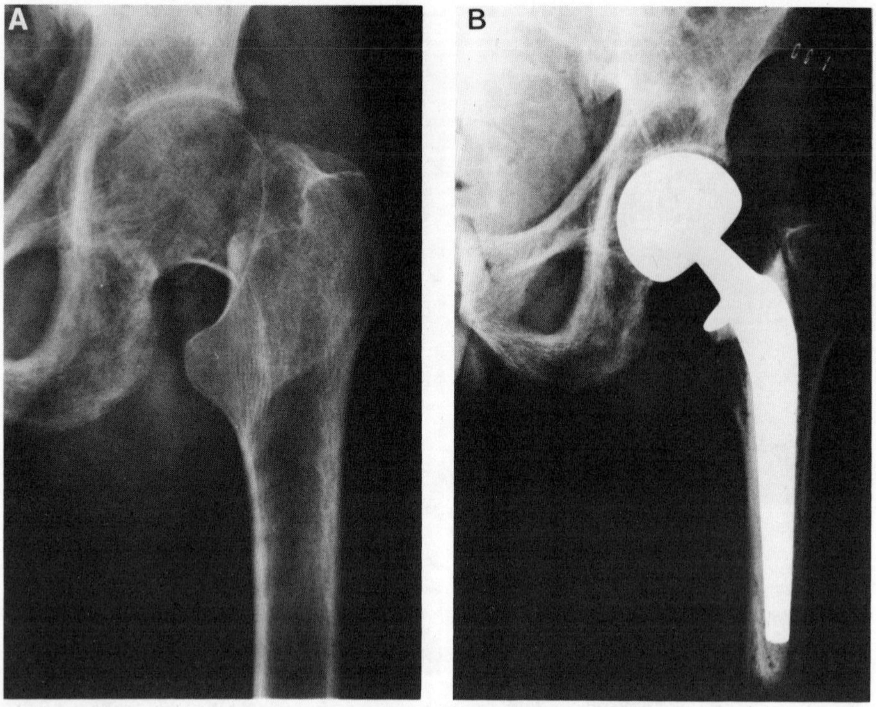

Figure 36-15. 76-year-old male without preexisting hip symptoms fell at home sustaining a displace femoral neck fracture (*A*). Pagetoid changes of the acetabulum were mild, and there were no significant degenerative changes. A cemented bipolar endoprosthesis was performed (*B*).

toms are present and/or acetabular involvement is extensive with secondary degenerative changes, total hip replacement is preferred.

Patients with spastic hemiplegia following a cerebral vascular accident are at increased risk for sustaining femoral neck fractures (276). These fractures usually occur on the affected side (189, 270, 276). This subgroup of patients may be problematic because of the presence of osteoporosis, spasticity, and/or contracture. As in Parkinson's disease, the degree of involvement may be quite variable, ranging from minimal spasticity without contracture in ambulatory patients to severe spasticity and contracture in nonambulatory patients. Therefore, the treatment approach must also be individualized. Nondisplaced fractures in ambulatory patients with minimal spasticity should be treated with internal fixation. Displaced fractures in ambulatory patients with minimal spasticity should be treated according to the protocol described previously in which age and posterior comminution are important factors. Patients with nondisplaced or displaced fractures who exhibit severe spasticity and contracture should undergo primary prosthetic replacement. Since the classic contracture is a flexion-adduction deformity, prosthetic replacement should be combined with muscle release to correct the deformity. In addition, the posterior approach should be avoided because of the potential for instability with flexion and adduction. Rather, an anterior approach is preferred to increase the stability of the prosthesis.

Complications

Complications following femoral neck fractures can be divided into three specific categories: (*a*) general complications in relation to comorbidities, surgery, or anesthesia; (*b*) complications following the use of internal fixation devices; and (*c*) complications following the use of primary prosthetic replacement. Each of these categories is discussed separately.

The age and medical fragility of this patient population increases the risk of postoperative complications. Pneumonia, congestive heart failure, myocardial infarction, cardiac arrhythmias, electrolyte imbalances, urinary tract infections, decubitus ulcers, and thromboembolism are serious complications that unfortunately occur with significant frequency. The incidence of clinically significant thrombophlebitis has been reported as 15% to 20%, while the incidence of radiographically documented thrombophlebitis has been reported as high as 50% (74, 118, 203, 228, 241). Fatal pulmonary embolism occurred in 4% to 7% of patients who did not receive thromboembolic prophylaxis (89). However, prophylactic anticoagulation using a variety of regimens has been effective in decreasing the incidence of thromboembolic complications. Urinary tract infection and decubitus ulcers have been reported in up to 30% of cases (148, 206). In one series, the presence of decubiti was associated with a 30% mortality (165). Many of these complications can be prevented by aggressive respiratory therapy and early surgery followed by rapid mobilization, judicious management of fluid and electrolyte replacement, and meticulous nursing care.

Complications following internal fixation of femoral neck fractures include loss of fixation, infection, nonunion, and osteonecrosis. Early fixation failure (within three months after surgery) occurs in 12% to 24% of displaced femoral neck fractues (16, 41, 136, 281). Important factors associated with early loss of fixation included age, inaccurate reduction, initial fracture type/displacement, presence of posterior comminution of the neck, and delay of surgery for more than seven days after injury (14, 16, 35, 187, 191, 256).

In the 1980s, infections following internal fixation of femoral neck fractures have been uncommon. Superficial infection has been reported in up to 5% of cases (240, 290). Deep infection has also been reported in up to 5% of cases (52, 240, 271, 290), although one large series of 300 patients reported no deep infections (288). Perioperative antibiotic prophylaxis has now become standard in the management of elderly hip fracture patients and is responsible in part for the low rates of infection (154).

Nonunion of femoral neck fractures (Fig. 36-16) is related to fracture type (54, 282, 288). In nondisplaced fractures, nonunion occurs in 0% to 5% of cases (16, 54, 282, 288). However, for displaced fractures, the incidence of nonunion has been reported from 9% to 35% (13, 16, 43, 52, 54, 271, 275, 282). Nonunions are more common following inadequate reduction and in the presence of posterior comminution (9, 14, 16, 47, 256).

The development of osteonecrosis (Fig. 36-10) following femoral neck fracture reflects the vulnerability of femoral head circulation to disruption. The incidence of osteonecrosis following nondisplaced femoral neck fractures has been reported to be as high as 15% but in general is approximately 5% to 8% (13, 16, 25, 188, 259, 282, 288). However, the incidence following displaced femoral neck fractures has been reported as 9% to 35% with most series reporting 20% to 35% (13, 16, 25, 52, 54, 175, 188, 282, 288). Factors associated with an increased incidence of osteonecrosis include inadequate reduction, delay of reduction and fixation, and use of sliding hip screws or nail-plate devices. However, not all osteonecrosis requires reoperation. In a large series of patients with osteonecrosis and late segmental collapse following displaced femoral neck fractures, 30% were disabled by the associated pain, 24% were symptom-free, and 46% had symptoms that were not disabling (16). In general, approximately one-third of patients developing osteonecrosis will require reoperation.

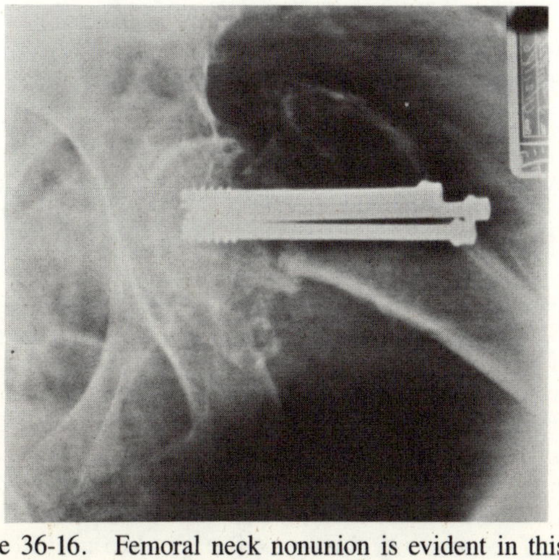

Figure 36-16. Femoral neck nonunion is evident in this 64-year-old female 7 months after internal fixation of a displaced femoral neck fracture.

Complications following primary prosthetic replacement for acute femoral neck fractures include infection, dislocation, and pain associated with acetabular erosion and/or prosthetic loosening. The incidence of infection has been reported from 2% to 20% (7, 46, 49, 310). The higher rates of infection were reported in earlier studies and reflect in part the fact that the population chosen for prosthetic replacement was generally older and more debilitated than most patients with femoral neck fractures. More recent series using mostly bipolar endoprostheses have reported infection rates of 2% to 8% (37, 47, 240, 303, 318). This can be attributed in part to patient selection and use of prophylactic perioperative antibiotics.

The incidence of dislocations following prosthetic replacement has varied from 1% to 10%, with the posterior approach associated with the higher dislocation rate as compared to the anterior approach (27, 49, 76, 138, 152, 179, 295, 318). Dislocations appear to occur less commonly after bipolar endoprosthesis when compared with hemiarthroplasty (27). However, closed reduction of a bipolar endoprosthesis is more difficult to achieve than with a hemiarthroplasty (Fig. 36-17).

Hip pain that develops following a prosthetic replacement may have a multitude of etiologies, many of which are unrelated to the prosthesis (257). The most important prosthesis-related causes of pain are acetabular erosion and prosthetic loosening. As noted previously, acetabular erosion was found to be a problem with early prosthetic designs. However, it appears to be less of a problem with the use of bipolar endoprostheses. In addition, cement fixation of the femoral component appears to reduce the incidence of postoperative pain associated with prosthetic loosening. Overall, the need for reoperation following prosthetic replacement is less than the inci-

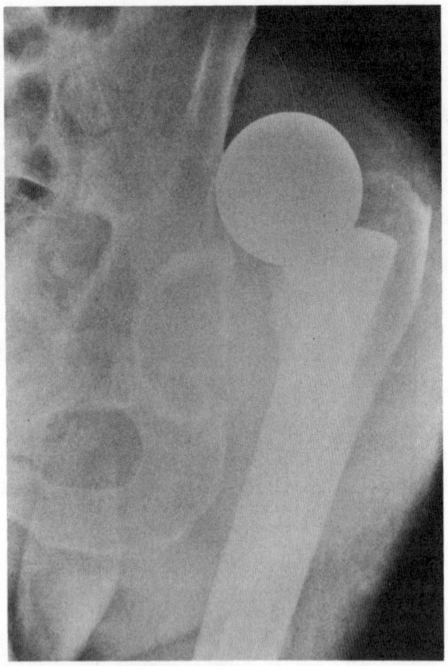

Figure 36-17. Dislocation of the bipolar endoprosthesis occurred 8 days after surgery. Closed reduction was successful, but redislocation occurred 1 week later. Closed reduction was not successful, and an open reduction was necessary.

dence of significant acetabular erosion and prosthetic loosening (27, 319).

Intertrochanteric Fractures

Intertrochanteric fractures occur in the region between the greater and lesser trochanters. They are extracapsular fractures indicating that the fracture line is distal to the anatomic limits of the capsule of the hip joint. The cancellous bone in this area is well vascularized. Consequently, the problems of nonunion and osteonecrosis encountered with intercapsular fractures are rarely a problem following intertrochanteric fractures.

Intertrochanteric fractures occur as a result of direct or indirect forces transmitted to the intertrochanteric area. This may result from a direct blow to the area of the greater trochanter or from indirect forces transmitted along the axis of the femur. Both mechanisms almost always occur in association with falls.

Many classification systems have been used for intertrochanteric hip fractures (11, 36, 90, 298). However, the the most important aspect of any classification system is determining the stability of the fracture pattern to a stable reduction. The key to a stable reduction rests in the ability to restore posteromedial cortical continuity. In stable fracture patterns, the posteromedial cortex remains intact, and a stable reduction can be obtained. Unstable fracture patterns are characterized by comminution of the posteromedial cortex. These fractures are inherently unstable but can be converted to a stable reduction if medial cortical apposition is obtained.

We prefer to classify intertrochanteric fractures into stable and unstable fracture patterns (Fig. 36-18). Therefore, the first step in the evaluation of these fractures is to differentiate stable and unstable fracture patterns. If a stable fracture pattern is present, then treatment will follow a specific protocol, which will be described. If an unstable fracture pattern is identified, a different protocol should be utilized, which will also be described.

Clinical Evaluation

Virtually all patients who sustain intertrochanteric hip fractures are unable to stand or ambulate following the injury. The range of clinical deformity of the involved lower extremity will vary depending upon the displacement and comminution of the fracture. Nondisplaced fractures may present with virtually no clinical deformity. Displaced comminuted fractures present with a classical shortened and externally rotated extremity. There is usually tenderness on palpation in the area of the greater trochanter. Range of motion of the hip will be painful and should be avoided. Following admission to the hospital, light skin traction should be used for the involved extremity, both for patient comfort and to avoid any additional injury.

The standard radiographic examination of intertrochanteric fractures includes an AP and cross table lat-

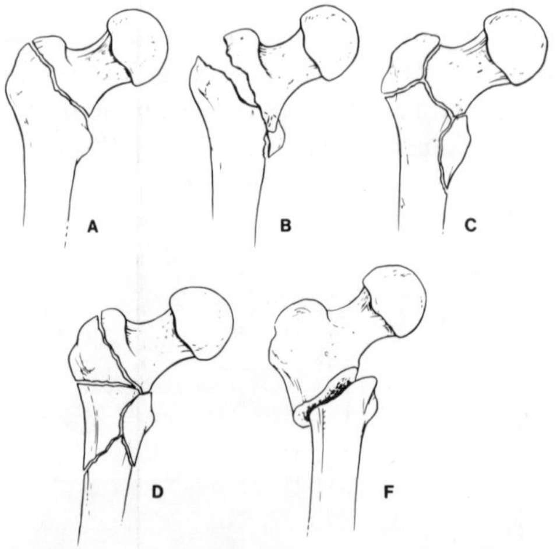

Figure 36-18. Classification of intertrochanteric fractures: **A** is a two-part fracture and is stable; **B** is also a stable pattern because the medial fragment is small and does not significantly compromise the posteromedial buttress; **C** represents an unstable fracture because of the large posteromedial fragment; **D** is an unstable intertrochanteric fracture with subtrochanteric extension; **E** is a reverse obliquity pattern and is also unstable because of the tendency for the shaft to displace medially. This classification is a combination of those described by Evans (90) and Kyle (166).

eral view of the hip. Because of patient discomfort, it is often impossible to obtain a lateral radiograph at the time of initial evaluation. However, it is important to have a complete radiographic evaluation prior to surgery. In unusual circumstances when a fracture is suspected but not identified on standard radiographs, technetium bone scanning will aid in identification of the fracture (93).

Treatment

The goal of treatment of intertrochanteric fractures in the elderly is prompt restoration to their pre-injury level of activity. The methods of obtaining this goal have changed dramatically over the past 50 years. Before suitable fixation devices were available, treatment was nonoperative, consisting of prolonged bed rest in traction until fracture healing occurred. This was then followed by a lengthy program of ambulation training. In elderly patients, this approach was associated with a very high complication rate including decubiti, urinary tract infection, joint contractures, pneumonia, and thromboembolic complications (91, 155, 166). In addition, fracture healing generally occurred with significant malunion and shortening because of the difficulty counteracting the deforming muscular forces with traction alone.

It soon became apparent that nonoperative management of these fractures resulted in an unacceptably high complication rate. It was also recognized that early mobilization of the patient was necessary to avoid the problems of prolonged recumbency. To achieve this, operative management consisting of reduction and stabilization of the fracture was necessary. Over the past 30 years, the techniques of operative fixation have changed significantly, and the fixation problems encountered earlier have largely been overcome. Currently, operative management has become the treatment of choice for intertrochanteric fractures because it allows early mobilization of the patient, thereby avoiding many of the complications that would result from prolonged bed rest.

Patients who sustain intertrochanteric fractures require prompt evaluation and management. In the vast majority of cases, surgery can be performed within the first 24 to 48 hours following admission. However, if the patient is unstable medically, delaying surgery until the problems are stabilized is essential. The goal of operative management is to achieve a stable fracture reduction and maintain it with internal fixation so the patient can be mobilized rapidly. The fracture fixation should allow weight-bearing ambulation as tolerated since non-weight-bearing or partial weight-bearing ambulation is difficult for the elderly. Achieving this goal is dependent on a number of factors including the fracture pattern, the stability of the reduction, and the method of fixation. For stable fracture patterns, achieving this goal is usually straightforward. However, for unstable fracture patterns it is much more difficult.

An important aspect of the treatment of intertrochanteric fractures is the choice of internal fixation device. Over the last 40 years, the available devices have undergone an important evolution. At the present time the sliding hip screw (Fig. 36-19) is the most commonly utilized device. This device allows controlled impaction at the fracture site, thereby increasing the stress on the implant, which further decreases the incidence of implant failure. Even though these devices are "forgiving" by allowing impaction at the fracture site, they must be inserted properly for this to occur. In addition, a stable reduction must be obtained at the time of surgery. Sliding hip screws are available in plate angles, varying from 125 to 155 degrees, of which 135 degrees is the plate angle most commonly used. Some authors have recommended the use of the 150-degree sliding hip screw, but thus far comparative studies have failed to show a significant advantage over the 135-degree device (205, 315). Other devices have also been used for the internal fixation of intertrochanteric fractures, of which flexible intramedullary nails have the largest experience (Ender nails) (Fig. 36-20). These devices are inserted in a retrograde manner under fluoroscopic guidance through portals in the distal femur. The proposed advantages of this procedure include decreased blood loss, decreased anesthetic and operative time, and reduced mortality (34, 163, 247). Excellent results with this device have been reported (304). However,

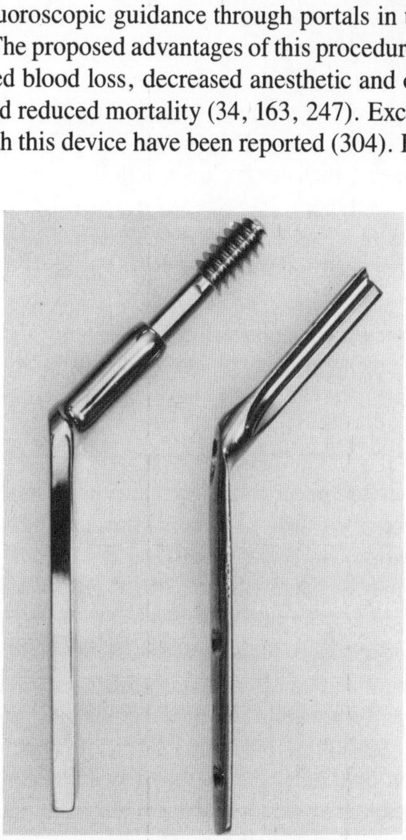

Figure 36-19. The fixed-angle Jewett nail (right) is compared to the sliding hip screw (left). The sliding hip screw allows impaction to occur while the Jewett nail does not.

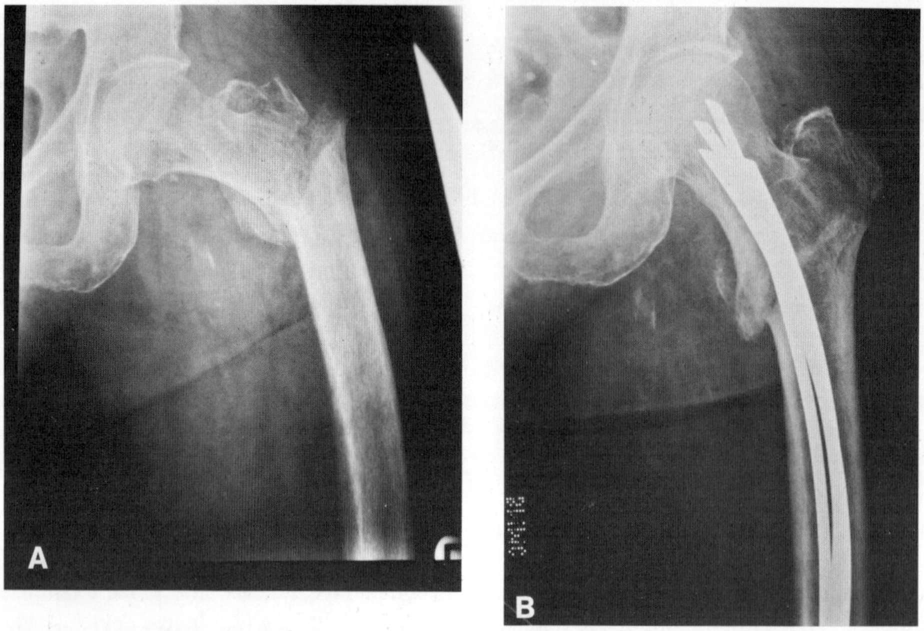

Figure 36-20. 82-year-old female with stable intertrochanteric fracture (*A*) treated by retrograde Ender nailing (*B*). The fracture healed uneventfully.

the majority of studies have shown a significant incidence of complications associated with their use, including rotational malalignment, supracondylar femur fractures, proximal migration of the nails through the femoral head, and backing out of the nails causing knee pain and stiffness (51, 55, 87, 120, 142, 146, 164, 236, 263). At present, it appears that flexible intermedullary nails are best utilized by surgeons experienced in their use. Some authors have reported satisfactory results using prosthetic replacement for comminuted intertrochanteric fractures in osteoporotic bone (244, 284, 285). However, this option has been used to only a limited extent, and thus far specific indications for its use have been difficult to define.

Treatment: Stable Fractures

Stable intertrochanteric fractures are those in which the posteromedial cortical buttress is intact and medial cortical apposition can be re-established (Fig. 36-21). These fractures may be nondisplaced or displaced. Nondisplaced fractures do not require reduction. Displaced fractures require reduction, which can usually be performed by closed manipulation. If unsuccessful, open reduction is necessary. We prefer to use the fracture table and image intensifier for all intertrochanteric fractures being treated by internal fixation (Fig. 36-22). It is important that the feet and ankles of both lower extremities be protected with soft padding when placed in the foot holders. This must be done in order to prevent any skin problems from excessive pressure. Closed reduction can be performed by gentle traction and either abduction or adduction, depending upon the position of the fragments. Closed reduction should be evaluated with the image intensifier on both AP and lateral views. Permanent AP and lateral views should be obtained at this time to evaluate the reduction and confirm the nature of the fracture pattern. At this point, the surgery is performed through a lateral approach. The lateral aspect of the proximal portion of the femur is exposed. Any manipulation of the fracture that is necessary to improve reduction can be performed at this time. We utilize the 135-degree sliding hip screw for virtually all intertrochanteric fractures. A few technical points should be emphasized. First, the guide wire and hence the position of the screw within the femoral neck and head should be in a central position. A superior and anterior position should be avoided because of the risk for "cutting out" through this weakened area of bone. Second, the screw should be inserted into the subchondral bone for best fixation. It should be located approximately ½ to 1 cm from the articular surface. Third, after the plate is inserted over the screw, the fracture should be impacted prior to fixation of the plate to the shaft. This impaction maneuver is necessary to enhance the stability of the reduction and to avoid excessive impaction postoperatively that may exceed the sliding capacity of the nail. Permanent AP and lateral radiographs must be obtained for accurate evaluation of the reduction and placement of the internal fixation device.

Postoperatively, patients should be out of bed to a chair the day after surgery. Ambulation begins the second

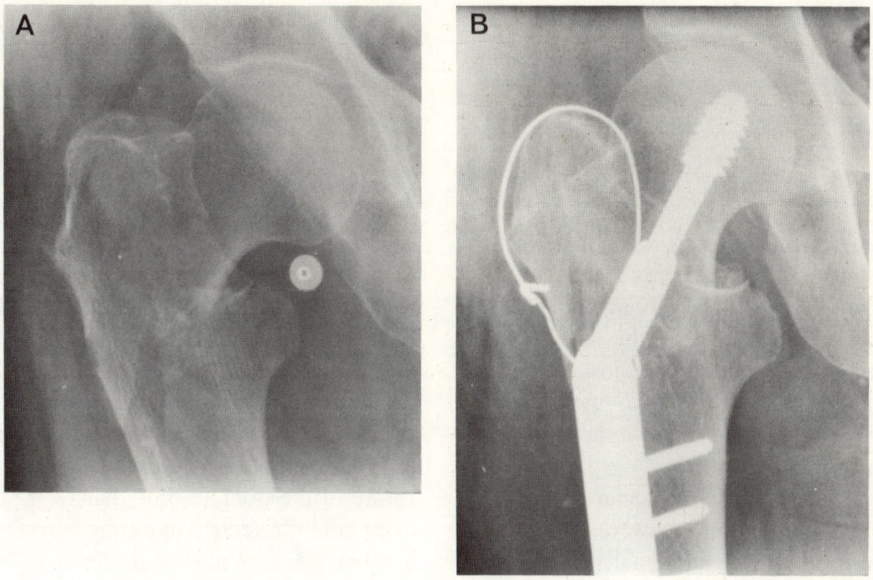

Figure 36-21. Stable intertrochanteric fracture pattern (*A*) treated by closed reduction and internal fixation using a 135° sliding hip screw (*B*). The cerclage wire was used to stabilize the greater trochanter fragment.

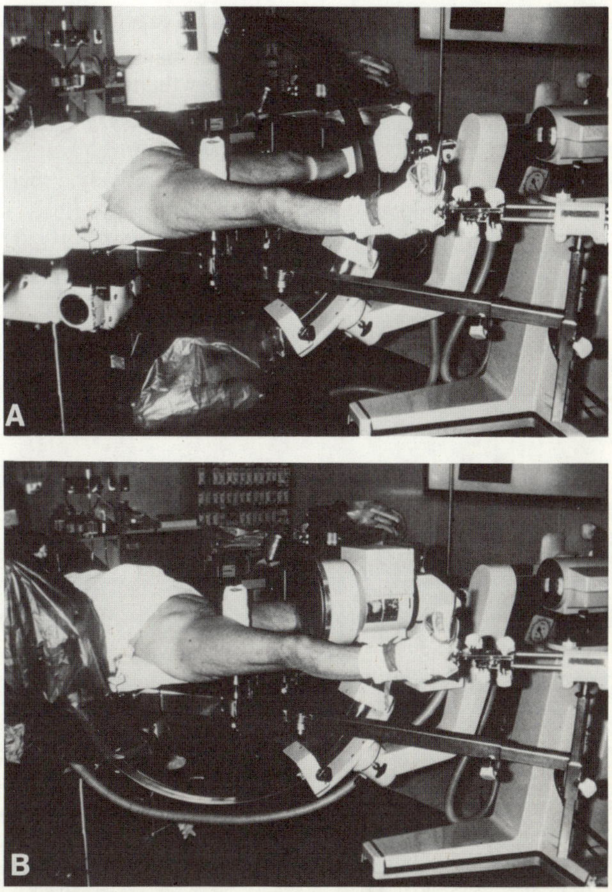

Figure 36-22. Standard operating room set up for open reduction and internal fixation of intertrochanteric fractures utilizing the fracture table and image intensifier. This allows excellent anteroposterior (*A*) and lateral (*B*) views during the procedure.

postoperative day with assistive devices as needed. Patients are allowed and even encouraged to bear weight as tolerated, since this is most compatible with optimal recovery.

Treatment: Unstable Fractures

Unstable intertrochanteric fractures are much more difficult to treat than stable fracture patterns (Fig. 36-23). They are characterized by loss of the posteromedial buttress. This comminution can extend into the subtrochanteric area, thereby increasing the degree of instability. In general, the goal of treatment of unstable intertrochanteric fractures is to convert the fracture to a stable reduction and obtain secure internal fixation.

The general approach for unstable fractures is as described for stable fracture patterns. However, different techniques for fracture reduction and internal fixation may be necessary. Closed reduction may be difficult to obtain because of the instability of the fracture, and open reduction is often necessary. Different reduction techniques have been developed over the years because of the high failure rate associated with the use of fixed angle nail plate devices. In general, these techniques resulted in a significantly lower complication rate when fixed angle nail plates were used. Examples of these reduction techniques include the Dimon and Hughston medial displacement osteotomy (Fig. 36-24), the Sarmiento valgus osteotomy, and the Wayne County lateral displacement (79, 155, 253, 255). In our opinion, the importance of these techniques has been significantly diminished with the development of the sliding hip screw. We prefer anatomic alignment with the sliding hip screw for the treatment of unstable intertrochanteric fractures. If the posteromedial fragment is large, then an attempt should be made to internally fix the fragment in a near anatomic position (Figs. 36-23 and 36-25). This aids in restoration of the posteromedial cortical support. Fixation of this fragment may be difficult, particularly if comminution is present. We have had most success utilizing one or two cerclage wires. It is important to recognize that an anatomic reduction of this fragment is not required. Rather the fragment should be brought back to the area of the posteromedial defect and secured in that position to provide an effective buttress to prevent a varus displacement. After this fragment is reduced and an acceptable reduction of the fracture is obtained, the sliding hip screw should be inserted as described. The unstable nature of the fracture often makes it necessary to manually hold the reduction during insertion of the internal fixation device. Once the device is inserted, the fracture should be impacted to obtain a stable position. This often results in a slight medial displacement of the shaft. It is important at this point to be certain that an adequate amount of sliding capacity remains. If this is not present, then a plate with a short barrel should be used to increase the sliding capacity. The plate should be securely fixed to the shaft. In comminuted fractures a longer plate is often necessary than is used for stable fractures (Fig. 36-26). It is important to have 8 to 10 cortices of fixation in the distal shaft fragment.

Postoperatively, management follows the same guidelines as described for stable fractures. Patients should be mobilized out of bed to chair on the 1st postoperative day. Ambulation begins the 2nd day after

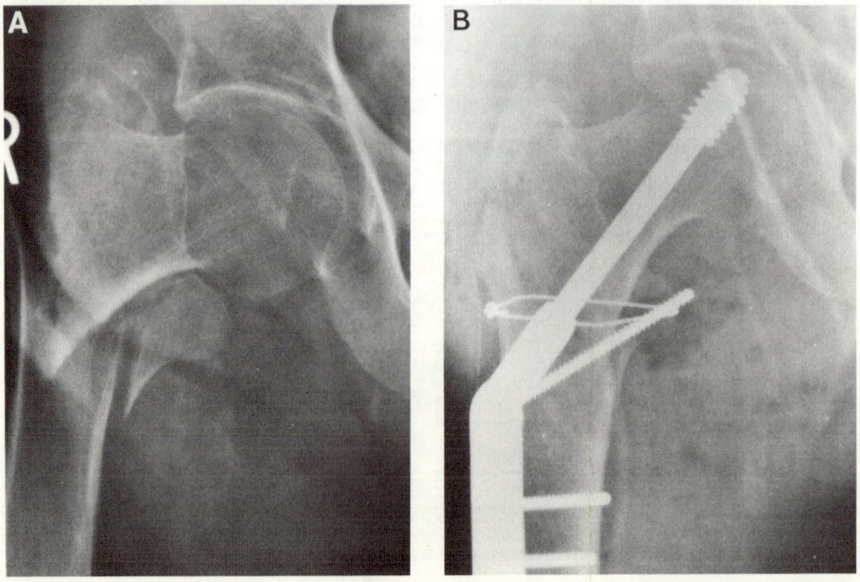

Figure 36-23. Unstable intertrochanteric fracture (*A*) in an 82-year-old female. The large posteromedial fragment was reduced to a "near-anatomic" position and fixed with a screw and cerclage wire (*B*).

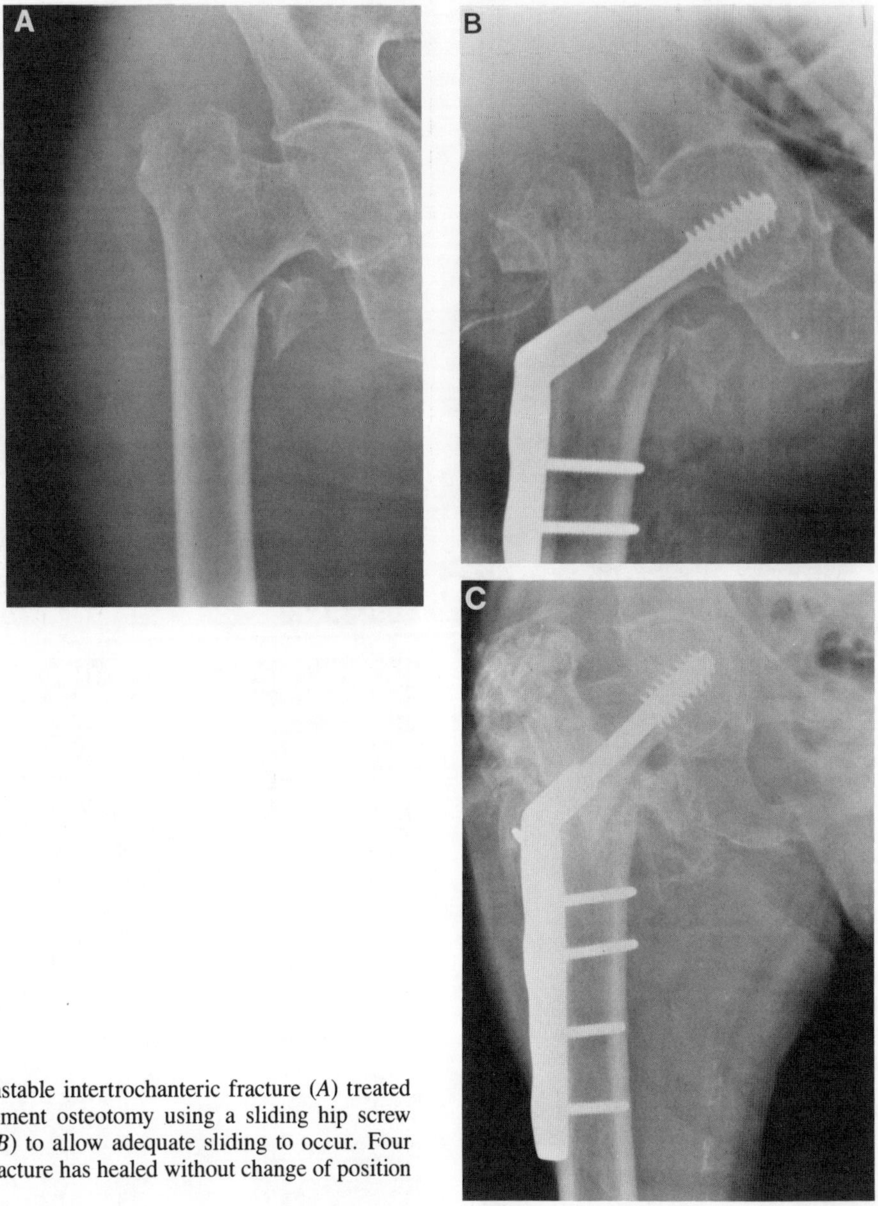

Figure 36-24. Unstable intertrochanteric fracture (*A*) treated by medial displacement osteotomy using a sliding hip screw with short barrel (*B*) to allow adequate sliding to occur. Four months later, the fracture has healed without change of position (*C*).

surgery. We allow all patients to be weight bearing as tolerated since this is most compatible with recovery of ambulation.

Complications

Complications of intertrochanteric fractures include both medical and surgical complications. These elderly patients may develop complications because of preexisting medical problems. In addition, urinary tract infections, decubiti, cardiopulmonary problems, and deep vein thrombosis occur with a frequency equal to that described for femoral neck fractures. Mortality following intertrochanteric fractures does not differ significantly from that associated with femoral neck fractures (4, 77, 197, 309). The incidence of wound infection has decreased significantly with the use of prophylactic antibiotics (132, 218, 294). Recent studies have generally reported an incidence of less than 3% (218). Risk factors for wound infection include urinary tract infection, decubitus ulcers, prolonged operative time, disorientation that interferes with proper wound care, and proximity of the incision to the perineum (17).

Complications most frequently encountered with the sliding hip screw include varus displacement of the proximal fragment, malrotation, and nonunion. Osteonecrosis, disengagement of the fixation device, and migration of the screw into the acetabulum are extremely uncommon occurrences (173, 184). Varus displacement following inter-

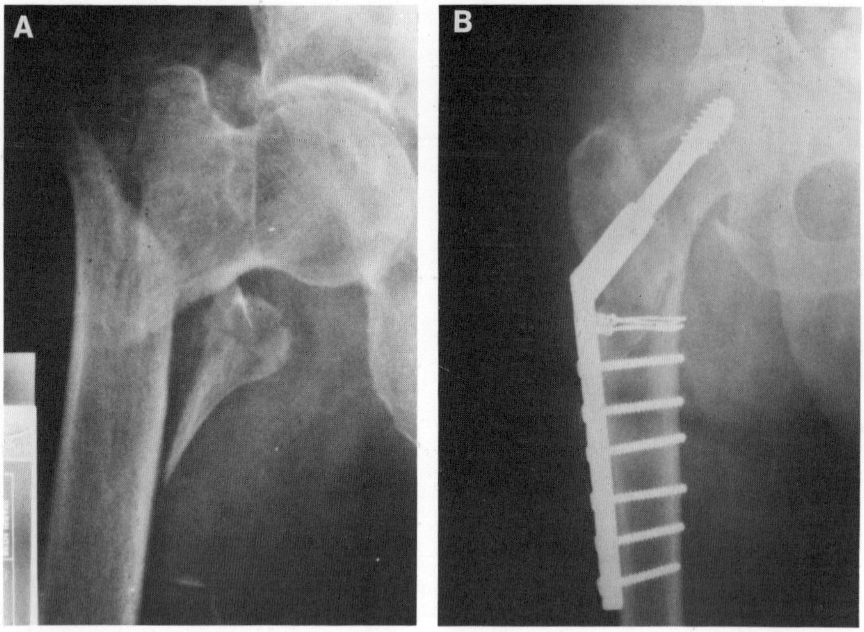

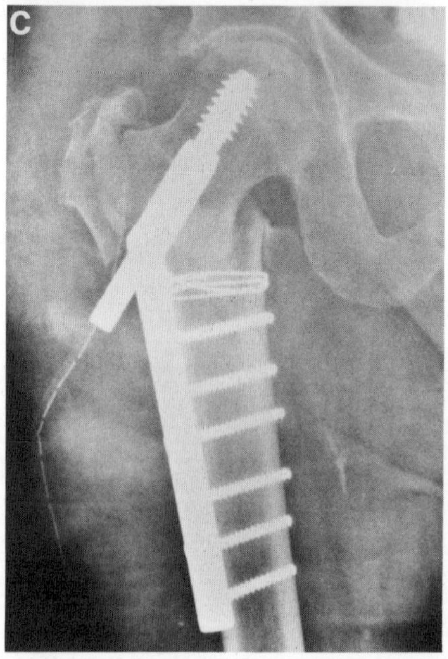

Figure 36-25. 90-year-old female with an unstable intertrochanteric fracture (*A*) treated by open reduction and internal fixation with cerclage wiring of the posteromedial fragment (*B*). Although a stable reduction was obtained at the time of surgery, additional impaction occurred postoperatively into a medial displacement position as shown on these radiographs taken 2 weeks after surgery (*C*). Additional impaction would have compromised the sliding capacity of the nail. This did not occur and the fracture healed uneventfully. (The suction drain became detached under the skin at the time of removal and was left in place).

nal fixation is associated with unstable fractures as a result of the lack of posteromedial support. Varus displacement usually results in the screw "cutting out" through the anterosuperior portion of the femoral head. This complication occurs as a result of different factors including: (*a*) placement of the screw into the anterosuperior aspect of the femoral head; (*b*) improper reaming, which creates a second channel; (*c*) inability to obtain a stable reduction; (*d*) excessive collapse of the fracture, such that the sliding capacity of the device is exceeded; (*e*) inadequate screw barrel engagement, which prevents sliding; and (*f*) severe osteoporosis, which precludes secure fixation. The best way to prevent postoperative loss of fixation and varus displacement is by achieving a stable reduction at the time of surgery with proper technical insertion of the sliding hip screw.

Malrotation deformities usually result from internal rotation of the distal fragment at the time of internal fixation of unstable fractures. This is a technical error that can be prevented with careful attention to the position of the extremity. This is different than the malrotation deformities that occur following the use of flexible intermedul-

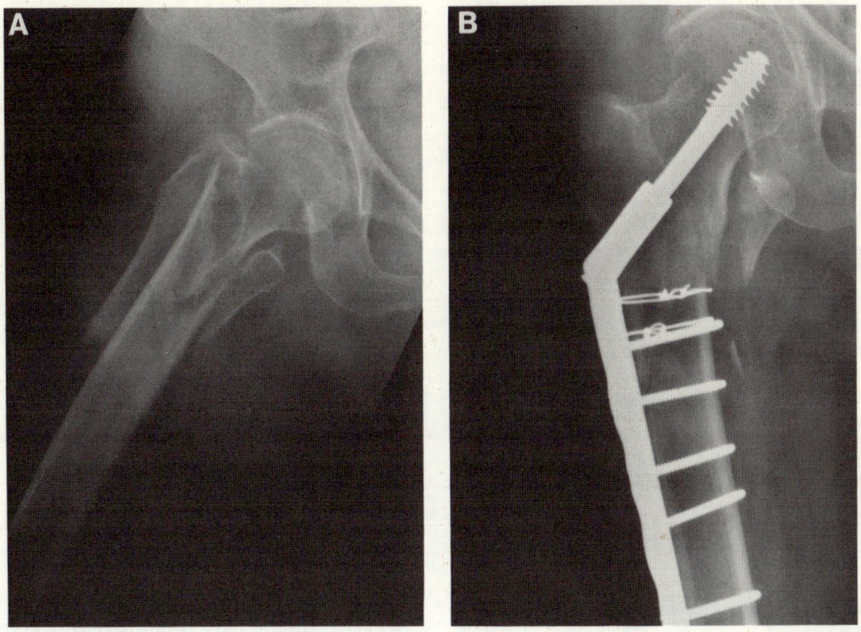

Figure 36-26. Intertrochanteric fracture with subtrochanteric extension in a 76-year-old male (*A*). Cerclage wires were used to stabilize the subtrochanteric component before insertion of a sliding hip screw with a long side plate (*B*).

lary nails, which occurs after insertion of the devices. Nonunion occurs in less than 2% of cases (185). In most elderly patients, conversion to a calcar replacement bipolar endoprosthesis is the treatment of choice.

Distal Radius Fractures

The distal radius has long been recognized as one of the most common sites of fractures in the elderly. Population-based studies of fracture frequency and distribution have shown that the rate of distal radius fractures increases dramatically with age. This increase is seen primarily in women, who show a greater than tenfold increase in fracture rate for the 55 and over age group as compared to 35- to 45-year-olds (5, 161, 219). These age-related rate changes parallel similar increases seen with proximal femur and proximal humerus fractures, and have been attributed to the effects of osteoporosis, which might be secondary to the hormonal changes of menopause (161). Also, other factors, such as the increased tendency of the elderly to fall due to poor eyesight, impaired coordination, and decreased muscular strength, have been implicated (21).

The typical distal radius fracture appearance, as described by Colles, is a shortened dorsally displaced distal radius with dorsal tilting of articular surface (Fig. 36-27) (63, 286). Many classification systems have been described for distal radius and ulna fractures. All are based on fracture geometry, degrees of displacement and comminution, and involvement of either the radiocarpal or distal radioulnar joint. One commonly used classification is that of Frykman, which is based on biomechanical and clinical studies (102) (Fig. 36-28). Types I to VIII are described, with Type I being purely extra-articular. Type III

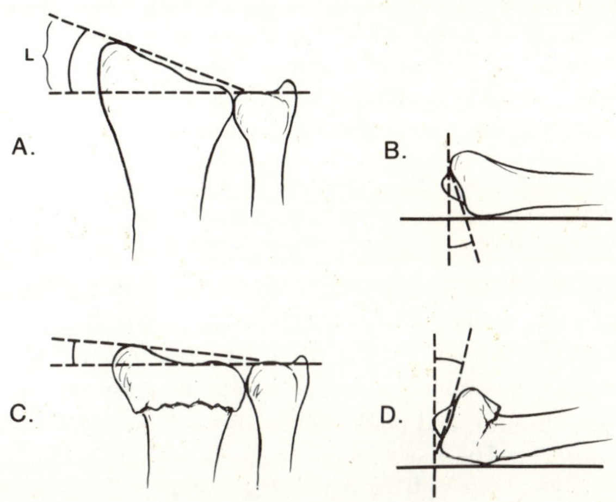

Figure 36-27. Significant radiographic measurements to determine adequacy of Colles' fracture reduction are radial length, radial inclination, and palmar tilt. Angles are measured relative to a line perpendicular to the radial shaft, at the level of the ulnar head. **A,** Normal *radial inclination* (tilt to the articular surfaces about 20 degrees as seen in the AP view. Radial length (**L**) is 1 cm distal to the ulnar head. **B,** Normal *palmar tilt* (of the articular surface) is about 10 to 15 degrees. **C,** Significant displacement and symptoms related to instability and loss of motion occur when radial length and radial inclination approach 0 or less, and the palmar tilt (**D**) of the radial articular surface is reversed to more than 10 degrees of dorsal tilt.

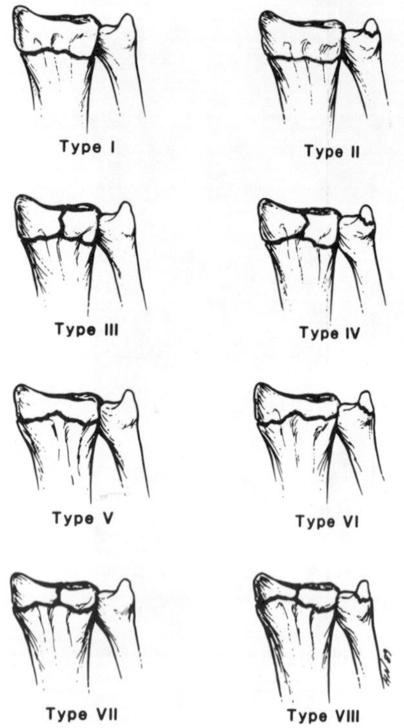

Figure 36-28. The Fryckman classification of distal radius fractures. The Type I fracture is a simple transverse fracture of the radius proximal to both the articular surface and the radial ulnar joint. Type III fracture is the same with an added intra-articular fracture line. The Type V fracture is a simple transverse fracture of the distal radius involving only the distal radioulnar joint, and a Type VII fracture involves both the intra-articular surface of the radius and the radioulnar joint. Fracture Types II through VIII are similar to Types I through VII with an additional fracture of the ulnar styloid.

has involvement of the radiocarpal joint, Type V the distal radioulnar joint, and Type VII involves both. Types II, IV, VI, and VIII correspond to Types I, III, V, and VII except that they have associated fractures of the ulnar styloid. In general, stable fractures are those with lesser degrees of comminution and displacement. Unstable fractures show marked comminution, radial shortening (usually more than 10 mm), and marked angulation of the distal radial fragment. The more severe fractures are intra-articular, involving the radiocarpal and distal radiounlar joints (Frykman Types III–VIII). Unstable and intra-articular fractures have a poorer prognosis. It has been estimated that comminuted, intra-articular fractures account for 15% to 25% of distal radius fractures seen in adults (65, 116). Also, studies show that the percentage of severe and displaced fractures in adults (all fractures combined, and Colles' fractures in particular) increases with increasing age (108, 311). Thus, the elderly account for a large portion of comminuted, intra-articular distal radius fractures.

Closed reduction and external fixation using casts and splints has been and still is considered the mainstay of treatment for distal radius fractures (223). The large majority of these fractures can be successfully treated by closed means. Reduction for distal radius fractures is assessed with anteroposterior and lateral radiographs of the wrist, specifically evaluating for restoration of normal length and angulation of the distal radius. However, reduction of these fractures can be difficult to maintain, especially in severely comminuted fractures with a poor cortical buttress, and often requires multiple reduction attempts. To achieve and maintain an adequate reduction in these unstable fractures, many operative methods have been advocated, including open reduction with internal or percutaneous fixation, various external fixator devices, and percutaneous pins incorporated in a plaster cast (Fig. 36-29).

Indications for operative fixation of distal radius fractures include open fractures, fractures with associated neurovascular compromise, inability to maintain an adequate reduction by nonoperative methods, and severely comminuted and displaced intra-articular fractures. Open reduction with internal plate fixation or percutaneous K-wire fixation is more commonly done in younger patients with displaced intra-articular fractures, where anatomic restoration of the joint surface is believed to decrease the incidence of late radiocarpal arthritis. In the elderly, although a congruous joint surface is important, shortening of the radius correlates best with a poor functional result. Therefore, the main goal of treatment is to maintain radial length and alignment (302). This is easily achieved by tension across the wrist by means of external skeletal fixation, relying on the soft tissue envelope of the wrist for the maintenance of the reduction. Bohler first described using external skeletal fixation for comminuted distal radius fractures in 1929 (29). Vidal coined the term *ligamentotaxis* (301), reporting that this method worked best for fractures about the wrist. Many orthopaedic surgeons have reported excellent results using various methods, all relying on this same principle of soft-tissue distraction and stabilization of the fracture.

The variations on the "pins and plaster" technique are the result of different pin placements used by different surgeons. All utilize one pin proximal (either radius or ulna) and one distal (in the metacarpals) to the fracture site incorporated in a short or long arm plaster cast. The method of Green (116) will serve as an example of this technique. After adequate general or regional anesthesia, linear traction is applied across the wrist using wire finger traps on the thumb and index fingers and 5 to 10 pounds of counter-traction to the arm. Gentle manipulation is performed, and radiographs are taken to confirm anatomic length of the radius. The hand and forearm are then prepped and draped. Smooth Steinmann pins, 2.3 mm in

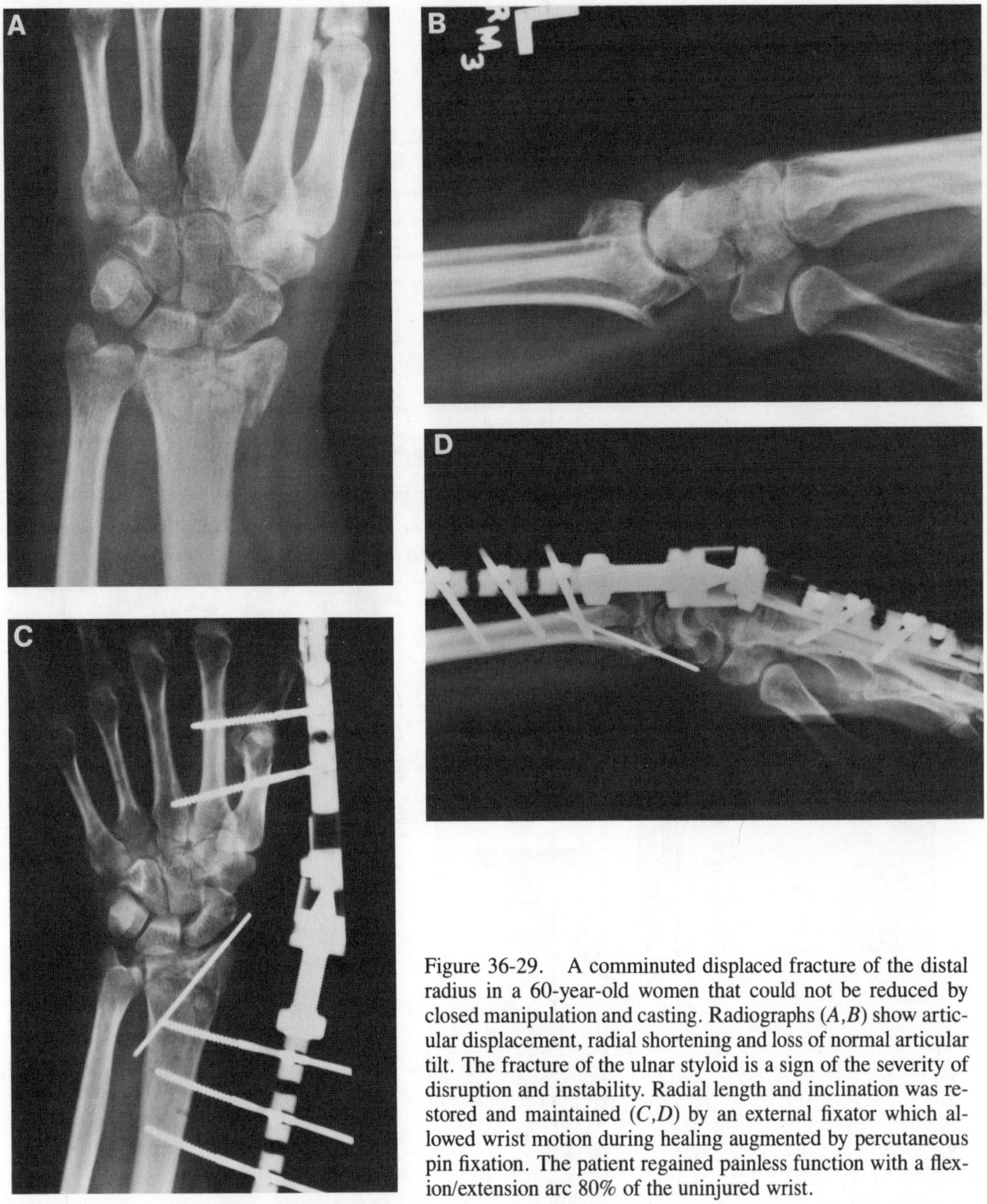

Figure 36-29. A comminuted displaced fracture of the distal radius in a 60-year-old women that could not be reduced by closed manipulation and casting. Radiographs (*A,B*) show articular displacement, radial shortening and loss of normal articular tilt. The fracture of the ulnar styloid is a sign of the severity of disruption and instability. Radial length and inclination was restored and maintained (*C,D*) by an external fixator which allowed wrist motion during healing augmented by percutaneous pin fixation. The patient regained painless function with a flexion/extension arc 80% of the uninjured wrist.

diameter, are used. The distal pin is placed in the second metacarpal just distal to the flare at its base, and is advanced so that it engages only the second and third metacarpals before exiting the skin dorsal to the other metacarpals. The thumb is adducted during pin placement to avoid injury to or contracture of the first interosseous muscle. The pin is bent dorsally where it enters the skin radially to allow for full range of motion of the thumb. The proximal pin is then inserted through the ulna from medial to lateral at least 6 cm distal to the olecranon tip. Tenting of the skin around the pin sites should be adequately released. Sterile cast padding is placed over the pin sites, and a short arm plaster cast is applied incorporating the pins with the wrist in neutral while traction is maintained. Final roentgenograms confirm the position of the pins and the fracture. The cast is then generously trimmed to allow unrestricted motion of the thumb, fingers, and elbow. At least 8 weeks of immobilization are thought to be needed for stabilization of a severely comminuted fracture. One variation on this method used at our hospital is placement of the metacarpal and proximal pins first (we use a radial half-pin), then applying traction via a sterilized traction bow attached to the distal pin with arm countertraction. Pin placement and reduction is then assessed by intraoperative roentgenogram prior to cast placement.

More recently, many orthopaedists have been using external fixator devices in place of a plaster cast (65, 66, 68, 207, 229, 301). This method allows for easy access to the skin and soft tissues, as might be needed in the case of an open fracture or associated soft-tissue injury. Various different frames and configurations are currently being used. Nakata studied the rigidity of four external fixators currently used, and found the small AO fixator to be twice as rigid as the other three (Ace-Colles, Roger Anderson, and mini Hoffman) (207). Cooney retrospectively examined results of four commonly used frames (not including the AO frame) and found satisfactory results in a majority of patients, independent of the type of fixator used (66). Pin type, pin placement, and frame configurations differ with the various fixators. Some are linear, such as the Hoffman C-series fixator, which utilizes two parallel pins in the second and third metacarpals and two parallel pins in the radius connected by a single bar (Fig. 36-30). The small AO fixator is a flattened quadrilateral configuration with four pins, two pins each placed parallel to the frame in the second metacarpal and radius, converging at an angle of 40 to 50 degrees to one another to increase their

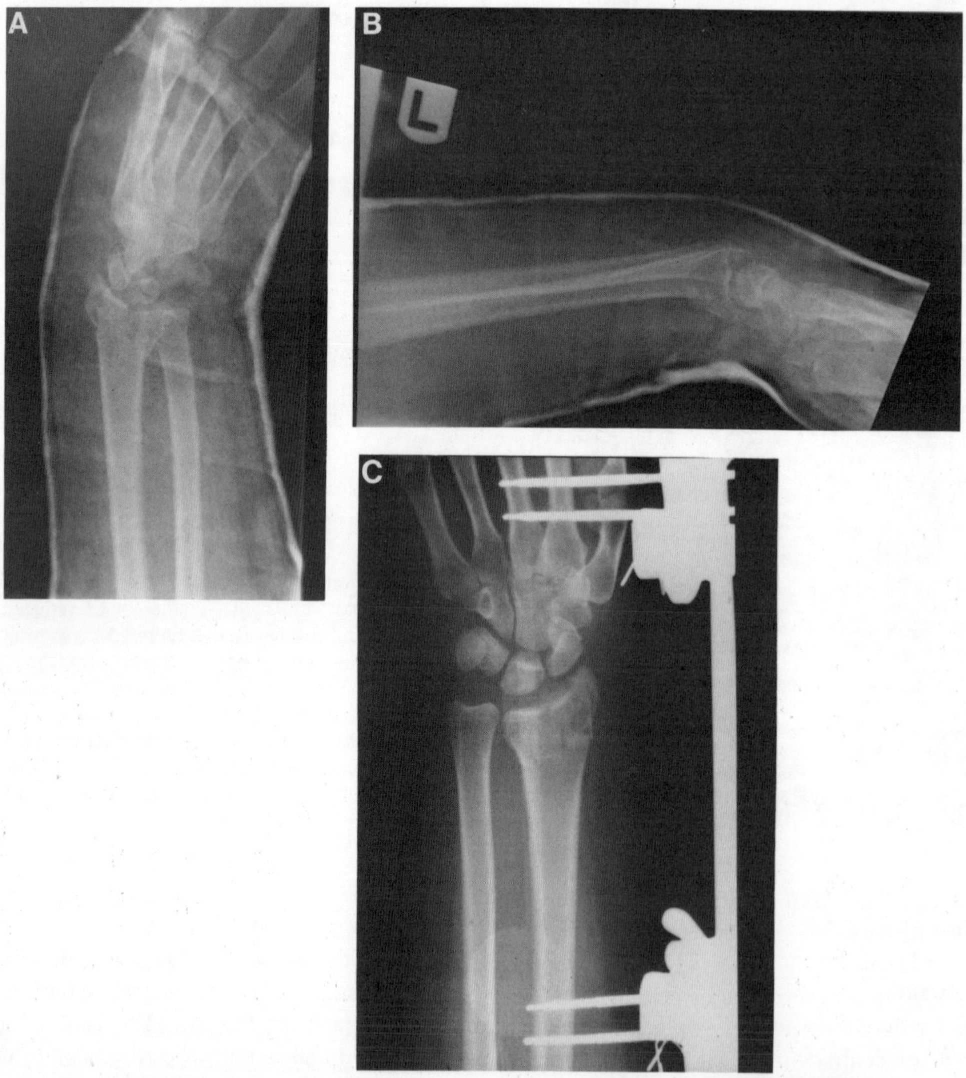

Figure 36-30. A severely comminuted fracture of the distal radius in a 63-year-old female. Pre-reduction radiographs (*A*,*B*) show residual volar angulation and shortening of the distal radius. The articular surface of the radius is also shown to be severely displaced. After reduction (*C*,*D*) with ligamentotaxis and application of external fixator, excellent alignment and radial length is achieved. Six weeks later (*E*,*F*), the patient has completely healed the fracture, and is ready for removal of external fixator.

holding power in the bone. Rectangular configurations, with pins placed at an angle to the rectangle, are used in the Roger Anderson, Ace-Colles, and mini Hoffman fixators.

Using these different skeletal fixation techniques, authors have reported good to excellent results in 70% to 90% of patients (66, 68, 116, 186, 207). In all of these studies, only patients with severely comminuted, unstable radius fractures were examined. However, closed treatment for similar fractures has not been reported for comparison. In Sarmiento's series, only six "severe" fractures were treated closed with functional cast bracing; 50% had good to excellent results (254). Fryckman reported good to excellent results in 75% of cases in his series, but noted poorer results for the subset of intra-articular fractures and fractures with residual shortening (102). It is the belief of the surgeons who perform external skeletal fixation for these unstable fractures, that this distraction ligamentotaxis achieves a more anatomic radial length than conventional closed treatment, and thus better functional results.

High complication rates have been reported for these severe wrist fractures treated with external fixation (50, 66, 67, 68, 116). Chapman et al. reviewed eighty cases of distal radius fractures treated by pins and plaster using Green's method (50). They reported 10 cases of carpal tunnel syndrome, 6 of which resolved spontaneously and 4 of which required surgical decompression. Pin tract complications were seen in one-third of patients. Pin loosening was most common (21%); more than half of these patients lost more than 5 mm of radial length when compared to the initial postoperative radiographs. Iatrogenic fractures occurred in 9% of cases (3 metacarpal, 4 ulnar), all of which were treated closed. Twenty percent of pins developed drainage, and 9% were diagnosed as pin tract osteomyelitis. In all, 16% required reoperation (for carpal tunnel syndrome, pin replacement, or sequestrectomy) or extended treatment in long arm casts. Cooney reported complications in 34% of patients treated by external fixation (66). Pin tract problems were seen in 14%, while carpal tunnel syndrome, reflex sympathetic dystrophy (RSD), arthrofibrosis, loss of reduction, and post-traumatic arthrosis were each found in 3% to 5% of patients. Three of the five cases of RSD, clearly the most serious complication, were associated with painful pin sites. Other complications reported included broken pins, delayed extensor pollicis longus tendon rupture, contracture of the third interosseus muscle, finger stiffness, Volk-

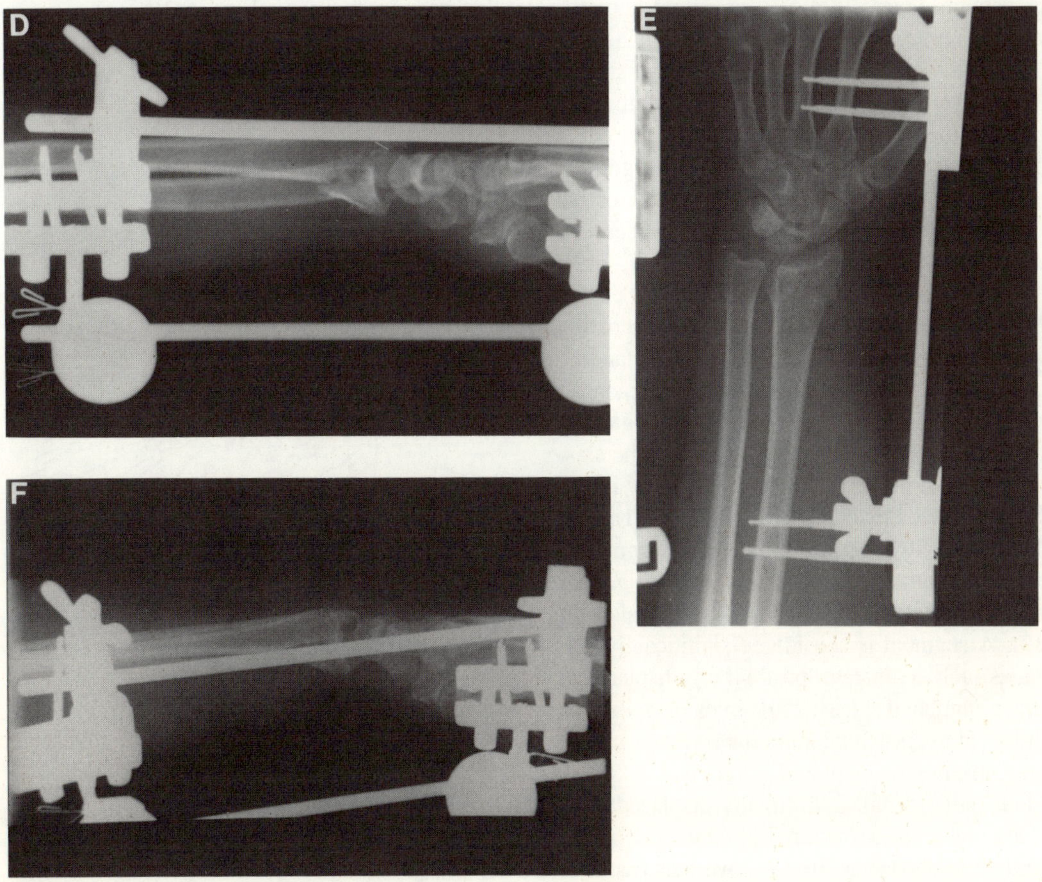

man's ischemia, and unrecognized associated injuries (67, 68, 207). Clearly, complications due to the operative procedure, such as pin loosening, infection, and iatrogenic fractures must be separated from complications of the injury itself, which are also seen in patients treated nonoperatively, such as carpal tunnel syndrome, tendon rupture, and RSD, when assessing complication rates for the specific treatment method.

In the elderly population, the overall level of function is often steadily declining. Any measure to improve the functional result of severely comminuted distal radius fractures in this population is very desirable. The large majority of these fractures continue to be successfully treated by closed reduction and cast immobilization. However, the use of external skeletal fixation, with reported good to excellent results of up to 85%, is becoming increasingly popular at our institution and throughout the orthopaedic community for the treatment of unstable, comminuted distal radius fractures in the elderly. Clearly, care in surgical technique must be taken to prevent complications of the procedure, but, in general, good results following this difficult fracture can be expected.

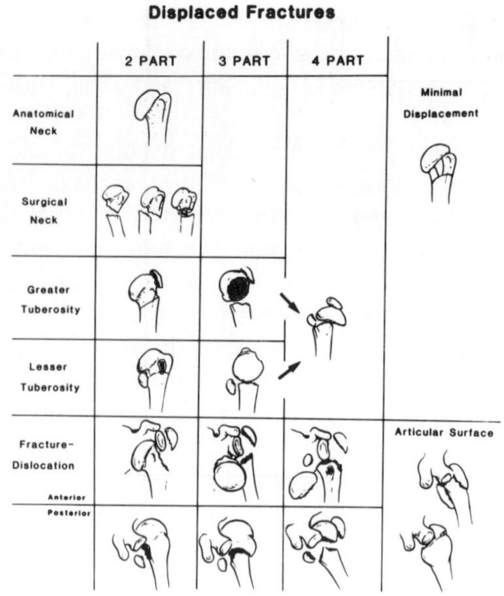

Figure 36-31. Neer classification of proximal humeral fractures (Modified from Neer, CS. 1970. Displaced proximal humeral fractures: I. Classification and evaluation. *J Bone Joint Surg* 52A:1077–1089.)

Proximal Humerus Fractures

In younger patients (ages 20 to 50), proximal humerus fractures are uncommon. Studies estimate their incidence to be approximately 40 per 100,000 person-years for the 40- to 49-year-old group (243). In this age group, they are more commonly the result of severe trauma, and occur equally in men and women. In the over 50 age groups, incidence rates rise dramatically, reaching peaks of 112 and 439 fractures per 100,000 person-years in men and women respectively for the 80+ age groups (137, 242). In people 75 and over, the proximal humerus is the third most common site of fracture (161), most often occurring secondary to minimal trauma, such as a fall from standing height. Only distal forearm and proximal femur fractures are more common. All three show the epidemiologic features of fractures associated with osteoporosis. The classification of proximal humerus fractures currently in use was described by Neer in 1970 (210) (Fig. 36-31). The proximal humerus is divided into four specific segments: (*a*) humeral head (with the articular surface), (*b*) greater tuberosity, (*c*) lesser tuberosity, and (*d*) humeral shaft (Fig. 36-32). A segment is considered significantly displaced (and, as such, a separate "part") if it is displaced at least 1.0 cm or angulated at least 45 degrees from its anatomic position. Thus, proximal humerus fractures can be described as minimally displaced ("one-part"), two-, three-, or four-part fractures. Minimally displaced fractures may have one or many fracture lines, but no segment is significantly displaced (Fig. 36-33). Two-part fractures occur at the anatomic neck, the surgical neck (Fig. 36-34), or the greater (Fig. 36-35) or lesser tuberosities. In three-part fractures (Fig. 36-36), one of the tuberosities remains in contact with the humeral head while the other is displaced, along with a surgical neck fracture. In four-part fractures (Fig. 36-37), all major segments are dis-

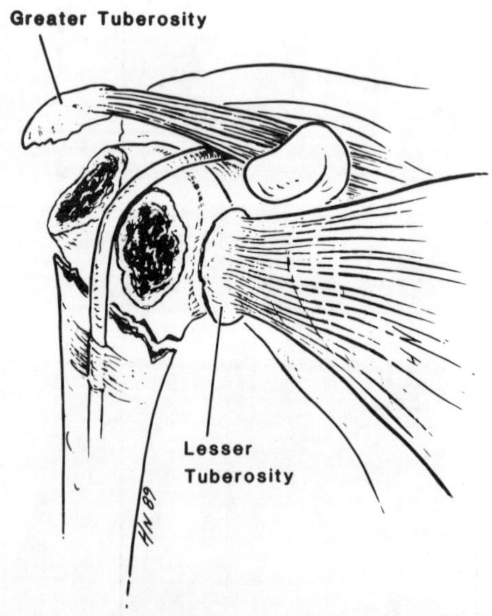

Figure 36-32. The four segments of the proximal humerus include the humeral head, greater tuberosity, lesser tuberosity, and humeral shaft. Lesser tuberosity fractures are displaced medially by the subscapularis. Greater tuberosity fractures are displaced superomedially or posteromedially by the supraspinatus or infraspinatus.

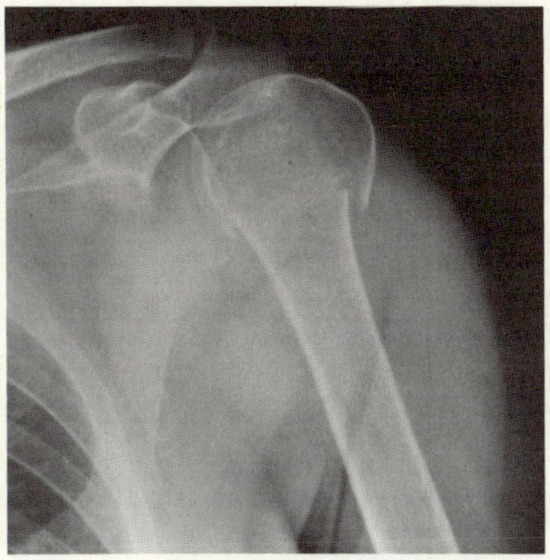

Figure 36-33. Although multiple fracture lines are evident, absence of significant displacement or angulation of the segments classifies this as a "one-part" fracture.

placed. Fracture-dislocations may also be two-, three-, or four-part. Anterior fracture-dislocations are always associated with greater tuberosity displacement, while posterior fracture-dislocations always have displacement of the lesser tuberosity (Fig. 36-38). Articular surface fractures make up the final group in this classification. These may be impression fractures, seen with acute or chronic dislocations, or "head-splitting" fractures, resulting from central impaction of the head on the glenoid. Fracture-dislocations and articular surface fractures are more commonly encountered in association with severe trauma, and are less frequently seen in the elderly.

The Neer classification is useful because it forms a basis for treatment of proximal humerus fractures. Minimally displaced fractures (Fig. 36-33), which account for 80% to 85% of all proximal humerus fractures, are usually stabilized by the intact surrounding soft tissue and periosteum or are impacted, so that early functional exercises can be instituted after a brief period of immobilization. In two-part fractures, closed reduction is often possible, followed by about 3 weeks of immobilization and initiation of a range of motion exercise program. However, specific types of two-part fractures require further discussion. Displaced anatomic neck fractures are often treated nonoperatively unless displacement is severe, in which case open reduction will be necessary. If osteonecrosis or a painful malunion results, prosthetic replacement may be indicated. Isolated lesser tuberosity displacement usually does not require open reduction, unless the fragment contains a large portion of the articular surface or blocks internal rotation. Isolated greater tuberosity displacements are associated with longitudinal rotator cuff tears, and require open reduction, internal fixation, and repair of the rotator cuff tear. This can be accomplished through a deltoid-splitting approach (213). Internal fixation of the greater tuberosity fragment can be accomplished by tension band suture or wire or screw fixation, depending on bone quality (Fig. 36-35).

Displaced surgical neck fractures can be either impacted and angulated (Fig. 36-39), separated (Fig. 36-34), or comminuted. All are treated by initial closed reduction, often under anesthesia and fluoroscopic evalua-

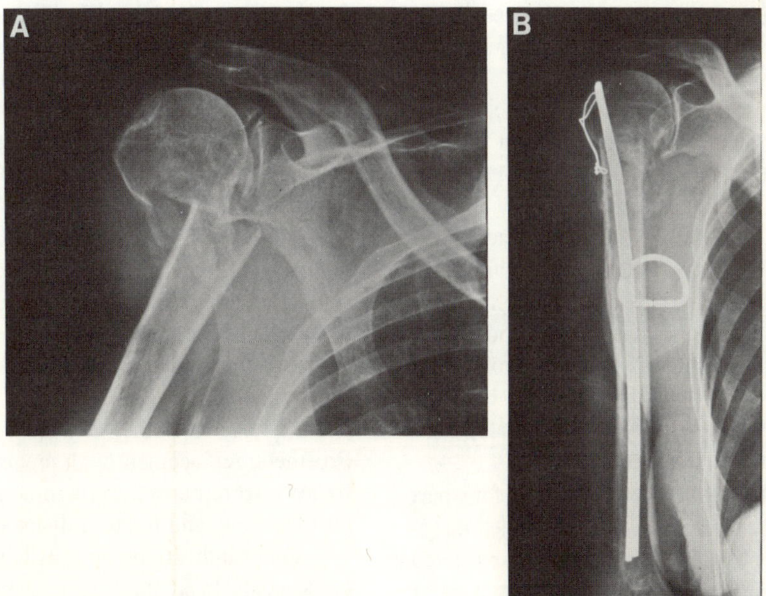

Figure 36-34. Completely displaced surgical neck fracture in a 68-year-old female (*A*). Four weeks following open reduction, Ender nailing and tension band wiring, callus formation is evident (*B*).

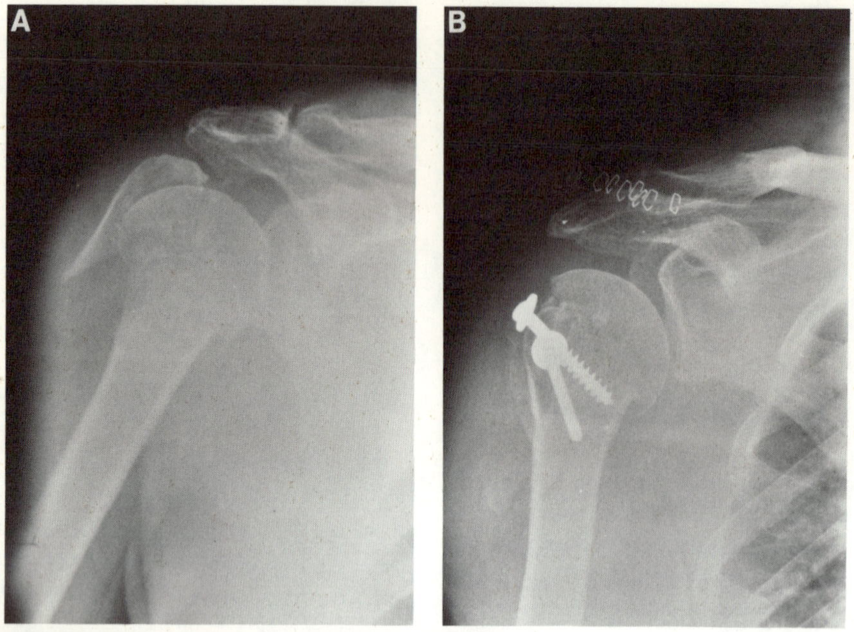

Figure 36-35. 66-year-old male sustained this displaced greater tuberosity fracture with a minimally displaced surgical neck fracture (*A*). Open reduction and screw fixation was performed (*B*). The longitudinal tear in the rotator cuff was repaired and mersilene tape was added as a tension band passed through the rotator cuff tendon and around the screw.

tion. If an acceptable and stable reduction is achieved, Velpeau immobilization should be used for about 3 weeks followed by a range of motion program (Fig. 36-39). If the reduction is unacceptable or unstable, internal fixation will be necessary. Neer recommends percutaneous pin fixation for 3 weeks, using a threaded Steinmann pin inserted anteriorly through the deltopectoral interval into the shaft and head (213). Intramedullary devices (Rush rods or Ender nails) may also be inserted in either an antegrade or retrograde manner (169).

If a two-part surgical neck fracture cannot be reduced by closed manipulation, open reduction will be necessary. A deltopectoral approach is used, and, after reduction, internal fixation is performed using a tension band figure-eight wire or suture around anterograde intramedullary fixation such as Rush rods or Ender nails (Fig. 36-34). A T-plate can also be used, but screw fixation in osteoporotic bone in the elderly is often suboptimal. Therefore, plate and screw fixation should be avoided for these fractures in the elderly with osteoporotic bone. A modified Zickel-type intramedullary device has also been used successfully for these fractures (204).

Results of closed treatment of three and four-part fractures have generally been poor. Neer examined three- and four-part fractures and fracture-dislocations treated closed, and reported satisfactory results in only 3 of 31 cases (211). These results were confirmed by Stableforth in both retrospective and prospective studies (280). Leyshon reported satisfactory results in over two-thirds of three-part fractures treated closed, but no satisfactory results in four-part fractures (172). He noted that satisfactory results tended to be in an older age group with fewer functional demands. The currently recommended treatment for displaced three-part fractures is open reduction and internal fixation through a deltopectoral approach, using either wire or nonabsorbable suture for tension band fixation (Figs. 36-36 and 36-40). Other methods that have been used include a tension band with intramedullary fixation, plate and screw fixation, or use of a modified Zickel device (58, 204, 211, 213). For elderly patients with three-part fracture-dislocations, prosthetic replacement with repair of the tuberosities and rotator cuff is generally preferred (213, 293).

For four-part fractures, results of open reduction and internal fixation have also been poor either because of loss of fixation or development of osteonecrosis (211). Although Mouradian reports good results using a modified Zickel device for four-part fractures and fracture-dislocations, he recommends this procedure only in "young, healthy patients whose reliability is judged above average" (204). Prosthetic replacement with repair of the tuberosities and rotator cuff remains the recommended procedure for four-part fractures and fracture-dislocations (Fig. 36-37).

Other indications for prosthetic hemiarthroplasty include acute head-splitting fractures or impression fractures that comprise greater than 40% of the articular surface and chronic fracture problems such as painful malunion with articular incongruity, osteonecrosis with

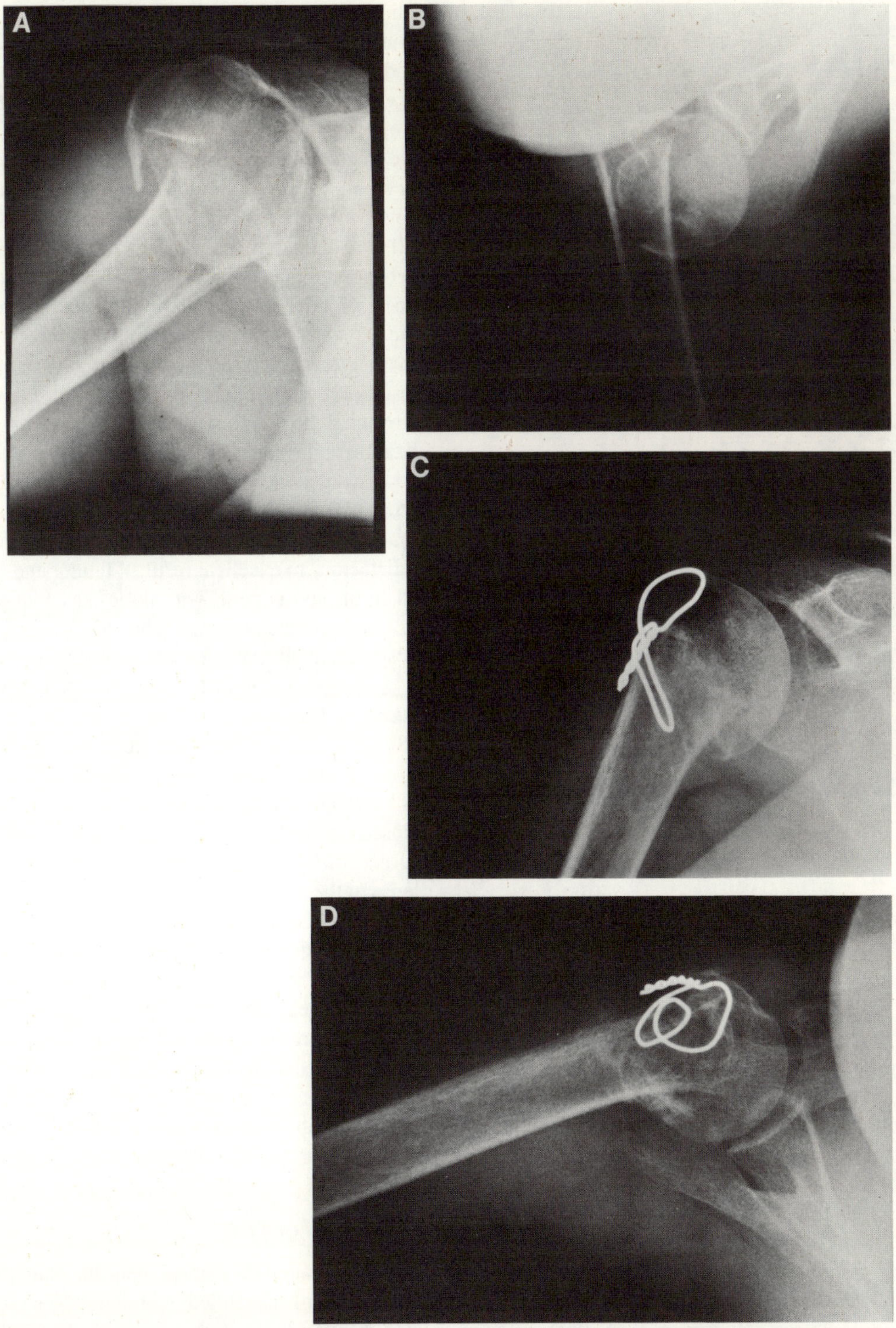

Figure 36-36. 69-year-old female with three part fracture with displaced greater tuberosity segment (*A,B*). Open reduction and tension band wiring was performed. Four months later, the fracture has healed in good position (*C,D*).

subchondral collapse and pain, and nonunion of surgical neck fractures with small, osteoporotic head fragments. The procedure can be performed through a long deltopectoral incision. The acromial and clavicular origins of the deltoid should not be disturbed. Adequate exposure can usually be obtained by abduction of the arm, but, if additional exposure is needed, the deltoid insertion on the humerus and/or the superior 1 cm of the pectoralis major

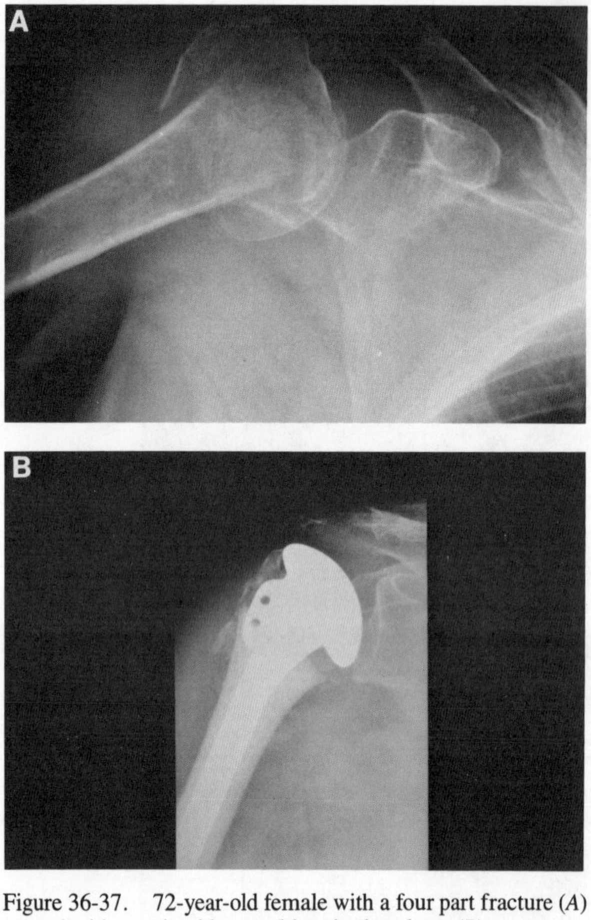

Figure 36-37. 72-year-old female with a four part fracture (*A*) treated with proximal humeral hemiarthroplasty (*B*).

insertion can be incised. Both should be repaired as part of closure. The fracture fragments are identified, taking care not to disturb the remaining soft tissue attachments. The humeral shaft can be prepared for the prosthesis. Care must be taken to maintain humeral length. Shortening of the humerus leads to deltoid weakness, inferior subluxation, and compromise of the operative result. The prosthesis should be placed in 30 to 40 degrees of retroversion. Cement is usually necessary for adequate stabilization of the prosthetic stem within the shaft. The tuberosities are then secured to the prosthesis and the humeral shaft using heavy nonabsorbable suture. Bone grafting may be necessary in cases of severe comminution to bridge a gap between the tuberosities and the shaft. The rotator cuff should be securely repaired, and the wound closed over suction drains. Early passive motion exercises are begun to prevent formation of adhesions. Active motion exercises should not be started for at least 6 to 8 weeks until the tuberosities have healed.

Regardless of the treatment method, elderly patients with displaced proximal humerus fractures require supervised physical therapy to optimize the functional results. The final outcome depends on the severity of the initial injury, the treatment method chosen, and the cooperation and motivation of the patient. Patients with minimally displaced fractures generally obtain good functional results. However, the disability time may be prolonged. Although the fracture may be clinically healed in 6 weeks, recovery of a painless arc of motion may take up to 6 months. Recovery of strength and coordination may take even longer (213). Adequately reduced two-part fractures can also expect good functional results (172). Poor results are usually due to inadequate repair of the rotator cuff (seen with greater tuberosity avulsions), nonunions, and malunions. In three-part fractures, Neer reported 19 of 30 satisfactory results for open reduction and internal fixation (211). He attributed the poor results to technical errors in tuberosity fixation and rotator cuff repair. Others have also reported good results with internal fixation for three-part fractures (204). Results for prosthetic replacement in three- and four-part fractures are quite good. Neer reported 39 of 43 satisfactory to excellent results. Tanner and Cofield found all 16 of their patients with three- and four-part fractures to have satisfactory pain relief (293). Active abduction postoperatively averaged 101 degrees.

Various complications are associated with proximal humerus fractures and their treatment (204, 211, 213, 280, 293). Joint stiffness due to bursal and capsular adhesions or articular incongruity occurs frequently. Nonunion of surgical neck fractures is often encountered following closed treatment (Fig. 36-41). It can also occur following surgery if fixation is inadequate. Osteonecrosis with collapse of the articular surface can result from two-part anatomic neck fractures and three- or four-part fractures (Fig. 36-42). Infections can occur following operative treatment. Malunion is more commonly seen following nonoperative treatment (Fig. 36-43), but can be found following operative treatment if loss of fixation occurs. Neurologic deficits of the axillary, median, radial, and ulnar nerves can occur as a result of the initial injury. Finally, myositis ossificans can occur, and is most often seen following fracture-dislocations of the proximal humerus.

Pathologic Fractures

Improved palliative management for patients with metastatic cancer has resulted in prolonged survival, but it has also resulted in an increased incidence of skeletal metastases and their complications. This is most evident in the elderly, where a growing population is experiencing a rising frequency of pathologic fractures secondary to metastatic disease, as well as from primary bone tumors, tumor-like lesions, and metabolic bone disease. Management of these different types of pathologic fractures follows similar principles, which are outlined below.

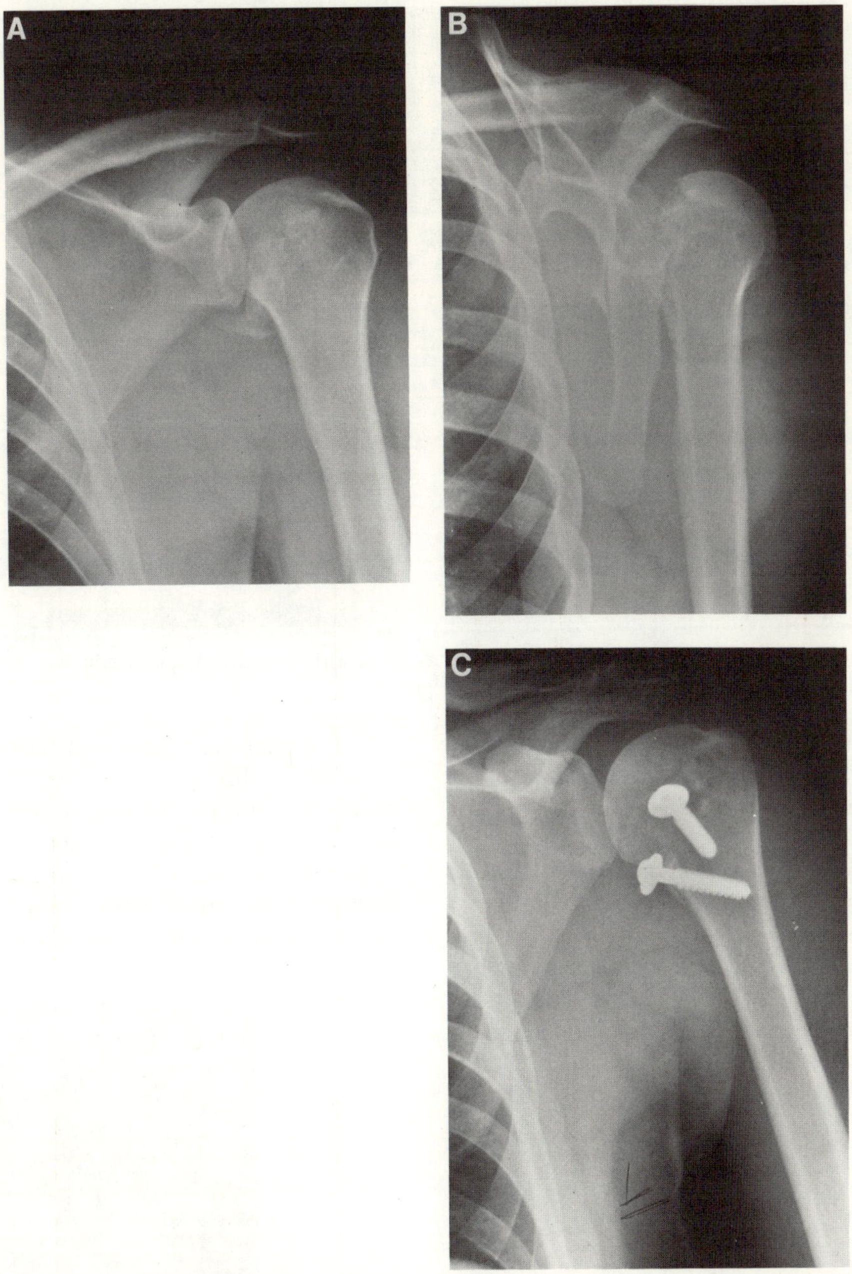

Figure 36-38. This two part posterior fracture-dislocation was recognized six days after injury (*A,B*). Following closed reduction, the shoulder was unstable. Open reduction and screw fixation of the lesser tuberosity fragment was performed to restore stability (*C*).

Pathologic fractures and impending fractures secondary to metastatic neoplasms are all too common in the geriatric population. Primary tumor sites that commonly metastasize to bone include breast, prostate, kidney, lung, thyroid, and stomach. Other cancers, including melanoma, uterus, cervix, adrenal, bladder, and testicular may also metastasize to bone (26). Tumors not of bone cell origin that occur in bone are myeloma and lymphoma. Most metastases are either osteolytic or mixed osteolytic-osteoblastic. Pure osteoblastic lesions are seen in prostatic adenocarcinoma, Hodgkin's disease, and carcinoid tumor. Although these blastic lesions are radiodense, they also weaken the structural integrity of the bone by disrupting the normal cortical anatomy and stress transmission. They predispose to pathologic fracture just slightly less than the osteolytic foci (122).

Bony metastases are most commonly found in the axial skeleton and proximal region of long bones. (Spinal metastases and their management will be discussed in the section on spinal surgery.) Of the long bones, the proxi-

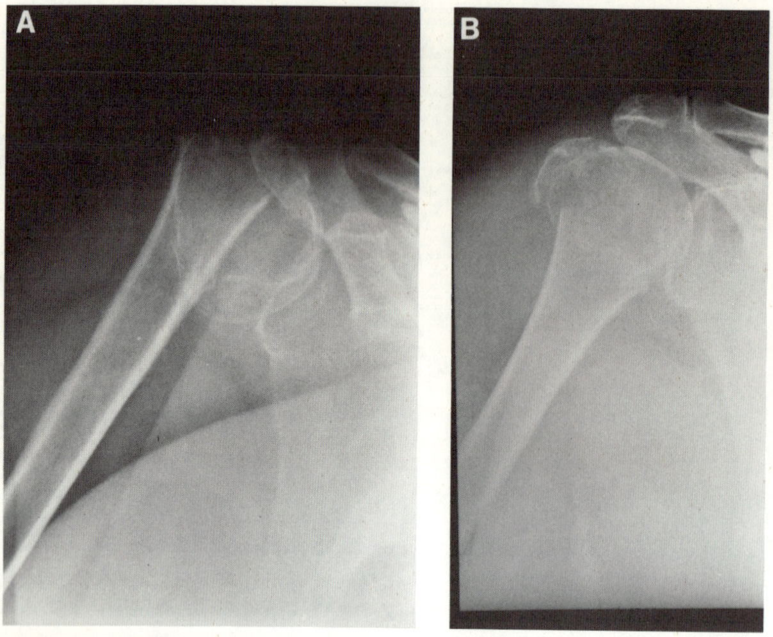

Figure 36-39. 71-year-old female with impacted and angulated surgical neck fracture (*A*). A closed reduction was performed (*B*). Mild residual displacement of the greater tuberosity was felt to be acceptable.

mal femur is by far the most commonly involved site. Other frequent locations include the femoral shaft, acetabulum, and humerus. Much less commonly, the tibia and forearm may be involved.

Long bone skeletal metastases most often present with pain. Pain is seen in two-thirds of patients with radiographically detectable lesions, but it may begin even before the lesion becomes detectable on standard radiographs (104). Pain associated with a large lesion may represent microfracture and indicate an impending fracture. Hypercalcemia is also encountered and is due to rapid bone destruction by tumor. It is usually treated by a calcium diuresis using saline, diuretics, or chemotherapeutic agents such as mithramycin, steroids, or neutral phosphates (104).

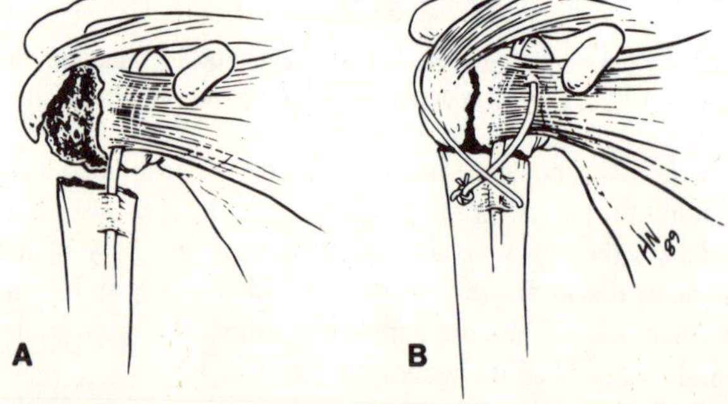

Figure 36-40. Technique of tension band wiring as described by Hawkins et al. for three part fractures (*A*). We prefer heavy nonabsorbable suture (No. 5 mersilene tape) over wire because it is easier to handle and tie (*B*).

The treatment of pathologic fractures caused by bony metastases is based on palliation. Resection for cure is done only for the rare isolated metastasis of an occult primary thyroid or renal carcinoma (26). The primary treatment goals are relief of pain and rapid return of function of the involved extremity. Radiation therapy is often used to treat painful metastatic lesions. Dosages depend on pa-

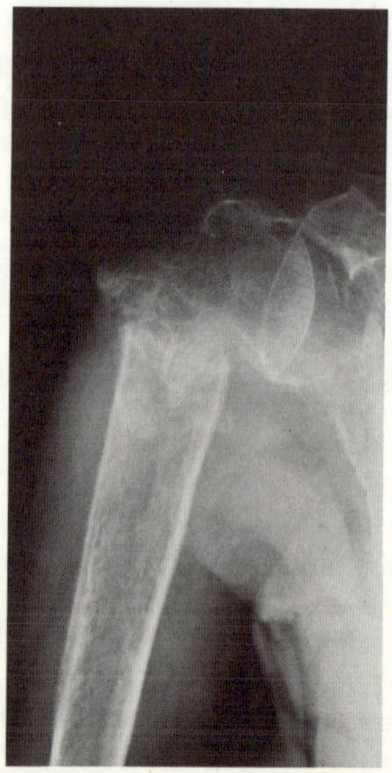

Figure 36-41. Atrophic nonunion of a surgical neck fracture. Note the marked osteoporosis of the proximal fragment.

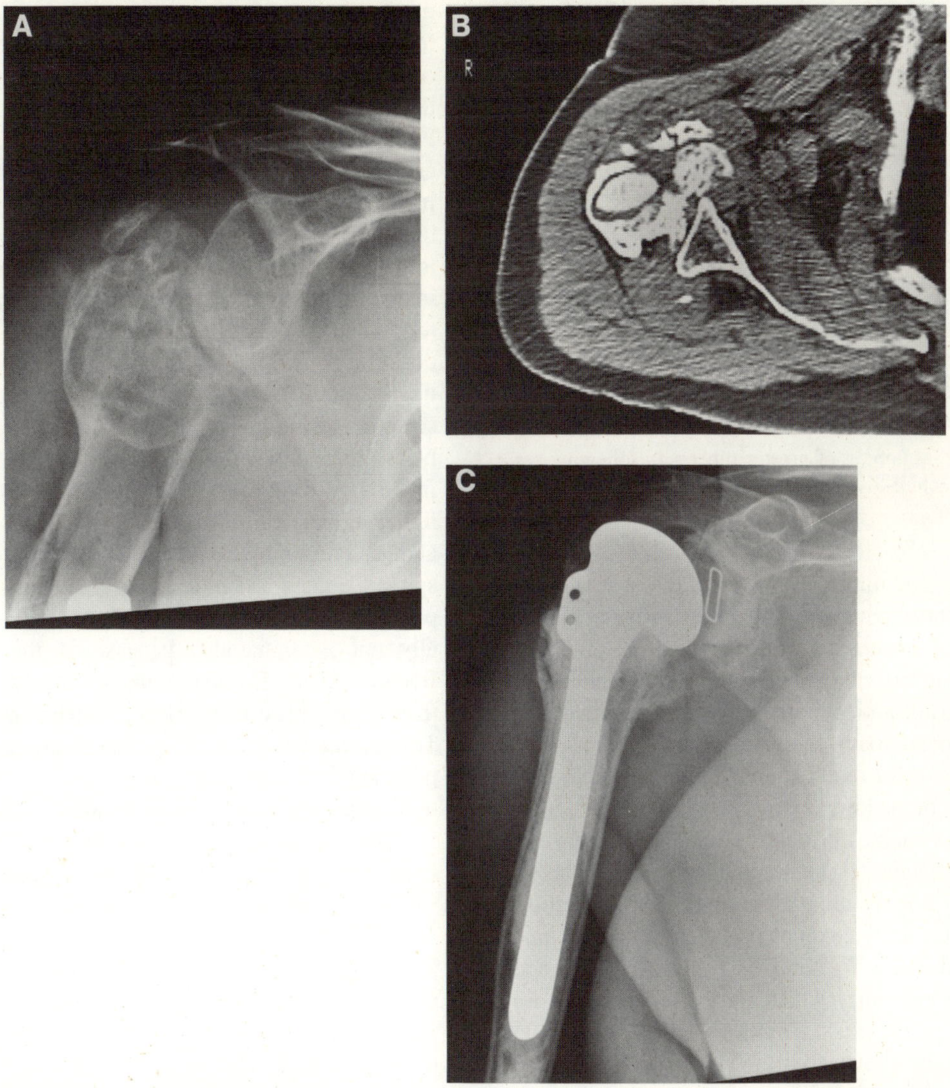

Figure 36-42. Osteonecrosis and collapse 14 months after open reduction of a four part anterior fracture-dislocation (*A*). Note the sequestrated appearance of the humeral head on CT scan (*B*). Total shoulder arthroplasty was performed because of severe pain and disability (*C*).

tient age, general condition, tumor type, and the extent of bony involvement. However, radiation produces a hyperemic response in the bone, maximal at 10 to 14 days, which actually weakens it, making it more susceptible to pathologic fracture. Radiation also disrupts the normal fracture healing process by interrupting the radiosensitive chondrogenesis step required for fracture healing by callus. Two thousand rads have been shown to control tumor progression at the site of pathologic fracture, but also have prevented bony union unless rigid internal fixation has been performed (32). Rigid internal fixation allows primary osteosynthesis, thus bypassing chondrogenesis and callus formation (32).

Studies of survival after pathologic fracture secondary to metastatic disease clearly indicate that it does not necessarily represent an impending terminal event. The mean survival after pathologic fracture in one series was 10.1 months (103). Twenty-three percent of patients survived more than 1 year. Survival in patients with bony metastases, especially secondary to breast cancer, can be prolonged. In a study of patients with disseminated breast cancer metastases limited to the skeleton, the median survival was 33 months and 5-year actuarial survival was 45% (267). In this group, aggressive management of pathologic fractures is certainly indicated.

Nonoperative management of pathologic fractures relies on immobilization of the injured part. In the upper extremity, the result is loss of use of one arm; for the lower extremity, this often means bed rest and traction. Nonunions are common, especially when radiotherapy is used

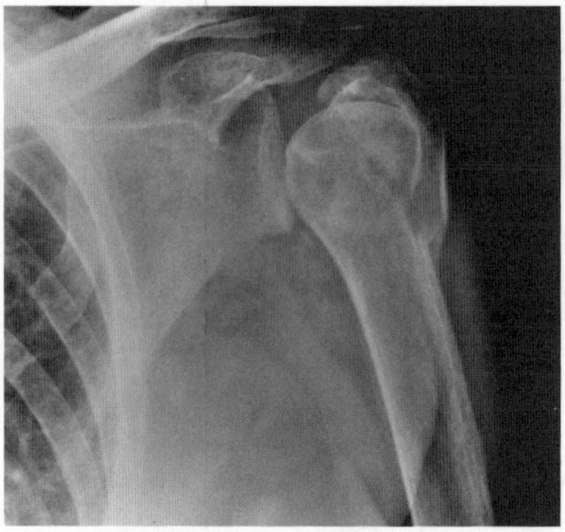

Figure 36-43. Malunion of greater tuberosity following two-part anterior fracture-dislocation resulting in painful, restricted range of motion.

to control pain and tumor progression. Bed rest is poorly tolerated by these patients, who often suffer complications including pneumonia, thromboembolic problems, and decubitus ulcers. Two complications of prolonged bed rest specific to this patient population are disseminated intravascular coagulopathy and malignant hypercalcemia (123). For all of these reasons, operative fixation of pathologic fractures of the lower extremities is indicated for any patient who is medically able to undergo surgery and whose life expectancy is greater than one month. The primary goals of surgery are early mobilization to facilitate general care. Operative fixation is also indicated for upper extremity pathologic fractures to allow early return of function of the extremity, which may be necessary for ambulation or to accomplish activities of daily living (104, 127). It has been shown to provide excellent pain relief after pathologic fracture of the humerus, and is also indicated after failure of closed treatment (127).

Before proceeding with operative intervention, a full medical and orthopaedic evaluation is mandatory. This is necessary to avoid iatrogenic fractures through unknown additional pathologic lesions while positioning a patient who is under anesthesia. This complication can and should be avoided by thorough preoperative evaluation. A total body bone scan should be done preoperatively, with standard radiographs of any suspicious areas, to assure that any other lesions at risk for fracture are not overlooked. When other lesions are found, special care must be taken with positioning of the patient in preparation for any surgical procedure.

Prophylactic internal fixation of impending pathologic fractures has been a controversial area. Keene and coworkers showed retrospectively that breast cancer metastases at risk of fracture cannot be identified by measurements obtained from standard radiographs (157). They found a high percentage (57%) of permeative lesions that could not be accurately measured, with more than half of the pathologic fractures occurring through these lesions. Fidler retrospectively reviewed 19 pathologic fractures, and noted greater than 50% cortical involvement by tumor in all but one case (96). He also found pre-fracture pain in only 10 of 19 patients, showing that pain is a poor indicator of impending fracture. He recommended prophylactic internal fixation for lesions involving over half of the cortex, whether or not the patient had pain. Most orthopedists currently use the indications for prophylactic internal fixation outlined by Harrington, which include: (*a*) a destructive lesion involving more than 50% of the cortical bone circumference; (*b*) a lytic lesion of the proximal femur larger than 2.5 cm; (*c*) a lesion of the proximal femur associated with avulsion of the lesser trochanter; and (*d*) a lesion of any size with persisting stress pain despite adequate radiotherapy (122) (Fig. 36-44). Prophylactic internal fixation of humeral metastases is generally not recommended because of the lower risk of fracture (99). However, many patients bear weight through the humerus by using a walker, cane, or crutches. This increased stress of the bone increases the risk of pathologic fracture, and should be considered an indication for prophylactic internal fixation (122).

The use of methylmethacrylate to augment internal fixation of pathologic fractures and impending fractures is well described in the orthopedic literature (81, 82, 99, 104, 122, 123, 127, 269). It is most useful in large lytic foci with significant bone loss and after tumor debulking (Fig. 36-44). The primary goal of stable fixation, to allow immediate pain-free weight bearing and immobilization, often cannot be achieved without bone cement to bridge cortical gaps and provide resistance to compressive forces. Methylmethacrylate does not interfere with postoperative radiotherapy, and fracture healing has been shown to occur by periosteal new bone formation (123).

The operative method and fixation used depends on the site of the lesion or fracture and the extent of tumor invasion and bone loss. Pathologic acetabular fractures are usually managed by total hip arthroplasty. Special acetabular components, such as the Harris-Oh protrusio shell, are often needed when extensive bony invasion by tumor and loss of structural continuity of the medial or superior acetabulum are found (125). Pathologic fractures of the femoral neck rarely unite, regardless of their displacement or method of fixation (104). They are best treated by cemented hemiarthroplasty (Fig. 36-45). Pathologic intertrochanteric fractures are usually managed by internal fixation with a sliding compression hip screw and sideplate with adjunctive methylmethacrylate

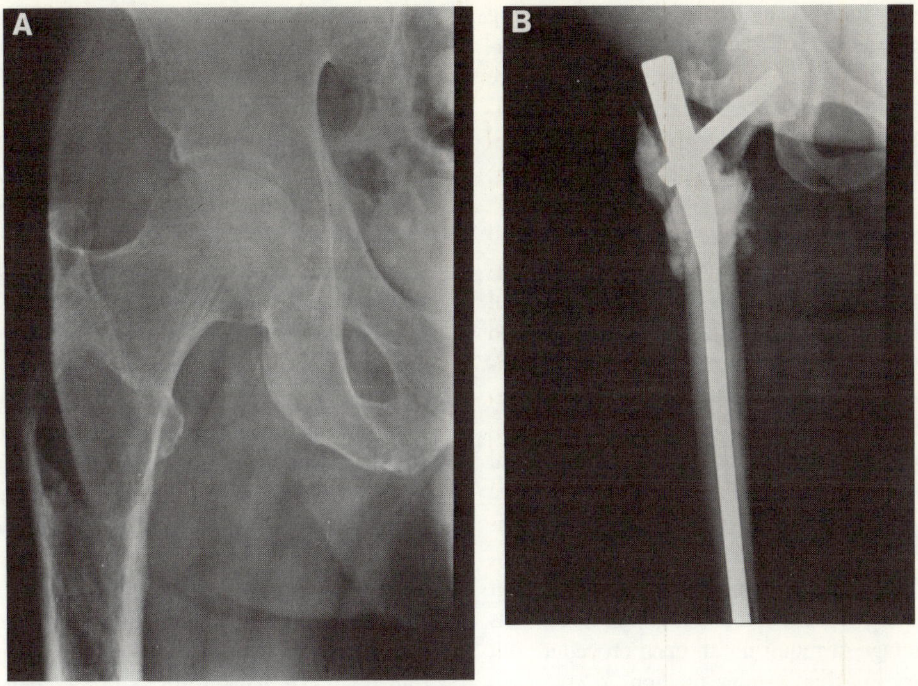

Figure 36-44. *A*, AP radiograph of the right hip in this 69-year-old male taken after a 3-month history of progressively worsening pain. Large radiolucent lesion of the proximal femur involves over 50% of the cortex and measures 3.5 cm in its largest diameter. *B*, Despite focal irradiation and chemotherapy for presumed metastatic thyroid cancer, the patient progressed to pathologic fracture necessitating methylmethacrylate augmented Zickel nailing of the proximal femur. Postoperatively, he regained independent ambulation and was alive without pain 3 years later.

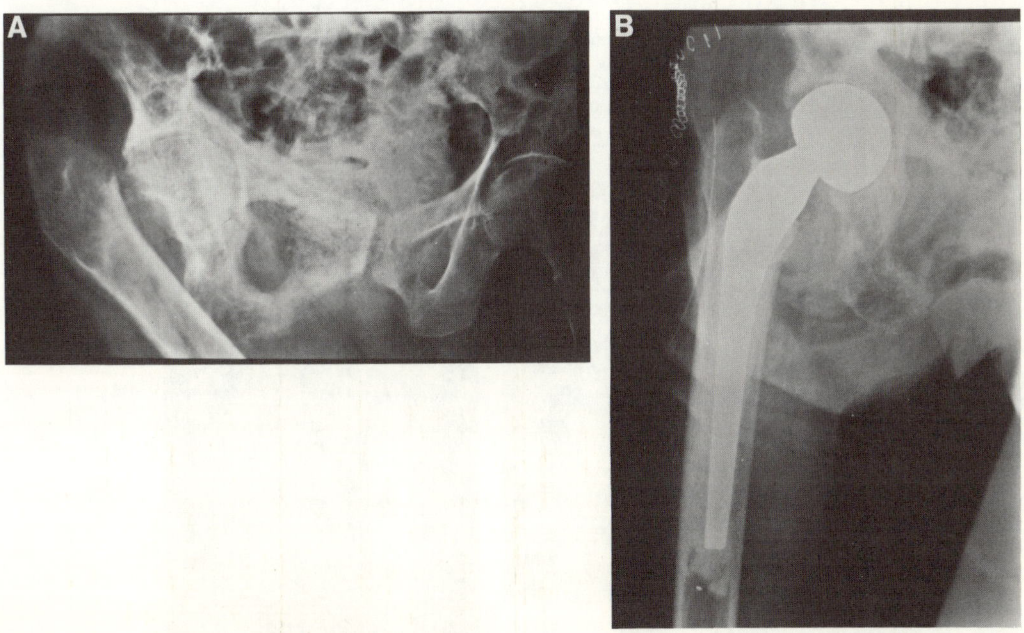

Figure 36-45. *A*, AP radiograph of the right hip in a 73-year-old female with Paget's disease following a fall. There is a displaced subcapital fracture through pagetoid bone. Notice the cortical enlargement and trabecular coarsening of the ipsilateral pubic and ischial rami. *B*, Cemented hemiarthroplasty was performed without complications, although at the time of surgery, bony bleeding was noted to be excessive.

after tumor curettage to fill any bony defects. Impending fractures of the femoral neck and intertrochanteric regions can usually be treated by hip screw and sideplate with bone cement. Some orthopedists recommend proximal femoral replacement with or without acetabular replacement for large intertrochanteric lesions (123) (Fig. 36-46).

Pathologic subtrochanteric fractures and impending fractures are commonly treated by closed or open intramedullary fixation using a Zickel nail with or without adjunctive methylmethacrylate. Diaphyseal lesions and pathologic fractures of the femur are treated by closed intramedullary nailing, using standard flexible or rigid devices. If shortening is likely due to extensive tumor invasion and bone loss, two options are available. First, a nail that can be locked both proximally and distally could be used. The locking screws, however, may be prone to fatigue failure if fracture healing does not occur. Secondly, the lesion or fracture can be exposed, and bone cement used after debulking of the tumor and involved bone. This has the disadvantage of requiring an open procedure but may be necessary to achieve stable fixation.

Pathologic humerus fractures are most common in the mid-diaphysis. They can be treated by intramedullary fixation, inserted anterograde or retrograde, with or without exposure of the lesion, tumor debulking, and the use of methylmethacrylate if needed (Fig. 36-47). Rush pins or Ender nails are often used for intramedullary fixation of the humerus. For proximal humeral lesions, bony destruction may warrant excision of the proximal humerus and cemented hemiarthroplasty.

Results of operative fixation of pathologic fractures and impending fractures have been excellent in terms of achieving the palliative goals of pain relief, mobilization, and return of function. Douglas examined the treatment of pathologic fractures, excluding those due to breast cancer, and found 91% of patients treated operatively had good pain relief, compared to only 59% of patients treated by irradiation, and 45% of patients treated by other nonoperative means (82). For lower extremity fractures, 63% of patients treated by internal fixation became ambulatory, compared to only 23% of those treated nonoperatively. For upper extremity fractures, function was restored in 50% of patients treated operatively as compared to less than 25% of patients treated nonoperatively. Harrington, using internal fixation with adjunctive methylmethacrylate for pathologic fractures and impending fractures, reported that 85% of patients had satisfactory pain relief, and 94% of patients who were ambulatory before fracture regained the ability to walk (127). He also noted that the rate of union depends in part on primary tumor cell type. Breast, prostate, myeloma, and lymphoma united more frequently than lung, kidney, and gastrointestinal tract metastases. Good results with internal fixation were also reported by Zickel, using his intramedullary device for pathologic subtrochanteric fractures

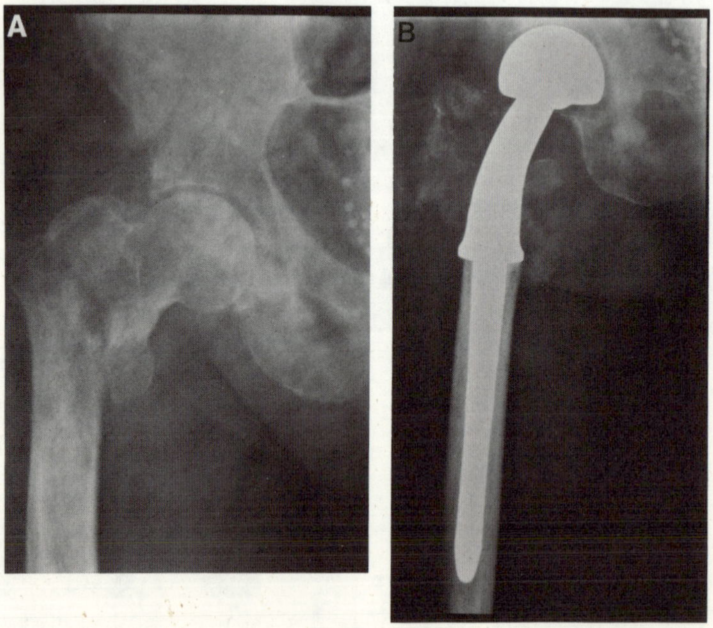

Figure 36-46. *A,* AP radiograph of the right hip showing intertrochanteric fracture through bone which appears to have a mixed lytic and blastic appearance in an 80-year-old male with known prostate carcinoma. *B,* Proximal femoral replacement with methylmethacrylate resulted in resumption of prefracture independent ambulation.

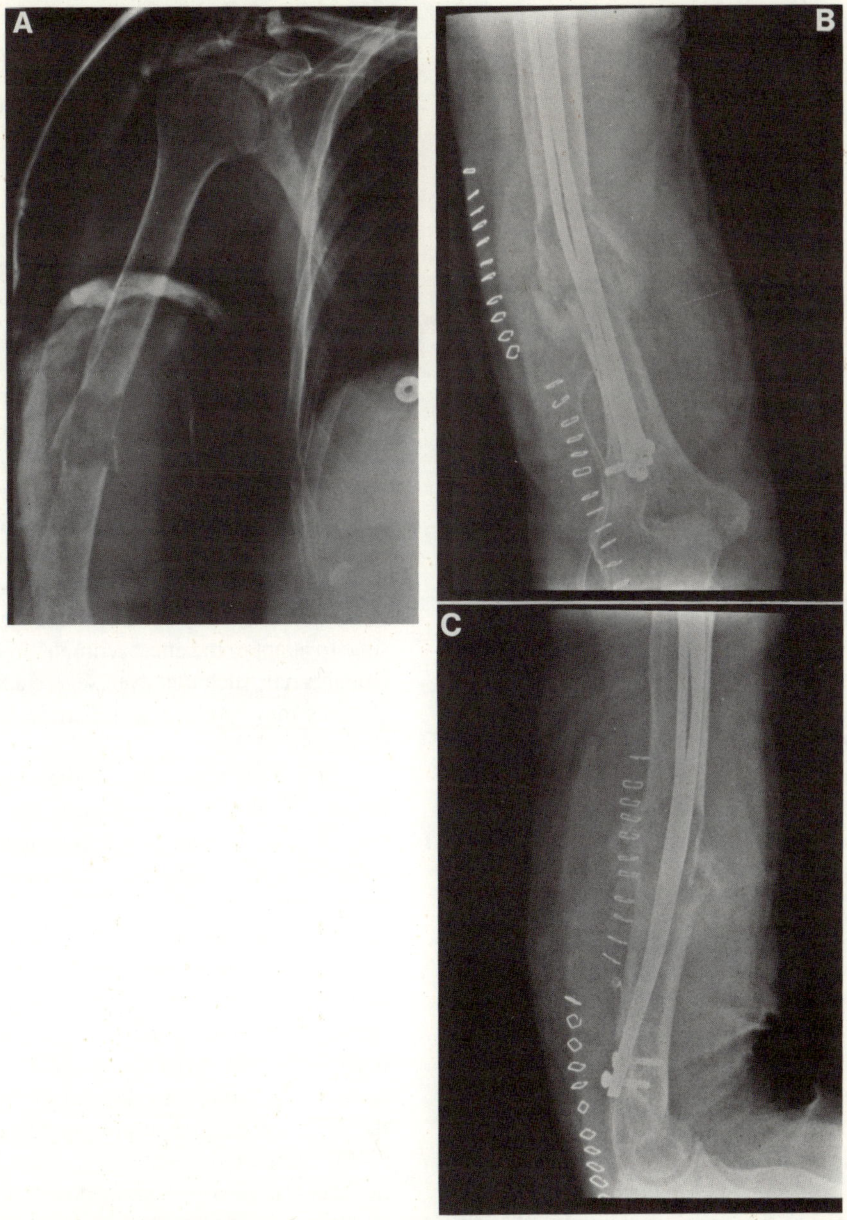

Figure 36-47. *A,* AP radiograph of the humerus in a 75-year-old female showing a midshaft fracture through an area of pathologic bone. This fracture occurred as a result of a fall. *B* and *C,* Fracture was treated by a retrograde Ender's nailing without cement. Intraoperative biopsy confirmed the presence of carcinoma, but workup failed to identify the primary lesion. Healing was evident clinically and radiographically at the time of the patient's demise 11 months following surgery.

(320). Dobozi, reviewing prophylactic flexible intramedullary nailing of impending pathologic femur fractures, reported 92% of patients ambulatory at discharge and 95% having marked pain relief (81). Excellent pain relief and improvement in function with internal fixation of pathologic fractures and impending fractures of the humerus has also been reported (269).

Complications of internal fixation of pathologic fractures or impending fractures are not uncommon, as might be expected in this debilitated patient population. Superficial and deep wound infections, thromboembolism, local tumor seeding, and delayed wound healing have been reported (127). Failure of fixation, iatrogenic fractures at the site of insertion of intramedullary devices, and persistent postoperative pain are all uncommon but can occur. Finally, excessive bleeding is sometimes encountered when dealing with vascular tumors, such as hypernephroma, myeloma, colon, and pancreatic carcinoma. A preoperative arteriogram to assess tumor vascularity and controlled arterial embolization using gelfoam for extremely vascular tumors should be considered in these cases (123).

Spinal Surgery

Spinal surgery in the elderly population is most commonly indicated for degenerative or metastatic disease of the vertebral column that results in severe pain, instability, or neurologic compromise. As the spine ages, a series of changes take place that result in decreased motion, an alteration of overall alignment, and a reduction in the space available for the passage of neural elements (277). Changes in the intervertebral disk include an increase in collagen and glycoprotein content and a decrease in water content and keratin sulfate as the nucleus pulposus shrinks and the disk becomes entirely fibrocartilage (277). Disk degeneration results in instability or hypermobility of the facet joints, which respond by hypertrophic overgrowth of the articular facets. The load-sharing properties of the synovial facet joints (18% in compression and 50% in shear and rotation) decrease with advanced degenerative changes (277). This increases the load across the intervertebral disks, resulting in additional degenerative changes and decreased mechanical efficiency. The vertebral bodies themselves show a decreased ability to transmit load secondary to the decrease in bone density that occurs with increasing age.

The venous drainage of the spinal column communicates with the intercostal and lumbar veins through a valve-less plexus, which allows two-way flow between the two venous systems (30). With increased abdominal pressure, such as during the Valsalva maneuver, venous blood can flow into the spinal column from the abdominal or pelvic viscera. This mechanism has been implicated as a cause of the high incidence of hematogenous metastatic and infectious spread to the spinal column. In addition, the highly vascular red marrow found in the vertebrae throughout life may also act as an excellent host environment for seeding of both tumor and infection.

The most common indications for spinal surgery in the elderly are: (*a*) decompression of degenerative lumbar spinal stenosis that causes significant pain and is unresponsive to nonoperative therapies; (*b*) decompression and/or stabilization of the spine for unremitting pain, neural compression, or instability secondary to metastatic disease; and (*c*) open or percutaneous vertebral biopsy for diagnosis and culture of spinal infections and for tissue diagnosis of unknown (usually metastatic) lesions. Each area will be considered separately.

Spinal Stenosis

Spinal stenosis is defined as a narrowing of the spinal canal, with a resulting decrease in the space available for the neural elements (10, 278). In the elderly population, this is almost always an acquired condition. Congenital and developmental spinal stenosis does occur, but usually in the younger patients. Acquired stenosis is most often due to degenerative disease of the spinal column. Other causes include spondylolisthesis, post-traumatic herniations of the nucleus pulposus in association with preexisting mild to moderate degenerative stenosis, Paget's Disease, and fluorosis (317). The lumbar spine is most often affected and will be the focus of this discussion. The structures of the vertebral column that are altered by degenerative changes and are responsible for the resulting stenosis include the facet joints (particularly the superior articular facet), laminae, pedicles, ligamentum flavum, and intervertebral discs (278). Disease progression is slow and insidious. As such, the neural elements have time to adapt to the encroachment on the space within the spinal canal, such that even severe acquired degenerative stenosis may produce surprisingly few neurologic manifestations (278).

Spinal stenosis can also be classified anatomically based upon the location of the spinal narrowing (278). It may be general (common with congenital stenosis) or localized to a specific spinal segment or group of segments. When localized, the regional position of the stenosis is classified into central (within the main spinal canal), lateral recess (in the region where the nerve roots pass laterally prior to exiting the spinal canal), or foraminal (as the nerve root exits the canal). A "far-out" stenosis has also been described, seen in spondylolisthesis, where the nerve root is compressed distal to the foramen, between the subluxed transverse process of L_5 and the sacral ala (314). Degenerative stenosis, with or without a herniated nucleus pulposus or spondylolisthesis, usually results in lateral recess or foraminal stenosis, and is often found on both sides of the spinal column. Paget's disease and fluorosis usually result in central or lateral recess stenosis (278).

Symptoms of spinal stenosis develop over many years. The primary symptoms are low back pain and stiffness (262, 278, 317). In the early stages, the pain and stiffness can often be relieved with mild activity. As the condition progresses, the pain becomes worse at night, and may occasionally awaken the patient. The pain is exacerbated by hyperextension and relieved by flexion of the lumbar spine. Pseudoclaudication or "neurogenic claudication" develops in up to 94% of patients (117). This is defined as a "discomfort" of the back and legs on standing or walking, relieved by rest. The "discomfort" is described as pain by 93% of patients, numbness by 63%, weakness by 43%, but most often as a combination of these manifestations (117). It is relieved by lying down, sitting, or flexing at the waist in about 85% of patients. Unlike claudication of vascular origin, the pain of pseudoclaudication may occur while simply standing still. When present with walking, it usually is not relieved by standing in place. The symptoms of pseudoclaudication occur bilaterally in 69% of patients.

The physical exam usually produces a paucity of specific findings related to the disease process. Patients may show decreased spinal motion and pain with extension of the lumbar spine. There may be weakness of the extensor hallucis longus, or sensory changes in a dermatomal distribution. The straight leg raising test and other tests of sciatic tension are usually negative. Stair climbing or similar exercise may increase symptoms, and make subtle physical findings more apparent. A positive "stoop test" is also consistent with spinal stenosis. In this test, the patient walks a specified distance until symptoms develop. The patient is then asked to flex forward at the waist. If the pain is relieved with flexion but recurs with extension, the test is positive. Referred pain to the back from other conditions must be ruled out by a thorough, complete physical exam. This is especially true in the elderly, where disorders of the hips, pelvis, and retroperitoneum are more common. Significant back pain in the elderly can also be psychogenic in origin, usually related to major depressive illnesses (277). Therefore, psychological assessment prior to any surgical intervention may be indicated.

The workup of spinal stenosis begins with standard radiographs of the lumbar spine. Degenerative disc disease and facet joint arthritis are noted in 70% and 62% of patients respectively, but these findings are not diagnostic (117). The main purpose of the standard radiographs is to exclude other pathologic processes in this region. Computed tomography scanning can be quite useful to delineate the bony anatomy (Fig. 36-48). However, findings must be closely correlated with the clinical picture. Studies have shown 35% to 50% abnormal findings in lumbar spine CT scans in asymptomatic subjects (277). Myelography currently is the most valuable study to examine the extent of stenosis and the degree of nerve root entrapment (Figs. 36-49*A* and *B*). Combining myelography with computed tomography provides a detailed examination of both the bony and soft-tissue contributions to the stenosis (Fig. 36-49*C*). Magnetic resonance imaging is becoming more popular for evaluating spinal stenosis, and will likely play a major role in assessing spinal stenosis in the future. Electrodiagnostic studies can be useful preoperatively to document the extent of neurologic in-

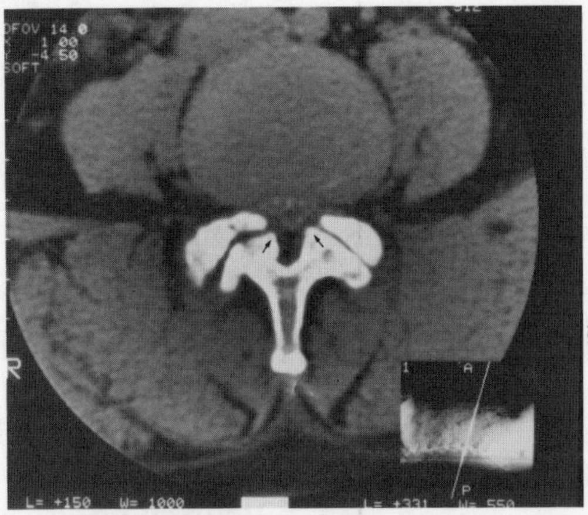

Figure 36-48. CT scan through the L_4–L_5 disc space in a 70-year-old male with persistent back pain shows bilateral hypertrophic facet joints. *Arrows* note hypertrophy of the superior facets, and overlying this, the hypertrophic inferior facets can be seen to be encroaching on the nerve root canals. Also note the arthritic nature of the right facet joint.

volvement. Abnormalities on EMG can be found in over 90% of patients, making it far more sensitive than a careful neurologic exam (117). Over 80% of patients have been found to have multiple levels of neurologic involvement.

Surgery is indicated in spinal stenosis only for those patients with increasing pain that affects quality of life and is unresponsive to nonoperative treatment. Rest, salicylates, or other nonsteroidal anti-inflammatory medications, lumbosacral orthoses, an appropriate exercise program, and education about posture and body mechanics form the first line of treatment. Epidural steroid injections, combined with decreased activity, can also be useful in providing symptomatic relief in up to 60% of patients (222). However, symptoms tend to recur after about 6 months. Repeat injections have been found to be less efficacious. Spinal stenosis due to Paget's disease often responds well to calcitonin therapy. Many patients obtain significant relief with these nonoperative treatment modalities. For those patients whose symptoms are not relieved, surgery can offer significant benefits.

The operative treatment of spinal stenosis is performed through a posterior approach, with the patient in the 'knee-chest' position (33). In this position, the abdomen hangs freely, decreasing the intra-abdominal pressure and decompressing the epidural veins, significantly lessening intraoperative blood loss. A midline incision is used with incision of the lumbodorsal fascia followed by a subperiosteal dissection of the spinous processes. The paraspinal muscles are retracted laterally. The spinous processes of the levels to be decompressed are identified and removed. Appropriate laminae and ligamentum fla-

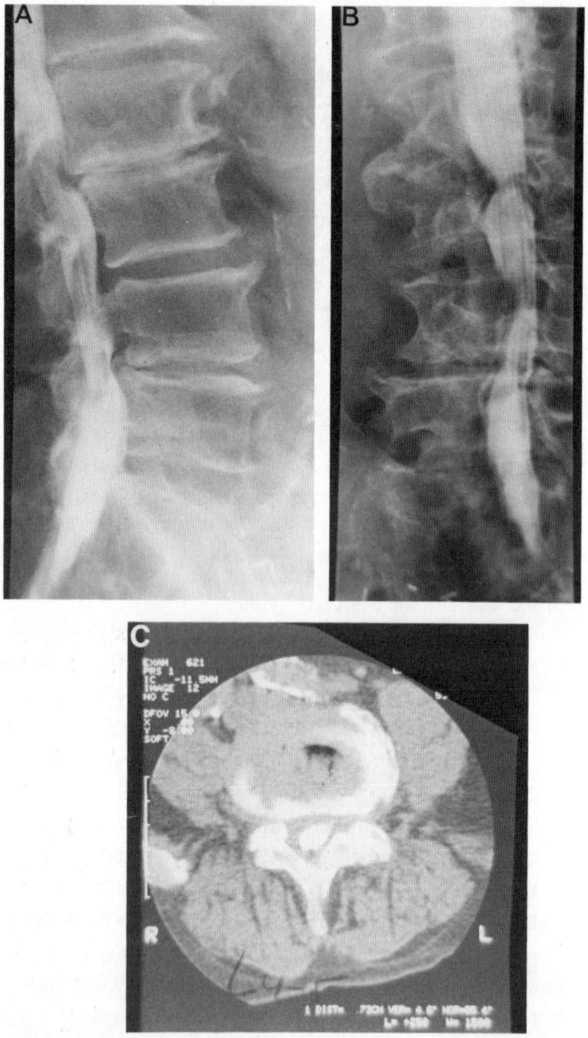

Figure 36-49. Lumbar myelogram in a 67-year-old black female with a long history of spinal claudication and progressive weakness of the right lower extremity. *A,* Lateral view showing annular bulging at L_2–L_3, L_3–L_4, and L_4–L_5 with stenosis throughout the L_4 level. *B,* An oblique view showing nerve root entrapment at L_4–L_5. *C,* CT scan following myelogram confirms the presence of hypertrophic facet and ligamentum flavum and blockage of nerve root on the right at L_4–L_5. This patient had marked pain relief and some increased sensation following multiple level lumbar laminectomy with partial facetectomies.

vum are then carefully removed, exposing the underlying dura.

If the stenosis is purely central, this posterior decompression may be all that is required. More commonly, however, there is significant nerve root compression at one or more levels caused by lateral recess or foraminal stenosis. This requires additional dissection and decompression (33). The course of the involved nerve roots in the lateral recesses are probed, and any excess ligamentum flavum or encroaching hypertrophic portions of the superior articular facets are carefully removed. The nerve root is again examined, and, if it fails to move freely, the foramen must be explored and decompressed. Commonly, the nerve root will be found to be trapped between the bulging annulus of a degenerated disc and the pedicle of the vertebra above. In this case, the lateral annulus can be excised or the inferomedial aspect of the pedicle can be removed. The nerve root may instead be trapped between the superior facet and either the posterolateral vertebral body or the pedicle above. In this situation, the nerve should be freed by excising as much of the involved superior facet as is necessary. Another pattern of foraminal stenosis may be encountered in which a degenerative spondylolisthesis has resulted in the nerve root being trapped between the upper aspect of a vertebral body and the advancing inferior facet of the level above. This is most commonly seen at the L_4-L_5 level, with symptoms of L_5 root compression. In this situation, decompression can be accomplished by excision of the involved aspects of the facet joint.

When an adequate decompression is completed, residual spinal stability must be carefully assessed. In most cases, lumbar spinal stability is not compromised, providing that at least one facet joint remains at each spinal level (33). For example, a unilateral total facetectomy or bilateral hemifacetectomies at the same level will not compromise stability. Bilateral total facetectomies, however, will render the spine potentially unstable. These patients should be stabilized by unilateral or bilateral lateral lumbar spinal fusion. However, in many elderly patients, their decreased activity level combined with disc space narrowing and the absence of motion at the operated level preoperatively may make fusion unnecessary.

Following complete decompression and fusion (if necessary), the use of an interpositional membrane such as a fat graft or Gelfoam is recommended to decrease the risk of epidural scar formation (278). Also, intraoperative monitoring of sensory evoked potentials has been used by some surgeons, who feel that prompt improvement in evoked potentials suggests adequate decompression (278).

The results following surgical decompression of lumbar spinal stenosis have generally been quite good with significant or complete relief of symptoms in 70% to 85% of patients (117, 208, 278). The results of surgery vary with the type of stenosis and the extent of disease. Patients with extensive disease, central stenosis, and severe degenerative joint disease of the spine generally do not show as much improvement compared to patients with localized, segmental, central and lateral stenosis (317). In one study with an average follow-up of 4 years, 84% good to excellent results were reported (117). Nasca reported 71% good results in 80 patients who underwent surgery for spinal stenosis, and noted that 13 of the 23 with fair and poor results were patients who had previous spinal surgery, including laminectomies, discectomies, and/or spinal fusions (208). Wiltse noted that the clinical result of pain relief following surgical decompression of spinal stenosis was better in the elderly than in the 30- to 50-year age group (314). Spengler, in his review of the subject, felt that surgical decompression of the lumbar spine for acquired degenerative stenosis will result in a good outcome in 85% of patients (278).

Complications of surgical decompression of lumbar spinal stenosis do occur and are similar to those found in lumbar disc surgery. However, there is a higher risk of nerve root laceration and dural tear in spinal stenosis surgery because of the concomitant degenerative disease and hypertrophic facets and ligamentum flavum, which alter the normal anatomy of the nerve roots and dural sac (317). Some consider persistent symptoms following surgery a complication; when this occurs, it is most commonly due to an inadequate decompression. Postoperative spondylolisthesis secondary to instability can be seen in 6% of cases after bilateral facetectomy, and in 15% of cases when three or more facets are removed without fusion (317). Other reported complications include hematoma formation, requiring drainage, and postoperative disseminated intravascular coagulopathy (208).

Metastatic Disease of the Spine

The spine is the most common site for skeletal metastases of malignant disease. On careful postmortem exam of the spine in cancer patients, vertebral column metastases are found in over 70% (104). Of these, 85% occur in the vertebral body, and only about 15% involve the posterior elements. The lumbar spine is most commonly affected. Spinal cord compromise, however, is most common in the thoracic spine, where the ratio of cord size to canal diameter is larger. The most common primary tumors producing spinal metastases include breast, prostate, lung, kidney, thyroid, bladder, colon, myeloma, and lymphoma.

Spinal metastases are commonly asymptomatic and require no local treatment. Symptoms occur with growth of the tumor, causing one of the following: (*a*) mass effect and necrosis within the vertebral body, with or without cortical breakthrough and invasion of local soft tissues anteriorly or laterally; (*b*) pathologic fracture secondary to bone destruction; (*c*) spinal instability, secondary to pathologic fracture, complete vertebral body destruction, or involvement of the posterior elements; or (*d*) involvement of neural structures, consisting most commonly of compression of the spinal cord or nerve roots. The most common presenting symptom is pain, which is often well localized, persistent, and worse at night (104) (Fig. 36-50). It is usually responsive, at least initially, to local radiation therapy. This is the primary form of treatment of spinal metastases, usually in combination with systemic chemotherapy or hormonal therapy. Symptoms of neural compression may represent radicular pain and dysfunction if due to nerve root compression. Motor dysfunction with later sensory changes followed by bowel and bladder dysfunction usually represents anterior cord compression. Both are usually amenable to emergent radiotherapy, especially when the compression is caused by direct impingement from a radiosensitive tumor. Systemic high-dose steroids, with a rapidly tapering schedule, are also used when the onset of symptoms is acute and cord edema is felt to be a factor. Gilbert et al. showed that radiation alone was as effective as decompressive laminectomy with or without radiation in the treatment of epidural spinal cord compression secondary to metastatic tumor (111). In both groups, just over 50% of patients regained the ability to walk following treatment. However, currently, posterior decompression (laminectomy) is usually not indicated for spinal cord compression secondary to metastatic tumor. This most often represents an anterior cord compression by tumor, vertebral body or intervertebral disc fragments, or severe kyphosis. Results following anterior decompression, and stabilization if necessary, are significantly better (see below).

Prior to surgical intervention, the exact location and degree of tumor involvement must be assessed, as well as any associated neurologic deficit. Computed tomography is helpful to define tumor location and extent of bony destruction, soft-tissue involvement, and neural impingement. Myelography is very useful in cases with potential for multiple levels of extradural compression. In cases of complete myelographic block, dye should be introduced more cephalad to define the upper limit of neural involvement. The medical condition of the patient must also be fully assessed. Anemia and particularly leukopenia and thrombocytopenia are common after chemotherapy and must be corrected preoperatively. If hypercalcemia is present (usually with rapidly destructive skeletal metastases), it must be corrected to avoid problems with cardiac arrhythmias. Finally, the patient's overall condition must be stable enough to undergo what may be an extensive surgical procedure, especially if the more physically demanding anterior decompression and stabilization is contemplated.

It is estimated that less than 10% of patients with confirmed spinal metastases require operative treatment (121). Most respond well to radiotherapy and usually succumb to the underlying disease before requiring spinal surgery. Indications for operative management of metastatic disease of the spine include: (*a*) progressive spinal cord compression by radioresistant tumor, by recurrent tumor in an area that has already received maximal irradia-

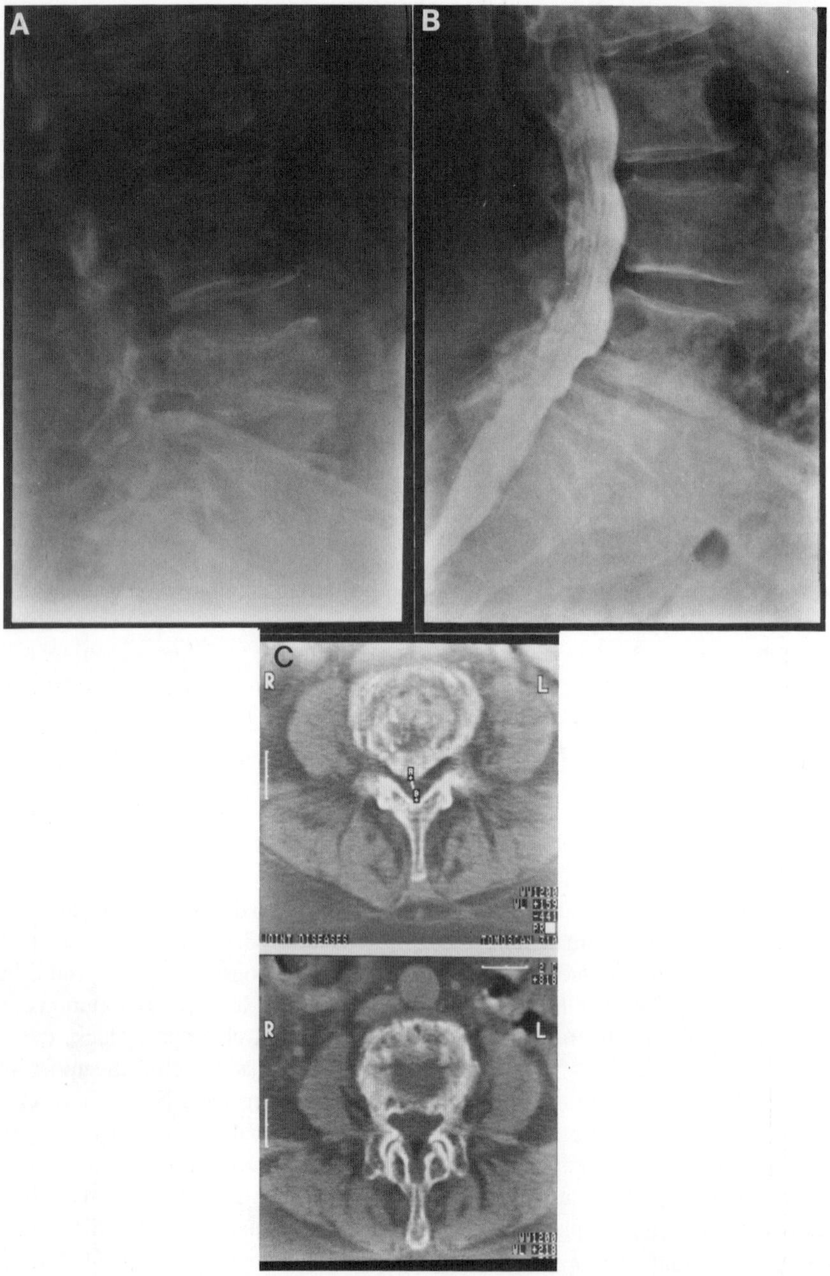

Figure 36-50. *A,* Lateral radiograph of the lumbar spine showing a destructive process of collapse in a 67-year-old female with the insidious onset of back pain without radiculopathy or evidence of nerve root involvement. *B,* Lumbar myelogram shows a normal dye contrast column with minimal extradural bulge at the L_3–L_4 interspace, just proximal to the pathologic fracture at L_4. *C,* CT scan without contrast demonstrates vertebral body destruction, but no evidence of canal impingement or cord compression.

tion, by bony fragments and extruded disc material, or by progressive kyphotic deformity; (*b*) progressive kyphotic deformity without neural compromise but with intractable pain either from mechanical causes or from instability due to destruction of the posterior elements; (*c*) progressive neural deterioration while receiving radiotherapy; and (*d*) spinal instability due to bony destruction by tumor or pathologic fracture (15, 97, 124, 268). Surgery may also be indicated if a histologic diagnosis of the primary tumor is lacking in the face of neural compression (268). Depending on the location of the lesion and the specific surgical indication, an anterior and/or posterior approach for decompression and/or stabilization may be warranted. The use of methylmethacrylate for vertebral body replacement after tumor debulking has been described (126). Spinal canal impingement generally requires decompression but may or may not need stabilization. Spinal cord compromise almost always results from anterior compression; therefore decompression requires an anterior approach with anterior or posterior stabilization if needed. Rare cases of circumferential "napkin-ring" cord compression by tumor require both anterior and posterior decompression and stabilization. Progressive kyphotic deformities with intractable pain are treated by anterior decompression and stabilization alone if the posterior elements are intact. If they are disrupted and shear-type instability is present, anterior and posterior stabilization will be required (124).

While straight midline approaches are used posteriorly for all levels of the spine, anterior approaches will vary based on the location of the lesion (97). In the cervical spine above C_4, a transoral approach is used. For cervical lesions below C_3, the anterior approach utilizes the avascular interval between the sternocleidomastoid and carotid sheath laterally, and the strap muscles, trachea, and esophagus medially. For lesions of the thoracic spine, the anterior approach can be performed with either a left or right thoracotomy. The side utilized is generally based on the pattern of tumor involvement and the individual surgeon's preference. Some surgeons, however, recommend always using a left-sided approach, to avoid any potential difficulties with mobilizing the vena cava. Anterior exposure of lower thoracic and upper lumbar lesions is accomplished by extending the thoracotomy distally, detaching the posterolateral corner of the diaphragm and continuing the dissection retroperitoneally as needed. For the lower two lumbar vertebrae, intraperitoneal dissection is often required, and supplementary posterior stabilization is recommended as a second procedure following anterior decompression and stabilization (97).

When an anterior approach is used, decompression is performed by resection of the tumor and the involved vertebral bodies. After spinal cord and nerve root decompression is completed, stabilization is performed, consisting of an interbody corticocancellous bone graft with external spinal immobilization until there is radiographic evidence of fusion. This technique is problematic because it requires prolonged immobilization, and the use of pre- or postoperative irradiation decreases the likelihood of bone graft incorporation. Currently, the preferred method of anterior stabilization utilizes an adjustable distraction device (such as a Knodt distraction rod) placed between the remaining vertebral bodies, incorporated in a methylmethacrylate vertebral construct (97). This provides immediate stability, obviating the need for postoperative immobilization. Cancellous autograft to fill the gap anteriorly is recommended if the patient's life expectancy is greater than 2 years.

Posterior decompression can be performed, via laminectomy. However, this approach is recommended only for decompression of tumor found circumferentially within the spinal canal (in combination with anterior decompression), for nerve root decompression, and for the uncommon metastasis primarily involving the posterior elements.

Posterior stabilization is often used to supplement anterior procedures, especially in the high cervical and lower lumbar regions. Above C_4, even after anterior transoral decompression, posterior stabilization is performed because of the risk of infection with transoral placement of internal fixation (97). Isolated posterior stabilization can be used in cases of spinal instability and pain without cord compression in the elderly patient who is a poor surgical risk for a major anterior procedure (Fig. 36-51). Many different methods of posterior stabilization are available. Harrington recommends wire stabilization for the cervical spine; for the thoracic and lumbar spine he recommends Luque-rod stabilization with sublaminar wiring extending three levels above and below the decompressed segments (124). Fidler recommends a bent, inverted Y-shaped plate for occipitocervical fusion in high cervical lesions and a rectangular rod construct wired to the laminae for the thoracic and lumbar spine (97). Methylmethacrylate stabilization along one side of the fixation with bone grafting along the opposite side has also been suggested. Newer devices, such as the Coltrel-Dubousset instrumentation, allow for pedicle hook or screw segmental fixation of the posterior thoracolumbar spine, and are becoming more popular among orthopaedic spine surgeons.

The prognosis for metastatic disease of the spine depends on both the pretreatment clinical course and the treatment method used. Barcena et al. reviewed many clinical series of patients with spinal metastases, and found that life expectancy and functional results after therapy are primarily dependent on tumor type (15). The rapidity of onset of muscular weakness also affects prognosis (30, 124). Rapid onset (less than 24 hours) of symptoms of neurologic compromise has a poorer prognosis, regardless of which treatment is used. Conversely, slowly developing deficits (over 7 to 10 days) respond more favorably to radiotherapy or decompression. Gilbert et al. compared functional results after radiation therapy alone and decompressive laminectomy with postoperative irradiation (111). They found no significant difference between the two groups: about 50% of surviving patients were ambulatory at 1 year. Operative results of anterior decompressions have been more encouraging. Harrington

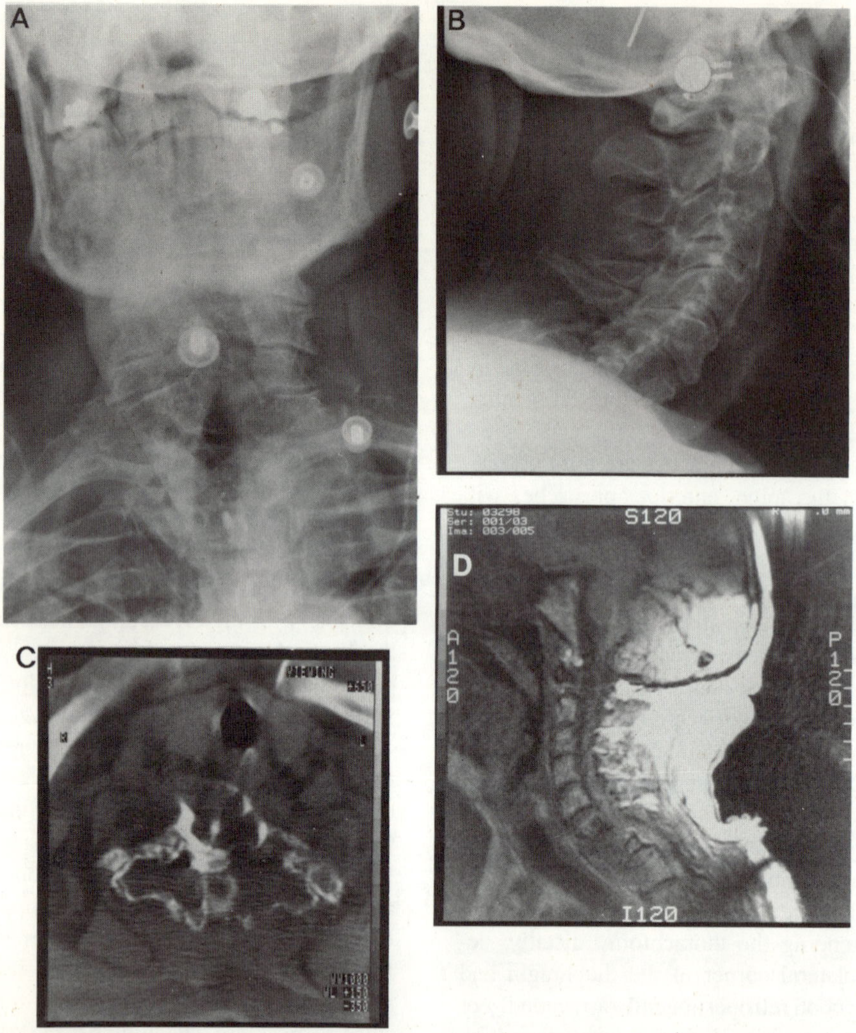

Figure 36-51. A 67-year-old male with a known history of multiple myeloma of the spine treated previously with chemotherapy and radiation therapy. Two years following treatment, the patient noted the sudden onset of left shoulder pain and numbness of the fourth and fifth digits in the left hand. *A* and *B*, AP and lateral views of the lower neck revealing vertebral body destruction at C_5 and C_6. *C*, CT scan showing diffuse myelomatous involvement of the vertebral body, as well as the posterior elements. *D*, MRI in the sagittal plane showing acute kyphotic deformity at C_6 and C_7 with vertebral body collapse and angulation and impingement of the neural cavity. *E*, Myelogram shows complete blockage at approximately T_2 level. *F* and *G*, Postoperative radiographs following posterior fusion, C_2–T_6 with decompression and segmental instrumentation using Drummond wires and Cottrell-Debousset rods from C_2–T_6 with methylmethacrylate augmentation and iliac bone graft. The patient had good relief of pain and the numbness of the fourth and fifth digits but had some persistent weakness of the left hand.

reviewed anterior decompressions and stabilization performed in 77 patients (121). Resolution of spine pain was found in over 90% of patients postoperatively. Of the 62 patients with a major neurologic impairment preoperatively, 42 made complete (26) or significant (16) improvement postoperatively. Siegal et al. found that while only 26% of their patients were ambulatory preoperatively, 80% were able to walk following vertebral body resection and anterior stabilization for malignant metastatic epidural compression (268). Preoperative bowel and bladder dysfunction was noted in 53% of their patients, with 93% regaining normal sphincter control postoperatively. Given the multitude of medical problems and the debilitated state of patients with metastatic cancer and the physiologic stresses of major spinal surgery, it is not unexpected that various complications have been reported with operative therapy of metastatic spine disease. Siegal et al. reported a 6% perioperative mortality for patients undergoing anterior procedures, due to pulmonary embolism, cardiac arrest, and bronchopneumonia (268). Other com-

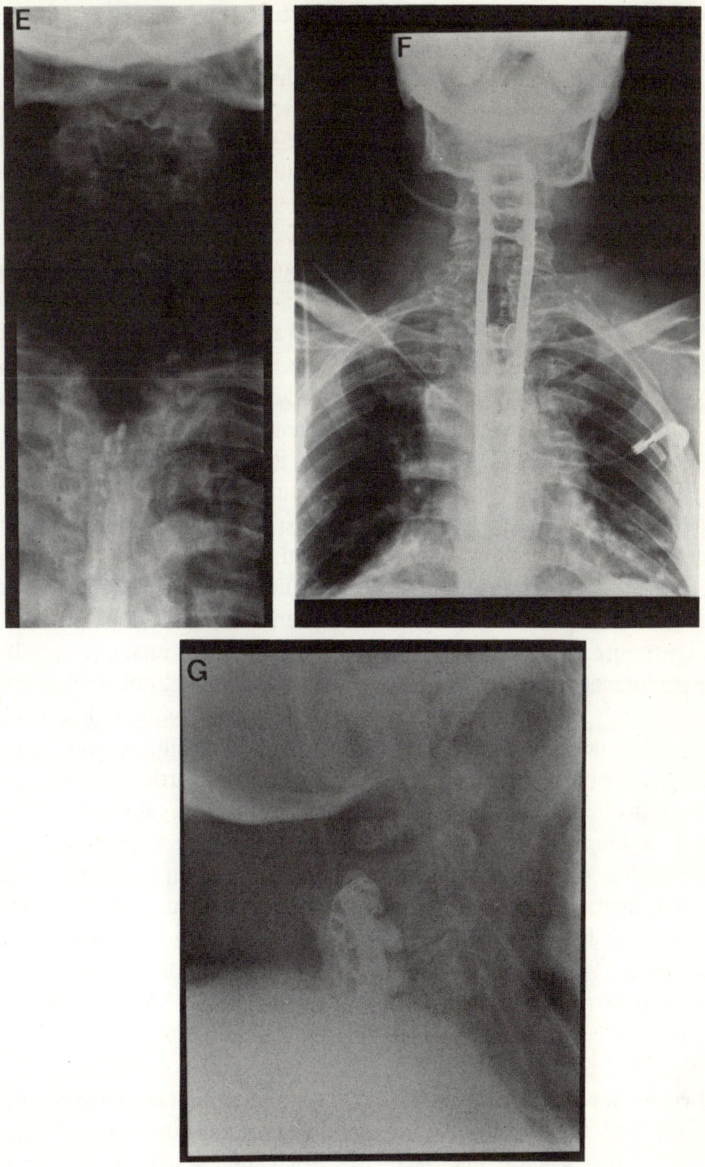

plications included wound infections, failure or dislodgement of fixation, CSF hydrothorax, transient neurologic deterioration, intercostal neuritis following thoracotomy, and disseminated intravascular coagulopathy (121, 268). Poor wound healing with dehiscence and infections was noted by Harrington to be a significant risk in patients who received previous high-dose radiation therapy (121).

Vertebral Biopsy

In our review of operative procedures performed on elderly patients, vertebral biopsy was relatively common. Biopsy of the spine can be performed either open or percutaneously (45, 246). Percutaneous biopsies are often done in the operating room under sterile conditions because of the risk of infection and because the discomfort of the procedure often requires significant sedation or general anesthesia. The two main indications for vertebral biopsy are: (*a*) to establish the diagnosis of vertebral osteomyelitis or disc space infection by obtaining tissue for microbiologic analysis, and (*b*) to obtain a histologic specimen of an unknown spinal lesion in order to establish a tissue diagnosis (most commonly performed for metastatic spine disease) (45, 247, 316). The decision of open versus percutaneous biopsy depends on the nature and location of the disease process, and the familiarity of the surgeon and pathologist with the procedures and specimens obtained.

The technique for percutaneous needle biopsy of the spine varies with respect to location of the biopsy site, both in the spinal column and within the specific vertebrae in question (45). In all cases, fluoroscopy is used to guide the biopsy needle. Many different needle systems are available, most of which utilize a 2-mm diameter biopsy trochar.

A pharyngeal approach with general anesthesia is used for biopsy of the first three cervical vertebrae. For C_4 to T_1, a lateral neck approach between the scalenus anterior and scalenus posterior is utilized. Vertebral bodies of T_2 to T_9 are biopsied from a posterior approach, with the needle introduced through a skin stab incision 4 cm to the right of midline. Special guide systems are available, which direct the needle at an angle of 35 degrees off the sagittal plane toward the midline. A smaller exploring needle is often used within the lumen of a larger biopsy needle, and both are always advanced under fluoroscopic control. For spinal levels T_{10} to L_5, a similar technique is used, with the needle introduced 6.5 cm from the midline at the level of the involved vertebra. Sacral lesions are generally not amenable to percutaneous biopsy and require open biopsy for diagnosis.

Open vertebral biopsies can be done via the standard anterior or posterior approaches previously described, depending on the location of the lesion to be biopsied. Other approaches can also be used for biopsy. Lower thoracic and upper lumbar vertebral bodies can be approached through a longitudinal incision lateral to the paraspinal muscles, dissecting along the plane between the erector spinae muscles and lumbar fascia (246). The transverse processes are transected or excised to allow visualization of the vertebral body. A retroperitoneal approach, using an anterolateral skin incision above and parallel to the inguinal ligament, can be used for the lower lumbar vertebrae (246). For lesions of the posterior elements, open biopsy is recommended, using a direct posterior approach (97).

Special care and planning must go into the choice of incision and approach for open biopsy of an unknown neoplastic lesion. It should allow enough exposure to provide a representative tissue sample, and should be at a site that could be included in an en block resection if later required (246).

It is generally agreed upon that open biopsy, although more invasive, affords a greater percentage of positive results. Boland et al. biopsied spinal lesions when they provided the first evidence of metastatic disease and found that percutaneous biopsy yielded positive results in 65% of lytic lesions and only 20% to 25% of blastic metastases, while open biopsy had a greater than 85% positive yield for both types of lesions (30).

Arthroscopy

Arthroscopy refers to the percutaneous endoscopic visualization of joint spaces. Originally conceived in 1918 by Tagaki in Tokyo and first used clinically by Watanabe in the 1950s, the technique did not become popular in this country until the early 1970s. Diagnostic arthroscopy employs this endoscopic visualization technique to make a diagnosis. Operative or therapeutic arthroscopy utilizes intra-articular surgical procedures in the absence of a formal arthrotomy, thereby potentially decreasing rehabilitation time and perioperative morbidity. Originally popularized for use in the acutely injured knees of young, active patients, arthroscopy has found many uses in various joints of patients of all age groups (143). In the elderly population, as in younger patients, the knee remains the most common joint for which arthroscopic techniques are used. The equipment, indications, operative procedures, results, and complications of knee joint arthroscopy in the elderly will form the basis of this section. Although becoming more frequently performed, arthroscopy of the shoulder, ankle, elbow, and other smaller joints is still a relatively uncommon procedure in the older age groups, where its benefits in impingement syndrome (shoulder), degenerative arthritis (ankle), and other joint disorders are still being evaluated.

Operative arthroscopy is usually performed as an ambulatory surgery procedure, but hospitalization is sometimes required for patients with bilateral procedures (for physical therapy and pain relief), for procedures that require hemovac drainage (such as a lateral patellar retinacular release for patellofemoral malalignment), and for immediate postoperative use of the continuous passive motion (CPM) machine.

Knee joint arthroscopy is performed with the patient in the supine position on the operating table (Fig. 36-52). Adequate anesthesia can be obtained using general, regional, or sometimes local techniques. The choice of anesthesia is made based on the preferences of the surgeon, the anesthesiologist, and the patient. In the elderly, concomitant medical problems often favor regional anesthesia. The procedure can be done with or without the use of an upper thigh pneumatic tourniquet to control the bleeding that can accompany certain arthroscopic procedures, such as abrasion arthroplasty and synovectomy. Many elderly patients have coexisting vascular disease; in these patients, a tourniquet should only be used when absolutely necessary to complete the procedure. Most arthroscopists place the distal thigh in a leg holder prior to prepping and draping the knee, to maintain control over the knee joint as well as to apply varus and valgus stresses as needed during the procedure.

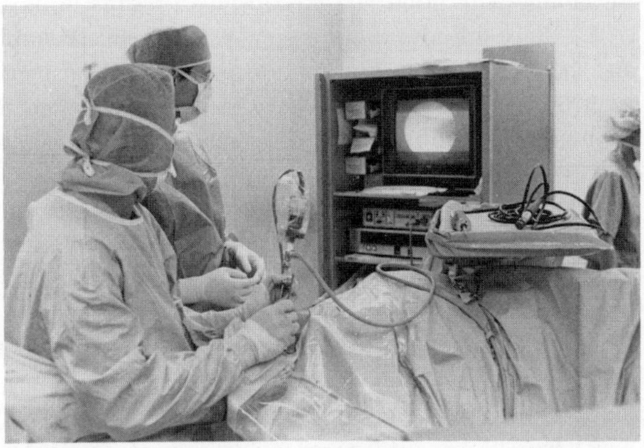

Figure 36-52. Arthroscopy of the knee is commonly performed with the patient in the supine position with the surgical knee draped free and manipulated by the surgeon during the arthroscopic procedure. As shown here, the surgeon has the arthroscope in his left hand and is using a probe in his right hand to examine the meniscus. The technique of triangulation is used with manipulation of instruments in both hands towards a central point, as viewed in the video monitor.

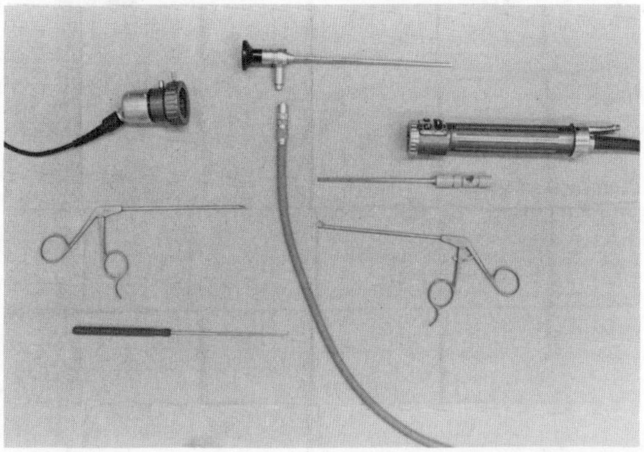

Figure 36-53. Commonly used arthroscopic instruments include (from top left in clockwise order) a miniature video camera, the straight viewing arthroscope, a motorized shaver for debridement, shaving, and abrasion, disposable blades used for the motorized shaver, a meniscal grabber used to hold a portion of the meniscal tear or to grab and remove loose bodies, the fiberoptic light source for the viewing arthroscope, a probe used to examine articular surfaces and menisci for signs of softening or tears, a biting forceps used to debride torn and degenerated menisci.

The arthroscope is a rigid endoscope, which is attached to a fiberoptic light source and often to a video camera to allow the procedure to be viewed on a nearby television monitor rather than directly through the arthroscope's eyepiece. Arthroscopes are available in outer diameters, ranging from 1.7 to 6.6 mm, with the 4 and 5 mm sizes most commonly used in knee joint arthroscopy. The viewing tip of the scope is angled, so that by simply rotating it within the knee the effective field of view is increased. Commonly used arthroscopes have angles of inclination of 30 and 70 degrees. Although some older arthroscopes had lumens in them to permit passage of operative instruments (operative arthroscopes), today the technique of "triangulation" is favored. This technique utilizes operative instruments passed through separate portals, and visualized by the viewing arthroscope. A wide variety of operative arthroscopic instruments are available to the surgeon to aid in the performance of many arthroscopic procedures (Fig. 36-53). Hand instruments include simple needles, probes, knives, scissors, grasping and basket (biting) forceps, curettes, rasps, and osteotomes. Motorized instruments also exist, where an outer stationary sleeve covers a rotating inner cutting blade, controlled by foot or hand controls and attached to suction. Various types of blades are available for cutting, shaving, and abrading of surfaces. Other specialized instruments are available for specific arthroscopic procedures, such as meniscal repair or cruciate ligament repair, but these procedures are rarely indicated in the elderly population.

The indications for knee arthroscopy in older patients fall into three main categories: for palliative treatment in degenerative joint disease, for treatment of acute internal derangements of the knee, with or without underlying arthritis, and for certain select patients following total knee arthroplasty with residual stiffness or pain (100, 101, 144, 151, 233, 239, 265, 279). Diagnostic arthroscopy as an isolated procedure is rarely done in this age group.

The most common indication for operative arthroscopy is for pain associated with degenerative knee joint arthritis (100, 233, 265). These patients often show diffuse radiographic changes in all three bony compartments of the knee. However, patients with minimal radiographic changes are even better candidates for arthroscopic debridement (Fig. 36-54). Most orthopaedic surgeons regard this as a palliative procedure with limited ability to slow the relentlessly progressive process of cartilage breakdown and joint destruction. A growing number of orthopaedists, however, believe that by correcting intra-articular mechanical problems (such as osteophytes and degenerative meniscal tears) in the early stages of the disease process, it can be significantly slowed, halted, and even possibly reversed (144, 233, 265). Some also believe that abrasion of severely degenerated cartilage and sclerotic lesions down to bleeding subchondral bone can stimulate repair. Indeed, follow-up arthroscopies in these cases have demonstrated a 2- to 3-mm thick fibrocartilage-like tissue covering areas previously arthroscopically abraded (151). Arthroscopic procedures for the degenerative knee

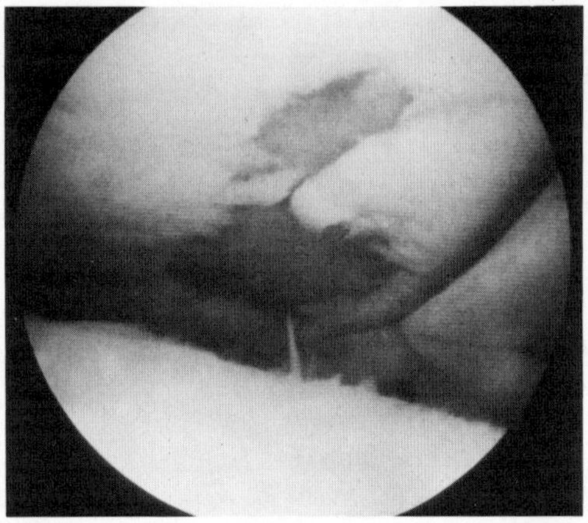

Figure 36-54. Arthroscopic view of grade IV chondromalacia of the femoral condyle. Note the two large areas where no cartilage is found, the sclerotic bone is visible. The miniscus is seen on the right and the tibial articular surface shows some fibrillar changes at the lower part of the view.

include joint lavage and debridement, and abrasion arthroplasty. Simple joint lavage has been noted to have a pain relieving benefit in these patients, probably by removing debris and relieving the joint of fluid high in lytic enzymatic activity and cartilage breakdown products. Thorough joint debridement involves removal of hypertrophic synovium, degenerated meniscal tissue, and obstructing osteophytes, along with a shaving chondroplasty of areas of significant chondromalacia, followed by copious joint lavage. In abrasion (eburnation) arthroplasty, degenerated, sclerotic areas are abraded down to subchondral bleeding bone to stimulate a repair response. This procedure is best indicated for inactive people with significant rest or night pain, and 8 weeks of protective weight bearing postoperatively is recommended (151). Orthopaedists are in general agreement that arthroscopy cannot correct joint instability or angular deformities, and elderly patients with these problems in association with degenerative arthritis would best benefit by total knee arthroplasty if medically stable.

The second indication for knee arthroscopy in the elderly patient is for an acute internal derangement, either in a previously normal knee or in a knee with underlying degenerative arthritis. Acute meniscal injury was originally thought to be a problem of the young, athletic knee, but as early as 1968, Eichenholtz and coworkers recognized the growing problem of acute injuries to the meniscus in the elderly (85). Half of the older patients with acute onset of joint line knee pain who had meniscal lesions could not recall any specific trauma prior to the onset of the pain. In addition to pain (found in 90% of cases), swelling was the other common symptom (48%), with locking and instability less common (20% each). These patients were treated by arthrotomy and open meniscectomy, with good late postoperative results in most cases. Since the advent of minimal partial meniscectomy and the use of the arthroscope to perform partial meniscectomies, excellent results have been reported for operative arthroscopic treatment of meniscal tears in the elderly (144, 233).

The third and least common indication for knee joint arthroscopy in the elderly is in select patients following total knee replacement (TKR) (101). Patients with suspected or proven loose bodies following TKR require removal of these loose bodies to prevent accelerated wear of the polyethylene components and further debris. These loose bodies are usually free-floating cement fragments, which have broken off from excessive cement mantles left in place during the arthroplasty. Another indication for arthroscopy following TKR is for lysis of adhesions and intra-articular scarring to improve the range of motion in the patient with postoperative stiffness. This indication has yet to be universally accepted for two reasons. First, the range of motion following TKR tends to gradually improve over the 1st year postoperatively. Surgeons should wait until the range of motion has sufficiently plateaued before proceeding with arthroscopic treatment. Second, many causes of decreased motion following TKR are extra-articular (such as a contracted quadriceps mechanism) and are not amenable to arthroscopic treatment. Patients with postoperative patellofemoral symptoms may benefit from an arthroscopic lateral retinacular release if patellar malalignment and tracking problems are diagnosed clinically. A newly described indication for operative arthroscopy following TKR is the presence of a large pseudomeniscus, which forms postoperatively in some patients and can be a source of pain and decreased motion due to impingement between the tibial and femoral components (101). Finally, a patient with a painful knee following knee replacement may benefit from a diagnostic arthroscopy if a full workup fails to reveal an etiology for the pain. Often, hypertrophic synovium is found, and the patient achieves at least some pain relief following arthroscopic synovectomy. If not, revision TKR is usually not indicated, as the results of revision for persistent pain of unknown etiology have been uniformly poor.

In arthroscopy of the knee, the joint is first approached anteriorly. After a sterile preparation and draping with the leg free and the operating table bent at the knee level, a cannula for fluid inflow is usually placed, most commonly through a stab wound in the medial suprapatellar area. The joint is then distended with an isotonic solution such as Ringer's Lactate, although a gas medium such as CO_2 can also be used. The arthroscope is then introduced, usually through an anterolateral approach, approximately 1 cm lateral to the patella tendon just below the level of the inferior pole of the patella.

From this entry site, a complete visual inspection of the joint compartments and suprapatellar pouch can be accomplished. While visualizing the anteromedial aspect of the joint, a spinal needle is used to locate the optimal position for an anteromedial portal, which is used for the introduction of a probe, other operative instruments, or the arthroscope, if a better view of the posterior aspect of the medial compartment or the anterior aspect of the lateral compartment is desired. After a thorough examination of the knee, specific areas of pathology are individually addressed. Any foreign bodies found are carefully removed using a hand-held grabber. Meniscal tears and irregularities are resected back to a smooth rim, using a combination of hand and motorized instruments as required. Hypertrophic synovium is resected using a motorized shaver. Cartilage displaying evidence of chondromalacia is shaved (if minimal changes are found) or abraded (for sclerotic lesions) as indicated. Intra-articular osteophytes are removed as well. Following these procedures, the joint is reexamined and a thorough lavage is performed. The portals are closed with simple nylon skin sutures or simple absorbable subcuticular sutures. Other operative approaches to the knee, such as the central approach through the patellar tendon, the midpatellar approaches (medial or lateral), the suprapatellar approaches, and the posteromedial and posterolateral approaches can be utilized as needed to address specific pathologies found in these areas.

The results of arthroscopic knee surgery in the elderly population are generally good, but they depend on the indication for the procedure and the degree of degenerative arthritis present at the time of surgery. Earlier studies of open meniscectomy in the older age groups for acute knee pain showed that the results varied significantly with the amount of preexisting degenerative changes. When minimal radiographic evidence of arthritis was present, good and excellent results could be expected in greater than 90% of patients (174, 177). Patients with moderate or marked preexisting arthritic changes had only a 21% chance of good or excellent results. Studies utilizing arthroscopic partial meniscectomy show similar trends. Jackson and Rouse reported 95% good or excellent results at an average follow-up of 2.5 years in older patients when no degenerative changes were associated with a meniscal tear, but only 80% good or excellent results if changes of degenerative joint disease were identified at the time of surgery (144). Rand looked at degenerative meniscal tears in patients with osteoarthritis and reported that 90% of patients reported subjective improvement if the knee had no preoperative radiographic evidence of osteophytes or subchondral sclerosis, while only 72% had improvement if either of these findings were present (233). For arthroscopic joint debridement of the degenerative knee, good or satisfactory results are reported in 70% to 80% of patients at 1- to-2-year follow-up (239, 265). In these patients, success is determined by relief of pain and increase in function. Reports of abrasion arthroplasty in patients whose arthritis was severe enough to make them candidates for TKR or tibial osteotomy show symptomatic improvement in 53% to 74% of patients at 1- to-2-year follow-up (100, 151). The results of arthroscopy post TKR are usually good if specific pathology (such as a loose body, intra-articular adhesions, or pseudomeniscus) is identified and corrected (101). Failure to locate any pathology as a cause of pain is usually associated with continued pain and a poor result.

Complications occur in arthroscopic surgery as with any surgery, but careful attention to detail can minimize their number and severity. Small utilized a questionnaire completed by 21 experienced arthroscopists and found an overall complication rate of about 1.7% (273). The most common complication reported was hemarthrosis (60%), followed by infections (12.1%), thromboembolic disease (6.9%), anesthetic complications (6.4%), instrument failure (2.9%), reflex sympathetic dystrophy (2.3%), ligament injury (1.2%), and fractures and neurologic injuries (0.6% each). It is likely that the actual rate of complications would be somewhat higher if less experienced arthroscopists were included. Sherman and coworkers reported a complication rate of 8.2%, based on a retrospective analysis of 2,641 cases, but this figure includes many "minor" complications, such as ecchymosis and delayed wound healing, which were not reported in the previous study (266). They also found that an age greater than 50 years and a tourniquet time over 1 hour were associated with significantly higher rates of complications.

Rotator Cuff Tears

Rotator cuff tears are frequently encountered in elderly patients. To understand the nature of this problem, its pathophysiology and the rationale for treatment, it is first necessary to understand the pertinent anatomy. The rotator cuff consists of the tendons of the supraspinatus, infraspinatus, and teres minor, which insert on the greater tuberosity superiorly and posteriorly, and the subscapularis, which inserts on the lesser tuberosity anteriorly (Fig. 36-55). Its most important function is to stabilize the humeral head against the glenoid as the arm is elevated (181). The rotator cuff tendons form half of the "force couple" with the deltoid, thereby allowing the powerful deltoid muscle to elevate the arm (178). If the stabilizing function of the rotator cuff is absent, there will be unopposed pull of the deltoid, driving the humeral head upward into the acromion. In this situation, abduction will not occur. This is the classical finding in a large

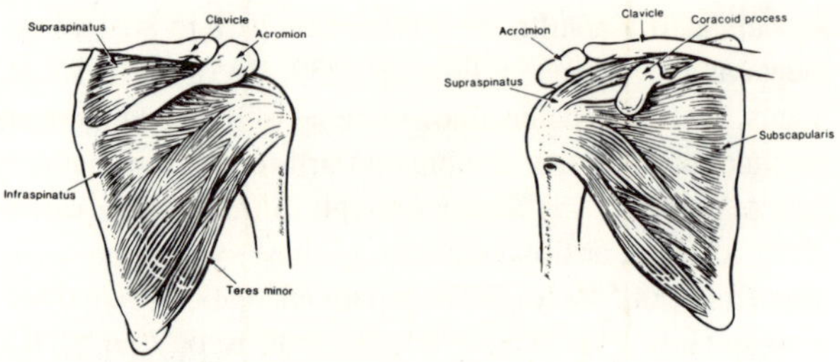

Figure 36-55. Musculoskeletal anatomy of the shoulder region.

rotator cuff tear. In addition, the rotator cuff is an important dynamic stabilizer of the glenohumeral joint (321). The inherently unstable bony configuration of the glenohumeral joint requires the strong dynamic stability provided by the rotator cuff. Therefore, a healthy intact rotator cuff provides the structural integrity and dynamic support that is essential for optimal shoulder function.

Aging produces changes which significantly weaken the rotator cuff tendons and make them more susceptible to injury (39, 69, 238). Codman identified an area near the insertion of the supraspinatus tendon where rotator cuff tears often originated (57). Moseley and Goldie identified a zone of avascularity that corresponded to this same area and termed this the *critical zone* (202). This was further delineated by Rathburn and McNab who performed microangiographic studies of the rotator cuff (212). They found a constant area of avascularity near the insertion of the supraspinatus tendon that was dependent upon the positioning of the upper extremity. Brewer studied the histologic changes in this area (39). He found inflammatory changes of the greater tuberosity with degeneration of the sulcus between the greater tuberosity and the articular surface. With time, disruption of the integrity of the attachment of the tendon to bone was evident. Brewer felt that these changes could be accelerated by repetitive overhead activity (39). This introduces another important factor in the effects of aging on the rotator cuff—mechanical impingement.

In 1972, Neer introduced the concept of impingement as a critical factor in understanding the etiology of rotator cuff tears (209). He felt that with forward elevation of the arm, the supraspinatus tendon was impinged upon by the structures of the coracoacromial arch. This specifically includes the anterior one-third of the acromion (exacerbated when osteophytes form in this area), the coracoacromial ligament, and the underside of the acromioclavicular joint. Repetitive overhead activity causes repetitive impingement, which leads to "wear and tear" of the supraspinatus tendon. Over time, this may result in disruption of tendon fibers, partial tearing, and eventually full thickness tears. This is the mechanism of the "attrition" type of rotator cuff tears that often occur with aging. The location of supraspinatus tendon involvement with impingement corresponds to the area of avascularity described previously (57, 202). The poor vascularity in this area makes it much more susceptible to degenerative changes and, more importantly, limits the healing potential for any tendon injury in this area. In this section, we will address the evaluation and management of rotator cuff tears in the elderly. Although the term rotator cuff tear includes both partial- and full-thickness tears, our discussion will specifically address full-thickness tears. Full-thickness tears are of much greater clinical significance in terms of pain and functional disability than partial-thickness tears.

Clinical Evaluation

The evaluation of the elderly patient with suspected rotator cuff tear requires a careful assessment for preexisting shoulder problems. Since almost all rotator cuff injuries in the elderly occur to an already compromised cuff (20, 59), it is essential to determine the presence and extent of any preexisting problems. Two types of rotator cuff injuries are most often accounted. The first is an acute injury superimposed on an area of chronic degenerative changes, and the second is a chronic "attritional" rotator cuff tear.

Most elderly patients with shoulder pain and suspected rotator cuff tears are able to describe an injury or activity that precipitated their acute shoulder problems (130). For some, it will be obvious, like a fall onto the outstretched arm, followed by pain and inability to raise the arm overhead. Others will report the onset of pain and a "tearing" sensation when doing some strenuous lifting, pushing, or pulling. Others will report the onset of pain following a simple everyday maneuver like pushing open a door or pulling open a window. These injuries most often result in an "acute on chronic" rotator cuff tear. There will be some patients who will not be able to describe an event or activity that precipitated their shoulder pain (221). However, they may describe the insidious but progressive onset of shoulder pain in the absence of a precipitating injury. These patients usually manifest the signs and symptoms of an attritional rotator cuff tear from chronic impingement (212).

Preexisting shoulder problems should be carefully assessed. Many patients will describe a history of previous "bursitis," which was treated with medication or steroid injection. Some will describe multiple steroid injections for treatment of similar problems. This is important to note because of the known detrimental effects of injected corticosteroids on rotator cuff tendons (305). It is also important to assess pre-injury shoulder function, particularly with respect to range of motion and performance of activities of daily living.

Upon presentation, patients most often complain of pain about the superior aspect of the shoulder that can radiate to the upper arm in the area of the deltoid insertion (38, 61). The pain is often worse at night and can interrupt sleep (38). Attempts at overhead elevation will often exacerbate the pain, and the patient may describe an inability to lift the arm overhead. Patients seen shortly after the injury will complain of more pain and disability than those who were evaluated weeks or months following injury. With time, the pain may subside but will continue to be exacerbated by shoulder elevation. Shoulder function may initially improve, although over time, a significant and progressive loss of function may be expected to occur.

Following a careful history, a complete physical examination should be performed. The first part is an examination of the cervical spine including a neurologic examination of the upper extremities. This will exclude the possibility of an underlying or associated cervical radiculopathy. The examination of the shoulder proceeds with inspection, particularly to note muscular atrophy that could be consistent with a chronic rotator cuff problem (Fig. 36-56). Palpation may elicit tenderness over the greater tuberosity. There may also be tenderness over the anterior acromion and acromioclavicular joint suggestive of preexisting impingement. Both active and passive range of motion should be assessed including forward elevation and internal and external rotation (Fig. 36-57). Loss of active range of motion compared to passive range of motion is an important finding suggestive of a rotator cuff tear. The "drop arm test" should be performed by passively elevating the arm overhead and asking the patient to slowly lower the arm to the side. In the presence of a large rotator cuff tear, the arm will drop to the side as it is lowered. However, a negative drop arm test should not be considered evidence of an intact rotator cuff. Many full-thickness rotator cuff tears will present with a negative drop arm test as well as full active forward elevation.

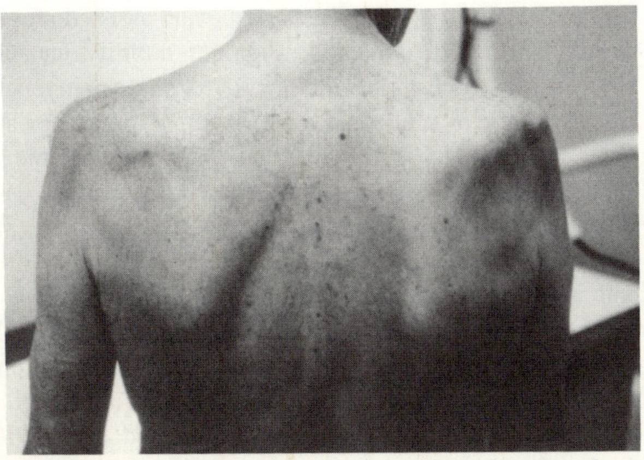

Figure 36-56. Rotator cuff atrophy is evident upon inspection of the left periscapular area compared to the right side. The supraspinous and infraspinous fossae have a concave appearance and the scapular spine is more prominent.

Assessment of strength in the rotator cuff and shoulder musculature should be performed carefully to identify any deficits that may be present. All three portions of the deltoid should be assessed as well as abduction and internal and external rotation. Strength testing should also be performed on the asymptomatic shoulder for comparison. Specific testing maneuvers are also helpful. The impingement test, consisting of maximum forward elevation with scapular stabilization or forward elevation to 90 degrees with internal rotation, recreates the impingement positions and will usually cause significant discomfort. Adduction of the arm across the chest will elicit pain secondary to degenerative changes at the acromioclavicular joint (322).

If the patient is having significant discomfort while the examination is being performed, the results may be unreliable. For example, active range of motion may be limited solely because of pain. In addition, apparent muscular weakness may be secondary to pain inhibition. Therefore, the lidocaine injection test is an important adjunct to the physical examination (38, 212). It consists of the injection of 8 to 10 cc of 1% lidocaine into the subacromial space. The exam should be repeated approximately 5 to 10 minutes after the injection. This will effectively remove the pain inhibited deficits and aid in identification of problems with the musculotendinous unit. It will also aid in identifying sources of pain not related to the subacromial space.

Radiographic evaluation can be helpful in identifying longstanding rotator cuff disease secondary to impingement. Significant findings include sclerosis or cyst formation about the greater tuberosity. There may also be sclerosis or osteophyte formation about the inferior and anterior aspects of the acromion along with calcification at the acromial attachment of the coracoacromial ligament (38, 61, 209, 212). Degenerative changes of the acromioclavicular (AC) joint with osteophyte formation at its inferior surface may also be present in chronic rotator cuff disease (38). An acromiohumeral distance of less than 6 mm is associated with full-thickness rotator cuff tears (69, 226, 308) (Fig. 36-58). Confirmation of the diagnosis of a full-thickness rotator cuff tear requires an arthrogram. This is performed by injecting contrast material into the glenohumeral joint. If the dye enters the subacromial space from the glenohumeral joint, the presence of a full-thickness tear is confirmed (Fig. 36-59). Ar-

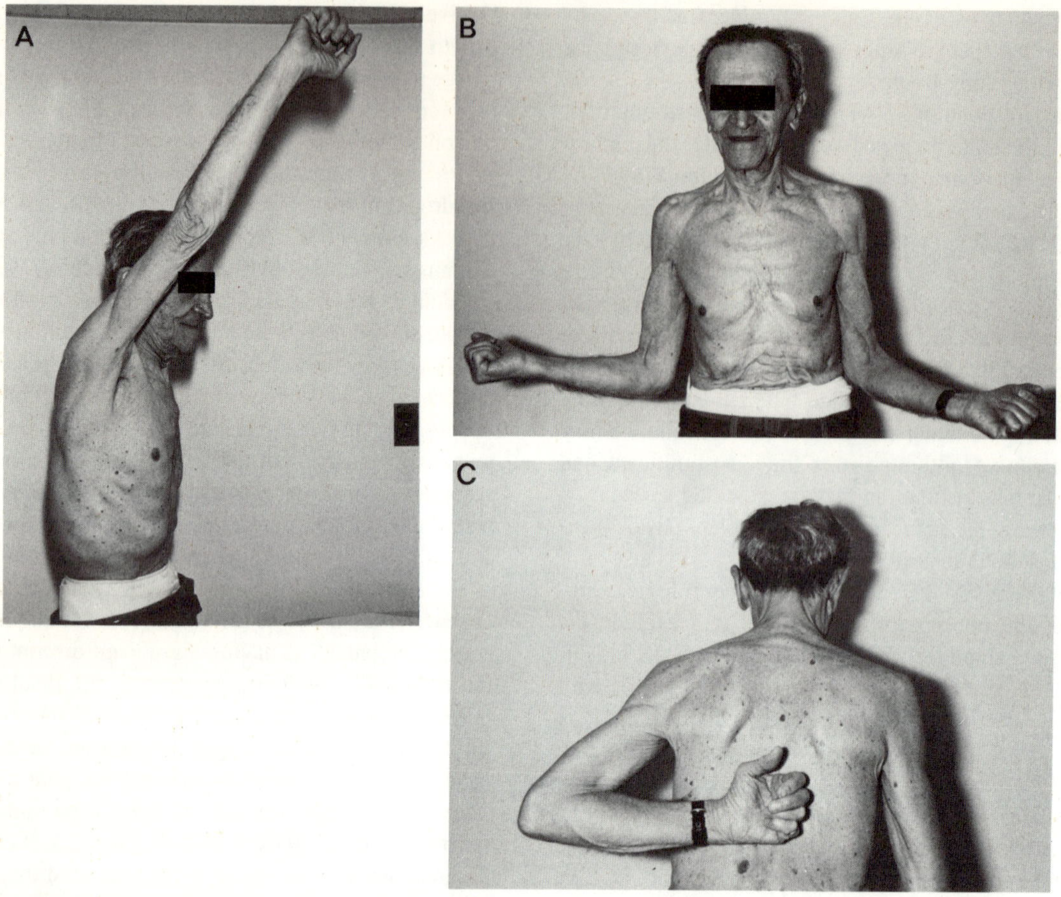

Figure 36-57. Assessment of active range of motion of the shoulder including forward elevation (*A*), external rotation (*B*), and internal rotation (*C*).

thrography has been the "gold standard" for the identification of full-thickness tears. Recently ultrasound and magnetic resonance imaging have also been used to evaluate for rotator cuff tears. However, standard arthrography remains the most common method of evaluation.

Treatment

The course of treatment chosen for the elderly patient with a rotator cuff tear depends on many factors. These factors include the specific functional requirements for the involved shoulder and upper extremity, the level of discomfort and disability, age of the patient, and the patient's expectations. In this section, the treatment approaches for "acute on chronic" and chronic rotator cuff tears are discussed. It is important to recognize that the treatment regimens to be discussed are meant to serve only as guidelines. The treatment approach for any specific patient must be individualized. Patients who fall into the category of "acute on chronic" rotator cuff problems usually present with the acute onset or an acute increase in shoulder pain following an injury. If the patient is within a week of the injury, treatment should be directed at obtaining pain relief. The patient should be placed in a sling for comfort but at the same time started on an assisted range of motion program to maintain shoulder mobility. Ice applied directly to the shoulder may provide some pain relief along with use of nonsteroidal anti-inflammatory medications. Mild analgesics can also be used, but medications containing narcotics should be avoided in the elderly. Patients should be reevaluated a few days later and again at about 2 to 3 weeks following the injury. If at that point the pain is subsiding and motion, strength, and overall function are improving, then the patient should be continued on the same treatment plan and a supervised rehabilitation program should be begun. However, if significant disability persists, then an arthrogram is indicated. If a full-thickness tear is present, surgical repair should be considered. However, before proceeding with surgical management, it is important to carefully consider the factors listed previously.

Rotator cuff surgery has the primary goal of obtain-

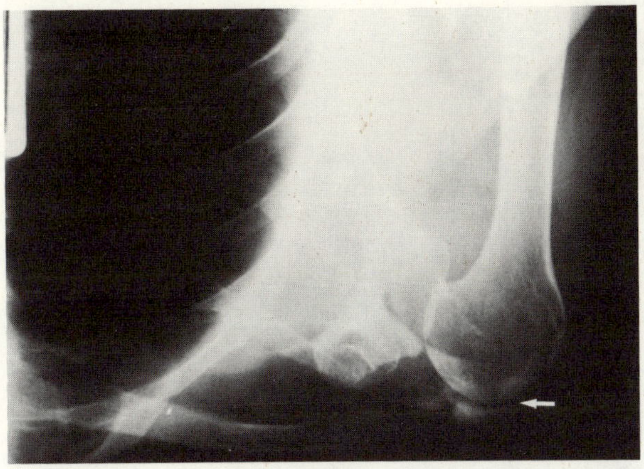

Figure 36-58. An acromiohumeral distance of less than 5 mm is suggestive of a full-thickness rotator cuff tear. In longstanding rotator cuff tears, the humeral head may articulate with the underside of the acromion, which developes a concave shape.

ing pain relief; improvement of motion is a secondary and much more unpredictable goal (20, 59, 61, 131, 221, 305, 307). In addition, one study found that the results of rotator cuff tears in patients over age 60 deteriorated over time (305). The patient's age and medical status as it impacts on the risk of surgery is also important. Some patients may be willing to accept their disability to avoid surgery, or they may be unacceptable surgical risks. These patients should be treated with the pain-relieving measures previously described along with a rehabilitation program directed at maintaining shoulder function. Patients who elect to undergo surgical management should have a clear understanding of the goals of surgery and the anticipated outcomes. Pain relief can be anticipated in 75% to 95% of patients undergoing subacromial decompression and rotator cuff repair (12, 59, 221, 305). However, improving the function and range of motion is less predictable (59). It is essential for the patient to have realistic expectations about surgery. A patient with unrealistic expectations will not be satisfied, regardless of the outcome.

Patients with significant shoulder pain and disability with a "chronic rotator cuff tear" should be treated with the pain-relieving measures described. In addition, a rehabilitation program directed at maintaining and improving range of motion and function should also be instituted. These patients have chronic "attritional" rotator cuff tears from longstanding impingement. In these patients, operative management should not be considered unless the patient has failed to respond to at least 6 months of nonoperative management. Here, once again, the goal should be pain relief, with restoration of motion being a less predictable outcome.

Operative Management

Operative management of rotator cuff tears include subacromial decompression and rotator cuff repair. Decompression of the subacromial space is mandatory to address the impingement process that is probably present in all "acute on chronic" and "chronic" cases. This consists of

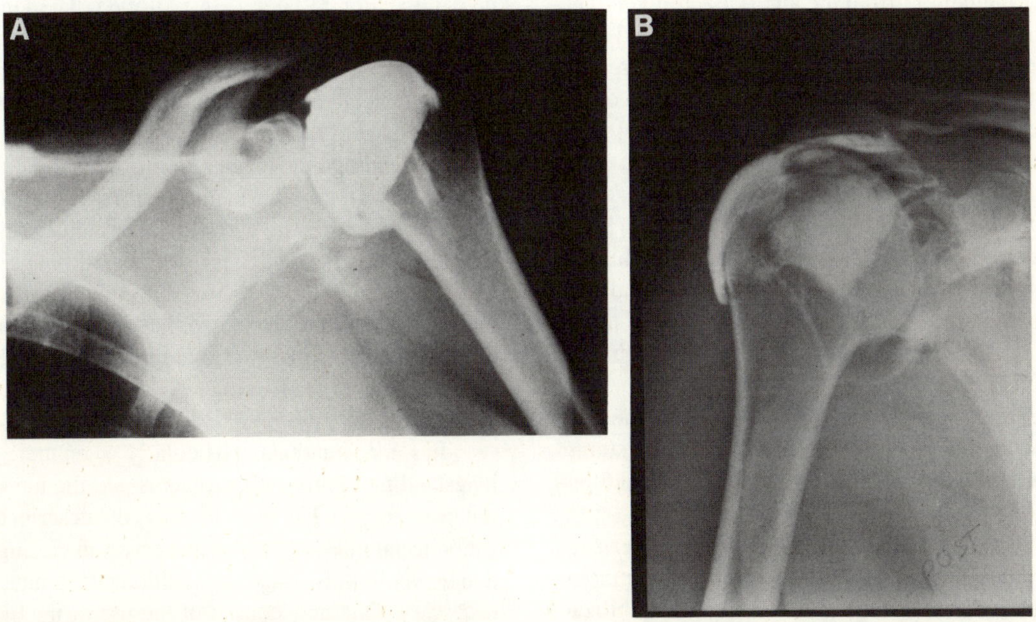

Figure 36-59. Arthrographic appearance of an intact rotator cuff (*A*). The contrast material is contained within the joint and outlines the underside of the rotator cuff. The presence of a full-thickness rotator cuff tear allows extravasation of contrast material into the subacromial space (*B*).

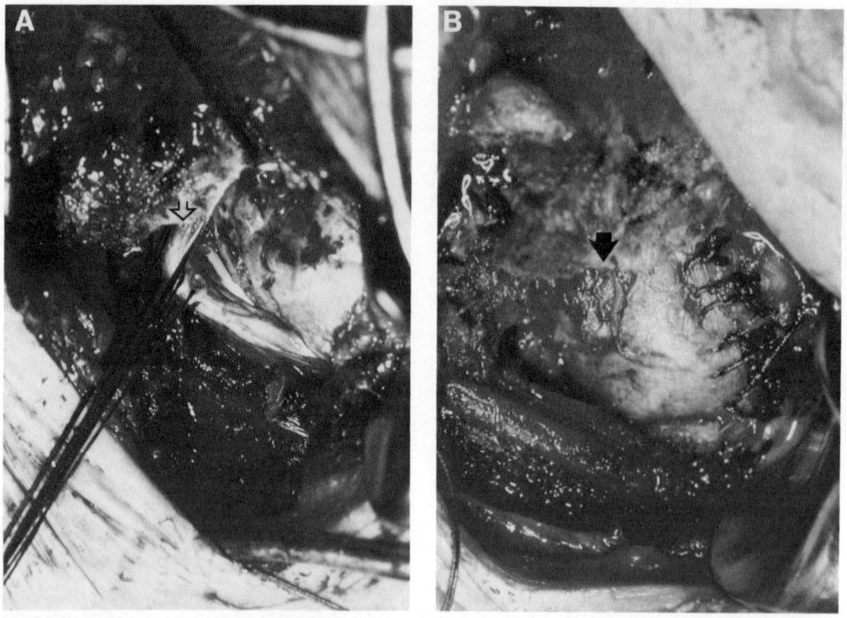

Figure 36-60. Rotator cuff tear in a 72-year-old male following a fall onto his outstretched arm (*A*). The sutures are in the lateral edge of the supraspinatus tendon. The biceps tendon can be seen under the tendon. The repair consisted of a combination of tendon-to-tendon and tendon-to-bone sutures (*B*). (*Arrow* indicates the anterior edge of the acromion.)

anterior acromioplasty, resection of the coracoacromial ligament, and excision of any osteophytes located on the inferior aspect of the acromioclavicular joint. A distal clavicle excision should be performed when symptomatic degenerative changes of the acromioclavicular joint are present. A superior surgical approach is utilized with detachment of the deltoid from the anterior acromion. The subacromial decompression is performed first. This improves the exposure of the rotator cuff. The type of rotator cuff repair used will depend on the size and location of the tear and the condition of the remaining tendons (61). It is important to follow the established treatment pinciples. First, the overlying subacromial bursa should be excised so that the tendon edges can be clearly visualized. Thickened and scarred bursal tissue can be confused with rotator cuff tendons if the anatomy is not clearly identified. Frayed tendon edges should be trimmed back a few millimeters to healthier tissue. The extent of the tear should be clearly delineated and traction sutures placed using a noncutting needle. As the needle is passed through the tendon, tension should be applied to confirm that the suture will not "pull out" following repair. After traction sutures are placed, the tendon should be mobilized (Fig. 36-60). This is first done by blunt dissection along the outer surface of the muscle into the supraspinous and infraspinous areas. In most cases, this will allow adequate mobilization for the tendon to be reattached laterally at the edge of the articular surface. If the tendon edges have retracted and significant scarring is present, additional mobilization will be necessary. This is accomplished by dividing the attachments of the underlying capsule at the glenoid rim. When the tendons can be advanced laterally to the desired point of reattachment, closure can be performed. Tendon to tendon repair is preferred but this is usually not possible. Most repairs are a combination of tendon to tendon and tendon to bone (Fig. 36-60*B*). The longitudinal portions of the tear should be repaired in a tendon to tendon fashion and the lateral edge reattached directly to bone. A cancellous bed should be made just medial to the articular edge of the greater tuberosity. Drill holes should be placed through the greater tuberosity and out the lateral cortex. Overlapping horizontal mattress sutures are then placed. The sutures are tied with the arm in 15–20 degrees of abduction as the tendon is drawn into the cancellus bed. The shoulder should be placed through a gentle range of motion to assess the security of the repair and to aid in the design of the postoperative therapy program. In some instances, an abduction splint will be necessary to protect the repair.

In some situations, particularly when there has been longstanding rotator cuff problems and the interval from injury to surgery has been lengthy, the described mobilization techniques will be unsuccessful in closing the tendon defect. In this situation, additional techniques will be necessary. This may consist of the use of the biceps tendon as a graft or transfer of the subscapularis or teres minor tendon superiorly (60, 61). Freeze-dried cadaver rotator cuff, as well as synthetic materials have also been used (215, 220, 230). In general, the simpler techniques have the best chance of success and are preferred compared to more complex techniques. When rotator cuff repair is complete, closure is performed. The most important aspect of the closure is a secure reattachment of the deltoid to the anterior acromion and lateral clavicle. This should be repaired directly to bone using nonabsorbable sutures. Skin and subcutaneous tissues are closed in a routine fashion. The upper extremity is then placed in a sling with Ace bandages used for additional Velpeau-type immobilization.

Postoperative management is determined by the nature of the repair. In general, active elbow, wrist, and hand motion is begun on the 1st postoperative day. Shortly thereafter a program of passive range of motion, specifically forward elevation and external rotation, is begun and is maintained for 6 to 8 weeks, depending on the size of the tear and the security of the repair. This is followed by an active range of motion program. Strengthening exercises are begun when active range of motion is comfortable. In general, recovery from rotator cuff surgery of this type requires at least 4 to 6 months.

Carpal Tunnel Syndrome

Of all hand operations in the elderly population, surgical release of the carpal tunnel for carpal tunnel syndrome is the most commonly performed procedure. Carpal tunnel syndrome refers to a compression neuropathy of the median nerve at the wrist (80, 227). It is the most common of all entrapment neuropathies of the upper extremity and represents a common orthopaedic problem in the geriatric age group. The carpal tunnel is formed by a dorsal bony arch (the carpal bones) connected by a dense volar ligamentous base formed by the transverse carpal ligament (Fig. 36-61). The limited volume of this rigid canal must accommodate the long flexor tendons and the median nerve as they pass into the hand. Any situation that compromises the available space within the canal can cause compression of the median nerve, resulting in local ischemia and nerve dysfunction. Slowly progressive nerve compression may go unnoticed or have only minor symptoms for quite a long time because the nerve is able to adapt to a slowly decreasing volume. However, when the compression becomes severe, certain classic symptoms are manifested.

The usual symptoms of carpal tunnel syndrome include hypesthesia or paresthesia in the distribution of the median nerve and weakness or loss of manual dexterity in the affected hand (80, 93, 227). The condition can present as shoulder or forearm pain, and proximal radiation of the pain to the elbow is not uncommon. The symptoms are often aggravated with use of the hand, and awakening from sleep with wrist pain and paresthesias in the fingers is commonly described. The classic teaching is that carpal tunnel syndrome is twice as common in women as in men, but new evidence suggests that the condition is more common in men than previously believed (93). About 50% of cases are found in the 40- to 60-year age group, with 30% of cases in patients over age 60 (227).

Diagnosis of carpal tunnel syndrome is based on the clinical presentation described above and several classic findings. The most constant finding is a sensory disturbance in the distribution of the median nerve distal to the wrist. Sensation over the entire fifth digit should be normal. Findings of sensory dysfunction in the fifth digit must alert the examiner to other possible conditions, such as: (*a*) involvement of the ulnar nerve in Guyon's canal, which is adjacent to the carpal canal (Fig. 36-61); (*b*) a peripheral neuropathy such as that seen in diabetes; or (*c*) involvement of the cervical roots on the affected side. Atrophy of the thenar muscles may be present and may be quite striking when compared to the unaffected hand. When thenar atrophy is present, it is usually preceded by hypesthesia for many months to many years. Two special tests used in the diagnosis of carpal tunnel syndrome are the Tinel's sign and the wrist-flexion test. A positive Tinel's sign is present when light percussion over the median nerve at the wrist causes a tingling sensation radiating distally into the hand (80). The wrist-flexion test, or Phalen's test, involves active maximum wrist flexion by the patient, which causes the median nerve to be compressed between the proximal edge of the transverse car-

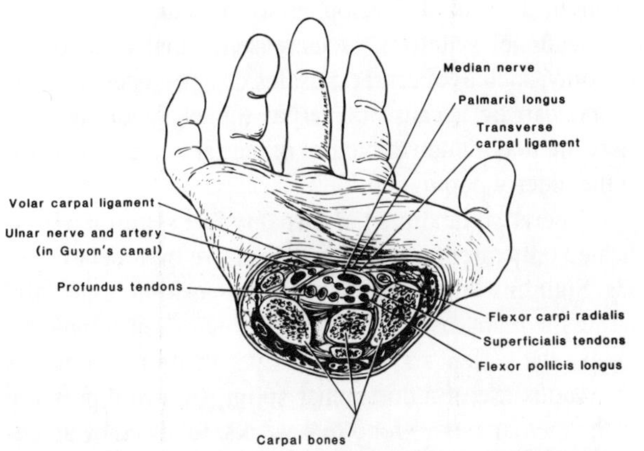

Figure 36-61. The carpal tunnel at the wrist. Contents of the tunnel include the superficial and deep flexor tendons, as well as the flexor pollucis longis tendon and the median nerve. The canal is bordered by the carpal bones along the dorsal radial and ulnar surfaces with the transverse carpal ligament covering the volar aspect. Release is done near the midline through the transverse carpal ligament. Also note the ulnar nerve and artery at the wrist in a separate enclosed space (Guyon's canal), which may show signs of entrapment as well.

pal ligament and the flexor tendons (227). The test is positive if, within 60 seconds, the previously described numbness or paresthesias are reproduced or exaggerated. A positive Phalen's test is believed to be strong evidence for carpal tunnel syndrome.

Electrodiagnostic studies are often useful in the diagnosis of carpal tunnel syndrome. In suspected cases, nerve conduction studies showing an increased latency between median nerve at the proximal wrist flexion crease and the action potential of the opponenes pollicis or the abductor pollicis brevis confirm the diagnosis (227). Electromyography can also be useful in differentiating carpal tunnel syndrome from thoracic outlet and cervical compression syndromes (115).

There are many etiologies for carpal tunnel syndrome (80, 93, 227). All result in compression of the median nerve due to a decrease in the available space within the carpal canal, either by the addition of abnormal structures or by the alteration of the normal anatomy. Benign tumors, such as ganglia and lipomas, can compete for space within the carpal tunnel and result in median nerve compression. Systemic illnesses associated with carpal tunnel syndrome include rheumatoid arthritis, diabetes mellitus, amyloidosis, multiple myeloma, thyroid imbalance (particularly myxedema), gout, and acromegaly. Carpal tunnel syndrome is also belived to have a traumatic origin in many cases. Minor repetitive wrist stress, seen in many patients who work with their hands using a particular wrist motion repeatedly, results in thickening of the transverse carpal ligament or chronic tenosynovitis of the flexor tendons. Following major trauma to the wrist, such as a Colle's fracture or carpal bone fracture or dislocation, the risk of developing an immediate or delayed carpal tunnel syndrome is increased. Finally, abnormal anatomy, such as aberrant muscles or a persistent median artery, can be a cause of carpal tunnel syndrome, but these are uncommon etiologies of carpal tunnel syndrome in the elderly population.

Operative treatment of carpal tunnel syndrome is indicated only after failure of nonoperative treatment methods. Splinting of the wrist in a neutral position, especially during the night, usually reduces and may even completely resolve the patient's symptoms. Eversmann recommends continuous use of a dorsoulnar splint, (to avoid pressure on the median nerve) for 3 to 4 weeks, followed by an additional 4 weeks of night splinting (93). He notes that even if the symptoms completely resolve with splinting, their recurrence with removal of the splint is an indication for operative treatment. Oral nonsteroidal anti-inflammatory medications and short courses of oral corticosteroids are sometimes prescribed, but their efficacy in carpal tunnel syndrome remains uncertain (93). Corticosteroid injection into the carpal tunnel is another commonly used method of nonoperative treatment. Series reporting on this technique show improvement of symptoms in 62% to 96% of patients, with recurrence rates varying from 8% to 94% (115). Green found that although most of the 81% of patients obtaining good relief of symptoms with injection showed recurrence of symptoms after about 2 to 4 months, 54% of these patients did not have recurrent symptoms severe enough to warrant operative treatment. He also noted that a good response to injection was an excellent prognostic sign, which correlated with a good surgical result even if the symptoms recurred. Gelberman et al. conducted a prospective trial of steroid injections and splinting, and found 22% completely symptom free at an average 18-month follow-up (110). They found that hands with mild symptoms and findings initially had the best response to injection and splintings.

Failure of nonoperative treatment or the return of significant symptoms following a trial of splinting, injections, or oral medication are all indications for carpal tunnel release. Surgical release may also be indicated for severe thenar atrophy and hand dysfunction in the absence of nonoperative intervention.

Decompression of the carpal canal is performed by release of the transverse carpal ligament. Various incisions, approaches, and methods of sectioning of the ligament have been described, and the specific details of the many different approaches are beyond the scope of this chapter. However, as an example, the incision recommended by Eversmann begins at the distal border of the transverse carpal ligament, extending proximally along the longitudinal crease of the palm, crossing the base of the palm ulnar to the long axis of the ring finger in a zigzag fashion, and continuing 3 cm proximal to the proximal wrist crease (93). After careful dissection and identification of the surrounding structures, including the palmar cutaneous branch of the median nerve, the transverse carpal ligament is carefully exposed, and sectioned in line with the underlying nerve and tendons. Others suggest removal of a thin strip of the ligament to be sure that the ends will not heal to one another. Many surgeons performing carpal tunnel releases recommend a more limited incision and exposure and a blind scissor release of the proximal aspect of the ligament through the more distal exposure (80). A median nerve neurolysis is performed if the median nerve appears abnormally scarred or if the patient displayed severe signs of median nerve compromise preoperatively. It is estimated that internal neurolysis of the median nerve is done in 10% to 15% of surgical releases of the carpal tunnel (93). This is a delicate procedure that should be performed under loupe magnification. Recently, however, others have stressed the importance of avoiding further surgery on the nerve if possible to prevent the possibility of increased postoperative scarring.

Some surgeons will compromise and perform a simple epineurotomy of the median nerve at the wrist, which acts as a "fasciotomy" of the nerve and can be helpful in cases of epineural scarring secondary to compression. Following the appropriate tissue releases, the skin is the only layer closed, usually with nonabsorbable simple sutures. The wrist is immobilized for up to 14 days, at which time progressive range of motion and strengthening exercises are begun.

Patients usually experience almost immediate relief of pain, and a rapid improvement in sensory deficits, provided that a neurotmesis or axonotmesis had not been present prior to surgery. Wrist swelling can be expected for up to 16 weeks following surgery. The return of muscle strength in the wrist and hand following carpal tunnel release can be prolonged, with only about 50% of preoperative grip strength present 6 weeks postoperatively, 75% by 8 to 10 weeks, and maximum grip strength only at 6 months or more (93). In general, the results of carpal tunnel decompression are good, with a significant relief of pain and paresthesias in up to 85% of cases (93, 153, 227). As might be expected, the results do correlate with the severity of median nerve pathology. Return of lost sensation and thenar muscle atrophy is quite variable. As mentioned previously, a good response to steroid injection of the carpal canal, even if temporary, does correlate with a good surgical outcome.

True complications specific to carpal tunnel surgery are not very common, but do occur. Phalen reported on 212 procedures, and noted no serious postoperative complications (227). In another report, MacDonald et al. reviewed 186 cases and noted a complication rate of 12% (180). In more than one-third of these, however, persistent symptoms and signs were attributed to incomplete division of the transverse carpal ligament. Of the other reported complications, damage to the palmar cutaneous branch of the median nerve was most common (4%), with cases of reflex sympathetic dystrophy, hypertrophic scar, palmar hematoma, bowstringing of the flexor tendons, and adherence of the flexor tendons responsible for the remaining 4%. It is clear that careful surgical technique using a longitudinal incision, adequate exposure, and appropriate postoperative care are all important in minimizing the complication rate of carpal tunnel surgery.

Bunions

Foot pain with an associated "bunion" deformity is a common complaint in the older population. Commonly, these patients describe a long history of a slowly progressive deformity. They often have a history of poor shoe wear, including "fashionable" shoes with narrow toe-boxes and high heels. These patients complain of foot pain with shoe wear and difficulty finding comfortable shoes. They often have an associated hammer-toe deformity of the second toe or an overriding of the hallux on the second toe. The term "bunion" refers to an enlargement or deformity of the metatarsophalangeal (MTP) joint of the first ray (183). It is most often caused by a hallux valgus, which is defined as a static subluxation of the first MTP joint with lateral deviation of the first toe and medial deviation of the first metatarsal (metatarsus primus varus) (183). The bunion deformity related to hallux valgus will be the focus of the remainder of our discussion. Other much less common causes of a bunion deformity include bursal enlargement, hallux rigidus, a ganglion cyst, and an arthritic first MTP joint with proliferative arthritic changes.

The etiology of an acquired bunion deformity in adults is believed to be related to both genetic factors and shoe wear. Ligamentous laxity and progressive stretching over time is felt to be the result of genetic predisposition, with progressive attenuation of the medial collateral ligament of the MTP joint resulting in a valgus deviation of the hallux and forefoot pronation (159). The muscles about the hallux act to accentuate the deformity because of the abnormal position of the phalanx. Bunions due to hallux valgus are predominantly found in the shoe-wearing populations of the world (182). Poor shoe wear creates abnormal mechanical forces across the joints of the first ray during ambulation and weight bearing act to maximize the morphologic expression of this genetic predisposition (159). A flexible flat foot, a positive family history, and a long first ray can all be associated with a bunion deformity later in life (261). Two-thirds of all patients surgically treated for their bunion deformities give a positive family history of the disorder. In series of surgically treated cases, the reported female:male ratio is 9:1 (261). This high female predominance is likely related to the use of shoes with a narrow toe-box and high heels. Long-term use of high-heeled shoes has been associated with a combined bunion deformity and a second hammer-toe.

The primary treatment of all patients with bunions is nonoperative. Most patients will have significant benefit by switching to more appropriate shoe wear, such as a rubber-soled low-heeled shoe with a wide toe-box, which relieves pressure over the medial prominence. Patients over age sixty often place less demands on their feet than younger, more active patients, and surgery can often be avoided. However, many older patients are quite active and have significant persistent pain despite appropriate shoe wear modifications, and surgery becomes necessary.

The main goal of bunion surgery is pain relief. The mere presence of a bunion deformity in an asymptomatic patient requesting a cosmetic improvement is not an indication for surgery (261). The possibility of turning an asymptomatic, unsightly deformity into a painful, cosmetically acceptable one is real and should be avoided at all costs. Another important goal of bunion surgery is to correct the deformities of the first ray and prevent a recurrence. To accomplish this, the surgeon must restore (*a*) the articular congruency of the joints of the first ray, and (*b*) the alignment of the first ray relative to the lateral aspect of the foot (261). Although cosmesis is not a primary goal of the surgery, accomplishing the goals outlined above will result in an improved cosmetic appearance.

The elderly patient indicated for bunion surgery (or any other type of foot surgery) should undergo a thorough preoperative physical exam including a complete peripheral vascular exam of the lower extremities. The absence of strong distal pulses in the dorsalis pedis and posterior tibial arteries may be indicative of vascular insufficiency, which could severely retard wound healing and significantly increase the risk of surgical complications (182). An arterial doppler examination should be performed comparing the ankle and brachial pulse pressures (the ankle/brachial index). This is important because arterial insufficiency may be present even if a palpable pulse is present. Patients with diabetes exhibit poor wound healing and an increased risk of infection even in the presence of good distal pulses because of small vessel disease. This must be considered carefully when contemplating any type of foot surgery. Diabetics may also have a falsely normal or elevated ankle/brachial index in the presence of vascular insufficiency, because of atherosclerotic hardening of the vessels.

In addition to the physical exam, radiographs of the feet (including A-P and lateral weight-bearing and non-weight-bearing views) are necessary to fully define the bony aspects of the deformity. In hallux valgus associated with a bunion deformity, by definition, valgus angulation of the MTP joint is greater than 15 degrees. Associated with this is a variable amount of metatarsus primus varus (defined as an intermetatarsal angle greater than 9 degrees) (159, 182). Severe metatarsus primus varus is more commonly encountered in adolescent hallux valgus. It is unclear at this time whether the metatarsus primus varus is a cause of the hallux valgus deformity or a result of it. Mann believes that in adolescents it is an initiating factor, but in the adult population it represents a secondary change (182). A valgus deformity of the interphalangeal joint of the great toe (hallux interphalangeus) is sometimes found as part of the first ray pathology and may also need to be addressed. As a general rule, the deformities should be corrected as close as possible to where they exist. Therefore, a full understanding of the anatomy of the deformity is important to choose the appropriate method of surgical correction (159).

Before discussion of some specific procedures in bunion surgery, some general principles about skin and joint capsule incisions should be mentioned. The recommended skin incision for most bunion procedures is longitudinal and medial, following the line of the first metatarsal and proximal phalanx. This results in a curved incision with a plantar concavity (261). This is felt to be a safer incision than the popular dorsal-curved incision for two reasons: (*a*) the dorsal-curved incision requires more undermining of skin to achieve exposure and presents a higher risk of wound complications, and (*b*) the dorsal-curved incision has a higher risk of injury to the dorsal sensory nerves of the first ray resulting in a sensory deficit or painful neuroma. The recommended MTP joint capsular incision is longitudinal and medial with subperiosteal reflection of the capsule both dorsally and plantarly (261). Closure of this incision must be done in a pants-over-vest fashion bringing the plantar capsule more dorsal, to derotate the tendon of the abductor hallucis from its abnormal plantar position (secondary to the forefoot pronation deformity commonly seen with hallux valgus). Mann recommends using a vertical capsular incision 2 to 3 mm proximal to the base of the proximal phalanx, with a second incision that parallels this incision proximally (with the distance determined by the amount of correction and excess medial capsule) connected by V-shaped dorsal and volar extensions (182, 183). A distally based long medial capsular flap has been used for many years but is currently not recommended for two reasons: (*a*) proximal reattachment is often compromised secondary to the attenuated proximal joint capsule, and (*b*) it fails to derotate the phalanx and abductor hallucis tendon insertion.

In the elderly population, a few specific factors must be considered when choosing the surgical procedure to be used for bunion correction. First is the vascular status of the foot. In a foot with a partially compromised blood supply, minimal corrective procedures are recommended. More extensive osteotomies and soft tissue reconstructions are relatively contraindicated. Second, the skin quality about the hallux must be carefully assessed. Poor skin quality or tense skin will often not accommodate large angular corrections without some type of shortening of the ray. In these cases, a Keller resection arthroplasty (see below) is often indicated (182). The presence of arthritis in the MTP joint is another important finding that is an indication for Keller arthroplasty, MTP joint arthrodesis, or MTP joint implant rather than a realignment procedure (159, 182, 183, 261). There are literally over one hundred specific operations described in the orthopaedic literature for correction of bunion deformities. Detailed descriptions of even the most commonly performed procedures are clearly beyond the scope of this chapter. However, it is important to understand the location of the correction and the major structures addressed in the more popular bunion operations.

Surgical procedures for correction of the bunion deformity with hallux valgus can be divided into six types. First is the simple exostectomy, where, after the surgical approach already described, an osteotome or microsagittal power saw is used to remove the medial eminence of the first metatarsal head followed by repair of the medial joint capsule (Fig. 36-62). Significant hallux valgus and metatarsus primus varus are not corrected by this procedure, and so it must be used in combination with other bony or soft-tissue correction in patients with these deformities.

Soft-tissue repair and reconstruction constitutes the second type of procedure used in bunion surgery. These procedures correct the hallux valgus deformity, and, to a lesser extent, the metatarsus primus varus. Mann recommends a soft-tissue repair that is a modification of the procedures described by DuVries, McBride, and Silver (182, 183). The main features of this repair include: (*a*) lateral release of the adductor hallucis insertion, (*b*) lateral capsulotomy of the first MTP joint, (*c*) suture approximation of the first and second MTP joints through a midline vertical incision in the first web space, (*d*) an exostectomy of the medial eminance, and (*e*) a medial capsule plication. Mann feels this procedure is indicated for hallux valgus deformities of less than 40 degrees with concomitant metatarsus primus varus of 15 degrees or less. For MPV greater than 15 degrees, he recommends an additional basilar metatarsal osteotomy. For hallux interphalangeus, a proximal phalanx osteotomy should be included (see below).

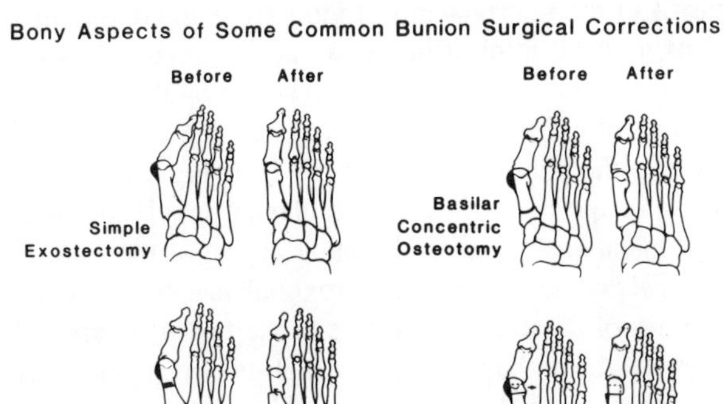

Figure 36-62. Schematic representation of the bony aspects of some of the more common surgical procedures done for bunion deformity (see text for details of specific procedures).

The third category of surgical procedure for bunion correction is the metatarsal osteotomies. Many have been described, and they can be broadly divided into proximal and distal metatarsal osteotomies. For proximal metatarsal osteotomies, various types of opening wedge, closing wedge, and concentric osteotomies have been described. These are indicated in patients of all ages with significant metatarsus primus varus, usually over 15 degrees (183). Mann recommends a basilar concentric osteotomy, done in the cancellous portion of the proximal first metatarsal approximately 1 cm distal to the metatarso-cuneiform joint, using a curved osteotomy saw (Fig. 36-62). The apex of the curved osteotomy is located proximally, and the metatarsal shift is angled and derotated as necessary and then stablized using a single smooth Steinmann pin or multiple K-wires for 4 to 6 weeks (Fig. 36-63). Multiple variations of distal metatarsal osteotomies have been described. The Mitchell procedures, described by Hawkins et al., is a double step-cut osteotomy through the neck of the first metatarsal which is usually done in patients less than 50 years old with moderate hallux valgus and an intermetatarsal up to 18 degrees (130) (Fig. 36-62). A chevron-type osteotomy has become quite popular (183). It is also commonly done in younger adults with moderate hallux valgus and mild metatarsus primus varus without a pronation deformity of the great toe. It involves a biplane horizontal osteotomy angled 60 degrees with its base proximally, followed by a lateral displacement of the metatarsal head of less than one-third the width of the metatarsal shaft (Fig. 36-62). It may be stabilized with a Kirschner wire, but this is usually not necessary.

The fourth type of procedure performed for bunion correction is an MTP resection arthroplasty, known as the Keller procedure (158). This was a very popular procedure in the past, but its indications have become more limited since the advent of newer operative techiques such as those already described. The procedure involves: (*a*) resection of one-third to one-half of the proximal phalanx through a dorsomedial skin incision and a proximally-based medial rectangular capsular flap, (*b*) a resection of the medial eminence of the metatarsal head, and (*c*) reattachment of the medial capsular structures and plantar plate with the attached sesmoids and tendons to the re-

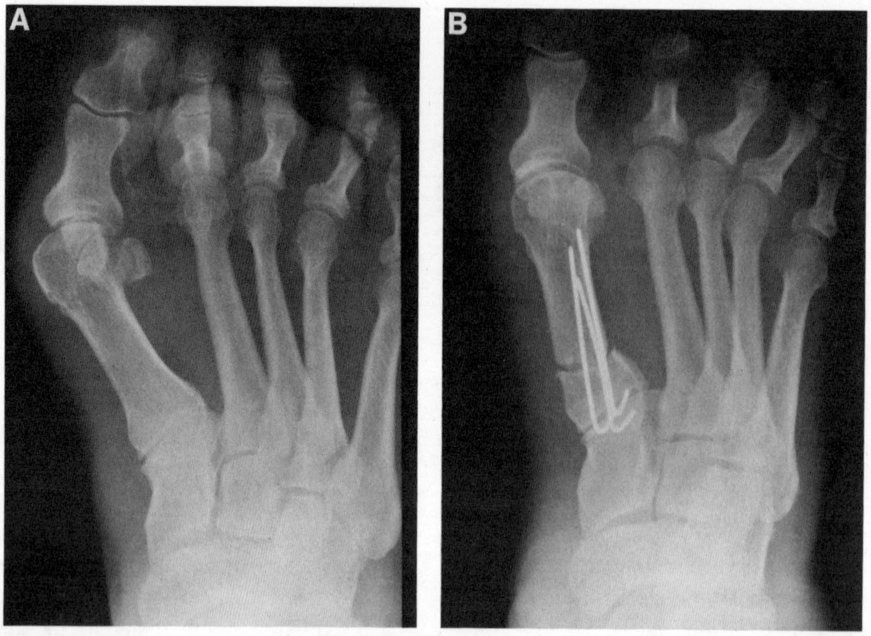

Figure 36-63. 61-year-old female with severe painful bunion deformity. *A*, This AP radiograph shows hallux valgus and metatarsus primus varus. The patient also had a cock-up of the second toe. *B*, Correction was performed using a basal concentric osteotomy fixed with percutaneous K-wires. The patient also had soft tissue correction of the hallux valgus and resection of the head of the second proximal phalanx.

maining proximal phalanx through drill holes on the medial and plantar diaphysis (Fig. 36-62). A smooth Steinmann pin is often used as a longitudinal intramedullary stabilizer, maintaining a 5 mm gap across the resected MTP joint for 4 to 6 weeks. Mann recommends use of this procedure only in elderly patients who will place minimal demands on the foot (183) (Fig. 36-64). This is not the procedure of choice for an active individual of any age, unless chronic skin problems prevent adequate correction of large deformities without significant shortening of the ray. Even in this case, arthrodesis may be preferred. The most common problem following a Keller procedure is significant metatarsalgia beneath the second and third metatarsal heads, due to the abnormal transfer of the weight-bearing load laterally in the absence of a stable first MTP joint. Push-off power is compromised, severely affecting rapid gait or running activities. This is more likely to affect active patients, which is why this procedure is not indicated even for elderly patients who remain active and place significant demands of their feet.

Arthrodesis of the first MTP joint has been described for the treatment of hallux valgus, but it is currently recommended only for use in bunion patients with: (*a*) associated rheumatoid arthritis of the MTP joints, (*b*) traumatic degenerative arthritis of the first MTP joint, (*c*) absence of the second toe, and (*d*) recurrent bunion deformities and hallux valgus (183). Arthrodesis, unlike a Keller procedure, maintains the length and stability of the first ray. Because of the increased stresses transmitted to the great toe and interphalangeal joint, an insensate foot and arthritis of the interphalangeal joint are both contraindications to MTP joint arthrodesis. The optimal position of fusion places the great toe in a position of about 10 to 15 degrees of valgus and about 15 degrees of dorsiflexion relative to the plantar surface of the foot (Fig. 36-62). Because of the normal 15-degree plantar angulation of the first metatarsal relative to plantar aspect of the foot, the optimal position of the fused proximal phalanx is about 30 degrees of dorsiflexion relative to the first metatarsal. In women who anticipate wearing high-heeled shoes, an angle of up to 45 degrees is desirable. The fusion is performed by removing the remaining articular cartilage of both sides of the joint followed by flattening of the surfaces. Stabilization is achieved using staples, crossed Kirschner wires, axial Steinmann pins, or a screw. Mann, using axial Steinmann pin fixation, reported a fusion rate of 98%, most of which healed in 10 to 14 weeks (183).

For bunions associated with hallux valgus of up to 30 degrees or for valgus deformity of the interphalangeal joint (hallux interphalangeus), a proximal phalangeal osteotomy and soft tissue correction (Akin procedure) can be performed. It involves a closing wedge osteotomy in the proximal metaphysis of the proximal phalanx along with excision of the medial eminence and a lateral capsular release of the MTP joint (3) (Fig. 36-62). This procedure maintains the congruity of the MTP joint, but it

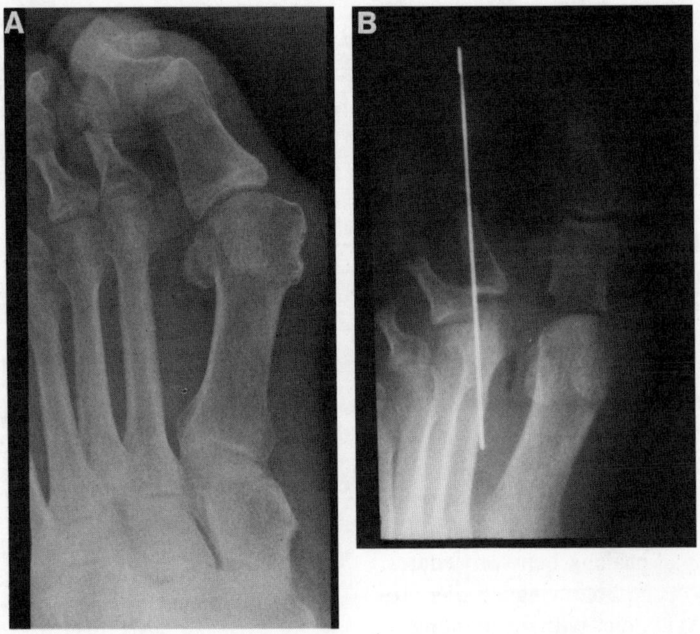

Figure 36-64. A 77-year-old female with a painful bunion deformity and overriding of the second toe. The patient was a household ambulator who ventured outside her apartment infrequently and placed minimal demands on her feet. *A*, Preoperative radiograph. *B*, Following Keller resection arthroplasty of the base of the first proximal phalanx. Also note the K-wires for fixation following resection of the second proximal phalangeal head for the lesser toe deformity.

does not correct any metatarsus primus varus. Therefore, a concomitant metatarsal osteotomy may also be necessary. A medial skin incision is used, but it is begun more distal than the standard incision. A small medially based wedge is removed from the base of the proximal phalanx approximately 7 mm distal to the MTP joint, using a needle-nosed rongeur or a small oscillating saw. Care should be taken to leave the lateral cortex intact. The osteotomy site is closed and fixed with either a 0.045 Kirschner wire exiting through the tip of the toe for 4 to 6 weeks or with sutures passed through drill holes in the medial side of the osteotomy site.

In a review of the rationale for the surgical treatment of bunions, Kenzora advocates the use of the soft-tissue corrections (Mann, Silver) or a Keller arthroplasty in the elderly (159). He feels that advanced age and low functional demands are implied by the term "elderly bunion" and that metatarsal osteotomies are contraindicated in the elderly because of the prolonged healing time, higher morbidity, and higher failure rate in this population, possibly related to the higher incidence of vascular disease, impaired immune response, and general atrophic changes associated with aging. Many patients over age 60 or 65 are quite active and place high demands on their feet in everyday life. In the absence of severe medical contraindications, many feel that these patients should be treated as other adults with painful bunions, and should be considered for procedures that include osteotomies to correct severe hallux valgus and severe metatarsus primus varus deformities (183, 261). Kenzora also states that in the elderly, if the MTP joint is arthritic, a silicone implant or Keller procedure should be performed (159). However, patients must be aware of the 25% failure rate of silastic MTP joint implants secondary to bone resorption, implant breakage and dislocation, unexplained pain, or lack of toe purchase (159). The salvage procedures for a failed implant include either an arthrodesis or Keller arthroplasty.

In general, good results and a high rate of patient satisfaction can be expected following surgical correction of symptomatic bunions. Mann, in his series of soft-tissue corrections, reported an 89% total satisfaction rate in his patients, with 7% "somewhat happy," and only 4% "very unhappy" (182).

Complications of bunion surgery, although uncommon, do occur. They can be divided into general complications and procedure-specific complications (183). Of the general complications, poor wound healing with or without skin necrosis can occur, especially in the elderly patient, if the vascular supply to the foot is compromised. Infection, both superficial and deep, is also more likely in association with poor circulation or diabetes. A preoperative vascular evaluation and the use of the midline medial skin incision will help limit these serious complication. Injuries to the cutaneous nerves of the hallux can occur, resulting in dysesthesia or anesthesia at the injury site and distally. The main complications of the soft-tissue procedures are loss of correction secondary to failure of the soft tissue repair or overcorrection with resulting hallux varus deformity. In Mann's series of soft-tissue corrections, an 11% rate of residual hallux varus was reported (182). For any of the procedures involving an osteotomy, loss of correction, malunion, and nonunion can occur. To avoid these complications, broad stable osteotomies should be utilized with adequate fixation and proper immobilization of the foot. A more common complication of metatarsal shaft osteotomies is significant shortening, which can cause metatarsalgia due to the transfer of weight-bearing to the second metatarsal head. Complications of metatarsal head procedures include instability of the MTP joint with resultant hallux varus. This commonly is the result of excessive resection of the medial eminence of the metatarsal head. Displacement of the metatarsal head resulting in malunion can occur following head osteotomies, as can osteonecrosis. With proximal phalanx bony procedures, similar complications also occur. Following a Keller procedure, instability of the MTP joint with resultant metatarsalgia and dorsal/valgus drift of the hallux is the most common complication. Following MTP joint arthrodesis, degenerative arthritis of the interphalangeal joint occurs in up to 40% of patients, but much fewer actually develop clinical symptoms (183). These degenerative changes appear to be related to a lack of valgus position of the hallux following arthrodesis.

Conclusion

Orthopaedic surgical procedures are commonly performed in the elderly. The vast majority of these procedures involve joint replacement for painful arthritic conditions, fixation of osteoporosis-related fractures, or corrective procedures for other chronic disabling conditions. The primary goal of most of these procedures is to relieve pain and disability and improve the "quality of life" goals that become more and more important as our population ages.

References

1. Abrami, G, and Stevens, J. 1964. Early weight-bearing after internal fixation of transcervical fracture of the femur. *J Bone Joint Surg* 46B:204–205.
2. Agarwal, N, Reyes, JD, Westerman, DA, et al. 1986. Factors influencing DRG 210 (hip fracture) reimbursement. *J Trauma*, 26:426–431.
3. Akin, OF. 1925. The treatment of hallux valgus: A new operative procedure and its results. *Med Sentinel* 33:678–679.
4. Alffram, PA. 1964. An epidemiological study of cervical and trochanteric fractures of the femur in an urban population. *Acta Orthop Scand* (Suppl) 65:1–109.
5. Alffram, P, and Bauer, G. 1962. Epidemiology of fractures of the forearm. *J Bone Joint Surg* 44A(5):105–114.
6. Amstutz, HC, Thomas, BJ, Kabo, M, et al. 1988. The Dana total shoulder arthroplasty. *J Bone Joint Surg* 70A.
7. Anderson, LD, Hamsa, WR, and Waring, TL. 1964. Femoral head prostheses. *J Bone Joint Surg* 46:1049–1065.
8. Arnala, I, Alhava, EM, Kivivuori, R, et al. 1986. Hip fracture incidence not affected by fluoridation. Osteoflurosis studied in Finland. *Acta Orthop Scand* 57:344–348.
9. Arnold, WD. 1984. The effect of early weight-bearing on the stability of femoral neck fractures treated with Knowles pins. *J Bone Joint Surg* 66A:847–852.
10. Arnoldi, CC, Brodsky, AC, Cauchoix, J, et al. 1976. Lumbar spinal stenosis and nerve root entrapment syndromes: Definition and classification. *Clin Orthop Rel Res* 115: 4–5.
11. Astrom, J, Ahngvist, S, Beertema, J, et al. 1987. Physical activity in women sustaining fracture of the neck of the femur. *J Bone Joint Surg* 69B:381–383.
12. Bankart, ASB. 1939. The pathology and treatment of recurrent dislocation of the shoulder joint. *Br J Surg* 26:23–29.
13. Banks, HH. 1962. Factors influencing the result in fractures of the femoral neck. *J Bone Joint Surg* 44A:931–964.
14. Banks, HH. 1974. Nonunion in fractures of the femoral neck. *Orthop Clin North Am* 5:865–885.
15. Barcena, A, Lobata, RD, Rivas, JJ, et al. 1984. Spinal metastatic disease: Analysis of factors determining functional prognosis and the choice of treatment. *Neurosurg* 15(6):820–827.
16. Barnes, R, Brown, JT, Garden, RS, et al. 1976. Subcapital fractures of the femur. *J Bone Joint Surg* 58B:2–24.
17. Barr, JS. 1974. Diagnosis and treatment of infections following internal fixation of hip fractures. *Orthop Clin North Am* 5:847–864.
18. Barrett, WP, Franklin, JL, Jackson, SE, et al. 1987. Total shoulder arthroplasty. *J Bone Joint Surg* 69A:865–872.
19. Barry, HC. 1967. Fractures of the femur in Paget's disease of bone in Australia. *J Bone Joint Surg* 49A:1359–1370.
20. Bassett, RW, and Cofield, RH. 1983. Acute tears of the rotator cuff. *Clin Orthop Rel Res* 175:18–24.
21. Bauer, Goran C. 1970. Epidemiology of fracture in aged persons. *Clin Orthop Rel Res* 17:219–225.
22. Beals, RK. 1972. Survival following hip fracture. Long follow-up of 607 patients. *J Chronic Dis* 25:235–244.
23. Beckenbauch, RD, and Ilstrup, DM. 1978. Total hip arthroplasty. *J Bone Joint Surg* 60A:306–313.
24. Bentley, G. 1968. Impacted fractures of the neck of the femur. *J Bone Joint Surg* 50B:551–561.
25. Bentley, G. 1980. Treatment of nondisplaced fractures of the femoral neck. *Clin Orthop Rel Res* 152:93–101.
26. Bhardwaj, S, and Holland, JF. 1982. Chemotherapy of metastatic cancer in bone. *Clin Orthop Rel Res* 169:34.
27. Bochner, RM, Pellicci, PM, and Lyden, JP. 1988. Bipolar hemiarthroplasty for fracture of the femoral neck. Clinical review with special emphasis on prosthetic motion. *J Bone Joint Surg* 70(A):1001–1010.

28. Bogoch, ER, Ovellette, G, and Hastings, DE. 1989. Failure of internal fixation of femoral neck fractures in rheumatoid arthritis patients. Paper #228, *Annual Meeting of the American Academy of Orthopaedic Surgeons,* February 11.
29. Bohler. 1956. *The Treatment of Fractures,* ed 5. vol. I. New York: Grune & Stratton.
30. Boland, PJ, Lane, JM, and Sundaresan, N. 1982. Metastatic disease of the spine. *Clin Orthop Rel Res* 169:95–102.
31. Bollett, AJ, Engh, G, and Parson, W. 1965. Epidemiology of osteoporosis. *Arch Intern Med* 16:191–194.
32. Bonarigo, BC, and Rubin, P. 1967. Nonunion of pathologic fracture after radiation therapy. *Radiology* 88:889–898.
33. Booth, RE, Jr. 1986. Spinal stenosis. *AAOS Instructional Course Lectures,* 420–435.
34. Bos, CFA, and Vanderlist, W. 1982. Ender nailing of trochanteric and subtrochanteric fractures in 146 patients. *Acta Orthop Belg* 48:811–822.
35. Boston, DA. 1982. Bilateral fractures of the femoral neck. *Injury* 14:207–210.
36. Boyd, HB, and Griffin, LL. 1949. Classification and treatment of trochanteric fractures. *Arch Surg* 58:853–866.
37. Bray, TJ, Smith-Hoefer, E, Hooper, A, et al. 1988. The displaced femoral neck fracture: Internal fixation versus bipolar endoprothesis results of a prospective, randomized comparison. *Clin Orthop Rel Res* 230:127–140.
38. Brehms, J. 1988. Rotator cuff tear: Evaluation and management. *Orthopaedics* 11(1):69–81.
39. Brewer, BJ. 1979. Aging of the rotator cuff. *Am J Sports Med* 7(2):102–110.
40. Brooker, AF, Bowerman, JW, Robinson, RA, et al. 1973. Ectopic ossification following total hip replacement. *J Bone Joint Surg* 55A:1629–1632.
41. Brown, T, and Court-Brown, C. 1979. Failure of sliding nail-plate fixation in subcapital fractures of the femoral neck. *J Bone Joint Surg* 61B:342–346.
42. Buchner, DM, and Larson, EB. 1987. Falls and fractures in patients with Alzheimer-type dementia. *JAMA* 257:1492–1495.
43. Calandruccio, RA, and Anderson, WE. 1980. Post-fracture avascular necrosis of the femoral head: Correlation of experimental and clinical studies. *Clin Orthop Rel Res* 152:49–84.
44. Callaghan, JJ, Dysart, SH, and Savory, CG. 1988. The uncemented porous-coated anatomic total hip prosthesis. *J Bone Joint Surg* 70A:337–346.
45. Carnesale, PG. 1987. General principles of tumors. In *Campbell's Operative Orthopaedics,* ed. 7. Ed, AH Crenshaw, 713–746. Toronto: C.V. Moseby Co.
46. Carnesale, PG, and Anderson, LD. 1975. Primary prosthetic replacement for femoral neck fractures. *Arch Surg* 110:27–29.
47. Cassebaum, WH, and Nugent, G. 1963. The predictability of bony union in displaced intracapsular fractures of the hip. *J Trauma* 3:421–424.
48. Ceder, L, Stromquist, B, and Hansen, LI. 1987. Effects of strategy changes in the treatment of femoral neck fractures during a 17 year period. *Clin Orthop Rel Res* 218:53–57.
49. Chan, RN, and Hoskinson, J. 1975. Thompson prosthesis for fractured neck of the femur. *J Bone Joint Surg* 57B:437–443.
50. Chapman, DR, Bennet, JB, Bryan, WJ, et al. 1982. Complications of distal radius fractures: Pins and plaster treatment. *J Hand Surg* 7(5):509–512.
51. Chapman, MW, Bowman, WE, Csongradi, JJ, et al. 1981. The use of Enders pins in extracapsular fractures of the hip. *J Bone Joint Surg* 63A:14–28.
52. Christie, J, Howie, C, and Armoir, P. 1988. Fixation of displaced femoral neck fractures: Compression screw fixation versus double divergent pins. *J Bone Joint Surg* 70B:199–201.
53. Coates, R. 1975. A retrospective survey of eighty-one patients with hemiarthroplasty for subcapital fracture of the femoral neck. *J Bone Joint Surg* 57B:256.
54. Cobb, AG, and Gibson, PH. 1986. Screw fixation of subcapital fractures of the femur—a better method of treatment. *Injury* 17:259–264.
55. Cobelli, N, and Sadler, A. 1985. Ender rod versus compression screw fixation of hip fractures. *Clin Orthop Rel Res* 201:123–129.
56. Cobey, JC, Cobey, JH, Conant, L, et al. 1976. Indications of recovery from fractures of the hip. *Clin Orthop Rel Res* 117:258–262.
57. Codman, EA. 1934. *The Shoulder.* Boston: Thomas Todd Company.
58. Cofield, RH. 1988. Comminuted fractures of the proximal humerus. *Clin Orthop Rel Res* 230:49–57.
59. Cofield, RH. 1985. Rotator cuff disease of the shoulder. *J Bone Joint Surg* 67A:974–979.
60. Cofield, RH. 1972. Subscapularis muscle transposition for repair of chronic rotator cuff tears. *Surg Gynecol Obstetr* 154:667–672.
61. Cofield, RH. 1981. Tears of the rotator cuff. *Instructional Course Lectures* 30:258–273.
62. Cofield, RH. 1984. Total shoulder arthroplasty with the Neer prosthesis. *J Bone Joint Surg* 66A:899–906.
63. Colles, A. 1814. On the fracture of the carpal extremity of the radius. *Edin Med Surg J* 10:182–186.
64. Collis, DK. 1977. Femoral stem failure in total hip replacement. *J Bone Joint Surg* 59A:1033–1041.
65. Cooney, WP, III. 1978. Current management of fractures of the distal radius and forearm: Experience with external pin fixation. In *External Fixation, the Current State of the Art,* Eds., AG Brooker, and CC Edwards, Williams & Wilkins, Baltimore. 83–124.
66. Cooney, WP. 1983. External fixation of distal radial fractures. *Clin Orthop Rel Res* 150:44–49.
67. Cooney, WP, Dobyns, JH, and Linscheid, RL. 1980. Complications of Colles' fractures. *J Bone Joint Surg* 62A:613–619.
68. Cooney, WP, Linscheid, RL, and Dobyns, JH. 1979. External pin fixation for unstable Colles' fractures. *J Bone Joint Surg* 61A(6):840–845.
69. Cotton, RE, and Rideout, DF. 1964. Tears of the humeral rotator cuff: A radiological and pathological necropsy survey. *J Bone Joint Surg* 46B:314–328.
70. Coughlin, L, and Templeton, J. 1980. Hip fractures in patients with Parkinson's disease. *Clin Orthop Rel Res* 148:192–195.
71. Coventry, MB. 1959. An evaluation of the femoral head prosthesis after ten years of experience. *Surg Gynecol Obstet* 109:243–244.

72. Coventry, MB, Bechkenbaugh, RD, Nolan, DR, et al. 1974. 2,012 total hip arthroplasties: A study of postoperative course and early complications. *J Bone Joint Surg* 56A:273–284.
73. Craxford, AO, and Stevens, J. 1979. Proximal femoral fractures in psychiatric patients. *Injury* 11:19.
74. Culver, D, Crawford, JS, Gardiner, JH, et al. 1970. Venous thrombosis after fracture of the upper end of the femur: A study of incidence and site. *J Bone Joint Surg* 52B:61–69.
75. Cummings, SR, Kelsey, JL, Nevitt, MC, et al. 1985. Epidemiology of osteoporosis and osteoporotic fractures. *Epidemiol Rev* 7:178–208.
76. D'Arcy, J, and Devas, M. 1976. Treatment of fractures of the femoral neck by replacement with the Thompson prosthesis. *J Bone Joint Surg* 58-B(3):279–286.
77. Dahl, E. 1980. Mortality and life expectancy after hip fractures. *Acta Orthop Scand* 51:163–170.
78. DeLee, JC. 1984. *Fractures and Dislocations of the Hip, Fractures in Adults,* ed. 2, Eds., CA Rockwood and DP Green, vol. 2, 1211–1357. Philadelphia: J.B. Lippincott.
79. Dimon, JH, and Hughston, JC. 1967. Unstable intertrochanteric fractures of the hip. *J Bone Joint Surg* 49A:440–450.
80. Ditmars, DM, Jr., and Hovin, HP. 1988. Carpal tunnel syndrome: Treatment, pitfalls, and failures. *Surgical Rounds Ortho* 37–53, October.
81. Dobozi, WR, Dronch, VM, Saltzman, M, et al. 1984. Treatment of impending pathologic fractures of the femur with flexible intramedullary nails. *Orthopedics* 7:1628–1685.
82. Douglass, HO, Jr., Shukla, SK, and Mindell, E. 1976. Treatment of pathologic fractures of long bone excluding those due to breast cancer. *J Bone Joint Surg* 58A(8):1055–1061.
83. Dove, J. 1980. Complete fractures of the femur in Paget's disease of bone. *J Bone Joint Surg* 62B:12–17.
84. Drinker, H, and Murray, WR. 1979. The universal proximal femoral endoprosthesis. A short-term comparison with conventional hemiarthroplasty. *J Bone Joint Surg* 61A:1167–1174, Dec.
85. Eichenholtz, SN, Jacobs, B, and Patterson, RL. 1968. Meniscus injuries of the knee in the elderly. *J Amer Geriatr Soc* 16(3):281–289.
86. el-Banna, S, Raynal, L, and Gerbtzop, A. 1984. Fractures of the hip in the elderly: Therapeutic and medicosocial considerations. *Arch Gerontol Geriatr* 3:311–319.
87. Elabdien, BS, Olerud, S, and Karlstrom, G. 1985. Ender nailing of pertrochanteric fractures: Complications related to technical failures and bone quality. *Acta Orthop Scand* 56:138–144.
88. Engh, G, Bollet, AJ, Hardin, G, et al. 1968. Epidemiology of osteoporosis II. Incidence of hip fracture in mental institutions. *J Bone Joint Surg* 50A:557–562.
89. Eskeland, C, Solheinik, H, and Skjorten, F. 1966. Anticoagulant prophylaxis, thromboembolism and mortality in elderly patients with hip fractures. A controlled clinical trial. *Acta Chir Scand* 131:16–29.
90. Evans, EM. 1949. The treatment of trochanteric fractures of the femur. *J Bone Joint Surg* 31B:190–203.
91. Evans, EM. 1951. Trochanteric fractures. *J Bone Joint Surg* 33B:192–204.
92. Eventor, I, Moreno, M, Geller, E, et al. 1983. Hip fractures in patients with Parkinson's syndrome. *J Trauma* 23:98–101.
93. Eversmann, WW. 1988. Entrapment and compression neuropathies. In *Operative Hand Surgery,* ed. 2, Ed., DP Green, 1430–1440. New York: Churchill Livingstone.
94. Fairclough, J, Colhoun, E, Johnson, D, et al. 1987. Bone scanning for suspected hip fractures. *J Bone Joint Surg* 69B:251–253.
95. Farmer, ME, White, LR, Brody, JA, et al. 1984. Race and sex differences in hip fracture incidence. *Am J Public Health* 74:1374–1380.
96. Fidler, MW. 1973. Prophylactic internal fixation of secondary neoplastic deposits in long bones. *Br Med J* 1:341–343.
97. Fidler, MW. 1987. Surgery for spinal metastases. In *Bone Tumor Management,* Eds., R Coombs, and G Friedlander, 246–255. London: Butterworth & Co.
98. Finsen, V, and Benum, P. 1986. The second hip fracture, An epidemiologic study. *Acta Orthop Scand* 57:431–433.
99. Flemming, JE, and Beals, RK. 1986. Pathologic fracture of the humerus. *Clin Orthop Rel Res* 203:258–260.
100. Friedman, MJ, Beras, CC, Fox, JM, et al. 1984. Preliminary results with abrasion arthroplasty in the osteoarthritic knee. *Clin Orthop Rel Res* 182:200–205.
101. Friedman, RJ, and McGinty, JB. 1983. Arthroscopy of total knee replacements. *Surg Rounds Ortho* 3(4):50–54.
102. Fryckman, G. 1967. Fractures of the distal radius including sequelae. *Acta Orthop Scand* Suppl 180:1–153.
103. Galasko, CSB. 1974. Pathologic fractures secondary to metastatic cancer. *J R Coll Surg Edin* 19:351.
104. Galasko, CSB. 1986. Skeletal metastases. *Clin Orthop Rel Res* 210:18–30.
105. Galasko, CS, Rushton, S, Sylvester, BS, et al. 1985. The significance of peak expiratory flow rate in assessing prognosis of eldery patients undergoing operations on the hip. *Injury* 16:398–401.
106. Gallagher, JC, Melton, LJ, Riggs, BL, et al. 1980. Epidemiology of fractures of the proximal femur in Rochester, Minnesota. *Clin Orthop Rel Res* 150:163–167.
107. Garden, RS. 1961. Low angle fixation in fractures of the femoral neck. *J Bone Joint Surg* 43B:647–663.
108. Garraway, WM, Stauffer, RN, Kurland, LT, et al. 1979. Limb fractures in a defined population. I: Frequency and distribution. *Mayo Clinic Proc* 54:701–707.
109. Gates, B, Fairbaum, A, and Craxford, AD. 1986. Broken necks of the femur in a psychogeriatric hospital. *Injury* 17:383–386.
110. Gelberman, RH, Aronson, D, and Weisman, MH. 1980. Carpal-tunnel syndrome: Results of a prospective trial of steroid injection and splinting. *J Bone Joint Surg* 62A(7):1181–1184.
111. Gilbert, W, Kim, JH, and Posner, JB. 1978. Epidural spinal cord compression for metastatic tumor: Diagnosis and treatment. *Ann Neurol* 3:40–51.
112. Goldberg, VM, Figgie, MP, Figgie, HE, et al. 1988. Use of a total condylar knee prosthesis for treatment of osteoarthritis and rheumatoid arthritis. *J Bone Joint Surg* 70A:802–811.
113. Gordon, PC. 1971. The probability of death following fracture of the hip. *Can Med Assoc J* 105:47–62.
114. Graham, J. 1968. Early or delayed weight-bearing after

internal fixation of trancervical fracture of the femur. *J Bone Joint Surg* 50B:562–569.
115. Green, DP. 1984. Diagnostic and therapeutic value of carpal tunnel injection. *J Hand Surg* 9A(6):850–854.
116. Green, DP. 1975. Pins and plaster treatment of comminuted fractures of the distal end of the radius. *J Bone Joint Surg* 57A(3):304–310.
117. Hall, S, Bartleson, JD, Onofrio, BM, et al. 1985. Lumbar spinal stenosis: Clinical features, diagnostic procedures, and results of surgical treatment in 68 patients. *Ann Int Med* 103:271–275.
118. Hamilton, HW, Crawford, JS, Gardiner, JH, et al. 1970. Venous thrombosis in patients with fractures of the upper end of the femur: A phlebographic study of the effect of prophylactic anticoagulation. *J Bone Joint Surg* 52B: 268–289.
119. Hanssen, AD, and Rand, JA. 1988. A comparison of primary and revision total knee arthroplasty using the Knematic Stabilizer prosthesis. *J Bone Joint Surg* 70A:491–499.
120. Harper, MC, and Walsh, T. 1985. Ender nailing for pantrochanteric fractures of the femur: An analysis of indications, factors related to mechanical failure and postoperative results. *J Bone Joint Surg* 67A:79–88.
121. Harrington, KD. 1988. Anterior decompression and stabilization of the spine as a treatment for vertebral collapse and spinal cord compression from metastatic malignancy. *Clin Orthop Rel Res* 233:177–197.
122. Harrington, KD. 1986. Impending pathologic fractures from metastatic malignancy: Evaluation and management. In *AAOS Instructional Course Lectures,* 35:357–381.
123. Harrington, KD. 1977. The management of malignant pathologic fractures. *AAOS Instructional Course Lectures,* 26:147–162.
124. Harrington, KD. 1986. Metastatic disease of the spine. *J Bone Joint Surg* 68A(7):1110–1115.
125. Harrington, KD. 1982. New trends in the management of lower extremity metastases. *Clin Orthop Rel Res* 169: 53–61.
126. Harrington, KD. 1981. The use of methylmethacrylate for vertebral body replacement and anterior stabilization of pathological fracture-dislocations of the spine due to metastatic malignancy. *J Bone Joint Surg* 63A(1):36–46.
127. Harrington, KD, Sim, FH, Enis, JE, et al. 1976. Methylmethacrylate as an adjunct in internal fixation of pathologic fractures. *J Bone Joint Surg* 58A:1047–1055.
128. Harris, WH. 1982. Revision surgery for failed, nonseptic total hip arthroplasty. *Clin Orthop Rel Res* 170:8–20.
129. Harris, WH, McCarthy, JC, and O'Neill, DA. 1982. Femoral component loosening using contemporary techniques of femoral cement fixation. *J Bone Joint Surg* 64A:1063–1067.
130. Hawkins, FB, Mitchell, CL, and Hendrick, DW. 1945. Correction of hallux valgus by metatarsal osteotomy. *J Bone Joint Surg* 27:387–394.
131. Hawkins, RJ, Misamore, GW, and Hobeika, PE. 1985. Surgery for full-thickness rotator cuff tears. *J Bone Joint Surg* 67A:1349–1355.
132. Hedstrom, SA, Lidgren, L, Sernbo, I, et al. 1987. Cefuroxime prophylaxis in trochanteric hip fracture operations. *Acta Orthop Scand* 58:361–364.
133. Higgins, RW, and Hughes, JL. 1983. Preliminary results of eighty-one hip replacements with the Bateman endoprosthesis. *Orthop Trans* 7:411–412.
134. Holbrook, TL, Barrett-Connor, E, and Wingard, DL. 1988. Dietary calcium and risk of hip fracture: 14 year prospective population study. *Lancet* 2(8619):1046–1049.
135. Holmberg, SH, Conrad, P, Kalen, R, et al. 1986. Mortality after cervical hip fracture. *Acta Orthop Scand* 57:8–11.
136. Holmberg, S, Kalen, R, and Thorngren, KG. 1987. Treatment and outcome of femoral neck fractures. *Clin Orthop Rel Res* 218:42–52.
137. Horak, J, and Nilsson, BE. 1975. Epidemiology of fractures of the upper end of the humerus. *Clin Orthop Rel Res* 112:250–253.
138. Hunter, GA. 1969. A comparison of the use of internal fixation and prosthetic replacement for fresh fractures of the neck of the femur. *Br J Surg* 56:229–232.
139. Hunter, GA. 1983. The rationale for internal fixation and against hemiarthroplasty in the hip. *Proceedings of the Eleventh Open Scientific Meeting of the Hip Society,* 34–41. St. Louis: C.V. Mosby.
140. Hunter, G, and Dandy, D. 1977. The natural history of the patient with an infected total hip replacement. *J Bone Joint Surg* 59B:293–297.
141. Insall, JN, Hood, RW, Flawn, LB, et al. 1983. The total condylar knee prosthesis in gonarthrosis. *J Bone Joint Surg* 65A:619–627.
142. Iwegbu, CG, and Patel, RJ. 1981. Difficulties and complications of the Ender method of treatment of trochanteric fractures of the femur. *Injury* 13:116–124.
143. Jackson, RW. 1983. Current concepts review: Arthroscopic surgery. *J Bone Joint Surg* 65A:416–420.
144. Jackson, RW, and Rouse, DW. 1982. The results of partial arthroscopic meniscectomy in patients over 40 years of age. *J Bone Joint Surg* 64B:481–485.
145. Jennings, JJ, Harris, WH, and Sarmiento, A. 1976. A clinical evaluation of aspirin prophylaxis of thromboembolic disease after total hip arthroplasty. *J Bone Joint Surg* 58A:926–927.
146. Jensen, JS, Sonne-Holm, S, and Tondevold, E. 1980. Unstable interbiochanteric fractures: A comparative analysis of four methods of internal fixation. *Acta Orthop Scand* 51:949–962.
147. Jensen, JS, and Tondevold, E. 1979. Mortality after hip fractures. *Acta Orthop Scand* 50:161–167.
148. Jensen, TT, and Juncker, V. 1987. Pressure sores common after hip operations. *Acta Orthop Scand* 58:209–211.
149. Jewett, EL. 1941. One piece angle nail for trochanteric fractures. *J Bone Joint Surg* 23:803–810.
150. Johnell, O, and Sernbo, I. 1986. Health and social status in patients with hip fractures and controls. *Age Ageing* 15:285–291.
151. Johnson, LL. 1986. Arthroscopic abrasion arthroplasty historical and pathologic perspective: Present status. *Arthroscopy* 2(1):54–69.
152. Johnston, CE, Ripley, LP, and Bray, CB. 1982. Primary endoprosthetic replacement for acute femoral neck fractures. *Clin Orthop Rel Res* 167:123–130.
153. Jones, JA, and Burton, RI. 1988. Carpal tunnel syndrome: Treatment, pitfalls and failure. *Surg Rounds Orthop* 2:37–53.

154. Jones, S, DiPito, JT, Nix, DE, et al. 1985. Cephalosporins for prophylaxis in operative repair of femoral fractures: Levels in serum, muscle and hematoma. *J Bone Joint Surg* 67A:921–924.
155. Kaufer, H, Matthews, LS, and Sonstegard, D. 1974. Stable fixation of intertrochanteric fractures. *J Bone Joint Surg* 56A:899–907.
156. Kavanagh, BF, Ilstrup, DM, and Fitzgerald, RH. 1985. Revision total hip arthroplasty. *J Bone Joint Surg* 67A:517–526.
157. Keene, JS, Sellinger, DS, McBeath, AA, et al. 1986. Metastatic breast carcinoma in the femur: A search for the lesion at risk of fracture. *Clin Orthop Rel Res* 203:282–288.
158. Keller, WL. 1904. The surgical treatment of bunions and hallux valgus. *NY Med J* 80:741.
159. Kenzora, JE. 1988. A rationale for the surgical treatment of bunions. *Orthopaedics* 11(5):777–789.
160. Kenzora, JE, McCarthy, RE, Lowell, JD, et al. 1984. Hip fracture mortality. *Clin Orthop Rel Res* 186:45–56.
161. Knowlden, J, Buhr, AJ, and Dunbar, O. 1964. Incidence of fractures in persons over 35 years of age: A report to the MRC working party on fractures in the elderly. *Br J Prev Soc Med* 18:130–141.
162. Kofoed, H, and Kofod, J. 1983. Moore prosthesis in the treatment of fresh femoral neck fractures. *Injury* 14:531–540.
163. Kuderna, H, Bohler, N, and Collon, DJ. 1976. Treatment of intertrochanteric and subtrochanteric fractures of the hip by the Ender method. *J Bone Joint Surg* 58A:604–611.
164. Kuokkanen, H, Korkala, O, and Lauttamus, L. 1986. Ender nailing of trochanteric fractures: A review of 73 cases. *Arch Orthop Trauma Surg* 105:46–48.
165. Kyle, RF. 1987. Trauma: Hip fracture. Orthopaedic Knowledge Update II, *AAOS* 357–368.
166. Kyle, RF, Gustilo, RB, and Premer, RF. 1979. Analysis of 622 intertrochanteric hip fractures: A retrospective study. *J Bone Joint Surg* 61A:216–221.
167. Laskin, RS. 1981. Total condylar knee replacement in rheumatoid arthritis. *J Bone Joint Surg* 63A:29–35.
168. Lausten, GS, Vedel, P, and Nielsen, P. 1987. Fractures of the femoral neck treated with bipolar endoprosthesis. *Clin Orthop Rel Res* 218:63–67.
169. Lentz, W, and Maser, P. 1980. The treatment of fractures of the proximal humerus. *Arch Orthop Traumat Surg* 96:283–285.
170. Lestrange, NR. 1979. The Bateman UPF prosthesis. A 48-month experience. *Orthopaedics* 2:373–377.
171. Lewinnek, GE, Lewis, JL, Tarr, R, et al. 1978. Dislocations after total hip replacement arthroplasties. *J Bone Joint Surg* 60A:217–220.
172. Leyshon, RL. 1984. Closed treatment of fractures of the proximal humerus. *Acta Orthop Scand* 55:48–51.
173. Lichtblau, S. 1986. A pitfall in the insertion of a sliding screw. *Bull Hosp Joint Dis* 46:60–62.
174. Lichtman, HM, Silver, CM, and Simon, S. 1966. Injuries to the medial meniscus of the aging patient. *JAMA* 196(2):164–166.
175. Linde, F, Anderson, E, and Hvass, I. 1986. Avascular femoral head necrosis following fracture fixation. *Injury* 17:159–163.
176. Lotke, PA, and Ecker, ML. 1988. Osteonecrosis of the knee. *J Bone Joint Surg* 70A:470–473.
177. Lotke, PA, Lefkoe, RT, and Ecker, ML. 1981. Late results following medial meniscectomy in an older population. *J Bone Joint Surg* 63A(1):115–119.
178. Lucas, DB. 1973. Biomechanics of the shoulder joint. *Arch Surg* 107:425–432.
179. Lunt, HRW. 1971. The role of prosthetic replacement of the head of the femur as primary treatment for subcapital fractures. *Injury* 3:107–110.
180. MacDonald, RI, Lichtman, DM, Hanlon, JJ, et al. 1978. Complications of surgical release for carpal tunnel syndrome. *J Hand Surg* 3(1):70–76.
181. Mack, LA, Matser, FA, Kilcoyne, RF, et al. 1985. Ultrasound evaluation of the rotator cuff. *Radiology* 157:205–209.
182. Mann, RA. 1983. Hallux valgus. In *AAOS Symposium on the Foot and Ankle,* Eds., RH Kiene, and KA Johnson, 159–176. St. Louis: C.V. Mosby.
183. Mann, RA, and Coughlin, MJ. 1986. Hallux valgus and complications of hallux valgus. In *Surgery of the Foot,* ed. 5. Ed. RA Mann, St. Louis: C.V. Mosby.
184. Manoli, A. 1986. Malassembly of the sliding screw-plate device. *J Trauma* 26:916–922.
185. Mariani, EM, and Rand, JA. 1987. Nonunion of intertrochanteric fractures of the femur following open reduction and internal fixation. *Clin Orthop Rel Res* 218:81–89.
186. Marsh, HO, and Teal, SW. 1972. Treatment of comminuted fractures of the distal radius with self-contained skeletal traction. *Am J Surg* 124:715–719.
187. Martens, M, Van Audelercke, R, Mulier, JC, et al. 1979. Clinical study on internal fixation of femoral neck fractures. *Clin Orthop Rel Res* 141:199–202.
188. Massie, WK. 1973. Treatment of femoral neck fractures emphasizing long term follow-up observations on aseptic necrosis. *Clin Orthop Rel Res* 92:16–62.
189. Matkovic, V, Kostiac, K, Simonovic, I, et al. 1979. Bone status and fracture rates in two regions in Yugoslavia. *Am J Clin Nutr* 32:540–549.
190. McClure, J, and Goldsborough, S. 1986. Fractures of neck of femur and contralateral intracerebral lesions. *J Clin Pathol* 39:920–922.
191. McCutchen, J, and Carnesale, P. 1982. Comparison of fixation in the treatment of femoral neck fractures. *Clin Orthop Rel Res* 171:44–50.
192. McLean, M. 1986. Total hip replacement and sciatic nerve trauma. *Orthopaedics* 9:1121–1128.
193. Meislin, R, and Zuckerman, JD. 1989. Management of infected total knee replacement. *Bull Hosp Joint Dis* 49(1):21–36.
194. Melton, LJ, Ilstrup, MS, Beckenbaugh, RD, et al. 1982. Hip fracture recurrence. A population-based study. *Clin Orthop Rel Res* 167:131–138.
195. Melton, LJ III, Wahner, HW, Richelson, LS, et al. 1986. Osteoporosis and the risk of hip fracture. *Am J Epidemiol* 124:254–261.
196. Merkow, RL, Sondry, M, and Insall, JN. 1985. Patellar dislocation following total knee replacement. *J Bone Joint Surg* 67A:1321–1327.
197. Meyn, MA, Hopson, C, and Jayasankar, S. 1977. Fractures of the hip in the institutionalized psychotic patient. *Clin Orthop Rel Res* 122:128–134.

198. Milgram, JW. 1977. Orthopaedic management of Paget's disease of bone. *Clin Orthop Rel Res* 127:63–69.

199. Miller, CW. 1978. Survival and ambulation following hip fracture. *J Bone Joint Surg* 60A:930–934.

200. Moore, AT. 1937. Fracture of the hip joint: Treatment by extra-articular fixation with adjustable nails. *Surg Gynecol Obstet* 64:420–436.

201. Morrey, BF, Adams, RA, Ilstrup, DM, et al. 1987. Complications and mortality associated with bilateral or unilateral total knee arthroplasty. *J Bone Joint Surg* 69A:484–488.

202. Mosely, F, and Goldie, I. 1963. The arterial pattern of the rotator cuff of the shoulder. *J Bone Joint Surg* 48B:780–789.

203. Moskovitz, PA, Ellenberg, SS, Feffer, HL, et al. 1978. Low dose heparin for prevention of venous thromboembolism in total hip arthroplasty and surgical repair of hip fractures. *J Bone Joint Surg* 60A:1065–1070.

204. Mouradian, WH. 1986. Displaced humeral fractures: Seven years' experience with a modified Zickel supracondylar device. *Clin Orthop Rel Res* 212:209–218.

205. Mulholland, RC, and Gunn, DR. 1972. Sliding screw plate fixation of intertrochanteric femoral fractures. *J Trauma* 12:581–591.

206. Mullen, JO. 1985. Relationship of admission mental status, hospital confusion, and mortality in hip fractures: A prospective study. *Presented at AAOS 52nd Meeting,* January 24.

207. Nakata, RY, Chand, Y, Matiko, JD, et al. 1985. External fixators for wrist fractures: A biomechanical and clinical study. *J Hand Surg* 10A(6) Pt. 1:845–851.

208. Nasca, RJ. 1987. Surgical management of lumbar spinal stenosis. *Spine* 12(8):809–806.

209. Neer, CS, II. 1972. Anterior acromioplasty for the chronic impingement syndrome in the shoulder. *J Bone Joint Surg* 54-A:41–50.

210. Neer, CS, II. 1970. Displaced proximal humerus fractures: Part I Classification and evaluation. *J Bone Joint Surg* 52A(6):1077–1089.

211. Neer, CS. 1970. Displaced proximal humerus fractures: Part II: Treatment of three-part and four-part displacement. *J Bone Joint Surg* 52A(6):1090–1103.

212. Neer, CS, II. 1983. Impingement lesions. *Clin Orthop Rel Res* 173:70–77.

213. Neer, CS, II, and Rockwood, CA, Jr. 1984. Fractures and dislocations of the shoulder. In *Fractures and dislocations of the Hip, Fractures in Adults,* ed. 2, Eds., CA Rockwood and DP Green, vol. 2, 675–986. Philadelphia: JB Lippincott Co.

214. Neer, CS, Watson, KC, and Stanton, FJ. 1980. Recent experience in total shoulder replacement. *J Bone Joint Surg* 64A:319–337.

215. Neviaser, JS, Neviaser, RJ, and Neviaser, TJ. 1978. The repair of chronic massive ruptures of the rotator cuff of the shoulder by use of a freeze-dried rotator cuff. *J Bone and Joint Surg* 60A:681–684.

216. Nicholas, JA, and Killoran, P. 1965. Fracture of the femur in patients with Paget's disease. *J Bone Joint Surg* 47A:450–461.

217. Nieminen, S. 1975. Early weight-bearing after classical internal fixation of medial fractures of the femoral neck. *Acta Orthop Scand* 46:782–794.

218. Norden, CW. 1983. A critical review of antibiotic prophylaxis in orthopedic surgery. *Rev Infect Dis* 5:928–932.

219. Owen, RA, Melba, LJ, Johnson, KA, et al. 1982. Incidence of Colles' fracture in a North American Community. *Am J Public Health* 72(5):605–607.

220. Ozaki, J, Fujimoto, S, Masuhara, K, et al. 1986. Reconstruction of chronic massive rotator cuff tears with synthetic materials. *Clin Orthop Rel Res* 202:173–183.

221. Packer, NP, Calvert, PT, Bayley, JIL, et al. 1983. Operative treatment of chronic ruptures of the rotator cuff of shoulder. *J Bone Joint Surg* 65B:171–175.

222. Paine, KWE. 1976. Clinical features of lumbar spinal stenosis. *Clin Orthop Rel Res* 115:77–78.

223. Palmer, AK. 1988. Fractures of the distal radius. In *Operative Hand Surgery,* ed. 2, Ed. DP Green, 991–1026. New York: Churchill Livingston Inc.

224. Pauwels, F. 1935. *Der Schenkelhalsbruch, ein Mechanisches Problem: Grundlagen des Heilungsvorganges, Prognose und Kausale Therapie*. Stuttgart: Ferdinand Enke Verlag.

225. Pellicci, PM, Wilson, PD, Sledge, CB, et al. 1985. Long-term results of revision total hip replacement. *J Bone Joint Surg* 67A:513–516.

226. Petersson, CJ, and Redlund-Johnell, I. 1984. The subacromial space in normal shoulder radiographs. *Acta Orthop Scand* 55:57–58.

227. Phalen, GS. 1966. The carpal-tunnel syndrome: Seventeen years' experience in diagnosis and treatment of six hundred fifty-four hands. *J Bone Joint Surg* 48A(2):211–228.

228. Pini, M, Spadini, E, Carluccio, L, et al. 1985. Dextran/aspirin versus Heparin/dihydroergotamine in preventing thrombosis after hip fractures. *J Bone Joint Surg* 67B:305–309.

229. Pool, C. 1973. Colles' fracture in a prospective study of treatment. *J Bone Joint Surg* 55B(3): 540–544.

230. Post, M. 1985. Rotator cuff repair with carbon filament: A preliminary report of five cases. *Clin Orthop Rel Res* 196:154–158.

231. Pugh, WL. 1955. A self-adjusting nail-plate for fractures about the hip joint. *J Bone Joint Surg* 37A:1085–1093.

232. Radin, EL. 1980. Biomechanics of the human hip. *Clin Orthop Rel Res* 152:28–34.

233. Rand, JA. 1985. Arthroscopic management of degenerative mensicus tears in patients with degenerative arthritis. *Arthroscopy* 2(4):235–258.

234. Rand, JA, and Bryan, RS. 1988. Results of revision total knee arthroplasties using condylar prostheses. *J Bone Joint Surg* 70A:738–745.

235. Rand, JA, Morrey, BF, and Bryan, RS. 1984. Management of the infected total joint arthroplasty. *Orthop Clin North Am* 15:491–504.

236. Raugstad, TS, Molster, A, Haukeland, W, et al. 1979. Treatment of pertrochanteric and subtrochanteric fractures of the femur by the Ender method. *Clin Orthop Rel Res* 138:231–237.

237. Ray, WA, Griffin, MR, Schaffner, W, et al. 1987. Psychotropic drug use and the risk of hip fracture. *N Engl J Med* 316:363–369.

238. Refior, HJ, Krodel, A, and Melzer, L. 1987. Examinations of the pathology of the rotator cuff. *Arch Orthop Trauma Surg* 106:301–308.

239. Richards, RN, and Lonergan, RP. 1984. Arthroscopic surgery for relief of pain in the osteoarthritic knee. *Orthopedics* 7(11):1705–1707.
240. Rodriguez, J, Herrara, A, Canales, V, et al. 1987. Epidemiologic factors, morbidity and mortality after femoral neck fracture in the elderly. *Acta Orthop Belgica* 53:472–479.
241. Rorbach-Madsen, M, Jakobsen, BW, Pederson, J, et al. 1988. Dihydroergotamine and the thromboprophylactic effect of dextran 70 in emergency hip surgery. *Br J Surg* 75:364–365.
242. Rose, HA, Hood, RW, Otis, JC, et al. 1982. Peroneal nerve palsy following total knee arthroplasty. *J Bone Joint Surg* 64A:347–351.
243. Rose, SH, Melson, J, III, Morney, BF, et al. 1982. Epidemiologic features of humeral fractures. *Clin Orthop Rel Res* 168:24–30.
244. Rosenfeld, RT, Schwartz, DR, and Alter, AH. 1973. Prosthetic replacement for trochanteric fractures of the femur. *J Bone Joint Surg* 55A:420.
245. Rothermel, JE, and Garcia, A. 1972. Treatment of hip fractures in patients with Parkinson's syndrome on Levodopa therapy. *J Bone Joint Surg* 54A:1251–1254.
246. Rothman, RH, and Simesne, FA. (Eds.) 1982. *The Spine,* ed. 2, 1024. Philadelphia: W.B. Saunders Co.
247. Russin, LA, and Sonni, A. 1980. Treatment of intertrochanteric and subtrochanteric fractures with Ender's intramedullary rods. *Clin Orthop Rel Res* 148:203–212.
248. Rydell, NW. 1973. Biomechanics of the hip joint. *Clin Orthop Rel Res* 92:6–15.
249. Rydell, NW. 1966. Forces acting on the femoral head prosthesis. A study on strain gauge supplied prostheses in living persons. *Acta Orthop Scand* (Suppl) 88:7–132.
250. Salvati, EA, Artz, T, Aglietti, P, et al. 1974. Endoprosthesis in the treatment of femoral neck fractures. *Orthop Clin North Am* 5:757–777.
251. Salvati, EA, Robinson, RP, Zeno, SM, et al. 1982. Infection rates after 3175 total hip and total knee replacements performed with and without a horizontal unidirectional filtered air flow system. *J Bone Joint Surg* 64A:525–535.
252. Salvati, EA, Wilson, PD, Jolley, MN, et al. 1981. A ten year follow-up study of our first one hundred consecutive Charnley total hip replacements. *J Bone Joint Surg* 63A:753–767.
253. Sarmiento, A. 1963. Intertrochanteric fractures of the femur: 150-degree-angle nail-plate fixation and early rehabilitation: A preliminary report of 100 cases. *J Bone Joint Surg* 45A:706–722.
254. Sarmiento, A, Pratt, GW, Berry, NC, et al. 1975. Colles' fractures: Functional bracing in supination. *J Bone Joint Surg* 57A(3):311–317.
255. Sarmiento, A, and Williams, EM. 1970. The unstable intertrochanteric fracture: Treatment with a valgus osteotomy and I-Beam nail-plate. *J Bone Joint Surg* 52A:1309–1318.
256. Scheck, M. 1980. The significance of posterior comminution in femoral neck fractures. *Clin Orthop Rel Res* 152:138–142.
257. Schon, L, and Zuckerman, JD. 1988. Hip pain in the elderly: Evaluation and diagnosis. *Geriatrics* 43:48–62.
258. Schutzer, SF, and Harris, WH. 1988. Deep wound infection after total hip replacement under contemporary aseptic conditions. *J Bone Joint Surg* 70A:724–727.
259. Scott, WA, Allum, RL, and Wright, K. 1985. Implant induced trabecular damage in cadaveric femoral necks. *Acta Orthop Scand* 56:145–146.
260. Scott, WN, Rubinstein, MA, and Scuderi, G. 1988. Results after knee replacement with a posterior cruciate substituting prosthesis. *J Bone Joint Surg* 70A:1163–1173.
261. Scranton, PE. 1983. Principles in bunion surgery. *J Bone Joint Surg* 65A(7):1026–1028.
262. Sculco, TP. 1985. *Orthopaedic care of the geriatric patient,* 185. St. Louis: C.V. Mosby Co.
263. Sernbo, I, Johnell, O, Gentz, G, et al. 1988. Unstable intertrochanteric fractures of the hip: Treatment with Ender pins compared with compression hip screw. *J Bone Joint Surg* 70A:1297–1303.
264. Sexson, SB, and Lehner, JT. 1988. Factors affecting hip fracture mortality. *J Orthop Trauma* 1:298–305.
265. Shahriar, H, O'Connor, RL, and Noltage, W. 1982. Seven years' follow-up on arthroscopic debridement of the degenerative knee. *Field of View* 1(1):1–7.
266. Sherman, OH, Fox, JM, Snyder, SJ, et al. 1986. Arthroscopy—"No Problem Surgery." *J Bone Joint Surg* 68A(2):256–265.
267. Sherry, M, Greco, FA, Johnson, DH, et al. 1986. Breast cancer with skeletal metastases at initial diagnosis: Distinctive clinical characteristics and favorable prognosis. *Cancer* 58(1):178–182.
268. Siegal, T, Tiqua, P, and Siegal, T. 1985. Vertebral body resection for epidural compression by malignant tumors. *J Bone Joint Surg* 67A(3):375–382.
269. Sim, FH, and Pritchard, DJ. 1982. Metastatic disease in the upper extremity. *Clin Orthop Rel Res* 169:83–94.
270. Sisk, TD. 1980. Fractures. In *Campbell's Operative Orthopaedics,* Eds, AS Edmonson and AH Crenshaw, St. Louis: C.V. Mosby.
271. Skinner, PW, and Powles, D. 1986. Compression screw fixation for displaced subcapital fracture of the femur: Success or failure? *J Bone Joint Surg* 68B:78–82.
272. Sledge, CB, and Walker, PS. 1984. Total knee arthroplasty in rheumatoid arthritis. *Clin Orthop Rel Res* 182:127–136.
273. Small, NC. 1988. Complications in arthroscopic surgery performed by experienced arthroscopists. *Arthroscopy* 4(3):215–221.
274. Soreide, O, Lillestol, J, Algo, A, et al. 1980. Acetabular protrusion following endoprosthetic hip surgery. A multifactorial study. *Acta Orthop Scand* 51:943–948.
275. Soreide, O, Molster, A, and Raugstad, TS. 1979. Internal fixation versus primary prosthetic replacement in acute femoral neck fractures: A prospective, randomized clinical study. *Br J Surg* 66:56–60.
276. Soto-Hall, R. 1960. Treatment of transcervical fractures complicated by certain common neurological conditions. *AAOS Instructional Course Lectures* 17:117–120. St. Louis: C.V. Mosby.
277. Spengler, DM. 1984. The aging lumbar spine. In *The Aging Musculoskeletal System,* Eds., CL Nelson and AP Dwyer, 103–112. Lexington, MA: D.C. Heath & Co.
278. Spengler, DM. 1987. Current concepts review—degenerative stenosis of the lumbar spine. *Spine* 69A(2):305–308.

279. Sprague, NF. 1981. Arthroscopic debridement for degenerative knee joint disease. *Clin Orthop Rel Res* 160:118–123.
280. Stableforth, PG. 1984. Four-part fractures of the humerus. *J Bone Joint Surg* 66B(1):104–108.
281. Stappaerts, KH. 1985. Early fixation failure in displaced femoral neck fractures. *Arch Orthop Trauma Surg* 104:314–318.
282. Stappaerts, KH, and Broos, PL. 1987. Internal fixation of femoral neck fractures: A follow-up study of 118 cases. *Acta Chir Belgica* 87:247–251.
283. Stauffer, RN, and Sim, FH. 1976. Total hip arthroplasty in Paget's disease of the hip. *J Bone Joint Surg* 58A:476–478.
284. Stern, MB, and Angerman, A. 1987. Comminuted intertrochanteric fractures treated with Leinbach prosthesis. *Clin Orthop Rel Res* 218:75–80.
285. Stern, MB, and Goldstein, TB. 1977. The use of the Leinbach prosthesis in intertrochanteric fracture of the hip. *Clin Orthop Rel Res* 128:325–331.
286. Sternbach, G, and Colles, A. 1985. Fracture of the carpal extremity of the radius. *J Emergency Med* 2:447–450.
287. Stromquist, B. 1983. Femoral head vitality after intracapsular hip fracture: 490 cases studied by intravital tetracycline labeling and TcMDP radionuclide imaging. *Acta Orthop Scand* Suppl 200, 54:1–71.
288. Stromquist, B, Hansson, L, Nilsson, L, et al. 1987. Hook pin fixation in femoral neck fractures: A two year follow-up study of 300 cases. *Clin Orthop Rel Res* 218:58–62.
289. Stulberg, BN, Insall, JN, Williams, GW, et al. 1984. Deep vein thrombosis following total knee replacement. *J Bone Joint Surg* 66A:194–210.
290. Svenningsen, S, Benum, P, Nesse, O, et al. 1984. Internal fixation of femoral neck fractures: Compression screw compared with nail-plate fixation. *Acta Orthop Scand* 55:423–429.
291. Swiontkowski, MF, Harrington, RM, Keller, TS, et al. 1987. Torsion and bending analysis of internal fixation techniques for femoral neck fractures: The role of implant design and bone density. *J Orthop Res* 5:433–444.
292. Swiontkowski, MF, Winquist, RA, and Hansen, ST. 1984. Femoral neck fractures in patients aged 12–49. *J Bone Joint Surg* 66A:837–846.
293. Tanner, MW, and Cofield, RH. 1983. Prosthetic arthroplasty for fractures and fracture-dislocations of the proximal humerus. *Clin Orthop* 179:116–128.
294. Tengve, B, and Kjellander, J. 1978. Antibiotic prophylaxis in operations on trochanteric femoral fractures. *J Bone Joint Surg* 60A:97–99.
295. Testa, NN, and Mazur, K. 1988. Heterotopic ossification after direct lateral approach and transtrochanteric approach to the hip. *Orthop Rev* 18:965–971.
296. Thomas, BJ, Salvati, EA, and Small, RD. 1986. The CAD hip arthroplasty. *J Bone Joint Surg* 68A:640–646.
297. Trippel, SB. 1986. Antibiotic-impregnated cement in total joint arthroplasty. *J Bone Joint Surg* 68A:1297–1302.
298. Tronzo, RG. 1974. Special considerations in management. *Orthop Clin North Am* 5:571–583.
299. Uden, G, and Nilsson, B. 1986. Hip fracture frequent in hospital. *Acta Orthop Scand* 57:428–430.
300. Van Demark, RE, Jr., Cabanela, ME, and Henderson, ED. 1980. The Bateman endoprosthesis. 104 arthroplasties. *Orthop Trans* 4:356–357.
301. Vidal, J, Buscaynet, C, and Connes, H. 1978. Treatment of articular fractures by "ligamentotaxis" with external fixation. In *External Fixation, the Current State of the Art,* Eds., AG Brooker and CC Edwards, 75–82. Baltimore: Williams & Wilkins.
302. Villar, RN, Marsh, D, Righton, N, et al. 1987. Three years after Colles' fracture: A prospective review. *J Bone Joint Surg* 69B(4):635–638.
303. Waddell, JP. 1984. Femoral head preservation following subcapital fracture of the femur. *Instructional Course Lectures* 33:179–190.
304. Waddell, J, Czitrom, A, and Simmons, EH. 1987. Ender nailing in fractures of the proximal femur. *J Trauma* 27(8):911–916.
305. Watson, M. 1985. Major ruptures of the rotator cuff. *J Bone Joint Surg* 67B: 618–624.
306. Watson-Jones, R. 1955. *Fractures and Joint Injuries,* ed. 4. Baltimore: Williams & Wilkins.
307. Weiner, DS, and McNab, I. 1970. Ruptures of the rotator cuff: Follow-up evaluation of operative repairs. *Can J Surg* 13:219–227.
308. Weiner, DS, and MacNab, I. 1970. Superior migration of the humeral head. *J Bone Joint Surg* 52B:524–527.
309. White, BL, Fisher, WD, and Laurin, CA. 1987. Rate of mortality for elderly patients after fracture of the hip in the 1980s. *J Bone Joint Surg* 69A:1335–1340.
310. Whittaker, RP, Abeshaus, MM, Scholl, HW, et al. 1972. Fifteen years' experience with metallic endo-prosthetic replacement of the femoral head for femoral neck fractures. *J Trauma* 12:799–806.
311. Wiener, F, Pospisil, M, and Franz, J. 1985. Treatment of Colles' fractures in elderly patients. *Acta Universitatis Carolinae Medica* 31(3/u):105–117.
312. Winter, WG. 1987. Non-operative treatment of proximal femoral fractures in the demented, non-ambulatory patient. *Clin Orthop Rel Res* 218:97–103.
313. Wiss, DA, Brien, W, Becker, V, et al. 1989. Subtrochanteric femur fractures: A comparison between the Zickel nail, 95° blade plate and interlocking nail. Paper #229. *Annual Meeting of the American Academy of Orthopaedic Surgeons,* February 11.
314. Wiltse, LL, Guyer, RD, and Spencer, CP. 1984. Alar transverse process impingement of the L5 spinal nerve: The Far-Out Syndrome. *Spine* 9:31.
315. Wolfgang, GL, Bryant, MH, and O'Neill, JP. 1982. Treatment of intertrochanteric fracture of the femur using sliding screw plate fixation. *Clin Orthop Rel Res* 163:148–158.
316. Wood, GW. 1987. Infections of the spine. In *Campbell's Operative Orthopaedics,* ed. 7. Ed., AH Crenshaw, 3323–3345. St. Louis: C.V. Mosby Co.
317. Wood, GW. 1987. Spinal stenosis. In *Campbell's Operative Orthopaedics,* ed. 3. Ed., AH Crenshaw, 3347–3353. St. Louis: C.V. Mosby Co.
318. Wood, MR. 1979–1980. Femoral head replacement following fracture: An analysis of the surgical approach. *Injury* 11:317–320.
319. Yamagata, M, Chao, E, Illstrup, D, et al. 1987. Fixed-head and bipolar hip endoprosthesis. *J Arthroplasty* 2(4):327–341.
320. Zickel, RE, and Marradian, WH. 1976. Intramedullary

fixation of pathological fractures and lesions of the subtrochanteric region of the femur. *J Bone Joint Surg* 58A(8):1061–1066.

321. Zuckerman, JD, and Matsen, FM. 1989. Biomechanics of the shoulder. In *Basic Biomechanics of the Musculoskeletal Systems,* Eds., M Nordin and VH Frankel. Philadelphia: Lea & Febiger.
322. Zuckerman, JD, and Shapiro, I. 1987. Geriatric shoulder pain: Common causes and their management. *Geriatrics* 42:42–58.
323. Zuckerman, JD, and Sledge, CB. 1985. Total joint replacement: Latest developments for the geriatric patient. *Geriatrics* 40(3):71–92.
324. Zuckerman, JD, and Stuchin, SA. 1986. Total joint replacement: Indications, management considerations and expected outcomes. *IM-Internal Medicine for the Specialist* 7(5):88–118.

37

Gynecologic Surgery in the Elderly

Stephen C. Rubin and Alan Rubin

The increase in the proportion of elderly persons in the United States population is a well-recognized phenomenon and is attributable to both an increase in life expectancy and a decrease in birth rates. At birth, the life expectancy of a female child in the United States is now 77 years, a dramatic increase from the early part of this century. At age 65, women have an additional 18.4 years of life expectancy, and those who reach the age of 75 years can expect to live to approximately age 86. Individuals over 65 years of age, less than 4% of the population at the turn of the century, represented 9.8% of the population in 1970, and 11.3% in 1980. More than 1% of our population is now over 85 years of age. Sixty-nine percent of these individuals are women; their life expectancy is now 5 years. According to the U.S. Census Bureau (1), by the year 2050 the over-85 age group is expected to constitute 5% of the population. Although acute medical illness occurs more commonly in the young, the incidence of virtually every chronic condition rises with age, and most are more common in the female. These conditions span the spectrum from minor nuisances to serious threats to health and life. For example, urinary stress incontinence is estimated to affect 5% to 20% of the elderly living in the community and 40% to 75% of those in nursing homes (2). Most gynecologic malignancies occur more commonly in the elderly. Lifshitz et al. (3) estimate that over 70% of the patients with vulvar, 40% with endometrial, 35% with ovarian, and 25% with cervical malignancy are over age 65. Hospitalized elderly women are more likely to undergo major surgery than their younger counterparts. Krauer (4) reported that although women over 70 years of age constituted only 5% of the patients on a gynecology unit, they accounted for 8.9% of the major surgery.

General Considerations

Essential to good medical care for the elderly is an understanding of preventive measures, chronic medical diseases, remedial therapy, and the social and psychologic influences of prolonged illness. Warshaw (5) outlines basic principles of good geriatric care as follows: (*a*) that the caregiver be familiar with scientific knowledge specific to medical problems of older people, (*b*) that success of care be measured by the restoration of functional capacity, (*c*) that sufficient time be allowed for healing and repair of older tissues, (*d*) that the constant concern should be to avoid iatrogenic illness, and (*e*) that one cannot care adequately for older patients without being concerned about the social, family, financial, and psychologic resources and support available to them.

Specific Considerations

Special care is required for the elderly who undergo surgery because of age-related changes in various organ systems as well as the more frequent presence of medical illnesses, particularly chronic ones. Although age-related physiologic changes are covered in detail elsewhere in this volume, the more important considerations will be mentioned here.

Cardiovascular Physiology

Although cardiovascular function in healthy elderly individuals is normal at rest, age-related changes lead to a diminution of the cardiovascular response to stress. These changes include decreased maximal heart rate, stroke volume and ejection fraction, as well as possible regional cardiac wall motion abnormalities (6). These reduced responses are due to decreased baroreceptor sensitivity, increased peripheral resistance, decreased tachycardic response to hypoxia, absent tachycardic response to hypercarbia, and probably decreased ventricular compliance. Maximal heart rate is decreased because of both structural changes in the sinoatrial node and decreased sensitivity to catecholamines. Thus, although resting cardiovascular function may be near normal in healthy elderly individuals, there may be a significant decrease in cardiovascular reserve. With meticulous perioperative management, however, age per se should not be a contraindication to surgery (7).

It should be remembered that arteriosclerosis-related hypertension and coronary artery disease affect more than 50% of women past 65 years of age. Patients who are at highest risk are those who have had: (*a*) prior myocardial infarction; (*b*) angina pectoris, which in the presence of hypoxia could lead to myocardial infarction intraoperatively; (*c*) congestive heart failure; and (*d*) arrhythmias. In these patients, elective operations should be deferred until medical therapy has been given and the patient's condition is stable and optimal. The importance of hemoglobin concentration, adequate oxygenation, and avoidance of hypotension cannot be overemphasized. Expertise in consultative cardiology coverage, anesthesia, and intensive care nursing are essential to decrease the risk of complications (8).

Pulmonary Physiology

Aging of the pulmonary system also is associated with multiple changes. There is intimal thickening and medial hypertrophy of the pulmonary vasculature and bronchial gland hypertrophy. There is an increased anteroposterior diameter of the chest with decreased chest wall compliance. Although there is an increase in lung compliance, there is a decrease in total lung-chest wall compliance. Lung volumes show a decreased forced vital capacity and decreased forced expiratory volume in 1 second, with an increase in residual volume and increased closing volume. There is a decrease in PaO_2 and decreased diffusing capacity. There is a decrease in hypoxic and hypercapnic ventilatory drive. These age-related changes in static lung volumes, mechanical properties, gas exchange, and control of ventilation lead to a decrease in baseline pulmonary function as well as pulmonary reserve, and consequently increase the risk of pulmonary complications in the elderly surgical patient (7).

In addition, pulmonary disease of the chronic obstructive type, such as emphysema, chronic bronchitis, and asthma, is seen more frequently in the patient over 65 years and predisposes her to an increase in respiratory problems following abdominal surgery. Obstructive lung disease is exacerbated by smoking, obesity, chronic alcoholism, and aging. Smoking causes changes that increase airway resistance, decrease surfactant activity, and alter alveolar macrophage activity. Anesthesia, which further insults the diseased lungs, and postoperative impairment of respiratory function predispose the patient to atelectasis and pneumonia. Restrictive pulmonary diseases, including pulmonary fibrosis, infiltrative lung diseases, and neuromuscular disorders, are also seen more frequently in the aged. These high-risk elderly patients must have preoperative pulmonary evaluation and therapy to enhance optimal function. Pulmonary consultation often is overlooked because the patient in deceptively comfortable at rest (9).

Renal Physiology and Body Composition

The aging process leads to significant decreases in weight and volume of the kidneys, a decrease in renal blood flow, glomerular filtration rate, and tubular length, and decreased concentrating and diluting capabilities of the tubules (10). There also is a diminished capacity to excrete acid. Thus, perturbations of sodium, potassium, and acid-base balance are handled less quickly and less completely in the elderly, although they can generally maintain relatively normal intravascular volumes and electrolyte concentrations in the basal state (7). In addition, the standard indices of renal function, including serum creatinine, urine output, and specific gravity, are less reliable for evaluation of renal function and intravascular volume status.

With aging there is a drop in total body water (TBW) calculated as a percentage of body weight (11). Although there are no specific age-related changes in blood, plasma, or total extracellular fluid volumes, intracellular volume does decrease with age. These changes not only influence fluid and electrolyte balance, but drug therapy as well, since drug doses may be influenced by relative proportions of body water and fat (7).

Fluid and Electrolyte Balance

Preoperative and intraoperative regulation of fluid and electrolyte balance is a vital part of the surgical management of the elderly patient. The most frequent problem in fluid balance preoperatively is hypovolemia. Preparations for tests (enemas, laxatives) and restricted oral intake may result in patients being taken to the operating room dehydrated. This in turn may lead to overhydration during operation to allay hypotension or to compensate for known preoperative dehydration, resulting in congestive failure of an already diseased heart. The problem may be made worse by poor communication between the surgeon and the anesthesiologist regarding clinical evidence of cardiovascular decompensation. Accurate and continuous monitoring of cardiovascular, renal, and respiratory functions is essential. It should be remembered that probably the most frequent electrolyte problem in the elderly patient undergoing operation is a lowered serum potassium level related to diuretic use, and that this is of particular significance in digitalized patients.

Digestive System

Age-related changes in the gastrointestinal and hepatobiliary systems do not ordinarily play a major role in the management of the elderly gynecologic surgical patient. The presence of hiatal hernia should be considered, since its incidence increases with age from 14% in women under age 30 to 58% in women over 60 (12), and it may increase the risk of aspiration during intubation. Symptoms of upper abdominal pain due to hiatal hernia may add concern and confusion to the postoperative management. In patients undergoing extensive pelvic surgery or very long operations, we have deemed it wise to attempt prophylaxis against gastrointestinal bleeding by use of H2 blockers and antacids via a gastric tube. However, recent evidence suggests that these may not be beneficial.

Surgical Morbidity and Mortality

In their excellent review, Polacek and Buchsbaum (7) have suggested that surgical morbidity and mortality in the elderly are influenced importantly by the increased frequency of concurrent medical disease, the nature of the surgical procedure, whether elective or emergency, operating time, and probably the age of the patient per se.

Of 4,038 patients admitted to a gynecologic teaching service of a medical school hospital, 432 were found to have serious medical complications (13). In patients undergoing surgery for gynecologic malignancy, Pierson et al. (14) found the incidence of major medical disease in women over 75 (mean 79.9 years) was 76% compared with 28% in a control group of women under 55 (mean 47.6 years) who were undergoing identical procedures for similar conditions. The most common problems of the elderly were hypertension (52%), arteriosclerotic heart disease (38%), and diabetes (20%). The most common problem in the control group was varicose veins. Similar results have been found in other series (15, 16). As would be expected, operative risk rises in proportion to the number and severity of medical problems (17).

Studies that have attempted to separate the higher than normal risk of surgery associated with coexistent medical complications in the elderly from the risk of age per se fail to demonstrate a clear association between age and risk of surgery (18, 19). Panayiotis et al. (20) found no increase in postoperative complications in patients over 65, as compared to a control group aged 40 to 55 years. In a study of patients undergoing major operations for gynecologic cancer, Pierson et al. (14) reported a complication rate of 1.12 per patient in a study group, averaging 79.2 years of age. This compares with a rate of 1.04 per patient in the control group, averaging 47.6 years.

In general, the elderly tolerate vaginal or vulvar surgery better than transabdominal surgery. In vaginal surgery, the decreased manipulation of the small bowel permits earlier return of normal gastrointestinal motility with less distention, hence less deterrent to deep breathing. Less distention and less pain may allow the use of less medication for pain relief, less sedation, more normal breathing, and earlier eating and ambulation. The percentage of surgical procedures done via the vagina in elderly gynecologic patients ranges from 54% to 85% (16, 20–22).

Emergency gynecologic surgery in the elderly is rare. In our experience, uncontrolled bleeding or an adnexal accident are the commonest causes. The three- to fivefold higher mortality associated with emergency surgery in the elderly is significantly contributed to by the underlying gynecologic pathology (18, 23, 24). In one series (16), there was a postoperative complication rate of 33% in "indicated" procedures, as compared to 19% in "elective" procedures.

It has been suggested that in addition to the influence of the type of procedures on operating time, the skill of the operator (house staff versus attending staff, for example), is a major determinant of operating time. Hence, it is difficult to determine whether operative time per se influences outcome. Several authors have reported that the duration of surgery is probably not related to morbitity or mortality in the elderly (23, 24). Such ideas are contrary to the concept that the longer the exposure of the abdominal field, the higher the incidence of infectious complications. In one study, the operating time in women over 75 years of age was slightly shorter than that of women under 55 (14).

There are studies reported in which the majority of elderly women had conduction anesthesia for gynecologic operations (14, 15, 20). However, up to 98% of gynecologic operations have been reported as performed on the elderly under general anesthesia with apparently equally good results (21). The choice of anesthetic technique is generally based on the patient's overall medical status, the type of surgery, and the preferences of the anesthesiologist, surgeon, and patient.

Indications for Gynecologic Operations in the Elderly

The major indications for operation are: (*a*) postmenopausal bleeding; (*b*) pelvic relaxation; (*c*) undiagnosed pelvic mass, most commonly adnexal; (*d*) urinary stress incontinence; (*e*) malignancy of the endometrium; (*f*) malignancy of the ovary; (*g*) malignancy of the cervix; and (*h*) malignancy of the vulva.

Postmenopausal Bleeding

Postmenopausal patients should always be asked specifically about vaginal bleeding. After having approximately 500 such episodes during a normal reproductive lifetime, some women are unaware that the normal postmenopausal genital tract produces no blood, and they will fail to volunteer this information.

The actual incidence of postmenopausal bleeding (PMB) is unknown and will vary widely, depending on the definition of PMB that is employed, the population in question, the use of estrogen replacement, and other factors. A rough estimate is that perhaps 10% of women will require evaluation for postmenopausal bleeding. A more important concern is the actual likelihood of malignancy in a patient with postmenopausal bleeding. Most recent series have reported that about 20% of women with postmenopausal bleeding will have malignancy as the cause. It is clear that the likelihood of malignancy increases with age in women with postmenopausal bleeding, so that the further away a woman is from her reproductive years, the more seriously this symptom should be viewed (25).

Pathophysiology

In the majority of cases of PMB, the bleeding originates in the endometrium and is related to estrogen stimulation or the lack of it. After menopause, when ovarian estrogen and progesterone production decline, the normal uterus becomes a quiescent organ. The endometrium becomes inactive, histologically showing small tubular glands and a dense, compact stroma, reflecting a lack of estrogen activity. This so-called atrophic endometrium is quite fragile and may occasionally break down and cause bleeding. It has been suggested that myometrial arteriosclerosis may be a cause of bleeding from the atrophic endometrium (26). It should be remembered, however, that the postmenopausal woman is not entirely devoid of estrogen. Although the postmenopausal ovary produces only insignificant amounts of estrogen, there is considerable estrogen production through peripheral conversion (in adipose tissue) of adrenal androgens. Thus, after menopause, estrogen levels are related to body weight, and in some women may be high enough to cause irregular bleeding from stimulation of the endometrium. Even hyperplasia or carcinoma may develop from prolonged unopposed estrogen stimulation.

The pathophysiology of the bleeding in non-endometrial causes of PMB is quite straightforward and is discussed where appropriate in the following section.

Etiology

The etiology of postmenopausal bleeding can be divided into malignant and nonmalignant causes. Although in the majority of women PMB will not be due to cancer, we will discuss the malignant causes first, since the others are generally not of serious consequence.

Malignant causes. Endometrial cancer is the most common of the malignancies found in women with PMB and should be the foremost concern of the clinician evaluating such patients. Endometrial adenocarcinoma is primarily a disease of postmenopausal women. The average age at diagnosis in this country is about 60 years, and age-specific incidence rates peak at about the same age. About three-fourths of patients with endometrial carcinoma will present with abnormal bleeding. Such bleeding usually occurs early in the natural history of this disease, and the low threshold of most physicians for evaluation of this bleeding is responsible for the fact that about three-quarters of the cases are diagnosed in stage I, when the disease is limited to the uterine fundus. In one study that attempted to quantitate bleeding, postmenopausal women who reported only staining were just as likely to have endometrial cancer as those who reported gross bleeding (27).

Certain factors have been associated with an increased risk of developing endometrial carcinoma. These include obesity, nulliparity, late menopause, diabetes, and hypertension. Clinicians have long been impressed with the association of obesity and endometrial cancer, and there are many studies that support this. Wynder et al. (28) have found that women who were 21 to 50 pounds overweight had a threefold increased risk, and those more than 50 pounds overweight had a 10-fold increased risk of developing endometrial carcinoma, as compared to women of normal or below-normal weight. The increased risk probably is due to the elevated estrogen levels that result from obesity. Nulliparity is another well-recognized risk factor. In Wynder's study, endometrial cancer rates in nulliparous women were twice as high as those for women with one child and more than three times as high as those for women with five or more children. Age at menopause tends to be higher in women who develop endometrial cancer. Kaplan and Cole, cited by MacMahon

(29) found a 2.4-fold increased risk of endometrial cancer in women whose menopause occurred at age 52 or older as compared to those undergoing menopause prior to age 49. This prolongation of "menstrual" bleeding is probably reflective of hormonal activity rather than an early sign of neoplasm, since late menopause was found to be a risk factor even in women who were in the 60 to 69 and 70 or more age groups at the time of diagnosis of endometrial cancer. The association of diabetes with endometrial cancer is less well established since many studies have had major methodologic flaws. Nevertheless, diabetes, whether diagnosed by history or by glucose tolerance testing, has been reported consistently as a risk factor for endometrial cancer. Hypertension has frequently been cited as a risk factor, but the data for this association are generally unconvincing.

Other risk factors for endometrial carcinoma include a history of postmenopausal estrogen replacement therapy, prior pelvic radiation, and conditions of endogenous estrogen excess, such as chronic anovulation and estrogen-secreting ovarian tumors.

Except for abnormal bleeding, patients with endometrial carcinoma will generally be totally asymptomatic and may have normal physical findings, including pelvic examination. Cervical Pap smears are usually normal in the presence of endometrial carcinoma, and this test must never be relied upon to exclude the diagnosis, which must be made by histologic sampling of the endometrium. Since cervical involvement by endometrial carcinoma alters the staging, treatment, and prognosis, histologic sampling from the cervix is also required. In addition to direct extension to the cervix and other pelvic structures, endometrial carcinoma may spread by other routes. In the last decade, gynecologists have gained a new understanding of the very real potential for lymphatic dissemination. In patients whose tumor appears clinically to be confined to the uterine corpus (stage I), approximately 10% will have spread to the pelvic and/or para-aortic lymph nodes (30). The disease also may spread by the hematogenous route, with the lungs being the most frequent site of metastases. Other important prognostic factors include the histologic grade of the tumor and the depth of penetration into the myometrium.

Patients with endometrial carcinoma should be managed by a physician experienced in gynecologic oncology. In the early stages, treatment is primarily surgical, with radiotherapy applied in selected cases depending on various prognostic factors. In advanced or recurrent cases, chemotherapy or hormonal therapy may be used for palliation.

Cervical carcinoma has in the past been prominent among the malignant causes of postmenopausal bleeding. The advent of Pap smear screening has allowed the diagnosis of cervical cancer in earlier stages and in younger women, so that the more recent literature reflects a ratio of endometrial to cervical cancer of approximatedly 5:1 in women with PMB.

Cervical carcinoma has the epidemiologic characteristics of a venereal disease and has recently been strongly associated with certain subtypes of the human papilloma virus (31), which also causes venereal warts. When the disease is locally advanced enough to cause abnormal bleeding, a gross cervical tumor is generally present, and a tentative diagnosis can be made by inspection and palpation. Of note is the fact that the sensitivity of the Pap smear is lower in gross cervical cancer than it is in early lesions, since the surface of the gross lesion may be covered with blood and necrotic debris, which obscure the cytologic diagnosis. For this reason, a normal Pap smear should never dissuade the physician from biopsying a visible cervical lesion.

Cervical cancer is a disease that tends to remain localized to the pelvis for a long period of its natural history, and this feature allows for effective therapy by local treatments such as radiation and surgery. Patients with early tumors who are acceptable surgical risks will be treated with radical hysterectomy and pelvic lymph node dissection. Patients who are poor surgical risks or who have advanced disease will generally be treated with radical radiation therapy. Chemotherapy may provide palliative benefit.

Among the more unusual gynecologic malignancies that may present as postmenopausal bleeding are carcinomas of the vagina or vulva (see section on vulvar cancer) and uterine sarcomas. An occasional patient with cancer of the fallopian tube or ovary may present with postmenopausal bleeding, as may patients with metastatic disease involving the genital tract.

Some patients may be unable to distinguish urethral or rectal bleeding from vaginal bleeding, and thus diseases involving the urinary and intestinal tracts may need to be considered.

Nonmalignant causes. In the majority of women who undergo evaluation for postmenopausal bleeding, no malignancy will be found. Histologic sampling from the endometrium most often (in about 27%) reveals an inactive or "atrophic" endometrium associated with the normal hypoestrogenic state after menopause. In some women, the postmenopausal endometrium may show evidence of estrogen stimulation. This may result from exogenous sources, from endogenous conversion of adrenal androgens in adipose tissue, or rarely from estrogen-producing tumors, such as granulosa cell carcinomas of the ovary. Prolonged estrogen stimulation unopposed by progesterone can lead to the development of endometrial hyperplasia, which has been reported in from 3% to 25% of women with PMB. Depending on the precise histologic features, some types of endometrial hyperplasia can be considered to be "premalignant." Other benign conditions that may cause endometrial bleeding include polyps (in about 6%), endometritis (including tuberculous), and rarely parasitic infections.

The epithelium of the lower genital tract in hypoestrogenic women is quite delicate, and minor inflammation of the cervix, vagina, and vulva may cause PMB. L-dopa has also been associated with PMB (32). Of note is the fact that women with benign PMB may be at a slightly increased risk of subsequently developing a genital malignancy (33) and thus deserve continuing close follow-up.

Evaluation

Careful inspection of the lower genital tract and bimanual and rectovaginal examination should be performed. It is important to remember that the normal postmenopausal ovary is shrunken and atrophic and usually is not palpable; thus to feel a "normal-size" ovary in a woman with PMB may be a sign of disease. A Pap smear should be performed to detect cervical abnormalities, but this should not be relied upon to rule out endometrial pathology. It is not unusual for the entire pelvic examination to be completely normal.

The cornerstone of the evaluation of PMB is histologic sampling of the endometrium and endocervix. This can conveniently be accomplished by fractional dilatation and curettage performed on an outpatient basis under either local or general anesthesia. A number of instruments have been devised to allow sampling of the endometrium in an office setting without the need for anesthesia. Some of these produce cytologic samples, while others produce specimens satisfactory for histologic processing. Although a vigorous endometrial biopsy is fairly accurate at detecting endometrial cancer, the sensitivity of many of the cytologic sampling techniques in detecting cancer is relatively low, and they are probably even less accurate at detecting precursor lesions, such as endometrial hyperplasia. Thus, although they may be useful in evaluating the endometrium in certain other circumstances, they cannot be recommended for evaluation of women with PMB.

Hysterectomy for Benign Conditions

Choice of Approach

Although vaginal hysterectomy has the advantages of lesser risk of morbidity, shorter period of illness, and far less pain, it is not a technique that is always feasible. In patients with a narrow subpubic angle and a narrow, tight atrophic vagina, it may be technically difficult or impossible. Likewise, if there are extensive pelvic adhesions as from previous surgery or inflammatory disease, particularly of the intestines, vaginal hysterectomy may be too hazardous. It may not always be possible to remove the adnexa via the vagina, because the vascular pedicles may be short and hold the ovaries so high in the pelvis as to be inaccessible from below.

Abdominal Hysterectomy for Benign Conditions

When abdominal hysterectomy for benign disease in the elderly is undertaken, a modified Richardson technique is preferred. Pelvic tissues in the elderly usually separate easily and with less bleeding than in premenopausal patients. Pushing the bladder down from the anterior cervix, making upward traction on the uterus, and dissecting the peritoneum off the cervix posteriorly serve to carry the ureters down and out of the operative field. The frequently weak, attenuated pelvic tissues of the elderly make it important to support the vaginal cuff as much as possible. In general, both tubes and ovaries should be removed with the uterus in the elderly patient undergoing hysterectomy for benign disease.

In the elderly, among the commonest indications for abdominal exploration would be adnexal masses that prove to be benign. In such instances, unless there is some medical contraindication to the additional surgery, the proper course usually is total hysterectomy with removal of the adnexa. If there should be extensive adhesions or other conditions that might make the surgery unduly prolonged or hazardous, then a lesser procedure might be indicated. It is well to keep in mind that postmenopausal involution and shrinkage of myomas takes place, so the sudden enlargement of the postmenopausal uterus can rarely be attributed to benign degeneration of a preexisting myoma and should be viewed with concern. Abdominal X-rays in the elderly woman with myomas will often show a characteristic pattern of calcifications.

Laparoscopy for the diagnosis of a pelvic mass in the elderly should rarely be performed, since one cannot accomplish therapy this way, and the steep Trendelenberg position and carbon dioxide insufflation required may be as stressful to elderly patients as a rapid, skillfully executed laparotomy with competent anesthesia support. Laparoscopy may on occasion be useful for distinguishing a pedunculated uterine myoma from an adnexal mass.

A left-sided pelvic mass may be a uterine myoma, adnexal pathology, or intestinal disease. Inflammatory bowel disease, diverticulitis, and malignancy can all produce a left-sided mass indistinguishable from an ovarian neoplasm on physical examination. Hence, a barium enema should be performed before exploring most patients with pelvic masses, particularly left-sided lesions. One should bear in mind the timing of the X-ray so that the bowel is not filled with barium at the time of surgery. Even a cystic, seemingly obvious left adnexal mass may upon occasion turn out to be a bowel lesion, and lack of proper preparation of the intestinal tract and proper operative consent can prove to be a handicap to proper care. Lower left-sided colonic pathology often will be adherent to the left adnexal structures, which may require removal at the time of surgery. Occasionally, the uterus must also be removed because of adherence or difficulty in exposure for the bowel surgeon. In such circumstances, both adnexa should also be removed. The additional surgery adds little increase in operative time or blood loss.

It should be remembered that the ovaries normally are atrophic and cannot be palpated even in a thin postmenopausal woman. In general, an ovary that is large enough to be palpated in a postmenopausal woman is abnormal and must be explained or explored. It must be pointed out that CT scans and ultrasound have limited accuracy in the detection of small pelvic masses, and may at times suggest masses that do not exist. This compounds the problems of the gynecologic surgeon who may at times be unable to palpate a mass demonstrated by these imaging techniques.

Vaginal Hysterectomy for Benign Disease

Except for prolapse or as part of surgery for pelvic floor relaxation, vaginal hysterectomy has a limited place in the elderly, where a small introitus and a narrow vagina may produce technical difficulties. It may occasionally be appropriate in the treatment of pre-invasive cervical lesions or atypical endometrial changes, provided that one is sure there is no invasive malignancy. Its advantages have been described at the beginning of this section. Further comments about vaginal hysterectomy will be found in the subsequent section on operations for pelvic relaxations.

Hysterectomy for Malignancy

Simple Abdominal Hysterectomy

Endometrial cancer is the most common of the female genital malignancies and the most common malignant indication for simple abdominal hysterectomy. The etiology, pathophysiology, and clinical features of the disease have been discussed previously in the section on postmenopausal bleeding.

The technique of simple abdominal hysterectomy for early endometrial cancer is similar to that used for benign conditions, with several modifications. On entering the peritoneal cavity, saline washings should be taken from the pelvis and submitted for cytologic analysis. Approximately 5% to 10% of patients with clinically early endometrial cancer will have malignant cells in such washings. Although their significance is unclear, there is evidence that this finding may markedly worsen prognosis. Some surgeons practice routine ligation of the distal ends of the fallopian tubes prior to beginning the hysterectomy to prevent dissemination of malignant cells during uterine manipulation. Since this does not add significantly to operative time or morbidity, it is probably worthwhile. Sharp tenacula should not be used to grasp a uterus containing a malignant tumor, again to decrease the possibility of escape of tumor cells.

The hysterectomy itself should be performed by the extrafascial technique, without incising the pubocervical fascia over the cervix. There has been much debate in the past over the need for occlusion of the cervical os prior to hysterectomy for endometrial cancer. Although various techniques have been devised for this purpose, including sutures, screws, and cervical obturators, it is generally considered unnecessary. Likewise, there is no demonstrated benefit to the removal of a vaginal cuff to decrease the incidence of local recurrence.

Depending on certain prognostic factors (including tumor grade and depth of myometrial penetration), on institutional treatment protocols, and on whether preoperative pelvic radiotherapy has been used, sampling of aortic and/or pelvic lymph nodes may be appropriate.

In patients explored for adnexal masses that are found to be malignant (ovarian or tubal cancer), the uterus should generally be removed, since it may harbor metastatic disease.

Simple hysterectomy may also be indicated in cases of pre-invasive or micro-invasive cervical cancer.

Radical Abdominal Hysterectomy with Pelvic Lymphadenectomy

The most common indication for this procedure is in the primary treatment of early (stage IB or IIA) cancer of the cervix. It is also used occasionally in the primary treatment of stage II endometrial cancer and rarely in the secondary treatment of cervical cancer that has failed primary radiotherapy (34). Since approximately equal cure rates for early cervical cancer can be obtained with combinations of external radiotherapy and brachytherapy, this extensive surgical procedure is not often employed in elderly women. There is no arbitrary age cutoff, however, and the choice of therapy is based more on the patient's physiologic condition than chronological age.

Radical hysterectomy as performed today differs from simple hysterectomy in several important aspects. Most importantly, a radical excision of the parametrium, that fibrofatty tissue extending laterally from the cervix and upper vagina to the pelvic side wall, is removed. This tissue contains vascular and lymphatic channels for the central pelvic viscera and is an important potential route of spread for tumors involving the cervix. Approximately the upper one-third of the vagina is removed as well, and the operation is combined with a complete pelvic lymphadenectomy, including the external iliac, obturator, and hypogastric nodal chains. The removal of the parametrium requires complete dissection of the ureter from its entry into the parametrial tunnel lateral to the cervix to the trigone of the bladder. This inevitably disrupts a portion of the segmental blood supply to the distal ureter, and is responsible for the small risk of ureteral fistula that follows the operation.

Prophylactic antibiotics have been shown to be of benefit, and most surgeons prefer to drain the pelvis using closed suction drains. With the use of these techniques, the rate of ureteral fistula, previously in the range of 10%, has fallen to approximately 2% (35). The other important complication specific to this operation is postoperative motor and sensory dysfunction of the bladder, which results from the necessary disruption of the autonomic nerve supply to the bladder during the radical dissection of the parametrium, uterosacral, and vesicouterine ligaments. Most gynecologic oncologists prefer to drain the bladder for 4 to 6 weeks following radical hysterectomy to allow time for recovery of bladder function. Rarely, postoperative bladder dysfunction will be severe enough to require long-term intermittent catheterization.

Radical Vaginal Hysterectomy

This operation, pioneered by Schauta in the early part of this century, is today primarily of historical interest. It allowed the satisfactory removal of the parametrium and upper vagina from below, and avoided an abdominal incision in an era when laparotomy carried substantial morbidity and mortality. More recently, it was combined with a bilateral extraperitoneal pelvic lymphadenectomy performed through groin incisions to provide essentially the same surgical treatment of early cervical cancer as can be accomplished with radical abdominal hysterectomy. With the development of modern antibiotics and anesthetic techniques, radical vaginal hysterectomy has been largely supplanted by the abdominal approach, and today few American surgeons are familiar with the technique.

Vulvectomy

Vulvar cancer is primarily a disease of elderly women. The majority of these tumors are of the squamous cell variety, with melanoma, adenocarcinoma, and sarcomas occurring much less frequently. This discussion will be restricted to the management of squamous carcinomas, although many of the same principles and techniques apply to the other histologic types as well.

Cancer of the vulva spreads primarily by lymphatic dissemination. It does so in a predictable, systematic fashion, involving initially the regional (inguinal and femoral) lymph nodes and secondarily the pelvic nodes. Although there are demonstrable lymph pathways from the clitoris and perineal body directly to the pelvic nodes, these are of little clinical significance, as pelvic nodal spread rarely occurs in the absence of groin node spread, even with centrally located lesions (36). The predictable pattern of spread and the tendency of the tumor to remain localized (or regionalized) for a relatively long period of its natural history make vulvar cancer a disease that lends itself well to surgical treatment.

Surgery is the treatment of choice for vulvar malignancies. The standard surgical treatment for invasive vulvar cancer is radical vulvectomy and bilateral inguinal lymphadenectomy. The vulvectomy includes removal of all vulvar tissue down to the inferior fascia of the urogenital diaphragm, including skin, subcutaneous tissue, superficial fascia, and the superficial vulvar musculature, including the bulbocavernosus, ischiocavernosus, and portions of the superficial transverse perineal muscles. If necessary to obtain clear margins, the distal urethra and vagina may be incorporated into an en bloc dissection. Generally, the vaginal walls and skin surrounding the operative site can be mobilized sufficiently to allow primary closure and satisfactory healing. Occasionally, mobilization of full-thickness skin flaps or myocutaneous flaps may be needed to cover large vulvar defects.

The groin dissection is most often performed in continuity with the vulvar dissection, removing the skin and subcutaneous tissues in the inguinal area and over the mons. A complete inguinal lymphadenectomy is performed bilaterally, cleaning out the femoral triangle, skeletonizing the femoral vessels, and removing a segment of the proximal saphenous vein. Recently, some have advocated performing the groin dissection through separate incisions with preservation of all or most of the skin in the groin to allow for better closure and healing (37).

There has been a trend in recent years toward modification of the radical surgical approach in cases of small superficially invasive vulvar cancers, with efforts made toward preservation of part of the vulva and less than full bilateral groin dissections (38, 39). Although further experience is needed, this approach appears promising. Vulvar carcinoma in-situ may be treated by wide local excision.

Pelvic Relaxation

Anatomy

The structures supporting the female pelvic viscera against the gravitational forces imposed when upright, as well as intra-abdominal forces associated with coughing, defecation, lifting, or even bending, may, with time, prove inadequate. Childbirth injuries, the gradual weakening of tissue with aging, and menopausal status can all contribute to a loss of support. Congenital weaknesses may also play a role. There are patients whose hymens had to be incised to gain room to surgically correct uterine prolapse.

The structures that can be involved in such relaxations are the levator ani muscle with its anterior (puborectalis), middle (pubococcygeus), and posterior (ileococcygeus) portions. Their names roughly approximate their origins and insertions. Weakness of this muscular support can lead ultimately to downward displacement of the pelvic viscera through the levator hiatus of the pelvic floor. The more superficially located muscles of the perineum, including the paired ischiocavernosus, bulbocavernosus, deep and superficial transverse perineal muscles, together with the external anal sphincter, form a second hammock-like supporting mechanism. This, however, is less important and by itself would be inadequate to prevent the continued downward displacement of the uterus, bladder, or rectum should the levator muscle supports fail. The uterosacral, cardinal, and round ligaments play a role in supporting the uterus by tending to maintain it in its proper axis to the vaginal canal, and so prevent gravity and increases in intra-abdominal pressure from forcing the uterus down the vagina. The uterosacral ligaments are of particular importance, for they should hold the cervix posteriorly, thus tending to keep the uterus perpendicular to the line of the vaginal canal and in a position over the muscular plate of the levator sling. The cardinal ligaments of Mackenrodt contain the blood vessels and lymphatics passing between the pelvic walls and uterus at the level of the cervix. They gain their important supportive strength for the uterus because of the condensation of fibrous and areolar tissue, the endopelvic fascia, which is reflected from the pelvic walls medially along the vascular, muscular, and peritoneal tissue planes running toward the central pelvic viscera. If the levator sling fails in the face of continued support from the cardinal ligaments, the cervix below the level of the cardinal ligaments can become markedly elongated because of the lack of support below this level.

Operations for Relaxation

Vaginal Hysterectomy

The surgical management of the clinical manifestations of failure of support, i.e., cystocele, rectocele, urethrocele, and enterocele, entail efforts to repair or overcome the weaknesses. In general, the patient with significant pelvic floor relaxation will be best served by combining vaginal hysterectomy with the repair, if the patient's medical condition is satisfactory and there is no surgical contraindication.

Detailed descriptions of surgical techniques can be found in any atlas of gynecologic surgery. Certain caveats bear mention.

Patients with a prolapsed uterus and cystocele often have no impairment of urinary continence. Unless due care is taken during repair to elevate the vesicourethral junction adequately, incontinence may result. With complete prolapse of the uterus and a large cystocele and rectocele, maintaining a well-supported vagina that is adequate for coitus can be a challenge. Identifying even badly attenuated uterosacral and round ligaments and shortening them considerably with fixation of the reconstructed vaginal vault to them can help achieve both these goals. Any time the cul-de-sac is opened, as it is with all vaginal hysterectomies, it is important to close any existing or potential hernial orifice. This is readily accomplished using a heavy mattress suture to approximate the sides of the cul-de-sac.

Fothergill (Manchester) Operation

In the past, gynecologists performed Sturmdorf amputations of the cervix and plication of Mackenrodt's ligaments (the Fothergil or Manchester operation) combined with an anterior repair for treatment of pelvic relaxation in elderly patients who were poor surgical risks and had an adequately supported, small uterus. This procedure assures good uterine support and a sufficiently long vagina for coitus. With the development of modern techniques of anesthetic and medical support, this operation has been largely supplanted by vaginal hysterectomy and repair, and is now mainly of historical interest.

Le Fort Operation (Colpocleisis)

Traditionally, this operation has been reserved for the poor-risk patient where coital function need not be preserved. It was felt that the lesser operative time and blood loss made it preferable in these patients. As with the Fothergill operation, it is now rarely performed. Its disadvantages include prolapse of the uterus along the surgically created vaginal channels (if left too large), inaccessibility for examination and treatment should bleeding develop (the uterus is "buried" behind the obliterated vagina), and, occasionally, urinary incontinence.

Anterior Colporrhaphy

Although repair of cystocele seems technically simple, recurrences are not uncommon. Efforts should be made to create good support while avoiding strangulation of tissue. It is of great importance to perform an appropriate preoperative evaluation to assure that infection, or more seriously, neurologic defects, are not responsible for the patient's symptoms. Along with urinary incontinence, symptoms of anterior vaginal relaxation may include a protrusion of the anterior wall with a sense of pelvic pressure and fullness. Inadequate bladder emptying with a cystocele may predispose to recurrent or chronic cystitis. It is important to remember that while stress urinary incontinence is not a symptom of cystocele per se, it may, however, appear as a result of a cystocele repair. Hence, it is essential to be sure that the bladder neck is well elevated during any repair. Further comments can be found in the section on urinary incontinence.

Rectocele and Lacerated Perineum

The chief symptoms of this condition are an uncomfortable protrusion of the posterior vagina and anterior rectal wall, sometimes associated with difficulty in evacuating the rectum. Posterior colporrhaphy and treatment of any old perineal laceration is readily, quickly, and relatively bloodlessly accomplished, with good symptomatic improvement to be anticipated. Too tight a posterior repair, together with the often ongoing tissue shrinkage accompanying aging, can make coitus difficult or impossible. Vaginal estrogen creams can help stem this process, and are often useful before and after surgery to improve the condition of the tissues and speed healing.

Enterocele

Enterocele is a hernial weakness occurring between the uterosacral ligaments just posterior to the cervix. It can be distinguished from rectocele (which it often accompanies) by rectovaginal examination. One can palpate the hernial sac, often containing small intestine, dissecting along the rectovaginal septum just anterior to the rectum. Treatment is as for any hernial defect: closure of the neck and amputation of the excess peritoneum. The vaginal approach to repair has been described in the section on vaginal hysterectomy; it should always be a part of this operation. If noted at abdominal surgery, the cul-de-sac can be plicated with a purse-string suture, with care to avoid the ureters (40).

Vaginal Inversion

Complete prolapse of the vagina can follow vaginal or abdominal hysterectomy. Careful attention to providing adequate vaginal support at the time of surgery is important to help prevent this problem.

Sacrospinous fixation as described by Randall and Nichols (41) is extremely useful but fraught with hazard for the inexperienced or unwary by virtue of possible injury to the pudendal vessels or nerve or the sciatic nerve.

Although sacrospinous fixation can be used for vaginal inversion, if a deep well-supported vagina is desired, we favor sacropexy placing a non-absorbable mesh from the apex of the vagina retroperitoneally to the sacrum (42). Fascia lata, preserved dura, and other materials have been suggested to reduce the occasional problem of erosion of the mesh material into the vaginal vault.

Mechanical Devices

There is an occasional elderly patient with symptomatic relaxation whose health is so precarious, or resistance to surgery so fixed, that nonoperative management must be employed. Under such circumstances, a pessary can serve well. The patient should be made aware of the necessity for its periodic removal and inspection of the vagina to check for possible vaginal erosion. Some patients can manage removal and washing of the pessary, and its reinsertion after douching, themselves. There are other cases of neglectful or mentally incompetent women whose pessaries after prolonged retention required anesthesia and a perineotomy for removal. Pessaries that are generally easiest to insert and remove are of the soft, hinged type. Rubber doughnut pessaries of the inflatable variety can be inflated and deflated with a needle and syringe to facilitate insertion and removal. Vaginal estrogen cream used in small quantities on a weekly basis helps the vagina tolerate the pessary and reduces malodorous discharge. Combining estrogen and sulfa-containing vaginal creams can also be helpful. Sulfa preparations can be used alone if an estrogen cream is contraindicated, as in women with previous breast cancer, endometrial cancer, stroke, myocardial infarction, or thromboembolic disorder. In the rare patient whose vaginal orifice is so gaping that retention of the pessary is difficult, stemmed or suction cup varieties may be of use. One can also under local anesthesia tighten thc introitus surgically so that thc pessary will be held in the vagina.

Urinary Stress Incontinence

Urinary stress incontinence may be defined as the involuntary leakage of urine with increases in intra-abdominal pressure, such as coughing, sneezing, lifting, walking, or even bending. Significant stress incontinence is unusual in nulliparous women. When encountered, it presumably is secondary to poor pubococcygeal muscle tone, congenital weakness, or deficient innervation of the pelvic floor muscle supports. It is much more common in women who have born children, and increases in incidence and severity with advancing age due to loss of muscle strength and tissue turgor following menopause.

True urinary stress incontinence probably occurs as a result of diminished support of the bladder neck and urethra. Hence, it can occur in the absence of significant prolapse or cystocele, where the weakness may be of the more posteriorly situated bladder base. Many older women hesitate to complain of urinary incontinence, out of embarrassment or fear that they will be told they need surgery, or because of the conviction that it is the price of advancing age.

Correction of urinary stress incontinence can provide dramatic relief to the elderly woman who has decided she must live with wearing pads or diapers to absorb her urine and has limited her social or physical activities because of incontinence. It is important to be sure that one is dealing with stress incontinence, because surgery when this condition does not exist or when another problem causing urinary problems coexists unrecognized, may worsen rather than improve the patient's symptoms. Thus, first considering the differential diagnostic possibilities and then applying appropriate diagnostic and therapeutic modalities, is essential. Green (43), who has contributed much to the subject of incontinence, provides the following list:

1. True stress incontinence (deficient anatomic support of the bladder neck and urethra).
2. Detrusor dyssynergia, the disorder that most frequently masquerades as stress incontinence but is psychosomatic and functional in origin 70% to 80% of the time. Although frequency and urgency are the hallmarks of this condition, there may be a pseudostress incontinence in roughly 50% of patients. (In this situation, the stress serves to activate the hyperactive detrusor mechanism present in these patients, producing an actual "voiding" type of leakage rather than the instantaneous and brief spurt associated with the anatomically incompetent urethrovesical continence mechanism that is responsible for true stress incontinence).
3. Pure urgency incontinence, which is most often due to a nonbacterial trigonitis and cystitis, which in turn may be secondary to an underlying trichomoniasis, candidiasis, severe endocervicitis, or, most often, atrophic vaginitis. The latter is associated with similar atrophic changes in the mucosa of the bladder and urethra, leading to marked urgency and precipitate, uncontrollable voiding.
4. Bladder neuropathies (diabetes, syphilis, multiple sclerosis, primary neurologic disorders or injuries), usually leading to an overflow type of incontinence, less often to an uninhibited detrusor type of leakage.
5. Abnormal drainage situations (ectopic ureter, urethral diverticulum, acquired vesicovaginal or urethrovaginal fistula).
6. Increased intra-abdominal pressure (e.g., tumors, ascites, pregnancy) may lead to a temporary stress incontinence.
7. Primary lesions (inflammation, calculi, tumors) of the bladder, urethra, or adjacent organs (e.g., uterus, ovary, rectosigmoid), nearly always resulting in an urgency type of incontinence or to an abnormal leakage due to secondary fistula formation.
8. Short urethra "total incontinence" syndrome (the abnormal shortening may be congenital or acquired, resulting in a length of less than 2 cm). Here, there is a continuous leakage, regardless of position or stress, although the symptom may be aggravated by stress.

Theories abound as to the physiologic aberrations or anatomic defects that will result in stress incontinence. Techniques abound to demonstrate the defect popular at any one time as the cause of the condition. Their popularity wanes as new studies proving them wrong appear. Hence, we will forego such discussions and present operations which have been used and are used successfully in management.

The vaginal approach is particularly useful if vaginal repair also is required. It can be quickly and easily accomplished with little blood loss. It is made more difficult if there has been a previous anterior repair or previous surgery for incontinence. In such cases, the success rate will be lower. In primary cases repaired by the vaginal route, the success rate is almost equal to that which can be achieved by abdominal or combined vaginal-abdominal approaches: 85% to 95%.

Kelly Urethral Plication

The Kelly urethral plication, although described in 1911, still remains an important method of repair. After opening the anterior vaginal wall, there should be wide mobilization of the posterior urethra and paraurethral fascia at the urethrovesical junction. Several mattress sutures (the original technique used vertical mattresses, but these bunch the tissue in the long axis of the urethra and tend to shorten the urethra, whereas lengthening is desired to help continence) of number 0 chromic or delayed absorbable suture generally are used (44). High placement of the sutures at the urethrovesical junction is important to elevate the posterior urethra and vesical neck to their normal retropubic position and improve the posterior urethrovesical angle.

Marshall-Marchetti-Kranz Procedure

This retropubic urethral suspension, first described in 1949 (45), also has stood the test of time. It is particularly useful where an abdominal approach is to be used for some other purpose. It also is more likely to achieve good results than a repeat Kelly plication after previous failure of or recurrence of incontinence following a Kelly plication. Even as a primary operation, this procedure or many of its modifications, has higher cure rates than a purely vaginal approach. Burch's (46) technique of suspending the paraurethral tissues and bladder neck to Cooper's ligament avoids trauma to the periostium that the original technique of suturing to the symphysis pubis engendered. Thus, the infrequent osteitis pubis that once was a bete noir is almost eliminated. However, overcorrection of the urethrovesical angle with resultant difficulty in bladder emptying is easier with the Burch modification. Placing sutures in Cooper's ligaments, as well as a single suture on each side into the retropubic periosteum is preferable, although in the aged the periosteum has a greater tendency to tear. Number 1 delayed absorbable sutures are recommended. Prophylactic antibiotics are given, since one may penetrate into the vagina with a suture and thus implant vaginal flora into the periosteum.

Modifications of these concepts include that popularized by Pereyra et al. (47) in which there is a limited vaginal dissection of the paraurethral areas on each side. Nonabsorbable sutures are passed retropubically on either side of the urethra at the urethrovesical angle, employing a special ligature carrier introduced through a small suprapubic skin incision. The sutures then are tied down snugly against the anterior rectus sheath. This can easily be combined with a vaginal repair and probably will give better results than a Kelly plication. It is recommended that the patient be cystoscoped following suture placement to be sure that no sutures penetrate the bladder as a result of the relatively blind suture placement used in this procedure.

Sling Operations

Sling operations for urinary stress incontinence make use of a strip of material placed under the vesical neck to elevate it. The sling is commonly attached to the rectus fascia. These operations are usually reserved for failures of urethral plication or retropubic urethropexy, although in these circumatances repeat surgery other than a sling procedure may offer good results. Slings using rectus abdominus fascia are easy to fashion and insert paraurethrally unless extensive previous urethral surgery has scarred and fixed the urethra severely. In such cases, a sling operation can prove difficult and bloody. It also may leave a weakened abdominal wall in an elderly female who has poor fascia, and rectus fascia may not be easily available if there has been previous lower abdominal surgery. In such cases, fascia lata may be used and works well. Synthetic materials have been advocated for use as slings but carry a considerable risk of infection and extrusion. Any sling that is placed too tightly below the urethra may result in urethral necrosis. In skillful hands, sling procedures can be a useful option in cases where other procedures have failed. We feel they have a limited place in the primary surgery of stress incontinence because they have higher complication rates than the other procedures described above.

Nonoperative Management of Urinary Stress Incontinence

Kegel exercises (repeated contracting of the pubococcygeal muscles) can produce some strengthening of the muscle and sometimes improve continence (48). The results in the elderly are not nearly as consistent or as marked as in younger women. Estrogen administration, either orally or vaginally, may improve urinary continence in the elderly woman, particularly if combined with Kegel exercises. However, symptomatic improvement with such techniques usually falls far short of that which can be accomplished surgically. Vaginal pessaries can be tried, but often give little help with urinary continence even though they may elevate the anterior vaginal wall.

Operations for Introital Stenosis

With aging and postmenopausal status, the introitus and vagina may become shrunken and stenotic to the point where coitus is difficult or impossible. Estrogens by any route can be used to help rejuvenate the vaginal mucosa so that it becomes thicker and more elastic. If this does not produce sufficient improvement, surgical enlargement of the introitus may be appropriate. This can be accomplished simply by making a midline episiotomy and repairing the incision from posterior to anterior to effect a widening of the introitus. Continued use of estrogens and regular intercouse (or use of dilators) is usually necessary to prevent recurrence of the stenosis.

Fistulas

Gynecologic fistulas in the elderly, not related to malignancy or surgery, most commonly occur between the intestinal tract and the vagina. They occur most often with diverticulitis, and hence most often involve the sigmoid or rectum. Inflammatory bowel disease also may produce intestinal-vaginal fistulas. Primary efforts are directed to the management of the intestinal disease. Some fistulas may close spontaneously, particularly with the use of total parenteral nutrition. Those that do not can usually be repaired transvaginally using a layered closure of absorbable sutures. If the underlying bowel disease is not well controlled, the risk of recurrence will be high. One must also be aware of the possibility of malignancy of the bowel (or genital organs) with fistula formation. Fistulas may also occur occasionally as a result of gynecologic surgical procedures.

The technique of repair will generally depend on the location of the fistula. For fistulas at the apex of the vagina, a partial colpocleisis of the Latzko (49) type is simple to perform and has a high rate of success. The repair is accomplished by denuding the anterior and posterior vaginal walls around the fistulous opening and sewing them together in layers, thus excluding the fistula from the vaginal lumen. The slight shortening of the vagina that results is usually of no consequence.

For fistulas located in the mid-vagina along the anterior or posterior vaginal wall, excision of the fistulous tract, wide mobilization of the surrounding tissues, and a layered closure generally serves well. For large fistulas, in the case of previous failed repair, or where the tissues have been irradiated, it may be necessary to mobilize a flap that can provide a new blood supply for the damaged area. This can be accomplished conveniently by developing a subcutaneous and muscular flap from the bulbocavernosus muscle in the labia majora, as described by Martius (50). This flap can be tunneled under the labia and placed in the bed of the fistula, with the vaginal wall closed over it. Bricker (51) has described an innovative abdominal approach to severe cases of post-irradiation rectovaginal fistula using the proximal colon as a pedical graft with re-establishment of intestinal continuity above the graft.

Fistulas located in the distal vagina are unusual in elderly women, since fistulas in this location most commonly occur as a result of obstetrical injury. When they do occur, they can be managed by complete perineotomy through the fistula, excision of the fistulas tract, and layered closure, with good results expected.

References

1. U.S. Census Bureau. 1983. *1980 Census of Population: General Population Characteristics*. Washington, DC: U.S. Government Printing Office.
2. Rowe, JW. 1985. Health care of the elderly. *N Engl J Med* 312:827.
3. Lifshitz, S, et al. 1982. Primary epidermoid carcinoma of the vulva. *Surg Gynecol Obstet* 155:59.
4. Krauer, F. 1983. Surgery in the postmenopausal woman. In *The Menopause*, Ed., HJ Buchsbaum. New York: Springer-Verlag.
5. Warshaw, GA. 1983. Hospital care for elderly patients. In *Advances in Research: Duke University Center for the Study of Aging and Human Development*, Ed., GL Maddox, 7:3.
6. Gerstenblith, G, Lakatta, EG, and Weisfeldt, ML. 1976. Age changes in myocardial function and exercise response. *Prog Cardiovasc Dis* 19:1.
7. Polacek, DJ, and Buchsbaum, HJ. 1986. Surgery in the aged. In *Strategies in Gynecologic Surgery*, Eds., HJ Buchsbaum and L Walton. New York: Springer-Verlag.
8. Chirico, A-M, and Rubin, A. 1967. Medical complications of pre- and postoperative care of the elderly woman. *Clin Obstet Gynecol* 10:481.
9. Schleuter, DP. 1985. Pulmonary evaluation. In *Operative Gynecology*, ed. 6. Eds., RF Mattingly and JD Thompson. Philadelphia: JB Lippincott.
10. Darmady, EM, Offer, J, and Woodhouse, MA. 1973. The parameters of the aging kidney. *J Pathol* 109:195.
11. Edelman, IS, Shulka, KK, Cohn, SH, et al. 1952. Further observation in total body water. I. Normal values through the life span. *Surg Gynecol Obstet* 95:1.
12. Pride, RB. 1966. Incidence and coincidence of hiatus hernia. *Gut* 7:188.
13. Bowers, PA, and Lindquist, JN. 1962. Preoperative and postoperative medical complications. *Clin Obstet Gynecol* 5:579.
14. Pierson, RL, Figge, PK, and Buchsbaum, HJ. 1975. Surgery for gynecologic malignancy in the aged. *Obstet Gynecol* 46:523.
15. Ellenbogen, A, Agranat, A, and Grunstein, S. 1981. The role of vaginal hysterectomy in the aged woman. *J Am Geriatr Soc* 29:426.
16. Tancer, ML, and Matseoane, SL. 1966. Gynecologic surgery in patients over 65. *Geriatrics* 21:189.
17. Hirsch, RA. 1982. An approach to assessing perioperative risk. In *Medical Care of the Surgical Patient*, Eds., DR Goldman, FH Brown, WK Levy, et al. Philadelphia: JB Lippincott.
18. Blake, R, and Lynn, J. 1976. Emergency abdominal surgery in the aged. *Br J Surg* 63:956.
19. Robbins, RE, and Budden, MK. 1972. Major abdominal surgery in patients over 70 years of age: Results during 1962 to 1966 compared with those during 1950 to 1959. *Can J Surg* 15:73.
20. Panayiotis, G, Ellenbogen, A, and Grunstein, S. 1978.

Major gynecologic surgical procedures in the aged. *J Am Geriatr Soc* 26:459.
21. McKeithen, WS. 1975. Major gynecologic surgery in the elderly female 65 years of age and older. *Am J Obstet Gynecol* 123:59.
22. Paldi, E, Peretz, A, and Pascal, B. 1966. Gynecologic surgery in geriatric patients. *Geriatrics* 21:131.
23. Marshall, WH, and Gahey, PJ. 1964. Operative complications and mortality in patients over 80 years of age. *Arch Surg* 88:896.
24. Young, HD, Tanga, MR, and Wellington, JL. 1971. Major abdominal surgery in the elderly: A review of 172 consecutive patients. *Can J Surg* 14:324.
25. Rubin, SC. 1987. Postmenopausal bleeding: Etiology, Evaluation and Management. *Med Clin N Am* 71:59.
26. Meyer, WC, Malkasian, GD, et al. 1971. Postmenopausal bleeding from atrophic endometrium. *Obstet Gynecol* 38:731.
27. Hawwa, ZM, Nahhas, WA, and Copenhaver, EH. 1970. Postmenopausal bleeding. *Lahey Clin Foun Bull* 19:61.
28. Wynder, EL, Escher, GC, and Mantel, N. 1966. An epidemiological investigation of cancer of the endometrium. *Cancer* 19:489.
29. MacMahon, B. 1974. Risk factors for endometrial cancer. *Gynecol Oncol* 2:122.
30. Boronow, RC, Morrow, CP, Creasman, WT, et al. 1984. Surgical staging in endometrial cancer: clinical-pathologic findings of a prospective study. *Obstet Gynecol* 63:825.
31. Reid, R. 1984. Understanding human papilloma viral infections. *The Colposcopist* 16:3.
32. Wajsbort, J. 1972. Postmenopausal bleeding after L-dopa. *N Engl J Med* 286:784.
33. Paloucek, FP, Graham, JB, and Randall, CL. 1967. Benign postmenopausal vaginal bleeding. *JAMA* 199:111.
34. Rubin, SC, Hoskins, WJ, and Lewis, JL, Jr.: Radical hysterectomy for recurrent cervical cancer following radiation therapy. *Gynecol Oncol* 27:316.
35. Hoskins, WJ, et al. 1976. Radical hysterectomy and pelvic lymphadenectomy for the management of early invasive cancer of the cervix. *Gynecol Oncol* 4:278.
36. Plentyl, AE, and Friedman, EA. 1971. Lymphatic system of the female genitalia. Philadelphia: WB Saunders.
37. Hacker, NF, et al. 1981. Radical vulvectomy and bilateral inguinal lymphadenectomy through separate groin incisions. *Obstet Gynecol* 58:574.
38. DiSaia, PJ, Creasman, WT, and Rich, WM. 1979. An alternative approach to early cancer of the vulva. *Am J Obstet Gynecol* 88:509.
39. Hacker, NF, et al. 1984. Individualization of treatment for Stage I squamous cell vulvar carcinoma. *Obstet Gynecol* 63:155.
40. Moschcowitz, AV. 1912. The pathogenesis, anatomy and cure of prolapse of the rectum. *Surg Gynecol Obstet* 15:7.
41. Randall, CL, and Nichols, DH. 1971. Surgical treatment of vaginal inversion. *Obstet Gynecol* 38:327.
42. Birnbaum, SJ. 1973. Rational therapy for the prolapsed vagina. *Am J Obstet Gynecol* 115:411.
43. Green, TH, Jr. 1977. *Gynecology,* ed 3. Boston: Little Brown & Co.
44. Mattingly, RF, and Thompson, JD. 1985. *Operative Gynecology,* ed. 6. Philadelphia: JB Lippincott.
45. Marshall, VF, Marchetti, AD, and Krantz, KE. 1949. Vesicourethral suspension. *Surg Obstet Gynecol* 88:509.
46. Burch, JC. 1968. Cooper's ligament urethrovesical suspension for stress urinary incontinence. *Am J Obstet Gynecol* 100:764.
47. Pereyra, AJ, et al. 1982. Pubourethral supports in perspective: Modified Pereyra procedure for urinary incontinence. *Obstet Gynecol* 59:643.
48. Kegel, AH. 1948. Progressive resistance exercise in the functional restoration of the perineal muscles. *Am J Obstet Gynecol* 56:238.
49. Latzko, W. 1942. Postoperative vesicovaginal fistulas. *Am J Surg* 58:211.
50. Martius, H. 1932. Vesicovaginal therapy especially by plastic transplantation of flaps. *Z Geburtsh Gynak* 103:22.
51. Bricker, EM, and Johnston, WD. 1979. Repair of post irradiation rectovaginal fistula and stricture. *Surg Gynecol Obstet* 148:499.

38

Otolaryngologic Surgery in the Elderly

Charles F. Koopmann, Jr.

The elderly patient presents unique problems to the otolaryngologist—head and neck surgeon. In dealing with disorders of the head and neck in this group of patients, special attention must be paid to specific factors involving wound healing, hearing, vestibular disorders, laryngeal changes, and the oral cavity, as well as head and neck oncologic differences.

Wound Healing

Wound healing is affected by several factors, which include the type of tissue under study, tissue specificity, mechanical factors, sexual differences, neurogenic factors, and nutrition. Aging affects the growth rate and multiplication of fibroblasts and the amount of soluble versus insoluble collagen, as well as the synthesis of this material. It is markedly affected by nutrition and endocrinologic changes. Both insoluble and soluble collagen, as well as elastin, are affected as an individual becomes older. Insoluble collagen will increase as age increases, while the soluble collagen content decreases with age. The quantity of elastic fibers decreases both in blood vessels and skin, but the absolute quantity of elastin will increase with age. Thus, as age increases the density or amount of collagen in most tissues will increase, while the lower fluid binding capacity causes the older connective tissue to shrink.

Doberauber (1), as well as Howes and Harvey (2), have found that younger animals form granulation tissue faster then older ones, with the metabolic reactions occurring earlier and in a more noticeable fashion in reparative tissue in young animals. However, the total amount of deposited collagen in connective tissue is larger in older animals than in younger ones after injury. Thus, the younger the animal, the more rapidly the wound will heal, with more organization of the collagenous structures in the scar. This rate of wound healing in relationship to age appears to be related to the functional ability of the individual cells. Schmitt and Beneke (3) found that in wound healing fibroblasts, collagen synthesis, and polysaccharides decrease as age increases.

Nutrition is extremely important in wound healing. The role of vitamins is essential to adequate wound repair. Vitamin A deficiency will result in a slowing of epithelialization and a decreased rate of collagen synthesis. Vitamin E (which is a free radical scavenger) will reduce or inhibit inflammation due to the inhibition of lipid peroxidase activity with resultant stabilization of lysosomes. Deficiencies of pyridoxine and thiamine may adversely affect collagen organization and thus the tensile strength of the wound. Vitamin C (ascorbic acid) is essential as a co-factor in collagen synthesis and affects fibroblast division. Zinc is necessary for the formation of RNA and DNA polymerases and cellular proliferation. Zinc will inhibit collagen-induced platelet aggregation, as well as mast cell degranulation. A deficiency of dietary zinc will reduce the immigration of macrophages and polymorphonuclear leukocytes into the tissue spaces, as well as reduce the collagen organization and the tensile strength of wound collagen.

Anti-inflammatory, nonsteroidal drugs, such as indomethacin, will stimulate wound healing and increase contractile strength, while colchicine will reduce the tensile strength of connective tissue but will stimulate collagen and noncollagen protein synthesis (4). Low serum albumin due to either liver disease, increased protein metabolism, or chronic disease states may contribute to poor wound healing in its own right but also because it is a major carrier of zinc. Thus, in the elderly patient who has poor dietary intake, both low serum albumin and zinc deficiency will adversely affect wound healing.

Finally, multiple endocrine factors will play a role in wound healing. In this age group, the main difficulty is diabetes mellitus. Diabetics will exhibit decreased tensile strength, will form less new collagen, and during periods of hyperglycemia, will have impairment of wound repair due to problems with phagocytosis. The ingrowth of new fibroblasts and blood vessels is also reduced in diabetics (Table 38-1) (5).

Otologic and Vestibular Manifestations of Aging

The aging process affects not only the cochlea and its auditory function, but also the external ear, the external auditory canal, the middle ear space, and the vestibular system. The skin of the external ear is exposed to ultraviolet rays from the sun, as well as to temperature extremes and to external trauma. Thus, the elderly patient may exhibit changes such as actinic keratosis, seborrheic keratosis, keratoacanthoma, and basosquamous cell carcinoma. The external auditory canal has two types of hair: minute vellus hair and tragi (larger hair seen laterally). The tragi become more prominent after the 3rd or 4th decade of life. The sebaceous glands found in the external auditory canal are affected by endocrine secretion. In both sexes, androgenic secretions are responsible for sebaceous gland activities. After the age of 50, there is marked reduction in the activity of these glands in females (after menopause), while in males there is only minimal reduction in most cases. The apocrine glands (cerumen) decrease in number in elderly patients. This leads to drier skin in the external canal, with a greater tendency for cerumen impactions and also dry scaling skin, which is subject to superficial infections. Pruritus of the external canal is not uncommon in the elderly and is best treated with topical preparations, which reduce the inflammation and itching. As these symptoms progress, there may be a superimposed otitis externa caused by *Pseudomonas aeruginosa*. In the early stages, this is well treated with topical antibiotic ear drops. However, in a small group of patients who are elderly and diabetic, this may progress to malignant or necrotizing otitis externa with secondary osteitis and osteomyelitis of the temporal bone. This is a potentially fatal disease that must be treated with parenteral antibiotics, as well as a debridement of the involved skin and bone. With the recognition of the severity of this disorder and with aggressive early management, the mortality has greatly decreased.

Table 38-1. Effects of hormones on wound healing

Stimulatory effect	Inhibition
STH	Corticoids
TSH	ACTH
Insulin	Thyroxin
Calcitonin	Diabetes
Estrogen	Hypophysectomy
Testosterone	Gestagens

STH, somatotrophic hormone; TSH, thyroid-stimulating hormone; ACTH, adrenocorticotrophic hormone.

From Chvapil M. and Koopmann C. 1982. Geriatric otolaryngology. *Otolaryngol Clin North Am* 15(2):264.

Finally, tumors of the external auditory canal will include squamous cell carcinoma, ceruminomas, and basal cell carcinomas. These patients frequently present with itching, bloody discharge from the ear, otalgia, vertigo, hearing loss, and occasionally facial paralysis. Most commonly, the optimal method of therapy for these tumors is aggressive surgical resection with postoperative radiation therapy. If the medical status of the patient does not allow surgical resection, then radiation therapy alone may assist in reduction of the tumor.

The middle ear is also affected by the normal aging process. The incudomalleolar and incudostapedial joints are synovial diarthrodial joints. Thus, connective tissue changes of the elderly affect the joints with fibrillation and vacuolation occurring, followed by hyalinization of the joint capsule with opacification of the articular cartilage and narrowing in the joint space. In the most severe cases, there may even become opacification of the joint capsule with fusions of part or all of the joint space. In their study, Etholm and Belal found that all temporal bones in patients who are 70 years of age showed moderate to severe arthritic changes with no sexual predilection. These changes will rarely affect sound transmission through the ear (6).

The most recognized changes occurring in the otologic system are those related to the cochlea (inner ear). The elderly patient most frequently demonstrates presbycusis, which may be defined as a progressive decline in hearing sensitivity due to the aging process. The majority of people in all parts of the world over 40 years of age show a varying degree of progressive sensorineural hearing loss most commonly seen at frequencies above 2,000 Hz. Multiple variables may account for this, including environmental noise, arteriosclerosis, smoking, emotional stress, genetic factors, cholesterol levels, and diet. Royster and Thomas found that black males had significantly better auditory thresholds then Caucasian males, especially in those 60 years or older (7). Rosen et al. found that a Sudanese tribe living in a silent environment, exercising daily, and eating a diet low in serum cholesterol had much better hearing then paired subjects from the United States (8).

In 1964, Schuknecht described four types of presbycusis (9). The first of these can be termed sensory presbycusis and involves atrophy of the Organ of Corti, more commonly known as the basilar turn. This is usually very slowly progressive, although it most commonly spares the speech frequencies. Metabolic presbycusis refers to potential defects in the biochemical or biophysical processes in the cochlea and is linked to atrophy of the stria vascularis. The audiometric pattern in this type of hearing loss is one of a relatively flat nature. This is usually a slow progressive hearing loss with excellent speech discrimination until the pure tone average becomes less than 45 to 50 decibels. There is little or no degeneration of cochlear neurons associated with this hearing loss in its early stages. The third type of hearing loss is neural presbycusis or neural atrophy. Here one finds loss of ganglion cells in the spiral ganglia, as well as degeneration of the neurons in the higher auditory pathways. The audiogram has a downward slope with a highly variable nature. This type of hearing loss will also be associated with phonemic regression, which refers to the fact that the patient may have a much poorer speech discrimination than one would expect from a pure tone audiogram. In this type of hearing loss, the Organ of Corti remains relatively unaffected while there is a loss of functioning neurons contributing to integration of speech understanding. Finally, the fourth type of hearing loss described is called mechanical presbycusis, which may be related to atrophy, thinning, or rupture of the basilar membranes. The audiogram in these patients shows a progressive hearing loss in the high frequencies with no abrupt drop (Fig. 38-1).

Hearing loss in the elderly patient is highly significant in the United States. Almost 50% of patients over 75 years of age experience hearing difficulties. This has a significant social as well as economic impact upon our society. It is also of importance in the management of these patients surgically since lack of cooperation in the postoperative period may be secondary mainly to poor hearing. Thus, it is essential that patients who need hearing assistance (such as hearing aids) be amplified as soon as possible after surgery. Elderly patients also display worse speech discrimination than younger patients with similar hearing problems. It has not yet been determined whether this is merely due to peripheral end organ disease or whether there is some related central auditory pathway deficiency in these elderly persons.

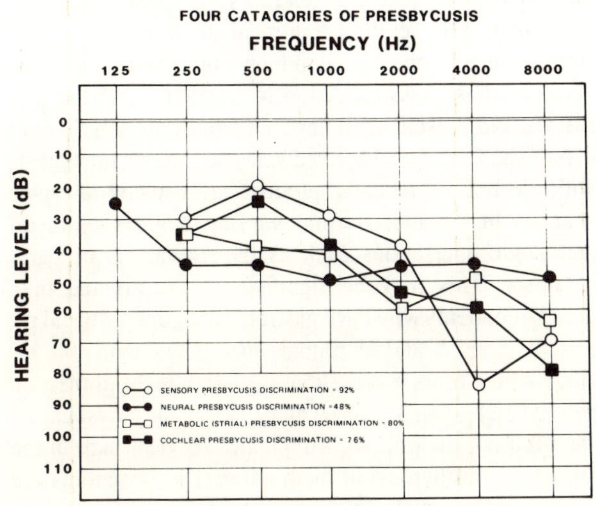

Figure 38-1. Four categories of presbycusis.

In the elderly patient with a significant hearing loss, it is important that some special consideration be made during communication. The speaker should attempt to get the person's attention before speaking, make his face visible and avoid covering his mouth while speaking. Reduction in background noise is helpful, as well as speaking slowly and distinctly. If a patient fails to understand an item the physician should attempt to paraphrase it rather than repeating it verbatim. Finally, multiple amplification or assistive devices are available including not only the standard hearing aid models, but also FM receivers or infrared receivers in some public facilities. These latter hearing assistive devices are extremely helpful for the elderly and are more common in our enlightened society (10).

The vestibular system may also be affected by the aging process. To understand the significance of reduction of the vestibular system sensitivity, one must realize that equilibrium is dependent upon the integration of input from the visual, vestibular, and proprioceptive systems. Most individuals can tolerate a reduction or loss in one of these systems, but when two or more are not functioning properly, the patient will have significant balance problems. The elderly are all affected by decreasing visual acuity due to degenerative changes such as cataracts. Thus, when visual input is reduced in addition to the vestibular or proprioceptive input (peripheral neural changes), severe disability may occur. The aging labyrinth has been shown to have a reduction in air cell count to as much as 40% in the cristae and 20% in the maculae (11). Bergstrom has estimated that there is a reduction in the primary afferent fibers after the age of 40, with the thick myelinated fibers at the cristae suffering the greatest loss (12). Schuknecht has suggested that there are four types of dysequilibrium related to aging (13). These include ampullary dysequilibrium, macular dysequilibrium, vestibular ataxia of aging, and cupulolithiasis. The latter, cupulolithiasis (also known as postural vertigo and benign paroxysmal postural vertigo), is described as dysequilibrium or vertigo caused by changing head position. He feels that this abnormality is caused by deposits of material along the pars superior in the ampulla of the posterior semicircular canal. This can occur not only from the inner ear vascular insufficiency, but also may occur after trauma or spontaneously. Finally, Krmpotic-Nemanic has described a reduction in the number of openings through which nerve fibers to the VIII nerve could pass in the internal auditory canal (14). He believes this causes vestibular problems as well as auditory problems due to vascular or neural insufficiency.

Unless vascular insufficiency is generalized, the treatment of age-induced vestibular postural vertigo is directed at avoiding the offending positions. The usual vestibular suppressants, such as diazepam, are rarely used in the elderly due to their slower metabolism of these drugs.

Rhinological Changes in Aging

The geriatric patient will show several problems relative to the nose and nasal cavity. Loss of internal moisture predisposes the patient to atrophic rhinitis. Hormonal changes, especially in females, will also cause loss of internal moisture, as well as a reduction in size of the inferior turbinates. The general changes in connective tissues—loss of hydration, atrophy of collagen, and a reduction in elastic fibers, as well as absorption of fatty tissue and increased fragility of blood vessels combined with arteriosclerosis—make the intranasal tissues highly subject to trauma; this can result in bleeding. The treatment of epistaxis follows the general principle of any other age group. Prior to initiating therapy, one must attempt to identify the bleeding site. Anterior epistaxis should be treated with cautery, either chemical (silver nitrate) or thermal. Light packing with 1/2 inch gauze or a hemostatic agent, such as oxydized cellulose (Oxycel), plus digital compression is also effective. If the bleeding is coming from the posterior nose and is severe, it must be treated with both anterior and posterior nasal packing. Posterior nasal packing predicates hospitalization since these patients are quite prone to hypoxia and arterial oxygen desaturation. Arterial ligation of either the ethmoidal arteries or the internal maxillary artery on the ipsilateral side is warranted if the bleeding persists. Occasionally, epistaxis may be treated with arterial embolization.

The nasal tip may be affected both cosmetically and functionally by changes associated with the aging process. The upper lateral cartilage will soften along its inferior or caudal margin in a fashion similar to the cephalic or superior portion of the lower lateral cartilage. Eventually separation occurs and the columella becomes retracted as the nasal tip becomes ptotic. This causes a reduction in nasal air flow and airway obstruction may occur. This problem can be treated nicely with nasal septoplasty with preservation of the cartilagenous septum in conjunction with the cartilagenous rinoplasty, where between 2 to 4 mm of the cephalic end of the lower lateral cartilage is resected as is the strip of the anterior or caudal portion of the nasal septum. This autogenous cartilage can be placed anterior to the nasal spine, and the skin over the nasal dorsum may be repositioned after undermining to allow elevation of the tip. This changes air flow patterns in the region of the nasal valve and is quite effective in improving the airway (15).

The elderly are as affected by similar inflammatory, allergic, and neoplastic disorders, in the nasal cavity and paranasal sinuses, as other age groups. The methods of treatment need not be altered due to age unless there is some concomitant overriding medical problem.

Laryngeal and Voice Changes in the Elderly

In general, the older patient does not have a specific phonatory disorder, although certain physiologic changes are related. Basically, speech is dependent upon the interplay between respiratory, oral, neuromuscular, and laryngeal factors. The elderly patient will commonly display a reduction in respiratory capacity due to a combination of atrophy of the respiratory muscles, a reduction in excursion of the rib cage, a loss of pulmonary compliance, and a reduction in vital capacity. These factors lead to a diminution of intra-oral pressure and reduction in volume.

The larynx also has specific changes associated with aging. The cricoarytenoid joint will show varied changes ranging from degrees of ossification, yielding fixation with reduction of vocal cord mobility, to relaxation with loss of arytenoid approximation and breathiness in the voice. In a rare instance, a patient may indeed have unilateral or bilateral vocal cord paralysis secondary to arthritic changes. This may lead to severe respiratory distress that will require treatment with either topical steroids or a tracheotomy and arytenoidopexy. The true vocal cords show a reduction in elasticity, and the thyroarytenoid muscles will have a decrease in muscle fiber mass. The false vocal cords display squamous metaplasia with decreased mucous production, causing atrophic changes in the mucosa and varying degrees of histopathologic aberrations such as hyperkeratosis or parakeratosis. This may be significantly exacerbated in a group of patients who have gastroesophagopharyngeal reflux. The signs and symptoms associated with this include hoarseness, a sensation of pharyngeal tightness, a paroxysmal cough, pharyngeal clearing, dysphagia, "heartburn", otalgia, and frequently cervical pain in the region of the thyrohyoid membrane. The symptoms are usually worse in the morning and are associated with physical findings of arytenoid erythema, granulomas, and point tenderness over the superior laryngeal nerve. Diagnosis is made by history, physical examination, and radiographic studies. The treatment is usually medical in nature, with elevation of the head while in bed, antacid therapy after meals and before bedtime, and resting the voice (16).

After the 6th or 7th decade, there appears to be a significant increase in hoarseness or dysphonia depending upon the sex of the patient. In the male patient, one finds an increase in the fundamental frequency of the voice with vocal fold atrophy (17). In female patients, there is vocal fold edema, hoarseness, and a lower fundamental frequency (18).

Senile bowing of the vocal cords is secondary to a loss of connective tissue and muscle atrophy with resultant poor approximation of the vocal cords. In severe cases, it may be necessary to consider phonatory surgery (still in the early stages of development). Chronic bronchitis and chronic cough will lead to edema of the vocal folds and vocal cords with resultant difficulty in speech. Dryness of the laryngeal mucosa (laryngitis sicca) is secondary to atrophy of the mucosal glands and may be made worse by smoking or alcohol. Hypothyroidism may manifest itself by ataxic dysarthria or dysphonia with low-pitched voice hoarseness. Finally, vocal tremor may occur due to hoarse qualities combined with the higher pitch and reduced strength of amplification with loss of glottic pressure. This must be differentiated from the pathologic changes associated with Parkisonism or from spastic dysphonia. The latter patients have excessive true vocal cord approximation without vocal tremor and can be treated with sectioning of an involved recurrent laryngeal nerve. Older patients with this dysarthria may indeed have improvement with either medical therapy or with active speech intervention. The administration of L-dopa for Parkinson's disease greatly reduces the dysarthria. In patients who have a loss of velopharyngeal function with hypernasal speech, one may find that palatal lift prosthesis or pharyngeal flap may be of assistance. Speech therapy will help the patient who requires a change in the pitch of voice, a change in articulation, or an improvement in laryngeal habits.

Disorders of the Oral Cavity

One of the most common complaints of the elderly patient relates to physiologic or pathophysiologic alterations in the mouth or oral cavity related to total changes, loss of taste, pain in the mouth or tongue, or dental difficulties. As is well known, the elderly patient will have an increased incidence of loss of dentition, with between 50% to 75% of the patients over 70 years of age being completely edentulous. This state is secondary to dental caries, periodontal disease, bruxism, and diminished salivary flow. There is a progressive loss of both maxillary and mandibular alveolar bone, which has been termed "senile atrophy" and may be associated with osteoporosis or physiologic skeletal bone changes. A dry mouth (xerostomia) is seen because of salivary gland fibrosis or atrophy. This contributes to dental caries, alteration in the taste of food, and a complaint of burning or oral discomfort. The xerostomia may be treated by increased fluid intake, stimulation of remaining salivary flow with sialagogues, or the use of artificial saliva.

As is seen in other parts of the body, the oral mucosa will undergo physiologic changes both in the epithelium and underlying connective tissue. The epithelium itself will become thinner with the prickle cell layer being specifically involved. In regions of denture use, parakeratosis and hyperkeratosis may be seen. Due to a thinning of the epithelium and a reduction of the vascular supply, the mucosal tissue becomes more susceptible to injury and has a greater degree of difficulty in repair.

Angular cheilitis may appear at the oral commissures either unilaterally or bilaterally. Its manifestations include erythema and cracking of the skin with occasional maceration (Fig. 38-2). The predisposing factors of this condition include redundant facial skin folds due to loss of connective tissue support, poor fitting dentures, pooling of saliva, loss of vertical height of the face, monilial infection, and possible systemic disorders, such as pernicious anemia or vitamin B complex deficiency. Treatment is directed at the underlying systemic deficiency, cleansing of the area, fitting of appropriate dentures, and the topical application of Nystatin cream or ointment.

Occasionally, angular cheilitis is associated with glossodynia (a burning sensation in the oral cavity or tongue). Most commonly, glossodynia has no definite etiologic source although it may be a manifestation of anemia (vitamin B_{12}, iron deficiency, or folic acid), peripheral diabetes mellitus, or xerostomia secondary to salivary flow deficiency. Local problems may include benign chronic migrating superficial glossitis, lichen planus, oral carcinoma, or denture irritation. If glossodynia is associated with dysgeusia (the altered sensation of taste) one may have a postviral neuropathy. Unless a specific cause can be found, the only therapy is reassurance of the patient that no major systemic problem exists. Occasionally, relief may be obtained using various types of mouthwashes.

Changes in the salivary gland function will lead to "dry mouth" syndrome, a very common complaint in the elderly. As one ages, the secretory rates of the salivary glands decrease and the viscosity of the saliva increases.

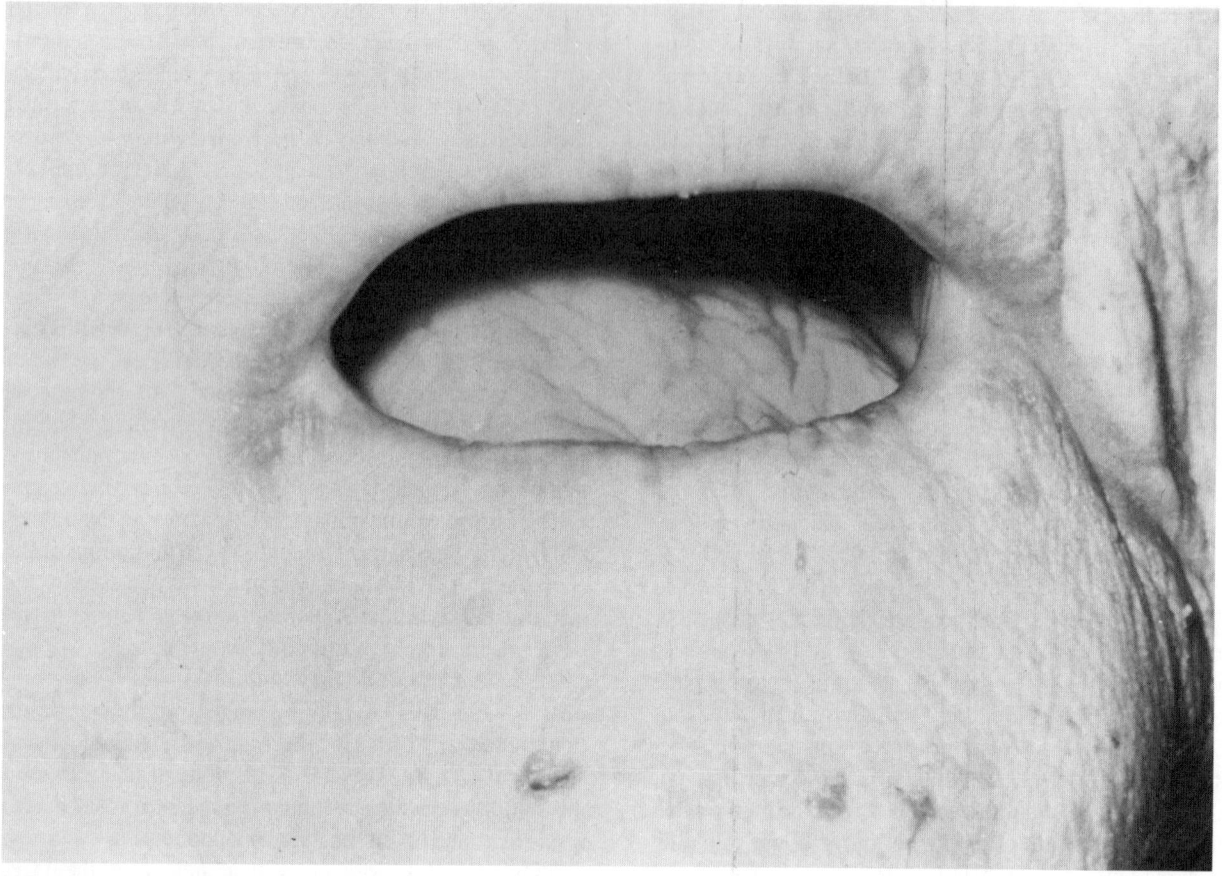

Figure 38-2. Angular cheilitis with erythema and cracking of the skin at the oral commissure. (Reprinted with permission from Koopmann, CF Jr. 1982. Geriatric otolaryngology. In *Otolaryngologic Clinics in North America,* Ed. CF Koopmann, Jr. Philadelphia: W.B. Saunders.)

This contributes to xerostomia, chronic sialadenitis, and a reduction in taste sensation. One can specifically find an increase in focal chronic and inflammatory changes in the submandibular gland in the geriatric population. Sjogren's syndrome (xerostomia, dry eyes, polyarthritis, salivary gland swelling) is also more prevalent in the aged. The loss of taste sensation is not only exacerbated by the decrease in salivation, but also by the reduction of taste buds in the tongue. Many patients complain of a salty or metallic taste. Hermal et al. found a decreased level of sensation to bitter, sour, and sweet taste in the elderly patient. He and his co-workers felt that removal of dentures improved taste reception (19).

Nicotinic stomatitis may occur in up to 10% of the elderly population, with a male predominance. The usual site of predilection is the palatal mucosa. In the early stages, there is erythema with papule formation, while more mature lesions are rough, white, and raised. Physiologic evaluation reveals acanthosis and metaplasia (Fig. 38-3). The lesions will usually resolve with cessation of the use of tobacco. If no improvement occurs, it may be necessary to biopsy the area to rule out underlying carcinoma.

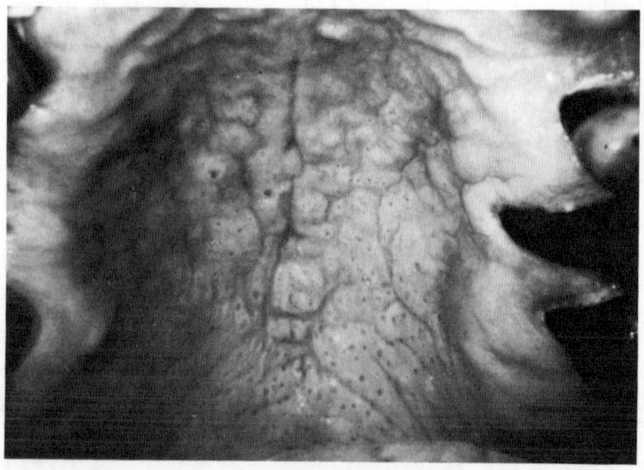

Figure 38-3. Nicotinic stomatitis of the hard palate. (Reprinted with permission from Koopmann, CF Jr. 1982. Geriatric otolaryngology. In *Otolaryngologic Clinics of North America,* Ed. CF Koopmann, Jr. Philadelphia: W.B. Saunders.)

Lichen planus is a chronic disease of the oral mucosa, which can be confused with carcinoma, especially in the older patient who has a cancer phobia. The etiologic basis of this disorder is uncertain, but it may be related to emotional stress, physical stress, or intake of certain drugs. Two forms of lichen planus exist, non-erosive and erosive (or bullous). Nonerosive lichen planus (Fig. 38-4) is usually asymptomatic. The majority of these lesions occur on the buccal mucosa (80%), although the tongue, lips, and palate may also be affected. The lesions are white or gray in color and are lacy or reticular in nature. Most commonly, the patients are symptom free, although some may complain of burning. Most are concerned about carcinoma. Erosive lichen planus is painful, and in the early stages, the lesions may be mistaken for herpetic disorders. These lesions are found to be associated with vesicles (with clear fluid present) and bullae. The bullous form of lichen planus must be differentiated from erythema multiforme, benign pemphigoid, syphilis, and nutritional deficiency states. The therapy is basically that of reassurance and relief of pain. The pain may be relieved by the application of 0.5% Dyclone or 2% Tetracycline mouthwash combined with steroid paste. If the medication is the inciting source, it should be discontinued or changed if possible.

Hyperkeratotic lesions are also a concern in this age group because of the fear of carcinoma. These lesions may include leukoplakia, frictional hyperkeratosis, verruciform hyperkeratosis, or frank carcinoma in situ or invasive squamous cell carcinoma. Frictional keratosis (Fig. 38-5) is secondary to irritation of the buccal mucosa or lip from chronic irritation from either dentures or trauma of the teeth. It can be compared to callous formation. Treatment is directed at removal of the inciting problem. If this does not succeed, then an incisional biopsy is warranted to rule out carcinoma. Verruciform keratosis is usually seen along the mandibular alveolus or buccal

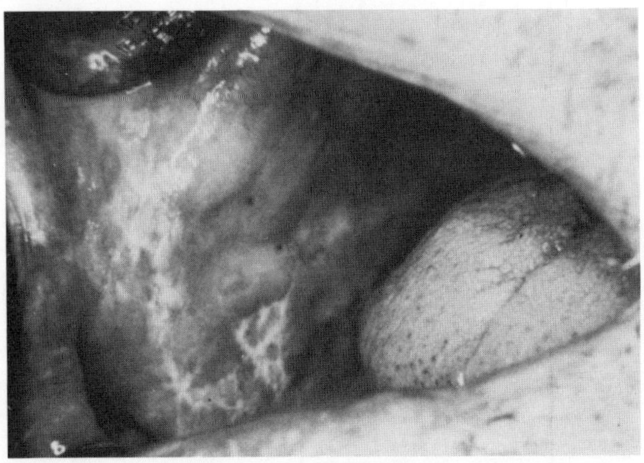

Figure 38-4. Nonerosive lichen planus of the buccal mucosa.

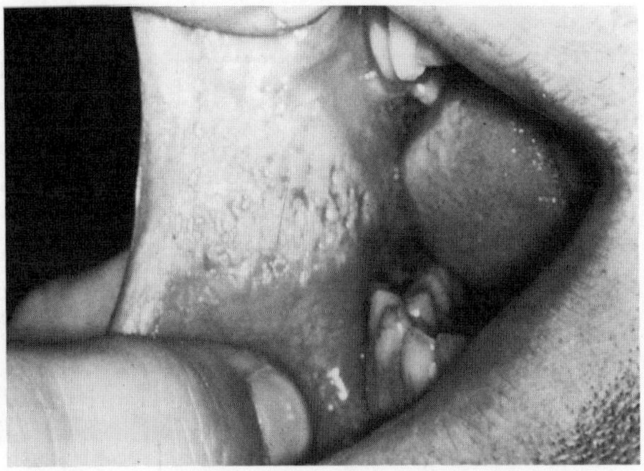

Figure 38-5. Frictional keratosis of the buccal mucosa.

mucosa (Fig. 38-6). It is entirely benign but may require surgical excision if symptoms are intolerable. The use of the carbon dioxide laser has been helpful in this disorder.

Actinic cheilitis (or keratosis) may be found around the vermillion border of the lower lip in patients who have a history of prolonged sun exposure. The lesions may be white and diffuse or may be midly ulcerated (Fig. 38-7). In areas that show any ulceration, it is essential to biopsy the tissue to rule out early invasive squamous cell carcinoma. If the lesion is entirely actinic keratosis then a "lip shave" should be performed. The remaining mucosa is then advanced to the vermillion cutaneous border. After surgery, the patient should be counseled concerning the use of sun screen preparation to give protection from ultraviolet rays.

Erythroplasia may be of three forms: homogeneous, interspersed with leukoplakia, or multifocal. These lesions are usually red and appear to be inflamed. They must be regarded with the highest index of suspicion for carcinoma since 90% are associated with either severe

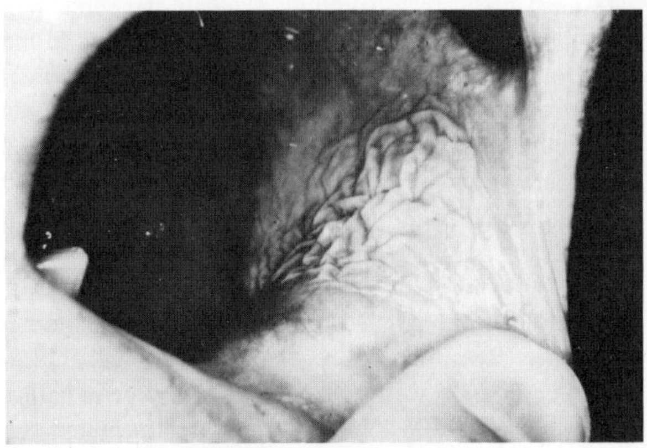

Figure 38-6. Verruciform keratosis of the buccal mucosa. (Reprinted with permission from Koopmann, CF Jr. 1982. Geriatric otolyngology. In *Otolaryngologic Clinics of North America,* Ed. CF Koopmann, Jr. Philadelphia: W. B. Saunders.)

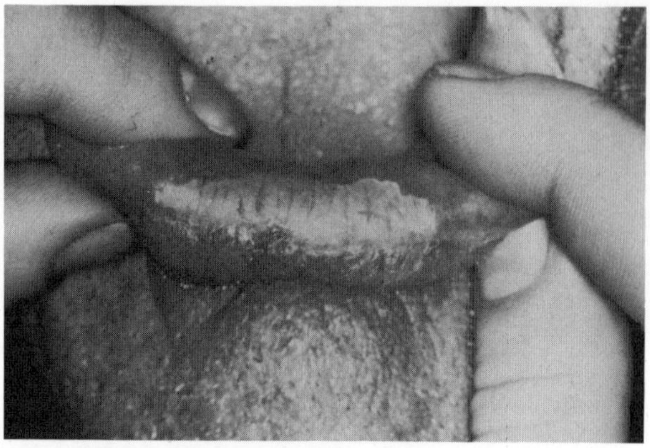

Figure 38-7. Actinic cheilitis of the lower lip. (Reprinted with permission from Koopmann, CF Jr. 1982. Geriatric otolaryngology. In *Otolaryngologic Clinics of North America,* Ed. CF Koopmann, Jr. Philadelphia: W.B. Saunders.)

dysplasia or carcinoma. If localized, an attempt should be made to excise them. In contrast, leukoplakia (white and flat lesions) is really not a specific clinical entity, but is used to describe a whitish area, which cannot be wiped off and has no specific classification, although the biopsies usually reveal either acanthosis, parakeratosis, or hyperkeratosis. This is most commoly seen in the buccal mucosa, gingiva, or floor of the mouth and may be near regions of invasive squamous cell carcinoma. The majority of these white lesions (90%) are benign, but a surgical biopsy is occasionally warranted (20).

Carcinoma of the vermillion of the lip and tongue makes up 22% to 30% of all cancers of the oral cavity, with the majority (95%) occurring on the lower lip. Squamous cell carcinoma will predominate in the lower lip and may be one of three types: ulcerative, exophytic, or verrucous. The exophytic type is the most common (Fig. 38-8). This is best treated with wide local excision. Care must be taken to carefully evaluate the submental and submandibular areas for potential metastasis. In the upper lip, basal cell carcinoma is more common (70%). Again, treatment is aimed at surgical excision. Metastasis is infrequent (5% to 10%) in carcinoma of the lip, and the 5-year survival may reach 80% for all patients.

Carcinoma of the tongue (Fig. 38-9) is a common form of carcinoma. It may occur in either the anterior (mobile) two-thirds of the tongue or the posterior one-third (base) of the tongue. The anterior location offers a much better prognosis. Early lesions (T_1 and small T_2) can be treated equally well with either surgery or radiation therapy. Surgical excision offers rapid treatment and can usually be performed with minimum mortality and morbidity. Especially well tolerated is surgical excision of lesions along the mobile anterolateral tongue. More advanced lesions such as T_2 and T_3 size masses are likely to

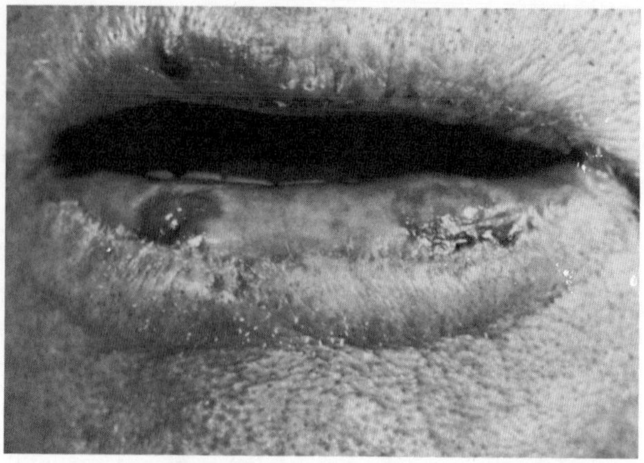

Figure 38-8. Squamous cell carcinoma of the lower lip.

have regional or distant metastasis. Thus, combined surgical and radiation therapy is recommended for these lesions. Also, chemotherapy may be useful in the T_3 lesions with large regional metastasis.

Carcinoma of the floor of the mouth (Fig. 38-10) may have deep extension or regional metastasis prior to the initial diagnosis. Superficial lesions can be treated with surgical excision and either primary skin grafting or with a regional myocutaneous flap. Larger lesions may require a partial mandibulectomy combined with radiation therapy and possibly adjuvant chemotherapy. For functional purposes, either myocutaneous flaps or free flaps with autogenous bone may be utilized.

Cutaneous Problems of Head and Neck in the Elderly

This section discusses a portion of the dermatologic problems encountered in the head and neck region in elderly patients. Some of these lesions are specifically age re-

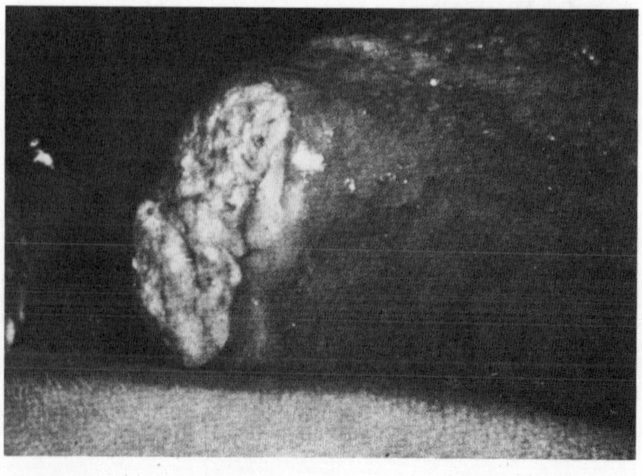

Figure 38-9. Squamous cell carcinoma of the mobile tongue.

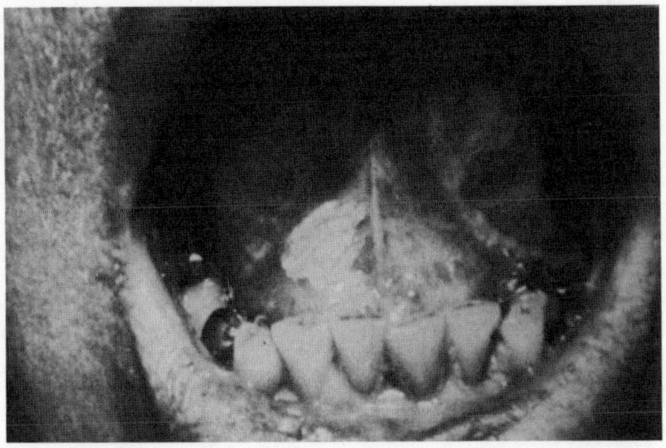

Figure 38-10. Squamous cell carcinoma of the floor of mouth.

lated, while others may be found at any age, although the incidence increases as the age increases.

Chronic exposure to ultraviolet light from the sun will most commonly cause damage to the cells of the epidermis (especially those cells involved with the production of keratin and melanin). The longer the duration of exposure, the more skin changes one sees. In the deeper layers (the dermis), changes can include wrinkling of the skin along with very thin skin, capillary fragility with easy bruisability, and telangiectasia. These changes can be reduced by protection of the skin by sun screens.

Seborrheic dermatitis has an increased incidence in elderly patients, especially those with any chronic debilitating state. These lesions (Fig. 38-11) are characterized by red, scaling lesions along the scalp margin, postauricular area, eyebrows, glabella, or nasolabial folds. These lesions must be differentiated from disorders such as psoriasis. The treatment for these lesions is one of a medical nature, whereby the patient is prescribed a medicated shampoo such as Selsun or advised to buy over-the-counter products such Neutrogena T-gel or Sebulex. If inflammation occurs, use of a topical fluorinated steroid cream or lotion, such as Valisone, is helpful.

Seborrheic keratosis is distinguished by sharp margination and flatness of lesions. These lesions may be dark brown or tan and can occur anywhere in the head and neck (Fig. 38-12). The differential diagnosis includes actinic keratosis or warts. Most lesions require no treatment, but if they are disturbing thc patient cosmetically one may either remove the lesions with cryosurgery, a shave excision, chemical peeling with phenol solution, or very rarely, by surgical excision.

Chondrodermatitis nodularis occurs on the helix of the ear and is commonly along the rim or the antihelix. These lesions are papular in nature and may have associated erythema, pain, and inflammatory changes. The differential diagnosis includes basal cell and squamous cell carcinoma. However, the pain associated with chondrodermatitis nodularis usually indicates the nature of the lesion. These lesions may be treated with steroid injection or occasionally steroid creams. If there is a concern about malignancy, an incisional biopsy may be warranted. When the lesion is along the helical rim, excision and primary closure can be carried out if the lesion does not respond to medical management.

Lentigo maligna can occur anywhere in the head and neck but is most commonly seen over the anterior face, such as the nasolabial crease region (Fig. 38-13). These lesions have distinct black pigmentation surrounded by brown to tan pigmentation. Lentigo maligna lesions can be considered a melanoma in situ and thus should be removed surgically. Most commonly, the lesion can be excised entirely with regional advancement flaps being utilized. Thus, complete surgical excision is recommended rather then cryotherapy. Malignant melanoma (Fig. 38-14) can again occur anywhere in the head and neck region. Lentigo maligna may indeed transform into lentigo maligna melanoma as in this example or melanoma may arise de novo. Any lesion that is felt to be a melanoma should be removed by total excision rather than incisional biopsy for fear of seeding the surgical area. Adequate

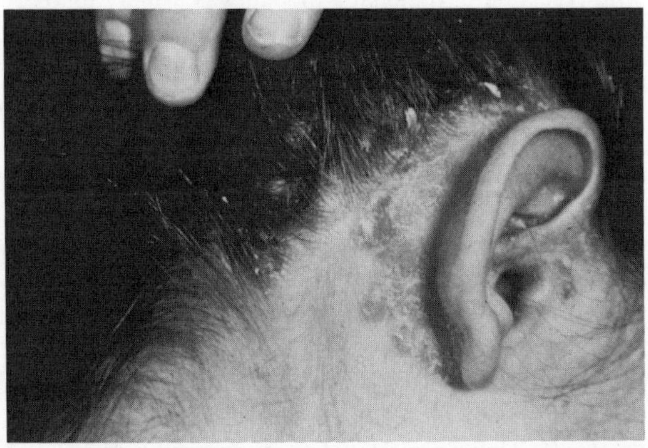

Figure 38-11. Seborrheic dermatitis of the postauricular area.

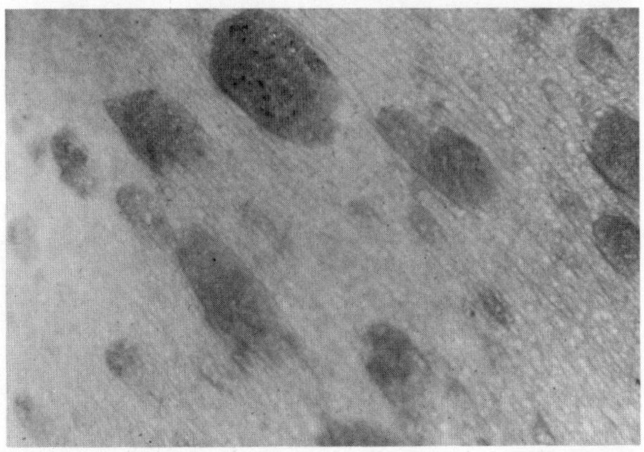

Figure 38-12. Seborrheic keratosis.

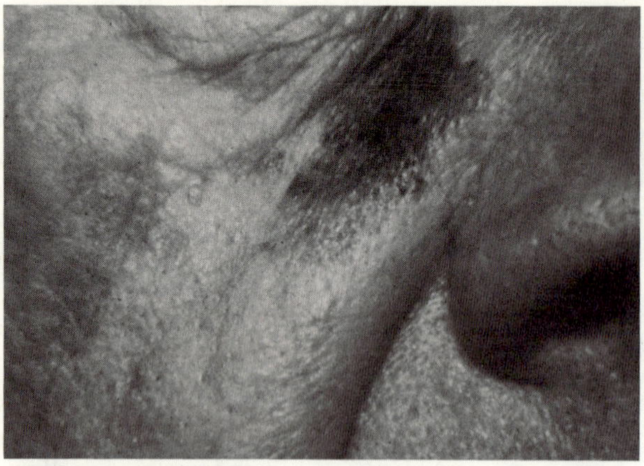

Figure 38-13. Lentigo maligna of the nasolabial fold. (Reprinted with permission from Koopmann, CF Jr. 1987. Head and neck surgery in the aged patient. In *Comprehensive Management of Head and Neck Tumors, Vol. 2,* Ed. SE Thawley and WR Panje. Philadelphia: W.B. Saunders.)

depth should also be taken so that not only can the tumor be totally removed, but the pathologist can adequately stage the lesion.

Keratoacanthoma are lesions that many consider benign, although they can be closely aligned with squamous cell carcinoma. Keratoacanthoma usually grows extremely rapidly in a matter of a few weeks, whereas squamous cell carcinoma usually grows more slowly. The central depression in a keratoacanthoma most commonly is filled with keratin (Fig. 38-15). These lesions should be totally excised so that the base can be examined microscopically since many lesions that appear to be benign have invasive squamous cell carcinoma at their base.

Basal cell carcinomas most commonly occur in sun-exposed areas. These lesions are usually flat and may have small telangiectatic vessels near the margins or on the surface. As the lesions become larger, they frequently ulcerate and will have a slightly elevated rolled border. These lesions usually grow very slowly and may be quite extensive prior to diagnosis and management. If function can be maintained, the optimal method of therapy for basal cell carcinoma would be surgical excision with rotation flaps, skin grafts, or cosmetic closure. In multiple areas or in regions where surgery would be functionally not indicated, radiation therapy can be utilized with high cure rates.

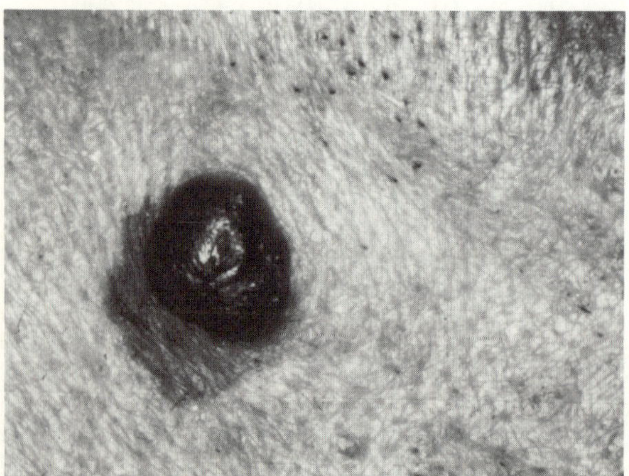

Figure 38-14. Malignant melanoma of the cheek.

Head and Neck Oncologic Surgery

Until the last 10 years, many medical and surgical specialists felt that the elderly should be treated in a different fashion for head and neck malignancies due to a supposed intolerance to the surgery. However, recent studies have failed to substantiate this philosophy.

Malignancies of the thyroid gland in the older patient are more likely to be less differentiated. If the lesion is considered one of the more favorable cell types (such as papillary or follicular), the tumor may be more aggressive. The most common complaint relative to thyroid malignancy is either enlargement of a pre-existing nodule in the thyroid gland or a lower cervical mass. Later symptoms include difficulty swallowing, hoarseness, cervical adenopathy, or airway obstruction. Cytologic aspiration and radioactive imaging are useful diagnostic tools in the differentiation of benign versus malignant lesions. If the lesion is malignant, surgical resection is most commonly the initial preferred treatment (21). In papillary and follicular carcinoma, a total or near total thyroidectomy with a modified neck dissection for clinically positive lymph nodes is advocated, followed by radioactive iodine ablation and thyroid hormone suppression. For patients with follicular carcinoma, a total or near total thyroidectomy with resection of regional lymphatics is usually followed by external radiation to the neck and mediastinum, plus thyroid hormone replacement therapy. Although anaplastic carcinoma carries an extremely dismal prognosis, the tumor should be resected with postoperative radiation therapy and thyroid hormone replacement utilized.

Carcinoma of the oral cavity may occur in the tongue, buccal mucosa, or retromolar trigone region. In small lesions of the mobile anterior two-thirds of the tongue without evidence of regional lymphatic spread, resection with primary closure or skin grafting is most commonly utilized. In lesions classified as T_2 or T_3, one must consider therapy for regional surgical spread, either overt or occult. Thus, a combination of surgical removal and

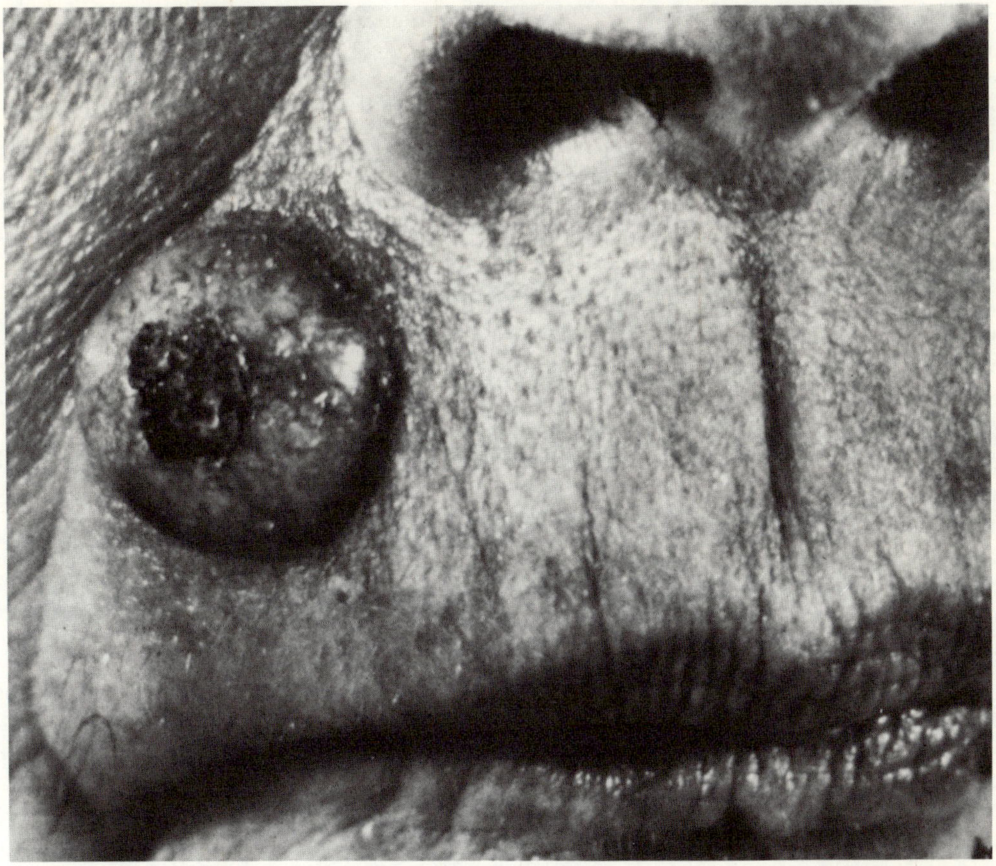

Figure 38-15. Keratoacanthoma of the upper lip. (Reprinted with permission from Koopmann, CF Jr. 1987. Head and neck surgery in the aged patient. In *Comprehensive Management of Head and Neck Tumors, Vol. 2*, Ed. SE Thawley and WR Panje. Philadelphia: W.B. Saunders.)

radiation therapy is most often utilized. In larger lesions, adjuvant chemotherapy may be useful. For carcinoma of the floor of the mouth and tongue lesions that require removal of part of the mandible, or for retromolar trigone or tonsillar carcinoma requiring surgical excision, the standard composite resection with the removal of a portion of the mandible followed by radiation therapy can be performed in the elderly patient. Johnson and co-workers (22) illustrated that the composite resection is a procedure well tolerated in the elderly patient. They found that the elderly experienced both major and minor wound complications with a similar frequency to their younger counterparts, including return to oral alimentation and discharge in approximately the same number of days. The elderly were more likely to suffer medical problems related to the surgery than were those in the younger age group. These investigators found that surgical morbidities such as fistula, wound infection or flap necrosis, carotid rupture, hematoma, or delay in alimentation were not increased in the elderly. Associated medical complications such as cardiac arrhythmias, pulmonary difficulties more serious than postoperative atelectasis, and gastrointestinal hemorrhage were slightly increased in the older population. However, their conclusion was that the composite resection offered not only a chance for cure, but also offered effective palliation with an acceptable complication rate in this age group and thus should not be withheld.

Laryngeal carcinoma is also seen more commonly in older patients. In lesions with mobile vocal cords, in the pyriform sinus, or small epiglottic lesions without cervical metastasis, radiation therapy can be quite well tolerated. However, in patients who have malignancies that should be treated with surgical excision (such as lesions with fixed vocal cords, larger pyriform sinus lesions, or supraglottic lesions with regional metastasis), conservation laryngeal surgery (either a vertical hemilaryngectomy or a supraglottic horizontal laryngectomy) with preservation of phonation or, in large lesions, a total laryngectomy may be necessary. Until the last 10 years, it was felt that conservation laryngeal surgery could not be performed in patients 65 years or older. However, Tucker in 1977 reviewed his experience with conservation laryngeal surgery in the elderly patient and presented a very strong case for preservation of vocal function in these patients (23). In his group, the total complication rate was approximately 11%. The vertical hemilaryngectomy patients and the majority of the supraglottic (horizontal) laryngectomy patients had no major surgical difficulties and had minimal pulmonary complications. There were no surgical mortalities. In the vertical hemilaryngectomy patients, there were no fistulas, carotid blowouts, skin break down, or delay in discharge. In the supraglottic lesions, there were two fistulas that were closed within 3 weeks of surgery, no carotid blowouts, no skin break down, and one delayed discharge. Thus, the complication rate of 11% in the older patients was totally acceptable, and the argument for withholding conservation procedures in the elderly due to an anticipation of high morbidity and mortality rate did not seem to be appropriate. Consequently, in carcinoma of the larynx, one should look at the patient as an individual, irrespective of age and, if the patient's cardiac and pulmonary status appear to be satisfactory, then a conservation laryngeal procedure is warranted. If the patient has extremely poor pulmonary function that would be made much worse with aspiration (as seen after supraglottic laryngectomies and occasionally after hemilaryngectomies), this patient may require total removal of the larynx.

Total laryngectomy is advocated for patients who have tumors that prevent preservation of vocal function or in patients whose medical status will not allow the risk of aspiration. John and Vaughan found that the elderly patient tolerates total laryngectomy well (24). Indeed, in patients who had postoperative mortality, the deaths were most commonly seen in patients who had preexisting severe cardiovascular disease. In 1977, Gall and co-workers found that laryngopharyngeal surgical complications had no relationship to age and sex (25). Thus, total laryngectomy appears to be a procedure tolerated well in the older age group. After total laryngectomy, the patient can be rehabilitated with either a voice button (Singer-Blume or Panje prosthesis), an electro-larynx, or esophageal speech.

McGuirt et al. reviewed complications of major head and neck surgical procedures in 162 patients over a 10-year period (26). They found that the incidence of surgical complications was no different for age groups above and below 70 years of age, although the medical complications were 8% higher in the more elderly patients. Thus, the evidence is clear that if the patient's pulmonary and cardiovascular status are satisfactory, age should not be a deterrent for major surgical extirpation for head and neck malignancies.

References

1. Doberauer, W. 1963. Zum Einfluss des Lebensalters Auf die heilung Kunstlicher Haut defekte. *Klin Med (Wein)* 18:199–204.
2. Howes, EL, and Harvey, SC. 1932. The age factor in the velocity of the growth of fibroblasts in the healing wound. *J Exp Med* 55:577–584.
3. Schmitt, W, and Beneke, G. 1970. Untersuchungen der Rindege websprolifertion in verschiedenen Lebensaltein. *Virchows Arch [Cell Pathol]* 5:351–364.
4. Boucek, RJ. 1984. Factors affecting wound healing. *Otolaryngol Clin North Am* 17(2):243–264.
5. Chvapil, M, and Koopmann, CF. 1982. Age and other factors regulating wound healing. *Otolaryngol Clin North Am* 15(2): 259–270.
6. Etholm, B, and Belal, A. 1974. Senile changes in the middle ear joints. *Ann Otol* 83:49–54.
7. Royster, LH, and Thomas, WG. 1979. Age effects hearing levels for a white nonindustrial noise exposed population (NINEP) and their use in evaluating industrial hearing conservation programs. *Ann Ind Hyg Assoc J* 40:504–511.
8. Rosen, S, Plester, D, El-Mofty, A, et al. 1964. Relation of hearing loss to cardiovascular disease. *Trans Am Acad Ophth Otol* 68:433–444.
9. Schuknecht, HF. 1964. Further observations on the pathology of presbycusis. *Arch Otolaryngol* 80:369–382.
10. Matkin, ND, and Hodgson, WR. 1982. Amplification and the elderly patient. *Otolaryngol Clin North Am* 15(2):371–386.
11. Engstrom, H. 1977. Structural changes in the vestibular epithelia in elderly monkeys and humans. *Adv Otorhinolaryngol* 22:93–110.
12. Bergstrom, B. 1973. Morphology of the vestibular nerve II: The number of myelinated vestibular nerve fibers in man at various ages. *Acta Otolaryngol* 76:173–179.
13. Schuknecht, HF. 1974. *Pathology of the Ear,* 388–409. Cambridge, MA: Harvard University Press.
14. Krmpotic-Nemanic, J. 1969. Presbycusis, presbystasis, and presbyosmia as consequences of the analogous biological process. *Acta Otolaryngol* 67:217–223.
15. Koopmann, CF. 1986. Geriatric Otolaryngology. In *Manual of Otolaryngology—Head and Neck Therapeutics,* Ed. AE Katz, 431–445. Philadelphia: Lea & Febiger.
16. Boone, DR, Bayles, KA, and Koopmann, CF. 1982. Communicative aspects of aging. *Otolaryngol Clin North Am* 15(2):313–327.
17. Hollison, H, and Shipp, T. 1972. Speaking fundamental frequency and chronologic age in males. *J Speech Hear Res* 15:155–159.
18. Honjo, J. and Jssiki, N. 1980. Laryngoscopic and voice changes of aged persons. *Arch Otolaryngol* 106:149–150.
19. Hermal, J, Schonwetter, S, and Samueloff, S. 1970. Taste sensation and age in man. *J Oral Med* 25:39–44.
20. Koopmann, CF, and Coulthard, SW. 1982. The oral cavity and aging. *Otolaryngol Clin North Am* 15 (2):293–311.
21. Simpson, WJ. 1982. Thyroid malignancy in the elderly. *Geriatrics* 37:119–127.
22. Johnson, JT, Rabuzzi, D, and Tucker, HM. 1977. Composite resection in the elderly: A well tolerated procedure. *Laryngoscope* 87:1509–1515.
23. Tucker, HM. 1977. Conservation laryngeal surgery in the elderly patient. *Laryngoscope* 87:1995–1999.

24. John, AC, and Vaughan, Ed. 1980. Laryngeal resection in patients of seventy years and older. *J Laryngol Otol* 94:629–635.
25. Gall, AM, Sessions, DG, and Ogura JH. 1977. Complications following surgery for cancer of the larynx and hypopharynx. *Cancer* 39:624–631.
26. McGuirt, WF, Loevy, S, and Krause, CJ. 1977. The risks of major head and neck surgery in the aged population. *Laryngoscope* 87:1378–1382.

39

Ophthalmic Surgery in the Elderly

Frank J. Weinstock

In spite of major technologic advances that have decreased the period of disability and improved visual restoration, ophthalmic surgery in the geriatric patient is still major surgery in terms of the eye. Because of these advances and the virtual elimination of hospitalization of eye patients, the effect of eye surgery on the total body is often minimal and therefore represents minor surgery with respect to the body as a whole. However, severe physical or ocular disability may result from an eye surgical procedure. The gravest outcomes are blindness and death.

The primary goals of most eye surgery are preservation and/or restoration of vision or to improve the functioning of the eye or its adnexa. Ophthalmic surgery is also carried out for preservation of life when a malignant lesion is present. Cosmesis is the primary goal in dealing with nonmalignant lid abnormalities or with ocular muscle surgery. The ophthalmologist may also be called to treat the eye complications of nonophthalmic surgical procedures or medical problems such as stroke. Such complications may include neurotrophic keratitis, corneal abrasions, precipitated angle-closure glaucoma, exposure keratitis, or ocular muscle paresis. Trauma may also affect the eyes of the geriatric patient and require the cooperation of the ophthalmologist in patient management.

This chapter begins with a discussion of general considerations in the ophthalmic surgery patient: preoperative, intraoperative, and postoperative. Discussions of specific procedures and eye problems then follow: cataract extraction, intraocular lens implantation, corneal transplantation, refractive surgery, glaucoma, retinal detachment and tears, other laser surgery, ocular motility, lids conjunctiva, oribit, eye problems in non-ophthalmic patients, and eye problems incidental to other surgical procedures.

General Considerations

Preoperative

For a number of reasons, the geriatric patient with eye problems often delays seeking the attention of an ophthalmologist. With decreased mobility due to age and possible poor vision, the older patient may find it difficult to get to the physician for necessary diagnosis and treatment. If unable to drive because of poor vision, the patient is dependent upon others for transportation and may or may not have access to easy public transportation. With decreased vision, the patient may not notice lesions of the eye or lids if they do not further affect his or her eyesight. A malignant lesion can therefore become quite large before the patient seeks help.

The presence of significant systemic conditions, such as cardiac decompensation, pulmonary problems, cancer, and dementia, may overshadow eye problems and cause them to be ignored. With decreased mentation or sensation, the elderly patient may not be aware of significant ophthalmic conditions, which show up as decreased vision, ocular irritation, or redness.

Because of the tremendous importance of vision in everyday life, denial of the visual decrease and other signs of cataract, glaucoma, and retinal detachment may be responsible for the individual not seeking care. The fear of blindness by Americans ranks second to their fear of cancer. This denial, coupled with the slow onset of visual deterioration of glaucoma and cataracts, may cause sufficient delay to the point that irreparable damage may have occurred. Consequently, all physicians must be aware of their role in detecting eye problems as early as possible. This is often relatively easily accomplished as a part of the history and physical examination, regardless of the specialty of the physician or the presenting problem of the patient. Once the problem has come to light, it may still be necessary to impress upon the patient the need for care. This is especially significant in the areas of glaucoma, retinal detachment, and malignancies. If the older patient does not understand, it may be necessary to involve a family member (a good idea in any case), nursing home staff member, or guardian.

Once the diagnosis is made and surgery is recommended, the indications, risks, and alternatives are discussed with the patient, the family, or the guardian (when indicated). Movies are often used as a part of preparing the patient. This discussion should be noted in the patient's office chart. A consent form should be obtained in the office in addition to what may later be obtained in the hospital or surgical facility; it is not unusual for the hospital to note the wrong eye or procedure. Although use of an operative consent form is considered essential, the forms used for consent for cataract surgery in the United States go into such detail that a certain number of patients read the forms and become so frightened that they refuse to have surgery. Sufficient time must be allowed for questions to be raised and fully answered.

The mechanics of the procedures as well as the preoperative and postoperative care should be discussed. The patient must also understand the potential for visual improvement. If the fundus cannot be evaluated due to a dense cataract, it may not be possible to give a definite prognosis. The possibility of macular degeneration or other limiting retinal conditions must be made clear to the patient and the family.

Financial considerations cannot be ignored since they are responsible for a number of patients refusing any surgery. Although most senior citizens have Medicare coverage and often additional insurance coverage, these usually do not provide completely cost-free care. Deductibles usually must be met. If the physician does not accept Medicare assignment, there will be additional expense to the patient. The surgical facility may also require a deductible or co-payment. To the patient on a limited income, these expenses may be frightening, if not overwhelming. Most eye surgery is elective, with third-party insurance carriers requiring a second opinion in many situations. In addition to the increased cost, this may be confusing to the patient and rarely will even frighten him or her sufficiently to result in cancellation of surgery.

Prior to the contemplated surgery, the patient should be evaluated by his or her primary care physician to determine if the surgery can be tolerated. In addition to the physical examination (usually a short examination), it is desirable to know how the patient's current medical status is with respect to his or her usual state of health. In addition to informing the ophthalmologist and the anesthesiologist about the medications being used, the primary care physician should answer the following questions. Is this the best that the patient has been? Is the patient stable? If diabetic, is the diabetes stable? If hypertensive, is this under control and stable? Is the endocrine status stable? If there has been a stroke, is there any residual defect? Are there any special instructions or any special tests that the primary care physician desires? It is the responsibility of the ophthalmologist to inform the primary care physician of the exact type of procedure to be performed, the anticipated type of anesthesia, and the location of the contemplated surgery.

Ophthalmic surgery can be carried out in the hospital, in an office surgical facility, or in a freestanding surgical facility. It is relatively rare to keep the patient in the hospital overnight except for retinal, vitreous, orbital, or some plastic surgery. Outpatient surgery is much less traumatic for the patient and is responsible for significant cost savings. If the surgery is not carried out in the hospital or hospital-type freestanding facility, it is important that quality and safety not be sacrificed in any way.

Intraoperative

The majority of surgical procedures are carried out under local anesthesia or under topical anesthesia, although some ophthalmologists prefer general anesthesia for almost all procedures. Those who use general anesthesia for cataract surgery and similar procedures prefer the complete control of the patient with the ability to avoid concern about the patient moving, coughing, or becoming uncooperative during the operation. In long operations, such as retinal detachment surgery, general anesthesia also avoids the problem of limited duration of action of a local injection.

With ambulatory surgery, it is often possible to avoid premedication or to significantly decrease the amount of systemic medications used. The psychologic and emotional preparation of the patient in the office in reference to understanding of his or her diagnosis and the details of the procedure will greatly affect the patient's attitude and the need for additional anesthesia. Many eye patients require no premedication or other systemic medication during the procedure. On the other hand, many ophthalmologists, especially for cataract surgery, will use small doses of Brevital or Pentothal intravenously to induce amnesia and render the patient unconscious for 1 to 2 minutes during the administration of the local anesthesia injection. This may expose patients to an additional risk, especially if adequate resuscitation personnel and equipment are not immediately available. No injections or medications should be taken lightly.

Because of potential systemic reactions from the local anesthesia, as well as other complications related to the patient's age and general condition, it is recommended by many that controlled anesthesia monitoring be used during most procedures carried out under local anesthesia. Whether or not an anesthesiologist is used, most local procedures require the use of oxygen, an intravenous line, and an electrocardiogram monitor. These may be avoided with minor lid and short outpatient procedures, however. Since the patient is covered with drapes with only an eye showing, it is necessary to be aware of the patient's general status during even the smallest procedure. Without proper monitoring, systemic disasters can easily occur without detection until it is too late.

For intraocular surgery, the local anesthetic used is either a retrobulbar or peribulbar injection of several cubic centimeters of anesthetic, usually containing epinephrine to decrease vascular egress of the anesthetic and hyaluronidase to facilitate diffusion into the local tissues. It must be remembered that the epinephrine may be responsible for causing tachycardia, cardiac irregularities, and/or systemic hypertension.

The retrobulbar injection (injection of the local anesthetic into the muscle cone behind the eye by a long No. 19-gauge needle through the lower lid) has been implicated in various untoward reactions, ranging from a localized retrobulbar hemorrhage to a more severe hemorrhage, which could compress the eye enough to cause total irreversible blindness. Injection into the sheath of the optic nerve may be responsible for optic nerve atrophy with loss of vision. Injection into the sheath may also allow the anesthetic to enter the central nervous system with resultant apnea, loss of vision, or other central nervous system effects. The peribulbar (injection of the local anesthetic through the upper lid via a long No. 25-gauge needle hugging the roof of the orbit) injection hopes to avoid these problems, but requires the use of a greater volume of anesthetic agent and more prolonged preoperative pressure on the eye. A retrobulbar injection may use 1 to 3 cc of anesthetic as opposed to 10 cc of a higher concentration of peribulbar anesthetic.

Following these injections, pressure is usually applied to the eye for 5 to 30 minutes to soften the eye and make the surgery safer in terms of cataract procedures. The pressure may be digital massage or it may consist of a bag of mercury or a more sophisticated cuff connected to a pressure gauge. Use of excessive pressure for an overly prolonged period of time rarely may result in closure of the central retinal artery with resultant loss of vision. During the application of ocular massage, the patient must be monitored for a significant slowing of the cardiac rate by stimulation of the oculo-cardiac reflex. This will normally revert to normal by stopping the massage or pressure.

It is not unusual for the patient to develop tachycardia with or without an elevation of blood pressure after injection of a local anesthetic agent containing epinephrine. Tachycardia and cardiac rhythm disturbances may also occur in a patient who is awake and has the need to void during the procedure. This may be misinterpreted as a serious cardiac problem if one does not communicate with the patient and realize that it is simply a need to void. For this reason, it is important that the patient void just prior to surgery.

The anesthetist should be aware of any eye medications that the patient may be using since eye drops are absorbed into the circulation and may have systemic effects for the patient. For example, anticholinergic drops used for the treatment of glaucoma may cause the patient to have prolonged apnea if succinylcholine is used. Steroid use is common in ophthalmology, and recent use should be communicated to the anesthetist. Beta-blockers may cause bradycardia and breathing difficulties (especially in asthmatic patients). Epinephrine drops may cause cardiac irregularities. Acetazolamide may cause significant electrolyte abnormalities. These side effects may cause confusion in interpreting the patient's condition during ophthalmic procedures if the anesthesiologist is not aware of the eye medications being used.

It is not unusual to use preoperative topical antibiotics for several hours or several days before the operation, but in general perioperative systemic antibiotics are not used.

The ophthalmologist wants to have total control of the patient. During procedures it is essential that the patient cooperate and not buck, since this type of movement may increase intraocular pressure and cause serious ocular damage if it occurs while the eye is open. The use of the operating microscope also requires a minimum amount of movement by the patient.

A highly trained assistant is desired, either another ophthalmologist or a specially trained nurse. Due to the delicate nature of some procedures, many ophthalmologists prefer another ophthalmologist as the assistant. This is particularly important if the patient has only one eye or has suffered a complication of cataract surgery in the first eye, whereby there has been a loss of vision. Unfortunately for the patient, Medicare and third-party regulations have essentially eliminated this practice.

Postoperative

With most procedures being performed under local anesthesia without overnight hospitalization, postoperative systemic complications have been almost eliminated. Resumption of activity is almost immediate with the patient not being confined to bed.

Postoperative medications are usually antibiotic or antibiotic-steroid topical medications. The patient wears an eye pad and shield for a short time. Often there are restrictions against heavy lifting and against sleeping on the side of the operation to avoid undue pressure on a newly operated eye. With retinal detachment surgery, the patient may be required to assume special head or body positions depending upon the location of the detachment.

The patient is then followed closely in the office. Due to the delicate nature of the surgery and the rapidity with which infections, glaucoma, and other complications may occur, it is essential that the ophthalmologist follow the patient carefully and be readily available if a change in vision or symptoms occur. If the patient is to be followed by someone other than the operating surgeon, it is essential that this person be an ophthalmologist who performs eye surgery or is familiar with the procedure that has been performed. Postoperative office visits evaluate the vision and success of the surgery and look for the presence of complications. This requires the use of the sophisticated ophthalmic equipment in the office. As in other types of surgery, the surgeon should follow his or her own patients and not delegate this responsibility to others.

Complications

The major complications of ophthalmic surgery are infection and loss of vision. Infection may occur early or late, even years later, and must be diagnosed and treated promptly. Loss of vision may result from retinal detachment, corneal decompensation, cystoid macular edema, intraocular hemorrhage, vascular occlusions, or glaucoma. Chronic uveitis and inflammation may be responsible for discomfort and sensitivity to light. Interference with functioning of the lids or extraocular muscles may be responsible for corneal exposure, double vision, or an unacceptable cosmetic appearance.

Specific Procedures

Cataract Extraction

Cataract extraction has become one of the most frequently performed surgical procedures in the United States and the most frequently performed outpatient surgical procedure. In 1989, over 1,000,000 cataract operations were carried out. In addition to these, over 150,000 laser procedures were performed on patients who have had cataract surgery in the past.

When the natural lens of the eye becomes cloudy or opaque, the term cataract is used to refer to this lens (Fig. 39-1). Since light must pass through the natural transparent lens and focus on the macula in order to obtain good vision, any decrease in the transparency of the lens will cause a change in vision. Depending upon the characteristics of the cataract and its location in the lens, the cataract will have a greater or lesser effect upon the patient's vision and visual performance.

The majority of individuals over the age of 60 years have some degree of cataract. However, the presence of a cataract is not synonymous with a need for surgery. Nine out of 10 patients with cataracts do not need surgery at the time of being seen. It is not possible to predict if a cataract will progress to the point of requiring surgery.

At the present time, there are no drops or medications that will prevent or reverse cataracts or slow their progression. The only treatment available is surgical removal when visual improvement is necessary.

After removal of the cataract, vision will be poor until an alternative lens system replaces the original lens. Such alternative lens systems include spectacles, a contact lens, primary placement of an intraocular lens, or secondary placement of an intraocular lens. The subject of

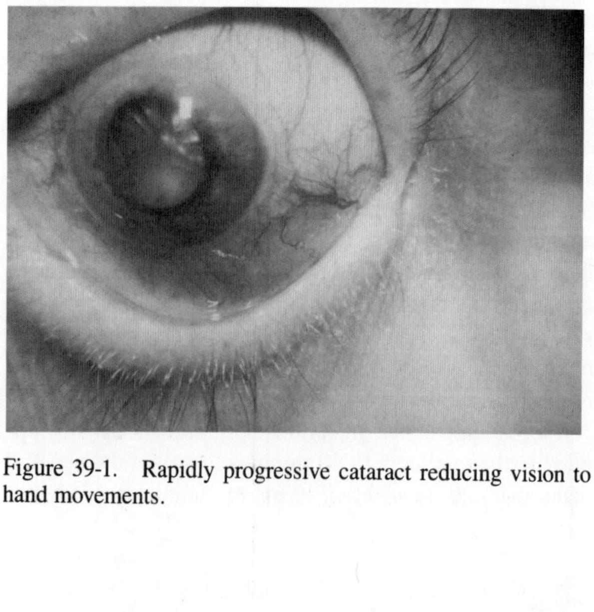

Figure 39-1. Rapidly progressive cataract reducing vision to hand movements.

visual correction after cataract removal will be amplified in the following section on intraocular lens implantation.

Indications

The main indication for surgery is the interference with the visual functioning of the patient. This is dependent upon the individual's visual requirements and cannot be reduced to a number such as 20/40, 20/60, etc. A senior citizen who drives and is still working in a job that requires 20/20 vision in each eye would obviously require surgery earlier than a bedridden patient in a nursing home who does not drive or read.

Depending upon the location of the opacity in the lens (e.g., cortical, nuclear, or posterior subcapsular cataract), it may cause greater or lesser interference with vision. The posterior subcapsular cataract especially may be disabling in spite of the fact that the vision in the usual testing situation in the ophthalmologist's office is quite good. For example, a patient may have 20/30 vision in the office and may be unable to read with normal illumination or to drive on a sunny day or at night due to the extreme glare produced by the cataract under these conditions. This information can be elicited by a careful history and confirmed by glare and contrast sensitivity testing. It is not unusual for the vision to be reduced to 20/200 or less with these special tests. These tests should only be used to demonstrate the disability, not to talk the patient into surgery. In the above situations, cataract surgery is elective and should be performed when the patient is having difficulties and desires surgery.

There are other situations in which cataract removal is indicated. If the patient has bilateral cataracts, with the vision in one eye being very poor and borderline in the other eye, surgery is indicated before the patient's better eye deteriorates to the point where driving and other tasks will be impossible. If the lens becomes very opaque and involves the outer capsule in addition to the central portion, it may be hypermature and may swell and become intumescent. This type of cataract may cause an acute glaucoma (Fig. 39-2) as a result of this swelling or may leak protein, causing uveitis. In these situations, emergency removal of the cataract may be necessary to reverse the glaucoma and uveitis.

If it is not possible to visualize the fundus, a B-scan ultrasound evaluation often can detect the presence of a retinal detachment, vitreous hemorrhage, or tumor. It is desirable to know this prior to the surgery; in some situations, this knowledge may encourage or contraindicate surgery. With diabetics and others in whom periodic fundus examinations are required, it may be necessary to remove the cataract to allow adequate visualization of the fundus and follow-up of the patient.

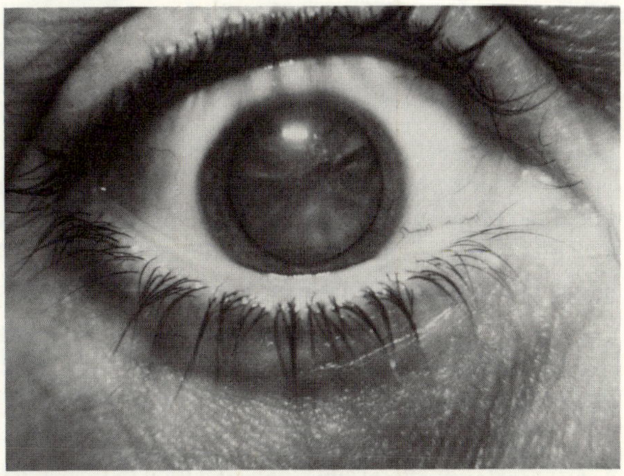

Figure 39-2. Hypermature cataract causing secondary glaucoma and decreased vision.

There are few contraindications to cataract surgery. Certainly, if a patient does not want surgery it should not be carried out. If a patient is functioning well and does not require improved vision, cataract surgery is not indicated. Rarely, systemic conditions may be severe enough to threaten an individual's life if any procedure is performed. If the patient has only one eye, surgery is usually delayed longer because of the greater effect potential complications would have on the patient's quality of life.

Operation

There are two prime methods of cataract extraction: intracapsular and extracapsular. Each requires an incision into the eye, following which the cataract is removed.

Extracapsular. With the extracapsular technique, a smaller incision is made into the eye, following which the cataract is removed by either a planned extracapsular method or by phacoemulsification.

The planned extracapsular method involves a slightly larger incision, followed by making an opening into the anterior capsule of the lens. The incision is enlarged, and the nucleus is removed by pressure or by the use of a loop. After this the wound is closed, and the cortical material is aspirated by a mechanical or hand suction method, leaving the posterior capsule intact for protection and for the positioning of a posterior chamber intraocular lens implant. The wound is closed with 10-0 sutures, and the patient is allowed to be up and around in a short time if stable.

With the phacoemulsification method, the incision is not enlarged, and the nucleus is broken up by high-speed ultrasound and aspirated from the eye. After cortical aspiration an implant is inserted. Usually the incision is enlarged from 3 mm to 6 or 7 mm to enable the insertion of the implant. Foldable and injectable implants are being developed, which would avoid the necessity of enlarging the incision. A smaller incision may decrease postoperative astigmatism and may allow the patient to carry out more vigorous activities immediately after surgery.

Over 90% of cataract surgery involves the implantation of an intraocular lens, since this provides the closest vision to what the patient experienced prior to the development of the cataract. Intraocular lens implantation procedures are discussed in the following section.

Intracapsular. Intracapsular cataract extraction (less than 10% of all cataract extractions) requires an incision into the eye, following which the lens is grasped with a cryoprobe (Fig. 39-3) and removed within the capsule in one piece, after having its zonular attachments weakened with alpha chymotrypsin (an enzyme). This requires a relatively large incision and removes the protective posterior lens capsule. This lack of a capsule will prevent the use of a posterior chamber intraocular lens and require an anterior chamber lens implant, the latter not as physiologic as a posterior chamber lens. If an implant is to be used, it could be placed in the anterior chamber immediately following the extraction. If an intraocular implant is not to be used, an iridectomy (an opening in the iris) is made and the incision is closed; the iridectomy appears to decrease the chance of postoperative pupillary block glaucoma. This procedure is rarely carried out in 1990.

Complications

Complications of cataract surgery may occur preoperatively, intraoperatively, and postoperatively.

Since we are dealing with an older population, patients may develop cardiovascular and other systemic problems prior to commencing the procedure. Occasionally, a reaction to preoperative drops may occur. This may be simply an ocular irritation, or there may be development of angle-closure glaucoma or a systemic reaction to medication, such as beta-blockers, sympathetic, or cholinergic drops. Patients must be monitored and observed carefully from the moment they enter the surgical facility and must not be left alone after having received preoperative medications.

Intraoperatively, rupture of the posterior capsule may allow loss of vitreous—which will prevent the use of a posterior chamber implant—may increase the risk of later retinal detachment, and may prevent the best vision from being attained. Hemorrhage may occur in the anterior chamber or in the vitreous. In patients with a friable vascular system an expulsive choroidal hemorrhage may occur, usually resulting in loss of the eye. Damage to the iris may also prevent the use of an implant due to lack of a supporting structure. During surgery or in the immediate postoperative period, blood pressure instability, chest pain, or cardiac rhythm disturbance may require that the patient be admitted to the hospital for observation and treatment of the systemic problem.

Postoperatively, the most devastating concern is infection in the form of endophthalmitis (Fig 39-4). This requires immediate recognition and action. Cultures from the conjunctiva, anterior chamber, and vitreous may be required. In addition, it may be necessary to perform a vitrectomy and remove the implant. Intensive topical and intravenous antibiotics may be supplemented with subconjunctival and intravitreal administration. A certain number of these eyes may be saved. Sterile inflammatory reactions may occur and must be differentiated from microbial endophthalmitis since they usually respond to steroid therapy. They present with ocular redness, decreased vision, photophobia, and pain.

Anterior chamber and vitreous hemorrhages usually resolve with time but may require surgical intervention, especially if an anterior chamber hemorrhage (hyphema)

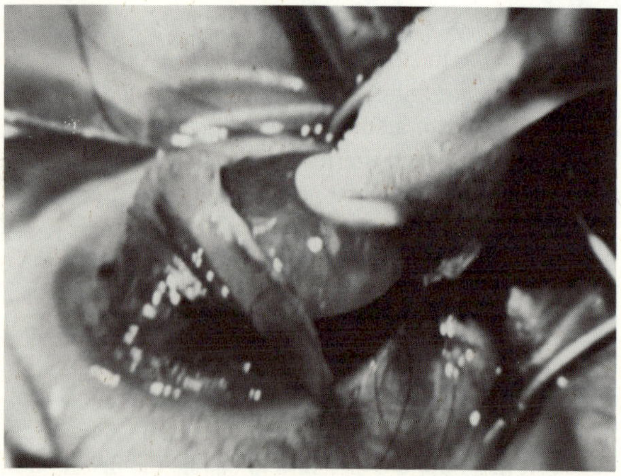

Figure 39-3. Extraction of mature cataract with cryoprobe.

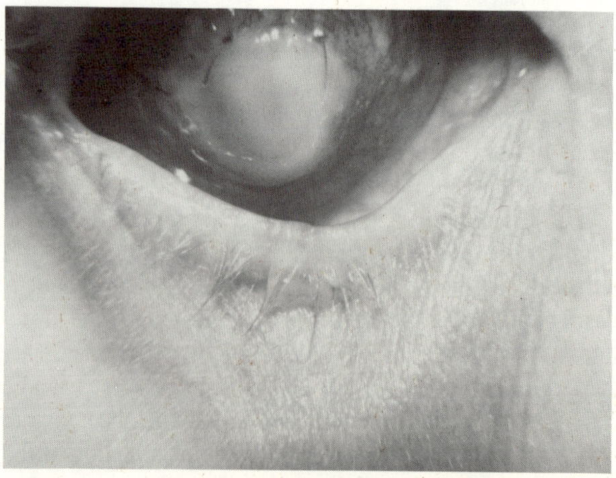

Figure 39-4. Postsurgical endophthalmitis (staphylococcus infection one day following surgery).

progresses to glaucoma and/or bloodstaining of the cornea. The delicate cornea may not withstand surgery and may develop a corneal dystrophy, thereby requiring a corneal transplant.

If retinal, optic nerve, or macular pathology was present prior to surgery, the visual outcome may be compromised. With very dense cataracts, it may not have been possible to visualize the fundus prior to the surgery.

A certain number of patients will develop cystoid macular edema, which will cause decreased vision. This edema will often resolve spontaneously and is treated with steroids and prostaglandin inhibitors. There seems to be a decreased incidence with posterior chamber lenses. Elevated intraocular pressure or glaucoma may occur acutely or after a variable length of time. Initially, it may be related to the use of Healon or steroids or to inflammation. This usually responds to topical medications. Retinal detachments may occur at any time and would require retinal surgery for correction. With time, vision may decrease simply from age-related changes, such as macular degeneration, diabetic vascular changes, or other retinal vascular changes.

With extracapsular surgery, the posterior capsule, which has been left in place, may opacify with resulting decreased vision. This would necessitate that the capsule be opened. Until recently, it had been necessary to take the patient to the operating room and to incise the membrane surgically. In addition to the expense to the patient, any surgical intervention exposes the patient to most of the potential complications of intraocular surgery listed previously. Modern treatment involves opening the membrane noninvasively by the use of the neodynium yttrium-aluminum-Garnet (Nd YAG) laser. This outpatient procedure avoids any incisions and may provide rapid complete restoration of vision. Laser posterior capsulotomy may be complicated itself by development of glaucoma, bleeding, retinal damage, or corneal damage in rare situations.

Postoperative Care

In general, the geriatric patient may resume normal activities after cataract surgery. These include ambulation, reading, watching television, etc. If the patient drives, this is usually allowed on an individualized basis. Ambulatory surgery allows the patient to return to his or her home or care facility within hours of surgery. Heavy lifting and strenuous sports are usually curtailed to a greater or lesser degree for 1 to 2 months, depending upon the size of the incision and the habits of the individual surgeon.

It is not unusual to see an essentially blind individual with severe sensory deprivation who has required constant nursing care become alert and able to care for himself or herself as soon as the dressing is removed, usually the morning after surgery.

Antibiotic-steroid drops are usually used for several weeks after surgery. A patch and eye shield are used at night with the eye uncovered during the day. The vision may be excellent immediately after surgery or may take a while to improve. Preexisting disease, such as macular degeneration, may prevent visual improvement to the degree that one would like. If macular degeneration is present, cataract surgery with use of an intraocular lens may allow the use of low-vision aids, which might give the patient the opportunity to read.

Summary

Modern cataract surgery is extremely successful and is carried out in a relatively painless manner. Rehabilitation is quick and effective. The surgery and instrumentation are highly technical and must not be underestimated. The postoperative care and observation are extremely important and must be carried out by surgeons who perform and are familiar with the procedure. These steps will prevent loss of vision and allow maximum restoration of vision.

Intraocular Lens Implantation

After removal of the cataract, vision will be poor until an alternative lens system replaces the original lens. Spectacles function quite adequately, but are thick and unsightly, cause much peripheral visual distortion, have a large peripheral blind spot, which might cause difficulties while driving or crossing the street, and cause the image size in the operated eye to be 15% to 20% larger than in the unoperated eye. If the vision in the unoperated eye is good, most patients cannot tolerate the difference in image size and will either wear a patch over one eye, elect to have no spectacle correction, use a contact lens, or request a secondary implant.

A contact lens on a daily or extended-wear basis will reduce this image size to 3% to 5% and improve the peripheral vision. Most patients are able to fuse these images. However, the patient must be capable of handling and caring for the contact lens. A major advantage of lens correction is the ability to use a bifocal contact lens and dispense with spectacles completely. Contrary to popular belief, a patient is not blind when the glasses or contact lenses are removed. Large-form vision and peripheral vision are still present.

The best visual correction, which most closely approximates the vision with the natural lens, is obtained by the use of an intraocular lens. With the use of an intraocular lens, spectacles are usually necessary for near vision correction (bifocals) and for some residual distance correction. Visual correction with spectacles or a contact lens is usually delayed until 6 to 8 weeks after surgery, whereas the use of an intraocular lens placed in the eye at the time of surgery may provide improved or excellent vision immediately after surgery.

Determination of the type of visual correction depends upon the individual patient. If a patient has had surgery on the first eye and is getting along well with spectacles, an implant is usually not used. Use of an implant in this situation will often require that the eye, which has had previous surgery, have another operation with secondary intraocular implantation to avoid the disturbing difference in image size. If a contact lens has been used with the first eye, an implant is usually used in the second eye.

As noted above, over 90% of cataract surgery involves the implantation of an intraocular lens since this provides the closest vision to normal. There are two broad classes of intraocular lenses in use today: the anterior chamber lens and the posterior chamber lens. These are named according to the lens location in the eye. Most surgery involves the implantation of a posterior chamber implant, with the anterior chamber implants reserved for those situations in which a posterior chamber lens cannot be used, namely for a secondary implant or when the supporting posterior capsule has been removed in an intracapsular extraction or has been damaged during extracapsular surgery. Some surgeons, however, do prefer an anterior chamber lens routinely. Iris plane or pupillary support intraocular lenses are rarely used today. These lenses are attached to the pupil by wedging the lens behind and in front of the iris or are clipped to the iris by loops (haptics), which go behind and in front of the iris. These lenses appear to have been associated with significantly increased complications over time.

Anterior Chamber Implants

The anterior chamber lenses may be implanted at the time of the cataract removal (primary implantation) or at a later date (secondary implantation). Anterior chamber implants are placed in the anterior chamber in front of the iris. They stay in place by being wedged in the anterior chamber with the haptics in the angle between the cornea and the iris. The loops (haptics) may be open or closed. The closed-looped haptics appear to have an increased complication rate of corneal decompensation and systoid macular edema, causing their use to be discouraged.

Patients who have had previous cataract surgery without the use of an implant may have severe visual problems as a result of the fixed spectacles, the difference in image size between the two eyes, or an inability to use contact lenses. If the patient has been wearing a contact lens, arthritis and other age related changes may make it difficult or impossible to handle and manage a contact lens. In these situations, an implant can be placed in the eye as a secondary procedure. This is similar to the original cataract operation except that it is unnecessary to remove the lens. After making an incision into the eye, an anterior chamber lens is usually used since most of these patients will have undergone an intracapsular procedure already. If an extracapsular procedure had been used and the posterior capsule is intact, a posterior chamber lens may be used as an option.

Complications of anterior chamber implants include hyphema, damage to the iris or cornea, and vitreous loss. Postoperative complications include hyphema, endophthalmitis, corneal decompensation, glaucoma, pupillary distortion, or capture and malposition of the implant.

Posterior Chamber Implants

Posterior chamber implants are placed in one of two locations behind the iris: either within the capsule or bag, which is left in place with the extracapsular techniques, or just in front of the capsular bag and posterior to the iris and the ciliary sulcus. It is held in place by the loops of the implant (haptics), which are wedged in place. Due to the extremely fine manufacturing techniques and extremely light weight of the implants, this wedging rarely causes pressure necrosis or extrusion.

Since the normal location of the lens is in the posterior chamber and since there appears to be a better tolerance of posterior chamber lenses, this is the preferred location for implant for most surgeons. However, placement of an implant in the posterior chamber requires that the surgeon learn extracapsular techniques, which are quite different from the intracapsular techniques that many surgeons learned during their initial training in ophthalmology. Since their development in the 1940s, implants have benefited from modern technology and have attained a high level of quality and sophistication. Many of the early problems of design and manufacturing have been eliminated. However, new designs are constantly being presented and must be carefully evaluated in order to assess short- and long-term effectiveness and safety. It is not unusual for complications to show up years after the implantation of the lens.

At the time of this writing, endocapsular cataract extraction is under evaluation. This entails making a small incision into the anterior chamber, after which a puncture is made into the lens. The nucleus and cortical material are then aspirated, leaving most of the capsule intact with minimal disturbance of the zonular attachments. Following this, the capsular bag is injected with a substance which will then act like a new lens to focus the light on the retina.

Complications of posterior chamber implants, in addition to those of cataract surgery in general, include dislocation into the vitreous or decentration. The power of the lens may then be under- or overestimated. A completely dislocated lens is usually left in the vitreous where it will cause no difficulty. For visual correction, an anterior chamber lens may be secondarily implanted or a contact lens may be used. Decentration may require surgical correction if symptoms of glare are not reduced or eliminated with miotic drops. Significant residual refractive correction may require using a contact lens or removing the implant and exchanging it for an implant of a different power.

Postoperative care after lens implantation procedures is similar to that after cataract surgery in general. After implant surgery, some patients may be able to dispense with glasses, but most will have some residual visual deficit and require glasses. Since there are no approved bifocal implants, almost all patients require glasses for reading. However, bifocal intraocular lens implants are currently under evaluation. Therefore, most patients still wear glasses after this surgery. Occasionally, the need for a large correction may require the use of a contact lens or may require exchanging the implant at a second operation for attainment of maximum vision.

Corneal Transplantation

When the cornea becomes opaque from injury, surgery, disease, or dystrophy from aging, it may be replaced with a cornea obtained from a recently deceased individual. Another indication is painful, bullous keratopathy. This is a breakdown of the corneal pump, whereby the cornea becomes edematous with epithelial blebs that periodically rupture, causing painful tearing of the eye.

With the growth of intraocular lens implantation and extracapsular surgery, there has been an associated increase in resulting corneal decompensation and dystrophy, which requires corneal transplantation. This may occur as a result of trauma, especially in the early learning phase, or as a reaction to an implant that cannot be tolerated by the eye. This is less common with the use of posterior chamber implants. Anterior chamber and iris plane implants, especially some of the earlier designs, may occasionally touch the cornea, causing it to break down.

Lamellar corneal transplants involve replacing the superficial portion of the cornea with a lamellar partial corneal thickness graft. Penetrating keratoplasty involves trephination to remove a full-thickness button of the majority of the cornea and replacement of it with a donor cornea. This is carried out with the help of the operating microscope and is extremely successful.

Postoperatively, activities are usually restricted and intensive topical drops are used to decrease inflammation and the possibility of graft rejection. The complications associated with cataract surgery apply to corneal transplants also. In addition, the concern for graft rejection is paramount. In this case, it is necessary to treat intensively with anti-inflammatory agents.

Refractive Surgery-Epikeratophakia-Keratomileusis

Refractive surgery deals with the alteration of the cornea to correct a refractive error. In the geriatric population, this surgery, still in its developmental stages, is almost exclusively used to correct the vision after cataract extraction when an intraocular lens was not implanted. In this situation, the thick glasses, besides being unsightly, may contribute to problems with peripheral vision and cause a difference in image size, which might be quite disabling if the other eye has not had cataract surgery. If one eye has had the cataract removed and the other eye has the natural lens, there is a 20% to 25% difference in image size between the two eyes, which will prevent fusion of images by the patient. To provide a natural image size, refractive surgery may be used in the place of a secondary intraocular lens implant.

Keratomileusis involves the use of expensive, sophisticated equipment, which is used to remove the cornea, freeze it, lathe it to the correct prescription and replace it in its original position. This is usually carried out under general anesthesia. After several weeks to several months, excellent vision might be obtained. If the refraction is not perfect, poor vision might result. Correction of the residual refractive error might require the use of glasses or contact lenses, or a repeat procedure.

Epikeratophakia (Fig. 39-5) uses a preserved corneal button ("living cornea") of a specific power, which is sutured to a cornea after removing a superficial lamella of cornea under local anesthesia. A major asset of this procedure is the fact that it is carried out on the surface of the eye and is not an intraocular procedure. Usually the vision takes several months to stabilize. If the prescription is not

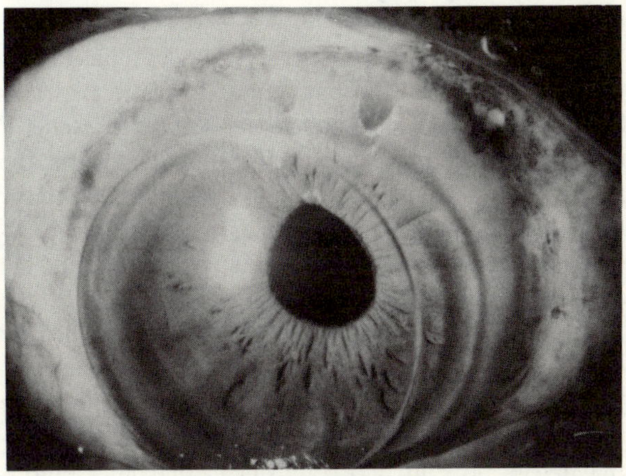

Figure 39-5. Epikeratophakia (for aphakia).

correct, glasses or a contact lens may be used for the residual correction. If the epi button does not take or is not tolerated, it may be removed completely with minimal scarring. Infections may require removal of the epi graft, but since the eye has not been opened, they usually are not as serious as an endophthalmitis.

Rapid ambulation is allowed with the use of topical eyedrops after refractive procedures.

The above procedures have not achieved widespread use.

Glaucoma

Glaucoma secondary to an intumescent cataract is rare (Fig 39-2). When it occurs, it is an acute, painful glaucoma of sudden onset. The treatment is cataract extraction.

A hypermature cataract may cause a phacolytic, acute glaucoma with severe uveitis. Treatment involves the use of topical steroids with cataract extraction, preferably with the uveitis under control.

Acute, angle-closure, narrow-angle glaucoma occurs in anatomically predisposed eyes. There is severe pain accompanied by visual decrease, a dilated pupil, severe conjunctival injection, and a high intraocular pressure. Initial treatment requires the lowering of the pressure by medical means, followed by a laser or surgical iridotomy (hole in the iris) to enable aqueous humor to pass from the posterior chamber to the anterior chamber, thus relieving the pupillary block. The medical means include intensive use of pilocarpine eye drops (1 drop of 2% or 4% pilocarpine every 15 minutes for 4 to 8 doses), drinking of 50% glycerol (1.0 to 1.5 mg per kg body weight), and use of 500 mg of oral or intravenous diamox. Occasionally, a 20% mannitol solution may be given intravenously (6 to 8 ml per kg body weight) over a 20- to 30-minute period. After the pressure is lowered and under control, pilocarpine eye drops are used until a definitive iridotomy is performed.

The Argon or YAG laser is used under topical anesthesia in the office or hospital setting to create the iridotomy. If a patient cannot cooperate and sit at the laser or if it is not possible to make an opening through the iris, the patient may be taken to the operating room, where, under local anesthesia, a surgical opening (iridotomy or iridectomy) is made in the iris after making an incision into the anterior chamber.

Rarely, laser iridotomies may be accompanied by bleeding, corneal injury, cataract formation from lens injury, or damage to the macula from poor focusing of the laser or eye movement on the part of the patient. Occasionally, the pressure may rise, which will require a surgical iridectomy to be carried out quickly in the operating room. Surgical iridectomy or iridotomy may be complicated by endophthalmitis, hyphema, corneal damage, or cataract. If the anterior chamber does not reform after surgery (a flat anterior chamber) and remains flat, a chronic glaucoma may occur. This may require that a filtering procedure be performed as discussed later.

Primary, open-angle, chronic simple glaucoma refers to a series of entities in which elevated intraocular pressure results in damage to the optic nerve with concomitant visual field loss. If medical treatment cannot lower the intraocular pressure sufficiently to halt the progressive ocular damage, laser trabeculoplasty or a filtering surgical procedure must be carried out for lowering of the intraocular pressure. The medical treatment consists of a combination of the following medications: pilocarpine, epinephrine, and beta-blocker drops, with or without systemic carbonic anhydrase inhibitors.

Laser trabeculoplasty or trabecular shortening involves the use of the Argon laser, under topical anesthesia in the office or hospital setting, to make 50 to 150 micron-size burns over 180 to 360 degrees of the trabecular meshwork via a special mirrored lens that allows visual access to the angle of the eye between the cornea and the iris. In cooperative patients, this is almost always used as a first procedure to try to avoid invasive surgery. Complications include bleeding, damage to the cornea, and damage to the iris. Occasionally, severe pressure rises, which may further damage the optic nerve and force a surgical filtering operation.

After laser trabeculoplasty, the preoperative medications usually must be continued. Occasionally, the pressure lowering may be sufficient to discontinue the use of antiglaucoma medications. The pressure-lowering effect of laser usually is not as great as that of surgery and may decrease with time. If the effect wears off, surgery should be carried out. Usually repeat laser trabeculoplasty is relatively ineffective and not indicated.

Filtering procedures take various forms that are meant to create an artificial channel to circumvent the blockage of aqueous outflow in the trabecular meshwork of the angle and allow the aqueous to filter under the conjunctiva. The most common form of operation is the trabeculectomy, whereby the conjunctiva is pulled back and a partial thickness of sclera is elevated, following which the lower remaining portion of sclera is removed with an opening being made into the anterior chamber and an iridectomy being made. The partial thickness flap is sutured and the conjunctiva is closed. Aqueous may then drain through the opening from the anterior chamber and percolate through the thin scleral flap under the conjunctiva where a fluid-filled bleb may be seen (Fig. 39-6).

Occasionally, a punch or a trephine may be used to remove a portion of the sclera. This type of operation may

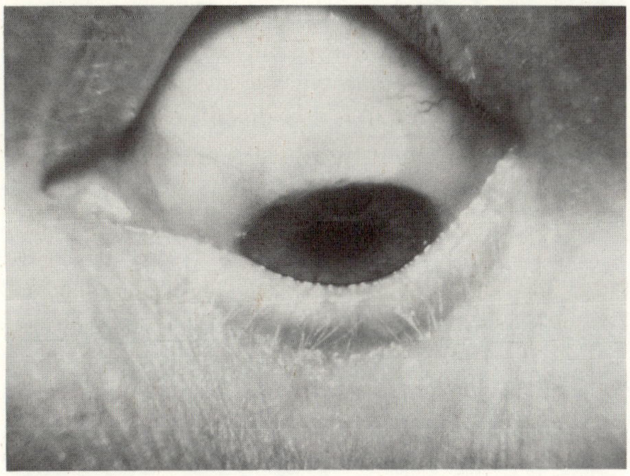

Figure 39-6. Well-functioning, filtering bleb post-trabeculoplasty (laser trabeculoplasty failed).

provide a greater pressure reduction. A multicenter clinical trial of the use of subconjunctival 5-fluorouracil is being undertaken to evaluate its efficacy in enhancing the formation of the filtering bleb.

Postoperative care after glaucoma surgery is similar to that of cataract surgery. As with other intraocular procedures, complications may occur, such as infection and bleeding (hyphema). Cataract formation and corneal damage may accompany this operation. If the anterior chamber does not reform, it may be necessary to reform it surgically. A prolonged flat anterior chamber may result in cataract formation or intractable glaucoma. Failure to get adequate lowering of pressure may require a repetition of the filtering procedure or opening of the filtration site with the YAG laser.

If the chronic glaucoma is accompanied by many blood vessels in the iris (rubeosis iridis), following central retinal vein occlusion or in certain diabetics, the standard filtering operations will not be successful since there will be intractable bleeding from these vessels. A continual search for a consistently reliable mechanical filtering valve has not been successful. Unfortunately, these valves will often close over with fibrosis, thereby allowing the pressure to rise to damaging levels.

Retinal Detachment And Tears

Interruption of the retinal integrity by a retinal tear or a retinal detachment presents itself to the patient with the sudden onset of "floaters," a curtain or veil descending on the vision or loss of a portion of the visual field. Examination with the ophthalmoscope reveals the presence of a retinal tear with a retinal detachment.

If the retina surrounding the tear is flat without fluid, it may be sealed off by surrounding the hole with "burns" from the Argon laser, which will "spot-weld" the area surrounding the tear. As with other laser procedures, this is carried out with topical anesthesia in the office or hospital setting, usually with excellent results.

If fluid causes a separation of the retina, it is not possible to seal this off with the laser. One of a variety of procedures must be carried out for the purpose of indenting the globe in order to bring the choroid and sclera closer to the elevated retina. An external explant or balloon may be placed over the eye or a plastic encircling band (Fig. 39-7) may be placed around the globe with particular pressure over the area of the tear and detachment. The fluid may be drained by a puncture wound through the sclera from the exterior of the globe. At this point the area surrounding the retinal tear may be treated by cryotherapy or diathermy over the sclera in an effort to seal the hole.

If the retinal detachment is caused by traction of the vitreous or vitreous bands internally, an internal approach may be added to the external approach. Vitreous surgery may require removal of the vitreous, cutting of vitreous bands, peeling of epiretinal membranes, endophotocoagulation, and the use of intravitreal gas (SF6), which expands two-fold to approximate the retina.

Vitreous surgery is a relatively recent advance in technology. It is used most frequently in diabetic patients who have developed vitreous hemorrhages with or without detachments. It has had remarkable success in restoring vision to patients who had been blind from vitreous hemorrhages that have not spontaneously cleared. Prolonged vitreous hemorrhages may be responsible for the development of vitreous bands and massive vitreous traction, which can produce a large vitreous detachment. There are indications that earlier intervention may prevent this vitreous traction and prevent future retinal detachments.

These retinal detachment and vitreous procedures are usually prolonged and are carried out under general

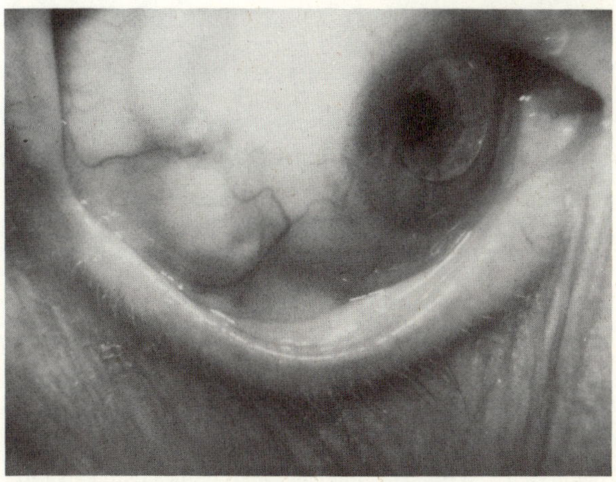

Figure 39-7. Retinal buckle visible through the conjunctiva.

anesthesia. Postoperatively, the patient may remain in the hospital for several days. Vision may be poor and require that the patient not drive. If subretinal fluid remains, it may be necessary for the patient to sleep in certain positions (sitting, lying on one side, etc.). Eye drops, usually antibiotic-steroid combinations and dilating-cycloplegic drops, are used for several weeks after surgery. Ambulation and activity will vary with respect to the location of the detachment and the results and the type of surgery performed. It is usually limited to some degree.

An alternative procedure of pneumatic retinopexy is being evaluated. This involves the treatment of the retinal break with transconjunctival cryotherapy, following which perfuoropropane (C3F8) is injected into the vitreous. The gas will expand fourfold to reapproximate the detached retina. This procedure may be carried out in an outpatient setting.

Complications of retinal and vitreous surgery include adhesions (Fig. 39-8), infection, anterior chamber and vitreous hemorrhages, corneal clouding, glaucoma, and redetachment of the retina. When extraocular muscles are temporally removed in order to place the scleral buckle, the patient may experience annoying double vision afterwards. Scleral buckles may extrude and have to be removed at a later date.

Retinal detachment surgery is extremely effective in producing anatomic reattachment of the retina. However, often the visual improvement is less than desired due to macular damage from a prolonged detachment or damage from preexisting disease.

Other Laser Surgery

In addition to the management of flat retinal detachments, laser energy is used to manage conditions in which retinal vasculature abnormalities occur. The prime situations are age-related macular degeneration and diabetes, in which hemorrhages, neovascularization, and macular edema may occur. One of various types of laser (the Argon laser is the most widely used) is used to either seal off vessels directly, wall off an area of leakage or, in diabetics, decrease the production of a vasoproliferative factor by panretinal laser photocoagulation (Fig. 39-9).

Laser therapy is amazingly effective and can decrease the risk of blindness by 25% to 50% in diabetics. Postoperatively, there is minimal interference with normal activities unless a concern for rebleeding requires the patient to avoid strenuous activities. Night driving should not be carried out if the patient has difficulty seeing at night. If the vision is not good, it may be necessary to discontinue driving altogether.

The risks of laser surgery are ineffectiveness, precipitation of glaucoma, damage to the macula, and increased retinal or vitreous hemorrhage. Especially in panretinal photocoagulation, in which 2,000 to 3,000 retinal burns may be placed around the circumference of the retina, blind spots (scotomata) and decreases in peripheral and night vision may occur.

Ocular Motility

Ocular motility disturbances result in double vision or a cosmetic disturbance. They result from direct damage to the ocular muscles from injury or disease or from central nervous disturbances such as stroke, diabetes, tumor, etc. Fortunately, most disturbances will resolve with time. If the muscle weakness and double vision do not resolve with time, or if there is a contracture of the contralateral muscle, extraocular muscle surgery may be required.

This surgery usually may be carried out with local retrobulbar anesthesia. Since traction on the muscles during the operation may induce the oculocardiac reflex of

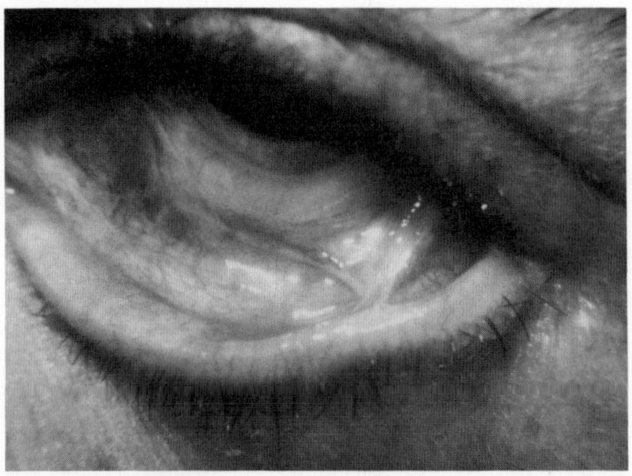

Figure 39-8. Symblepharon (adhesions of the conjunctiva following retinal detachment surgery).

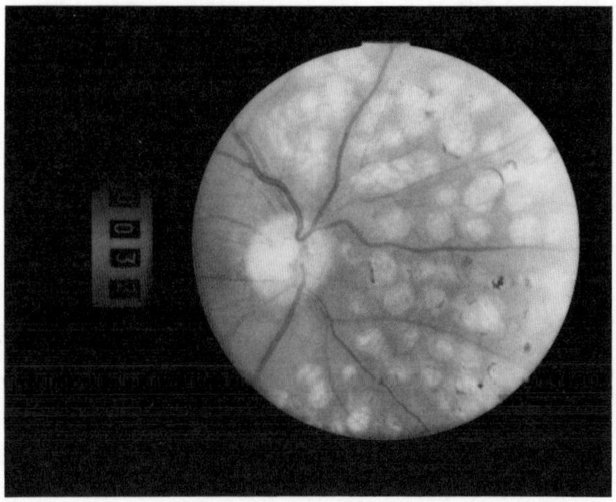

Figure 39-9. Laser photocoagulation areas in the retina.

cardiac slowing, it is important to monitor the patient closely with the assistance of an anesthesiologist.

Careful preoperative measurements of the ocular deviation are taken. Surgery is not carried out until the deviation is stable. Each ophthalmologist has a formula for the amount of surgery to be carried out. The extraocular muscles are reached by making an incision through the conjunctiva and Tenon's capsule. The overacting muscle is isolated with a muscle hook, after which it is weakened by severing it from the globe and reattaching it to the globe by suturing it several millimeters behind its original insertion. The opposing muscle, which is too weak, is isolated and strengthened by excising several millimeters and resuturing this tighter muscle to its original insertion.

Postoperative care is minimal with the patient resuming normal activities and usually using a steroid eye drop four times a day for 1 to 2 weeks. Driving should not be undertaken until the double vision disappears.

Surgery may cause the deviation to be undercorrected, and still exist, or to be overcorrected to go in the opposite direction. For example, an inturning eye (esotropia) may continue to turn in or may turn outwards (exotropia) following surgery.

Infections are extremely rare. Since this is an extraocular procedure there is usually no effect upon vision. Due to the thin sclera, however, it is possible to perforate the sclera when suturing the muscle to the globe, thereby causing a retinal hole or detachment or a choroidal detachment.

When the eyes are realigned, the patient may experience transient or permanent double vision from the new position of the eyes.

Botulinum toxin is now an approved method of weakening the overactive muscle by injecting a minute amount of botulinum toxin, under careful monitoring, in the muscle. There have been minimal lasting side effects.

Lids

The lids and adnexa require surgical treatment in instances of tumors, exophthalmos, infections, and age-related abnormalities of lid position. In addition to the cosmetic and potential malignant aspects of lid lesions, they may be responsible for severe symptoms. Accurate approximation of smooth lids to the cornea is necessary for clear vision. Lesions and distortion of the lids may interfere with the normal lid function and cause redness of the eyes, irritation or severe pain, or a significant decrease of vision by damaging the cornea directly by irritation or indirectly by allowing exposure and dryness of the cornea to occur.

Chalazia (Fig. 39-10) are granulomatous reactions of the meibomian glands in the edges of the lids. If they do

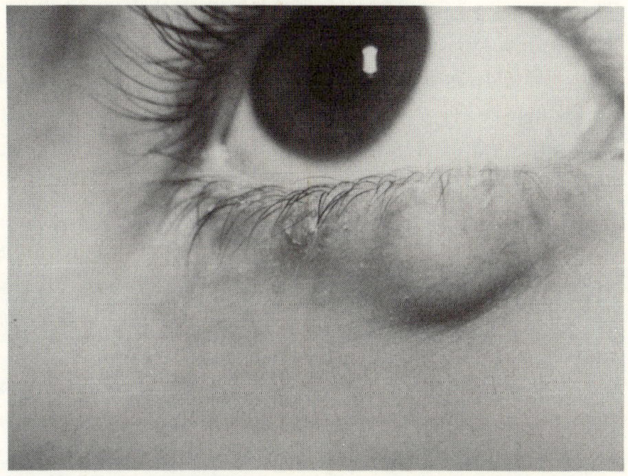

Figure 39-10. Chalazion.

not respond to warm compresses and antibiotic or antibiotic-steroid topical medication, a mass of varying size may remain. Although these rarely have any effect upon vision, they may be uncomfortable and unsightly, thereby requiring excision. This is carried out in the office or outpatient setting after infiltrating the area with a small amount of xylocaine, placing a clamp over the involved area of the lid, inverting the lid, and opening and draining the chalazion from the posterior surface of the lid without the use of sutures. A tight patch is usually placed over the lid overnight to prevent bleeding.

Basal cell and squamous cell carcinomas, as well as many other benign and malignant primary and secondary neoplasms, may occur in the lids (Fig. 39-11). These are removed by excision, as opposed to cautery, in order to send a specimen to the laboratory for diagnosis and for examination to be sure that the lesion margins are free of the tumor. Of particular concern in the geriatric patient is the lack of pain and the inability to verbalize on the part of many patients, causing these growths to be overlooked.

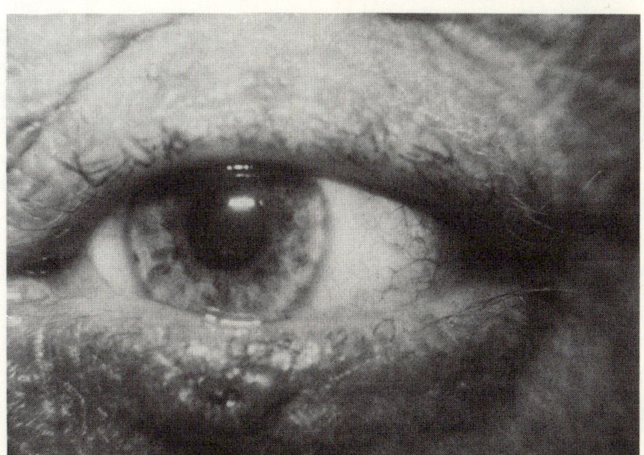

Figure 39-11. Basal cell carcinoma of the lower lid.

The lids must be examined routinely as a part of the physical examination.

Excision is made sufficiently large to encompass the entire lesion. The Moh's technique of continually monitoring the margins until they are free of tumor cells is excellent. When the tumor is sufficiently large, there may be interference with the adequate functioning of the lids, causing entropion or cosmetic notching and shortening. With highly malignant lesions such as squamous cell carcinomas, radical removal of the lids, and possibly the eye, may be recommended.

Malpositions of the lids occur as entropion (inturning) (Fig. 39-12), ectropion (outturning) (Fig. 39-13), lagophthalmos (inadequate closure), and ptosis (drooping). Ptosis may interfere with the ability to see due to covering of the pupillary axis. It may occur with age and injury or after a stroke or surgery. If it interferes with the ability to see, corrective surgery is carried out under local or general anesthesia. The procedure depends upon the degree of ptosis.

Blepharochalasis or "baggy eyelids" with redundant skin may cause visual interference, with the lids actually hanging in front of the visual axis. The cosmetic appearance may be extremely disturbing to the patient. Surgical correction involves excision of the excess skin and any prolapsed fat with strengthening in the underlying septum and muscle.

Lid surgery may induce scarring whereby cicatricial ectropion or entropion may occur. Lesions involving the lid margin may result in notching of the lid with cosmetic disfigurement and possible interference of lid function in maintaining the integrity of the cornea. Malignant lesions may not be completely excised, thereby requiring additional excision or radiation treatment if the lesion is sensitive.

Ptosis surgery may result in an undercorrection with no significant improvement. Overcorrection may result in poor lid closure and exposure of the eye with keratitis. Any lid surgery may be complicated by infection. The most dreaded complication is significant bleeding, which may exert pressure on the globe and result in central retinal artery closure and blindness. Meticulous attention to hemostasis is essential during surgery, followed by postoperative monitoring to detect any potential bleeding.

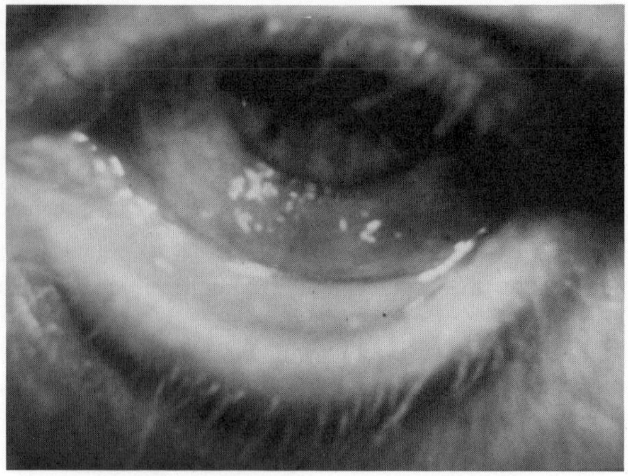

Figure 39-13. Ectropion.

Conjunctiva

Conjunctival lesions may be mistaken for conjunctivitis or completely ignored (Fig. 39-14). A pinguecula (small, yellow, elastic, raised degenerative lesion) nasal to the cornea is only excised if it becomes large and symptomatic—a rare situation. A pterygium may extend from the conjunctiva onto the cornea (Fig. 39-15). If it is enlarging, symptomatic, and encroaching sufficiently upon the cornea, it should be removed. This is done under microscopic control in the operating room after local infiltration of anesthetic. A lamellar keratectomy is carried

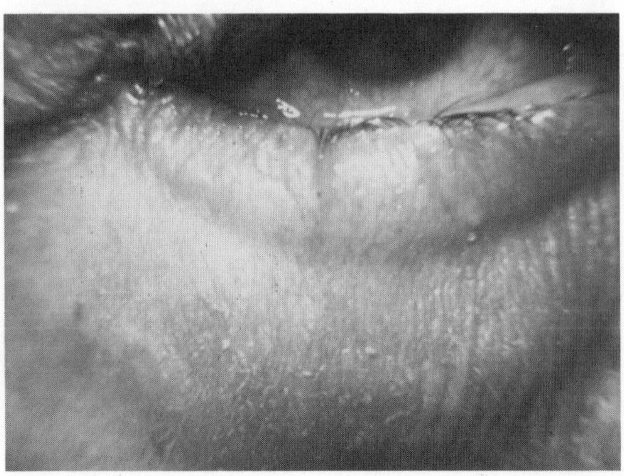

Figure 39-12. Entropion.

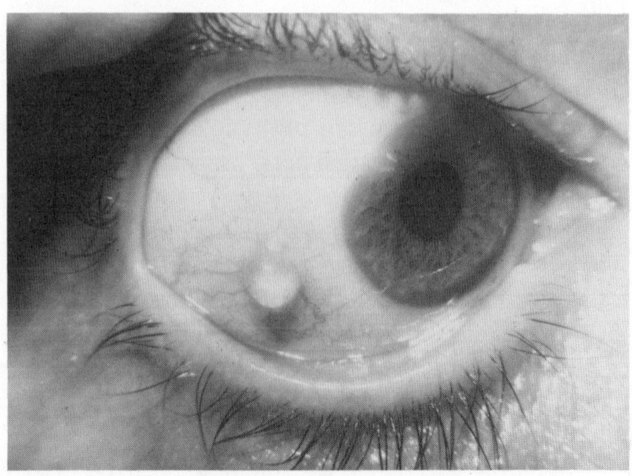

Figure 39-14. Lymphocele.

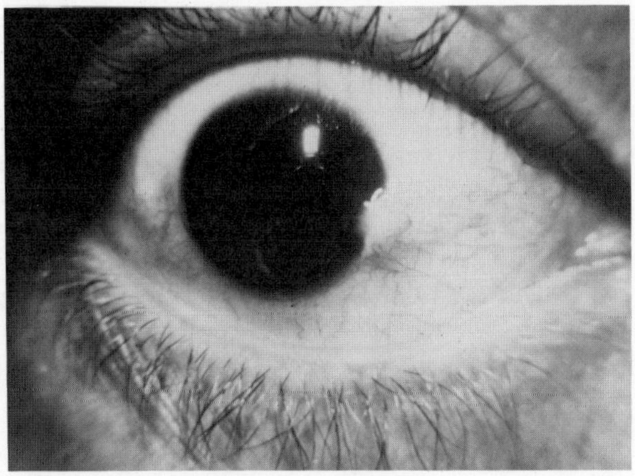

Figure 39-15. Pterygium.

out on the cornea, followed by dissection and excision of the conjunctival component. A patch is placed over the eye overnight. The major intraoperative complication is perforation of the cornea. Postoperatively, the pterygium may recur and require removal and possibly radiation therapy.

Tumors of the conjunctiva require removal if they are enlarging or if malignancy is suspected. Highly malignant tumors may require removal of the eye and orbital exenteration. Bleeding may occur but is of little significance. Excision of large amounts of conjunctiva may cause scarring and retraction, which may be cosmetically disfiguring or may produce limitation of ocular movement.

Orbit

Primary and metastatic tumors, as well as pseudotumors and other inflammatory masses, of the orbit may occur. They may arise in any of the orbital structures or migrate into the orbit from the adjacent sinuses or central nervous system. As with other tumors, some will be sensitive to radiotherapy or chemotherapy. Others will require surgery, usually under general anesthesia.

The approach to orbital tumors depends upon the location in the orbit. If they are relatively anterior, they may be approached anteriorly through the conjunctiva or the lids. If the tumor is posterior, a lateral approach, requiring the removal of a piece of the lateral portion of the bony orbit, or a superior approach through the roof of the orbit may be necessary.

Postoperative care allows for immediate resumption of ambulation and activity. Complications include damage to the eye or to the optic or other nerves in the orbit, damage to the extraocular muscles, or hemorrhage. Postoperatively, infections may occur and require intensive systemic antibiotic therapy. Hemorrhage may occur after surgery and cause sufficient pressure to occlude the central retinal artery resulting in blindness. Recurrence of the tumor and metastasis are significant concerns for the malignant tumors.

Choroidal Melanomas

The surgical management of these tumors is changing. Until recently, the diagnosis of a choroidal melanoma resulted in immediate enucleation of the eye. Although tumor dissemination may occur, alternative treatment modalities are being evaluated. A conservative approach of observation is followed by many ophthalmologists, especially in the very old patient. Newer techniques of radiation therapy are being evaluated as a means of causing tumor regression, with the ability to save the globe and maintain useful or residual vision. The major concern is incomplete removal of the tumor with postoperative spread of the tumor. During enucleation seeding of the tumor may occur.

Enucleation

Enucleation (removal of the entire eye) is carried out for malignant lesions or for blind, painful eyes where medical therapy has failed to provide comfort. Usually the pain in a blind eye (from absolute glaucoma, from degenerative phthisis or from decompensation following eye surgery) may be controlled by giving the patient a retrobulbar injection of about 3 cc of 50% alcohol in the office. The cosmetically unaesthetic blind eye remains. If the alcohol injection is not effective, if there is concern that the blind eye may harbor a tumor, or if the patient is concerned about the poor cosmesis, the eye may be removed.

This surgery may be carried out under local, retrobulbar anesthesia, but many ophthalmologists prefer general anesthesia, feeling that this is better tolerated psychologically. The eye is isolated by making an incision through the conjunctiva around the cornea, isolating and removing the extraocular muscles and severing the optic nerve with long scissors. Cold packs are used for hemostasis, after which the conjunctiva is closed over an orbital implant. A conformer (colored "artificial eye") is placed between the lids in order to match the other eye.

Complications include hemorrhage, possible perforation of the eye, and damage to the eyelid. If the reason for enucleation is the presence of a tumor, there may be seeding of the tumor during the procedure or there may be later spread due to incomplete removal of the tumor. Later, the socket may sink, the implant may extrude, and ptosis (drooping) of the upper lid may occur.

It is important to recognize the chronically painful eye in the poorly communicative older patient to make him or her as comfortable as possible.

Retrobulbar Alcohol Injection

An alternative to enucleation of a blind painful eye is a retrobulbar injection of alcohol. In the office or at the bedside, a retrobulbar 19-gauge needle is used to inject 2 to 3 cc of 2% Xylocaine into the muscle cone. Leaving the needle in place, the syringe is removed and replaced with a syringe containing 5 cc of 50% absolute alcohol. Two to four cubic centimeters are injected into the muscle cone. Normally, there is immediate complete relief of pain. For several hours following the procedure, the patient may have a headache. There may be transient third nerve weakness with ptosis and exotropia. Retrobulbar hemorrhage may occur. The length of effect of the injection of pain relief varies. Occasionally, it may be necessary to repeat the injection if the pain recurs. If the injections do not provide sufficient pain relief, it may be necessary to enucleate the blind, painful eye.

Eye Problems in Nonophthalmic Patients

A patient may require non-ophthalmological surgery but have an ocular problem that the surgeon may wish to have corrected during the same hospitalization or while the patient is already anesthetized if possible. This would result in a significant effort and cost savings for the patient. From the standpoint of a nursing home or extended care facility or the third-party provider, it is important to decrease days away from the facility or in the hospital as much as possible. Duplicate payments for two facilities or loss to one may be significant.

With minor lid procedures and extraocular procedures, it may be possible to perform the eye surgery while under the same anesthetic. This would require prior coordination with the anesthesiologist, since it would be necessary for the ophthalmologist to have access to the head area. It would also require that trained ophthalmic nurses are available for the procedure. In general, the ophthalmic procedure is carried out before or after the general surgical procedure in order to have better control and order in the operating room.

Since many procedures may be performed under local anesthesia, it may be relatively simple to perform the ophthalmic procedure at another time during the hospitalization. With intraocular procedures (e.g., cataract, glaucoma, etc.), it is preferred that they be carried out at a separate time in an eye operating room to minimize the chance of infection from the general surgical procedure. With cataracts, it is usually required to have a complete office evaluation, including refraction and ultrasound, in order to determine the need for surgery and determine and order the correct implant. Since these are usually outpatient procedures, unless there are significant transportation and mobility problems, it may be best to arrange for the intraocular procedure to be performed during a different hospitalization.

Trauma (e.g., falls, auto accidents, etc.), may involve multiple systems. In acute blood loss and other life-threatening situations, it is important to be aware of the eye and to evaluate it for potential damage, which might require immediate care in order to preserve vision. The ophthalmologist must then coordinate the eye care with the general physical care. Each situation is individualized.

Eye Problems Occurring Incidental to Other Surgical Procedures

Many patients come to surgery with contact lenses in place. There are many types of contact lenses available—hard, soft, gas-permeable, daily wear, extended wear, etc. Each has a specific handling method and care regimen. In general, contact lenses should be removed by the patient and kept in the contact lens case with the appropriate soaking solution.

If the patient has not removed the contact lenses prior to surgery, a determination must be made as to the desirability of leaving them in or removing them. In general, it will do no harm to leave the lenses in place for up to several hours. The main concern is to avoid getting any toxic solution on the lenses during surgery. If the anesthetist opens and closes the lids periodically, this should be sufficent to keep the lenses and the cornea lubricated.

If it is desired to remove the lenses, rigid lenses (hard or gas-permeable) may be removed with a contact lens suction cup, whereas soft lenses are grasped between the fingers and removed. Generally, the hard and gas-permeable lenses are thicker and smaller and do not cover the entire cornea; the larger, thinner soft lenses are more difficult to see and usually extend onto the sclera.

If the lenses are removed, it is essential to place them in a container which is marked "Right Eye" or "Left Eye," with the appropriate lens placed in the appropriate container. Inexpensive contact lens cases are available, or paper or medicine cups may be used. The lenses must be hydrated since some of them will dry out and be damaged. Balanced salt solution from the eye room or sterile nonpreserved contact lens saline is used for the container to keep the lenses moist. The labeled container should accompany the patient after leaving the operating room.

The most frequent ocular problem following other surgical procedures is irritation from a corneal abrasion. This may occur from the patient inadvertently rubbing his or her eye when awakening or from the anesthetist or the mask during the procedure. Special concern must be taken to protect the eyes during general anesthesia and to avoid touching the eye when opening the lids to monitor the pupils. Also, the mask must be positioned carefully to avoid touching the eye or putting pressure on the eye.

If it is felt that the lids may be open during the procedure, the cornea should be protected by the use of an ocular lubricant. Since they diffuse over the corneal surface to give protection and still allow the pupils to be seen clearly, 2.5% methylcellulose drops are preferable. Ointments provide protection but often prevent a clear view of the pupils or the fundus. A piece of tape from the upper lid going to the cheek is usually adequate to avoid exposure of the cornea with its resulting exposure keratitis.

Following surgical procedures involving the V or VII cranial nerve, exposure or neurotrophic keratitis may occur. These require intensive lubricant-type medications and may require a tarsorrhaphy. In a tarsorrhaphy, the edges of the lids are denuded and then sutured together to avoid the exposure. Occasionally, the lids are reopened at a later date if lid function is expected to be adequate.

Corneal abrasions usually respond to tight patching for 1 to 2 days with complete relief of symptoms. Under no circumstances should topical anesthetics be used for relief of pain. A collagen shield, which spontaneously dissolves within 24 hours, may be used in conjunction with a tight patch to decrease pain and speed healing. They are only used during ocular evaluation since prolonged use of topical anesthetics may result in severe corneal damage and blindness. Although corneal abrasions usually resolve without incident, they may become chronic in the form of recurrent corneal erosion. This condition of poor healing of the cornea results in recurrent irritation of the eye and breakdown of the corneal surface. Repeated patching, corneal debridement, and use of ointments may be required.

Especially in neurosurgical and orthopedic procedures in which the patient may require positioning in the face down position, special care is necessary to avoid pressure on the eye. Prolonged pressure on the globe may result in closure of the central retinal artery and blindness. If the artery does close, there is no adequate treatment to restore vision. The best treatment is prevention.

In a patient with an eye that has a shallow anterior chamber and an anatomical predisposition, angle-closure glaucoma may be precipitated by pupillary dilatation, which may be related to systemic medications, such as atropine, or to pupillary changes during the various stages of anesthesia. Prompt recognition is important for institution of the treatments discussed earlier in this chapter.

Upon awakening or afterwards, patients may complain of painless loss of total or partial vision. This may be coincidental to the procedure or directly related. Following carotid or other vascular surgery, emboli to the eye or brain may be responsible for this. Following facial or neurosurgical procedures, double vision may occur from involvement of the ocular nerves or from damage during the procedure. The double vision may be immediately eliminated by patching either eye until the patient is evaluated. Usually time is necessary for resolution of the double vision if it is to recover.

Ocular problems may precede the surgery, especially in trauma and neurosurgical patients, but may not have been diagnosed. This presents a potentially difficult medicolegal situation that, often, could have been avoided. In any of the above situations, it is important to have an evaluation by the ophthalmologist as early as possible. In addition to management of the specific problem with possible relief of pain and/or possible maintenance or restoration of vision, the involvement of the ophthalmologist may make the patient and family feel more comfortable and may avoid medicolegal problems in the future.

Summary

Eye problems in the elderly are frequent but are also frequently amenable to amelioration, usually in an outpatient setting and often under local anesthesia. All who care for geriatric patients should learn to talk to their patients about visual problems and to examine the eyes. Correction of these common disorders may result in dramatic improvement in quality of life.

40

Oral and Maxillofacial Surgery of the Elderly

Nalton F. Ferraro and R. Bruce Donoff

As the specialty of oral and maxillofacial surgery changes, so changes the services and treatments that it can offer the elderly. But a knowledge of operations and treatment certainly is not enough when they are applied to any specific group in the population. The treatment must be viewed from a perspective that includes the biologic, psychologic, and social changes in the elderly, the risks versus benefits of the treatment we offer, and the natural history of the ailment that we treat.

With this perspective two important things happen: the elderly patient will not be put at risk simply because an innovation is available, and at the same time elderly patients will not be denied treatments that can substantially improve the quality of life simply because "they are too old" to undergo treatment. A constant tension, then, is created between the surgeon's wanting to intervene and "leaving well enough alone." Even in nonelective treatments, the pressure to simply compromise in the elderly is present. At times compromise is appropriate and sometimes it is not necessary. We will be coming back constantly to this point as specific aspects of surgery are discussed.

At first mention of oral surgery in the elderly, one thinks of dental extractions and a few procedures to help dentures fit better (preprosthetic procedures). It is important to underscore that while this forms an important cornerstone of our treatment of the elderly, it is by no means all that is offered.

Oral Health of the Elderly

The dental needs of the elderly were and are significant. In a study of the population over 65 years, the National Center for Health Statistics showed that 46% were edentulous and of the remaining group 50% had periodontal disease (1).

Another study from Canada, looking at 250 residents of a long-term care institution aged 64 to 95+ years, showed that 43% were on medicines that have oral side-effects (anticholinergics, antihistamines, sedatives, hypnotics, phenothiazines) (2). Complaints and symptoms in that population included denture difficulties, chewing difficulties, oral hygiene difficulties, mouth dryness, restricted opening, toothaches, temporomandibular clicking, clenching and bruxing, and oral ulcers.

A recent study by the U.S. Department of Agriculture Human Nutrition Research Center on Aging at Tufts University "found that tooth loss was a better predictor in inadequate nutrition than demographic factors such as living alone or being homebound" (3). The group, however, pointed out that edentulism has declined 10% in the past decade.

Generalizations that are broadly accepted regarding the mouth and face of the elderly include:

1. loss of teeth
2. atrophy of the oral mucosa
3. increased cervical caries
4. atrophy of the orofacial musculature
5. alteration in the amount and composition of saliva
6. wear of the hard tissue
7. decreased sense of smell and taste

Baum (4) investigates these generalizations and refutes some of them, but there are other studies that reinforce these generalizations.

For example, Shklar (5) studied 300 oral mucosal biopsies and noted some significant differences over the age of 60, among them thinner epithelium, increased keratinization, increased epithelial glycogen, and atrophy of the salivary gland tissue.

The alveolar bone undergoes osteoporosis, with decreased osteoblast activity. Interestingly, it is noted to be similar to the antianabolic activity noted with corticosteroid, estrogen deprivation, and radiation. "In aging, the equilibrium shifts towards resorptive activity because the activity of the osteoblastic cells is depressed. Then, the antianabolic activity produces bone resorption. The endosteal surfaces of bone are more sensitive to metabolic influences than the periosteal surfaces, and extensive bone loss occurs primarily within the tissue rather than at the surface" (6). This results in osteoporotic bone, which is less resistant to trauma, inflammation, or disease.

Tissue healing is often depressed in old age, "particularly in the restoration of alveolar bone following injury or surgical intervention" (7).

Shklar (6) also emphasizes some oral disorders associated with old age: attrition of teeth, chronic periodontal disease, xerostomia, mucositis and mucosal atrophy, leukoplakia, and malignant disease. In association with the xerostomia, salivary gland stasis and infection, and root caries should be added.

Silverman (8) called attention to some ailments that can be very distressing to the elderly. Burning mouth is such an example, possibly related to depression, medicines, and oral candidiasis.

The above are mentioned as examples of relatively common complaints in the elderly. For some of these, of course, there is no surgical cure. This is all the more reason to understand the complex changes and needs in these patients. For example, the use of artificial saliva or liquid dietary supplement in a patient with dry mouth who is undergoing oral surgery may make recovery and hygiene easier. Another example: one patient with sore mouth and ill-fitting dentures may benefit from a preprosthetic procedure, whereas another patient with denture complaints and burning mouth may need treatment for depression and, at least initially, not preprosthetic surgery.

Medical Considerations in the Elderly Oral Surgical Patient

The Federal Council on Aging notes that 86% of older adults have at least one chronic disease (9). This is particularly important for the oral and maxillofacial surgeon to note because in very few specialties do patients come in and present themselves for a surgical procedure with only a brief referral note. Often the patient may have had to secure transportation and make other arrangements for the appointment, and they are very disappointed if the procedure is not going to be done that day. "Doctor, I was so hoping you could do the extractions today."

The best advice here is be loathe to compromise regarding the patient's overall health. Know the patient's history, his or her medicines, and idiosyncracies. This means a good history from the patient, exam, vital signs, communication with the family, patient's physicians and dentist, and review of the medical record.

It is this insight that will enable the best oral surgical care to be given. One must know about the severity of the patient's medical history. The patient may overstate or understate. There may be important issues regarding compliance, care at home, and follow-up. Only when these are known can the decision regarding when, where, and how to treat a patient be made accurately.

When doubt occurs as to whether a patient should be treated in an office setting or hospital, one should choose the hospital, even though expense and administrative details are increased.

Local anesthesia will usually be preferred, but some authors such as Laskin (10) state "age alone is not necessarily a contraindication to carefully used sedation techniques or even general anesthesia, provided dosage is properly adjusted.

Because amide-type local anesthetics are transformed within the liver, potentially significant increase in half-life can occur in older patients (9). The range that is used for most outpatient oral surgical procedures (100 to 200 mg of lidocaine) is quite safe.

Bennett (11) notes that in patients with heart disease, the total amount of epinephrine used for vasoconstriction should be limited to 0.04 mg (4 cc of a 1:100,000 solution). The question regarding epinephrine use in certain patients is essentially unresolved and will be until total endogenous production perioperatively (which is probably significant) can be compared to the exogenous total. Epinephrine as vasoconstrictor should be avoided in patients with known significant tachyarrhythmias, hyperthyroidism, or uncontrolled hypertension, as well as those on monoamine oxidase inhibitors, guanethidine, or reserpine. Other patients of concern should be discussed with the physician involved.

A high index of suspicion should be kept for certain clinical situations that might predispose a patient to complications even with a relatively minor oral surgical procedure. These include:

1. The patient who is recovering from a myocardial infarction within the last 6 months
2. Any evidence at all of unstable and changing angina
3. Aortic stenosis
4. Decreased pulmonary reserve, wheezing, smoking, any patient who has tachypnea as they are sitting in

the office or when they are speaking, evidence of low exercise tolerance, e.g., walking up one flight of stairs

5. Evidence of significant cardiac arrhythmias that are not well controlled with medicine
6. Less than well-controlled hypertension—blood pressure greater than 160/100
7. Evidence of congestive heart failure with distended neck veins, peripheral edema
8. Evidence of any unexplained neurologic events (blackouts, unexplained fall, temporary loss of vision, clumsy hand, slurred speech, new headache, sensory deficits, or neuralgias)
9. Severe rheumatoid disease with jaw hypomobility, cervical disease
10. Use of multiple medicines, especially if they include diuretics, digoxin, phenothiazines, tricyclic antidepressants, antihypertensives, anti-arrhythmics, steroids, insulin, aminophylline, sympathomimetics, anticoagulants
11. Less than well-controlled diabetes with episodes of hypoglycemia or diabetic ketoacidosis
12. Evidence of malnutrition and dehydration with poor skin turgor, recent weight loss
13. Evidence of hyperthyroidism (can be subtle in the elderly)
14. Evidence of depression, alcoholism, drug abuse, or other psychiatric disease
15. Severe osteoporosis

Specific Oral and Maxillofacial Problems and Their Treatments

Dental Pathology, Extraction, Alveoloplasty

Whatever else oral and maxillofacial surgeons do, the elimination of pain and infection caused by hopelessly carious or periodontally involved teeth is a most important function. While nutrition can be maintained in the edentulous, it is the chronically infected patient with toothaches who is at great risk.

The elderly tolerate removal of teeth quite well. If several need to be removed, sometimes it is best to stage them in the outpatient setting; but for some patients, especially if there are associated medical problems, hospitalization is necessary.

Several points of advice:

1. Loose teeth: the vast majority are secondary to periodontal disease, but unusual bone loss or gingival change could represent metastatic disease or other infiltrative lesions.
2. Associated alveoloplasty should be conservative, but sharp spots should be eliminated since remodeling of the bone takes a substantial length of time.
3. Extraction of one standing molar in thinned maxillary alveolus can result in fractures of large sections of the maxillary alveolus. Removal of such teeth should be done with minimal force.
4. Impacted teeth without associated pathology (e.g., cysts) are often very difficult to remove and, in fact, finding a plane between the tooth and sclerotic bone might not be possible. Such teeth are best left alone, unless they are imminently interfering with a prosthesis. Impacted teeth without associated pathology should not be blamed for facial pain until other sources are ruled out.
5. Ecchymosis is common after multiple extractions, especially if mucoperiosteal flaps must be developed or if aspirin products have been taken. The patient should be warned regarding this.
6. Communicate freely with the prosthodontist regarding the prosthetic requirements.

Odontogenic Infection

Odontogenic infections certainly occur at any age, but there are special considerations in the elderly. Some have already been mentioned. The mucosal changes, the bony changes, and the fragility of the tissue will certainly affect spread of infection.

Makinodon and Kay (12) discern a "decline in immunologic vigor." These authors note that this is a characteristic of aging mammals and has been observed in humans and experimental animals including the mouse, rat, hamster, guinea pig, rabbit, and dog. The salivary changes have a deleterious effect since saliva does perform some immunologic and bacterial inhibitory functions.

There is an increase in root caries with increased *Streptococcus mutans,* lactobacillis, filamentous bacteria, and diphtheroids. Deep periodontal pockets contain multiple anaerobes. Also, adults over 50 years are more prone to suprainfection (e.g., candidiasis) (13).

The likelihood is also high that the patient may be dehydrated and malnourished as a baseline, and there will often be associated medical problems, with less reserve.

These factors can result in the spread of infection in a rather alarming fashion. The unilateral submandibular infection becomes a Ludwig angina quickly. One author has seen a periapical infection from a lower incisor track along the space of the body of the mandible and cause a life-threatening parapharyngeal and parotid space infection. The organism was a coagulase-positive *Staphylococcus.*

The treatment of infection, then, must be decisive. Antibiotics and timely surgical intervention, correction of dehydration without causing fluid overload or hyponatremia, and correction of uncontrolled underlying medical problems (e.g., diabetes) are all crucial.

General anesthesia and intubation often need to be performed under very adverse circumstances. The airway may be compromised with the added concerns of poor toleration of hypoxia and myocardial depressant drugs. Also, the fragility of the tissues can add to the problems. A recent report discusses retropharyngeal abscess and hematoma in an elderly woman on anticoagulants following esophagoscopy and endotracheal intubation (14). Early anesthetic consultation is important.

The surgical approaches for drainage of infection are the same as for younger patients. In the patient with facial swelling and deep infection, but endentulous mouth, a careful clinical and radiographic exam must be made to rule out tumors, impacted teeth with cysts, or other pathologic entities such as ameloblastoma, occult pathologic fractures, or salivary gland disease. Three examples from the author's experience illustrate this point. A patient presented with a pterygomandibular space infection from an infected dentigerous cyst in the ramus. Another elderly patient presented with a full-blown Ludwig angina secondary to an obstructed submandibular salivary gland from sialolithiasis (Fig. 40-1). A third patient was admitted with trismus and parapharyngeal infection secondary to an invasive squamous cell carcinoma of the pharynx.

The more uncommon infections are well covered by Topazian (13), including fungal infections, which can develop at any age but certainly are of great concern in the elderly, especially if there is concurrent disease such as diabetes.

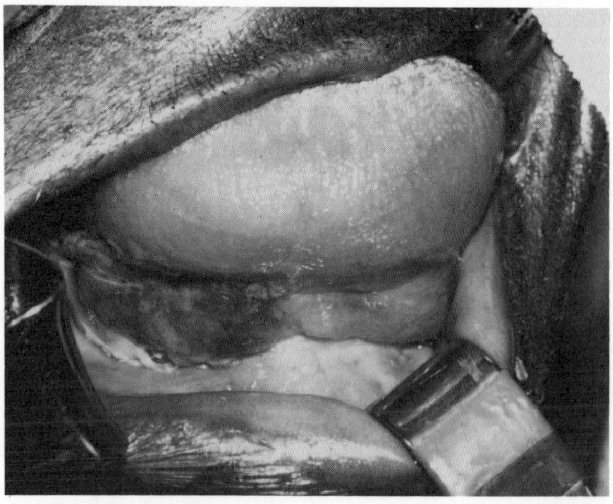

Figure 40-1. Swelling of the tongue and floor of mouth in Ludwig's angina.

Aspergillosis with sinus, nasal, and orbital involvement can present with nasal discharge, sinusitis, and facial swelling.

A particularly fearsome disease is mucormycosis (phycomycosis). The symptoms and signs may involve the maxilla, the palate, nose, and sinuses with ulcerations, swelling, and frank necrosis. It can extend intracranially rapidly. Dehydrated, acidotic patients (especially diabetics) are at risk.

Another infection that must be mentioned is erysipelas, which can often involve the face and is a rapidly spreading streptococcal cellulitis. The spreading pink or red infection has sharply demarcated borders on the skin. Toxic and constitutional symptoms and signs are common, and patients can be very ill. Group A beta-hemolytic streptococcus is implicated, and treatment is with antibiotics.

Osteomyelitis of the Jaws

Acute osteomyelitis can occur as a sequel to odontogenic infection. Pain, swelling, erythema, and possibly drainage can be seen. The radiographic picture will include rarefaction and sequestration. Treatment will include antibiotics, transoral debridement, sequestrectomy, and decortication with closure of mucosa over drains (15). At times, resection must be carried out. A continuity defect can be stabilized with intermaxillary fixation or external skeletal pin fixation. Hyperbaric oxygen therapy may be of some use.

Any of the oral flora can be implicated. Particular attention must be paid to the oral anaerobes, *Staphylococcus* and *Actinomyces israelii*. Actinomycosis can be indolent, producing swelling, osseocutaneous sinus tracts, and osteolysis.

Sclerosing osteomyelitis affects females more than males, especially after the age of 50 years. The cause may be an infected tooth. Rather than rarefaction and drainage, a sclerosis of the affected bone occurs. The symptoms can include pain with enlargement of the affected jaw. Removing the focus of infection is primary treatment. Decortication might be needed . . . but observation may be all that is needed. An acute exacerbation requires long-term antibiotic therapy after biopsy and culture.

Osteoradionecrosis of the Jaws

Radiation for head and neck tumors results in several tissue changes locally. The end result is that the tissues become hypovascular, hypocellular, and hypoxic (16). Tissue repair and anabolism cannot keep pace with catabolism. Minor trauma to the tissues around the jaws does not heal, and exposed bone results. Marx's work (16) shows that osteoradionecrosis is not a primary infection but an ischemic process (Fig 40-2). Superficial infection with bacteria is secondary and is often only colonization; therefore, antibiotics are not the key to treatment.

Prevention is most important. Removal of a questionable tooth or teeth in the line of radiation should be done at least 2 weeks in advance of radiation. Maintenance of the teeth afterward with regular dental care, fluoride, and meticulous avoidance of denture sores is a must.

Both the Marx study (16) and the M.D. Anderson (17) study show that osteoradionecrosis of the jaws is preceded in two-thirds of the cases by extractions or denture sores.

Once the jaws have been irradiated, especially if greater than 6,000 rads or implants have been used, tooth removal carries the hazard of leaving nonhealing bone and mucosal wounds. If teeth must be removed, pretreatment with hyperbaric oxygen and antibiotics may be very helpful (18).

Treatment of established osteoradionecrosis involves hyperbaric oxygen, debridement, and local resections.

Osseocutaneous fistulae, pathologic fractures, and large areas of involved bone almost always necessitate resection. Reconstruction can be done with bone grafts and adjunctive hyperbaric oxygen (18) or with microvascular free flaps to bring in bone (19) and/or soft tissue.

Salivary Gland Disease

The salivary glands atrophy with age. The acinar cells of the glands can become hyperchromatic and the acini are replaced by connective or adipose tissue with a decrease in glandular tissue. Less saliva is produced (6). The decreased flow coupled with dehydration leads to stasis and obstruction with and without stone formation.

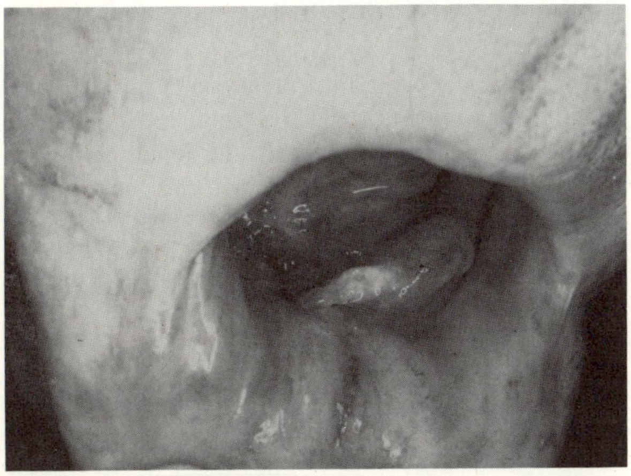

Figure 40-2. Exposed bone of the mandibular symphysis in osteoradionecrosis.

Parotid or submandibular gland swelling of relatively rapid onset, perhaps with increased tenderness during meals, is consistent with obstruction. The examination of such patients includes careful palpation of the tissues in the preauricular area and overlying the posterior ramus and angle of the mandible. Stensen's duct can be palpated on the cheek by rolling the finger over the masseter muscle. At times, a stone within Stensen's duct may be palpable. The deep lobe of the parotid gland is palpated intraorally at the level of the anterior tonsillar pillar. The submandibular gland is best palpated bimanually with a gloved finger in the lateral floor of the mouth and the second hand underneath the gland in the submandibular region. The whole of Wharton's duct may be palpated in the floor of the mouth. The sublingual gland is in the floor of the mouth along Wharton's duct. Areas of greatest density of minor salivary gland tissue are the mid- and posterior palate, the lower lip, and the retromolar pad.

Plain films such as posteroanterior view of the head, panorex, or radiographs of the cheek with an intraoral film may be used to delineate parotid stones, and occlusal film of the floor of the mouth is excellent for detecting stones in the submandibular duct. Forty percent of the stones in the parotid gland are radiolucent compared to 20% of submandibular stones (20). Of all salivary stones, 10% occur in the parotid gland and 83% in the submandibular gland (21) (Fig. 40-3).

The search for stones, therefore, will be more rewarding in the submandibular gland. Computed tomography (CT) scans will help delineate the gland, degree of enlargement, masses present, and stones. Sialography will demonstrate duct anatomy, obstructions, and condition of the parenchyma, but it should not be performed in the acutely inflamed gland.

Obstruction must be relieved, and a combination of methods is needed. Rehydration, instrumentation and di-

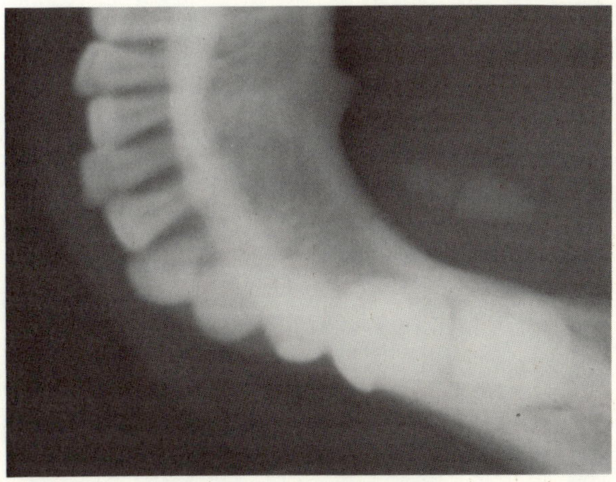

Figure 40-3. A submandibular sialolith.

latation of the duct, and sialolithectomy are the cornerstones of therapy. Hard, sour, sugarless candies may be used to help stimulate salivary flow. Stasis and obstruction lead to retrograde bacterial invasion and infection, with all the sequelae of septic sialadenitis. Already mentioned was a Ludwig angina secondary to submandibular sialolithiasis.

Septic parotitis can be a severe disease in the elderly, with great toxicity, inanition, extension of infection into the neck and chest, and death. Severe pain, tenderness, erythema, fever, and leukocytosis are the hallmarks of the illness. Pus may or may not be expressible from Stensen's duct (Fig. 40-4). The presentation is a debilitated, relatively dehydrated elderly patient often on diuretics, antihistamines, or anticholinergics. Sometimes, the patients are postoperative, hospitalized patients.

Many bacteria have been implicated, but one must always cover for *Staphylococcus* infection since this is a common organism and is associated with high morbidity. Twenty percent of the patients have bilateral disease (13).

Aggressive, supportive care and antibiotics are mandatory. The decision to operate can be difficult since fluctuance rarely develops early in the parotid with its dense fibrous septae (22). Stensen's duct may not offer adequate drainage. In a patient who is worsening, despite adequate treatment, the gland must be directly drained.

Hemenway and English (22) review three reports on techniques of operative drainage. Lilienthal (23) in 1917 described developing a skin flap (similar to parotidectomy) and then making multiple incisions in the gland parallel to the branches of the facial nerve and Stensen's duct. The fascia posteromedial to the mandible was opened, and the wound was packed.

Blair and Padgett (24) described a similar approach, safeguarding the facial nerve by puncturing the gland with a blunt forceps. The wound was packed open. Perzik (25) notes that swelling, hyperemia, edema, and fever were his

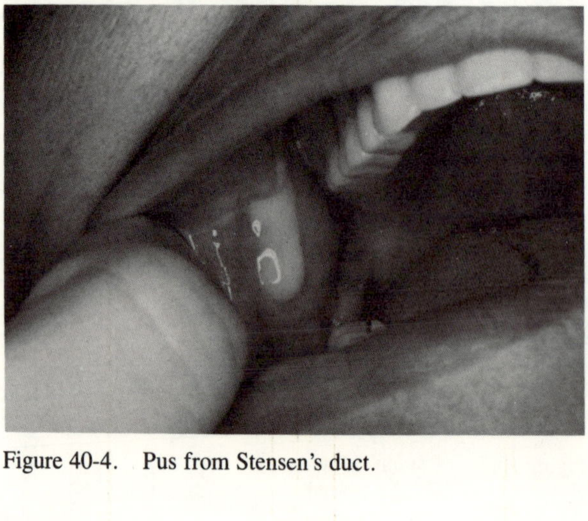

Figure 40-4. Pus from Stensen's duct.

indications to operate. A cloudy serum is present at this point within the gland and paraglandular spaces. His procedure included drainage of the surrounding fascial spaces.

After submandibular space drainage and treatment of the acute submandibular gland infection, intermittent swelling and tenderness of the gland may continue, necessitating removal; this can be made more difficult because of surrounding postinflammatory scarring. The earlier removal of an intermittently obstructing submandibular gland may be the more prudent and easier option.

Other Conditions of the Salivary Glands

Recurrent parotitis may herald Sjögren's syndrome. The full-blown disorder involves keratoconjunctivitis sicca, xerostomia, and another rheumatoid disease, often rheumatoid arthritis. Shearn (26) reported that parotid swelling can recur 2 to 24 years before the onset of ocular or systemic disease; the mean was 9 years. The dry mouth can aggravate denture wearing and caries. The swelling may be intermittent, but a gradual enlargement of the gland occurs (27). The sialogram pattern is quite characteristic of sialectasis that can progress from punctate to globular to cavitary to destructive pattern (20).

Minor salivary gland biopsy, usually the lower lip glands, is usually advocated to help confirm the diagnosis of Sjögren's syndrome. Bertram and Hjorting-Hansen (28) reported that 85% of a group of patients with Sjögren's syndrome exhibited minor salivary gland changes similar to those seen in major glands. The lower lip glands are subject to low-grade inflammation from lip biting or dentures; therefore, biopsy of the parotid gland has a theoretical advantage. The parotid gland would also show formation of epimyoepithelial islands, which do not develop in the minor glands.

One technique used by the author for parotid gland biopsy utilizes a 1.5-cm incision just behind the inferior attachment of the auricle. The dissection is carried anteriorly through the parotid fascia into parenchyma; at this point it is lateral to the facial nerve trunk. It is emphasized that this technique is not indicated for tumor biopsy but only for diffuse bilateral enlargements as seen in Sjögren's syndrome or sarcoidosis. Caution should also be exercised regarding new enlargement of an already enlarged gland in a known Sjögren's syndrome patient; it could represent lymphoma (29).

Benign lymphoepithelial lesion, Mikulicz's disease, is probably related to Sjögren's syndrome. In both cases, the patient's salivary tissue becomes antigenic. Parotid and/or submandibular salivary gland enlargement with some discomfort and xerostomia is noted. Histology shows orderly lymphocytic infiltration replacing acini with persistence of islands of epithelial cells (30, p. 243). At times, excision has been used for persistent gland enlargement. Radiation therapy is no longer used for Sjögren's syndrome or Mikulicz's disease.

Sialosis (sialadenosis) is a noninflammatory, nonneoplastic, bilateral parotid enlargement. The condition can be seen with cirrhosis, diabetes, ovarian and thyroid insufficiency, alcoholism, and malnutrition. Enlargement of acinar cells with loss of granules and fatty infiltration of the gland occurs (21, p. 101). There is no specific treatment, but parotid biopsy may confirm the diagnosis.

Oncocytosis, a replacement of ductal or acinar epithelium by oncocytes, occurs with aging. There is no known pathologic significance (21, p. 102).

Necrotizing sialometaplasia is a benign inflammatory reaction of salivary gland tissue that mimics a salivary gland malignancy. Abrams (31) first reported the condition in 1973. The mechanism appears to be an ischemic necrosis. The palate is the most common location, but other intraoral sites of minor salivary gland tissue, such as cheek, lip, and retromolar pads, have been involved. The parotid location has also been reported (30, p. 253). The lesion presents as an ulcer, often preceded by a swelling. It may require debridement but is generally self-limited. It is mentioned because it can be confused with a malignancy.

Tumors of the salivary glands are a topic well covered in the literature (21). There are some very important clinical statistics that must be borne in mind when one is examining a patient with a salivary gland mass.

The mass may be located wherever there is salivary tissue. Ectopic gland, however, has been found in the nasopharynx and even centrally within the jaws.

Eighty percent of salivary tumors occur in the parotid, 5% to 10% in the submandibular gland, less than 1% in the sublingual gland, and 10% to 15% percent in the minor glands (32). However, the incidence of malignancy by site is 20% parotid, 40% submandibular gland, and 70% sublingual gland (33). A salivary mass in the palate has a 50% chance of being malignant (34).

Oral Pathologic Entities of Particular Concern in the Elderly

Cutaneous and Mucocutaneous Lesions

Solar or actinic keratoses often affect the skin of the face and lips. Sun exposure is an important etiologic factor. The lower lip is by far the most affected. Significant keratotic changes and/or a blending or obscuring of the red lip-skin border is precancerous and responds to vermilionectomy (lip shave), followed by measures to protect the lip from further sun (hat visors, sun screens). Ulcerations may represent epidermoid carcinoma. Smoking, especially pipe smoking, is also an etiologic factor (35).

Keratoacanthoma occurs on the cheeks, nose, dorsum of the hands, and the lips. It develops an umbilicated or crateriform appearance and rarely has a diameter greater than 1.5 cm. It develops quickly and can remain 4 to 8 weeks. It is important because of its clinical histologic similarity to squamous cell carcinoma (10).

Angular cheilitis (perléche) is a wrinkling and maceration of the corners of the mouth (Fig. 40-5). It can progress to deep fissuring that stops at the mucocutaneous junction. Symptoms of dryness and a burning sensation at the corners of the mouth may be present. Suggestions regarding etiology include decreased vertical height because of tooth loss or lack of denture height, infection with *Candida albicans* (*Staphylococcus* and *Streptococcus* have also been cultured), and riboflavin deficiency (30, p. 556).

Lichen planus is a disease seen in skin and has an oral counterpart (Fig. 40-6). The majority of patients with dermal lichen planus have associated oral lesions (36). A study by Andreasen (37) showed that only 44% of 115 patients with oral lichen planus had skin lesions.

Oral lichen planus is characterized by gray or white lacelike lesions, in reticular, linear, or annular patterns, on the oral mucosa, particularly over the cheeks. It is often seen in high-strung individuals. It can be erosive and ulcerative. Particular mention is made of lichen planus because there is some evidence that long-standing lichen planus, especially the erosive type, can undergo malignant transformation (38). Close monitoring is necessary for long-standing lichen planus patients with a low threshold to biopsy ulcerations or other transformations of clinical concern.

Leukoplakia is a white patch on the oral mucosa. It can occur anywhere in the mouth, but typically on the

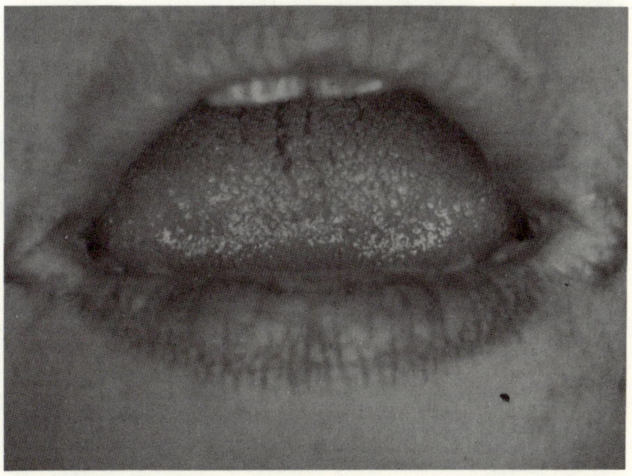

Figure 40-5. Angular cheilitis.

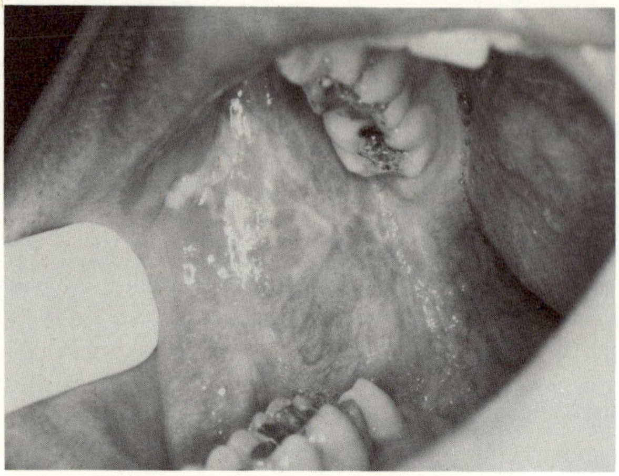

Figure 40-6. Lichen planus of the cheek mucosa.

buccal mucosa and lateral tongue (Fig. 40-7). It can range from delicate to rather thick lesions. The term specifically excludes all definite entities exhibiting white lesions (for example, lichen planus, syphilitic mucous patches, white sponge nevus), and refers to a hyperkeratosis of the mucosa. Of concern is the histologic appearance of dysplasia in some white lesions and therefore the possibility of cancerous transformation.

Etiologic factors include tobacco, alcohol, and chronic irritation from jagged teeth, ill-fitting dentures, possibly vitamin A deficiency, and syphilis. The presence of *Candida* is a frequent finding with leukoplakia. Renstrup (39) reported finding epithelial atypia in 56% of patients who showed candidal invasion. The *Candida*-leukoplakia relationship is not fully established. One cannot determine which white lesions are dysplastic on the basis of clinical appearance; even spot biopsies may miss areas of dysplasia. Small lesions can be entirely excised, and large lesions that have dysplasia can be treated by multiple staged excision procedures, sometimes with skin grafting. Cryosurgery and laser therapy can remove the lesions very well; however, cryosurgery and laser treatment of whole areas can destroy the histopathologic evidence. Assuming multiple incisional biopsies do not show dysplasia, lesions can be followed clinically at frequent intervals. Cytologic examination with Papanicolaou smear and vital staining (toluidine blue) have also been advocated. However, in any of these three methods, there is the chance of missing areas of dysplasia.

Most importantly, the patients must stop using tobacco products, stop drinking alcohol, and repair teeth and dentures.

Erythroplakia, a red atrophic lesion, has a much higher chance of being precancerous. Any erythroplakic lesion that does not involute 2 to 3 weeks after stopping an irritant must be removed. Erythroplakia in the floor of the mouth is particularly prone to cancerous transformation, and these lesions must be treated quickly and aggressively. Surgical excision, cryosurgery, or laser therapy may be used.

Malignant Tumors

Squamous cell carcinoma is the most common malignant tumor of the oral cavity (Fig. 40-8). Over 65% of the tumors are diagnosed between 50 and 79 years of age (40). Etiologic factors are the same as those mentioned for leukoplakia and actinic keratosis. Krolls and Hoffman (40) report the distribution of oral cancer as given in Table 40-1.

The usual presentation is an ulcer, painless or painful, often with slightly raised borders. Despite the accessibility of most of the oral cavity for examination, patients often present with tumors in an advanced stage. Despite advances in surgical resection, radiation, and chemotherapy, oral cancer still has an uncertain prognosis, particularly with larger lesions. Local recurrences,

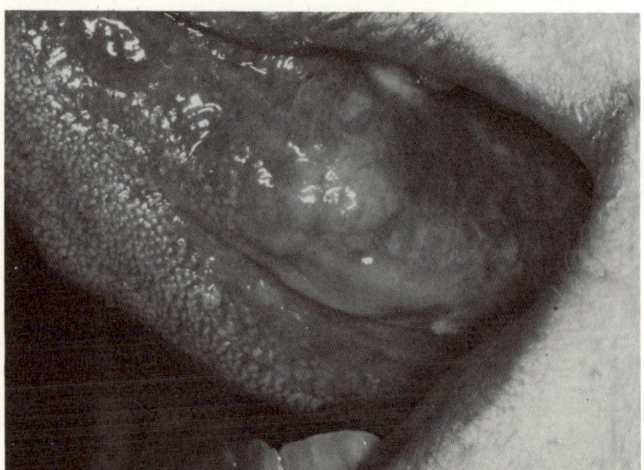

Figure 40-7. Leukoplakia of lateral border of tongue.

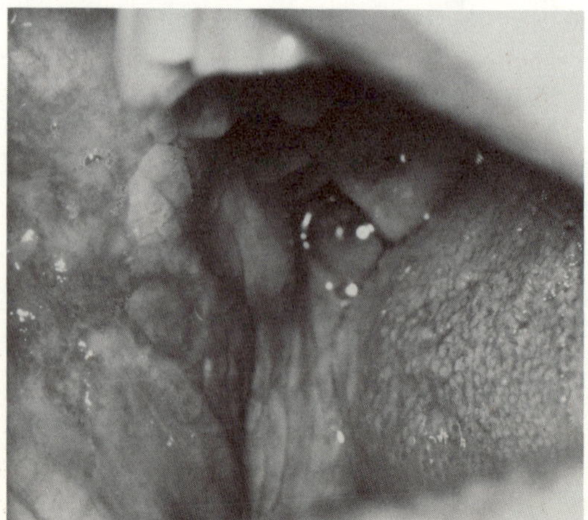

Figure 40-8. Squamous cell carcinoma of cheek.

Table 40-1. Anatomic distribution of oral cancer

Including lower lip	Excluding lips
Lower lip—38%	Tongue—38%
Tongue—22%	Floor of mouth—30%
Floor of mouth—17%	Gingiva—11%
Gingiva—6%	Palate—9%
Upper lip—4%	Tonsil—8%
Buccal musoca—2%	Buccal mucosa—3%
Uvula—0.5%	Uvula—1%
Tonsil—5%	

From Krolls and Hoffman (40).

field cancerization, neck metastases, and continuation of destructive habits (for example, smoking) can be seen.

Verrucous carcinoma is generally slow growing, exophytic, papillary, and initially superficial. The mean age of occurrence is 60 to 70 years. Seventy-five percent are present in males. Usually they occur on the buccal mucosa, gingiva, or alveolar ridge. An etiologic factor is tobacco chewing and snuff dipping. Treatment is generally by surgical excision.

Disease of the Jaws

Fibrosarcoma can be seen in old age (41). Periosteal fibrosarcomas develop outward from the bone and produce a soft-tissue mass, often ulcerated and adherent to the underlying bone. Radiolucency can be seen.

Primary interosseous carcinoma is rare and usually occurs in the mandible and presents as a radiolucency. The majority of cases are diagnosed in the 6th and 7th decades (42, p. 42), and the prognosis is poor. Carcinoma can also develop in long-standing odontogenic cysts. Poorly differentiated lymphomas can be seen within the jaws, causing pain and loosening teeth (Fig. 40-9, A-C). Multiple myeloma can involve the jaws, with swelling, loosening of teeth, and sensory changes (for example, paresthesia in the mental nerve distribution). Radiographs show lytic lesions, but expansion of the bone is not seen.

Other tumors that are metastatic to the jaws include thyroid, lung, renal cell, and breast cancers. Prostate cancer can also be metastatic to the jaw, exhibiting radiopaque metastases within the bone. The other tumors are generally radiolucent. Certainly, when there are osteolytic lesions in an older age group, these metastatic lesions must be considered.

Benign Lesions of the Jaws

Dentigerous cysts associated with impacted teeth may develop insidiously over a long period of time. They cause bone expansion and destruction, but maxillary cysts may be difficult to delineate on plain film. They can be noted incidentally on radiographic exam or noted on clinical

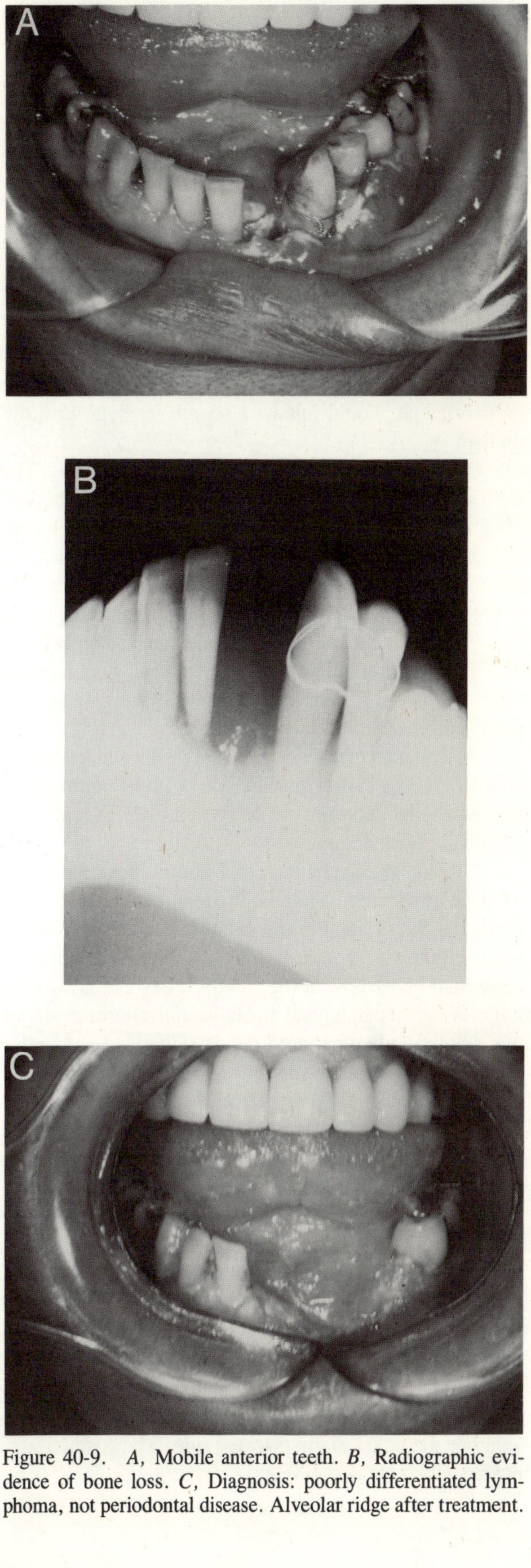

Figure 40-9. *A*, Mobile anterior teeth. *B*, Radiographic evidence of bone loss. *C*, Diagnosis: poorly differentiated lymphoma, not periodontal disease. Alveolar ridge after treatment.

exam because of bone expansion. Infection, swelling, and pathologic fracture also can bring the patient to attention.

Marsupialization of a large cyst may be tried to decrease its size, but enucleation with primary closure of the mucosa is done very readily and is tolerated well by the older patient. If the wound dehisces, then packing will be needed as it heals. The risk of pathologic fracture may necessitate a blenderized diet for several weeks.

The finding of a giant cell lesion either on the gingiva or within the jaw raises the possibility of hyperparathyroidism, and tests for serum calcium, phosphorus, and alkaline phosphatase levels and parathormone levels are needed to rule this out. The presentation may be a jaw radiolucency. Loss of the lamina dura around the teeth on radiograph should initiate a search for hyperparathyroidism.

Paget's disease of the bone can enlarge the jaws. The teeth may spread, and radiographically there will be loss of lamina dura and development of periapical radiolucencies, but osteosclerosis then occurs, with its characteristic cotton-wool appearance on radiograph. Hypercementosis at the roots may occur. The maxilla is more frequently involved than the mandible, and there can be frontal bossing. The serum alkaline phosphatase level may be very high. Giant cell lesions can be seen in the patient with Paget's disease.

After dental extractions, expect prolonged healing of the sockets with Paget's disease. Partial resections may be needed so that dentures can be accommodated if there is significant bone enlargement (42, p. 180).

Ameloblastoma, which is a benign but locally aggressive tumor more common in the mandible, may be of particular importance in the elderly. The average age of presentation is 38.9 years (42, p. 82), but they can persist, recur, and be present in the elderly. They can grow very large. A recent patient had ameloblastoma of the posterior mandibular body diagnosed the day Charles Lindbergh's baby was kidnapped. She had multiple aspirations and curettages over a 50-year period. Finally, she was definitively treated at 83 years of age with a resection of the ramus and mandibular body to the canine tooth in order to obtain adequate margins. The decision to remove the tumor was based on the likelihood of invasion into the parapharyngeal and infratemporal spaces and to the base of the skull, which would have escalated the complexity of surgical resection. There was also a likelihood of pathologic fracture and major infection. Because of the patient's wishes and the added morbidity involved, bone reconstruction was not done, and the patient is functioning perfectly well with a denture that has a guide plane to prevent jaw deviation to the resected side. The cosmetic appearance is quite acceptable.

Surgical treatment generally ranges from a marginal resection to a full resection. Curettage might be justified on some occasions, but complete removal is compromised. Resection can be well tolerated by the elderly patient, unless the symphysis must be resected, and then reconstruction is absolutely necessary.

Maxillofacial Trauma in the Elderly Patient

The elderly patient is subject to the same facial injuries that happen to younger patients. They are injured as motorists or pedestrians. While altercations are uncommon, assaults on the elderly happen with alarming frequency. This can be in the context of robbery or family strife. Falls are of particular concern because one must ensure that the fall was truly the result of a slippery sidewalk, a crack in the sidewalk, or some other impediment, and not attributable to a medical problem, for example transient ischemic attacks or heart block.

Care must be taken to rule out cervical spine injuries, neurologic trauma, or chest/abdominal/extremity injuries. Anticipation of airway problems because of dissecting hematomas and swelling, stupor, foreign bodies (such as dentures and teeth), loss of tongue support from symphysis or bilateral mandibular body fractures is important. Intubation under controlled circumstances may be necessary. Unless shock is present, facial fracture patients generally do well in the semisitting position.

Rarely do bleeders from soft tissue injuries need to be clamped. Packing with moist sponges with the head somewhat elevated (if blood pressure allows) will control most bleeding.

Examination of the Facially Injured Patient

The eyes must be inspected for obvious trauma and laceration, and ophthalmologic consultation should be obtained if there is any question at all. In examining the upper midface, the cheekbones are checked for symmetry and prominence; with a fracture, there may be flatness. There will be ecchymosis and subconjunctival hematoma. Tenderness will exist along the points of fracture, and intraoral palpation may reveal crepitus from sinus wall fracture. On opening the mouth, there might be hypomobility because of impingement of the zygoma or the zygomatic arch on the coronoid process of the mandible. The mobility of the globe should be examined to see if there is decreased range of motion and diplopia.

The nasoethmoidal area needs to be examined. The root of the nose and medial canthi may be injured in a high-level LeFort fracture or in an isolated fracture. The maxilla needs to be examined for dental alveolar trauma and degree of mobility. This mobility may be apparent at the LeFort I level where the alveolar portion of the maxilla is mobile, at the LeFort II level where the maxilla and nose are mobile, and at the LeFort III level where the whole midface is mobile. Fractures of the nose and injury to the nasal septum including hematoma must be evaluated. The mandible should be evaluated by bimanual palpation. The patient should be asked if there is any numbness of the lower lip, chin, and upper lip. Ecchymosis on the floor of the mouth, lacerations of the mucosa, and displacement of any teeth must be noted. Pain in the preauricular areas, limitations of opening, and deviation with opening should all be noted.

Teeth—Dental Alveolar Segments and Gingiva

If significant periodontal disease exists, it is best to remove the mobile, luxated, or avulsed teeth and not attempt to splint them. They do not heal well and morbidity is increased because such teeth remain infected and tender and thus increase the chances of soft tissue infection (for example, infection of the lip that is lacerated or crushed at the time of dental alveolar trauma). This is a judgment call, and while strategically placed teeth and maintenance of alveolar bone helps prosthetic rehabilitation, chronically infected teeth and bone are of no help.

Fractured teeth with firm roots may be left, and if the pulp is exposed it may be extirpated. These teeth may be of use in overdenture construction.

Injuries to the mouth while dentures are in place often result in deep lacerations in the oral vestibule, particularly the upper labial vestibule. These lacerations must be carefully explored for foreign bodies and meticulously repaired in layers with resorbable sutures.

Mandibular Fractures

Simple unilateral subcondylar fractures may be treated by observation and blenderized diet alone if the patient is edentulous or if the natural teeth occlude normally and there is no significant pain. Gentle jaw opening exercises help overcome jaw deviation to the side of the fracture and hypomobility.

Bilateral subcondylar fractures with a tendency to open bite, unilateral subcondylar fractures with malocclusion in the natural dentition, and condylar fracture with significant pain may need a short period of intermaxillary fixation (2 weeks). Even a small tendency for open bite and loss of vertical dimension secondary to bilateral condylar fractures can be tolerated in the edentulous patient and intermaxillary fixation can be avoided. The subsequent ridge relationship changes can be treated in the denture construction.

A nondisplaced unilateral body fracture or angle fracture without mobility or mucoperiosteal tearing in the edentulous patient can be treated by blenderized diet and close observation with frequent radiographs. Good compliance is absolutely necessary.

In the edentulous patient, mild to moderately displaced body fractures, symphysis fractures, and bilateral body fractures have significant impact on the airway and swallowing. The floor of the mouth can be markedly swollen. These fractures can be treated by modifying the dentures if available, or making Gunning splints after impressions of the ridge are taken and then wiring the maxillary splint to the maxilla with peralveolar, piriform rim, and circumzygomatic wires. The lower splint or denture is held with circum-mandibular wires. The patient is then placed into intermaxillary fixation. Healing may take place more slowly than in the young patient, requiring 6 to 8 weeks of fixation (43). In a report on mandibular fracture in the geriatric patient, an editor's note stated that bilateral fractures of the severely atrophic, edentulous mandible with minimal displacement and no intraoral tearing of the mucoperiosteal covering may be treated without intermaxillary fixation (44).

If absolutely necessary, the edentulous body can be opened for internal fixation, but as Bradley (45) has demonstrated, the atrophic mandible has the great majority of its blood supply coming from the periosteum. Stripping of the periosteum to perform an open reduction with internal fixation may result in ischemic necrosis of that portion of the mandible. Wires, plates, and pins may be used for internal fixation (Fig. 40-10). They may have to be removed after healing if they cause discomfort related to the denture. Meticulous handling of tissues and antibiotic coverage are needed in managing these difficult fractures. A method involving supraperiosteal reduction and placement of wires without stripping of the periosteum can be used.

External pin fixation with Joe Hall Morris type systems and acrylic bars for stabilization also can be useful in treating edentulous mandibular fracture.

There will be those fractures that occur in such a dra-

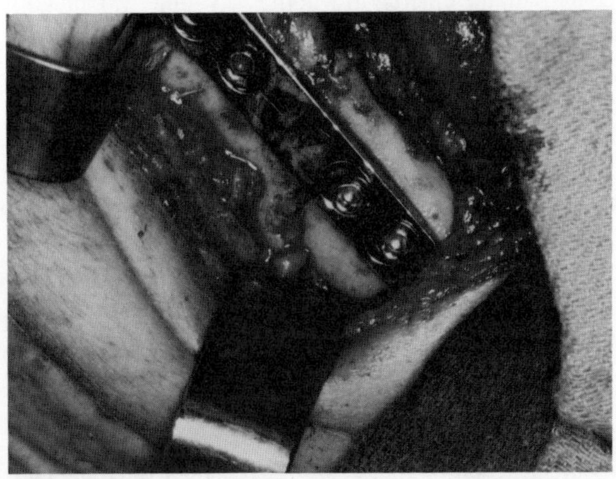

Figure 40-10. Mandibular ramus fracture reduced and fixated with a plate.

matically atrophic mandible (sometimes less than pencil thickness) that healing may not take place and bone grafting may be necessary.

Maxilla

Maxillary fractures at the LeFort I level in the edentulous patient need not be fixated if they are not grossly mobile with significant impaction or other displacement. In the edentulous patient LeFort II and LeFort III fractures also need not be fixated if the mobility is slight and the only reason to fixate them is related to the occlusion.

All other LeFort II, III, nasoethmoidal, and zygomatic injuries should be repaired if there is any significant functional or cosmetic deficit and the patient's condition allows general anesthesia and repair. Maxillofacial plating systems of small dimensions and self-tapping screws make open reduction and quite rigid internal fixation of midface fractures feasible. These systems can be used with and without intermaxillary fixation as clinical situations dictate. Occasionally the plates may need to be removed after healing if they interfere with denture fit.

The patient may decline repair at times. For example, a mildly displaced zygoma fracture without significant orbital floor disruption, no ocular findings, and no hypomobility may not be repaired if the patient is not concerned about cosmetic deformity.

Temporomandibular Joint Disease and Facial Pain

Temporomandibular joint (TMJ) problems are often associated with facial pain and, conversely, facial pain is often associated with TMJ problems. It is significant to note, however, that they are not one and the same. If tunnel vision prevails and the TMJ is blamed for facial pain without proper workup, then serious and potentially lethal pathology can be missed. This is true at any age but particularly in the elderly, in whom many entities, including tumors, can result in facial pain and/or headache.

The TMJ is at the center of great controversy regarding the types of symptoms it produces, the etiologies of the various TMJ disorders, and the modes of treatment. It is important to take a rational balanced approach and avoid the extremes that currently can be found.

The TMJ is a diarthrodial synovial joint with a fibrocartilage disc that separates upper from lower joint space. The condyle rotates in the lower joint space and then moves anteriorly with its disc (translates) on an inclined plane (the articular eminence). The TMJs are ultimately connected to the teeth, so there is some relationship between the occlusion and joint position, and because of the mandible's unique shape, one TMJ cannot function independently of the other.

Internal derangements involve an abnormal relationship of the condyle with the disc and the glenoid fossa. The disc can be displaced, usually anteromedially, when the jaw is closed and reduces to its normal or near-normal position as the jaw opens. A preauricular click with or without pain can be heard or felt. The jaw can temporarily lock when the disc does not reduce, and then it can permanently lock as the disc no longer reduces. The jaw opening may be limited to 25 mm intraincisally with preauricular pain and a feeling of fullness or blocking. The disc changes morphologically in a permanent fashion. Its posterior attachment can be stretched and also permanently changed.

In 50% of patients with internal derangements, there is no definite past history linked to the onset of the internal derangement. In the rest there is a history of trauma (often mild) or situations where the jaw is manipulated, such as wisdom tooth removal or general anesthesia. These patients often date their symptoms from that time (N.F. Ferraro, unpublished data).

As the disc thins it may perforate, and then crepitus may be heard or palpated (46). Without the protective function of the disc, degenerative changes may occur, with breaking, thinning, and erosive changes of the condyle. Condylar changes probably also occur without frank perforation of the disc. It is not clear how many elderly patients with osteoarthritis went through the internal derangement progression as described.

A divergence of clinical observations exists. It is clear that the psychologic factors in TMJ dysfunction are very important (47). Even when objective pathologic findings exist, the psychologic factors must be considered (48). The role of occlusion is not clear. According to Pullinger and colleagues (49), "there is general agreement that the etiology of temporomandibular joint disorders includes structural abnormalities, stress induced muscle hyperactivity, and overloading from trauma. The role of occlusal factors remains unclear, perhaps because of varying adaptive capacities among individuals."

Muscle hyperactivity, bruxing, and clenching can be seen in a population of tense, stressed individuals. That this muscle activity can directly lead to internal derangements is not proven, but the association is undeniable.

Psychologic management, stress reduction, biofeedback, and medicines, such as tricyclic antidepressants and muscle relaxants, are all part of therapy. Surgery alone, even in the face of a clinically apparent and radiographically demonstrated internal derangement, can be doomed to fail. In many of these patients, the preauricular pain is associated with pain and tenderness in the muscles of mastication, especially the temporal area. Also present are other somatic complaints, including shoulder, neck, and back pain, and colitis (50, 51).

Does the older patient with a crepitant painful TMJ

represent the end stage of a younger, tense, muscle-hyperactive patient who had developed an internal derangement? It is an intriguing question, but the answer is not clear.

Attempts to tie TMJ complaints simply to occlusion have not been successful. Costen (52) reported pain and several ear symptoms, and hypothesized a mechanism based on overclosure of the mandible with posterior condylar displacement because of loss of all the teeth or posterior teeth. Many of his symptom associations have been disproved, but the relationship of lack of vertical support of the jaw because of loss of teeth and TMJ symptoms remains an important question. There are those patients who are improved after denture support is provided.

A survey of completely edentulous patients revealed that 25% had TMJ symptoms (53). The group studied numbered 220 patients of whom 138 had dentures; the mean age was 63 years. Specific TMJ pain was seen in 3%, noise in 11%, subluxation or dislocation of the condyle in 1%, and headache, earache, or facial pain in 14%. Sixty-two percent of the patients had clinical signs, including noise, deviation of the jaw, and tenderness.

Treatment of the elderly patient with TMJ dysfunction, internal derangement, and degenerative joint disease is mainly nonsurgical. Ensuring that dentures fit well and have good vertical dimension, providing a bite splint or night guard for patients with natural dentition, gentle range-of-motion exercises, soft diet, gentle heat or gentle physical therapy, and the use of nonsteroidal anti-inflammatory agents if they are tolerated are all treatment modalities that work. Symptoms often remit in a cyclical pattern. Rarely, an intra-articular steroid injection is indicated.

Care must be taken to investigate the psychologic factors—loneliness, separation, anxiety, and depression may be part of the clinical picture. Symptoms will often remit after these are treated.

Sometimes surgery is indicated to reposition a meniscus or resurface a condyle. Many procedures have been described. These include high condylectomy, condylar shave, meniscus plication, and replacement of the meniscus with alloplastic materials or temporalis fascia or dermis; in rare instances a condyle-fossa prosthesis or bone graft reconstruction is indicated. There has been significant concern regarding alloplasts in the TMJ. Significant wear, fragmentation, and foreign body reactions, sometimes severe, have been noted.

Rheumatoid disease, especially rheumatoid arthritis and scleroderma, can cause joint symptoms and eventual joint destruction. There can be hypomobility and open bite because of loss of vertical height in the condyle. Almost always, the patient is known to have rheumatoid arthritis and is being treated by a rheumatologist; rarely will TMJ symptoms be the initial presentation. If the patient has severe functional deficits, such as hypomobility and open bite, arthroplasty with bone grafts, temporalis flaps, and alloplasts can be performed. TMJ replacement prostheses are available. Care must be taken regarding the use of condylar prostheses without a fossa replacement since there are cases of erosion into the middle cranial fossa in rheumatoid patients in whom such procedures were performed. In scleroderma, the condition of the soft tissues usually prevents a total TMJ replacement or adequate surgery.

Another entity which is important is condylar subluxation and dislocation. Subluxation is the displacement of the condyle out of the fossa with mouth opening but immediate reduction upon closing of the mouth. In dislocation the condyle is anteriorly displaced out of the fossa when the mouth opens. It is in front of the articular eminence, and the patient cannot reduce it. This is seen in the older patient population, usually due to extrapyramidal disease or tardive dyskinesias often brought on by the use of haloperidol and phenothiazines. Tremors, dyskinesia, and rigidity of the facial and jaw musculature can be seen in Parkinson's disease. The acute problem can be treated with diphenhydyramine. If the patient's drug regimens can be changed, this may help, but often the tardive dyskinesia is a very late and not totally remitting finding.

There are multiple surgical procedures to prevent the dislocation. Placing the patient in intermaxillary fixation may help temporarily but is often not a long-term cure. Scarifying the temporalis tendon via an intraoral approach has been used with some success. There is also an operation to flatten the articular eminence so that the patient can open widely but not lock out of position. The Dautrey procedure, which down-fractures the posterior aspect of the zygomatic arch to provide a mechanical block for dislocation, relies on there being some flexibility in the bone and may not be the ideal procedure in an old patient with brittle bone. Placing an alloplast on the eminence to block the condylar opening has been done, as has the use of surgical tape to prevent the condyle from translating too far anteriorly.

TMJ pain must be viewed in the broad sense, otherwise important pathology can be missed. Mizukawa et al. (54) reported TMJ pain from breast carcinoma metastatic to the condyle; multiple myeloma and poorly differentiated lymphoma have also been implicated in the TMJ. The proper radiographs include transcranial views, panoramic views, CT scans and magnetic resonance imaging, if necessary. This is an imperative adjunct to the clinical exam and history.

TMJ pain is part of the broader constellation of facial and head pain. As mentioned above, much of TMJ pain is related to the muscles and is very similar or in a continuum with muscle contraction headache. It is risky to assume that headache is a result of the TMJ without the proper workup, so liberal consultation with a neurologist is important. The same is true for ear symptoms; ear pathology must be ruled out before the complaints are related to the TMJ.

A careful search for causes of facial pain must be made when any doubt exists. This includes not only neurologic consultation, but assessment of the base of the skull, the infratemporal fossa, the pterygomaxillary space, the nasopharynx, the oropharynx, the hypopharynx, the sinuses, and the teeth. This is often a combined effort, including the oral and maxillofacial surgeon, the otolaryngologist, and the radiologist.

Of particular concern is the existence of sensory changes in any of the trigeminal distributions. Hypesthesia, paresthesia, and anesthesia should be taken as evidence of a neoplasm along the nerve until proven otherwise.

One must also have a high index of suspicion for giant cell or temporal arteritis. In the classic case, the superficial temporal artery is pulseless, tender, and hard. Variations certainly exist. Because there can be temporal tenderness, it may be confused with TMJ disease. Vague constitutional symptoms may be present, such as headache, flu-like symptoms, myalgias, fatigue, anorexia, and weight loss (55). Temporal arteritis affects the medium-sized arteries and produces an occlusive endarteritis. In the head and neck, the most important involvement is the ophthalmic arteries, with resultant blindness. Lingual necrosis has also been seen. The erythrocyte sedimentation rate can be very elevated, and steroids are needed for treatment.

Facial neuralgias may be classic (for example, classic tic douloureux), but they can be atypical and not related to dental pathology or other definite head and neck sources. We must bear in mind the diagnosis of psychogenic pain in these patients. It is a significant problem because persons 65 years and older continue to commit suicide at a higher rate than any other age group in the United States. Depression, alcohol, and chronic pain are usually related (56). There are several neurosurgical procedures that are performed above the level of the base of the skull for facial neuralgias, but at times a nerve is treated peripherally. Alcohol injection has classically been used, but cryosurgery (57), other chemicals (58), and radiofrequency lesions (59) have been used with reasonable success. In general, atypical neuralgias are not successfully treated by operative means, whether it is a dental extraction or a neurolytic lesion. The careful combination, then, of a thorough search for a source of the pain plus psychologic and pain management group consultation is stressed.

Preprosthetic and Reconstructive Surgery

Preprosthetic Surgery

After teeth are lost, the alveolar process of the maxilla and mandible undergo resorption. The results are:

1. A reduction in height of the residual ridge
2. An increase in interarch distance
3. A relatively prognathic mandible in profile
4. In the coronal plane, the maxillary arch becomes narrower and the mandibular arch wider as resorption progresses (60) (Fig. 40-11, *A* and *B*).

There can develop such anatomic problems that dentures cannot be made or worn comfortably. The field of preprosthetic surgery deals with the surgical preparation of the mouth for the most ideal prosthetic replacement. This can involve standard denture replacement or complex replacements following ablative surgery for tumors. It is best to bear in mind that no prosthesis is ideal compared with the natural dentition. Dentures are not a substitute for teeth, but a substitute for not having teeth. Careful consultation between the oral and maxillofacial surgeon and the prosthodontist is necessary before preprosthetic surgery is performed (61).

Common Alveolar Ridge Modification Procedures

Teeth and roots should be retained when possible since the alveolar bone is thus preserved. Vital root submersion is of questionable value.

Once teeth are removed, alveoloplasty should be done to smooth sharp edges of the alveolus and remove severe bulges, undercuts, and irregularities; however, care must be taken to avoid removing too much alveolus. Some work is being done regarding the placement of hydroxylapatite cones in the sockets to help retain alveolar height (62, p. 61).

Redundant soft tissue from the ridge can be trimmed with a blade or electrocautery. Papillary hyperplasia of the ridge and palatal mucosa and the pedunculated epulis fissuratum in the vestibule are two types of tissue response seen under dentures. Denture reline may help but often excision is needed.

The maxillary tuberosity area may have soft-tissue enlargement both in height and width; the denture flange, then, cannot fit well into the vestibule. Wedges of soft tissue can be removed to reduce the tuberosity bulk. At times, the maxillary tuberosity enlargement involves bone and maxillary sinus, so a more complex reduction procedure is needed. Such a method is described by Kreger et al. (63).

Palatal torus may not need removal unless it has significant undercuts, irregularites, or irritation. Removal must be done carefully after adequate reflection of the pal-

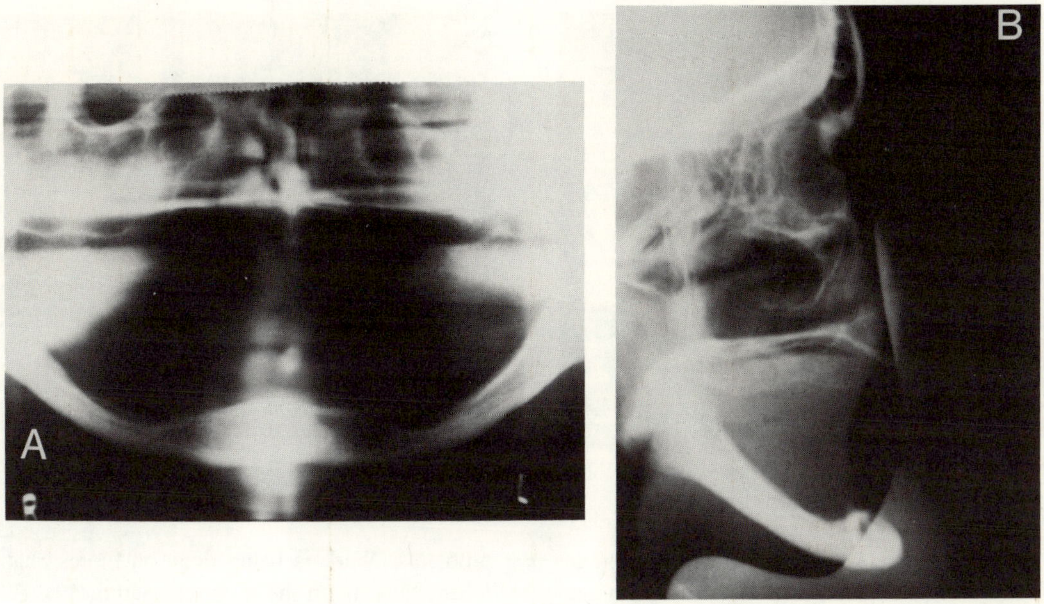

Figure 40-11. *A*, Panoramic jaw radiograph showing mandibular atrophy. *B*, Lateral radiograph also showing atrophy and prognathic appearance of mandible.

atal mucoperiosteum. Large tori should be removed after division into small sections to prevent fracture and perforation into the floor of the nose, with the potential for oronasal fistula.

Mandibular tori are generally bilaterally symmetrical and on the lingual aspects of the mandible at the canine premolar region. Adequate retraction and protection of the delicate tissues at the floor of the mouth are needed to safely remove lingual tori. A maxillary or mandibular frenum or a lingual frenum that is very close to the crest of the ridge may be contributing to denture instability and frenectomy may be needed.

Vestibuloplasty

When there is adequate height of the alveolar bone, but an unstable soft-tissue base, vestibuloplasty may be necessary. Potential tissue problems include:

1. Movable soft tissue on the ridge
2. Muscle attachments that are high on the crest of the alveolar ridge
3. Shallowness of the labial and buccal vestibules
4. On the lingual side of the mandible, crestal position of the mylohyoid muscle without much depth to the floor of the mouth.

There are many vestibuloplasty procedures currently practiced. In general, all the techniques involve inferiorly repositioning muscle attachments on the mandible and superiorly repositioning them on the maxilla. The raw periosteal surface is then:

1. Allowed to heal by secondary epithelialization,
2. Covered with a pedicled mucosal flap,
3. Covered with a skin graft, or
4. Covered with a mucosal graft (60) (Fig. 40-12, *A* and *B*).

Secondary epithelialization techniques undergo rapid and total relapse, plus healing of a raw surface is prolonged.

If a graft is used, it can be sutured into position, held by bolsters or a fabricated stent. A variation of the second technique has been advocated by Obwegeser (60). This works well in the maxilla and involves making a submucosal tunnel and a supraperiosteal tunnel on the lateral maxillary ridge and incising the intervening layer of tissue that contains the bulk of the muscular attachments. The mylohyoid attachment can also be lowered on the floor of the mouth.

With ridge atrophy, the mental foramen and nerve occupy a more crestal position and may produce pain because of the overlying denture. The mental nerve may also have to repositioned.

Augmentation of the Atrophic Ridge

When the absolute amount of atrophy has reached a point where soft tissue repositioning is not enough, augmentation of the ridge itself is needed. At first glance, replacing the lost bone with onlay grafts would seem to be the method of choice, but studies have shown that onlay bone grafts can undergo rather dramatic resorption, up to 100% in 3 years (64, 65). Both ribs and iliac crest have been used; however, there is concern about donor site mor-

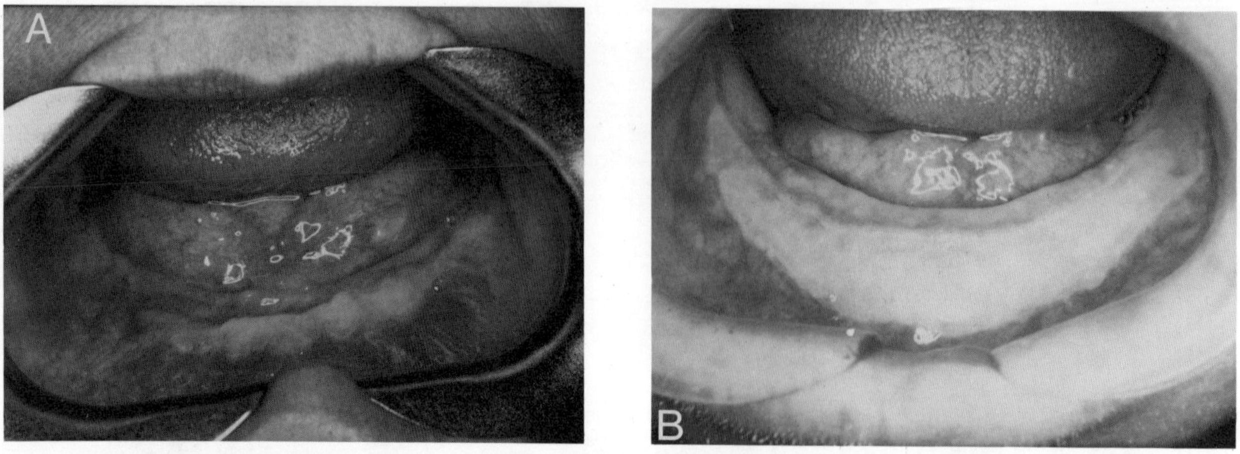

Figure 40-12. *A*, Poor ridge height for denture support in the mandible. *B*, Similar ridge after split-thickness skin graft vestibuloplasty.

bidity in the older patients. Allogeneic freeze-dried cadaver bone has been used. It resorbs very slowly but generally needs to be used with autogenous bone graft for any significant osteogenic potential. The techinque of interpositional bone grafting, then, was proposed in hopes that resorption of the graft could be slowed.

LeFort I maxillary osteotomy for down-fracture with inferior positioning and interpositional bone grafting has been advocated for the maxilla (66). Allogeneic bone has been studied as a interpositional graft by Frost et al. (67). Some resorption can be expected, but results are satisfactory. If bone plates are used, they usually have to be removed because of irritation under the denture. The same theory has applied in the mandible, with various visor and sandwich osteotomies that raise part of the osteotomized mandible and interpose bone grafts. These procedures carry some morbidity to the inferior alveolar nerve and risk of mandibular fracture. These techniques are well reviewed by Tideman et al. (60).

Following the augmentation procedures, vestibuloplasty is almost always necessary. The benefit to the patient must be weighed against the extent of these procedures and the need for donor bone. The use of banked allogeneic bone, of course, reduces the morbidity. Studies are being done regarding the efficacy of banked bone alone, and the answers are not yet in. Bone substitutes, of course, are very welcome and several are being used. Proplasts and Silastic have been used in the past, but deformation and extrusion have occurred.

Hydroxylapatite from a sea coral has been widely tested and is marketed in various forms for various uses. It is well incorporated into the recipient bone because it is porous (68) but does not remodel. It is available as ceramic-like granules and blocks. Granules have been placed along maxillary and mandibular ridges for augmentation, but migration and displacement have been problems. Work is being done on bioresorbable carrier tubes that contain the hydroxylapatite (69). Blocks have been onlaid to the ridge with good increase in height and width, but dehiscence of the mucosa has occurred, possibly because of the inability of hydroxylapatite to remodel with loading (Fig. 40-13).

Implants to replace teeth have been tried over the years. Linkow (70) was a pioneer in the use of various shaped metal blades that were inserted into the maxilla and mandible and then had dentures and bridges fastened to posts that protruded through the mucosa. Fibrous healing around the implant-bone interface occurred and implant mobility was a problem.

Subperiosteal implants are large, custom-made metal frameworks that fit over the maxillary or mandibular ridges. They are made from impressions of the ridges that are taken after elevation of mucoperiosteal flaps to expose the bone. The frameworks are placed using the same dissection at another operation. They also have posts perforating the mucosa that can act as denture and bridge supports. These implants are reasonably successful but require extensive dissection under general anesthesia. Commercial services can now fabricate subperiosteal implants from a template constructed on the basis of a CT scan of the jaws. This eliminates the first operation for taking impressions.

The mandibular staple bone plate designed by Small (71) is placed by a subsymphyseal incision, and it has three or five pins that engage the mandible in precisely drilled holes, and two transosteal pins or posts that perforate the mucosa. These pins provide stability for a tissue-borne denture and prevent its lateral displacement. The staple has been carefully studied; if meticulously placed with careful prosthetics and follow-up, it performs very well. Placement requires a general anesthetic, but duration is short and the dissection is superficial. The man-

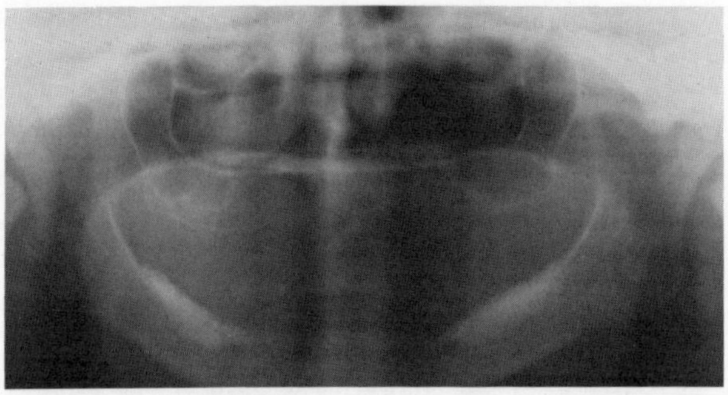

Figure 40-13. Radiopaque hydroxylapatite to augment the atrophic mandibular ridge.

dibular staple design has recently been modified. The new compression design is screwed into the inferior border of the mandible instead of being tapped in. It has two or four transosteal pins that can be loaded vertically; therefore, it can fully support fixed bridgework. Prior to this the mandibular staple's function had to be limited to preventing lateral displacement of prostheses. Tideman (60) refers to a transmandibular implant developed by Bosker and van Dijk.

A well-tested innovation involves implants placed transorally that integrate with bone so that there is an implant-bone interface without intervening fibrous tissues. These implants are technique sensitive and costly but involve little morbidity in placement. Branemark (72) is credited with the careful formation of this type of implant and the careful long-term follow-up. These implants can quite successfully provide posts to bear dentures and bridges (72, 73), (Fig. 40-14). Any of the implants require great patient cooperation and hygiene and may not be advisable if there is significant systemic disease that can predispose to infection. They recently have been used successfully in irradiated bone, bone grafts, and in other places in the facial skeleton (e.g., for prosthetic eyes, ears, and hearing aids). Osseointegrated implants involve little morbidity compared with bone grafts and large subperiosteal implants.

Other Reconstructive Procedures

After maxillary resection, a decision will have to be made whether the patient is going to have a bone–soft-tissue reconstruction or wear an obturator prosthesis. The older, debilitated patient often does very well with an obturator. Resection of the mandibular symphysis must be reconstructed, or great morbidity ensues with difficulty in breathing, swallowing, and speaking. Techniques of reconstruction may use metallic plates, bone grafts with metal or Dacron trays, block bone grafts, or autogenous bone grafts with allogeneic bone cribs.

There is less of a need to reconstruct the posterior mandibular resection (ramus and posterior body), but if

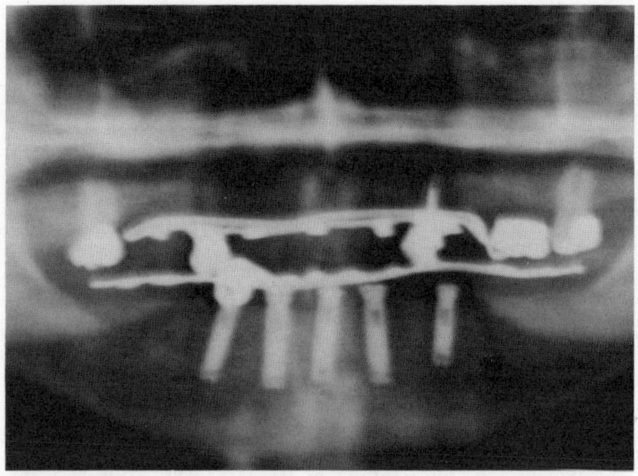

Figure 40-14. Osseointegrated mandibular implants for denture support.

the patient is vigorous enough, bone graft reconstruction can improve function, stop deviation, and improve contour and sense of well-being.

Conclusion

The oral surgical needs of the elderly patient and the treatments and operations that are available have been surveyed here. We have covered the full spectrum of surgery from extraction of the painful tooth to reconstruction of a resected mandible. Each patient's case, however, must be taken separately, for there are those patients who are so fragile that the extraction of a tooth may require a great deal of advanced planning, and then there are those elderly patients who are so vigorous that a reconstruction can be tolerated and allow them to function with an enhanced sense of well-being.

There is no question that, on the clinical side and in the laboratory, there is considerable effort being devoted to providing reconstructive and augmentation procedures that will be predictable with less morbid donor sites. The goal is maximum gain with minimum amount of surgery. We must also remember that there is much that the oral and maxillofacial surgeon treats that does not require operation. Unfortunately, many of these maladies are very difficult to treat indeed. The patient with chronic facial pain, with burning tongue, or with one of the various oral ulcerative diseases will be very grateful for what help they can receive. Providing some comfort for these patients will bring great satisfaction to the practitioner.

The discipline of oral and maxillofacial surgery has many treatments that are not elective—for example, the removal of hopelessly carious teeth or the drainage of a life-threatening infection—but there is also much within the discipline that is elective, and it is surgery that is designed to improve function and sense of well-being. The use of these surgical techniques in the elderly population requires careful consideration of each patient's needs and health, a sense of perspective, and meticulous technique when the surgery is performed.

References

1. Burt, BA, et al. 1985. Periodontal disease, tooth loss, and oral hygiene among older Americans. *Community Dent Oral Epidemiol* 13:93–96.
2. MacEntee, M, et al. 1985. Oral health in a long-term care institution equipped with a dental service. *Community Dent Oral Epidemiol* 13:260–263.
3. Papas, AS, and Hefferren, JH. 1987. Nutrition and preventive needs of older adults. *Spec Care Dent* 7:13–14.
4. Baum, BJ. 1981. Research on aging and oral health: An assessment of current status and future needs. *Spec Care Dent* 1:156–165.
5. Shklar, G. 1966. The effects of aging upon oral mucosa. *J Invest Dermatol* 47:115–120.
6. Shklar, G. 1979. Oral pathology in the aging individual. In *Geriatric Dentistry,* Eds., CJ Toga, et al. Lexington, MA: Lexington Books.
7. Davis, M, et al. 1972. The effect of age on extraction wound healing in Syrian hamsters. *J Dent Child* 39:384–389.
8. Silverman, S. 1987. Geriatrics and associated oral problems. *Spec Care Dent* 7:11.
9. Malamed, S. 1987. Anxiety and pain control in the older patient. *Spec Care Dent* 7:22–23.
10. Laskin, DM. 1985. Oral surgery in the geriatric patient. In *Clinical Geriatric Dentistry,* Eds., HH Chauncey, et al. Chicago: American Dental Association.
11. Bennett, CR. 1978. *Local Anesthesia and Pain Control in Dental Practice,* ed. 6. St. Louis: CV Mosby Co, p. 160.
12. Makinodon, T, and Kay, MMB. 1979. Immunologic changes in aging and their possible significance to geriatric dentistry. In *Geriatric Dentistry,* Eds., CJ Toga, et al. Lexington, MA: Lexington Books.
13. Goldberg, MH. 1981. Infections of the salivary glands. In *Infections of the Oral and Maxillofacial Region,* Eds., RG Topazian and MM Goldberg. Philadelphia: WB Saunders.
14. Carmody, TJ, and Wergowski, GL. 1983. Retropharyngeal abscess and hematoma in an elderly woman following esophagoscopy and endotracheal intubation. *J Am Gerontol Soc* 31:499–500.
15. Hjorting-Hansen, E. 1970. Decortication in treatment of osteomyelitis of mandible. *Oral Surg* 29:641–655.
16. Marx, RE. 1983. Osteoradionecrosis: A new concept of its pathophysiology. *J Oral Maxillofac Surg* 41:283–288.
17. Daly, TE, and Drane, JB. 1973. Management of teeth related to the treatment of oral cancer. National Cancer Conference Proceedings 7. New York: American Cancer Society, p. 147.
18. Marx, RE. 1983. Osteoradionecrosis: A new concept in the treatment of osteoradionecrosis. *J Oral Maxillofac Surg* 41:351–357.
19. Donoff, RB, and May, JW. 1982. Microvascular mandibular reconstruction. *J Oral Maxillofac Surg* 40:122–126.
20. Rubin, P, and Holt, JF. 1957. Secretory sialography in diseases of the major salivary glands. *Am J Roentgenol* 77:575–598.
21. Rankow, RM, and Polayes, IM. 1976. *Diseases of the Salivary Glands.* Philadelphia: WB Saunders.
22. Hemenway W, and English, J. 1971. Surgical treatment of acute parotitis. *Postgrad Med* 50:114.
23. Lilienthal, H. 1917. A method of incising parotid abscess without injury to the facial nerve distribution. *Am J Surg* 31:101.
24. Blair, VP, and Padgett, EC. 1923. Pyogenic infections of the parotid glands and ducts. *Arch Surg* 7:1–36.
25. Perzik, SL. 1962. Surgical management of acute parotitis. *Arch Surg* 85:247–251.
26. Shearn, M. 1971. *Sjögren's Syndrome.* Philadelphia: WB Saunders.
27. Mandel, L. 1976. Inflammatory disorders. In *Diseases of the Salivary Glands,* Eds., RM Rankow and IM Polayes. Philadelphia: WB Saunders.
28. Bertram, U, and Hjorting-Hansen, E. 1970. Punch biopsy of minor salivary glands in the diagnosis of Sjogren's syndrome. *Scand J Dent Res* 78:295.
29. Collins, RD, and Ball, G. 1986. Sjogren's syndrome. In *Clinical Rheumatology,* Eds., GV Ball and WJ Koopman. Philadelphia: WB Saunders.
30. Shafer, WG, Hine, MK, and Levy, BM. 1983. *A Textbook of Oral Pathology,* ed. 4 Philadelphia: WB Saunders.
31. Abrams, AM, Melrose, RJ, and Howell, FN. 1973. Necrotizing sialometaplasia: A disease simulating malignancy. *Cancer* 32:130.
32. Eneroth, CM. 1971. Salivary gland tumors in the parotid gland, submandibular gland, and the palate region. *Cancer* 27:1415–1418.
33. Rankow, RM. 1973. Surgical decisions in the treatment of major salivary gland tumors. *Plast Reconstr Surg* 51:514–523.
34. Batsakis, JG. 1972. Neoplasms of the minor and lesser major salivary glands. *Surg Gynecol Obstet* 135:289–298.
35. Widmann, BP. 1950. Cancer of the lip. *Am J Roentgenol Radium Ther Nucl Med* 63:13.
36. Shklar, G, and McCarthy, PL. 1961. The oral lesions of lichen planus. *Oral Surg* 14:164.
37. Andreasen, JO. 1968. Oral lichen planus. I. A clinical evaluation of 115 cases. *Oral Surg* 25:31.
38. Stillman, MA, Bart, RS, and Kopf, AW. 1973. Squamous cell carcinoma occurring in oral lichen planus. *Cutis* 11:486.
39. Renstrup, G. 1970. Occurrence of candida in oral leukoplakias. *Acta Pathol Microbiol Scand* 78:421.
40. Krolls, SO, and Hoffman, S. 1976. Squamous cell carcinoma of the oral soft tissues: A statistical analysis of 14,253 cases by age, sex and race of patients. *J Am Dent Assoc* 92:571.
41. Bernick, S. 1948. Growth of the gingiva and palate. II. Connective tissue tumors. *Oral Surg* 1:1098–1108.
42. Pindborg, JJ, and Hjorting-Hansen, E. 1974. *Atlas of Diseases of the Jaws.* Philadelphia: WB Saunders.
43. Rowe, NL, and Williams, J. 1985. *Maxillofacial Injuries,* vol 1. London: Churchill Livingstone.
44. Degnan, EJ. 1970. *J Oral Surg* 28:438–442.
45. Bradley, JC. 1975. A radiological investigation into the age changes of the inferior dental artery. *Br J Oral Surg* 13:82.

46. Graham, GS, Ferraro, NF, and Simms, DA. 1984. Perforation of the temporomandibular joint meniscus: Arthrographic, surgical, and clinical findings. *J Oral Maxillofac Surg* 42:35–38.
47. Rugh, JD, and Solberg, WK. 1976. Psychological implications in temporomandibular pain and dysfunction. *Oral Sci Rev* 7:3.
48. Denman, SB. 1980. Psychologic testing and evaluation. In *Current Advances in Oral Surgery,* Ed., WB Irby, vol 3. St. Louis: CV Mosby.
49. Pullinger, AG, Seligman, DA, and Solberg, WK. 1988. Temporomandibular disorders. Part II: Occlusal factors associated with temporomandibular joint tenderness and dysfunction. *J Pros Dent* 59:363–367.
50. Feinman, C, and Harris, M. 1984. Psychogenic facial pain (Part I). The clinical presentation. *Br Dent J* 156:165–168.
51. Feinman, C, and Harris, M. 1984. Psychogenic facial pain (Part II). Management and prognosis. *Br Dent J* 156:205–208.
52. Costen, JB. 1934. A syndrome of ear and sinus symptoms dependent upon disturbed function of the temporomandibular joint. *Ann Otol Rhinol Laryngol* 43:1–15.
53. Sakurai, K, et al. 1988. A survey of temporomandibular joint dysfunction in completely edentulous patients. *J Prosthet Dent* 59:81–85.
54. Mizukawa, JH, et al. 1980. Metastatic breast adenocarcinoma of the mandibular condyle: Report of case. *J Oral Surg* 38:448–451.
55. Sullivan, RJ Jr. 1986. Occult temporal arteritis. *J Am Geriatr Soc* 34:812–813.
56. Blazer, DG, Bachar, JR, and Manton, KG. 1986. Suicide in late life—review and commentary. *J Am Geriatr Soc* 34:519.
57. Zakrzewska, JM, Nally, FF, and Flint, SR. 1986. Cryotherapy in the management of paroxysmal trigeminal neuralgia. *J Maxillofac Surg* 14:5–7.
58. Sokolovic, M, et al. 1986. Peripheral streptomycin/lidocaine injections in the treatment of idiopathic trigeminal neuralgia. *J Maxillofac Surg* 14:8–9.
59. Gregg, JM, et al. 1978. Radiofrequency thermoneurolysis of peripheral nerves for control of trigeminal neuralgia. *Pain* 5:231.
60. Tideman, H, Anker, A, and Arvier, J. 1986. Major preprosthetic surgery. A review. *Aus Dent J* 3:403–414.
61. Kelly, EK. 1966. The prosthodontist, the oral surgeon, and the denture supporting tissues. *J Pros Dent* 16:464–477.
62. Scott, RF, and Olson, RAJ. 1986. Minor preprosthetic procedures. In *Reconstructive Preprosthetic Oral and Maxillofacial Surgery,* Eds., RJ Fonseca and WH Davis. Philadelphia: WB Saunders.
63. Kreger, T, Kent, K, and Samit, A. 1984. Crestal ostectomy and lateral wall compression for management of the enlarged pneumatized tuberosity. *J Oral Maxillofac Surg* 42:835–838.
64. Davis, WH, et al. 1975. Long-term ridge augmentation with rib graft. *J Maxillofac Surg* 3:103–106.
65. Fazili, M, et al. 1978. Follow-up investigation of reconstruction of the alveolar process in the atrophic mandible. *Int J Oral Surg* 7:400–404.
66. Farrell, CD, Kent, JN, and Guerra, LR. 1976. One-stage interpositional bone grafting and vestibuloplasty of the atrophic maxilla. *J Oral Surg* 34:901–906.
67. Frost, DE, Fonseca, RJ, and Burkes, EJ. 1982. Interpositional homologous grafts to the maxilla. *J Oral Surg* 40:776–784.
68. Piecuch, JF. 1986. Augmentation of the atrophic edentulous ridge with porous replamineform hydroxyapatite (Interpore-200). *Dent Clin North Am* 30:291–304.
69. Shen, K, and Gongloff, RK. 1986. Collagen tube containers: An effective means of controlling particulate hydroxyapatite implants. *J Prosthet Dent* 56:65–69.
70. Linkow, LI. 1968. Prefabricated prostheses for intraosseous implants. *J Prosthet Dent* 20:367–375.
71. Small, IA. 1975. Metal implants and the mandibular staple bone plate. *J Oral Surg* 33:571–584.
72. Branemark, PI, et al. 1977. *Osseointegrated Implants in the Treatment of the Edentulous Jaw. Experience from a 10 Year Period.* Stockholm: Almquist & Wiksell International.
73. Adell, R, et al. 1981. A 15-year study of osseointegrated implants in the treatment of the edentulous jaw. *Int J Oral Surg* 10:387–416.

41

Surgery in Centenarians

Mark R. Katlic

The 100th year of life holds a certain mystique, perhaps because the centenarian is as close to immortality as a human can be. Daily, local newspapers and national television show the names and visages of individuals celebrating their hundredth birthdays, setting a challenge for the population at large. More and more, the population appears to be meeting that challenge.

The United States Census Bureau (1) reported that 32,194 people were age 100 years or older in 1980. There are estimates, however, that the number may reach 100,000 by the year 2000 (2). It stands to reason that as our gross population increases and life expectancy lengthens, the absolute number of centenarians will climb. Inevitably, surgeons will see larger numbers of these most senior citizens.

History

Since the early 1900s, surgeons have written about operations in the elderly, but the definition of "elderly" has changed. One early report described 167 operations performed in patients older than 50 years (3), and even two decades later prominent surgeons were teaching that "an elective operation for inguinal hernia in a patient older than 50 years was not justified" (4). In 1937, Brooks reported a series of 293 procedures in patients 70 years or older (5), and during the past 50 years, most authors have considered patients above the ages of 60 to 70 years as being elderly (6, 7). Studies now show that good results can be obtained in octogenarians and nonagenarians (8), even with complex vascular (9, 10) and cardiac operations (11, 12).

Most papers devoted to centenarians per se are case reports. Welch and Whittemore (13), for example, presented a 100-year-old woman who recovered uneventfully from abdominoperineal resection of rectal carcinoma. Prostatic surgery in this age group was discussed by Mayock and Burns (14). This author more recently reported a series of major and minor procedures in six patients aged 100 to 104 years, all of whom survived (15) (Table 41-1). The two cases below are from that series.

Illustrative Cases

Case A

A 100-year-old woman fractured her right hip in a nursing home fall. She had a history of myocardial infarction, congestive heart failure, aortic stenosis, arthritis, and hiatus hernia and had previously undergone cataract surgery, cystocele repair, and open reduction internal fixation of a left hip fracture. Open reduction internal fixation of her new fracture was performed under general anesthesia. During her 2nd postoperative week, she developed acute gangrenous cholecystitis, requiring emergency cholecystectomy. This was complicated by left lower lobe pneumonia, which resolved with antibiotic treatment, and by a localized intra-abdominal abscess, which was successfully treated with percutaneous drainage and antibiotics. Six weeks after admission she returned to her nursing home.

Protruding Enders rod pins in her right leg led to pin removal under local anesthesia 8 months later.

At 101 years of age, she underwent elective endoscopic resection of a rectal villous adenoma containing carcinoma in situ. Postoperative bleeding from the resection site mandated suture ligation under general anesthesia. She returned to her nursing home, where she later died, 2 weeks before her 103rd birthday.

Table 41-1. Clinical summary of centenarians undergoing an operation

Patient No./Sex	Patient Age, yr	Medical problems	Operation	Status	Anesthesia	Complications	Death	Follow-up
1/M	100	Old myocardial infarction, sick sinus syndrome with pacemaker, congestive heart failure, prostatectomy, cataract extraction, gout, arthritis, chronic renal failure	Pacemaker generator replacement	Urgent	Local	None	No	Died, age 102 yr. congestive heart failure
2/F	100	Old myocardial infarction, left radical mastectomy (13 yr), arthritis	Excision of right femoral head, cemented Moore prosthesis	Urgent	General	None	No	Died, age 102 yr. cerebrovascular disease
3/M	100	Hypertension, severe peripheral vascular disease, prostatectomy, chronic lung disease	Above-knee amputation	Urgent	General	None	No	Died, age 101 yr. "old age"
4/F	100	Old myocardial infarction, congestive heart failure, aortic stenosis, cataract extraction, cystocele repair, left hip open reduction internal fixation, arthritis, hiatus hernia	Open reduction, internal fixation of right-hip fracture	Urgent	General	Acute gangrenous cholecystitis, protruding Enders rod pins	No	Alive, age 102 yr
			Cholecystectomy	Emergency	General	Pneumonia, resolved; abdominal abscess, percutaneously drained		
			Removal of Enders rod pins	Elective	Local	None		
	101		Colonoscopic resection of villous adenoma	Elective	Local	Bleeding excision site		
			Suture ligation of bleeding rectal polypectomy site	Emergency	General	None		
5/F	101	Congestive heart failure, atrial fibrillation, blind, basal cell carcinoma of face excised, adult-onset diabetes	Right inguinal herniorrhaphy	Elective	Local	None	No	Died, age 102 yr. congestive heart failure
6/M	104	Squamous cell carcinoma of neck excised, basal cell carcinoma of nose excised and irradiated	Gastroscopy with biopsy	Emergency	Local	None	No	Died, age 105 yr. gastric carcinoma

Case B

A 101-year-old woman was ambulatory and independent at home but suffered from a large right inguinal hernia. Her past history included congestive heart failure, atrial fibrillation, adult-onset diabetes mellitus, blindness, and resected basal cell carcinoma of the face. Elective right inguinal herniorrhaphy was completed under local anesthesia in the outpatient surgical unit. Postoperatively, stating that she would "rather wear out than rust out," she took a 3-month cruise around the world and later lectured at a local college geriatrics course. On the penultimate day of her life she completed a political poll. She died of congestive heart failure at age 102.

Speculation

Centenarians are as likely to survive surgery as are their offspring, and one may speculate that they are even more likely to do so. Individuals who have endured 10 decades of life's labors enter a select group whose physiologic resilience is greater than that of many who are chronologically younger.

Certainly all that has been learned from the preceding chapters must be applied to the 100-year-old patient: optimal preoperative preparation, gentle handling of tissues, meticulous technique, compulsive attention to every detail of postoperative care. It is not unreasonable to hypothesize, though, that the century-old patient who has not already succumbed to a myocardial infarction or pulmonary embolus is unlikely to do so, even in the perioperative milieu. Studies of nonagenarians tend to support this: neither pneumonia nor atherosclerosis with myocardial infarction was a major cause of perioperative death in the recent Mayo Clinic series (8). Similar data in centenarians are presently unavailable but will accumulate soon if the epidemiologists are correct.

Mere survival to the centenary indicates that one has been tested by life and has been found exceptionally fit. Elective surgery should not be deferred nor emergency surgery denied the centenarian on the basis of chronologic age.

References

1. U.S. Census Bureau. 1983. *1980 Census of Population: General Population Characteristics, United States*. Washington, DC: GPO.
2. Windom, RE, 1988. From the Assistant Secretary for Health. *JAMA* 259:2201.
3. Smith, OC. 1907. Advanced age as a contraindication to operation. *Med Rec (NY)* 72:642–644.
4. Ochsner, A. 1967. Is risk of operation too great in the elderly? *Geriatrics* 22:121–130.
5. Brooks, B. 1937. Surgery in patients of advanced age. *Ann Surg* 105:481–495.
6. Linn, BS, Linn, MW, and Wallen, N. 1982. Evaluation of results of surgical procedures in the elderly. *Ann Surg* 195:90–96.
7. Keller, SM, Markovitz, LJ, Wilder, JR, et al. 1987. Emergency and elective surgery in patients over age 70. *Am Surg* 53:636–640.
8. Warner, MA, Hosking, MP, Lobdell, CM, et al. 1988. Surgical procedures among those ≥ 90 years of age. *Ann Surg* 207:380–386.
9. Harris, KA, Ameli, FM, Lally, M, et al. 1986. Abdominal aortic aneurysm resection in patients more than 80 years old. *Surg Gynecol Obstet* 162:536–538.
10. Cogbill, TH, Landercasper, J, Strutt, PJ, et al. 1987. Late results of peripheral vascular surgery in patients 80 years of age and older. *Arch Surg* 122:581–586.
11. Rich, MW, Sandza, JG, Kleiger, RE, et al. 1985. Cardiac operations in patients over 80 years of age. *J Thorac Cardiovasc Surg* 90:56–60.
12. Tsai, TP, Matloff, JM, Chaux, A, et al. 1986. Combined valve and coronary artery bypass procedures in septuagenarians and octogenarians: Results in 120 patients. *Ann Thorac Surg* 42:681–684.
13. Welch, CE, and Whittemore, WS. 1954. Carcinoma of the rectum in a centenarian. *N Engl J Med* 250:1041–1042.
14. Mayock, PP, and Burns, CN. 1955. Prostatic surgery in centenarians. *J Urol* 74:546–548.
15. Katlic, MR. 1985. Surgery in centenarians. *JAMA* 253:3139–3141.

Index

Page numbers followed by t and f indicate tables and figures, respectively.